HANDBOOK OF AMBIENT ASSISTED LIVING

Ambient Intelligence and Smart Environments

The Ambient Intelligence and Smart Environments (AISE) book series presents the latest research results in the theory and practice, analysis and design, implementation, application and experience of *Ambient Intelligence* (AmI) and *Smart Environments* (SmE).

Volume 11

Recently published in this series

Vol. 10. J.C. Augusto et al. (Eds.), Workshop Proceedings of the 7th International Conference on Intelligent Environments
Vol. 9. B. Gottfried and H. Aghajan (Eds.), Behaviour Monitoring and Interpretation – BMI – Well-Being
Vol. 8. R. López-Cózar et al. (Eds.), Workshop Proceedings of the 6th International Conference on Intelligent Environments
Vol. 7. E. Mordini and P. de Hert (Eds.), Ageing and Invisibility
Vol. 6. G. van den Broek et al. (Eds.), AALIANCE Ambient Assisted Living Roadmap
Vol. 5. P. Čech et al. (Eds.), Ambient Intelligence Perspectives II – Selected Papers from the Second International Ambient Intelligence Forum 2009
Vol. 4. M. Schneider et al. (Eds.), Workshops Proceedings of the 5th International Conference on Intelligent Environments
Vol. 3. B. Gottfried and H. Aghajan (Eds.), Behaviour Monitoring and Interpretation – BMI – Smart Environments
Vol. 2. V. Callaghan et al. (Eds.), Intelligent Environments 2009 – Proceedings of the 5th International Conference on Intelligent Environments: Barcelona 2009
Vol. 1. P. Mikulecký et al. (Eds.), Ambient Intelligence Perspectives – Selected Papers from the First International Ambient Intelligence Forum 2008

ISSN 1875-4163 (print)
ISSN 1875-4171 (online)

Handbook of Ambient Assisted Living

Technology for Healthcare, Rehabilitation and Well-being

Edited by

Juan Carlos Augusto

University of Ulster, UK

Michael Huch

VDI/VDE-IT, Germany

Achilles Kameas

Hellenic Open University, Greece

Julie Maitland

National Research Council of Canada, Canada

Paul McCullagh

University of Ulster, UK

Jean Roberts

Phoenix Associates, UK

Andrew Sixsmith

Simon Fraser University, Canada

and

Reiner Wichert

Fraunhofer-Allianz Ambient Assisted Living, Germany

IOS Press

Amsterdam • Berlin • Tokyo • Washington, DC

ISBN 978-1-60750-836-6 (print)
ISBN 978-1-60750-837-3 (online)
Library of Congress Control Number: 2011942612

Publisher
IOS Press BV
Nieuwe Hemweg 6B
1013 BG Amsterdam
Netherlands
fax: +31 20 687 0019
e-mail: order@iospress.nl

Distributor in the USA and Canada
IOS Press, Inc.
4502 Rachael Manor Drive
Fairfax, VA 22032
USA
fax: +1 703 323 3668
e-mail: iosbooks@iospress.com

PRINTED IN THE NETHERLANDS

To Axel and María
J.C.A.

Handbook of Ambient Assisted Living
J.C. Augusto et al. (Eds.)
IOS Press, 2012

Foreword

What is the state of healthcare worldwide today?

Some things are certain. We know that the worldwide population is aging dramatically. We know that the cost of care in most countries is rising rapidly, fueled by the introduction of effective but expensive new drugs and equipment. We know that in many countries there will be far fewer medical professionals to care for people who are sick, and we know that as people live longer, they will be required to manage a greater number of chronic conditions for longer periods of time. We know that in some countries there is resistance to paying for additional care. We know that many industrialized health systems are biased toward "sick" care, helping people once they develop a problem, versus helping people stay well throughout their lifespan and minimizing the onset of conditions that are costly to treat and diminish quality of life. We know that individuals now survive traumatic events such as a heart attack or stroke that would have killed them in the past – a medical success story – but then live until old age when the cost of care skyrockets.

In short, we know that all of these pressures mean that we must change the way we deliver healthcare. We need better, more holistic, life-long care at lower cost.

It is for these reasons that the scientific and engineering contributions described in the Handbook of Ambient Assisted Living: Technology for Healthcare, Rehabilitation and Well-being are so important and timely. Innovative use of new technologies may be the only way to provide care affordably, and to scale that care to hundreds of thousands or millions of people, as our societies adapt to the changes mentioned above. The 45 technical chapters presented here together summarize achievements of an accomplished group of researchers around the globe taking a wide-range of approaches to improving health using technology. The chapters provide a thought-provoking framework in which to consider how healthcare might – and must – change in the future. I anticipate that this volume will inspire other researchers to explore how technologies ranging from in-home sensors to wearable systems to game-like interfaces might be used for elder care, wellness promotion, assistive aids, early diagnosis, coping systems, and rehabilitation. In ten or twenty years, the work described here is likely to be mainstream – incorporated into the way we receive daily care and taken for granted. We won't think twice about sensors in our homes or worn on our bodies to help our computers keep us healthy, and we will expect that computers help us to better manage our care when we get sick. Today, however, the research described here is pushing the limits of what we can do with technology and shows the value of transdisciplinary work that merges the latest advances in computing with solid medical research and practice.

Here's to a healthy, technology-aided future.

Stephen Intille
Ph.D., Assoc. Prof., College of Comp. and Inf. Science & Dept. of Health Sciences,
Bouve College of Health Sciences, Northeastern University, Boston, MA, USA

Contents

Ambient Assisted Living in Gerontology

Smart Homes as a Vehicle for Ambient Assisted Living

Novel Developments and Visions for the Area

Indexes

Ambient Assisted Living in the Health Space

Handbook of Ambient Assisted Living
J.C. Augusto et al. (Eds.)
IOS Press, 2012

doi:10.3233/978-1-60750-837-3-3

AAL in the Health Space – A Reflection

Jean ROBERTS*
Phoenix Associates UK

Abstract. Exemplars of operational AAL deployment in the healthspace are relatively few but increasing. This short reflective piece considers the reasons why, notes underpinning drivers for the future, outlines the increasing research-based activity and sets the context for the following papers that consider the current field from different perspectives across the globe. Firstly research-based (O'Kane, O'Donoghue, Gallagher, Aftab, Casey and Courtney), then Zayas-Caban and colleague propose a methodology for design and implementation, followed by a description of operational piloting (MacGinnis). The next two papers look at progress – in Taiwan (Tsai-Ya and Jenn-Hwan) from the historic development forwards, and comparatively (Shao-Huai and Jui-Chen) in Japan describing a novel incentivisation model. Both of these papers make observations that could be applied globally, as do all the contributors in this section. Wild and Boise then conclude the section by focusing on attitudes to and uses of AAL for a particular target group of potential recipients of assistive technology, Older Persons. Evaluated AAL practical applications are emerging in the health space but the pace of roll-out could be speeded up if frequently observed constraints and some practical lessons learnt from deployment, which have been brought into focus by these papers, were addressed more effectively. There are however some additional refreshing and emerging European and global eHealth initiatives that look set to also facilitate progress.

Keywords. Reflection, context, health, welfare, lifestyle, AAL, professional, end-user

Introduction

The following six papers ably demonstrate the range of activity in assisted / ambient (AAL) technology developments in health; from specialized research developments to operational deployment and user acceptance of the concept of AAL. However, whilst these contributions showcase very interesting examples, it must be recognized that the depth of activity in the health space globally is becoming more significant. Other locations where activity is ongoing were approached but pressures of other commitments meant they were not able to document their activity at this time. Many limitations currently exist to widespread deployment; these are touched on in the papers. O'Kane et al look at an alert scorecard that will support clinicians in determining when a clinical condition may be escalating into a critical phase; 'creating future opportunities for sensor development, Ambient Assisted Living, assessing the impact of therapies, and improved data quality. But possibly the most significant opportunity is the production of prediction models for patient deterioration that are based on actual patient data'. This support to professional practice is not intended to usurp professional judgment but to work in conjunction to reduce risks engendered by competing pressures in a complex

*Corresponding Author: Jean Roberts. E-mail: jean@hcjean.demon.co.uk.

health environment. Zayas-Caban and Marquard broaden the concept of consumer informatics to include assistive technology, and propose a pragmatic methodology by which to evaluate applications and reduce unintended consequences. As Macginnis states when describing the NHS England deployment of telehealth solutions, there is a slower operational uptake in England than could be potentially useful. This reluctance is felt to be replicated elsewhere because of a mix of factors discussed below. Tsai-Ya and Jenn-Hwan review progress in Taiwan indicating that a growing pressure for expenditure on health from an increasing elderly population is bringing about a wide range of government-supported projects; deploying AAL from specialist hospitals to home situations. This paper also makes welcome recognition that education of healthcare practitioners and lay end-users is most beneficial; as is close liaison with the developing industry sector. Shao-Huai and Jui-Chen outline developments in AAL from 2000 onwards and introduce a novel rental scheme for deployment of relevant technologies. They report legislatively prescribed qualification for assistive technology coordinators as part of effective roll-out. They highlight a note of caution that care delivery will be put at risk through an increasing scarcity of carers that can be minimized by deploying AAL in certain circumstances. To conclude this section, Wild and Boise close this section by consideration of the receptivity of a key target group, older persons, to the technologies described. A strong message to involve end-users – caring professionals, patients and families – in design and development of AAL is crucial to effective roll-out; but also to respect the ethical need to 'balance privacy with perceived need' in introducing innovative AAL support.

The AAL opportunities in the health space, represented in part by the initiatives described in this section, can be identified for citizens' use (independent living and improving quality of life); in institutions such as acute hospitals and tertiary care facilities (both public and private); and to enable trans-national activity (supra-specialist services, and patient/client monitoring which improves mobility). The range spans traditional ICT-enabled assistance to the emerging introduction of embedded / non-invasive, personally configurable, adaptive and anticipatory ambient technologies. The contributions in this section focus on health. Other areas where AAL affects general well-being – such as edutainment and infomedia provision, are considered elsewhere in this book.

The Presidential Declaration from the eHealth Ministerial conference (Budapest, 2011) acknowledges that 'appropriate use of ICT solutions in chronic disease management, in particular self-management, self-treatment and continuous remote monitoring, results in health gains by enabling patients to continue to live independently and to improve their quality of life'. Additionally 'wider use of ICT in healthcare is a fundamental condition to the development and implementation of innovative care solutions, as well as the introduction of new generation applications and innovative care models [and] efficient patient pathways'. It is high level recognition like this that may just make the difference in escalating research and development and the outcomes of roll-out in 2011/2012 and beyond. These aspirations are also supported by patients' rights as expressed in the European Cross Border Healthcare Directive (Article 14). Impetus also comes from 'A Digital Agenda for Europe (Key Action 13)' to promote 'deployment and usage of modern accessible on-line services' [including smart homes and online health] by 2020 achieving 'widespread deployment of telemedicine services'.

The expectations of end-users of health-related AAL solutions are changing frequently. Factors affecting the developments include increased distributed relocation for work (on a permanent or temporary basis), longer career lifetimes and higher expectations for (post-retirement) quality of unconstrained international mobility. These challenges put pressure on care delivery bodies to provide more fluid telehealth support and make readily available tools for day to day self-management of clinical conditions, with back-up of expert reassurance in periods of heightened concern or clinical escalation.

1. Operational Deployment Projections

1.1. Context

The aim of the 230-member Continua Alliance (a non-profit, open industry organization of healthcare and technology companies) to establish an 'eco-system of interoperable personal health systems and empower people and organizations to better manage their health and wellness' ably describes the scope of current activity. The European Disability Forum welcomes product deployment but the requirement for 'Nothing for us, without us' is coupled with a wish to be involved in defining user needs and product validation; a crucial part of acceptance testing. In a recent statement the chairman of the UK Local Government Association community wellbeing board, said: 'Investing in technology like [gadgets for the elderly] has been proven to reduce the need for hospital admission, GP referral, home help, day care and residential care'. Mestheneos observed (World of Health IT Europe (WoHIT), 2011) that 'Older people cannot be seen as a homogenous group' but that telemedicine *can* contribute to daily checks for patients with chronic diseases and can reassure their carers, especially those who cannot be there 24/7.

1.2. Quantification

Research by one UK local authority has shown modern technology could save its health system £7.5m a year. If expanded across England and Wales, this would represent savings of £270m – and extra years of independence and dignity for users.

The self-care website of the digitally-aware city of Espoo in Finland (www.espoo.fi/omahoito) gives guidance on how to deploy technology and improve the quality of life of its residents who have a diabetic condition, and projects that savings, expressed as a measure of the disease burden, of 0.3 QALYs can be made. Lehtovuori (WoHIT, 2011) values this at over one thousand Euros.

The range of clinical conditions that an be supported also includes those with mental health challenges. Kordy of Heidelberg (WoHIT, 2011) reports that post-hospitalisation by the 'Internet-Chat-Bridge' project (www.psyres.de) resulted in 80% patient satisfaction from the interactions with technology and significant sustainable therapeutic gains after one year, which were quantified at over 1 million Euro per thousand patients over usual [traditional] treatments.

1.3. Tools and Technologies

The technologies that could bring this about are many and various. These include the electronic pill dispenser which has been projected to save thousands of pounds a year, to the personal satellite locator which reduces day care costs by approximately

250 Euros a week. Other projects like Care-lab (de Ruyters and Pelgrim) can contribute to improved health status through nutritional guidance (for instance for diabetes sufferers and the obese), drug regime alerts and vital signs monitoring whilst being commercially promoted as lifestyle aids.

Project DREAMING (elDeRly fRiEndly Alarm handling and Monitoring, www.dreaming-project.org) encapsulates much of the current potential of AAL in its aim to 'keep elderly people in their home environment as long as their physical and mental conditions allow this'. However, it is recognised that this goal cannot be achieved with technology alone, but in conjunction with non-technology based services which are essential for supporting the autonomy of elderly people (such as visits by community nurses and social workers, psychological support, delivery of hot meals and shopping, special transportations for people with limited mobility, house cleaning). The current impressive list of technologies employed in this project includes motion, humidity, door open/close sensors, intelligent weighing scales, EKG monitors, fall and gas alarms; water and smoke detectors.

Gergely (WoHIT, 2011) suggests that approximately 86% of deaths can be attributed to chronic diseases, and that an integrated 'care space' should include Intelligent Agents which could support 'virtual visits [to clinical practitioners]' to attempt to reduce this figure. Facilitating extended independent living through [remote] vital signs monitoring and other AAL tools would be beneficial to [many of] the six hundred million older persons world wide, suggest research collaborators (www.continuaalliance.org). Poettgen's observations (WoHIT, 2011) indicate that by 2050 nearly 30% of Europeans will be over 80 years old, making increased demands for care. The majority will be of the digital generation who are already 'always online and connected' to augmented ehealth, telehealth services in addition to their social/workspace. Accessibility, affordability and usability (including digital literacy) are key to creating societal inclusivity of older persons. A further important consideration to be resolved is where legal liability might rest if assistive technologies fail.

1.4. Discussion

Constraints on roll-out include end-user attitudes, perceived costs, concerns about the current reorganisations of physical health and care authorities and the policies and responsibilities of any new bodies formed. Coupled with financial and economic pressures, common to many countries globally – investments however attractive are entered into very cautiously at present. Even providing a safe living environment and reassurance of health status to an individual in (sheltered) home environments is considered too expensive overall, with additional complications in some countries. These may relate to reimbursement issues (both capital and on a recurring revenue basis) or to a legislative framework which (still in some countries) only recognizes face-to-face clinical consultations.

The European view is also mirrored in America where suggestions that increased patient involvement and collaboration [in deploying health IT] in addressing chronic health issues can also bring down costs. Buchanan of eMids Technologies asserts that 'Chronic diseases brought on by poor lifestyle choices are difficult to handle, but health IT provides a clear avenue for enterprising organizations to develop innovative disease management solutions to address the issue'. However the transition from predominantly direct patient interaction to incorporating technological assistance is not readily accepted by all citizens' / patient groups; nor limited by work situation, age, challenges to abilities or gender.

Lessons learned from the practical assessment and caution raised in the following papers indicate that AAL cannot be seen as a universal panacea. Assistive technology and self-management should be seriously considered to reduce the pressures on human caring resources and pervasive financial stringency. Not everyone welcomes the technology with open arms but involvement in their design and development may improve understanding of AAL capability and increase acceptance of deployment in the health space over time.

2. Market Scope

Utilization of AAL in the health space is also curtailed, as it is the wider AAL domain, by 'the present infancy of the AAL market in which development is perceived as still very uncertain' (AALIANCE, 2010). The focus from published material is mainly on sustaining a quality of life of the older person, with additional tools being made available to sustain independent living for those with physical and mental challenges.

2.1. Research Opportunities

All the areas listed above have underpinning research developments such as those described by the European projects AALIANCE (www.aaliance.eu), the Danish / Netherlands-led Care-Lab projects, BETTER (looking at physical rehabilitation assistance for improved gait (www.iai.csic.es/better) and through various interworking networks established through EU-funded Framework 6 and 7 project collaboration. AALIANCE is interesting in that it contains partners from both the commercial world and academia which should make transition from research into practical application somewhat less problematical. In some cases the disjunction between academic and economically viable solutions remains wide and what were potentially useful ideas do not get exploited fully. Limited researcher time may be available for maintaining a multi-national information knowledge exchange platform because 'it might distract R&D staff from their core activities'; this short term strategy is understandable in the current restricted climate but could prove problematic longer term.

The research stimulus for AAL research crosses boundaries between EU programmes and objectives, notably those of Ageing Well, Policy Support, ICT Cooperation and the generic FP7 framework. Whilst this provides increased numbers of opportunities, it could be seen to add complexity to the exploitation of concepts into marketable products and solutions. This collaborative working on projects or in knowledge exchange is extremely positive but may 'grey' the boundaries further between health, welfare and lifestyle improvement.

3. Conclusion

The most significant challenges to AAL roll-out in the health space are a fluid care delivery environment, lack of detailed policies for recognition and reimbursement where AAL solutions are deployed, and incomplete business case evaluations of pilot initiatives. Citizens' perceptions and lack of awareness of the potential of AAL can limit pressures for their utilization. Some logistical gaps in the effective transition from research into practice also come into play; which could be reduced by increased high level sponsorship of the operational deployment of AAL solutions.

The initiatives described in the following section and the activity indicated above demonstrate what can be done and give a window into further use in the future. Evaluation outcomes and the generation of benefits projections will become more compelling as AAL deployment in its widest sense increases.

Handbook of Ambient Assisted Living
J.C. Augusto et al. (Eds.)
IOS Press, 2012

doi:10.3233/978-1-60750-837-3-9

Electronic-Early Warning Scorecard: An Intelligent Context Aware Decision Making Approach for Patient Monitoring

Tom O'KANE[a], John O'DONOGHUE[a,*], Joe GALLAGHER[b], A. AFTAB[b], Aveline CASEY[b] and Garry COURTNEY[b]
[a]*Health Information Systems Research Centre, University College Cork, Cork, Ireland*
t.okane@ucc.ie
[b]*St. Luke's General Hospital, Kilkenny, Ireland*

Abstract. It is now well established that many patients in hospital can suddenly become acutely ill but experience delayed recognition of their physiological deterioration resulting in late referral to critical care, or in some cases death. In recent years there has been significant growth in the use of scorecards to assist with the detection of increasing patient morbidity, but even though a scorecard may be well-constructed and its parameters carefully chosen, the usefulness of any scorecard is only as good as the accuracy and timeliness of the data that is used to populate it.

The scorecard in this chapter referrers to the Modified Early Warning Scorecard (MEWS) which is a paper-based clinical scorecard, intended to provide clinicians with an early warning of acute patient deterioration. While this paper based approach is a significant advance in patient care, major data capture and processing deficiencies still exist.

To overcome these limitations an electronic-Modified Early Warning Scorecard (e-MEWS) was designed and developed in collaboration with the staff at St. Luke's General Hospital, Kilkenny, Ireland. The e-MEWS is an intelligent rule-based clinical decision support system designed to automatically perform frequent wireless monitoring of a patient's vital signs, and to record and process the data to calculate and display a MEWS score and other valuable patient information.

This research demonstrates how an existing real-world paper based approach can be greatly enhanced through the application of intelligent Clinical Decision Support Systems (CDSS). In turn the adoption of wireless Body Area Network (BAN) technologies within a clinical environment highlights how Ambient Assisted Living (AAL) solutions can play a significant role in patient care delivery.

Keywords. Early warning scorecard, MEWS, CDSS, BAN

Introduction

There is a growing body of evidence that many patients in hospital become acutely ill, experience late referral to critical care, or unfortunately die due to delayed recognition of their physiological deterioration or mismanagement of the patient's care. Numerous studies have shown that such adverse outcomes are frequently preceded by abnormal vital signs in the hours prior to a catastrophic event such as coronary arrest, death, or

*Corresponding Author. John O'Donoghue. E-mail. John.ODonoghue@ucc.ie

late admission to a high dependency unit [11,20,26]. Such was the stimulus for the development of the Early Warning Scorecard (EWS) [22], and later Modified Early Warning Scorecards (MEWS) [33].

Paper based EWS are now in widespread use in many hospitals and feature prominently in the NICE Clinical Guideline 50 of the NHS in the UK [24]. They are, in effect, paper-based decision support dashboards[1] designed to help clinicians identify as early as possible those patients who are most at risk of suffering an adverse event. St. Luke's General Hospital, Kilkenny, Ireland, is a 299 bed facility and part of the Irish Health Service Executive's (HSE) South East region. It serves a catchment area of approximately 87,500 people and provides a range of healthcare services including medicine, surgery, obstetrics and gynaecology, paediatrics, and psychiatry. The paper based MEWS system is used within all the acute care wards as part of normal patient monitoring procedures [12]. This study was conducted as a joint investigation between researchers from the Health Information Systems Research Centre, University College Cork, Ireland, and their clinical colleagues in St. Luke's Hospital to examine how we might improve the paper-based MEWS system and advance patient care delivery.

1. Related Work

1.1. Clinical Decision Support Systems (CDSS)

Early Clinical Decision Support Systems (CDSS) stemmed from research into probabilistic and statistical algorithms to develop 'expert systems' that could 'think' like a physician when confronted with a patient [21]. However, investigators soon realised that these systems could provide much more by way of support to assist clinicians with decision making, and thus modern CDSS began to emerge [5].

Knowledge-Based CDSS typically have three components. First, a knowledge base consisting of information compiled by experts – provides the reference back-drop for decision making. Second, an inference engine containing the rule sets for combining the knowledge base with the information provided to the system (e.g. patient data). Third, a communications mechanism – simply a way of getting data into the system and getting results to the user [6].

To enable CDSS to work effectively and efficiently as possible, various tools and techniques have been developed. Scorecards, although not a new idea, are one of the decision support tools that have seen renewed enthusiasm due to advances in technology. They are essentially dashboards of information through which it is possible to rapidly ascertain the status of a given situation and they have gained wide acceptance in many applications.

Two important factors must always be stressed in the construction of scorecards: the content of the scorecard (i.e. what it is telling the user) and the context in which it is used (i.e. why it is important to consider this data and what actions will result). Thus, justifying the inclusion of a metric within a scorecard only makes sense if it can be shown that the metric will contribute to the effectiveness, reliability or timeliness of the decision making [1]. For CDSS these concerns have special significance as clinicians will not be motivated to use the system if it is only seen to exacerbate the increasingly time-pressured patient care process [5].

---

[1] A dashboard may be viewed as means to display a number of key operational measures through a computer interface to inform and assist decision makers in a clear and concise manner [9].

Modified Early Warning System Observation Score (MEWS) Parameters							
Score	**3**	**2**	**1**	**0**	**1**	**2**	**3**
Pulse (b.p.m)	<40	41–50	51–55	56–100	101–110	111–139	>140
Systolic Blood Pressure	<80	81–90	91–100	101–180	181–199	>200	
Respiratory Rate	<8			9–20	21–25	26–29	>30
Oxygen Saturation %	<85%	85–89%	90–94%	≥95%			
Temperature (°C)		<35.0	35.1–36	36.1–37.5	37.6–38.5	>38.5	
Canadian Neurological Scale (CNS) Level Alert, Verbal, Pain and Unresponsive (AVPU)	Unresponsive	Responds to Pain	Responds to Voice	Alert	New Agitation/ confusion		
Glasgow Coma Scale (GCS)				15	14	9–13	≤8
Urine Output	<10mls/hr	<30mls/hr	<50mls/hr				

Figure 1. Modified early warning scorecard (MEWS) St. Luke's hospital, Kilkenny, Ireland.

A final point is that CDSS, such as the electronic-Modified Early Warning Scorecard described in the following section, are there to enhance and support the human who is ultimately responsible for the clinical decisions, not to replace them [6].

1.2. Modified Early Warning Scorecard (MEWS)

There are many varieties of Early Warning Scorecards (EWS) in use throughout the world e.g. [10,27,29,31]. They differ in their composition (in terms of the vital signs to be collected) and in their construction (in terms of the number of scoring zones and the vital sign ranges within those zones). There is no general consensus on EWS content or construction, and arguing the relative merits of one versus another is beyond the purview of this chapter. Therefore, since there is no widespread agreement on the composition of the EWS, this study will reference the Modified Early Warning Scorecard (MEWS) deployed in St. Luke's Hospital, Kilkenny as an exemplar.

The MEWS is simply a reference table which associates individual vital signs parameters (e.g. heart rate, respiratory rate, etc.) with a 'score' (0, 1, 2, or 3), which is representative of the physiological derangement from a normal range. As [30] points out, they are not a panacea for accurate patient assessment and should be used judiciously in conjunction with clinical assessment, that is the clinical staff members tacit knowledge should be used in conjunction with the MEWS outputs.

In the sample MEWS chart from St. Luke's (see Fig. 1), the normal range for any given vital sign is shown under the '0' score column and the increasing deviation from the normal range is shown under the '1', '2' or '3' score columns.

By simply summing the individual vital signs MEWS scores an aggregate MEWS result is produced. Thus, for example, a patient presenting with a pulse of 108, systolic blood pressure of 140, a respiratory rate of 24, blood oxygen of 96%, a temperature of 37degC, a urine output of 60 mls/hr, and assessed as 'Alert', would have an aggregate score of 2 (score 1 for pulse & 1 for respiratory rate).

Depending upon the MEWS action protocols operating within the hospital, a rising aggregate MEWS score will trigger some corresponding action by clinical staff. By this means patient deterioration can be detected and clinical interventions enacted much

MEWS Score	Action
1	Inform registered nurse for patient review.
2	Inform registered nurse for patient review. Increase frequency of observations to at least 4 hourly.
3 (in any single parameter)	Contact appropriate doctor for immediate review. Increase frequency of observations to hourly.
3 or more	Contact appropriate doctor for immediate review. Increase frequency of observations to hourly.
If Canadian Neurological Scale (CNS) is increased by 2 or more regardless of the other observations.	Contact appropriate doctor for immediate review. Commence neurological observations.

Figure 2. MEWS action protocol St. Luke's hospital, Kilkenny, Ireland.

earlier, thereby avoiding a serious increase in patient morbidity. The MEWS action protocol in use in St. Luke's is provided in Fig. 2, and thus the action suggested for our hypothetical patient with a score of 2 would be to "Inform registered nurse for patient review and increase the frequency of observations to at least 4 hourly".

MEWS models and their pre-determined action protocols are intended to be used in general ward settings to indicate those patients who may need to be elevated to the Coronary Care Unit (CCU) or Intensive Care Unit (ICU), and there is some anecdotal evidence to show that earlier intervention triggered by the MEWS leads to earlier referral to ICU/CCU but shorter stays in those facilities. In Sections 1.3 and 1.4 of this chapter mobile technologies and body area networks will be discussed respectively as they act as the main information technology components in transforming the paper based MEWS into the e-MEWS DSS system.

1.3. Mobile Technologies

A mobile computing device is designed to help facilitate information transparency, data integration and provide expedient communication capabilities and computing services to assist individuals to carry out their day to day activities [17,19]. Mobile computing technologies such as smart mobile phones, and other handheld computing devices hold a great deal of promise in terms of their organisational relevance [32]. Applications of mobile technology in the healthcare context can be recognised as an enabling technology [2,18], which have been applied in several countries across a number of healthcare disciplines.

[16] hypothesise that mobile technologies are widely available and can play a primary role in healthcare at the regional, community, and individual levels. Currently active m-health technologies include the use of handheld devices to collect community health information; using smart mobile phones to deliver healthcare information to practitioners and their patients [3]. However, [28] highlight that m-health is not just the use of mobile phones for health related purposes or the mobility of both patients and health professionals. Instead, the authors put forward that a mobile environment incorporates self-organising systems and components along with mobile devices, tools and sensors. M-health technologies, therefore, include smart handheld devices with computational capabilities and/or wearable computing devices to monitor a patient physiological and 'location in space'. All of which aim to support clinical staff or caregivers to provide optimum or near optimum patient care. Patient physiological vital-signs and 'location in space' data is collected in this project through the usage of wireless Body Area Network (BAN) technologies.

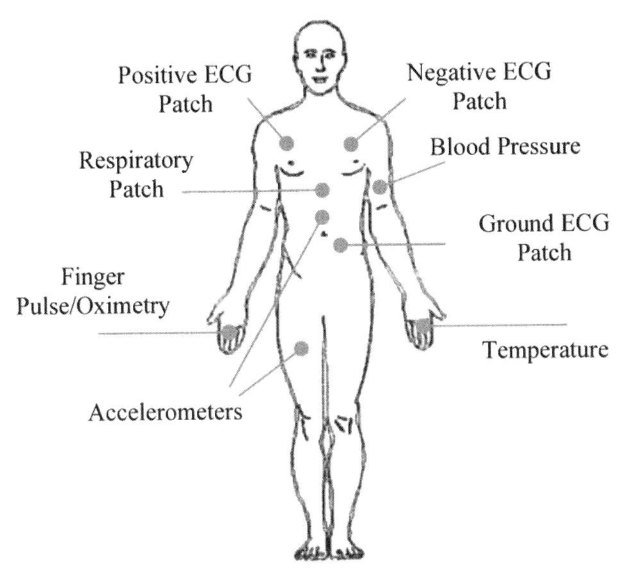

Figure 3. Body area network sensor configuration.

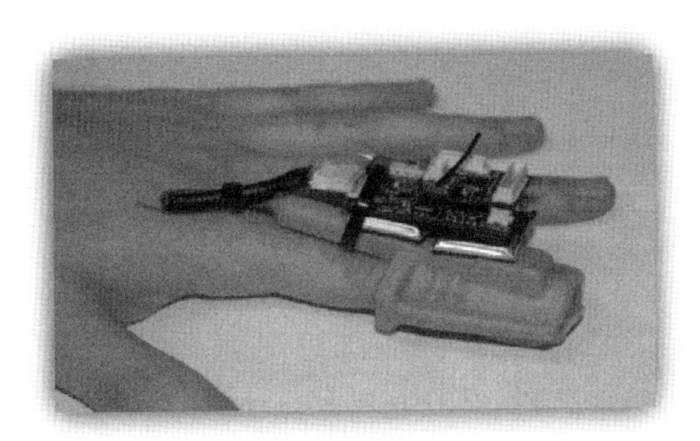

Figure 4. A wireless Pulse/Sp02 finger sensor as part of the BAN.

1.4. A Body Area Network

Wireless BAN's are a recent and exciting development in patient monitoring. It is through recent technological advances in integrated circuitry, sensor miniaturisation, and wireless technology has enabled the development of wearable, intelligent, low power devices such as the BAN. A number of sensors may be combined to monitor a patient from a number of areas of interest (see Fig. 3) e.g. which provide wireless real-time data on a range of physiological variables [7,15,25,7] with an example of a finger Pulse/Sp02 sensor in Fig. 4.

With a BAN the sensors are worn by the patient and the information they collect is then wirelessly transmitted to a base station for processing and analysis. While BAN's can collect significant amounts of data, great care must be taken to ensure the quality of the information is preserved and this is a major challenge for all wireless systems of this nature. In addition to this there are some vital signs that are difficult to collect au-

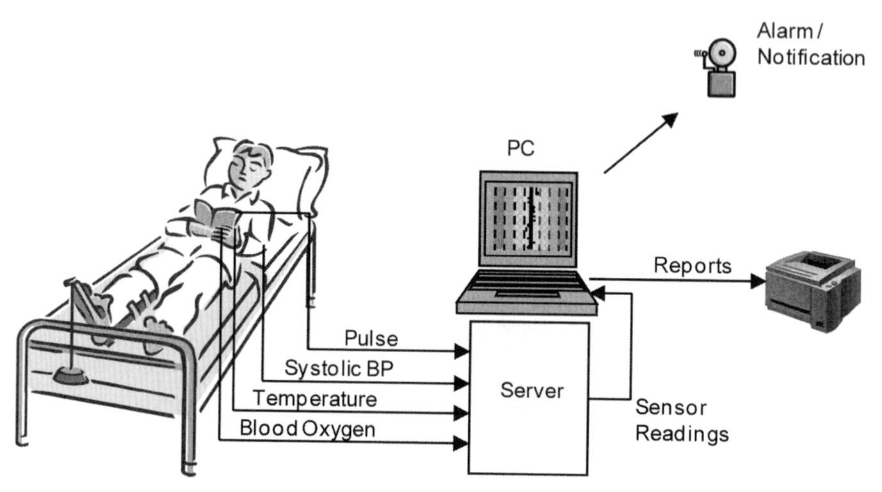

Figure 5. A single patient e-MEWS system configuration.

tomatically using BAN's, the most obvious being the patient's level of consciousness or urine output.

The e-MEWS project is using wireless BAN technologies that were developed at the Tyndall National Institute, Cork, Ireland, under the Science Foundation Ireland, National Access Program [23]. Currently the BAN is capable of monitoring pulse/ Sp02, ECG, body temperature and body movement (accelerometers). Future developments will include automatic capture of, Blood Pressure, and Respiratory Rate.

2. The e-MEWS System

Given the current restrictions of the paper-based version of MEWS, an electronic-Modified Early Warning Scorecard (e-MEWS) has been developed. The e-MEWS is an intelligent CDSS designed to automatically perform frequent wireless monitoring of patient's vital signs, record and process the data to display a MEWS score and other valuable patient information.

The system consists of two separate subsystems: first, the sensors which are worn by patients, where data is transmitted wirelessly to a base station connected to a laptop computer, and second, the e-MEWS software where the patient data is recorded, stored, processed and displayed. The most basic e-MEWS system configuration for a single patient is presented in Fig. 5.

Calls for the development of automatic patient monitoring systems are growing [4,8,13,14,24] however the authors of this chapter would argue that while a great deal of work has been completed on the monitoring aspects of systems, less attention is paid to the data processing of the patient data and hence decision making aspects associated with the collected data are less obvious.

The individual e-MEWS user interface scorecards have a number of major features including manual data recording, oxygen flow monitoring, summary reporting, and comparative analysis between vital signs. However, the substantive part of the user interface is the e-MEWS trend plots (see Fig. 6). These five vertical plots are at the

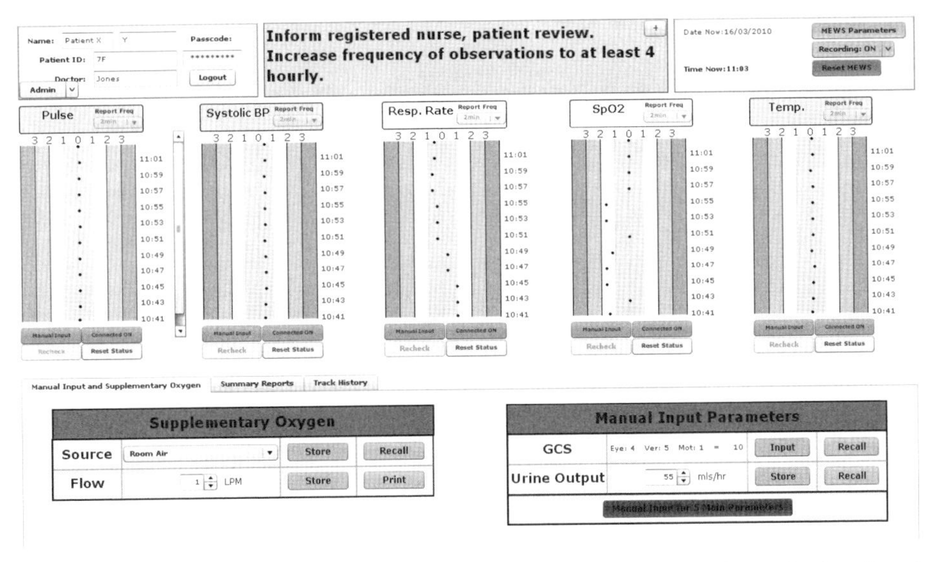

Figure 6. e-MEWS Graphical User Interface (GUI) with individual vital sign trend plots. Pulse, Systolic and Temp have a combined score of 0. With Respiratory (1) and SPo2 (1) having a combined score of 2, resulting in an action protocol 2 highlighted in amber on the centre top of the display.

heart of the e-MEWS system. They allow the ward staff to see at a glance the current MEWS status of any of the individual vital signs parameters indicated by the backlit colour of the header block; Green = 0, Yellow = 1, Orange = 2 and Red = 3. The overall MEWS score is displayed at the top of the e-MEWS Graphical User Interface (GUI) to inform the staff of the patients overall state of health in relation to their vital-signs, CNS/GCS and urine levels.

3. The MEWS Process

There are many reports on the growing use of early warning scorecards for initiating earlier interventions. However such benefits can only be realised if two major issues are addressed: first, collecting vital signs data at a sufficiently high frequency to detect patient deterioration, and second, the data processing is done correctly to yield accurate information and knowledge about the patient.

Presented in Fig. 7, is a high level overview of the e-MEWS architecture and the key levels of interaction between hospital staff and patients with the e-MEWS System. On the left hand side are BAN devices that communicate various vital sign data streams which feed into the e-MEWS system (steps 1–3). These patients may be residing in a hospital ward or at home. The presented patient datasets within the e-MEWS system are accessible by clinical staff within the hospital or to external consultants. Hospital staff, who provide direct patient care have the capability to update the patient's clinical record through the e-MEWS Graphical User Interface (steps 4 & 5). The e-MEWS will process this information and inform the hospital staff member of the patient overall MEWS reading (steps 6 & 7) as the patients EWS reading changes the frequency of the BAN readings can be altered automatically e.g. a high MEWS score will have higher sampling vital sign rate than a lower MEWS score. This global access

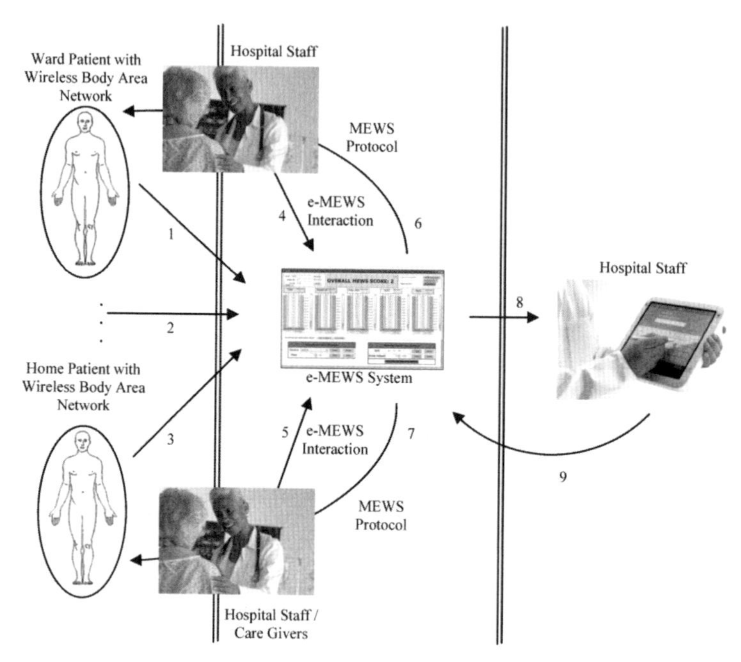

Figure 7. e-MEWS interaction.

approach helps to ensure that all hospital staff, are well informed and help to obtain a higher degree of awareness regarding the "known patient context" and their well-being. The e-MEWS system and its integration as part of the patient care process is designed to overcome the existing paper based limitations. This is primarily achieved by increased and intelligent patient vital sign capture through BAN technology and improved data processing. Both of which provide the hospital staff with more time to provide direct patient care.

3.1. Staff Feedback on the e-MEWS System Process

A total of 71 staff members at St. Luke's General Hospital made up of nurses (junior & senior) and clinical doctors were surveyed before and after using the e-MEWS prototype. The objective of this survey was to ascertain the usefulness of the e-MEWS system from 4 key perspectives 1) Effectiveness of the paper based system, 2) the advantages of the e-MEWS system over existing paper based system 3) e-MEWS usability and data modification and 4) e-MEWS usability and navigation.

3.1.1. Effectiveness of the Paper Based MEWS

Staff members were asked to respond to the following statement "The paper based MEWS scorecard improves patient care?" With an associated likert scale of 1 = Strongly agree, 2 = Agree, 3 = Neither agree or disagree, 4 = Disagree, 5 = Strongly disagree. This resulted in 45.65% and 26.08% strongly agree and agree respectively cf. Fig. 8. The remaining 26.08% and 2.17% neither agree or disagree or disagree. This is significant in that over quarter of the clinical staff felt that the paper based MEWS has little or no effect on patient care delivery.

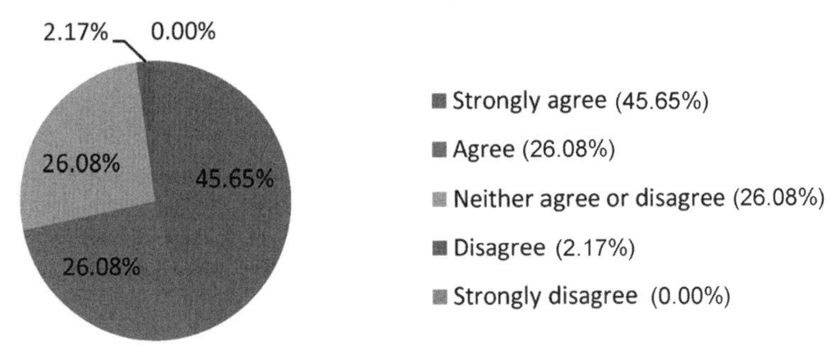

Figure 8. MEWS scorecard improves patient care findings.

Table 1. Advantages of the e-MEWS system findings

Aspect	Percentage
Accuracy & maintenance of patient data	38.77%
Reduction in paperwork & time savings	28.57%
Ease of use	18.36%
Interpretation of trends and MEWS Score	10.20%
Fewer opportunities for cross infection	4.08%

After further analysis of this 28.25% cohort it was discovered that the majority of this group was made up of clinical doctors and senior nurses. Senior nurses would have built up a great deal of understanding as to how to care for and monitor a patient. This tacit and explicit knowledge provides them with a higher degree of confidence when assessing a patient's mental and physical condition. Junior nurses tend to look at the raw vital signs as their primary indicator; whereas their levels of tacit knowledge may not be as mature.

3.1.2. Advantages of the e-MEWS System Over Existing Paper Based System

Based on the feedback to this question, five key areas of interest were identified by the hospital staff, as presented in Table 1. Accuracy was mentioned by just over 38% of the respondents. This was attributed to "*Data is displayed & easy to see*" and "*Tidy and easy to change*". Initially the hospital staff assumed that their workload would double as they would have to enter patient data onto the paper notes and the e-MEWS system. However once they realised that the e-MEWS would replace the paper notes over 28% indicated a reduction in paperwork and time saving "*Hopefully it will mean less time used on paperwork and more time on patient care*" and "*Less time consuming than the paper based approach. Less paper being used so less chance of documentation being lost*".

Just over 18% of the hospital staff indicated an 'ease of use' when using the e-MEWS system "*It is very easy to read and make changes to the patient data*" and "*Easier to read*". However, it is worth noting a number of the staff comments such as "*Lack of computer access*" and "*System training required*" as these are issues which all hospitals must take into account when deploying such systems. The patient vital sign trended plots and calculation of MEWS scores were also highlighted by 10+% as "*At a glance you can see what the MEWS score is, whereas on paper it would have to be*

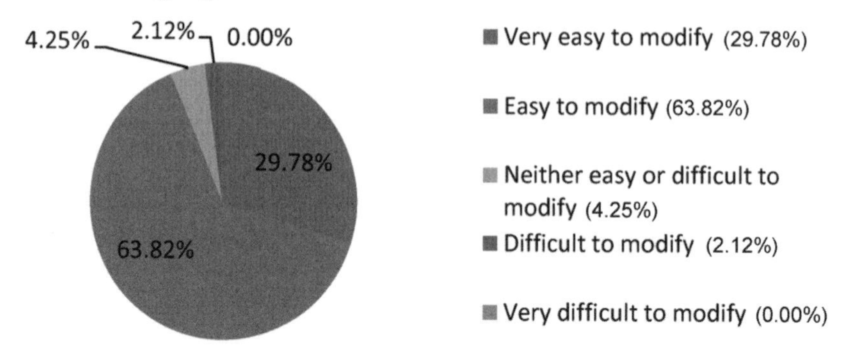

Figure 9. e-MEWS usability and data modification.

filled in and added up" and "*more attention to trend likely*" to result in a more accurate understanding of the patient's condition.

3.1.3. e-MEWS Usability and Data Modification

Over 93% of the respondents found that it was 'very easy to modify' or 'easy to modify' patient data within the e-MEWS system (see Fig. 9) stating that it is "*Less time consuming than the paper based approach*" and "*main advantages: 1) Time saving 2) Paper saving and 3) Legible, neat, clear viewing + reviewing*". This level of confidence is very important as it clearly highlights that staff are ready to make a complete transition from paper based MEWS to e-MEWS. For the remaining 6+% of staff members training and familiarity with computers were the primary obstacles "*Not enough training for all staff (mainly locum staff)*" and "*Yes with certain medical personnel that wouldn't be computer literate. Otherwise with education it should fit in with existing ward practices*".

3.1.4. e-MEWS Usability and Navigation

A total of 91+% of the respondents indicated that is was 'very easy' to 'easy' when navigating the e-MEWS system (see Fig. 10) stating "*Once familiar with e-MEWS may be quicker, save time*" and "*Tidy and easy to change*". A number of the respondents highlighted that if the e-MEWS trend plots could be "*Displayed horizontally (if possible) on display screen – Easier to visualise high and low recordings. Most monitors in use display on the horizontal.*" and "*Maybe join the dots!*" within the trend plots. These comments tie in with existing ICT systems across most hospitals. Future iterations of the e-MEWS project will factor in these comments to reduce potential confusion when reading the patient's vital signs.

4. Conclusions and Further Research Opportunities

Ward patients frequently show signs of deterioration many hours before they experience a catastrophic event. MEWS systems have been used widely to try and detect patient deterioration, but crucially they rely on frequent patient monitoring and accurate

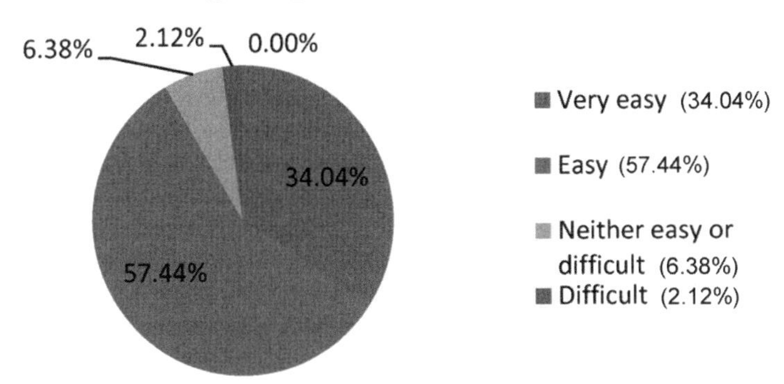

Figure 10. e-MEWS usability and navigation.

data processing. Unfortunately there are serious issues with both of these requirements. We have shown how, through the development of the e-MEWS system, these difficulties can be overcome. Coupling a decision support system (DSS) in the form of the MEWS with wireless monitoring provides a major extension of system capability and a significant advance in patient care.

The deployment of the e-MEWS system in St. Luke's Hospital provided us with a unique opportunity to see firsthand how such a system performs 'out of the lab' and in a real-world environment. The insights which all hospital staff provided were of tremendous value as they highlighted numerous strengths and weaknesses. What was most encouraging from an AAL perspective was how open the vast majority of staff where to new technologies. The e-MEWS system is made up of two key components 1) wireless patient monitoring and 2) visualisation of patient MEWS scores in a DSS dashboard fashion. Individually each of these elements were a major operational change over the existing paper based approach. The rapid rate of adoption by staff to the e-MEWS system is very promising as it indicates that AAL solutions have the potential to be realised within a complex real-world healthcare environment.

This research creates future opportunities for sensor development, Ambient Assisted Living, assessing the impact of therapies, and improved data quality. But possibly the most significant opportunity is the production of prediction models for patient deterioration that are based on actual patient data.

References

[1] F. Adam and J-C. Pomerol, Developing practical decision support tools using dashboards of information, in: *Handbook on Decision Support Systems, International Handbook on Information Systems Series*, Burstein and Holsapple, eds, Springer-Verlag, London, 2008.

[2] E. Ammenwerth, S. Graber, G. Herrmann, T. Burkle and J. Konig, Evaluation of health information systems – problems and challenges, *International Journal of Medical Informatics* (2003), 125–135.

[3] A. Anta, S. El-Wahab and A. Giuffrida, *Mobile Health: The Potential of Mobile Telephony to Bring Health Care to the Majority*, Inter-American Development Bank, Washington, DC. 2009.

[4] R. Bellomo, Delayed MET activation: Incidence and cost, http://rapidresponsesystems.org/downloads 2009/Copenhagen_delayed_Bellomo.pdf, Austin Hospital, Melbourne, 2009, [online].

[5] E.S. Berner, Clinical Decision Support Systems: State of the Art, U.S. Dept. Of Health and Human Services, Pub. No. 09-0069-EF, Rockville, MD, June 2009.

[6] E.S. Berner and T.J. La Lande, Overview of Clinical Decision Support Systems, in: *Clinical Decision Support Systems – Theory and Practice*, 2nd edn, E.S. Berner, ed, Springer, New York, 2007, pp. 3–22.
[7] M. Chen, S. Gonzalez, A. Vasilakos, H. Cao and V. Leung, Body area networks: A survey, *Journal of Mobile Networks and Applications* (2010), Springer.
[8] M. DeVita, Medical emergency teams: Deciphering clues to crises in hospitals, *Critical Care* **9** (2005), 325–326.
[9] S. Few, Information Dashboard Design, ISBN 0596100167, Publisher: O'Reilly, 2006.
[10] D. Goldhill, A. McNarry, G. Mandersloot and A. McGinley, A physiologically-based early warning score for ward patients: The association between score and outcome, *Journal of Anaesthesia* **60** (2005), 547–553, Wiley Online Library.
[11] D. Goldhill, S. Singh, M. Tarling, L. Worthington, A. Mulcahy, S. White and A. Sumner, The patient at risk team: Identifying and managing seriously ill ward patients, *Anaesthesia* **54** (1999), 853–860.
[12] J.D. Groarke, J. Gallagher, J. Stack, A. Aftab, C. Dwyer, R. McGovern and G. Courtney, Use of an admission early warning score to predict patient morbidity and mortality in treatment success, *Emergency Medical Journal* **25** (2008), 803–806.
[13] D. Jones, B. Bates, S. Warrillow, H. Opdam, D. Goldsmith, G. Gutteridge and R. Bellomo, Circadian pattern of activation of the medical emergency team in a teaching hospital, *Critical Care* **9** (2005), 303–306.
[14] D. Jones, R. Bellomo, S. Bates, S. Warrillow, D. Goldsmith, G. Hart and H. Opdam, Patient monitoring and the timing of cardiac arrests and medical emergency team calls in a teaching hospital, *Intensive Care Medicine* **32** (2006), 1352–1356.
[15] E. Jovanov, A. Milenkovic, C. Otto and P. de Groen, A wireless body area network of intelligent motion sensors for computer assisted physical rehabilitation, *Journal of Neuro Engineering and Rehabilitation* **2** (2005).
[16] J. Kahn, J.S. Yang and J.S. Kahn, Mobile Health Needs and Opportunities, in: *Developing Countries, Health Affairs*, 2010, pp. 252–258.
[17] N. Kearney, L. Kidd, M. Miller M. Sage, J. Khorrami, M. McGee, J. Cassidy, K. Niven and P. Gray, Utilising handheld computers to monitor and support patients receiving chemotherapy: Results of a UK-based feasibility study, *Supportive Care in Cancer* **14**(7) (2006), 742–752.
[18] J. Kjeldskov, M. Skov, B. Als and R. Hegh, Is it worth the hassle? Exploring the added value of evaluating the usability of context-aware mobile systems in the field, *Journal of Mobile Human-Computer Interaction (MobileHCI)* (2006), 529–535, Springer.
[19] L. Kleinrock, Breaking loose, *Communications of the ACM* **44** (2001), 41–45.
[20] H. McGloin, S.K. Adams and M. Singer, Unexpected deaths and referrals to critical care of patients on general wards. Are some cases potentially avoidable?, *Journal of the Royal College of Physicians* (1999), 255–259.
[21] R.A. Miller, Medical diagnostic decision support systems – past, present, and future: A threaded biography and brief commentary, *Journal or the American Medical Informatics Association* **1** (1994), 8–27.
[22] R.J.M. Morgan, F. Williams and M.M. Wright, An early warning scoring system for detecting developing critical illness, *Critical Intensive Care* (1997), 100.
[23] NAP, (2010) www.tyndall.ie/nap.
[24] NHS: National Institute for Health and Clinical Excellence (NICE) (2007) NICE Guideline 50 – Acutely ill patients in hospital: Recognition of and response to acute illness in adults in hospital, [online], www.nice.org.uk/CG050.
[25] T. O'Donovan, J. O'Donoghue, C. Sreenan, D. Sammon, P. O'Reilly and K. O'Connor, A context aware wireless body area network (BAN), in: *Proceedings 3rd International Conference on Pervasive Computing Technologies for Healthcare*, London, 2009.
[26] S. Parissopoulos and S. Kotzabassaki, Critical care outreach and the use of early warning scorin systems; A literature review, *ICU and Nursing Web Journal* **21** (2005), 1–13.
[27] R. Paterson, D.C. MacLeod, D. Thetford, A. Beattie, C. Graham, S. Lam and D. Bell, Prediction of in-hospital mortality and length of stay using an early warning scoring system: Clinical audit, *Journal of Clinical Medicine* **6** (2006), 281–284, Royal College of Physicians.
[28] P. Pharow and B. Blobel, Mobile health requires mobile security: Challenges, solutions, and standardization, in: *eHealth Beyond the Horizon – Get IT There*, S.K. Andersen et al., eds, IOS Press, 2008, pp. 697–702.
[29] D.R. Prytherch, G.B. Smith, P. Schmidt, P.I. Featherstone, K. Stewart, D. Knight and B. Higgins, Calculating early warning scores – A classroom comparison of pen and paper and hand-held computer methods, *Resuscitation* (2006), 173–178.
[30] T. Roberts, The 'Early Warning Score': Is it the right tool for the job?, *British Journal of Anaesthesia and Recovery Nursing* **9** (2008), 75–78.

[31] J. Rylance, T. Baker, E. Mushi and D. Mashaga, Use of an early warning score and ability to walk predicts mortality in medical patients admitted to hospitals in Tanzania, *Journal of Transactions of the Royal Society of Tropical Medicine and Hygiene* **103** (2009), 790–794, Elsevier.
[32] H. Scheepers and R. Scheepers, The implementation of mobile technology in organizations: expanding individual use contexts, in: *Proceedings of the International Conference on Information Systems*, 2004.
[33] C. Stenhouse, S. Coates, M. Tivey, P. Allsop and T. Parker, Prospective evaluation of a modified early warning score to aid earlier detection of patients developing critical illness on a general surgical ward, *British Journal of Anaesthesia* **84** (1999), 663.

Handbook of Ambient Assisted Living
J.C. Augusto et al. (Eds.)
IOS Press, 2012

doi:10.3233/978-1-60750-837-3-22

Using Human Factors to Guide the Design and Implementation of Consumer Health Informatics Interventions

Teresa ZAYAS-CABÁN[a,*] and Jenna L. MARQUARD[b]
[a] *Agency for Healthcare Research and Quality, Rockville, MD, USA*
[b] *University of Massachusetts Amherst, Amherst, MA, USA*

Abstract. The use of consumer health informatics (CHI) interventions is proliferating rapidly with little consensus about how CHI interventions should be designed or implemented. While CHI interventions have been shown to improve clinical outcomes, barriers to their use remain. This chapter describes a well-developed conceptual model for program evaluation and suggests how it can be used to guide the design and implementation of CHI interventions, with the goal of supporting the intended outcomes of these interventions and minimizing the unintended outcomes. The chapter then provides an overview of how knowledge from three human factors domains can inform the CHI interventions design and implementation components of the evaluation model. By integrating human factors principles and methods into the evaluation model, developers can reduce barriers to use and minimize resulting unintended consequences of CHI interventions.

Keywords. Consumer health informatics, human factors, design, implementation, evaluation

Introduction

The development of consumer health informatics (CHI) applications, defined by Jimison et al. as "electronic information and communication technologies that patients/consumers use to improve their medical outcomes and/or participate in their health care decision-making process" (page 9), has dramatically increased over the last decade [25]. At the same time, the use of CHI interventions – health care interventions that leverage the use of CHI applications, along with devices that monitor symptoms and other observations – is proliferating rapidly [25]. National initiatives for the adoption and meaningful use of health information technology (IT) include monetary incentives for meeting "patient engagement" requirements [5]. Federal agencies and private foundations, such as the Agency for Healthcare Research and Quality (AHRQ) and the Robert Wood Johnson Foundation (RWJF), are funding projects to demonstrate the feasibility and efficacy of using CHI interventions to aid "laypeople" – individuals not formally trained as health professionals – as they engage in health promotion (e.g., nutrition and physical activity), self-care (e.g., prevention activities), and disease man-

*Corresponding Author: Teresa Zayas-Cabán, PhD, Senior Manager, Health IT, Agency for Healthcare Research and Quality, 540 Gaither Road, Room 6115, Rockville, MD, USA 20850. E-mail: Teresa.ZayasCaban@ahrq.hhs.gov.

agement (e.g., diabetes and asthma control) activities [38,43,50]. Ideally, CHI interventions will address deficiencies in today's acute-care-centric U.S. health care system, by effectively promoting and improving laypeople's health and well-being while preventing acute care episodes. If successful, CHI interventions could thereby increase health care quality while reducing health care costs. The Institute of Medicine proposed 10 rules to guide the design of the health care system [23]. Two of the rules are particularly relevant to the topic being addressed in this chapter. The first rule states that care must shift from being based primarily on office visits to being based on "continuous healing relationships" (page 67) and the third rule states that patients – instead of professionals – must take control of their care [23].

In response to these initiatives and the broad consensus of the health care community that CHI interventions will be an essential part of the future health care system, health care providers, health IT vendors, and commercial hardware and software designers are rapidly developing health IT applications and devices to be used as part of CHI interventions. These applications and devices, whether provider-based portals where laypeople can view laboratory results, or glucometers that send blood sugar readings to a clinic through a smart phone, allow laypeople to carry out health care activities in their locations of daily living (LDLs) such as homes, workplaces, parks, exercise facilities, and grocery stores.

Ambient assistive living (AAL) technologies are essential components of broader CHI interventions. For instance, a 'smart home' might collect data via sensors about laypeoples' activities of daily living. These data could serve as an essential input to a falls prevention CHI intervention. Like CHI interventions, AAL technologies can support laypeople by improving their health and well-being (e.g., supporting independent living) while preventing acute care episodes. Additionally, because of the aging population and the resulting growth of chronic health problems, a significant number of CHI interventions are designed to support older individuals. A falls prevention CHI intervention, for instance, may send community-based nurses sensor data from laypeoples' homes and data collected via computer-based cognitive assessment tests. Based on these data, the nurse may contact individuals (s)he believes are at risk of falling. Based on the information gleaned during the follow-up telephone calls, the nurse may decide to visit the individual's home to make physical changes to the environment or perhaps change the individual's medications.

Given the rapid development of health IT applications and devices, there is little consensus about how CHI interventions should be designed and implemented, or how they should be evaluated. In a review of AHRQ-funded CHI projects, Zayas-Cabán and Dixon found that CHI intervention designers typically did not start their development with a broad design evaluation framework in mind, and did not include human factors and human-computer interaction principles and methods in their design process [51]. While the current technology-centered approach can be successful, it may also lead to CHI intervention designs that add too much to laypeople's existing work, increase their frustration, and lead to errors, misuse, and/or disuse of the interventions, thereby negating some of the potential benefits of the interventions [32,51]. While there exist established models and approaches that can guide the evaluation of CHI interventions, these models and approaches have not been broadly applied in this field [14,53].

In this chapter we describe a well-developed conceptual model for program evaluation and suggest how this model can be used by the CHI community to guide the evaluation of CHI interventions. After describing this model in greater detail, we provide an overview of intended outcomes that have been used to evaluate CHI interven-

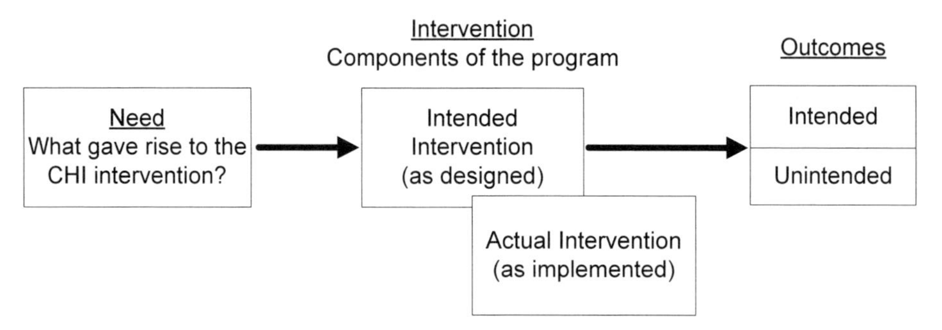

Figure 1. Conceptual model for program evaluation.

tions to date. We also outline a brief case example to demonstrate the intervention evaluation components in the context of the design and implementation of a CHI intervention. The value of this evaluation model is largely in defining the *relationships between* CHI intervention design, implementation, and related outcomes. The evaluation model does not, however, provide explicit guidance for the design and implementation of CHI interventions in a way that improves intended outcomes and reduces unintended outcomes.

The field of human factors can provide the explicit guidance necessary for identifying clinicians' and laypeoples' needs, and for informing the design and implementation of CHI interventions. We therefore provide an overview of the three human factors domains and give examples demonstrating instances where these methods have been used to identify negative CHI intervention design and implementation components, and instances where CHI interventions have had unintended outcomes.

1. Conceptual Model for Evaluating the Impact of CHI Interventions

The conceptual model for program evaluation shown in Fig. 1, with respect to CHI interventions, consists of three main components:

1. Identifying a problem or need faced by clinicians and/or laypeople,
2. Designing and implementing the components of the CHI intervention, and
3. Measuring the intended and unintended outcomes of the CHI intervention.

The conceptual model shown in Fig. 1 is based on generally established approaches for field research and program evaluation [16,42]. It requires clear definitions of the existing need that the CHI intervention should meet and details the CHI intervention design and implementation components. The conceptual model also requires clear definitions of the intervention outcomes, whether intended or unintended. This model is clearly beneficial to designers as they consider the downstream consequences of their needs assessment and design and implementation choices.

For instance, in their review of CHI projects, Zayas-Cabán and Dixon found that most CHI interventions were initiated based on clinical problems or needs rather than on laypeople's problems and needs [51]. This choice in framing the problem or need as clinical likely has a significant impact on the design and implementation of the intervention. Because laypeople may view clinical problems or needs differently from CHI intervention designers or clinicians, the implementation of the intervention may deviate from the intended design of the intervention and therefore may result in a significant number of unintended outcomes.

1.1. CHI Intervention Outcomes Measured to Date

CHI interventions will ideally improve health care quality, and thereby improve the health and well-being of laypeople using the interventions. The Institute of Medicine proposed six aims for improvement of health care quality [23], stating that the U.S. health care system should strive to provide care that is:

1. Safe – "avoiding injuries to patients from the care that is intended to help them" (page 39);
2. Effective – "providing services based on scientific knowledge to all who could benefit and refraining from providing services to those not likely to benefit" (page 39);
3. Patient-centered – "providing care that is respectful of and responsive to individual patient preferences, needs, and values and ensuring that patient values guide all clinical decisions" (page 40);
4. Timely – "reducing waits and sometimes harmful delays for both those who receive and those who give care" (page 40);
5. Efficient – "avoiding waste, in particular waste of equipment, supplies, ideas, and energy" (page 40); and
6. Equitable – "providing care that does not vary in quality because of personal characteristics such as gender, ethnicity, geographic location, and socioeconomic status" (page 40).

Accordingly, the majority of the studies evaluating the impact of CHI interventions have focused on outcomes that can demonstrate measurable changes in the health or well-being of their users (e.g., clinical outcomes) or in factors that may influence clinical outcomes.

Recent syntheses of the CHI literature illustrate the types of outcomes typically examined in these evaluations, with example outcomes from these syntheses shown in Table 1. As shown in Table 1, clinical outcomes focus on measurable changes in the health of a patient. For an elderly diabetic patient, a given CHI intervention may significantly reduce fasting blood glucose levels or produce a significant change in average glycated hemoglobin (HbA1C) values. Other measurable outcomes include process outcomes (e.g., whether the intervention aids the provider in ensuring that the patient receives an annual foot exam), relationship-centered outcomes (e.g., whether the intervention aids the primary care provider and the patient in discussing and agreeing on a shared care plan for the patient), economic outcomes (e.g., whether the intervention is cost-effective), and intermediate outcomes (e.g., whether the intervention increases the patient's knowledge about diabetes and how to manage it).

However, even though the design and implementation of CHI interventions can impact patient adoption, these features are often not examined. As Jimison et al. found, outcomes related to the design and implementation of CHI interventions are typically reported as "secondary findings, and not part of the primary study design" (page 30) [25]. Jimison et al. found a total of 129 articles for inclusion in their review of CHI intervention studies, and while 70 studies included outcomes related to clinical effectiveness, 31 evaluated use, 54 evaluated usability, 52 evaluated barriers to use, and 60

Table 1. Commonly examined outcomes in the evaluation of consumer health informatics interventions

Process Outcomes	Intermediate Outcomes	Relationship-Centered Outcomes	Economic Outcomes	Clinical Outcomes
• Health care utilization [15,25]. • Receiving appropriate treatment [15,25]. • Therapeutic adherence [14,15,25].	• Health behaviors [14,15,25]. • Health knowledge [14,15,25]. • [Patient] self-management [14,15,25].	• Access to medical or health information [15]. • Patient-clinician communication [14,15]. • Shared decision-making [14,15].	• Access to care [25]. • Health care costs [14,15,25]. • Intervention cost-effectiveness [14,15,25].	• Disease status [14,15,25]. • Functional status [15,25]. • Quality of life [14,15,25].

evaluated drivers to use [25]. Similarly, Gibbons et al. found a total of 162 articles addressing the outcomes of CHI interventions, but only 31 of these articles evaluated issues related to design and implementation of the intervention [15].

Moreover, while robust methods are often used to measure the outcomes listed in Table 1 (e.g., randomized controlled trials, cohort studies, trials with a case series or before-after designs, and cross sectional studies), in many cases, findings regarding the design and implementation of CHI interventions come from epidemiologic studies addressing rates of use of interactive CHI interventions or from nonvalidated surveys conducted to assess the perceived usefulness and/or usability of an intervention. While randomized controlled trials may not be appropriate, formal, robust studies intended to evaluate the design and implementation of these interventions are needed.

1.2. Example of a CHI Intervention

To better illustrate these concepts in the context of a CHI intervention, Table 2 details the program evaluation components for an example CHI intervention based on a real implementation. The intervention was developed based on a known clinical problem: *poor management of a specific complex condition that results in a high rate of hospitalization and deaths and high health care costs*. Based on this clinical problem, the intervention components in the left column of Table 2 appear to be well construed. The intervention provides direct support to patients with the chronic illness, and supports patient-provider communication. Again, AAL technologies often serve as key components of CHI interventions, which are frequently designed to support older individuals with chronic illnesses. While AAL technologies are not included in this intervention, one potential key outcome for this intervention would be to support patients' abilities to live independently. While patient vital signs were relayed to providers via a Web site in this study, vital signs could instead be monitored and transmitted (perhaps more effectively) via wearable sensors.

While the desired outcomes shown in the center column of Table 2 are all beneficial, they all likely depend on factors related to patients' uptake and use of the intervention. As shown in the right column of Table 2, there were significant barriers present during the implementation of the intervention, all of which likely affected patients' uptake and use of the intervention – which then limited the effectiveness of the intervention.

The intervention barriers detailed in this example of a CHI intervention are quite typical [14,15,25,51]. However, many of these barriers, and their subsequent effects on

Table 2. Program evaluation components for an example of a consumer health informatics intervention

Intervention	Desired Outcomes	Intervention Barriers and Unintended Outcomes
• Self-management system with decision support. • Patients provide vital signs to doctors through a Web site. • Doctors access the information through the Web site to monitor and treat patients.	• Improvements in patients' access to care. • Improvements in patients' quality of care. • Improved clinical outcomes 1. Fewer significant clinical episodes. 2. Lower mortality rates. • Reduction in costs of care due to fewer: 1. Physician visits. 2. Hospitalizations. 3. Hospital length of stay (LOS). 4. Emergency room visits. • Improved patient involvement in and satisfaction with care. • A delivery model that can be replicated.	• Intervention implementation experienced delays because vendor staff did not test the system adequately. • Patients failed to install the devices, requiring home visits by staff members. • Patients did not have existing technology in their homes to support the system. • Vendor IT support was limited and inconsistent. • Clinic staff was overwhelmed by the volume of data sent by patients. • Clinical staff did not proactively log on to the Web site. • Clinical staff did not file the data into the patient's medical record.

the intervention outcomes, could likely be minimized by carefully taking human factors design principles into account throughout the intervention design and implementation process.

2. Human Factors Domains

While the conceptual model shown in Fig. 1 provides an overarching way to structure the relationships between CHI intervention design, implementation, and related outcomes, it does not provide explicit guidance for the design and implementation of CHI interventions in a way that improves intended outcomes and reduces unintended outcomes. The field of human factors can provide the explicit guidance necessary for identifying clinicians' and laypeoples' needs, and for informing the design and implementation of CHI interventions by enabling designers to understand "interactions among humans and other elements of a system" in order to "optimize human well-being and overall system performance" [24].

Although human factors methods are typically applied to industrial systems, we have outlined how all human factors domains: physical ergonomics, cognitive ergonomics, and organizational ergonomics (or macroergonomics), can be used to guide the design and implementation of CHI interventions [47,52,53]. As detailed below, accounting for the key attributes of these three domains in CHI design and implementation will ensure that CHI interventions account not only for users' physical constraints and their cognitive tasks and needs, but also for the context in which CHI interventions are expected to be used.

2.1. Physical Ergonomics

Physical ergonomics encompasses both the physical characteristics of the users and their work environment. Therefore, to be used successfully, CHI interventions must fit both the physical characteristics of the individual and the existing physical environment. To date, the study of physical ergonomics within health care has largely focused on health care professionals – most often addressing musculoskeletal problems of nursing staff resulting from tasks such as lifting patients – or on the physical working environment in health care organizations [1,20].

CHI intervention users – especially those with chronic illnesses – may possess a variety of diminished physical capabilities. For example, users may have some form of reduced vision making them less able to see fine details on devices or interfaces, or diminished contrast sensitivity that impairs their abilities to differentiate levels of brightness on displays. Some users will be unable to distinguish between certain colors (e.g., they may have red-green color blindness), whereas others might have a portion of their field of view completely blocked [6]. Users may also have reduced hearing function. They may be unable to detect whether a noise, such as a reminder beep from a device, is present. They may be unable to discriminate speech from background noise, or discern the direction from which a sound originates [6].

CHI intervention users may also have reduced motor function. A user may have trouble with locomotion: walking, stepping up or down, or balancing. A user may have limited range of motion in his/her arms or limited dexterity, including limited ability to push, pinch objects between two fingers, grip something with the whole hand, or complete tasks that require two hands [6,17].

Physical ergonomics also addresses the characteristics of the physical work environment. Whereas health care workers tend to work in environments designed to deliver health care (e.g., clinics, surgery centers), users of CHI interventions perform health work in varied locations of daily living (LDLs), primarily private residences, where physical conditions limit the interventions that can be used. Additionally, the growth of mobile computing devices requires that CHI interventions be used in dynamically changing LDLs. Where an intervention in a traditional health care setting might include the redesign of the physical environment, designers of CHI interventions have less control over the redesign of LDLs such as individuals' homes, communities, and workplaces, in which CHI interventions may increasingly be used due to the growth of mobile computing devices. In fact, any physical redesign (e.g., railings, ramps) of LDLs is dependent upon the individuals' willingness and ability to make these changes, as well as the availability of outside resources to support these changes.

CHI interventions require laypeople to interact physically with CHI applications and related devices. Designers of CHI interventions would benefit by understanding the physical abilities and limitations of possible users. For guidance on users' physical abilities and limitations see [6,11,12,39,41]. In addition, designers need to consider whether the technologies will fit within the physical LDLs in which laypeople will use them. See [1,2,13,26,37,40] for guidance on the design of physical devices and environments.

2.2. Cognitive Ergonomics

Cognitive ergonomics focuses on aiding individuals as they complete tasks alone or in teams. Like physical ergonomics, cognitive ergonomics in the domain of health care has largely focused on aiding health care professionals as they complete demanding tasks [27,54]. While the types of health work laypeople engage in may not be as time sensitive as professional health care tasks, laypeople's health work is unpaid, and their training in completing this type of work is likely nonexistent or minimal. Additionally, laypeople tend to possess different skill sets, motivations, and capabilities than do health care professionals. Thus, CHI interventions used by laypeople require different design considerations.

As with their physical characteristics, laypeople may have diminished cognitive function, including diminished perception, attention, memory, and/or learning abilities. CHI interventions may be developed specifically because the user has cognitive function loss – an example would be a medication reminder system for an Alzheimer's patient. Communication barriers, whether because of language differences, literacy levels, or visual and hearing impairments, may also affect laypeople's use of CHI interventions [6].

The design and implementation of CHI interventions must account for how the technologies fit with or support individuals' macrocognitive functions [30]. Naturalistic decision-making studies show, for instance, that laypeople often make decisions based on their previous experiences and not by comparing options in a structured way [8,29,30]. Designers of CHI interventions must account for laypeople's potentially heuristic, experience-based styles of decision-making.

Laypeople's sensemaking regarding their current health status and predictions about their future health status will likely influence both their decision-making and behavior changes. Their sensemaking will also influence what CHI interventions they use, if any, and how they use these CHI interventions to make decisions and change their behaviors. People who believe that their health conditions result purely from genetic makeup will likely make different choices and engage in different behaviors from those who believe that their conditions result from their previous choices and behaviors. Identifying laypeople's sensemaking strategies may help identify those individuals who will benefit most from the use of CHI interventions.

Many CHI interventions are aimed at helping laypeople engage in planning, adaptation, problem detection, and communication tasks. Designers of CHI interventions would benefit by understanding how laypeople currently perform these tasks and how devices and applications are likely to fit or support these cognitive tasks. See [4,9,10,21,22,31,33,34,36,44–46] for guidance on cognitive ergonomics assessment methods.

2.3. Macroergonomics

Macroergonomics focuses on the analysis and design of work, including "any form of human effort or activity, including recreation and leisure pursuits" (page 1) [19]. While much health work occurs in health care settings and is conducted by clinicians, office and hospital staff, and other health care professionals, laypeople also engage in health work to maintain and manage their health. Macroergonomics addresses both the type of work laypeople might engage in, their workflow (i.e. the flow of information, people, and artifacts across space and time), and their work system (i.e. the social, workflow, organizational, and environmental conditions under which work is performed). Not only is laypeople's health work different from health care workers' care work, so are their workflows and work systems.

Work system design can include implementing a technological change within a particular health care process; for example, implementing a bar-coded medication administration system – a technological change within the medication administration process [3]. Such a change will have a significant impact on how nurses do their work, and will require training and effective engagement of staff throughout the change process. Similarly, a CHI intervention that an individual uses to manage his/her health and health care is a technological change that will have an impact on the work system, the household in this case. For example, a CHI intervention for patients managing diabetes will impact how and when they draw their blood sugar and how they adjust insulin levels and meals, among other things. These changes, whether creating new health care processes or redesigning existing processes, must account for the fit between the technical change and the household work system.

Like physical and cognitive design and implementation considerations, macroergonomic work system design and implementation must include both (1) understanding the current work system to guide the design of appropriate solutions, and (2) understanding the impact of the chosen CHI intervention on the work system.

Several work system aspects of a household must be considered when designing and implementing CHI interventions. Proper CHI design rests on understanding how tasks are carried out – including where they occur and the resources used. Health work is information-based, and the tools and technologies used by individuals to carry out health work vary – from calendars to keep track of appointments to devices to keep track of personal observations such as blood sugar or blood pressure. In addition, the sociocultural and socioeconomic characteristics of the individuals involved in health work are also relevant to CHI intervention design. Education level, for example, may affect both IT and health expertise. CHI interventions may need to fit or support a range of general and health literacy levels. Furthermore, an individual's ability to manage his or her health is greatly influenced by external factors such as having easy access to the providers that prescribe prevention or treatment plans, and having sufficient resources available in the individual's community.

Finally, how individuals manage their health may be influenced by their household structure, which can range in complexity from an individual who lives alone and makes all the decisions about his/her care; to a family of four where the mother is the primary health manager and keeps track of everybody's appointments and health regimens; to a single adult taking care of an elderly parent and making most of the health care decisions for the parent but taking into account her preferences; to a network of relatives across residences, who share health care responsibilities and decisions. All of these structures vary in their degree of formalization of how health care tasks are carried out and how decisions are made, and in their degree of centralization – whether decisions are made individually, or collectively with parents or adult children.

Many CHI interventions are aimed at supporting laypeople in their health and health information management work. Designers of CHI interventions would benefit by understanding the ways laypeople currently perform tasks to support health and health information management, the individuals who may aid them in doing so, and the resources used in the process. See [7,18,19,28,48–50] for guidance on macroergonomics assessment methods.

3. Barriers to Use and Unintended Consequences of CHI Interventions

As previously discussed, how a CHI intervention is designed and implemented can influence its outcomes, with poor design or implementation rendering CHI interventions ineffective or suboptimal. Even if an intervention is shown to be effective in improving clinical and related outcomes, if its design or implementation poses significant barriers to use, an unintended consequence may be that the intervention is not broadly adopted and used.

While not common for all CHI interventions, some studies have employed human factors methods in the design and implementation of CHI interventions. As noted by Zayas-Cabán and Dixon, projects incorporating user needs into the design of the CHI intervention have focused on users' (1) informational needs to manage a particular condition (i.e. ensuring that the content to be provided or user data to be collected by the CHI intervention is clinically relevant), (2) desired functionalities, (3) physical abilities or limitations (e.g., using a broad range of blood pressure cuff sizes to fit all users), (4) cognitive abilities and skills (e.g., selecting a device that could be easily used with minimal instructions), (5) variations in care plans (e.g., ensuring that the intervention includes asking patients with multiple comorbidities for relevant information), and (6) preferred device models (e.g., ensuring that the intervention provides for upload of data from different glucometer models) [51]. Methods for ascertaining these needs included guidance from clinicians, general knowledge about the patient or user population, and focus groups. Often, however, CHI interventions have not been designed and implemented with a clear understanding of actual user needs and their current health promotion, self-care, and disease management activities.

Methods commonly used to evaluate the design or implementation of a CHI intervention include measuring the patterns of usage of the intervention, its perceived usefulness, and/or its perceived or actual usability. Jimison et al. found that adoption and use of a CHI intervention is typically measured in one of three ways: "(1) the usage of technology by subjects over a specified time interval, (2) the change in technology usage by subjects over time, and (3) the absolute or relative usage of specific functions compared to one another, within a particular technology application" (page 22) [25]. Data sources for assessment of subjects' usage typically include Web log data (e.g., number of logins, time spent using the intervention once logged in) and surveys to collect self-reported information on intervention use.

Evaluation of the perceived usefulness of the intervention generally involves the use of focus groups and surveys or interviews. These methods typically are intended to ascertain users' perceptions of the intervention; for example, perceived benefits of use or barriers to use; as well as users' perceived efficiency in using the intervention. The usefulness of the intervention is very dependent on how the intervention is implemented, and a poor implementation may impact users' perceived usefulness of the intervention [25].

Evaluation of the usability of an intervention can include the use of surveys or more structured usability tests. Jimison et al. found that, of the few studies designed specifically to evaluate the usability of an intervention, most used "protocol analysis with 'talk aloud' techniques" (page 26) [25].

We categorized the barriers to use and the unintended consequences of CHI interventions currently identified in the literature, grouped by the three human factors domains. Table 3 includes the three issues that have been identified in the literature as physical barriers to the use of CHI interventions [14,15,51].

Elderly users in one of the projects described by Zayas-Cabán and Dixon encountered difficulties in using the scale that was part of the CHI intervention, as they could not stand on the scale long enough to measure their weight [51]. Similarly, Gibbons et al. found in one study that upper extremity weakness and decreased mobility affected users' abilities to easily use the intervention [14]. In addition, Gibbons et al. found that in one study limited hearing and vision prevented users from effectively interacting with the intervention's interface [14]. These examples show how important it is to con-

Table 3. Physical barrier to use of consumer health informatics interventions

No.	Barrier to Use
1	Limited dexterity, locomotion, and reach and stretch capabilities [14,15,51].
2	Limited hearing [14,15].
3	Limited vision [14,15].

Table 4. Cognitive barriers to use of consumer health informatics interventions

No.	Barrier to Use
1	Intervention supported novice users but not expert users [25].
2	Lack of perceived benefit [14,15,25].
3	Lack of trust in the system [14,15,25].
4	Lack of usability [14,15].
5	Language barriers [15].
6	Limited literacy, numeracy, and/or health literacy [14,15].
7	Cognitive impairment (e.g., caused by dementia, developmental disabilities, or head injuries) [14,15].
8	Low technology literacy, confusion with the technology, or limited technical proficiency [14,15,25].

sider the functional tasks required to effectively use the intervention, and how those tasks compare with the target user population's physical abilities and limitations.

Table 4 shows eight types of cognitive barriers to the use of CHI interventions identified in the literature. CHI interventions may need to support a wide range of users with diverse levels of experience with technology [14,15,25]. These interventions should be designed so that users can easily install and use the applications and devices on their own.

In addition, if users do not perceive a benefit to the intervention, they are unlikely to use it and therefore cannot benefit from it. In particular, if the intervention provides health advice or guidance that differs from users' prior experiences, they may not believe the system and may therefore not follow its guidance. Issues of literacy, numeracy, and health literacy can be significant barriers to use. For instance, to adjust their dietary intake, diabetic individuals must interpret numerical blood glucose levels and reason about what these numbers mean. Therefore, in designing an intervention, it is important to account for the variations in levels of literacy and numeracy within the target user population.

As shown in Table 5, eight different types of macroergonomic barriers to the use of CHI interventions have been found in the literature [14,15,25,51]. Many CHI interventions depend, for example, on a clinician's ability to access information uploaded to the system and provide timely feedback to the patient. As shown in the table, if clinicians are not interacting with the system, laypeople may be discouraged from further using it.

Interventions that create additional work for users, such as extensive data entry, may be seen as cumbersome, hindering adoption and use. Critical to the adoption of these interventions, however, is how they fit within the context in which they will be used. This includes, for example, ensuring that users have ready access to the technology needed to access the intervention, and/or that the intervention is compatible with the technology that individuals already use in their daily lives. For example, as noted by Zayas-Cabán and Dixon, a barrier to use for one intervention was that the CHI intervention was not compatible with voice-over Internet protocol (VOIP) or with cellular phones [51]. Similarly, another Web-based system required broadband Internet access to efficiently access the system. Dial-up users were at a disadvantage compared to

Table 5. Macroergonomic barriers to use of consumer health informatics interventions

No.	Barrier to Use
1	Clinicians are unresponsive or do not interact with the system [25,51].
2	Current resources, infrastructure, or systems do not support use of the intervention [14,15,25,51].
3	Intervention creates additional work [14,15].
4	Intervention does not fit user's lifestyle or clinician's workflow [14,15,25,51].
5	Privacy and data security concerns [14,15].
6	Reimbursement for interaction with the patient via the intervention is insufficient [15,25].
7	Technological malfunctions and/or poor IT support [25,51].
8	Technology is too cumbersome (e.g., manual data entry) [14,15,25].

those who used broadband. This problem will grow as more individuals use varied mobile devices to connect to the Internet, as opposed to utilizing home-based or location-specific connections.

A total of 19 unique barriers to use or unintended consequences of CHI interventions have been identified across the three human factors domains. Several of these relate to cognitive issues. In particular, the user's primary language (English), current computer and Internet use, and positive beliefs about CHI have been shown to positively influence adoption [35]. Many of the barriers found to CHI intervention use were macroergonomic, and they are consistent with barriers to use of clinical information systems [32]. The diversity of these barriers and their potential to influence adoption and use of CHI interventions highlights the importance of incorporating human factors approaches into the design and implementation of CHI interventions.

4. Conclusion

The increased development of CHI interventions is expected to support new models of care and improve health care quality. While CHI interventions have been shown to improve clinical, process, and other outcomes, their adoption and use may be hindered by poor design or implementation. To ensure that these interventions are adopted and used, and that they meet their goal of improving health care quality, it is important to evaluate both the design and implementation of CHI interventions.

Laypeople have distinct needs and abilities that may differ from those of professional health care workers. In addition, they perform health work in environments very different from those of health care workers. The field of human factors can reduce barriers to the effective use of CHI interventions and minimize unintended consequences, by offering concepts and methods to identify unique user needs and by guiding the design and implementation of the interventions.

Acknowledgements

The authors thank Kevin Chaney, MGS, Amy Helwig, MD, MS, and David Meyers, MD from the Agency for Healthcare Research and Quality for their valuable advice on this document. The authors also thank Marion Torchia for her editorial support. The opinions expressed in this chapter are those of the authors and do not reflect the official position of the Agency for Healthcare Research and Quality or the U.S. Department of Health and Human Services.

References

[1] C.J. Alvarado, The physical environment in health care, in: *Handbook of Human Factors and Ergonomics in Health Care and Patient Safety*, P. Carayon, ed., Lawrence Erlbaum Associates, Mahwah, NJ, 2007, pp. 287–307.
[2] R.L. Brauer, *Safety and Health for Engineers*, John Wiley & Sons, Hoboken, NJ, 2006.
[3] P. Carayon, Human factors and ergonomics in health care and patient safety, in: *Handbook of Human Factors and Ergonomics in Health Care and Patient Safety*, P. Carayon, ed., Lawrence Erlbaum Associates, Mahwah, NJ, 2007, pp. 3–19.
[4] S.K. Card, T.P. Moran and A. Newell, *The Psychology of Human-Computer Interaction*, Lawrence Erlbaum Associates, Hillsdale, NJ, 1983.
[5] Centers for Medicare & Medicaid Services Department of Health and Human Services, Medicare and Medicaid programs, electronic health record incentive program, *Federal Register* (2010), 44314–44588.
[6] J. Clarkson, R. Coleman, I. Hosking and S. Waller, eds, *Inclusive Design Toolkit*, Cambridge Engineering Design Centre, UK, 2007.
[7] E. Coakes, D. Willis and R. Lloyd-Jones, eds, *The New Sociotech: Graffiti on the Long Wall*, Springer-Verlag, London, 2000.
[8] B. Crandall, G. Klein and R. Hoffman, *Working Minds: A Practitioner's Guide to Cognitive Task Analysis*, MIT Press, Cambridge, MA, 2006.
[9] S.J. Czaja, N. Charness, A.D. Fisk, C. Hertzog, S.N. Nair, W.A. Rogers et al., Factors predicting the use of technology: Findings from the center for research and education on aging and technology enhancement (CREATE), *Psychol. Aging* **21**(2) (2006), 333–352.
[10] F.T. Durso, R.T. Nickerson, S.T. Dumais, S. Lewandowsky and T.J. Perfect, eds, *Handbook of Applied Cognition*, John Wiley & Sons, Chichester, UK, 2007.
[11] M. Evamy and L. Roberts, *In sight: A guide to design with low vision in mind: Examining the notion of inclusive design, exploring the subject within a commercial and social context*, RotoVision SA, London, 2004.
[12] A.D. Fisk and W.A. Rogers, Health care of older adults: The promise of human factors research, in: *Human Factors Interventions for the Health Care of Older Adults*, W.A. Rogers and A.D. Fisk, eds, Lawrence Earlbaum Associates, Mahwah, NJ, 2001, pp. 1–12.
[13] D. Gardner-Bonneau, Designing medical devices for older adults, in: *Human Factors Interventions for the Health Care of Older Adults*, W.A. Rogers and A.D. Fisk, eds, Lawrence Erlbaum Associates, Mahwah, NJ, 2001, pp. 217–236.
[14] M.C. Gibbons, R.F. Wilson, L. Samal, C.U. Lehmann, K. Dickersin, H.P. Lehmann et al., Consumer health informatics: Results of a systematic evidence review and evidence based recommendations, *Transl. Behav. Med.* **1**(1) (2011), 72–82.
[15] M.C. Gibbons, R.F. Wilson, L. Samal, C.U. Lehmann, K. Dickersin, H.P. Lehmann et al., Impact of consumer health informatics applications, Report No.: 188, Agency for Healthcare Research and Quality, Rockville, MD, 2009 (prepared by Johns Hopkins University Evidence-based Practice Center under contract no. 290-2007-10061-5).
[16] D. Grembowski, *The Practice of Health Program Evaluation*, SAGE, Thousand Oaks, CA, 2001.
[17] E. Grundy, D. Ahlburg, M. Ali, E. Breeze and A. Sloggett, Disability in Great Britain: Results from the 1996/97 disability follow-up to the Family Resources Survey, Department of Social Security Research Report, Report No.: 94, Corporate Document Services, London, 1999.
[18] H.W. Hendrick and B.M. Kleiner, *Macroergonomics: An Introduction to Work System Design*, Human Factors and Ergonomics Society, Santa Monica, CA, 2001.
[19] H.W. Hendrick and B.M. Kleiner, *Macroergonomics: Theory, Methods, and Applications,* Lawrence Erlbaum Associates, Mahwah, NJ, 2002.
[20] S. Hignett, Physical ergonomics in health care, in: *Handbook of Human Factors and Ergonomics in Health Care and Patient Safety*, P. Carayon, ed., Lawrence Erlbaum Associates, Mahwah, NJ, 2007, pp. 309–321.
[21] E. Hollnagel, ed., *Handbook of Cognitive Task Design*, Lawrence Erlbaum Associates, Mahwah, NJ, 2003.
[22] F.A. Huppert, Designing for older users, in: *Inclusive Design: Design for the Whole Population*, J. Clarkson, R. Coleman, S. Kates and C. Lebbon, eds, Springer-Verlag, London, 2003, pp. 30–49.
[23] Institute of Medicine, *Crossing the Quality Chasm: A New Health System for the 21st Century*, National Academy Press, Washington, DC, 2001.
[24] International Ergonomic Association, What is ergonomics?, 2000 [cited 2011 March 23], available from: http://www.iea.cc/01_what/What%20is%20Ergonomics.html.

[25] H. Jimison, P. Gorman, S. Woods, P. Nygren, M. Walker, S. Norris et al., Barriers and drivers of health information technology use for the elderly, chronically ill, and underserved, Report No.: 175, Agency for Healthcare Research and Quality, Rockville, MD, 2008 (prepared by the Oregon Evidence-based Practice Center under contract no. 290-2002-0024-9).
[26] W. Karwowski. *Handbook of Standards and Guidelines in Ergonomics and Human Factors*, Lawrence Erlbaum Associates, Mahwah, NJ, 2003.
[27] A. Kirlik, *Adaptive Perspectives on Human-Technology Interaction: Methods and Models for Cognitive Engineering and Human-Computer Interaction*, Oxford University Press, New York, 2006.
[28] B.M. Kleiner, Macroegonomics: Work system analysis and design, *Hum. Factors* **50**(3) (2008), 461–467.
[29] J.L. Marquard and P.F. Brennan, Are we crying wolf? Lay people may be more willing to share medication information than policy makers expect, *J. Healthc. Inf. Manag.* **23**(2) (2009), 26–32.
[30] J.L. Marquard and P.F. Brennan, Using decision scenarios to evaluate laypeople's computer-mediated medication information sharing choices, in: *9th Bi-annual International Conference on Naturalistic Decision Making (NDM9)*, 23–26 June 2009, British Computer Society, London, UK.
[31] N. Mead, R. Varnam, A. Rogers and M. Roland, What predicts patients' interest in the Internet as a health resource in primary care in England?, *J. Health. Serv. Res. Policy* **8**(1) (2003), 33–39.
[32] National Research Council, *Computational Technology for Effective Health Care: Immediate Steps and Strategic Directions*, National Academies Press, Washington, DC, 2009.
[33] J. Nielsen, *Usability Engineering*, Academic Press, San Diego, CA, 1993.
[34] D.A. Norman, *The Design of Everyday Things*, Basic Books, New York, 2002.
[35] C.K. Or and B.-T. Karsh, A systematic review of patient acceptance of consumer health information technology, *J. Am. Med. Inform. Assoc.* **16**(4) (2009), 550–560.
[36] C.K.L. Or and B.-T. Karsh, The patient technology acceptance model (PTAM) for homecare patients with chronic illness, in: *HFES 50th Annual Meeting October 16–20*, Human Factors and Ergonomics Society, San Francisco, CA, 2006, pp. 989–993.
[37] W.F.E. Preiser and E. Ostroff, *Universal Design Handbook*, McGraw-Hill, New York, 2001.
[38] Robert Wood Johnson Foundation, Project HealthDesign: Rethinking the power and potential of personal health records, 2009 [cited 2011 March 30], available from: http://www.projecthealthdesign.org.
[39] W.A. Rogers, B. Meyer, N. Walker and A.D. Fisk, Functional limitations to daily living tasks in the aged: A focus group analysis, *Hum. Factors* **40**(1) (1998), 111–125.
[40] M.S. Sanders and E.J. McCormick, *Human Factors in Engineering and Design*, 7th edn, McGraw-Hill, New York, 1993.
[41] A.R. Tilley and H. Dreyfuss Associates, *The Measure of Man and Woman: Human Factors in Design*, John Wiley & Sons New York, 2002.
[42] W.M.K. Trochim and J.P. Donnelly, *Research Methods Knowledge Base*, 3rd edn, Atomic Dog Publishing, Mason, OH, 2006.
[43] US Department of Health and Human Services, Ambulatory safety and quality: Enabling patient-centered care through health IT, 2006 [cited 2011 March 30], available from: http://grants1.nih.gov/grants/guide/rfa-files/RFA-HS-07-007.html.
[44] V. Venkatesh and H. Bala. Technology acceptance model 3 and a research agenda on interventions, *Decision Sciences* **39**(2) (2008), 273–315.
[45] K.J. Vicente, *Cognitive Work Analysis: Toward Safe, Productive, and Healthy Computer Based Work*, Lawrence Erlbaum Associates, Mahwah, NJ, 1999.
[46] C.D. Wickens and J.G. Hollands, *Engineering Psychology and Human Performance*, 3rd edn, Prentice Hall, Upper Saddle River, NJ, 2000.
[47] C.D. Wickens, J.D. Lee, Y. Liu and S.E. Gordon, *An Introduction to Human Factors Engineering*, 2nd edn, Pearson Prentice Hall, Upper Saddle River, NJ, 2004.
[48] T. Zayas-Cabán, Assessing the distributed nature of home health information management to inform human factors design, in: *HFES 49th Annual Meeting September 26–30*, Human Factors and Ergonomics Society, Orlando, FL, 2005, pp. 1747–1751.
[49] T. Zayas-Cabán, Introducing information technology into the home: Conducting a home assessment, *AMIA Annu. Symp. Proc.* (2002), 924–928.
[50] T.Zayas-Cabán and P.F. Brennan, Human factors in home care, in: *Handbook of Human Factors and Ergonomics in Health Care and Patient Safety*, P. Carayon, ed., Lawrence Erlbaum Associates, Mahwah, NJ, 2007, pp. 883–897.
[51] T. Zayas-Cabán and B.E. Dixon, Considerations for the design of safe and effective consumer health IT applications in the home, *Qual. Saf. Health Care* **19**(Suppl 3) (2010), i61–i67.

[52] T. Zayas-Cabán and J.L. Marquard, A holistic human factors evaluation framework for the design of consumer health informatics interventions, in: *HFES 53rd Annual Meeting October 19–23*, Human Factors and Ergonomics Society, San Antonio, TX, 2009, pp. 1003–1007.
[53] T. Zayas-Cabán, J.L. Marquard, K. Radhakrishnan, N. Duffey and D.L. Evernden. Scenario-based user testing to guide consumer health informatics design, in: *AMIA Annu. Symp. Proc.*, 2009, pp. 719–723.
[54] C.E. Zsambok and G.A. Klein, *Naturalistic Decision Making*, Lawrence Erlbaum Associates, Mahwah, NJ, 1997.

Handbook of Ambient Assisted Living
J.C. Augusto et al. (Eds.)
IOS Press, 2012

doi:10.3233/978-1-60750-837-3-37

The National Health Service in England – Moving to Mainstream Use of Ambient Assisted Living Technology

George MACGINNIS*
PA Consulting and Continua Health Alliance

Abstract. The UK has been an early adopter in the use of ambient assisted living technology for social care and this experience has helped to shape the approach to the use of technology in healthcare. The National Health Service (NHS) in England has benefited from a series of policy measures, supported by grant funding, that have resulted in a significant uptake of ambient assisted living technologies in both health and social care. Over the period 2005–2010 the NHS has moved from a few small scale pilots toward a situation where a growing proportion of local health authorities have implemented some form of service, and a few have moved on to plan or deploy technology on a large scale.

The paper examines the operational use of assisted living technologies, highlighting the pivotal place of the 'Whole System Demonstrators' which have been established to generate the evidence needed to support a move towards mainstream adoption. It also examines a number of other operational implementations of assisted living to identify trends in the technologies and draw out lessons for the deployment and use of these technologies as mainstream services.

Keywords. Telehealth, telecare, long term condition, whole system demonstrator, NHS, standards, continua health alliance

Introduction

The UK has been among the early adopters in the use of ambient assisted living technology to deliver better healthcare. The National Health Service provides universal coverage, free at the point of need and funded by tax which offers an opportunity to take a longer term view of health outcomes. Evidence based guidelines for clinical care are established by NICE, The National Institute for health and Clinical Excellence, and steps have been taken to move payments for primary care from an activity to an outcomes based model. Policies supportive of the use of ambient assisted living technology have been in place for some years and the near-universal coverage means that the NHS ought not to suffer from the fragmentation that holds back competitive payer-provider systems.

Yet the mainstream use of ambient assisted living technology in healthcare in the UK is not inevitable. Evidence that the benefits seen in early trials can be scaled and realised at a whole-system level remains weak, payment systems have yet to positively encourage the adoption of ambient assisted living technology and healthcare reforms that promote greater competition and patient choice mean that fragmentation is a factor.

* Corresponding Author: George MacGinnis, E-mail: george.macginnis@paconsulting.com

This is particularly true where the payer might not always be beneficiary of the services. The increasing number of initiatives and the growing size of each suggest that the NHS has been able to capitalise on its structural advantages. This chapter will looks at the operational deployment of ambient assisted living technology for the NHS in England. It will:

- Examine the policy context, in particular the move towards preventative models of care, supported by rewards for outcomes.
- Chart the growing adoption and use of technology, and the pivotal place of the 'Whole System Demonstrators' in furthering adoption.
- Consider the impact of new technologies on the pace of adoption.

The focus for this chapter will be the NHS in England, which covers 52M people (around 84% of the population of the UK). It will also briefly consider significant initiatives elsewhere in the United Kingdom. However, it should be noted that responsibility for healthcare in the UK is devolved regionally and as a result there will be some organisational and policy differences.

1. Ambient Assisted Living – Some Definitions

The interest in the use of ambient assisted living technologies in the NHS stems largely from the use of assistive technologies in social care to support independent living for vulnerable, often older people. Terminology in this field is not stable, and similar terms are often used to convey different meanings so, for clarity, this article will use the following definitions:

Telehealth. Telehealth involves delivering healthcare at a distance using electronic means of communication. Typical services involve patients measuring their vital signs at home and this data being transmitted via a Telehealth monitor to a clinician. Most early services have focussed on collecting biometric data from patients, but increasingly telehealth services are expanding to include a wider array of functionality such as interactive educational content, support for medications adherence, patient reminders and remote consultations via voice and video links.

Telecare. Telecare involves the continuous, automatic and remote monitoring of real-time emergencies and lifestyle changes over time in order to manage the risks associated with independent living. Typical devices include personal alarms, falls monitors, bed & chair sensors and movement detectors.

Most telecare services start with an emergency service ethos – providing a rapid response to an alarm. As the technology and infrastructure develops, telecare applications are becoming increasingly sophisticated to include:

- Location based services, such as wearable GPS devices to support care of people with dementia.
- Integration with home automation to provide holistic solutions to support independent living for those with disabilities and
- Systems which track activities of daily living and can provide an assessment for the quality of life of an individual living independently.

The broad spectrum of telehealth and telecare services is illustrated in Fig. 1.

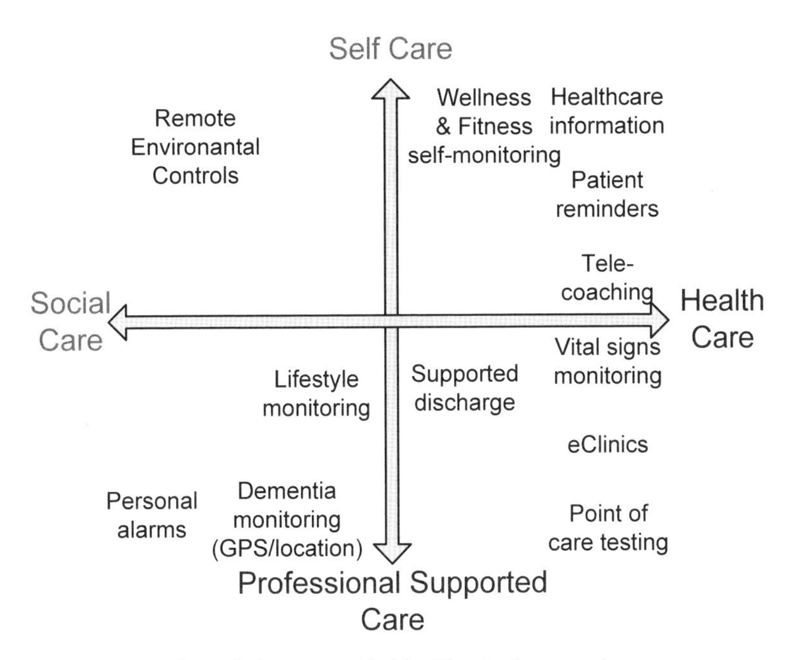

Figure 1. A spectrum of telehealth and telecare services.

Telemedicine. Telemedicine is the delivery of healthcare at a distance using electronic means of communication – usually from one clinician to another e.g. a non-specialist GP undertaking an ECG on a patient suspected of heart disease and the transfer of that data electronically to another specialist clinician for discussion/comment.

A range of clinical applications will benefit from the increasing availability of point of care testing devices aimed at both consumer and professional use. There are likely to be significant synergies arising from an alignment with technology standards for connected personal and connected clinical devices. These include:

GP Kiosks. A number of systems are available to automate check in for appointments. Some systems offer advanced features where patients can self administer tests (e.g. blood pressure, weight) and answer screening questionnaires (e.g. smoking cessation).

Public Health Kiosks. NHS Choices, the Department of Health's public-facing website, has conducted pilots with health-check kiosks that incorporate biometric tests and answers to questions. There is interest from the NHS in kiosks placed in public areas and pharmacies as a way of helping to identify early risk factors, such as hypertension.

Home Video Consultation. There is increasing interest in the use of home video consultation to extend the scope and availability of patient coaching services. Airedale NHS Trust has pioneered a service with technology that links to a TV set. The Scottish Centre for Telehealth has sponsored research in this field, including the use of video conferencing technology for pulmonary rehabilitation classes.

Specialist monitoring and screening services. Point-of-care testing (POCT) provides diagnostic tests at or near the site of patient care. Advances in electronics mean that increasingly complex tests can be conducted at the bedside (in hospital) or in the community. Testing may be conducted by clinicians or patients themselves. Examples of services include:

- HBA1c testing for diabetics. This is a blood test required every 3–6 months for patients with good control of their diabetes, and more frequently for others.
- Blood coagulation ('PT/INR') testing for patients on Warfurin. Point of care testing devices exist and electronic interface standards for this type of device are being developed in IEEE, and there are plans for adoption by the Continua Health Alliance (see [6,23]).
- 12-lead ECG testing with remote interpretation by a specialist to provide community based cardiac screening and assessment.
- Digital photography for monitoring of wound healing and skin conditions. There is also interest in the use of moving images, for instance films to show walking-gait and joint flexion.

While cost, usability and data quality (e.g. device calibration) issues may mean that some point of care testing devices remain exclusively for clinical use, the technical implications remain very similar for patient operated devices. All involve a need to capture data from devices, associate it with a person and pass the results to an electronic health record.

2. Policy: Shaping the Environment

This section provides the wider policy context for the adoption of ambient assisted living technologies. The use of ambient assisted living technologies by the NHS in England is in line with drivers common to all developed economies. The use of technology provides a key element of the response to rapidly rising demand for health care at a time when it is becoming increasingly hard to generate the financial and human resources to meet the demand. Demographic and lifestyle changes have created aging populations and an increasing prevalence of lifestyle related long-term conditions, such as diabetes. Another facet of declining fertility rates and aging populations is that the proportion of people in the workforce able to deliver care is declining, making existing approaches to care unsustainable. The Scottish Government have predicted that if the current trends continued unchanged, by 2020, 40% of all school leavers would be needed to join the caring professions [1]. These challenges require new models of care. Those that focus on prevention rather than treatment have shown most promise. These typically require patients, or more generally citizens, to be more active participants in managing their health and wellness. Aside from the technical issues of opening up health information systems to consumer access, this poses significant questions around culture, education and inclusion.

The adoption of ambient assisted living technologies in the UK is unusual in comparison to developments in other health systems. In the UK developments in the NHS have often been promoted, and in some cases led, by social care. This can in part be explained by the way state-funded health and social care have evolved in the UK. Historically, health and social care were managed by the same government department. Today, the Department of Health remains responsible for both health and social care although it has lost some of the former responsibilities for social security payments (such as unemployment benefit). While policy at the top level is united under a single ministry, responsibilities are devolved in different directions. The National Health Service (NHS) provides healthcare which is free at the point of need, funded by general taxation, while local authorities have the responsibility for delivering social care which is subject to more complex eligibility criteria. The dividing line is complex, particularly when it comes to care for older people and other vulnerable groups, and recent policies have focused on the need for both services to work together to deliver more coherent person-centred care packages.

Recent interest in the use of ambient assisted living technologies was driven by two key policy documents. It should be noted that at the time of publication of these documents the term telecare was used in an all-encompassing sense and the use did not differentiate between telecare and telehealth:

- In 2004 the Audit Commission (a publicly funded independent body responsible for ensuring that public money is spent economically, efficiently and effectively) produced a review, 'Older people: Implementing telecare' [31], highlighting the positive results from a limited number of trials. However, the document also noted that Telecare services generally involved multi-agency and multidisciplinary working, and would need effective partnership working to deliver mainstream services. As a result the document called for "better co-ordination of telecare implementation at both national and local levels and for more integrated guidance to support local implementation". The move towards greater use of telecare was seen to offer benefits in terms of:
    - Reduced emergency admissions.
    - Reduced lengths of stay.
    - Improved quality of life for patients, including extending the time that vulnerable (often older) people can remain in their own home.
    - Improved quality of life for carers.
- In a response to the Audit Commission report, the Department of Health published 'Building Telecare in England' [8] in July 2005. A key thrust of this strategy was to promote the use of telecare by social services to monitor people at home as an alternative to residential care. Residential care was seen as expensive, often led to a poor quality of life and frequently contrary to the user's wishes. To 'pump prime' telecare services, the Government made £80 million (approximately US $120 million) available as a grant to local authorities in England for investment in 'Preventative Technology' over the two years from April 2006. The funding was intended to increase the numbers of people who benefit from telecare by at least 160,000 older people nationally. In what may be seen as a brave move, this funding stream was not allocated specifically for this purpose. In retrospect, it does appear to have been used as intended. In some areas municipal authorities, in partnership with the NHS, used the grant to invest in new telehealth services, seeing the provision of healthcare at home as a logical extension of the move away from the use of residential care by social services.

In early 2006, in a related development, the Department of Health published the policy document 'Our health, our care, our say: a new direction for community services' [13]. This signalled a landmark shift in healthcare policy, moving debate on the future of the NHS away from an internal focus on the process of healthcare delivery, typified by concerns over hospital 'waiting lists', towards a focus on achieving better

Table 1. Telecare evidence assessment published by Department of Health taken from (Barlow et al., "Building an evidence base for successful telecare implementation").

Focus of telecare scheme included in systematic review	Evidence on:	
	Individual outcomes, i.e. clinical or Quality of Life improvement	Systemic outcomes, i.e. economic impact or impact on processes
Specific application, e.g. telecare aimed at patients with diabetes	Relatively good, growing – numerous individual studies on which to build systematic reviews	Limited, problematic – poor specification of assumptions, lack of robust data
General application, e.g. aimed at a heterogeneous population ('frail older people')	Largely anecdotal, growing – not yet peer reviewed	Virtually un-researched – based on simulation modelling with limited data

outcomes through delivery of improved preventative care services. The White Paper set out a vision to provide people with good quality health and social care services in the communities where they live, detailing a range of actions to achieve this, including the use of remote monitoring technologies.

A review of evidence at about the same time[1] (see also [27]) noted that while there was growing evidence of effectiveness in terms of individual outcomes, there was a gap in the quality of evidence on systemic outcomes (see Table 1). This was influential in setting the direction for the NHS. The 'Our health, our care, our say' White Paper promised a number of Whole System Demonstrators (WSDs) "to explore the possibilities opened up by truly integrated health and social care working, supported by advanced assistive technologies". The outcome of these demonstrators, discussed later, is therefore a key milestone on the way to mainstream adoption.

The 2008 NHS review conducted by Lord Darzi [11] reaffirmed previous commitments to the use of ambient assisted living technology, particularly for patients with long term conditions. There were numerous references to the use of technology in documents relating to the review, including 'The Primary and Community Strategy' [12] and 'Delivering Care Closer to Home' [10]. The Carers' Strategy [9], also published at that time, contained the statement '*Tele-care to be viewed as integral not marginal*' [9, Annex A, Section 3.3]. Three aspects of the Darzi review are noteworthy in the context of driving adoption of ambient assisted living technologies:

- The review proposed a focus on three interrelated themes: prevention, improved quality and innovation. In particular, the innovation theme aimed to highlight the poor record in spreading new ideas. A number of measures that were introduced as a result have had a positive impact on adoption of assisted living technologies by the NHS. Regional ('Strategic') health authorities acquired a statutory duty to promote innovation, which can be seen as a key stimulus for their subsequent role in promoting large-scale deployments.
- As part of the review each of the 9 regional bodies in England (SHAs) produced a strategy. These varied widely in their mention of services using ambient assisted living technologies, suggesting that even after 2 years the policy message had yet to percolate through even at this relatively high level.

[1] Care Services Improvement Partnership, *Building an evidence base for successful telecare implementation – updated report of the Evidence Working Group of the Telecare Policy Collaborative chaired by James Barlow*, published by Department of Health, London, November 2006. Key aspects of this analysis were subsequently published in: J.G. Barlow, D. Singh, S. Bayer, A systematic review of the benefits of home telecare for frail elderly people and those with long-term conditions, *Journal of Telemedicine and Telecare* **13** (2007), 172–179.

- A commitment to develop a national ‘Patient Prospectus’ indicated that patient choice would be an important part of the approach to the use of ambient assisted living technologies. The Patient’s Prospectus is intended to provide patients with long-term conditions with information about the choices which should be available to them locally and to enable them to self-care in partnership with health and social care professionals. The review included a commitment that:

  ‘*The prospectus will set out the choices that should be available for self care ... include details of ... the technologies that are available to help people monitor conditions in their own homes*’ [12, Section 4.28].

  The implementation of the Prospectus (see [33]), which was published on the NHS Choices website, falls somewhat short of this promise. This is a reflection of the fact that the services are not yet universal, in part due to technical constraints as current offerings in the market lack the interoperability needed to enable patient choice.

The quality, prevention and innovation themes have been picked up as important drivers for improvements in the NHS that have helped to promote adoption of ambient assisted living technologies. In a move seen as a direct response to growing budgetary pressures on the NHS, the Department of Health established the QIPP programme, where QIPP stands for Quality, Innovation, Productivity and Prevention. ‘QIPP’ became a benchmark for testing new ideas and driving changes to deliver some of the most ambitious cost savings expected of any healthcare system in the developed World.

The QIPP theme has been carried through the change of Governments in 2010. The White Paper ‘Equity and excellence: Liberating the NHS’ set out the new coalition government’s vision for the future of the NHS and reaffirmed the commitment to a wider QIPP programme aimed at enabling the NHS to make significant efficiency savings, which could then be reinvested back into the service to continually improve quality of care. NHS funding is expected to remain flat in real terms over the next 4 years from 2011/12, while meeting healthcare inflation and rising demands requires around 4% ‘efficiency’ gains each year in the same period.

The 2010 policy shift also proposed some radical changes to the way the NHS is managed. Regional and local health authorities are to be abolished and replaced by a system of clinical commissioning in which GP’s are expected to form collaborative with other clinicians to drive the purchasing of acute and community care services. There will be a National Commissioning Board to provide strategic guidance. It is not clear how the reform will affect the adoption of ambient assisted living services; as the most likely outcome appears to be commissioning consortia that are smaller than the current arrangements and may find it hard to generate the up-front investment needed to establish new services. In these circumstances, some central support for this rapidly emerging and innovative range of services is likely to be required.

So far this section has charted the main policies that have directly influenced the adoption of ambient assisted living technologies by the NHS. A number of wider moves also mean that the NHS is positioned to remain an early adopter of these preventative services:

- The NHS has moved towards outcomes-based payments which provide rewards for improved quality and more preventative models of care.

- The Quality and Outcomes Framework for General Practice provides the basis for rewarding effective preventative care, although the indicators do not reflect the real possibilities. For instance the indicator for coronary heart disease only requires a record of blood pressure in the previous 15 months [32]. There is no additional incentive for the more frequent monitoring possible with AAL technology.
- In recent changes to the Payment by Results mechanisms for hospital care, the 'Commissioning for Quality and Innovation' mechanism now provides commissioners (payers) with the ability to alter reimbursement to reflect good practice. Taking this a stage further, a recent announcement indicated that hospitals will be made responsible for reducing the number of emergency re-admissions following treatment, and support treatment at home, as part of a single payment' [19].

- A reform of community service provision is underway. Part of this reform involves establishing effective management and payment mechanisms for community services. This is a key enabler, offering new business models that would underpin an expansion of community services by rewarding performance. Another aspect of the changes will see community services move from being directly managed by local health authorities. There is no single template for this change, and services are variously moving to join acute trusts, mental health trusts or setting up as stand-alone entities. While it is too early to understand the impact of these changes, it seems likely that those moving to acute trusts will be well placed to maintain the drive to adopt ambient assisted living technology as their parent Trusts represent large health businesses with established professional and technical infrastructure. The new tariff scheme gives them an incentive to develop new community based services.
- The NHS has established an eHealth infrastructure that provides a platform for connected health solutions. Electronic health record systems are used throughout general practice and there is increasing deployment in other environments including community services. Shared summary records are being deployed, allowing for the sharing of care plans and other information between different providers.

3. NHS Adoption – Moving to Scale

The adoption of ambient assisted living technologies by the NHS has reflected the strongly supportive policies that have been set out by the Department of Health. Much of the focus has been on the three WSD sites which have accounted for around 1,500 telehealth units deployed by the NHS. By mid 2010, the total deployment of telehealth equipments in the NHS in England was estimated to be around the 5–10,000 units. This contrasts with the adoption of ambient assisted living technology in social care. The Department of Health estimates there are up to 1.6 million users of telecare. A large proportion are users of pendant alarms in residential care schemes, around 400,000 individuals benefit from an advanced telecare package, designed to support independent living at home. This package typically involve the use of a pendant alarms and other sensors, such as falls monitors and remote smoke alarms, and can extend to more complex arrays of sensors.

While this scale of telehealth deployment is significant in European terms, it is still small when compared to some of the leaders in the US. For instance, the Veteran's Administration now deploys upwards of 40,000 telehealth units. Adoption by the NHS represents around 2% of the currently addressable market. There are currently around 15 million people with a diagnosed long term condition in England [14], but this figure can lead to over-optimistic projections. The evidence for remote monitoring technologies is largely confined to high intensity users whose condition is in some way life limiting, and this is reflected in the way technology has been deployed by the NHS. These patients offer the potential for relatively short-term returns on investment in assisted living services, mainly through avoiding emergency episodes. Around 10% of the total population with a long term condition, or 1.5 million, would be classed as intensive users of services and these people represent the immediate opportunity for active monitoring. Applying a factor for uptake suggests that a realistic estimate of the addressable market would be around 1/3rd of potential, or around 500,000 users.

The following sections set out:

- How the pace and scale of adoption by the NHS is increasing.
- The pivotal place of the WSDs, and the learning that is coming from them.
- Some of the wider experiences from across the NHS that will help shape thinking on mainstream operational deployments.

3.1. Adoption Has Started to Rise Rapidly

While the main Department of Health focus has been on generating robust evidence through the WSDs, the Department's Care Network found that 58 of the 151 local health authorities (Primary Care Trusts) in England have either established or plan some form of telehealth operation, as illustrated in Fig. 2[2]. In many cases, partnerships involving health and social care have used funding from the Preventative Technology Grant to purchase the equipment. For the most part these operations are small scale, involving less than 50 patients at any one time, and reflect an appetite to experiment with new ways of working.

A few areas have started to establish services as a mainstream offering and deploy at a significantly larger scale, typically around 500 to 1,000 units. Deployments of this size are mainly centred on the WSD sites and a group of 12 early adopters chosen by the Department of Health to form the WSD Action Network.

There are indications of a step-change in the scale of NHS implementations. The Regional Strategies produced in the Next Stage Review included significant commitments to telehealth implementation. Three of the nine regional health authorities in England have made some high profile moves, and others have also started to show interest behind-the-scenes:

- Yorkshire and Humber SHA have plans to develop a regional tele-monitoring infrastructure [2] with an investment in infrastructure linked to local QIPP plans. The SHA has initiated 9 separate projects covering a wide range of aspects of assisted living, including telemonitoring for diabetes, chronic obstructive pulmonary disease (COPD) and heart failure, telemedicine for stroke care, telecoaching for supported discharge, dementia, medications adherence, social

[2] Published as a Google Map at http://maps.google.co.uk/maps/ms?hl=en&ie=UTF8&msa=0&msid=100406857045032193451.00047bfad6341183c8523&z=6.

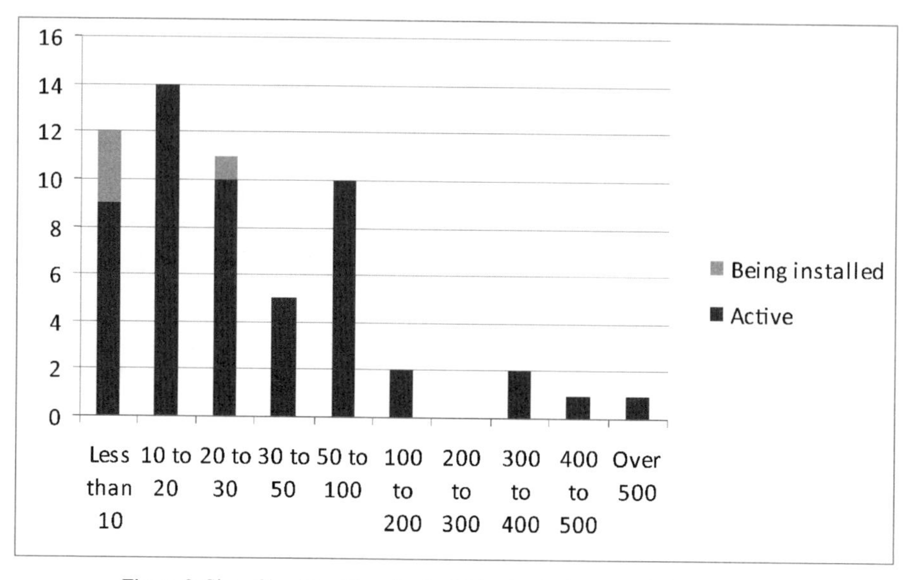

Figure 2. Size of local health authority telehealth deployments in January 2010.

networking for wellness and behavioural support and e-consultations. Within the region, the NHS North Yorkshire and York Primary Care Trust has separately announced plans [4] for an implementation involving 2000 systems, similar to those used in Cornwall's WSD, and targeting similar patients.

- West Midlands SHA have established a telehealth programme and have forged strong links with the Medilink West Midlands industry association.
- The South West SHA regional plan included a commitment to build on the work done in Cornwall by expanding the use of telecare, telemedicine and assistive technology in three or more health communities by 31 March 2011.

The following sections highlight examples of the operational deployment of ambient assisted living technologies in the NHS, covering the Whole System Demonstrators and other leading initiatives. The examples have been selected to illustrate the scale of adoption and the range of technologies in use.

3.2. Whole System Demonstrators

The most significant development in the period 2005–2010 has been the creation of the WSDs. These were established by the Department of Health to explore the possibilities opened up by truly integrated health and social care working supported by advanced assistive technologies such as telehealth and telecare. The demonstrators aim to provide a better understanding of the level of benefit associated with such developments and to help fast track future change by addressing the key implementation barriers in providing solutions for the wider NHS and Social Care.

Scale was an important driver in the design of the Demonstrators. Three sites were selected to participate in the programme, Kent, Newham and Cornwall. Together these sites represent a combined population of around 1 million residents. All three demonstrators involve local partnerships between health and social care and they provide an interesting mix of challenges, illustrated in Table 2.

Table 2. Whole system demonstrator sites.

Cornwall	Newham	Kent
• The poorest County in England, with a dispersed rural population • Population of >500,000 with a significant influx of temporary residents during the summer holiday season • 46% of the population live in settlements of <3,000 people • 99.1% White British • 10.3% of the population are aged 65+; 7.2% 75+ and 2.6% 85+ • 21% of the population report a limiting long term illness	• One of the most deprived areas in the UK • Population of 270,442, and increasing at a higher rate than the London average • 2nd most diverse population in the UK – >68% Black and minority ethnic; Over 140 languages spoken as a first language • 8.5% of the population are aged 65+ • 17.3% of the population have a limiting long term illness • Highest death rate from stroke and COPD • Highest diabetes rate in the UK • 2nd highest CHD rate in London	• Combination of rural and urban populations • Population of 1.37 m (excluding Medway) • 3.5% Black and minority ethnic • 17.3% of the population are aged 65+; 8.4% 75+ and 2.2% 85+ • Within the target population, individuals report having an average of 1.6 of the three target conditions of HF, COPD, Diabetes

The focus of the WSDs is on individuals with COPD, Heart Failure and Diabetes, and adults with social care or health and social care needs at risk of hospital admission. In addressing the needs of these groups, two main assisted living technologies were used:

- Telehealth patient remote monitoring systems with a range of devices, tailored to fit individual needs, to measure blood pressure, blood glucose, pulse & oxygen saturation and weight.
- Telecare packages comprising at least a personal alarm and remote smoke detector with options for a range of other commercially available devices such as pill dispenser, falls monitor and flood detector.

The design of the services at each of the sites, including the selection of commercial partners, was under local control while the overall objectives and evaluation, including research design and patient/client selection were set centrally.

The partnership arrangements reflected the somewhat unique position of the UK, where telecare services were already established to provide an alternative to residential social care. In the Kent and Newham demonstrators, the lead partner was the local authority (social care), while in Cornwall it was led by the NHS Primary Care Trust. All three demonstrator sites had already established mainstream telecare services that, apart from the recruitment of participants for the evaluation, remained largely unchanged. Newham's social care service had previously experimented with telehealth, and Kent's social care service was running what had, until the WSDs, been the largest implementation of telehealth in England (with 250 patients enrolled in remote monitoring). This existing service provided the basis for the WSD telehealth service in Kent. The other two sites established new telehealth services and selected different technologies.

Responsibility for monitoring at each site was split between the two service offerings, with the NHS monitoring telehealth patients and adult social services looking after telecare users. The Demonstrators did set off with the intention of investigating users who would require integrated packages involving both telehealth and telecare services. Eligibility criteria meant that very few patients fell into this overlap group and, due to constraints of research design which was based on randomising by GP practice, investigation of the joint group was dropped.

The sites implemented broadly similar operational models for the telehealth. These were based on a centralised nurse-led team responsible for delivery of the core monitoring service. The services varied slightly in responsibilities for home visits and the way that the services linked into other aspects of primary and community care. All the demonstrator sites involved working with GPs to identify and enrol patients, and had to link back to GPs and community health teams for following-up response. This arrangement validated the value of a centralised team for delivering the service.

The research design was a cluster randomized control trial involving 6000 clients across the 3 sites, with a roughly equal split between telecare and telehealth, and between intervention and controls. The intervention period was 1 year, after which all those in the control groups would be offered an intervention. In addition, around 400 carers also participated in the research.

The evaluation, which is being delivered by a consortium of 7 leading UK institutions, will examine to what extent the WSD model of care:

- Promotes individuals long term well-being and independence.
- Improves individuals and their carer's quality of life.
- Improves the working lives of staff.
- Is more cost effective.
- Is more clinically effective.
- Provides an evidence base for future care and technology models.

The study period came to an end in 2010, and the results are due to be published in 2011. In anticipation of the formal evaluation, due to be published in early 2011, it is possible to draw some lessons from the experience gained by the Demonstrators sites in implementing telehealth at scale.

3.2.1. The Demonstrators Have Addressed the Needs of Patients for All Three Target Conditions

The Demonstrators recruited patients from each of the three target long term condition groups, with a bias towards heart failure and COPD. Provisional figures, released at the end of the recruitment period, are shown in Table 3. Recruitment was based on two criteria. The first was that the patients had a diagnosed condition as defined using the Quality and Outcome Framework criteria[3]. In all cases additional physical co-morbidities may be present and these individuals were still eligible. Initially a second criteria was also applied, requiring at least one 'unplanned' event in the last 12 months in relation to their long term condition. Eligible events were an unplanned hospital admission, intermediate care/rapid response service use, a treatment following call out of Ambulance services or an Accident & Emergency visit. However, due to data quality issues the unplanned event criteria was later made optional.

---

[3] The assessment criteria used for the Whole System Demonstrators were:

- Heart failure – diagnosis confirmed by echocardiogram or by a specialist assessment.
- Type 1 or 2 diabetes – with HbA1C of 7.5 or greater in the previous 15 months.
- Chronic Obstructive Pulmonary Disease (COPD) – diagnosis confirmed by spirometry and FEV1 is less than 70% of predicted normal and FEV1/FVC ratio is less than 70%.

Table 3. WSD telehealth patients by disease.

Condition	% of total
Diabetes only	20%
COPD only	38%
HF only	27%
Diabetes & COPD	5%
Diabetes & HF	4%
COPD & HF	4%
ALL 3 LTCs	2%

Source: Harborn F, 'Current Status Update' presentation to WSD Action Network Roadshow, Bristol, 10 September 2009.

The relatively smaller cohort for diabetes is interesting, given the high general prevalence of diabetes as a condition. It may be explained in part by the different demographic profile of diabetes patients. Most people recruited onto the telehealth part of the Demonstrators were older and their conditions would fall into the UK definition of 'limiting' (conditions that affect day-to-day activity). In contrast, many diabetics are not limited in the same way until late on in the disease progression, when significant – effects become manifest through co-morbidities. The Newham site intended to establish a separate service for diabetics using a smart-phone based solution that has been successfully implemented elsewhere in the UK. However this part of their service was implemented late on and at the time of writing no information was available on their experience with the alternative solution.

Qualitative evidence, mainly in the form of case studies published by the trial sites, suggests that patients in all three disease groups benefited from the telehealth intervention. The case studies also highlight patients with a number of co-morbidities, indicating that the services were able to meet the more complex needs of these patients. An indication of the overall success is given by the decisions in both Cornwall and Kent to run their services on beyond the trial period. At the time of writing no decision had been taken by Newham.

In Cornwall, the PCT reported successes with equipment being used to diagnose postural blood pressure drop in prevention of falls [25]. Trials are underway or planned to assess whether the scope of the telehealth service in Cornwall could be extended to include support for stroke patients, prevention of falls and management of urinary tract infections.

3.2.2. Telehealth Patients Required Long Term Support

At all three sites monitoring has been provided as a long-term service, with participants enrolled for at least a full year. The number of people who left the service during the course of the 1-year trial was relatively small. Early figures on people who chose to leave after equipment had been installed identified the top reasons for leaving as (a) not wanting electrical equipment in the house, (b) not able to operate the equipment (c) 'family issues'.

The long term provision is, in contrast to practice in many US operations, where services are typically offered for up to 60 days post-discharge, and also different from the design chosen for the service in Northern Ireland, which is based on 13-week packages of care. This preference for WSD patients to be long-term users of the service could be interpreted as creating a dependency, and that is understood to be part of the reason for the different approach taken in Northern Ireland. However, the recruitment

Table 4. Patient recruitment.

Item	Total	Remarks
GP practices	239	From a total of nearly 350 practices
Patient invitation letters	27,000	
Initial Assessment Home Visits	>9,000	
Patients on trial	<6,000	

Source: Harborn F, 'Current Status Update' presentation to WSD Action Network Roadshow, Bristol, 10 September 2009.

criteria suggest that the patients would probably remain relatively high intensity service users as a result of their limiting conditions. Cornwall considered a 'step down' strategy where patients who were generally stable would be moved onto a light-touch service, but at the time of writing this approach had not been implemented.

3.2.3. Integrated Care Pathways Are Essential for Delivering at Scale

Patient recruitment took significantly more effort, and longer to achieve, than originally anticipated. The degree of effort is illustrated in Table 4 showing the numbers of patients invited and follow-up visits conducted in recruiting patients. This is an experience common to most early telehealth operations where, despite apparently significant populations that should fit with the criteria, it proved both difficult to identify those at risk, and to secure their agreement to receive the service.

The most significant dynamic in patient recruitment was the enlisting of GP practices. The difficulty recruiting patients was surprising, particularly given the expected prevalence of the target conditions. The total combined population for the demonstrators was nearly 1 million, which would have meant that there would be in the order of 30,000 patients with an eligible condition[4]. To achieve a fully recruited trial involving around 20% of the eligible patients required nearly 70% of the GP practices in the three areas to be enlisted as referring practices, and recruitment took nearly 18 months.

Part of the recruitment issue would be addressed by better case finding tools. While the original design called for the use of the Combined Predictive Model[5], a case finding tool that draws on both GP and acute care datasets, none of the sites were in a position to use it in this way. As a result, there was a high reliance on local disease registers which were often not as accurate as had been hoped. It was originally thought that most of the eligible people on the trial would be known to a wide range of services. As recruitment progressed and the sites were forced to look for new referral routes it became clear that there was significant unmet demand [17].

As well as technical constraints limiting the use of case finding tools, data quality issues in clinical records were also a factor. The Department of Health anticipated that it would not be too difficult to find eligible people from current records, however in some cases disease registers were not accurate [17], and significant variations in GP's electronic health records made it difficult to identify patients at risk. For instance, anecdotal evidence from the research team suggested that large numbers of patients with a recorded diagnosis of COPD did not have the results of the spirometry tests required to make that clinical diagnosis entered on their clinical record. In addressing these

[4] Based on a prevalence of 30%, of which around 10% would be considered 'high risk' and have life limiting conditions within the eligible groups.

[5] For further information on the Combined Predictive Model see the King's Fund website: http://www.kingsfund.org.uk/current_projects/predicting_and_reducing_readmission_to_hospital/.

shortfalls, it was also found that front line services did not routinely share data. New data sharing agreements had to be established to support integrated working, particularly between community primary care teams, GPs and adult social care services.

The research and ethical constraints were a significant contributing factor in the recruitment difficulties. Limitations on the role of clinicians in patient recruitment go a long way in explaining the low uptake. No active 'selling' of the service to participants was permitted. The effect of this became very clear in the case of telecare, where all the sites had existing services. While no published or validated data is available, one person involved in the process suggested that refusal rates for people offered telecare went from less that 10% in a the existing service to over 90% as a result of the trial process. In particular it was believed that the additional requirements to start with establishing research consent agreement whilst also not raising patient expectations by explaining the anticipated benefits would explain the differences.

A significant challenge facing all the sites was the design and implementation of effective chronic care pathways so that the new telehealth services formed part of an integrated care delivery system. At the start of the WSDs it was recognised that a key requirement would be for clinical and professional input into care pathway design. Each of the sites probably under-estimated the complexity of the project management task. Those that were led by social care providers (Newham, Kent) would have faced more difficulties securing the clinical leadership required. None of the sites established any significant direct involvement of acute hospital services.

A complex recruitment process may also influence the drop out rate and has implications for the way telehealth services are integrated into care pathways. The Department of Health identified 12 steps in the patient recruitment process, only 3 of which specifically related to evaluation requirements, as shown in Fig. 3. This patient recruitment process involves a range of different agencies and requires careful orchestration to avoid unnecessary delays which are a contributing factor to potential users dropping out.

3.2.4. Benefits Are Being Achieved with Relatively Simple Technology

The timescales for the WSDs meant that the sites were limited to off-the-shelf solutions with little scope for technology enhancements or integration into other local systems. Each of the Demonstrator sites chose slightly different telehealth solutions, providing some opportunity to look at the impact of different technologies. All involved monitoring of vital signs using a range of devices as well as asking the patients questions on a regular basis. All three solutions were 'fixed' hub devices, linked to standard telephone or domestic broadband connections. In technology terms, the biggest difference was at Newham, which used a solution based on set-top box technology with a capability to provide additional interactive educational content.

Patient education was thought to be a key part of a telehealth service, and the WSDs provided an opportunity to look at how different technologies could affect that aspect of the services. Newham selected an interactive set-top box based system with support for educational content, while the other sites used telehealth hubs with more basic capabilities. The Newham experience has been reported as positive, but has also highlighted both language and content challenges with the delivery of patient information programmes over telehealth systems. Video content was initially available in English and some European languages, whereas the population of Newham was ethnically diverse with a large proportion of non-European languages spoken as a first language.

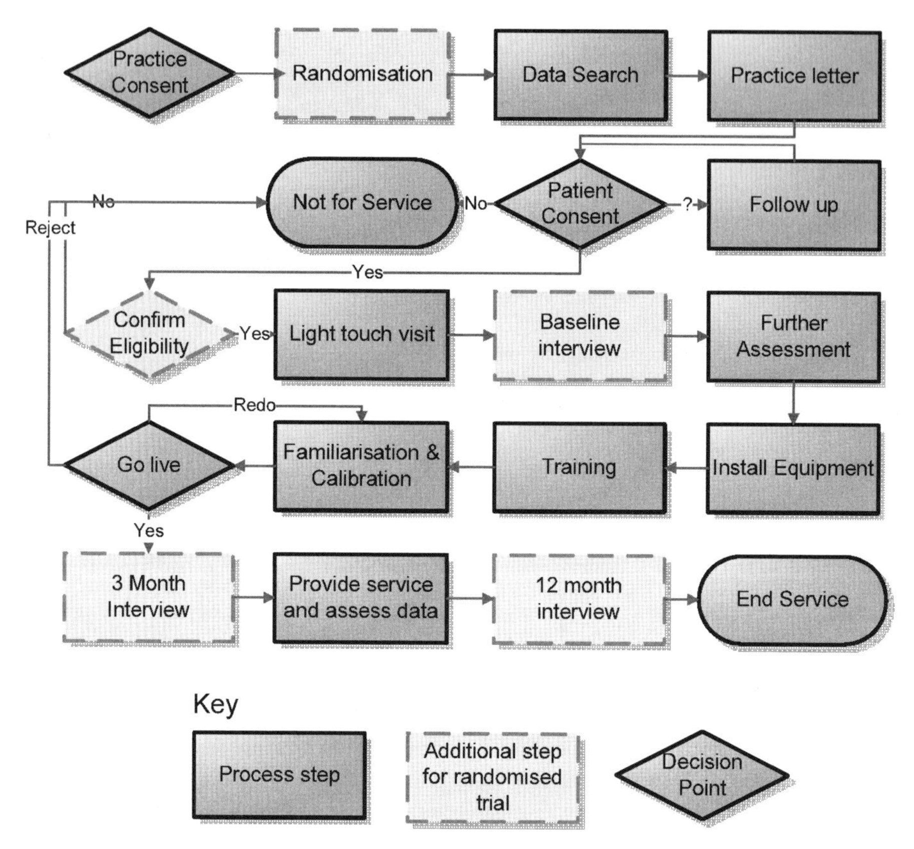

Figure 3. Whole system demonstrator patient pathway.

Cost and research constraints served to limit use of the system to people who spoke English or had a carer who would be able to help. Content was also problematic, limited both in scope and variety. Some patients have also been reported as commenting on the relevance of content, for instance including suggestions for more exercise that were not suitable for wheelchair users or noting that they had already seen the video in question. This highlights a need for services intending to use more interactive capabilities to put in place the capability to develop fresh content and deliver it with a more personalised approach.

3.2.5. Further Technology Integration Is Required for Large-Scale Deployments

In adopting off-the-shelf telehealth technologies, the WSDs were forced to accept that the telehealth data would not be integrated into existing clinical record systems. In particular, in the UK all general practitioners use electronic health records. Various approaches were taken to address this, based in part on local preferences. In some cases GPs or their practice staff accessed the information by using the remote monitoring system, but would then manually transcribe the data they deemed needed into their clinical record system. In other cases, data was sent in hard copy or by fax with referral notes.

The Department of Health funded a separate technology activity as part of the WSDs that developed a proof of concept demonstrator for integrating the systems deployed in Newham. The demonstrator is based on data messaging guidelines developed by the Continua Health Alliance and uses health informatics industry-standard HL7 formats. The base work was further developed by the NHS to include guidelines for the implementation of the interface that addressed information governance concerns, and involved a number of key features:

- Support for a 'telehealth referral' business process, allowing monitoring staff to raise reports which also controlled the flow of reports, and therefore the anticipated workload, to general practitioners. There were three report types created:
    - Routine – scheduled reports to ensure general practitioners were kept informed of patient progress.
    - Information reports – raised by exception to report incidents of note, such as patients starting medication according to pre-agree protocols.
    - Action reports – referrals to a GP that would be prioritised by their system appropriately.
- Provision to allow clinicians to review incoming data and decide which would be accepted as part of the formal clinical record. There was flexibility for clinicians to accept none, some or all the incoming data, thus allowing them to maintain control of the quality of data in their record.
- The ability to tailor the timing and content of the messages to individual patient and clinical requirements. An interesting aspect of this was the need to support multiple 'thresholds', so that not every telehealth 'alert' would result in a GP referral. For instance, a GP may set a monitoring threshold for a telehealth nurse intervention at a lower level than the threshold for notification of the GP.

The proof of concept demonstrator was developed with significant local clinical input and the result has attracted favourable comments when exposed to wider clinical audiences. The Department of Health's Information Directorate went on to develop other aspects of the workflow integration, including setting out requirements to be able to support messaging back from a GP in a 'Clinicians Response Message'. These additional interactions have yet to be implemented.

3.3. Wider Adoption of Assisted Living Technologies in the NHS

With healthcare policy broadly supportive towards the use of assisted living technology, and with some central funding and support, there was an expectation that health authorities would begin to establish local telehealth services. One area of concern was over the strong emphasis that the Department of Health placed on establishing evidence from the WSDs. A Kings Fund report, Technology Adoption in the NHS [20], which looked more generally at issues of technology adoption, contained this specific warning:

> *"Trials can hold up national roll-out: at its worst the NHS can find itself in a state of permanent trial, with each new trial delaying a larger-scale roll-out. For example, the Whole System Demonstrator programme is a two-year telecare pilot that will establish an evidence base for telecare in a UK context. Although this is a highly valuable and important piece of work, local services are to a certain extent holding back until its results are published."*

The figures presented earlier on the number and size of different telehealth schemes in England suggest that this risk appears to have been averted. The parallel Preventative Technology Grant given to local authorities provided some of the mitigation, with several local authorities funding, or part funding, small initiatives with local NHS partners. Another key aspect was central support provided through the WSD Action Network (WSDAN) to share learning and support other sites.

The WSDAN was established in July 2008 and provided an open, online resource for evidence on telecare, telehealth and the management of long-term conditions. Run jointly by The King's Fund and the Department of Health, the Network also supported 12 pro-active local partnerships in health and social care in action research. The aim of the action research was too understand the barriers faced by organisations implementing telehealth and telecare on a smaller scale and without the constraints of a randomized controlled trial or the additional resources associated with one of the main WSD sites. The WSDAN's value has extended beyond the original remit to support action research, becoming a key forum for the exchange of ideas both within the sites and more generally with others NHS organisations.

The following sections illustrate the broad range of services being considered by NHS Trusts, highlighting:

- How new service models are evolving that address issues of scalability, including support for wider adoption and improving the economic case by reconfiguring the care pathway. Illustrated by the examples from Barnsley, Kent and NHS Direct / NHS South East Essex.
- The increasing convergence between ambient assisted living and other services for patients in the community. Illustrated by the Birmingham Own-Health and Airedale examples.
- Increasing use of technology to support better clinical services in the community – illustrated by the Cumbria and North Lincolnshire examples.
- Use of technology to improve awareness and access to healthcare, as illustrated by the NHS Choices work on health kiosks.

3.3.1. Barnsley

A study run in Barnsley in 2006, from the Acute Hospital Trust, involved installing telehealth at home for 42 chronic heart failure patients. Patients were recruited through heart failure clinics and monitoring was conducted by nurses from the clinic.

The interim report [3] on the trial is interesting for the information it reveals on the nature of telehealth monitoring. The report noted that interventions from the monitoring staff generally fell within four categories:

- Regulating medicine.
- Changing medication (adjusting doses).
- Advice.
- Dealing with cross morbidity including referrals.

The report also captures some interesting statistics on the monitoring workload. After an initial period in which modifications of the questions and alert settings were made, clinicians reported 20–30 minutes per day were required to review the website data for the 42 patients and respond accordingly. On average, the monitoring generated 173 alerts and four key medical interventions per week.

The Barnsley report illustrates experience that has been reported elsewhere, in particular the high proportion of alerts that do not lead to a medical intervention. Anecdotal evidence suggests that a significant part of this workload involves following up missing or apparently anomalous readings. While these follow-up calls do provide an opportunity to maintain active contact with patients, they represent low value work for staff with advanced clinical skills, such as community matrons. In larger operations there should be opportunities to exploit alternative arrangements for this first-line, non-clinical triage, or data-cleansing, work.

3.3.2. Kent – Telehealth Pilot

In a forerunner to participation in the WSDs, Kent County Council established a 'Telehealth Evaluative Pilot' in partnership with local health authorities. The pilot involved deploying telehealth solutions to 250 patients in the period 2005–2007. Eligibility was based on a diagnosis of at least one of 3 conditions, Chronic Obstructive Pulmonary Disease, Coronary Heart Disease or Diabetes Mellitus and included patients with these and other co-morbidities. At that time it was the largest deployment of telehealth remote monitoring systems in the UK by a significant margin. The pilot has generated some interesting findings [18] on organisational models, sustainability and benefits.

The Kent pilot evolved with two main care models. One based on GP practices where the monitoring of patients was undertaken by a practice nurse and a more centralised model in which community matrons or specialist nurses took on the role for monitoring patients as part of their caseload. In both cases a central administrative team handled issues with logistics, training and ongoing support for patients in the use of the equipment.

The evaluation report notes some differences in the results achieved through the various care delivery models, with generally better outcomes resulting from the more centralised matron models. The analysis highlights a tendency for monitoring in devolved operations to become more intermittent, typically every 3 days or twice a week. In contrast, the specialist community matrons generally reviewed the results daily and used the results to prioritise their appointments. There were some exceptions where the individual matrons had very high clinical caseloads, and where the telehealth patients represented a small proportion of the total caseload in which the frequency of monitoring dropped. The frequency and reliability of the monitoring is likely to be a significant factor in explaining the different results. Centralised services offer the potential to apply greater scrutiny on the delivery of this initial triage of readings and to dedicate sufficient resources to the task. A high caseload is also important for developing and maintaining the clinical and IT skills used in remote monitoring.

The Kent pilot produced some evidence on the sustainability of the telehealth service. The report notes that nearly 3 years after recruitment finished in July 2007, 159 out of the original 250 patients (63%) were still active on the programme.

The economic evaluation of the Kent pilot provided significantly positive results, with savings per patient in the range £1038 to £2718 (£1878 mean cost) over a 12 month study period. However, when the full costs of infrastructure were factored in the mean cost saving per patient reduced to just £568. Scale, and the ability to apportion infrastructure costs over a larger user base, is therefore an important economic driver and suggests that bold moves are required by organisations seeking to implement telehealth as part of a cost containment strategy.

3.3.3. NHS Direct / SE Essex

Centralised services have a key role to play in the move to large-scale monitoring operations and feature in a number of the planned large-scale implementations, notably those in North Yorkshire (1000+ users planned) and Northern Ireland (5000+ users). While this NHS Direct example lacked the sort of information systems integration developed for Newham's WSD, it does highlight how third parties could facilitate telehealth services through logistic and monitoring support. In many cases, local authorities already have a significant logistic capability for community equipment and operate monitoring centres although those centres may lack some of the clinical capabilities NHS Direct were able to offer in the South West Essex service.

NHS South East Essex and NHS Direct established a telehealth service which is noteworthy for the way in which it has addressed some of the logistic issues that have beset many of the other NHS implementations. The initial project went from an initial approval for the project to having 65 patients being monitored in only seven months.

The project had four main aims

- Improve patient's understanding of their condition, and how they can manage and cope with symptoms better.
- Improve the way healthcare staff prioritise their workload through effective use of patient vital signs data.
- Create case management capacity as a result of more informed home visits and interventions.
- Reduce the number of hospital admissions through effective case management.

To achieve this, patients with a primary diagnosis of Chronic Obstructive Pulmonary Disease (COPD) regularly recorded agreed data in their own homes. This information was monitored by NHS Direct staff who provided initial support, and advice if required. After examining the information against agreed protocols, NHS Direct would then alert the community teams to make a decision upon the appropriate level of intervention required.

The key factor in achieving the significant rate of patient recruitment was the way the service was provided as a 'turn-key' solution, where the more complex and technical aspects were handled through a central service without the need for significant change in working practices by community-based clinical staff. NHS Direct managed centrally the complexities of equipment deployment and IT skills needed for routine monitoring. This left the community nurses free to focus on their caseload. The NHS Direct internal evaluation report [29] is available through a third-party website.

3.3.4. Birmingham OwnHealth

NHS Birmingham East and North operate their OwnHealth (see [15]) service in partnership with NHS Direct and others[6] for people with long term conditions. It is a telephone-based service providing one-to-one advice and support by a designated care manager to help patients manage their condition. It operates in several languages, including English and Punjabi, suggesting that this form of coaching may be particularly

[6] Birmingham OwnHealth is a partnership of NHS Birmingham East and North, UK Pfizer Health Solutions and NHS Direct. Pfizer Health Solutions is a group within Pfizer Limited that operates independently of Pfizer's medicines business.

suitable as a complement to other forms of telehealth where support for multiple minority languages is not technically feasible or economic.

Another aspect which sets this form of telehealth service apart from others is the scale and breadth of services that have been delivered. In its first 4 years, the OwnHealth service supported over 6000 patients[7], significantly more than any other NHS organisation has achieved through a remote monitoring service. It also supports a wider range of chronic conditions than is typical, including diabetes, coronary heart disease, heart failure, chronic obstructive pulmonary disease (COPD), high blood pressure, stroke or TIA ("mini stroke"), chronic kidney disease as well as people who are aged over 65 with a range of conditions giving rise to more complex needs.

Having started as a purely telephone-based service, OwnHealth has expanded to include the use of remote monitoring technologies. The service now offers remote monitoring support, through the same call centre, to patients with chronic obstructive pulmonary disease (COPD) or heart failure.

3.3.5. Airedale

Airedale NHS Trust is one of a number of NHS Trusts looking to use video conferencing with patients at home to deliver care services. The work draws on Airdale's experience of providing telemedicine services to prisons. Tele-conferencing facilities had traditionally required expensive equipment and dedicated (and costly) communications links.

The Tele-health Consultation System is a TV-based video telephony solution, developing interactive e-learning applications for the service. It uses a set-top box with integral microphone, and a high quality webcam. It connects to a domestic television, which acts as the display. The set top box provides good quality video over a domestic internet connection. The service supports secure video calls over the internet and the delivery of streamed educational content.

This work started off as a research project using available technologies to develop an affordable and easy-to-use in-home two-way video technology for patient to clinician consultations and supply of health information [30]. It has now moved from research into a commercial service which is offered by NHS Airedale through a national framework procurement agreement [5].

Home video conferencing is attracting increasing interest in the UK for other applications, including home rehabilitation classes for orthopaedic and pulmonary patients.

3.3.6. Cumbria – Cardiac Monitoring

The North West regional health authority established a telemedicine service involving 12-lead ECG examinations in community settings such as GP practices and established NHS Walk-In Centres. The service uses specially adapted equipment that transmits the readings to a centralised interpretation service over standard telephone lines. The interpretation service is staffed by cardiac physiologists who are able to interpret the traces and respond back to the surgeries within 30 minutes, with a recommendation in one of the following four courses of action:

- Those within the norm – no further action.
- Check patient again after a suitable time interval.

[7] Dr. Richard Mendelsohn quoted in '*Your Own Health*' newsletter, Issue 2, February 2010.

- Refer to Cardiology Clinic.
- Emergency referral via A&E.

The Centres were recruited with the support of the local cardiac network. An independent audit of the project conducted by Ipsos Mori reported a substantial reduction in the number of referrals to Cardiology Clinics which in itself released capacity within the Acute Trusts. It also found that there was a high degree of acceptance among primary care physicians. The service provider, Broomwell Healthcare, now reports that, in a 4 year period from 2006, the service has handled 50,000 examinations with an estimated saving of 32,000 hospital referrals.

There is increasing interest in similar services elsewhere in the UK. In Scotland, Aberdeen Royal Infirmary has been operating a service for remote highland and island communities, as well as for the offshore oil industry. The technology used in this service creates a file attachment which is sent using the NHSmail secure email service for interpretation by staff in the hospital's Accident and Emergency department.

3.3.7. North Lincolnshire e-Clinics

A one year pilot of 'eClinics' in North Lincolnshire was established in 2009 to offer access to mental health support and treatment through an online NHS therapy clinic [28].

The trial was a partnership between Rotherham, Doncaster and South Humber Mental Health NHS Foundation Trust and the North Lincolnshire Council Digital Inclusion Unit. The eClinic approach aims to increase access to psychological therapies, extending the reach and availability of help for those who need it.

The e-clinics are a phone and web-based service that provides low intensity psychological interventions for people in primary care who have depression, anxiety, panic attacks and phobias, via the medium of live dialogue over the internet. Users of this service can talk directly to a trained mental health clinician, either through visiting the website (www.eclinic.org) to arrange an appointment, or through visiting the site to 'drop in' on scheduled e-clinics. Access to the E-Clinic is either through self-referral on the website, via a GP or through a mental health clinician.

The technology partner, British Telecom, provided a secure chat room and booking facility. This allows mental health professionals to host Internet and email based therapy sessions, organise internet chat room discussions and manage interactions in a controlled environment.

The use of the e-clinics is an interesting development that extends the use of information technology for assisted living in healthcare, and could open the way for the use of a range of online assessment and self-support tools. Following a successful trial and evaluation, Rotherham, Doncaster and South Humber Mental Health NHS Foundation Trust have re-designed the technology platform and launched a mainstream eClinics service called Talkingsense.org.

3.3.8. NHS Choices – Health Kiosks

There is growing interest in the use of health kiosks for two main applications: maximising the use of telehealth equipments installed in semi-public environments such as day-care centres, and in providing a health screening and educational capability.

NHS Choices (The Department of Health public-facing website, www.nhs.uk) and Directgov [24] (a pan-government initiative to provide a single citizen portal for online services) jointly fund pilot work to determine the optimum ways of reaching the digitally excluded population. This involved providing access to NHS Choices content via kiosks deployed in strategic locations such as community centres, health centres, an older care charity's shops, prisons, probation hostels and citizens advice bureaux.

NHS Choices piloted the use of interactive health kiosks in four private companies in Derbyshire to help the local NHS to work with employers in addressing health issues in the workplace. Employees were able to check their blood pressure, weight, body fat content and other aspects of their health by standing on a set of scales and following instructions on a computer screen.

One issue with health kiosks is a lack of integration into the healthcare system. The need to establish patient identity both reliably and securely is a barrier to using information from kiosks. Multi-user remote monitoring systems may provide some form of secure identity and log-on, but public access kiosks are by their nature not open to such solutions.

An increasing number of GP surgeries now have some form of kiosk for patients to check-in on arrival. One solution available on the market addresses the integration issue by enabling patients to complete self-testing similar to the public kiosk approach, but with the information sent to their electronic patient record.

3.4. The UK Devolved Regions

The devolved regions of Scotland, Wales and Northern Ireland have all looked to support the adoption of ambient assisted living technologies. These Regions are interesting, partly because they have different management arrangements from the NHS in England, including closer integration with social care. Due to their smaller scale, the devolved regions are sometimes able to be more agile in implementing innovative services. Of particular note is that both Scotland and Northern Ireland have established dedicated centres to promote the use of telehealth technology.

3.4.1. Scotland

The Scottish Centre for Telehealth (SCT) was established on the recommendation of the Kerr Report (20 year plan for Scotland's NHS, published in 2005) [26]. It has initially focused on fostering telemedicine services to support remote highlands and island communities, including video-consultations for minor injuries and the use of video conferencing for pulmonary rehabilitation classes. More recently it has sponsored telehealth research, including a 400-patient telehealth trial in West Lothian. In a recent change, SCT has been moved into NHS24, the central health contact centre operator. The move is seen as providing a better base than SCT to provide pan-Scotland services, and signals a shift from being a largely research and development organisation to one focused on large-scale operational delivery.

3.4.2. Wales

In Wales, the Welsh Assembly Government is supporting a number of initiatives in telecare and telehealth. For NHS Wales, the National Service Improvement Demonstrator Projects have been established to "Provide and test a sustainable, affordable generic chronic conditions management service model". The demonstrator in Carmarthen has a particular focus on health informatics and includes a small-scale 'Better Breathing' field trial involving deployment of telehealth monitoring solutions for COPD patients.

3.4.3. Northern Ireland

In Northern Ireland the 'European Centre for Connected Health' (ECCH) was established in 2008 to promote improvements in patient care through the use of technology in health and social care and to fast track new products and innovation in the health and social services.

For integrated care Northern Ireland has the advantage of one health and social care agency with responsibility for the planning, delivery, finance and regulation of health and social care.

ECCH is currently engaged in a procurement process for the "Remote Telemonitoring Northern Ireland" (RTNI) service. This will provide remote monitoring as a managed service to support the case management of patients with chronic disease. It will initially focus on heart failure, COPD, and diabetes and the target is to secure access for some 5000 patients with these conditions by 2011.

Northern Ireland started with ambitious plans for an integrated and interoperable technical solution. The resulting procurement process has proved to be complex and lengthy. At the time of writing the procurement process had taken nearly three years and seen a significant de-scoping of the original ambitions. While it is still too early to draw conclusions, this experience suggests that there are limits on the scale of 'mainstream' operations arising from technical constraints, particularly interoperability, and in the lack of agreed professional standards which makes negotiations across multiple provider organisations difficult.

3.5. Emerging Applications

This review would not be complete without a brief look at applications that are available now and which are poised to have an impact on the adoption of ambient assisted living technologies by the NHS.

3.5.1. mHealth

mHealth is a broad term that covers the use of mobile technology to deliver healthcare. In the context of ambient assisted living its potential stems from the near universal access to mobile phones, and their increasing sophistication.

The T+ Medical smart-phone based monitoring solution for diabetes has been used for several years in trials and small scale services in the NHS. Other solutions are now coming on the market. South Birmingham PCT have established a mobile phone based telehealth remote monitoring service and plan to deploy it to around 1000 users.

SMS messaging is now being used for a wide range of services, such as appointment reminders. The Meteorological Office have developed a service to provide SMS reminders and warnings including cold weather, heat-wave, UV and the Healthy Outlook® forecast alert service for COPD patients (see [16]).

3.5.2. Personal Health Records

With the widespread adoption of electronic health records, and the creation of the shared summary care record, the motivation for patients to have their own electronic personal health records is somewhat different in England than it is in the US, where most of the solutions have been developed. The NHS does have a personal health record offering, HealthSpace, and has recently extended the capability to provide patients with secure access to their summary care record, enable them to communicate securely with their GP and manage some transactional services such as requesting repeat prescriptions.

In the future it is likely that HealthSpace and other personal health records will provide a platform that will interface with medical and other devices to help patients manage their own health and wellness.

3.5.3. Lifestyle Monitoring (Activities of Daily Living)

The monitoring of activities of daily living, also known as lifestyle monitoring, is an enhancement to telecare systems that offers the potential to make monitoring more predictive. Various early experiments in the technology have highlighted the complexities involved and while there are some commercial solutions in use, it is not clear that the technology is sufficiently sophisticated to provide a reliable alarm system without excessive numbers of 'false-alerts'.

One interesting application of this technology has been in its use as an assessment tool by professionals who are planning a care package. The 'Just Checking' system, which is in active use in a number of areas (see, for instance, [21]), offers an 'out of the box' solution with door motion and room motion (PIR) sensors that are simple to install and remove. The system is typically installed for 2–6 weeks to provide a snapshot of how a person is using their home – which may include sleep/wake patterns and use of rooms. It avoids the issues with continuous lifestyle monitoring by not seeking to generate an automatic alert Instead it provides a relatively simple dataset that can be used as the basis for further investigation.

3.5.4. Telecare / Telehealth Convergence

There is growing interest in the potential for convergence between the health and social care aspects of ambient assisted living. There are a number of drivers for this. Both appear to align with the high level policies with to care for patients, or people, closer to home. Care services are increasingly forming multi-disciplinary community teams to provide holistic services, and it is logical that many of those considered vulnerable and thereby eligible for telecare support are also likely to have one or more chronic condition.

Convergence offers a number of clear logistic advantages, reducing the number of 'touch points' for patients, sharing equipment logistics and monitoring infrastructure. In some cases the line between telehealth and telecare is becoming increasingly blurred – such as in dementia care and in the use of lifestyle monitoring technologies which rely on telecare infrastructure to provide an early warning of a medical exacerbation. Policies in Scotland, Wales and Northern Ireland are actively promoting convergence, and several telecare services in England offer a telehealth service as well.

While ambitions and some early adopters point to a longer term potential for convergence, there remain a number of factors that militate against this trend. One is in the different driving philosophy for the two types of service. Telecare services has been established to meet a need to respond quickly, while the telehealth proposition only really works if coaching and self-care aspirations can be achieved. This means the services have divergent drivers and there are dangers in assuming convergence will happen early. Technology is also a barrier to convergence, as the lack of standards for interoperability would prevent a 'best of breed' approach in selecting technology for additional services. There are also risks that in a declining financial climate and at a time of significant reorganisation in primary care, 'converged' services will lose out.

3.5.5. Point of Care Testing

Developments in point of care testing technologies mean that devices that are considered medical may reach the consumer market. This is already true for devices like blood pressure and blood glucose monitors. The next wave of devices is likely to include pulse-oximetry, INR (blood coagulation), cholesterol and even ECG. Device regulators have also started to take an interest in smartphone applications, as devices like the iSteth [7] offer widespread use of capabilities once the preserve of clinicians, who were the only people who could afford expensive medical stethoscopes.

A new range of devices is coming on the market.

- Monica®, an ambulatory and non-invasive foetal monitoring device developed in Nottingham, is now being used in trials in Germany. Intended for clinical use, it is likely that there would be demand for a consumer solution.
- A growing range of devices developed for the fitness market offer new possibilities for health services, such as the ability to prescribe and monitor an exercise regime as part of a wider health programme, whether for weight-loss or to develop lung capacity in asthma.
- DNAe make a point of care testing device for genetic profiling that could support the more wide-spread use of personalised medicines.
- Health 'apps' for smart phones are further extending the possibilities.

4. Conclusions

The use of ambient assisted living technology by the NHS in England is set against a wider background of supporting policy, central funding for key initiatives and a strong legacy from social care, where use of technology to support people to live independently is now mainstream. Successive healthcare policies over the past 5 years have served to establish and reinforce a focus on prevention. This is driven both by payments that reward providers for good outcomes and the professional frameworks that govern front-line delivery.

The main focus in the past 5 years has been on the quest for better evidence that the early promise of services using ambient assisted living technologies can be realised on a whole health-system basis. Early movers are, by and large, just moving to the scale where sustainability may be achieved, with overhead costs apportioned over greater numbers of users.

Most services, and as a consequence most of the evidence, relate to relatively high risk individuals who are already high intensity users of health services, and thus where short term savings may be achieved. Nevertheless, this is not an easy equation, as releasing cash savings also require the removal of capacity from other parts of the healthcare system, typically from hospitals.

The focus on intensive users has important implications for the sort of technologies that have been used. The users have tended to be older people, often over 75, who have complex needs, mostly involving limiting long term conditions which provide a significant motivation to use the services. Significantly, most of this group are not routine users of information technology. As a result, most telehealth services use bespoke technology with simplified interfaces, such as touch screens, and have relatively restricted interactive capabilities. While these technologies serve the need of the target population, whose conditions would generally be considered 'life-limiting', they are less attractive to other groups of patients with chronic conditions where convenience and lifestyle 'fit' would be more important.

There is interest in moving beyond the high risk cohort and looking at the potential to support the medium risk group of users. This group comprises around 15–20% of patients, and accounts for a further third of the total expenditure on long term conditions[8]. Preventing those in this group from becoming high intensity users offers the potential for benefits, although it also involves a longer-term payback. Many of the patients in this group will not have limiting long term conditions, so providing services that match their needs and lifestyle will be important. Patient recruitment is also likely to be more difficult, requiring careful targeting and coherent care pathways. Effective case-finding tools, such as the Combined Predictive Model, will be important to ensure services are targeted, and complementary capabilities, such as provision of effective educational and motivational support are likely to be needed to ensure the benefits are sustainable. Targeting this group will therefore probably represent a second wave of service implementations, driven by low cost telehealth technologies that could take advantage of pervasive infrastructure, such as smart phones and lower cost delivery models. This second wave may be driven by wider policies such as the plans for personal budgets for long term conditions which could give patients some discretion to use NHS funds to purchase their own telehealth services, and would require the market to offer consumer-friendly solutions involving interoperable technologies based on effective technical standards.

There are also likely to be selective moves to address the needs of low risk individuals. The case for investment here is more difficult, as the returns may be extremely long term. In the Department of Health model, this is largely a domain for self-care, and focus may be on tools that support that, such as enabling self monitoring through personal health records. There are still some areas where the NHS might provide technology.

Titration of medication regimes is another opportunity for remote monitoring technologies that would become relevant to much larger groups of patients, and perhaps not only those with long term conditions. Research conducted by Birmingham University, the TASMINH2 Project [22] looked at the impact of self monitoring on the management of hypertension. The results point to significant improvements and the study concluded that self-management of hypertension in combination with telemonitoring of blood pressure measurements represents an important new addition to control of hypertension in primary care. The main impact of the telemonitoring was considered to be faster titration of medication regimes. There are already some NHS community-based services for INR monitoring of patients on anti-coagulants. As both communications and medical device technologies become more pervasive, it should be possible to exploit the potential for similar services for a much wider range of medications.

As the NHS learns new ways of working and puts in place the infrastructure to interact with patients in the community, this will open up new possibilities such as monitoring higher maternity cases, more effective monitoring of patients on discharge from hospital, and even providing better palliative care services for people who want to be cared for at home.

The evidence from the WSDs is eagerly awaited, and is expected to trigger a step change in the way the NHS uses ambient assisted living technologies.

---

[8] Sources: 1. *Supporting People with Long Term Conditions*, Department of Health 2005. 2. *Self Care – A Real Choice*; Department of Health 2005.

Glossary

Abbreviation	Term	Definition
A&E	Accident and Emergency	NHS term for services that assess and treat patients with serious injuries or illnesses.
COPD	Chronic obstructive pulmonary disease	Chronic obstructive pulmonary disease is the name for a collection of lung diseases including chronic bronchitis, emphysema and chronic obstructive airways disease. People with COPD have trouble breathing in and out. This is referred to as airflow obstruction. Breathing difficulties are caused by long-term damage to the lungs, usually because of smoking.
ECCH	European Centre for Connected health	Launched in 2008, it was been established to promote improvements in patient care in Northern Ireland through the use of technology in health and social care and to fast track new products and innovation in the health and social services.
ECG	Electrocardiogram	ECG is a test that measures the electrical activity of the heart
GP	General Practitioner / General Practice	The term used in the NHS for a primary care physician
HF	Heart Failure	Heart failure is a term used to describe a serious condition when the heart is having trouble pumping enough blood around the body. It usually occurs because the heart muscle has become too weak or stiff to work properly.
INR	International normalized ratio	A measure of blood coagulation. It is used in the management of warfurin treatment.
IEEE	Institute of Electrical and Electronics Engineers	IEEE is a professional association dedicated to advancing technological innovation and excellence. It's role includes publication of technical standards. Originally based on US professional institutions, IEEE has become a global leader in technical standards and by 2010 had over 395,000 members in 160 countries.
LTC	Long term condition	A long term condition is one that can not be cured but can be managed through medication and/or therapy. There is no definitive list of long term conditions. Conditions such as, diabetes, asthma, coronary heart disease, chronic obstructive pulmonary disease (COPD) and mental health issues can all be included as a long term condition.
NHS	National Health Service	The world's largest publicly funded health service, funded through taxation and providing healthcare free at the point of use for anyone who is resident in the UK.
PCT	Primary care Trust	NHS PCT is a local health authority which has its own budget and sets its own priorities At the time of writing there were 151 primary care trusts in England although they are due to be replaced by a system of GP commissioning of services through local clinical groups.
QIPP	Quality, Innovation, Productivity and Prevention	QIPP is a programme of reform for the NHS working at a national, regional and local level to support clinical teams and NHS organisations to improve the quality of care they deliver while making efficiency savings that can be reinvested in the service to deliver year on year quality improvements.

Abbreviation	Term	Definition
SCT	Scottish Centre for Telehealth	The Scottish Centre for Telehealth (SCT) was established in 2006 to support and guide the development of telehealth for clinical, managerial and educational purposes across Scotland. See www.sctt.scot.nhs.uk.
SHA	Strategic Health Authority	Regional health authority for the NHS in England. At the time of writing there were 9 SHAs. They are due to be replaced by an NHS Commissioning Board that will make allocations to GP commissioning consortia.
TIA	Transient Ischemic Attack	A transient ischaemic attack is a change in the blood supply to a particular area of the brain, resulting in brief neurological dysfunction that persists for less than 24 hours. It is often colloquially referred to as "mini stroke".
VC	Video conferencing	
QIPP	Quality, Innovation, Productivity and Prevention	QIPP is a programme of reform for the NHS working at a national, regional and local level to support clinical teams and NHS organisations to improve the quality of care they deliver while making efficiency savings that can be reinvested in the service to deliver year on year quality improvements.
WSD	Whole System Demonstrator	The Whole System Demonstrator (WSD) programme is a two year research project funded by the Department of Health to find out how technology can help people manage their own health while maintaining their independence.

References

[1] L. Adams, Crisis fears: 40% of school leavers may be forced to care for elderly, *HearaldScotland* (13 Oct. 2009).
[2] F. Barr, Yorks and Humber plans telehealth hub, *ehealthInsider* (15 April 2010).
[3] S. Brownsell et al., Telemonitoring chronic heart failure: Interim findings from a pilot study in South Yorkshire, *The British Journal of Healthcare Computing & Information Management* **23**(8) (October 2006).
[4] S. Bruce, North Yorks spends £3.2 m on telehealth, *ehealthInsider* (9 June 2010).
[5] Buying Solutions, Telecare, Telehealth and Telecoaching framework agreement, www.buyingsolutions.gov.uk/categories/ICT/telecare/.
[6] Continua Health Alliance website, www.continuaalliance.org.
[7] Daily Mail Reporter, iStethoscope: The iPhone app which is already replacing the real thing in hospitals, *Daily Mail*, London (31st August 2010).
[8] Department of Health, Building telecare in England, London, July 2005.
[9] Department of Health, Carers at the heart of 21st century families and communities: A caring system on your side, a life of your own, London, 10 June 2008.
[10] Department of Health, Delivering care closer to home: Meeting the challenge, London, 8 July 2008.
[11] Department of Health, High quality care for all: NHS next stage review final report, London, 30 June 2008, ISBN 978-0-10-174322-8.
[12] Department of Health, NHS next stage review: Our vision for primary and community care, London, 3 July 2008.
[13] Department of Health, Our health, our care, our say: A new direction for community services, London, 2006.
[14] Department of Health, Raising the profile of long term conditions care: A compendium of information, London, January 2008, Gateway reference 8734.
[15] http://birminghamownhealth.co.uk.
[16] http://www.metoffice.gov.uk/health/.

[17] S. Johnson, Department of Health Director of Long Term Conditions, Learning from the Whole System Demonstrator projects, presentation to sustaining innovations and new technologies for managing long term conditions event at the King's Fund London, 9 July 2009, http://www.wsdactionnetwork.org.uk/past_events/sustaining.html.
[18] Kent County Council, *Promoting and Sustaining Independence in A Community Setting. Kent Telehealth Evaluative Development Pilot: A Study into the Management of People with Long Term Conditions*, 2010, www.kent.gov.uk/telehealth.
[19] A. Lansley, Health Secretary sets out ambition for a culture of patient safety in the NHS, Department of Health Press Release, 8 June 2010.
[20] A. Liddell, S. Adshead and E. Burgess, *Technology in the NH STransforming the Patient's Experience of Care*, The King's Fund, London, 2008.
[21] London Borough of Sutton service information at: http://www.sutton.gov.uk/index.aspx?articleid=8714
[22] R. McManus et al., Telemonitoring and self-management in the control of hypertension (TASMINH2): A randomised controlled trial, London, *The Lancet* **376**(9736) (17 July 2010), 163–172.
[23] B. Moorman, Medical device interoperability: Standards overview, *IT WORLD* (March/April 2010), 132–138.
[24] NHS Choices, NHS Choices annual report 2009, London 26 June 2009.
[25] NHS Cornwall and Isles of Scilly, Annual Report and Accounts 2009/10, 22 Sep. 2010.
[26] NHS Scotland, *Building A Health Service Fit For the Future*, Scottish Executive, May 2005, ISBN: 0-7559-4669-3.
[27] G. Paré, M. Jaana and C. Sicotte, Systematic review of home telemonitoring for chronic diseases: The evidence base, *Journal of the American Medical Informatics Association* **14**(3) (May/June 2007), 269–271.
[28] Rotherham Doncaster and South Humber Mental Health NHS Foundation Trust, Annual report and summary financial statements 2009 / 2010, p. 14.
[29] A. Single and G. Donnelly, 'At home, not alone' COPD Telehealth Project Final Evaluation, NHS Direct East and NHS South East, February 2010.
[30] Technology Strategy Board, ALIP1 ADI100D TVPhone, An assisted living innovation platform project, www.assistedlivingplatform.org.uk.
[31] The Audit Commission, Implementing telecare, London, 2004, http://www.audit-commission.gov.uk/nationalstudies/health/socialcare/Pages/olderpeople6.aspx.
[32] The Health and Social Care Information Centre, Quality and outcomes framework achievement data 2009/10, 20 Oct 2010, see p. 34, CDH 5.
[33] Your health, your way: Your NHS guide to long-term conditions and self care, published on the NHS website at: http://www.nhs.uk/Planners/Yourhealth/Pages/Telecare.aspx.

Handbook of Ambient Assisted Living
J.C. Augusto et al. (Eds.)
IOS Press, 2012

doi:10.3233/978-1-60750-837-3-67

Telehealthcare Development & Effectiveness in Taiwan

Tsai-Ya LAI* and Jenn-Hwan TARNG
Service Systems Technology Center, Industrial Technology Research Institute, Taiwan

Abstract. This article is introducing the current development of telehealthcare and reviewing the past history and effect in Taiwan. Since 2006, the government has deployed several projects to facilitate the development of telehealthcare, which including U-Care (2006), 10 year projecton long term care (2007), Taiwan 12 construction project (2008), and six emerging industries (2009). The currently running project, Telehealthcare Service Development Program, started in 2007. This project is targeting Diabetes Mellitus and the population with Hypertension and also developing two models of service delivery, a Homecare/Community service model and an Institutional Care service model. Seven services are delivered in Homecare/Community service model, which are tele-physiological monitoring, member health management, tele-consulting, tele-health education, medication safety services, living resource referral, and emergency management; five services are delivered in Institutional Care service model, which are tele-consultation, tele-physiological monitoring, tele-visiting for family members, medication safety services, and tele-health education. The significant benefit outcomes for members in this project relate to hospitalization rate, ER admission rate, self-care monitoring, institutional infection rate, unexpected readmission rate, and redundant medication rate, and also the acceptance rate and satisfaction for both members and caregivers and reductions in the burdens on members' family are also relatively high. In the future, development of telehealthcare service will rely on amendment of the current legislation/decree by government, incentivizing of the services by healthcare/insurance providers, and introduction of new business models by all involved industries.

Keywords. Telehealthcare, integrated service model, information exchange standard

Introduction

Since 1985, a medical network, mental medical network, and emergency medical network have been incrementally implemented in Taiwan to balance the distribution of medical resources and to provide medical care accessibility. National health insurance (NHI) was also implemented in 1995 with the NHI coverage rate over 99% [2], thereby lowering the economic barrier to receive medical service. Health care infrastructure in Taiwan was rated the 13th among 55 countries over the world in the "World Competitiveness Yearbook" of the IMD Business School, Switzerland [6]. What underpins the advancement of Taiwan's health care is a unitary health care system and insurance with

* Corresponding Author: Tsai-Ya Lai. E-mail: rose_lai@itri.org.tw.

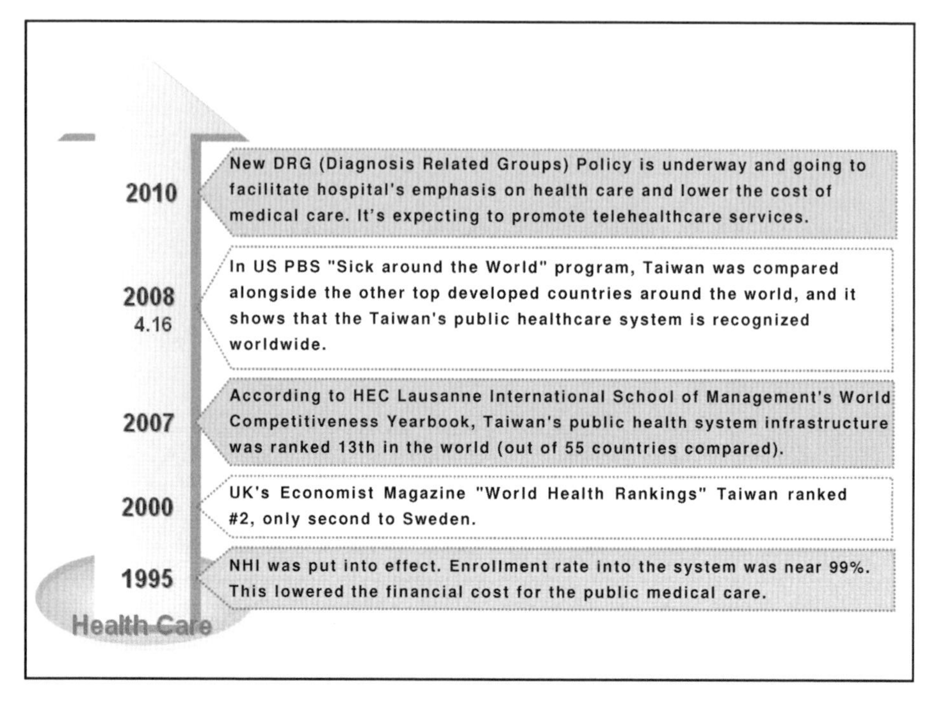

Figure 1. Health care development in Taiwan by NHI. IEK, ITRI (2009/12) [7].

sound medical and epidemiological information, which proves to be extemely valuable for disease study and prevention.

In 2010, people above 65 years old represented 10.74% of the population in Taiwan [4]. Under the global influence of low birth rates, aging in Taiwan is expected to rank the second highest in speed around the globe [3]. In 2008, the overall health care expense has reached 42 billion NT dollars, with 62.9% spent on public health. The health care expense for people over 60 years old is 4.5 times compared to that of others, and represents 44% of the overall health care expense [1].

As the need for long-term care increases along with the growth of aging population, it is imperative to plan in advance the long-term care human resources and service delivery models. Current service delivery models are mostly labor-intensive, yet technology-barren, thereby unable to cope with the rising problems of the aging baby-boom generation. In addition, the increasing health care cost has created a heavy financial burden upon the NHI system. We are in urgent need of a health care service model with high efficiency and sound effectiveness. Therefore, technology-enhanced health care service provides an important avenue for future sustainable development.

The comparative advantage of the health care industry in Taiwan includes sound medical systems and high efficiency, high medical care availability and accessibility, as well as high medical quality and lower cost when compared to Europe, US and Japan. On the other hand, Taiwan also possesses competitive advantage in the ICT industry. In 2008, the Economist Intellegence Unit (EIU) rated Taiwan as the 2nd place in IT industry competitiveness among 66 countries over the world [5]. The leading edge in ICT industry also benefits the development of a technology-enhanced health care industry. In addition, Taiwan's government has invested in innovation of the health care service.

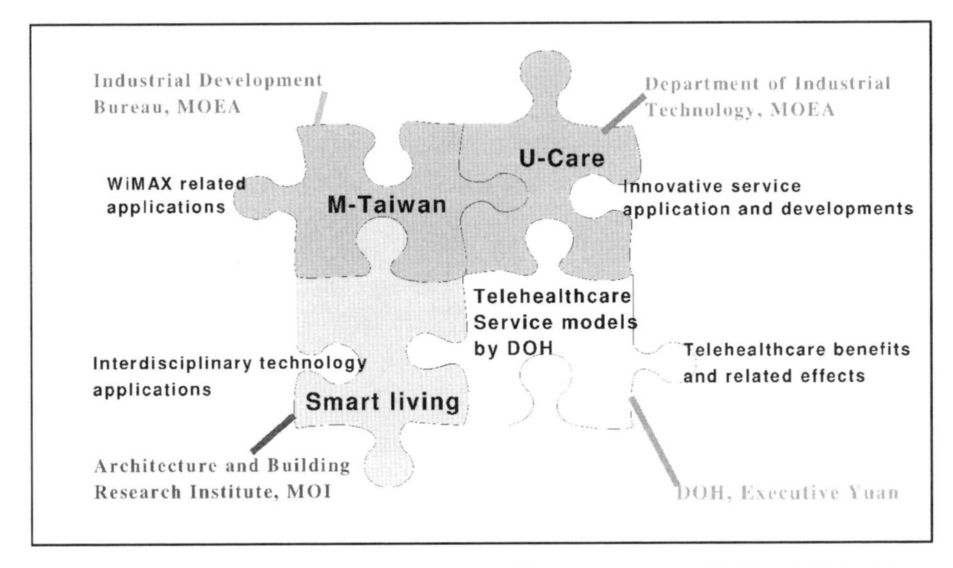

Figure 2. Devotion status in telehealthcare industry of Taiwan government. IEK, ITRI (2009/12) [7].

Under the sponsorship of the government, programs such as M-Taiwan, U-Care, and Telehealthcare have deployed many leading innovative initiatives.

The Department of Technology in Ministry of Economic Affairs (MOEA) has implemented the U-care project from 2006 to 2009 to encourage private enterprises to invest in device and system development while at the same time examing the feasibility of related business models. The Department of Health (DOH) also started the telehealthcare pilot program in 2007 to assess telehealthcare efficiency and feasibility for future dissemination. The Industrial Development Bereau in MOEA has been encouraging the application of WiMAX on telehealthcare since 2009, in the hope of providing a solution to the elderly care needs. Moreover, the Architecture Research Institute in the Ministry of the Interior (MOI) also has the "Smart Living" project to apply cross-border technologies on telehealthcare in either home space or other scenarios.

Regarding industry input, various government-sponsored telehealthcare trials have successfully invited industries' attention and therefore related investment in the R&D of new devices and systems. According to a research report published by Industrial Technology Research Institute (ITRI) in December 2009, many medical equipment suppliers have been investing in portable devices development. These suppliers include Aescu Technology, ApexBio, Chinese Care, Foxconn, Delta, Health & Life, Mesure Technology, Mytech Technology, Quanta, Leadtek TaiDoc, and Tatung. Netown, Qisda, and Compal Communication have been developing presentation interfaces. There are also companies focusing on monitoring home health devices, especially those specializing in emergency services, including Lifeline, Mennonite, Philips Lifeline and Sum-Gain.

At the system's service end, ITC companies often invest time into system development directly, given different needs for tailored functions and services for varied projects. ITC companies developing integrated systems include Techgroups, Nan-Kai University of Technology, Inqgen, NCHC, ITRI, Inventec, Cablesoft, Mayaminer, MiTAC, Elan, VODTEL, Universal Technology, Hitron Technologies, Formosa

Technologies, Aiontech, SYSTEX, La Spring Biotech, AVCON6, Unisage Technology, Advantech, GolbalNet Electronics, KTop Computer, K.Y.I.C.T, Lifememo, ACME Portable Corp, Chain Sea Information Integration, Chung-Hwa Wideband Best Network and Taiwan Foxconn. However, that these systems are mutually exclusive and disconnected engenders implications for future application and dissemination.

Finally, the system's operational end can be divided into two categories. The first category is operation centers providing medical care service, mainly composed of such hospitals as Far Eastern Memorial Hospital, Cheng Hsin General Hospital and National Taiwan University Hospital. Their goal is to provide high quality and professional medical service. The second category is operational centers that provide other related services, including SECOM and SKS Securities focusing on offering safety services.

1. Service Models

1.1. Telehealthcare Service Development Program, Department of Health, Executive Yuan, Taiwan

The speedy growth of an aging population in Taiwan has not only brought forth urgent long-term care needs but also imposed a growing burden upon National Health Insurance. Therefore, Executive Yuan has decided to promote "Strategic Service Industry in Taiwan" in the "Executive Yuan Industry Strategy Meeting 2003" and stipulated the "THIS" project which encompasses Telehealthcare, Health Tourism and Integrated Medical System; Telehealthcare development in Taiwan began ever since then. Recent government policies and statements, such as "10 Year Project on Long Term Care" in 2007, "Taiwan Twelve Construction Projects" in 2008, and "Six Emerging Industries" in 2009, all focused on smart medical care, which further entails development of telehealthcare, improvement of quality and efficiency of medical service, and reduction of the costs of long-term care.

1.1.1. Overview

Department of Health, Executive Yuan, has been promoting the "Telehealthcare Service Development Program" since 2007. During the pilot period (2007/5~2010/12), Industrial Technology Research Institute (ITRI) has been responsible for incorporating partners from the care, safety and ITC industry to build "Home/Community Telehealthcare Services" and "Institutional Telehealthcare Services," and to perfect a seamless care service network supported by an ITRI-constructed open "Telehealthcare Information Platform" to collect, connect, exchange, and standardize information streams. At the same time, ITRI-initiated Project Management Office is responsible for integrating and coordinating projects. Trial operation of the service had been rolled out since January 2008 to recruit members and provide related services, with the total budget of 110.35 million NT dollars. Objectives of the project include:

1.1.1.1. Establish local telehealthcare service models and encourage medical institutions to improve health/living quality of people.

1. Establish and promote home/community and institutional telehealthcare service models tailored to health care needs arising from local environments (Ex. Metropolitan areas, rural villages, mountainous areas or faraway islands).

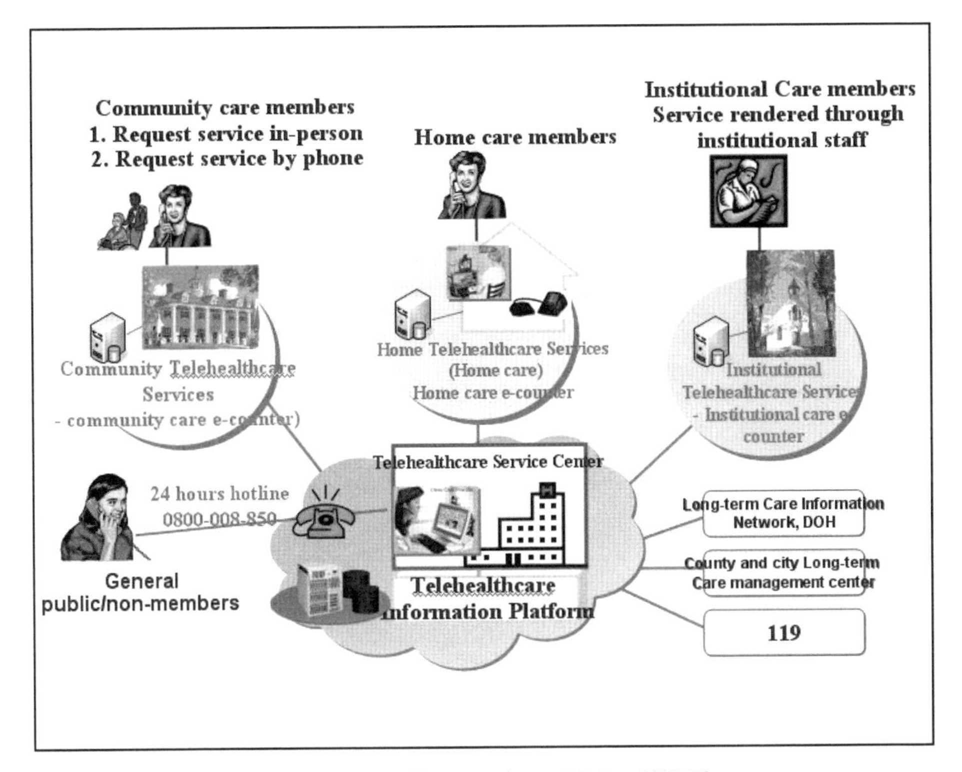

Figure 3. Telehealthcare service model, June 2008 [8].

2. Incorporate relevant industries and professionals in societal and health policy fields to establish a feasible service business model, to conduct cost-benefit analysis, and to set service charge rates and subsidy mechanisms.
3. Integrate and connect existing resources (for example, community medical groups and long-term care management centers), discuss with the hospitals currently providing telehealthcare service the possibility of partnership in order to integrate back-end information and furthermore upgrade the effectiveness of the telehealthcare service.

1.1.1.2. Promote the Telehealthcare Industry: Bring together medical care providers, medical equipment suppliers, the system integration industry, and information software industry to develop new service business models, invite other industries and talents to join the force, realize information platform interfaces to provide innovative telehealthcare pilot platforms connected with a variety of medical facilities and equipment.

1.1.1.3. Draft and promote patient health records and telehealthcare information exchange standards in order to build a health information exchange environment with worry-free privacy protection.

1.1.1.4. Education and Training: Implement telehealthcare inter-disciplinary training for human resources from various fields. Provide on-the-job telehealthcare training for institutional telehealthcare service staff.

Table 1. Telehealthcare service: Target clients and core services [8]

Model	Home/Community	Institute
Target Client	– Diabetes, Hypertension – Mild & Moderate Disability – Mild Denmentia – Elderly who lives alone – Care giver for chronic disease patients	– Residents of Nursing Home, Care Facilities and Disability Care Centers – Care providers of above intstitutes
Core Services	– Community Center/ Health Station – Member Health Management – Medication Safety Service – Living Resource Referral – Tele-physiological monitoring – Tele-consultation – Tele-education – Emergency services	– Tele-consultation – Tele-physiological monitoring – Tele-visiting – e-learning – Medication Safety Service

1.1.1.5. Hold International Seminars: Promote international cooperation in telehealthcare service and technology. Participate in international advocacy on technology-enhanced care and resource sharing; also invite foreign professionals to share experience and exchange ideas.

1.1.2. Current Status

1.1.2.1. Service Target Clients and Core Services

Target clients of the "Telehealthcare Pilot Project" are sorted by disease diagnoses. The service is mainly aimed at meeting the needs for selfcare and management for those patients diagnosed with diabetes, hypertension or dementia. The "Home/Community Telehealthcare Model" covers seven service items among the core service items of the "Telehealthcare Pilot Project." There are also five items in the "Institutional Telehealthcare Model".

Community Center or Health Station: Telehealthcare stations are set up in the members' communal space, or health stations are set up inside the communities for basic physical examinations, health workshops, and on-site/remote health consultations.

Tele-physiological monitoring: a 2-in-1 blood sugar and pressure meter is provided at community center or set up at members' home. It will record, store, and transmit blood pressure, blood sugar and pulse monitoring results. Members can use the information for selfhealth management. Records will also be sent back to the hospital for prescription reference or diagnosis assistance. Case managers can express concern and provide care service needed if any abnormality is found.

Member Health Management: A professional medical team is brought together to carry out a complete assessment on member's physical, mental, and social health management status. Individual care plans will then be established, tracked/documented and adjusted accordingly. Case managers will visit members actively to understand and help with their health management. Health records will be compiled individually so members can receive individualized personal or family care.

Tele-consultation: Services are available at member's home, community centers or health stations, so members can perform teleactivities such as video consultation and online health courses. In this way, a more complete and personalized health consultation service can be provided according to an individual member's care or medical problems. Residents can enjoy a complete health care service in their own neighborhood.

(1) Home/Community Telehealthcare Services

Tele-education: Trainings on care-giving techniques are provided for members and care givers. Professional medical staff can also share health information through group workshops or home videos in the community. Video consultation, phone calls, visits and health brochures are also available for members and families if personal health consultation is needed.

Medication Safety Services: A service that conbines institutionalized and community medical systems to create an auto-prescription mechanism to facilitate a community pharmaceutical medi-care program; including: complete medication record (includes chronic and other prescriptions), professional prescription instruction by pharmacists and medicine safety workshops, drug interaction assessment reminders, in order to raise public awareness about prescription safety.

Living Resource Referral: With the cooperation with 'living service' providers, various living resources referrals are provided to the members such as company information on the internet, living service subscription and living agency support services. Service includes: meal delivery, house keeping, hospital escort/walking/leisure activities, medication assistance, transportation service, bathing assistance, shopping assistance and aid equipment rental.

Emergency Services: Emergency consultation and doctors appointments are available if the system status shows emergency, hospitalization or abnormal values. Case managers will give home caring visits to relieve the anxieties of members and family, and also to assist with communicating with the doctor.

(2) Institutional Telehealthcare Services

Tele-consultation: The medical team in nursing homes can arrange consultation sessions with professional medical staff at the hospital for members through telehealthcare mechanisms such as video equipment and via integration with the information platform. Doing so is likely to save members' time in travelling, utilize medical resources efficiently, and improve the quality of life of patients. The management of medical records on video consultations will be established through an e-counter.

Tele-physiological Monitoring: Information on blood pressure, body temperature, blood oxygen, ECG, pulse and blood sugar are measured by an all-in-one biomonitor, and then conveyed to the e-counter for information storage and analysis. Caregivers can therefore monitor an individuals' health condition, take reference this way, and, when needed, give alert notification as basis for telehealthcare instruction and management.

Tele-visiting: Member's family and nursing centers will agree on a time schedule for vidio-visiting, during which members and their family can see and chat with each other. This service is especially convenient for families who live overseas because they can see their family when they are off work without having to travel all the way to the nursing centers.

Medication Safety Services: Pharmacists and doctors at the hospital will provide prescription instruction and medicine safety guides for patients. Personal basic information and medication history will also be developed so pharmacists and doctors can discuss substantively about patient medication safety through the remote platform.

E-learning: One-way or two-way job training and disease education courses such as infection control, principles of antibiotics use, needle-prick prevention and patient safety by a professional hospital medical team are available for medical staff at nursing homes through remote media thanks to the convenience brought by the internet. Medical staff of the institutes can have job training and take online courses at the institute, or download recorded courses on the e-counter system to enrich their knowledge on caregiving.

1.1.2.2. Equipment and Systems

Client terminals, measuring equipment, caregiver terminals and manager terminals are connected through an ADSL network by the telehealthcare service for information exchange and transmission. The service is a web-based design with improved accessibility and easy maintenance.

In terms of physiological measurement, the 2-in-1 blood pressure/sugar meter is used at home or in community health stations for home/community care service. Data measured will be sent back to the the system for processing and management through a home gateway chosen by each unit. The 4-in-1 biomonitor is used at institutional care facilities since more measurement is required there, patients have more severe disability conditions and monitoring requirements are also more complicated there. Measurement includes pulse, blood pressure, blood oxygen and ECG for comprehensive physiological information.

1.2. "Innovative Technology Health Care Service Program (U-Care)" by Ministry of Economic Affairs

1.2.1. Overview

The Ministry of Ecnomic Affairs has been promoting the "Innovative Technology Health Care Service Program" since 2006. The purpose of the program is to organize a health care service and also provide opportunities for emerging industries. The Department of Technology within the Ministry of Ecnomic Affairs estimate the growth rate of the industry will reach 17% and the production value will also reach 2.215 trillion NTD.

In order to solve problems like an aging population and declining birthrate, and to respond to the development trends of "Health Promotion" and "Disease Control", the Department of Technology in MOEA has been encouraging medical institutions to cooperate with ICT industry to generate a new method of operation. New operation methods should bring medical equipment and ICT together into applications, to develop innovative health care services, and support the long-term care system of MOI and the medical system of the DOH.

There are three stages for the "Innovative Technology Health Care Service Program". The first stage is the "U-Care Flagship Prgram for seniors" aiming at elderly seniors; it provides home, emergency, institutional or community care service for senior members. The second stage is to build a chronic disease service system aiming at chronic disease patients and their lives; life and recreational services for senior members are also included in this stage. Finally, the third stage of "Innovative Technology Health Care Service Program" will expand the parameters of the health care service system into, for example, employees' health management. A comprehensive and sound health care service industry roadmap is being built gradually through this program.

There are 12 applications for the first stage "U-Care Flagship Prgram for seniors" and a total of 32 units are involved (including 23 tech units, 8 medical units and 1 welfare unit). 7 projects have been approved with a total funding of 340 million NTD, of which 220 million is sponsored by companies and 120 million by the government. These projects were launched online at the end of 2008, including wireless biomonitor system and home care service in Changhua for seniors with diabetes and hypertension. In terms of institutional care, health management villages have been providing high quality service for senior members. So far, physiological signal collection and life management service planning & testing have been established; hardware and software solutions are also under construction.

At the second stage – chonic disease service system and patient life & recreation service program, 49 applications were received and 89 units are involved (including 46 technical units, 36 medical units and 7 welfare units). Five development cases and twelve planning cases were approved with a total funding of over 3 billion. Chronic disease management services available include "Integrated Diabetes Care Center", "Tailored Stroke Health Management" and an "Integrated Fitness Care Center".

Lastly, in the third stage aimed at the expansion of health care service system, there were four units approved at the end of 2009, including "B2B enterprise health management service", "National chronic disease e-pharmacy service", "Integrated long-term care health management service" and "Community elderly seniors digital health care service".

1.2.2. Current Status

1.2.2.1. Major Participating Institutions: Major participants are large institutions, such as Chang Gung Memorial Hospital, Taichung Veterans General Hospital, E-Da Hosipital, Changhua Christian Hospital and China Medical University Hospital. Other participants include security service companies (Taiwan Secom Co., Ltd.), ICT companies (Far Eastone Telecommunications Co., Ltd, Farnet Technologies Co., Ltd, HamaStar Technology Co., Ltd and Chunghwa Wideband Best Network Co., Ltd.), nursing care facilities (Senior welfare service center in Yunlin, Quixotic Implement Foundation), pharmacy chain stores (Maywufa Company Ltd.) and the health examination institution (Gsharp Corporation).

1.2.2.2. Target Client: Chronic disease patients, elderly seniors, people with disabilities at home or institutes, enterprise employees and other people who pay attention to their health.

1.2.2.3. Core Services: Ubiquitous health care services with innovative health care processes delivered through ICT.

1.2.2.4. Apparatus and Equipment Used:

1. Physiological Signal Sensor: Blood sugar meter, weight scales, blood pressure meter, thermometer and ECG machine.
2. Signal Transmission Interface: Sensor to hub–Infrared ray, USB, RS232, Bluetooth, RFID and Wi-Fi. Hub to server: Internet and mobile communications.
3. Computation: ICT platform, CRM, and HIS.

1.2.2.5. Data / information collected: Physiological and other life signals.

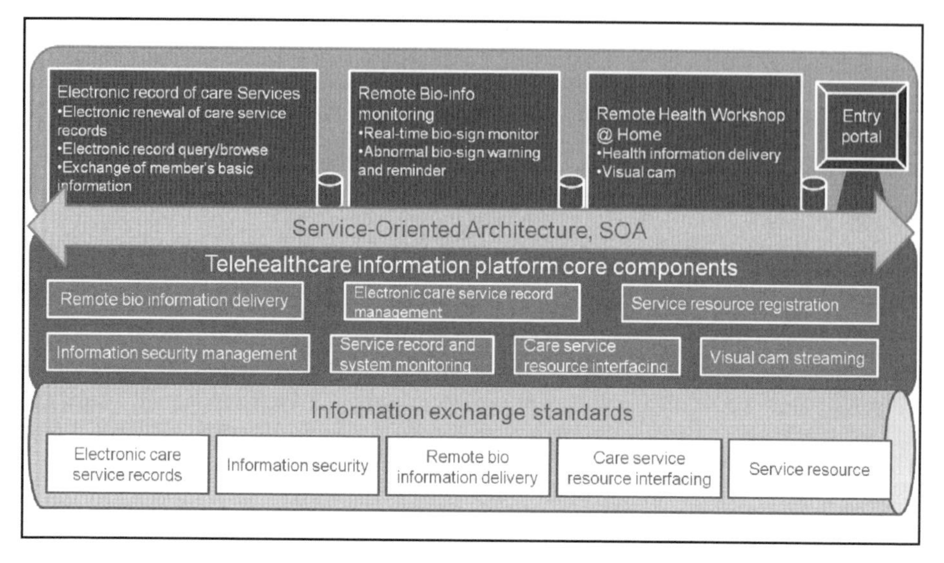

Figure 4. Information platform system infrastructure [8].

2. Technology Insights

2.1. "Telehealthcare Service Development Program," DOH

The telehealthcare information platform is an information infrastructure designed to advance seamless care services. The platform is responsible for integrating the information and service resources of three care models: home, community and institution. With such integration, resources are used wisely, integration complexity and redundance of care service system and external information system are reduced greatly, and operation efficiency of care management and service transport system is also raised significantly. Furthermore, it is also a development platform for innovative care service applications. It builds open remote bio-info transmission mechanisms and progresses the drafting and application of related standards.

2.1.1. Single Sign-on Portol

A single sign-on portal for care information and service resource acquisition is set for members, service providers and general public to acquire authorized care information.

2.1.2. Electronic Care Record Service

An electronic care record form is available for indexing the records function. Service providers can apply for a member's e-care record to fully understand their health condition for better continuous care service.

2.1.3. Care Resource Records Service

A care resource information database has been built to integrate all the service resource information from different service models; a care and living resource sharing environment is also available for all care models to provide media information for the general public.

2.1.4. Information Interfacing Service

The information interfacing channel of the long-term care information web is built to provide an intersection between the information platform and the long-term care system in each of the care models. Discharge preparation information and case assessment information can be acquired through this service for better continuous care service.

2.1.5. Tele-physiological Information Transmission System

An open and remote physiological information capture, transmission and management mechanism has been established. The physical information captured on a client terminal will be sent to the information platform through a gateway and over the internet. The information platform will encrypt the physical information received and send them to the care service system in standardized form for storage, analysis and management.

2.1.6. Remote Health Course and Education Platform

Remote health courses and an education platform are established for members, families and medical staff who need professional health education and want to share care experiences. Besides, integration of digital home technologies can also facilitate remote health courses at home for innovative care model development.

2.1.7. Information Platform Core Operation Service

Safety control mechanism such as identity confirmation, communication safety and privacy protection are established through dimensions such as the management process, physical security and technical safety mechanisms with international standards as public key infrastructure and internet safety standard WS-security. Information exchange safety and personal privacy are thus firmly protected.

2.2. Ministry of Ecnomic Affairs – U-Care Program

Remote biomonitor techniques: Various home or station physiological measurement services, such as blood pressure, blood sugar, body temperature and weight, are provided for patients and community residents. Measurement outcomes are sent to the gateway through RFID, infrared ray, USB, Bluetooth or RS232, and then sent to the health care center (hospital terminal). Through information collection, management, analysis and storage, suitable patient physical information is provided for the development of different innovative health care service models.

Information techniques: The information and communication technologies or ICT platform, integrated information system and related applications have been developed, including an integrated health care and health management service platform, health risk assessment system, patient or community resident self-health assessment system, mutil-function biomonitor service platform, integrated health examination system, health information system and operation benefit assessment system.

Table 2. Effectiveness of telehealthcare service [8]

Care Model	Idicator Subject	2008/1	2008/6	2009/10
Home/Community	Average hospitalization rate	6.11%	2.26%	2.87%
	Emergency revisits rate	4.29%	2.34%	2.39%
	Measure rate of blood sugar/pressure	53.8%	84.4%	86.6%
	Abnormal rate of blood sugar/pressure	–	47.16%	40.04%
Institutional	Density of nosocomial infections	–	12‰	2.36‰
	Rate of revisits	–	11.9%	9.55%
	Rate of repeat treatment	63.6%	20.7%	0.51%

3. Effectiveness Analyses

3.1. Quantitive Performance

3.1.1. Quantitive Performance of Telehealthcare Service

In the home/community telehealthcare model (refer to Table 2), average hospitalization rate has decreased from 6.11% to 2.87% and the revisit rate to the emergency room has also decreased from 4.29% to 2.39% after 22 months of participation in the program. The blood pressure and blood sugar measurement rate has increased from 84.4% to 86.6% and the abnormal rate of blood sugar/pressure has also decreased to the expected 40.04%. In the institutional care model, density of nosocomial infections (decrease 80.3%~87.3%), rate of unexpected revisits (decrease 19.74%), and repeat treatment rate (decrease 97.5%) have improved significantly.

3.2. Qualitative Benefits

Survey results from participants, family and caregivers based on “Telehealthcare Pilot Project” are described by DOH, Executive Yuan [8].

3.2.1. Member/General Public Satisfication and Acceptance Survey

The professional team for the second category “telehealthcare effectiveness indicators establishment and assessment” of “Telehealthcare Pilot Project” has established the cognition and acceptance of telehealthcare service survey with professionals from medical, care and ICT fields. During the time of “Telehealthcare service and quality improvement project”, cognition and acceptance of telehealthcare service survey has been revised based on previous phone survey results and delivered to members at the end of project.

3.2.1.1. Telehealthcare Service Cognition and Acceptance
Consideration of two services provided by telehealthcare project: telephysiological monitoring and tele-consultation, cognition and acceptance of telehealthcare service of general public and participants are compared. In general, participants have actually used the telehealthcare service; therefore their cognition is higher than the general public (telephysiological monitoring: 77.2% vs. 7.4%–12.9%); their attitute is also more

Table 3. Telehealthcare service cognition and acceptance [9,10]

	Telehealthcare Pilot Project: Survey of General Public			Telehealthcare Service & Quality Improvement Project
	20–49 yo, normal	>50 yo, normal	>50 yo, dementia	
N	4035	2005	2009	639
Heard about the service	9.5%	7.4%	12.9%	77.2%
Life is more secure	67.3%	69.5%	61.2%	84.8%
Easier access to care service	71.8%	71.9%	61.6%	84.8%
Secure personal information	34.8%	28.4%	41.2%	79.1%
More interaction with medical staff	62.8%	71.6%	56.1%	79.8%
Need or not	12.6%	4.5%	29.5%	56.3%
Possible futer use	50.0%	57.4%	29.5%	–
Have used before	–	–	–	60.3%

Table 4. Telehealthcare service cognition and acceptance [9,10]

	Telehealthcare Pilot Project: Survey of General Public			Telehealthcare Service & Quality Improvement Project
	20–49 yo, normal	>50 yo, normal	>50 yo, normal	
N	4035	2005	2009	639
Heard about the service	15.6%	23.2%	22.2%	77.4%
Easier access to care service	64.3%	61.4%	52.5%	74.0%
Improve care quality	62.0%	61.0%	52.9%	74.2%
More interaction with medical staff	64.7%	68.8%	53.9%	74.5%
Accept the service or not	40.1%	37.8%	34.8%	–
Awkwardness of lacking real person contact	–	–	–	61.8%
Need or not	6.6%	2.5%	21.8%	55.6%
Possible futer use	44.1%	50.7%	25.3%	–
Have used before	–	–	–	53.3%

positive ragarding the perceived effects on health brought about by use of the telehealthcare service.

3.2.2. Family Satisfication and Care Burden Survey

In general, family members (n = 320) have an 89.2% satsfication (Table 5) toward telehealthcare services, which has exceeded the expected goal of 80%. By examining care models and operation units separately, family members in individual cases under the institutional care service have fewer chances to feel the direct influence brought by telehealthcare service. In the future, more effectiveness information and publicity activities should be released, so that the family can understand the value of the telehealthcare service.

Table 5. Telehealthcare effectiveness in the end of 2009 [9]

Positive response rate	Home/Community			Institution	Total
	WangFung	TMCH	YonhGeng	Hsiao Chung-Cheng	
Telehealthcare Satisfication	95.4%	99.2%	72.3%	62.3%	89.2%
Burden reduced: money	1.2%	75.5%	35.3%	32.0%	41.7%
Burden reduced: time	9.3%	92.6%	41.2%	37.8%	53.3%
Burden reduced: phsychological pressure	31.4%	89.3%	52.9%	42.3%	60.3%

In terms of the change in the burden of care of the family members, telehealthcare exerts not much of an influence on financial side; only 41.7% of the family agrees that telehealthcare can save money on care service. 53.3% of the family agrees that telehealthcare can save time spent on care, and 60.3% of the family agree that telehealthcare service can relieve their psychological pressure arising from caring their family members. However, families under the home care model at WangFang Hospital rarely think they received any benefit in terms of time and money. With further investigation, it was discovered that these families have never done any self-health care management on chronic diseases before; therefore they had not previously neededto spend money on supplies and assistance. After they acquire the telehealthcare service, all the equipment and test strips have become an extra cost for them. This discovery tends to indicate that the time and money spent cannot be the standard baseline for comparison with pre-telehealthcare and simple values cannot be used to judge the effectiveness of telehealthcare services.

3.2.3. Telehealthcare Pilo Project Caregiver Satisfaction and Acceptance Survey

There were 40 service providers participating in this survey in 2008 and 67 in 2009. In general, although the satisfaction rate was only 65% before the project was launched, it raised to 92.5% after the implementation of "Telehealthcare Service and Quality Improvement Project." Future supportive willingness has also increased from 82.5% one and half a year ago to 95.4%. It is clear that the adjustment in service procedure and system equipment has met the purpose of enlisting more caregivers in the provision of telehealthcare service.

Conclusion

After about two years of promotion of telehealthcare services, the satisfaction rate has reached 90% for individual cases, families and service providers, thereby indicating that telehealthcare service has reached some level of high quality. However, the general public still has limited knowledge about telehealthcare services. It is therefore imperative for officials-in-charge and executive experts to devote more resources to promotion, publicity and education, so as to inform the general public of the benefits that telehealthcare service can bring about.

According to the survey, about 50% of the general public and case participants consider themselves in need of telehealthcare service in the future. This number offers an important reference for the assessments of future resource inputs and industry impact. In addition, limited by current regulations, the telehealthcare service is handicapped in its response to individual needs. Cases in point are limitations imposed upon remote diagnosis or remote prescription. The amendments of regulations are therefore needed in order to reach better responsiveness and wider scope for the application of the telehealthcare service. In the future when a telehealthcare service is widespreaded, it can be applied to a wider scope of disease, with the age range of users also expanded beyond 50 years old, particularly in regard to home health care.

The Tw-DRGs implemented in 2010 are likely to lower the hospitalization days; therefore, those are also a possible driving force for telehealthcare dissemination. Incentives-equipped and acceptable cost or payment methods will be the key to telehealthcare service dissemination. With a higher telehealthcare service use rate, the medical and social costs can be lowered. The industry value produced is likely to let the government adjust payment policy (telehealthcare service payment or subsidy), a new telehealthcare service business model (for example, payment accessibility), and the financial system.

Telehealthcare service effectiveness has increased with improved system links within the telehealthcare service due to dissemination and integration. Through the application of such technology as cloud computing, huge amounts of information can be transmitted and computed simultaneously. Health care service is likely to become virtualized/ dynamic/ expandable, with changes to the operation profit model and the establishment of a sound industry network.

References

[1] Bureau of National Health Insurance, National Health Insurance Executive Summary of 2008, Department of Health, Executive Yuan, Taipei, Taiwan, 2010.
[2] Bureau of National Health Insurance, National Health Insurance Executive Summary of 2009, Department of Health, Executive Yuan, Taipei, Taiwan, 2010.
[3] Council for Economic Planning and Development, Population Estimation of Taiwan 2008 to 2056, Executive Yuan, Taipei, Taiwan, 2008/10.
[4] Department of Statistics, Statistics of Population in Taiwan (2010/12), Ministry of the Interior, 2011/1/8.
[5] Economist Intelligence Unit, IT Industry Competitiveness 2008, Economist Intelligence Unit, 2008.
[6] IMD Business School, World Competitiveness Yearbook (WCY) 2007, IMD Business School, Switzerland, 2007.
[7] Industrial Technology Research Institute, Health Care Development in Taiwan by NHI, Industrial Technology Research Institute, Hsinchu, Taiwan, 2009.
[8] Industrial Technology Research Institute, Telehealthcare Pilot Project Annual Executive Report: Section II – Service Development and Implementation, Department of Health, Executive Yuan, Taipei, Taiwan, 2008.
[9] Industrial Technology Research Institute, Telehealthcare Service & Quality Improvement Project Annual Executive Report, Department of Health, Executive Yuan, Taipei, Taiwan, 2009.
[10] National Taiwan University, Telehealthcare Pilot Project Annual Executive Report: Section I – Research & Evaluation, Department of Health, Executive Yuan, Taipei, Taiwan, 2008.

Handbook of Ambient Assisted Living
J.C. Augusto et al. (Eds.)
IOS Press, 2012

doi:10.3233/978-1-60750-837-3-82

Study on Future Trend of the Elderly Care from the Aspect of Assistive Technology Rental System in Japan

Shao-Huai LEE[a] and Jui-Chen HUANG[b,*]
[a]*School of Geriatric Nursing and Care Management, Taipei Medical University, Taiwan R.O.C.*
[b]*Department of Health Business Administration, HUNGKUANG University, Taiwan 43302, R.O.C.*

Abstract. As Taiwan steps into an aging society, it faces problems of shortage of caregivers in aging society and an increased variety of care demands for elders, even those with serious disabilities. Considering Japan has similar cultural background as Taiwan, this study attempted to introduce an assistive technology rental system in Japan, where long-term care insurance and a rental service of assistive technology has been implemented since 2000. The use of assistive technology could reduce the caregivers' burden, and help elders to become more independent and active. As a result, Japan, the first aging country in the world, is able to reduce the waste of medical resources for the end of life.

Keywords. Long-term care insurance, rental system of assistive technology, aging society

Introduction

In response to the rapid aging trend in Taiwan, the Executive Yuan is actively planning the long-term care insurance, which is expected to be implemented in 2012. Among the countries implementing long-term care insurance around the world, such as the Netherlands, Germany, Japan and Korea, Japan shares similar historical and cultural features with Taiwan; hence, Japan is regarded as the main destination for official visits from social welfare departments or health administration departments of Taiwan. Japan has become a super-aging society, with 22.1% aged population (Ministry of Health, Labor and Welfare, Japan, 2008). Under such an aging trend, the Japanese government implemented long-term care insurance in April 2000, and provided emergency medical service for patients' rehabilitation at home. By providing "aging in place" service, the public's needs in terms of medical and health assistance can be satisfied.

The long-term care insurance provided by the government can help to achieve the goal of realizing "aging in place" in care institutions and homes. There are 12 items covered by the insurance: 1) home care service; 2) home bathing service; 3) home nursing service (known as hospital discharge planning service in Taiwan); 4) home

*Corresponding Author: Jui-Chen Huang, Assistant professor, Department of Health Business Administration, HUNGKUANG University, Taiwan. E-mail: juichen@ms17.hinet.net.

rehabilitation service; 5) day rehabilitation; 6) home care management instruction (by doctors and pharmacists); 7) day service; 8) short-term stay service (Respite Care Service); 9) short-term stay care service; 10) care for residents in specific institutions; 11) purchase service of specific assistive technology; 12) assistive technology rental service. The 12th item (assistive technology rental service) aims to help the elders to be independent, thus reducing the burden of caregivers.

In Taiwan, care services are human-oriented, and caregivers are the center of the care services, including doctors, nurses, long-term caregivers, and guardians, who utilize their professional skills to provide "high-quality" care. However, because of the variety and complicated types of disability, as well as the demand for better care quality, the human-based service is becoming overloaded. In Japan, there are many substitute instruments that can help the disabled to be independent and reduce the loading of long-term care. This paper attempts to introduce the assistive technology rental system of Japan.

1. Support of Assistive Technology Rental System for Independent Living of the Disabled

The physical conditions and strength of the elderly, disabled and ill patients are changeable over unpredictable periods, thus, the functions of assistive technology should be flexible. Moreover, assistive technology is improving constantly, thus, the assistive technology should be changed periodically, making the rental system more advantageous and economical. In early times, the rental of assistive technology was limited and not pervasive, and simply borrowing or transfer could not fully satisfy users' demands. As a result, the technology was only sometimes effectively used, and even was sometimes unused. In 2000, when the Japanese government implemented the long-term care insurance system, and developed the national assistive technology rental system, assistive technology began to have a larger market and developed rapidly.

The ownership of the assistive technology was guaranteed by the insurance companies with the competent authority (Japanese government), and the suppliers do not have to undertake the risk of loss when providing the services. Therefore, companies are more willing to provide rental services. In Taiwan, there is no such service available, and it is difficult for users to guarantee the devices.

In order to promote an assistive technology rental service, the Japanese government pays for 90% of the rental fee, whereas users only pay for 10%, making the service charge affordable. Since 90% of the fee is paid by the government, it is simple and convenient for service providers to collect the fees. In cases where the remaining 10% is not collected, the impact on the service providers is minimal. At present, Taiwan is unable to provide such service, and the charges are collected individually, thus bringing high costs and risks to the service providers. The coverage on assistive technology in long-term care insurance is limited, and is allocated based on the evaluation of the physical and mental conditions of the users. Moreover, with lack of designated organizations and related measures, the development of the rental system is limited. If such system could be open to the free market, the restrictions would be reduced.

2. Current Supply of Assistive Technology in Japan

At present, the disability care is in the charge of care managers of the long-term care insurance, who evaluate the cases' disability level and qualification, and then design specific care plans. In the care plan, if assistive technology is needed, assistive technology coordinators, occupational therapists (OT) and physical therapists (PT) with professional backgrounds in assistive technology will select suitable assistive technology from stores or manufacturers, and sign the rental agreement with the suppliers. For those who qualify for the long-term insurance program and reside in Japan, the National Health Insurance Association subsidizes 90% of the rental fee to the suppliers. The Japanese government also regulates that the service suppliers should appoint two coordinators on assistive technology in each service location.

The legal business scope of "assistive technology rental offices and assistive technology stores", as regulated by the Long-term Care Insurance Act, includes:

- Rental of assistive technology.
- Sales of specific assistive technology.
- Rental of long-term care and prevention assistive technology.
- Sales of specific long-term care and prevention assistive technology.

3. Professional Qualification of Assistive Technology Assessment – Assistive Technology Coordinators

The qualification has been established by the Ministry of Health, Labor and Welfare, and implemented within the long-term care insurance program since 2000, with 11 years of history to date. The purpose of certification is to select experts who can recommend assistive technology that are suitable for the elderly needs, and choose caregivers who can meet the expectations of the elderly and their families. As users' physical conditions may change, service providers are required to make home visits regularly in order to provide appropriate assistance. According to the regulations of the Long-term Care Insurance Act in Japan, "assistive technology rental offices and assistive technology stores" must appoint two assistive technology coordinators in order to ensure proper and safe service.

In order to be qualified as assistive technology coordinators, candidates must attend training course and internship, totaling 6 days and 40 hours. The training institutes are required to have sufficient display space for assistive technology, so that the students could recognize and subsequently operate assistive technology. The course contents are shown in Table 1.

Table 1.

Subjects	Time
Knowledge related to the elderly health and welfare	2 hours
Knowledge related to long-term care and assistive technology	20 hours
Basic knowledge of long-term care industries	10 hours
Practical courses related to assistive technology	8 hours
Total	40 hours

Long-term Care Insurance Act No. 2, Rule 22–33. (No. 269 announcement on March 31, 2006)

Certification course content (subjects):

1) Social Welfare Theory.
2) Social Protection Theory.
3) Public Support Theory.
4) Regional Welfare Theory.
5) Psychology.
6) Sociology.
7) Law.
8) Basic Medicine.
9) The Elderly Welfare Theory.
10) The Disabled Welfare Theory.
11) Children Welfare Theory.
12) Social Welfare Support Technique.
13) Introduction of Long-Term Care.

According to the regulations of the Long-term Care Insurance Act, the same qualification as "assistive technology coordinators" refers to below:

- Completion of level 1 and 2 courses of Home Helper.
- Completion of basic course of long-term care staff.
- Public health nursing personnel.
- Nurse specialists and nurses.
- PT.
- OT.
- Social workers.
- Long-term care welfare workers.
- Artificial limb technicians.

According to the regulations of the Long-term Care Insurance Act, duties and authority of assistive technology coordinators are below:

- Assistive technology coordinators in service providers under the long-term care insurance program.
- Home visits and suggestions for usage of assistive technology.
- Explanation on the specifications and information of assistive technology.
- Regular examination of assistive technology used by cases.
- Assistive technology adjustment according to cases' situations.
- Instruction of use.
- Repair of assistive technology.

In addition, in order to manage and improve the competences of assistive technology coordinators, the National Assistive Technology Coordinators Association is founded which establishes 10 guidelines of ethics, in order to:

1) Comply with related regulations.
2) Make evaluation based on an equality principle.

Table 2.

Courses and qualification	Subjects	Studying time	Examination	Ranking	Remarks
Assistive Technology Planner	Tech-aid Association	100 hours (including e-learning course)	Yes	None	Subjects of courses are assistive technology coordinators.
Assistive technology selector	Assistive Technology Supply Association of Japan	40 hours	Yes	None	Subjects of courses are the workers in the association
Welfare living Environment Coordinator	Tokyo Business and Industrial Association	According to ranking	Yes	1–3	Candidates should be qualified in level 2 in order to take the exams of level 1. Anyone can take exams of level 2 and 3.
Assistive technology suppliers conferences	Silver Service Promotion Association	45 hours	No	None	Subjects of courses are the workers in the association

* National Association of Assistive technology coordinators, 2011

3) Meet obligations for the confidentiality of cases.
4) Be responsible for providing detailed explanation.
5) Be prohibited to receive illegal returns and benefits.
6) Use the cases' information well.
7) Cooperate with people of other occupations.
8) Increase the prevalence of assistive technology.
9) Continue to improve their professionalism.
10) Contribute to the society.

The association has its own proposal layout for developing an "individual support plan". In addition, the form helps care managers to access and share the information about cases, and increases the efficiency of providing assistive technology.

Moreover, in order to enhance their skills, assistive technology coordinators can participate in training offered by local governments and private institutes, and take certification exams for improved professional competence. The channels of courses and certificates are shown in Table 2.

4. Targets and Kinds of Assistive Technology Use

The rental items of assistive technology sponsored by the long-term care insurance system and the related disability levels to which they apply are shown below:

4.1. Scope of Assistive Technology Rental (Specific Items Covered by the Long-Term Care Insurance in Japan)

Items	Support 1, 2~Disability 1	Disability 2–5	Description of Structure and Functions
Wheelchair		○	Self-pushed wheelchair, normal power wheelchair and standard care wheelchair
Accessories of wheelchair		○	Wheelchair seat cushion, power support device and various accessories of wheelchair
Care bed		○	One of conditions below: 1. Care bed with flexible angles of the back and end of the bed 2. Care bed with flexible heights
Accessories of care bed		○	Accessories such as railings and mattress
Bedsore prevention device		○	One of the conditions below: 1. Air bed with inflator or air pressure adjustment device 2. Body water bed for pressure reduction by water
Body turning and removable assistive technology		○	Air beds which change the body positions, not including the supportive air beds
Armrest	○	○	DIY; not manufacturing
Sloping plate rail for elevating and descending of wheelchair	○	○	DIY; not manufacturing
Walker	○	○	One of conditions below 1. Walker with wheel and handrail 2. Four supports for stable body moving
Walking stick	○	○	Underarm stick, four-feet stick for one hand and upper arm, four-feet stick for one hand and lower arm, stick for elbow joint disability
Wandering sensor for the elderly with dementia		○	Outdoor sensor system for the elderly with dementia according to Item 15, Article 7 of Long-term Care Insurance Act
Body hoist (not hoisting devices)		○	Assistive removable hoist include demountable, fixed and partially removable ones which can help the patients with difficulty to move

Moreover, because of concern for personal health, deformation after long-term use and various psychological effects, the government does not recycle rented assistive technology. For "specific assistive technology" the government provides the devices to people in need by grants (100,000 Yen every year). The users purchase the devices first and apply for grants with invoice from local governments and district offices. The government will pay 90% of insurance.

4.2. Scope of Selling Assistive Technology (Items Paid for and Covered by the Long-Term Care Insurance)

Items	Description of Structure and Functions
Sitting toilet seat	One of conditions below: 1. Removable toilet seat on squat toilet 2. Elevated toilet seat on Sitting toilet 3. Electric elevated assistive toilet seat 4. Removable toilet, urinal and all kinds of portable bedpan (indoor)
Special urinating technology	Urine collector and portable urinal. Convenient devices for caregivers.
Bathing assistive technology	Maintenance of sitting position and assistive technology in and out of bathtub. One of the conditions below: 1. Bathing chair 2. Falling prevention armrest beside bathtub 3. Falling prevention armrest in bathtub 4. Assistive bathing platform (on the top of bathtub) 5. Assistive footrest in bathroom 6. Assistive footrest in bathtub
Simple equipped bathtub	Air, folded, removable objects which are not manufacturing
Body hoist (hoisting devices)	Hoisting devices which fit the users and can be combined with body hoist

4.3. Disinfection and Recycling of Rental Assistive Technology

The long-term care insurance in Japan does not specify disinfection of rented assistive technology. thus, users do not know the cleanness of technology. The Silver Service Association then established the standards for the cleaning and disinfection of assistive technology. The association was founded in 1987 by businesses in the care service industries, and followed consensus ethical guidelines. In July 1989, the "Silver Mark" certification was established, and five home services, namely 1) home care service; 2) home bathing service; 3) purchased service of specific assistive technology; 4) assistive technology rental service; and 5) home food delivery service, were included in the "Silver Mark". Specific guidelines were established for on-site and factory visits, and conforming companies were granted with the "Silver Mark" for consumers' identification.

5. Concept of Assistive Technology in Taiwan

In Taiwan, the public, even professional workers, regard assistive technology as medical articles. In May 1999, the Ministry of Economic Affairs, Ministry of Health, Labor and Welfare (Department of Health and Ministry of the Interior) and Department of Labor Affairs of Japan collectively established the Assistive Technology Act, and promoted the concept of assistive technology. Private groups and research institutes were authorized to found the Assistive Technology Day Promotion Association in Japan, and Assistive Technology Day was set on October 1 every year. Thus, the society would recognize the importance of assistive technology for the disabled elderly and physically and mentally disabled. The definition of assistive technology in Article 2 of the Assistive Technology Act in Japan states that "assistive technology is the devices and supplementary tools to train the functions of the elderly with declining physical and mental states and difficulties in daily living, as well as the convenient devices for physically and mentally disabled". The function and positioning of assistive technology are to "support independent living and reduce work load of long-term care". Therefore, they are the important devices for caregivers and the disabled. Moreover, assistive technology can meet the residual functions of the elderly, the disabled and other patients, and they can reduce the work load of daily living. The caregivers and relatives in Taiwan are mostly healthy people. However, because of difference of age and background, they have different competences in caregiving. In addition, the job of caring is similar to 3K (dirtiness, danger and hard work), and is not considered to be a professional skill. The service quality is thus low and the caregivers have low intentions to work. As a result, physical strength and time is wasted during caregiving, thus affecting caregivers' physical, mental states, and life. The high turnover rate of personnel requires caregivers to learn to adapt to new patients constantly. Assistive technology can make up for the gap in caregiving. In Taiwan, care is based on "manpower" that is useful and flexible. The advantages and disadvantages of manpower are explained below.

Advantages of manpower care:

- Personal competence and empathy.
- Flexible functions and all-purpose.

Disadvantages of manpower care:

- Limited strength, easily overloaded.
- Unable to work continuously, need time to rest and sleep.
- Long-term care functions must be learned. Patients and long-term caregivers need time to adapt to each other.
- Long-term caregivers have their own life, and cannot provide around the clock services.
- Humans have emotional and physical changes, and thus are not constantly stable and reliable.
- Interaction between people requires tolerance, otherwise, argument may occur.
- Manpower care is not economical and the cost is high.
- Interaction may be difficult to control.

Even healthy people rely on tools, such as using shovels for digging, and using vehicles for transportation, in order to save time and strength. Long-term care service also needs assistive technology to make the care process easier, and prevent possible occupational injury.

6. Influence of Foreign Caregivers in Taiwan

Twenty years ago, Taiwan started importing foreign caregivers from Southeast Asia for elderly care. Currently, there are at least 160,000 foreign caregivers for patients with serious clinical conditions in Taiwan. These caregivers are from different countries with different backgrounds, and most of them grew up in villages without professional training in nursing. If assistive technology can replace 10–20% foreign caregivers in Taiwan, the effect will be significant.

Factors to be considered when using assistive technology:

- Physical conditions, figures, and personal perceptions of users.
- Adaptation and enhancement of affected physical function.
- Physical state and independent function.
- Types and levels of disability and responses to changes.
- Remedy for the residual functions.
- Effective use of the residual functions.
- Remedy for the substitute functions.
- Universal Design: it can be used for different types of disabled situations and it can be turned into common tool for use by most of slightly disabled or healthy people.
- Negative effect and risk.

7. Analysis of Supply and Demand Market of Assistive Technology in Taiwan

- National pension provision in Taiwan is low, with a relatively short history (it began in 2005) and is not popular.
- Long-term care insurance system is not implemented.
- There is no subsidy for assistive technology rental. Procurement of assistive technology is based on the product life, instead of users' physical and mental changes and functions needed.
- Users' disability is judged by doctors, PT and OT, without concern for the elders' needs for assistive technology, no care managers are appointed.
- Lack of explanation for the possible functions of assistive technology.
- Traditional assistive technology supply in Taiwan is under the classification of medical instruments and is restricted.
- The assistive technology industry alliance in Taiwan consists of many companies, but they operate individually, and form the market by holding long-term exhibitions. They are not as unified as department stores and they compete with each other.
- Customers must separately deal with selection, trial, cleaning and repair after rental. Although it is called a platform, it lacks the function and drive: limited numbers of assistive technology coordinators.
- Guarantee of assistive technology is based on deposit of the same amount, thus increasing users' burden.
- The charge and cost are high, and only high-price assistive technologies are rented.

- Concept of frequent cleaning and maintenance of assistive technologies: logistics systems in Taiwan are not popular and they necessarily apply to all medical equipment, including disposable articles.
- Manpower care is the mainstream and assistive technologies are not valued: manpower service for long-term care is only a rental system.
- Significant influences of techniques and financial factors: most people can accept them; and they lacks reorganization and explanation. It is difficult to transfer second-hand assistive devices. In fact, second-hand assistive devices highlight the problem of suitability for other users. As users have different physical and mental states, function disabilities, and residual abilities, random transfer might lead to the problem of suitability. Users cannot select and try the (second hand) devices in the same way as when purchasing new ones. Currently, in Taiwan, the second-hand devices are from private transfers, and the models and sizes are different, thus cannot meet the customers' needs. Therefore, the public has negative impressions of second-hand assistive technology.

8. Conclusions

In conclusion, assistive technology rental system in Japan is led by the government which provides at least 90% subsidy; hence, service providers and the public can use assistive technology comfortably. Regarding after-service of assistive technology, the third party institution is in charge of testing, disinfection, and cleaning. In Taiwan, there are many conferences related to assistive technology, health medicine exhibitions and the elderly exhibitions. The assistive technology companies in Taiwan may be involved in the following situations:

- Many assistive technology companies overly emphasize the advantages of their products; however, they do not indicate the disadvantages and remarks, and users might be misled.
- Taiwan does not implement long-term insurance system as in Japan, thus, when renting assistive technology, the users need to pay a higher rental fee for temporary use. The total rental fee for one year is equal to the amount for purchasing the devices.
- When renting assistive technology, in order to avoid the risk of loss or fraud, users must pay a deposit, usually in the form of check in Taiwan. Although it is not cash payment, the expenditure and risk may be considerable when the users move or die, and there is the need for litigation.
- If the amount of monthly rent is low, delivery cost and personnel cost will be relatively high. Unless these costs are paid by users, rental companies may encounter a loss.
- In the current assistive technology supply market in Taiwan, there are a few items for rent, including vehicles for long-distance use, wheelchairs, oxygen generators, and special mattresses.
- The policy of assistive technology rental is restricted by the government, and the opinions of experts, which tend to neglect users' difficulties.

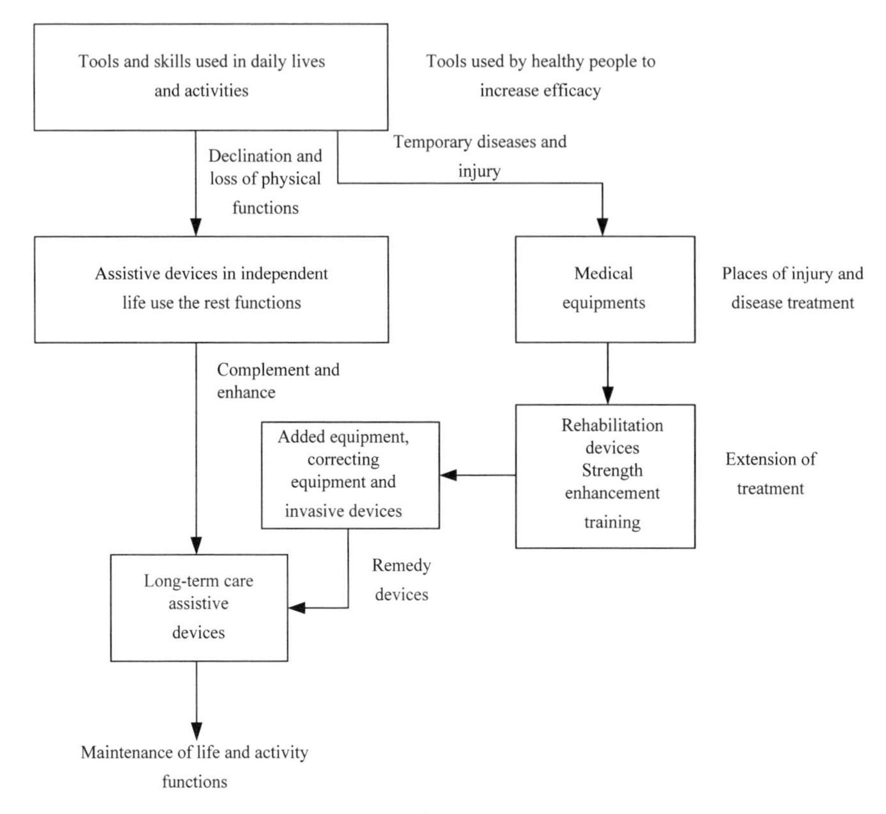

Figure 1.

9. Suggestions

Assistive technology in Taiwan is still treated as medical instruments. The division between medical instruments and assistive technologies is illustrated in Fig. 1.

Based on the above, assistive technologies are useful tools that can help users to become more independent in living, and reduce the work load of caregivers. Medical demands should be assessed by medical personnel for the guarantee. In Taiwan, many concepts and terms are defined ambiguously, thus, the public and even professionals are still uncertain about assistive technologies.

Analysis of the future market for assistive technology.

In Taiwan, there is no specific survey and estimation of the market for assistive technology. Using the patients with serious clinical conditions who employ foreign caregivers as an example, the basic function of assistive technology is to "support independent living and reduce work load in long-term care". In using assistive technology, 10–30% functions of long-term care can be replaced. If 10% of users in Taiwan used assistive technology to replace foreign caregivers, the cost for hiring 170,000 foreign caregivers, 60 billion NTD/year (30,000 NTD/month (including placement fee, monthly health insurance charge, food, lodging, salary, overtime salary, employment fund from government, bonus, etc.) × 170,000 × 12 months) could be saved. It could be estimated that the demand for assistive technology in Taiwan will be above tens of billions NTD.

According to the governmental policy in Taiwan, long-term insurance is expected to be implemented in 2012, with the aim to reduce the work load of long-term care. By reviewing the long-term insurance policy in Japan, the government and service providers could refer to related experiences. The companies can then provide appropriate services that benefit the users. The government can then implement supervision and assessment measures to select qualified service providers for the users.

References

[1] Conference of current situation and prospect of long-term care assistive technology, Welfare Organization for the Elderly, Taiwan, R.O.C., 2010.06.24.
[2] Conference of development trend of potential assistive technologies and key techniques, Industrial Development Bureau, Ministry of Economic Affairs, 2009.11.05.
[3] Conference of directions of assistive technology service in long-term care insurance plan, Welfare Organization for the Elderly, Taiwan, R.O.C., 2009.09.11.
[4] Conference of international standard of care equipments, Department of Industrial Technology, Ministry of Economic Affairs, 2009.05.01.
[5] Conference of key techniques of assistive technology design, Industrial Development Bureau, Ministry of Economic Affairs, 2009.05.04.
[6] Conference of law making of assistive technology act, Welfare Organization for the Elderly, Taiwan, R.O.C., 2010.05.18.
[7] Conference of marketing strategy and design application of medical equipments, Industrial Development Bureau, Ministry of Economic Affairs, 2010.06.25.
[8] Conference of medical care development and trend of assistive vehicle innovative operating model, 2009.05.02.
[9] Conference of planning of barrier-free environment and assistive technology use, Welfare Organization for the Elderly, Taiwan, R.O.C., 2009.05.04.
[10] Conference of promotion plans of care equipment rental service 2, Welfare Organization for the Elderly, Taiwan, R.O.C., 2008.11.21.
[11] Development and issue of assistive technology rental business under long-term care insurance system in Japan, France Bed Medical Service, Chief of business department, Terada.
[12] Information of Taipei international invention and technical trading exhibition, 2009.09.
[13] S.C. Liang, Assistive technology service in long-term care insurance system of Japan, Friend of Assistive Technology, 25.
[14] New regulation of assistive technology subsidy, multi-functional assistive technology resource center of Ministry of the Interior, 2008.11.
[15] Selection principle of the elderly assistive technology, Welfare Organization for the Elderly, Taiwan, R.O.C., 2010.06.25.
[16] Study on the elderly industry in Taiwan and long-term care development from successful experience of international assistive technology exhibition in Japan, Welfare Organization for the Elderly, Taiwan, R.O.C., 2008.05.01.
[17] Technology plan of Department of Health, Executive Yuan – classification database of medical equipments.

Handbook of Ambient Assisted Living
J.C. Augusto et al. (Eds.)
IOS Press, 2012

doi:10.3233/978-1-60750-837-3-94

In-Home Monitoring Technologies: Perspectives and Priorities of Older Adults

Katherine WILD* and Linda BOISE
Layton Aging and Alzheimer's Disease Center, Oregon Health and Science University, OR, USA

Abstract. A burgeoning area of investigation in the wake of advances in in-home technology has been the application of those new technologies to enhance the health and independence of older adults without the constraints and expenses of the traditional health care system. Increasingly, researchers are using home monitoring and assistive technologies to identify changes in health and behavior in home settings, and to facilitate successful adaptation to those changes. The successful application of assistive and monitoring technologies depends on receptivity of potential users, i.e. the older adults, family members, health care providers and others. In this chapter, we will review the current state of research in older adults' perceptions, attitudes, and priorities regarding in-home technology designed for health monitoring and/or maintenance of independence. Further, we will summarize current thoughts regarding ethical issues in the application of these technologies to older adults as end users.

Keywords. Older adults, attitudes, focus groups, ethical issues

Introduction

Advances in health and communications technology come at a time of dramatic worldwide increases in life expectancy and skyrocketing health care costs [21,28]. A burgeoning area of investigation has thus been the use of new technologies to enhance the health and independence of older adults without the constraints and expenses of the traditional health care system. Increasingly, researchers are using home monitoring and assistive technologies to identify changes in health and behavior in home settings, and to facilitate successful adaptation to those changes. Research in this area has ranged from single-home demonstration projects [1,11] to deployment of monitoring technology in multiple community-based homes [18,27]. Technological monitoring and intervention studies have included measurement of single health parameters [22,40] and ubiquitous in-home sensor systems [26,41]. The latter, also known as "smart home" technologies, have been reviewed in use with healthy older adults [20] and Alzheimer's disease patients [10].

With the aging of the population, the total number of seniors living alone has risen, with approximately one of every three noninstitutionalized older adults now living alone [8]. Despite the challenges of increased frailty and morbidity, most older adults desire to remain at home and the majority do live at home [25]. However for older adults to remain at home safely, methods to detect cognitive and physical decline that put them at risk must be in place. Many existing and potential technologies under de-

*Corresponding Author: Katherine Wild. E-mail: wildk@ohsu.edu.

velopment for the maintenance and/or supervision of health and independence offer promise. These range from blood pressure monitors and falls detection to "lifestyle monitoring" that detects changes in behavior patterns [7,25].

Ultimately, the successful application of assistive and monitoring technologies depends on receptivity of potential users, i.e. the older adults, family members, health care providers, and others. In recognition of the importance of user receptivity, a second wave of research has focused on the investigation of the attitudes and perceptions of older adults and their families as potential recipients of in-home monitoring technology. In recent years, much has been learned from older adults about how they might respond to such systems. In focus groups, interviews [3,18,20,23,34,35,42,45], and questionnaire-based research [13,16], older adults have generally expressed willingness to adopt new in-home technologies. Repeatedly, the notion of older adults as "technophobes" has been refuted across various populations and assistive devices.

In this chapter, we will review the current state of research in older adults' perceptions, attitudes, and priorities regarding in-home technology designed for health monitoring and/or maintenance of independence. Research in this area includes references to assistive technology [33], smart homes [19], and home-based monitoring, among others. While there is significant overlap, the terms are not interchangeable. Assistive devices generally refer to those that enable a person to perform a task that they would be otherwise unable to do, or enhance the ease with which it is performed [33]. Smart homes, as defined by Demiris et al. in their early work [19] are "residences equipped with technology that enhances safety of patients at home and monitors their health conditions" (p. 88). Home-based, or in-home technologies may refer to assistive devices, ubiquitous monitoring systems, or some combination thereof. In this review the terminology used will reflect that of the respective authors. Following the trajectory of this work over the past decade, we will first consider the more qualitative findings of focus groups, followed by survey methodologies including interviews and questionnaires. Summaries of our own research will illustrate the advantages and limitations of each methodology. Finally, we will offer an overview of the ethical issues regarding the use of technology with older adults.

1. Synopsis of Methodologies

Qualitative data collection methods such as focus groups are an effective approach for gaining in-depth insights and are especially valuable when there has been limited prior research in an area. In focus group methodology, small numbers of participants are convened to consider a particular issue in a relatively open-ended format [44], typically following a discussion guide under the direction of a moderator. Thus focus groups are a particularly efficient means for exploring attitudes and gaining understanding of issues from the point of view of the research participant. The format of focus groups may yield more comprehensive data than individual interviews through the interactions of participants [38]. They tend to reveal similarities and differences in attitudes through directed discussions among target populations, and quickly identify themes for further consideration by more quantitative methods. It is fitting, therefore, that much of the initial work in investigating older adults' attitudes about technology has been based in focus group methodology.

Nevertheless, qualitative approaches have been criticized for their lack of scientific rigor both in design and data analysis. Focus groups, by virtue of their sample size and selection processes, may be subject to biases that skew findings. For example, participants in focus groups about technology may be inherently more interested and more likely to be "early adopters" than a typical cross section of older adults. Investigator biases may lead to misinterpretation or misplaced emphases in the process of content analysis and identification of themes and concerns. Additionally, most analyses fail to distinguish among participants' comments, risking overrepresentation by more vocal participants [37]. However, with rigorous design and systematic analysis, these limitations can be minimized without losing the richness of data generated by a qualitative approach.

While focus group research has served to define the broader scope of older adults' attitudes and perceptions, survey methodology can provide the opportunity for a more detailed analysis of preferences and barriers toward use of in-home technologies. Further, the larger sample sizes in these more quantitative studies allow comparisons across of subgroups of users, whether based on age, gender, cognitive status, or other personal traits. As will become apparent, even among older adults there is no "average user" of technology [39], and possible differences in attitudes may be more readily identified by means of survey research. The risk of this methodology, particularly in the early phases of research, is that potentially important variables may be excluded from consideration in the process of instrument development.

Semi-structured interview studies have yielded a body of data in an intermediate position between the qualitative nature of focus group findings and more readily quantified responses to structured questionnaires. These studies have generally involved face-to-face interviews based on a questionnaire format, with opportunity for open-ended discussion of key points (e.g. [33]). Reported findings generally consist of a combination of content analysis for recurrent themes, and statistical analyses of quantifiable data.

2. Focus Group Studies

2.1. Prospective Users

With in-home monitoring technology is in its infancy, much of the early research on user attitudes was by necessity based on potential scenarios for future applications. Qualitative studies have tended to present participants with systems and devices with which they had no prior familiarity or experience, and sought their opinions in the context of "what if." In one of the earlier efforts, older adults were shown a range of devices in a demonstration home, and asked to comment about the specific devices as well as the concept of the smart home in general [34]. While the authors caution that their results should be interpreted in the framework of the participants' imagined use of the technologies, they found that most positive comments related to maintaining independence, while most negative statements concerned the potential intrusiveness of the devices. Surprisingly, while privacy issues were raised, security concerns were minimal. In a series of focus groups with residents of a continuing care facility, Demiris et al. [19] found that positive attitudes toward in-home sensors were based on perceived needs that overrode privacy concerns under defined circumstances. Maintaining quality of life and independence were priorities; to this end detection of falls and other emergency situations, and monitoring of physiological parameters were cited as potentially useful technologies.

More recent work has echoed these earlier findings, that is, that older adults are willing to accept in-home technology under certain conditions that remain fairly consistent across studies. The relationship between relinquishing privacy and meeting perceived needs has been a recurring theme. While privacy concerns are repeatedly raised, these concerns rarely outweighed a pragmatic willingness to trade privacy for potential benefits [15,20,35,42,43]. The importance for older adults of clearly defined personal benefits with assurances of affordability, reliability, and control by user has been well documented [23]. However, not all aspects of assistive and monitoring technology are equally accepted. Uniformly, video monitoring has been poorly received despite otherwise high levels of acceptance of in-home sensors [20,23,32,35,42]; worn devices were also generally negatively rated [19]. Based on their focus group work, Steele et al. [42] identified themes that seem to determine acceptance of in-home sensor technology among older adults. Independence and quality of life were the most commonly cited benefits, while prominent among concerns associated with sensors were cost and specific user and design preferences. Among these latter, embedded sensors were preferable to wearable sensors; ease of use and unobtrusiveness also affect acceptance.

The utility of proposed technologies has been the basis upon which assessments are made and attitudes formed. Perceived need, however, is a subjective and personal metric; while many older adults express positive attitudes about technology for some hypothetical "other," an acknowledgement of one's own need may represent a sign of frailty or disability [15]. Thus the use of technology is more readily understood and accepted as an intervention in emergency situations such as falls or other safety issues. Early detection of physical or cognitive decline is less frequently described as a current need; in most cases participants acknowledge the possibility of a future need for such an application, or they identify acquaintances that might benefit. Older adults who have not been personally exposed to in-home monitoring technology tend to resist considerations of their own needs in the present [45]. Thus investigation of the attitudes of older adults who have actual experience with various technologies offers an important perspective on which to base future research.

2.2. Current Users

Much of the research with actual users of in-home technology has been quantitative and is reviewed below. However, in one study community dwelling older adults participated in focus group discussions concerning their likes and dislikes regarding a range of technologies in current use [36]. In assessing everyday technologies from cell phones and televisions to blood glucose monitors, positive statements outpaced negative statements. Convenience, support for activities, and specific features such as design elements dominated the "likes" statements, while expense, effort, and features such as complexity and unreliability were cited as problems of technology. The authors conclude that older adults' attitudes are determined by multiple factors related to both the ease of use as well as the perceived benefit or utility of a device, which should be applied to future technology applications.

2.3. Our Study

2.3.1. Aims

In an effort to obtain preliminary feedback on the merits and drawbacks of in-home monitoring technology at the earliest stages of implementation, we conducted a series of focus groups with older adults prior to their having any direct experience with the intended applications. The intent of our study was to obtain feedback from older adults on home monitoring independent of specific applications or products. In focusing on unobtrusive monitoring, we were describing sensor systems and technologies that provide the capacity to continuously track and interpret motor and cognitive activity in the home. The goal of this project was to explore themes and to assess positive and negative responses to unobtrusive in-home monitoring from the perspectives of both the elderly and their family members, as potential users. For the present purposes only the responses of the older adults will be summarized.

2.3.2. Methods

Subjects were men and women who were at least 65 years of age, in stable health and showing no signs of dementia. Twenty-three older adults agreed to participate; the average age was 80.6 years (range = 66–91). In each of three separate focus groups, participants viewed a series of slides describing various aspects of monitoring in the home. For example, technologies promoting personal health and wellness were displayed with links between monitors in the home and potential recipients of the information, to demonstrate the general configuration of an in-home system. Other slides that were presented as examples of potential technology applications displayed methods of tracking motion through the household, monitoring of computer-based activities such as e-mail and game playing, and data derived from sleep sensors placed in beds. The slides were meant to generate discussion of these and other possible uses of in-home monitoring.

The following questions guided this section of the discussion: (a) How, if at all, would you use monitoring systems such as those presented? (b) What kinds of activity would you like to have monitored (e.g., behavioral, physiological)? All questions were open- ended to allow for greater depth of response. Participants were encouraged to offer positive and negative reactions to monitoring. Finally, the format of outgoing monitoring information and potential recipients of the information was explored. Figure 1 presents one of the slides that was shown to stimulate discussion. In this graph, summaries of activities that could be monitored are displayed in various formats. For example, the "walking activity" graph compares the distances walked by two hypothetical residents over time. Each quadrant was explained to participants and questions were answered before proceeding to discussion of the content. Again, reactions to and opinions on each slide were solicited by facilitators from participants and centered on the following discussion questions: (a) Do the data show information that is meaningful to you? (b) How, if at all, would you like to have such data about yourself disseminated and to whom (e.g., family members, physician, others)?

2.3.3. Results

Content analysis of the interview transcripts identified a number of recurring themes. These themes centered on how participants viewed their own current and projected needs and the needs of other older adults. An overarching theme in much of the discussion was the desire for older people to remain in their own homes. As focus group participants discussed this desire, safety was the chief concern; of particular interest was monitoring that would identify and respond to immediate needs, such as falls. Although there was an overriding interest in the potential for monitoring to enable older adults to stay in their home longer, some participants discussed the concern that there comes a

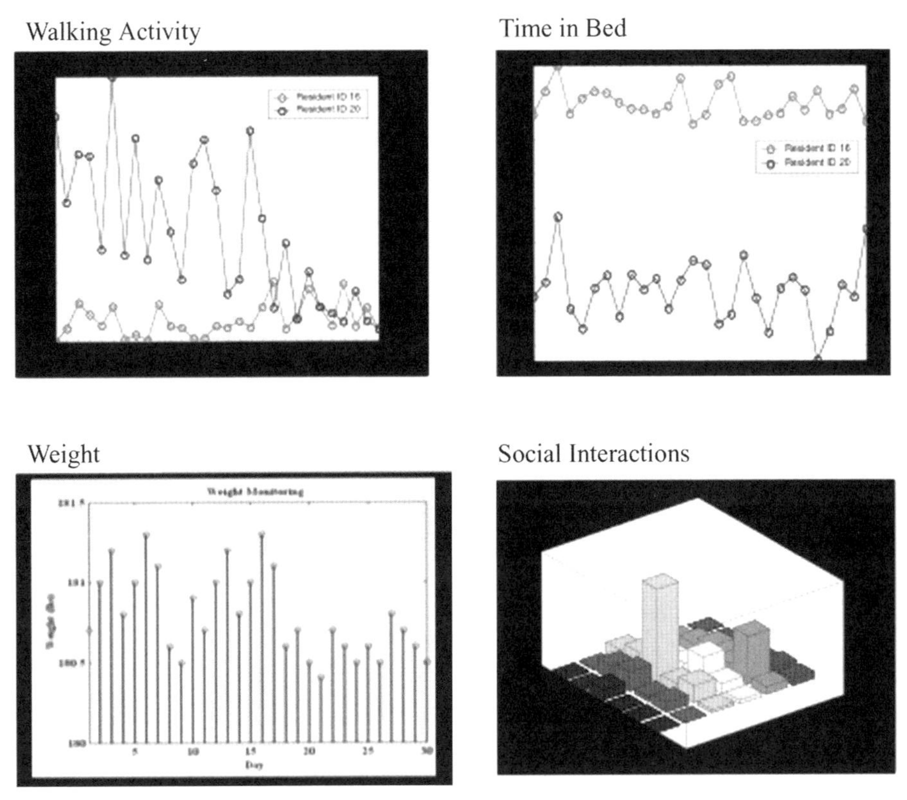

Figure 1. Focus group slide displaying different activity summaries.

time when remaining in the home is not the best option. Thus, although independence was an important theme in all groups, it was specifically acknowledged by some participants that people sometimes remain in a home setting longer than is appropriate. They felt that monitoring could enable family members to gain a more accurate understanding of problems that the elder was experiencing in his or her day-to-day activities. "I've seen lots of families where parents were in their home too long," commented one family member.

Many participants discussed the value of monitoring to detect gradual decline over time that might be otherwise difficult to detect. Often, this was mentioned in the context of cognitive decline. The participants were especially attentive to the potential benefits of monitoring for addressing issues of dementia. A number described personal experience with dementia in relatives or friends and were aware of the kinds of situations where monitoring would be beneficial. Dementia, however, also raised special concerns with respect to setting up and implementing a home monitoring system. Several participants expressed concerns related to the cognitively impaired person's acceptance of monitoring, as succinctly noted by one older woman: "Most people who really need it don't want it and wouldn't accept it." It was difficult for many of the participants to see themselves as persons with deteriorating cognitive function and the consequent need for monitoring of their activities. Although they could discuss persons they had known who had developed Alzheimer's disease, when asked about the possibility of such monitoring for themselves, their responses were frequently negative.

Older adults in this study were unanimous in their expressed desire to maintain control of data collected from any monitoring system. Within this parameter, however, there was considerable variability in the specifics of acceptable data sharing. In general, there was recognition of how useful monitoring data could be for family members, especially for those living at a distance. Nevertheless, while some participants assumed that family members should have access to all information to be kept apprised of their health status, others were reluctant to "worry" or "burden" their children. Although most participants thought their health care providers could receive regular updates based on the monitoring information, there was a widely held perception that medical professionals had little time to devote to perusal and analysis of such data. Nonetheless, some participants suggested that monitoring by others was more important than self-monitoring or monitoring within the household. The following comment was from an older participant: "Well, really, if you're going to do this (monitoring), except for sharing it with yourself, that's what it's for, isn't it really? People that love you and are responsible for you want to know how you're doing and so it just makes sense that if you're going to do this, that's who it would be for." Although focus group participants were aware of the potential for misuse of the data, most of the discussion suggested that privacy was not a major concern as long as there were proper controls in place. In general, privacy was a secondary issue if the monitoring was deemed useful with respect to safety, maintaining independence, and health.

2.3.4. Limitations

The participants in this study represented people with more computer experience than a random sample of the current U.S. population of elders would show. Therefore, caution in generalizing to the elderly population at large is warranted. One of the reasons for this recruiting strategy was to minimize the need for long, explicit, and possibly biased explanations – participants already had some idea of what computers are capable of and also were presumably more aware of the potential limitations and privacy issues than people with little or no experience. In addition, it is anticipated that computer users are likely to be early adopters of in-home assistive technology. This is a rapidly changing environment. Elders who may currently be considered early adopters will likely in the near future represent a more mainstream cohort; in an exploration of advanced applications of in-home technology, therefore, this seemed a reasonable approach. Finally, there was an explicit attempt to begin the focus group sessions with non- specific examples to elicit the key topics and themes from the participants, rather than introduce specific topics or devices. Although this may have produced some initial confusion among participants with regard to the possibilities of in-home monitoring, the tradeoff in not spending inordinate time on the pro's and con's of particular products was deemed worthwhile.

3. Survey Studies

3.1. Prospective Users

The American Association of Retired Persons (AARP) surveyed awareness of and attitudes toward home safety and personal health and wellness devices in over 900 older adults [2]. Despite a limited awareness of new technologies, respondents expressed willingness to use devices in the pursuit of safety and prolonged independence in their homes. Nevertheless, over 80% of this sample reported cost as a barrier to use, while over half (59%) were concerned with the potential stigma associated with use of assistive devices such as fall detectors, activity monitors and alarms. Demographic variables including age, gender, and income influenced respondents' willingness to employ specific technologies; for example women were more likely than men to consider use of electronic safety monitoring devices.

Mann and colleagues [31] interviewed 71 older adults regarding their hypothetical acceptance of a series of health care monitoring devices. Ratings of usefulness of devices ranged from 93% for a medication compliance monitor, to less than 2% for a thermometer that automatically sends information to a designated other. Eighty-eight percent of the respondents felt that the family of devices would relieve worry for family members. Tellingly, when given the opportunity to elaborate, comments by participants suggested that positive views of the devices were based on their usefulness for some other person, leading the authors to suggest that the questionnaire responses may not reflect actual willingness to deploy the devices in their own homes. In a similar design, 147 participants in four age groups (<50, 51–65, 66–75, >75) were asked to respond to representative assistive technologies based on their perceived usefulness, likelihood of personal acceptance, potential risks in using the device, and preferred recipients of monitoring data [32]. The researchers found no differences by gender or age, with generally universal acceptance of all devices with the exception of a videophone system; an emergency call system and continuous health monitoring were rated most positively. In terms of data dissemination, physicians received the highest rating, followed by relatives, professional caregivers, and participants themselves. Main concerns about technology related to intrusiveness and possible abuse of data by third parties. Significantly, fears of data security breaches were more common among the younger respondents, suggesting that older adults may be more technologically naïve and would benefit from additional education prior to actual acceptance of devices in their homes.

One hundred healthy older adults, in responding to a questionnaire evaluating preferences for electronic memory aids, voiced similar attitudes [13]. Concerns and potential barriers to use of various devices were related to fear of making mistakes/being too complicated. Attributes related to appearance were more variable, with some older adults preferring smaller, more portable and less obtrusive devices, while others wanted larger devices due to problems with vision and manual dexterity, and fear of losing a possibly expensive apparatus. The authors conclude that their findings demonstrate the importance of a flexible and individualized approach to technology design, given the variability of needs and concerns voiced by their participants.

3.2. Current Users

Demiris et al. [18] describe older adults' responses to living with sensor technology designed to detect changes in daily activity patterns in a retirement facility. Nine residents were interviewed regularly over a span of six months. Based on these interviews, the researchers identified three phases following the installation of smart home technology. First, users experience a process of familiarization, wherein the technology is assessed and initial feedback given. A period of adjustment follows, in which the technology becomes less novel but is still a target of curiosity and attention. Finally, in the phase of integration, the technology has become a seamless part of daily living. The authors suggest that to successfully achieve full integration, older adults as end users of technology must be included in all phases of design and implementation.

As the body of research in this area matures, investigations have begun to focus on the particulars of both the devices and potential users as determinants of acceptability of in-home technology. Among the former, key traits relating to "usability" have been identified fairly consistently. Appearance, efficiency, and ease of use were highly rated traits in a large sample of older adults and their family carers as part of the Assisting Carers using Telematics Interventions to meet Older persons' Needs (ACTION) project [3]. In rating that program's user interface, respondents were able to have early input to the final design in a process the authors described as essential to ultimate acceptance of any in-home assistive technology.

A series of in-depth interviews with community residing older adults revealed generally positive responses to basic assistive technology devices such as smoke detectors, alarms, and entry phones [33]. Based on their findings, the authors propose a model of assistive technology in which the interaction between perceived need and attributes of the technology determines ultimate acceptance. As have others, the authors note the possible discrepancy between one's subjective sense of need and the evaluations of significant others such as adult children or health care providers. Prominent among the attributes expected of the technology were reliability and ease of use.

User characteristics have been shown to play an equally important role in affecting older adults' interactions with assistive technology. Employing a series of questionnaires about attitudes toward computers and use of technology in a large cohort spanning the ages of 18–91, Czaja et al. [16] were able to identify demographic variables related to use of currently available technologies. They report that education, age, ethnicity, and cognitive ability predicted general use of technologies such as cellular phones and automatic teller machines. Additionally, self-rated computer anxiety and computer efficacy were strongly associated with technology use. Gender differences were found such that older women had more anxiety and lower self-efficacy with regard to computers, and used fewer types of technology than older men. While these results may represent particular generational attitudes towards devices that are relatively new in their experience, the relentlessly increasing complexity of everyday technology is a consideration for all cohorts as they age. As this study demonstrated, the interaction among demographic and psychological factors plays an important role in determining acceptance and use of a broad range of technologies.

In a recent review, studies of technology and older adults were evaluated in terms of the technology acceptance model (TAM) [12]. In this model, perceived usefulness and perceived ease of use are the primary factors determining actual usage. A database search yielded 19 studies that applied the TAM to empirical studies of technology use by older adults. They found that in general, perceived usefulness was related to the technology's capacity to improve quality of life and independence. Unlike younger users, older adults voiced less interest in newer, high tech products for their own sake. Relatedly, perceived ease of use was a critical factor in acceptance; older adults, while aware of the potential benefits of technology, do not assume that they can overcome the barriers of device complexity and their own anxiety in order to attain those benefits. Thus, perhaps more for older adults than the general population, personal characteristics were found to be important variables external to the technology itself. Demographic, social, and psychological factors, and life events all interact with user interfaces to determine ultimate use and success with technology. Changes in vision, sensation, auditory perception, mobility, and cognition dictate certain preferences and hindrances to older adults' willingness to employ in-home technology. Finally, the effects of the well-documented lack of self-efficacy and increased anxiety, combined with the social isolation of aging whereby support is less available, are additional hurdles to overcome. The authors of this review call for additional studies with actual use data, and for assessment of changes in acceptance over time.

3.3. Our Study

3.3.1. Aims

In order to gain better understanding of the attitudes and perspectives of older adults towards home monitoring while having systems operating in their homes, we developed and administered a survey as part of the Intelligent Systems for Assessment of Aging Changes Study (ISAAC) carried out by the Oregon Center for Aging and Technology [25]. ISAAC is an NIH-funded study that utilizes continuously active, unobtrusive technologies to detect change in functions that lead to loss of independence, specifically cognitive impairment and problems with mobility.

3.3.2. Methods

The survey, the ISAAC Technology Survey (ITS), was developed and refined largely from data previously gathered in focus groups [45]. It assessed research volunteers' attitudes toward the unobtrusive home and computer monitoring used in the study, and their willingness to have information obtained from monitoring shared with family members and health providers. It was administered to 153 community-residing ISAAC research participants.

3.3.3. Results

Figure 2 displays ratings of the importance of monitoring nine health activities and behaviors. Physiologic monitoring was rated as very important by the highest percent of respondents, followed by risk of falls and medication management. There were no group differences based on age (<85 vs. >85) or race. We found that men were significantly more concerned than women regarding possible misuse of home monitoring data, and were more likely to feel that information "could be given to people or organizations that have no right" (81% vs. 59%, $p = 0.02$) and that information "could be given to people or organizations that would use it in a harmful way" (81% vs. 62%, $p = 0.04$) [5].

We then analyzed data from baseline and Year 1 surveys and report on changes in attitudes following one year of experience with in-home monitoring. In addition, we investigated differences in attitudes according to age, gender, cognitive status, and ethnicity. One hundred twenty-one participants have completed the baseline and Year 1 surveys to date. Table 1 reports participants' perspectives on having information from in-home activity or computer monitoring shared with others and their perspectives on the risks of monitoring. The reported percentages represent the proportion of participants who "strongly agreed" or "agreed" with the statements. As shown, a strong majority agreed at both time points with the statement, "I do not mind being monitored unobtrusively in my home." Also, participants at baseline were overwhelmingly willing to have their activity monitoring information shared with their doctor (92%), spouse (90%) and family members (83%); there were no significant changes over time in participants' willingness to share this information. Despite the general receptiveness to being monitored, a number of participants expressed concerns about privacy and about the risks of monitoring/computer use. At baseline, about two-thirds reported being con-

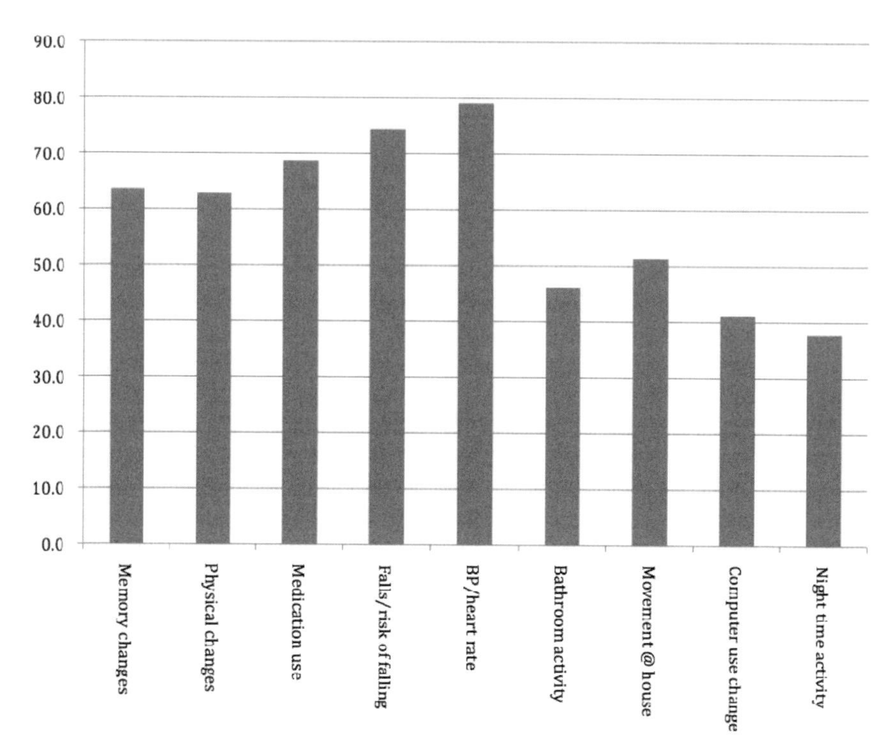

Figure 2. Percentage of participants responding that monitoring was "very important" in each of nine health indicators or behaviors.

Table 1. Attitudes regarding privacy concerns and sharing of monitoring information

	Baseline	Year 1	p-value
I am concerned my info could be given to people that don't have a right to it[a]	59%	84%	<0.0001
I am concerned my info could be given to people that would use it to harm me	61%	89%	<0.0001
I am willing to have information from activity monitoring shared with…[b]			
…my doctor	92%	88%	NS
…my spouse	90%	81%	NS
…other family members	83%	75%	NS

[a] Proportion reporting "Concerned/Very Concerned"
[b] Proportion reporting Agree/Strongly Agree

cerned that their information could be exploited, i.e., that it could be "given to people that don't have a right to it" or that it could be "given to people who would use it to harm you." The proportion of participants who reported these concerns increased significantly at Year 1, to 84% and 89% for those items.

Group differences in change in attitudes after a year of monitoring, based on age, gender, and cognitive status, were analyzed. At baseline, male participants were significantly more likely than female participants to be concerned that their information could be given to people who may use it to harm them. At Year 1, this gender difference had disappeared with high proportions of both men and women reporting concerns about the potential harms of monitoring. Nearly all participants with mild cognitive impairment (MCI) (96%) reported willingness at baseline to have activity monitoring shared with family members, significantly more than participants with normal cognition. At Year 1, this difference was no longer evidenced, as participants with MCI resembled those with intact cognition at this time point. Similarly, the proportion of participants with MCI who reported that they didn't care who had access to information from in-home or computer monitoring was significantly higher at baseline than participants with normal cognition (30% vs. 11%) but declined at Year 1 to the same proportion for both groups (10% vs. 11%). Interestingly, a significantly higher proportion of persons with mild cognitive impairment than those with normal cognition reported at both time points that they would not mind being videotaped to monitor their movement around the house. The difference between these two groups increased significantly at Year 1 due to a decline in willingness to be videotaped for participants with intact cognition.

3.3.4. Conclusions

Overall, the results from this technology survey suggest that the older adult participants in this study tended to set boundaries around what was acceptable with regard to monitoring. These participants in a home monitoring study were highly receptive to the sharing of the data for research purposes, and they were generally receptive to the idea of sharing information with others. The matter of sharing of information with family members and doctors is an important matter not only for technology studies but also for programs serving older adults. In our earlier focus group research, we found less willingness to share information with family members than with doctors. This was less apparent in the survey reported here; comparable proportions of study participants were willing to have information shared with a spouse or other family members as they were with their doctor. One possible explanation is that the experience of the participants in being monitored over time increased their general comfort with monitoring and with sharing information with people they know, such as family members. Nonetheless, even these "early adopters" expressed a high level of concern about perceived risks of sending information over the Internet, especially after a year's participation in this study. As research and development moves ever closer to these real-world settings, research is certainly needed to better understand how older adults, the primary beneficiaries of these technologies, view home monitoring and its risks. Over the next several years, we will be interested to see how continued participation in ISAAC and other technology studies influences attitudes toward monitoring and concerns about potential risks, as well as perceived benefits.

4. Ethical Considerations

In-home technologies in the older adult population have been increasingly applied to both research and practice settings. The interdisciplinary nature of these efforts calls for particular attention to ethical considerations that may or may not overlap across the fields of engineering, geriatrics, and social sciences. Further, the inclusion of potentially technology-naïve users warrants careful review of all projects and devices to ensure that benefits outweigh risks and discomforts. To this end, many have called for the application of ethical guidelines to all interactions between older adults and technology research and development [4,9,17,24,29,30]. The areas of concern generally fall into four domains: 1) informed consent, 2) equal access, 3) privacy, and 4) user-centered design.

4.1. Informed Consent

The findings from our study of changes in attitudes following exposure to in-home ubiquitous monitoring revealed an increase in privacy concerns over the course of one year. We wondered, based on these data, whether the increase in concerns was driven by greater familiarity with the potential risks of data transmission via the Internet following personal experience. The inclusion of relatively inexperienced older adults in technology research requires, then, that the process of informed consent ensures adequate understanding of the implications of one's participation. Over a decade ago, Bauer [4] noted that truly informed consent must include an explanation of the unique benefits and burdens of technology to allow for autonomy in decision-making by research subjects or patients. Drawing from gerontology practices where decision-making capacity is routinely assessed in seeking consent for research, the field of gerontechnology needs to adopt a similar stance in order to secure informed consent. Cantor [9] coined the phrase "no information about me without me" to highlight the importance of empowering older adults to make their own decisions regarding consent to monitoring technologies. Barriers to acceptance such as obtrusiveness, invasion of privacy, potential breaches in confidentiality, and inconveniences of malfunction should be realistically evaluated. As our data show that attitudes may change with time, consent needs to be viewed as an ongoing process. Demiris [17] and others [9] have described continuing assent as a requisite component of technology research, whereby the possibility of altered preferences based on additional experience and information is routinely assessed. Applications outside the research setting need to build in the same protections by providing control of important aspects of devices or systems in the hands of the user, thus obtaining continuing consent implicitly.

As in-home technology frequently relies on the participation or cooperation of family members, paid caregivers, or health professionals, the issue of informed consent has been expanded to include these significant others. The debate over whose consent must be obtained is not trivial; co-habitants in a single home, remote family members, and residents in care facilities may all be affected, and may all have different attitudes about the benefits and drawbacks of in-home technology. When an older adult participant is frail, or of questionable decisional capacity, whose consent takes priority? In separately held focus groups, we found that older adults and their family members frequently expressed incompatible preferences for monitoring technologies [45]. Preserving older adults' autonomy while securing their safety requires careful consideration of informed consent processes.

4.2. Equal Access

Issues of access to technology have implications for research as well as long-term implementation of assistive devices. In research, subtle influences on both participants and recruiters may direct selection of study subjects. Demiris [17] cautions against widening the "digital divide" through iniquitous study recruitment. The additional education and outreach necessary to ensure equal access to research by all segments of society should not be seen as an obstacle in these studies. Discrepancies in access to technology have been documented based on income, geographical location, age and education [45]; responsibly conducted research should make every effort to reduce rather than magnify these imbalances. Magnusson and Hanson describe factors influencing participation in the ACTION trial [29]. They found that potential subjects were drawn to their project as a means of using technology to which they would otherwise not have access, and viewed their inclusion in the study as a privilege. In many such projects, the opportunity to temporarily own a computer or assistive medical device may overwhelm any reservations about participating in research. It is the investigator's obligation to make certain that the technology itself does not become the focus, but remains a tool in service of some larger goal.

In research as well as in practice, the economic considerations of access to technology and its benefits present additional ethical obligations. In research, the withdrawal of monitoring systems or assistive devices at conclusion of a protocol can leave participants in difficult circumstances. A newly developed reliance on remote monitoring or in-home reminders and adaptive tools may leave older adults unprepared for their absence, and might cause additional anxiety or disability. In practice, the affordability of technology in the home may present a significant barrier to long-term implementation; one of the most frequently voiced concerns of elders is the cost of in-home technology [42,45]. While in the long run home-based interventions may be financially viable, on an individual basis the additional financial burden may pose an insurmountable obstacle to some segments of the older adult population. In his review of issues related to the use of monitoring technologies in the elderly, Kang [24] calls for large-scale studies to evaluate cost-effectiveness of these interventions.

4.3. Privacy

Bauer [4] draws a distinction between physical and informational privacy. In the former, assistive technology may enhance some aspects of physical privacy while disrupting others. The introduction of certain devices or monitoring systems may reduce the older adult's reliance on health care providers or caregivers and minimize physical presence of others in the home. At the same time, Bauer warns against the potential for medicalizing the homes of older adults, and in so doing "dissolving the thin membrane that separates our public and private lives" [4]. An additional threat to physical privacy is the seemingly inevitable introduction of additional personnel responsible for interacting with the technology and ensuring its seamless performance.

Informational privacy is of particular relevance in the older adult population, where the hazards of data transmission may be less appreciated. In contemporary cohorts of older adults, lack of technical expertise or experience can lead to misunderstandings about the nature of risks to privacy. Concerns about video monitoring [24] and even video communication [29] by older adults indicate that there are boundaries to acceptance of in-home assistance; the implications of these findings for more subtle forms of information sharing are less clear. While many have demonstrated that older adults tend to be willing to sacrifice privacy for independence [14,42,45], our experience with changes in attitudes following exposure to in-home monitoring suggests that lack of adequate understanding may be contributing to the relative indifference to issues of privacy. Given the realities of ubiquitous flow of data over the Internet, breaches to that privacy may be inevitable and must be adequately explained to potential research participants and users of technology.

Confidentiality in the context of in-home technology applications describes the ability to control the sharing of data about oneself. Older adults have consistently articulated their desire to be able to determine with whom they share information [14]. These preferences vary, with some participants expressing reluctance to include family members while others have no such concerns. Health care providers are generally viewed as within the realm of acceptable recipients of monitoring data; however the practicality or utility of such data sharing is not universally evident to older adults, whose attitudes may best be summed by one focus group participant's comment: "Ask my doctor if he'll use it. If he felt like he needed it to monitor me, I would be receptive to it" [45]. While older adults have expressed idiosyncratic and at times divergent opinions regarding who has access to their information, they are resolutely uniform in their insistence on personal control of this access. Cantor [9] and others have underscored the importance of reviewing confidentiality issues in both research and more general use settings prior to installation of technology.

4.4. User-Centered Design

The multidisciplinary nature of developing in-home technology for older adults provides ample opportunity for translating research findings from one area of expertise to another. Certainly, the needs and concerns of older adults require an approach to design and implementation that appreciates the issues of aging.

Bouma [6] uses the term "inclusive design" to describe the goal in development of products and services, that all members of the target population attain the expected benefits. In order to achieve this goal he calls for a methodology that includes direct participation by representatives of the intended user group. Only by identifying and respecting the needs of end users can the field move toward successful and wide-based deployment of in-home technologies [17,30]. The combined effects of frailty, sensory limitations, and lack of experience with technology call for an integrated approach among engineers, gerontologists, and end-users. Mahoney et al. [30] expand the concept of usability to include a family-centered approach that recognizes the involvement of important others in the older adult's care. As in-home technology begins to augment care of frail elders, the daily burden on family members may be reduced. However, it is the responsibility of providers of technology to ensure an understanding of its capabilities and limits by all involved parties. By participating in discussions in all phases of design, older adults can be better prepared for the realities of technology use in the home, and avoid the dangers of over-reliance or under-utilization of ostensibly useful devices.

Conclusions

Researchers in the field of attitudes and perceptions towards in-home monitoring technology by end users, specifically older adults, have uniformly described the importance of including them in all phases of design and implementation. It has been well established that, while a digital divide still exists between younger and older technology users, the idea of older adults as technophobes no longer appears to hold true. We have shown that there is general agreement in findings across studies, regardless of methodological approaches and technology applications, that older adults have clear preferences in terms of usability, control, privacy, and confidentiality. These preferences cannot be assumed to be invariant, as attitudes have been shown to differ both within groups and within individuals depending on changing circumstances and needs. Finally, we review some of the ethical issues that are beginning to be addressed in this field. Although the expectations and attitudes of older adult cohorts may evolve as lifelong exposure to technology becomes the norm, it remains the obligation of researchers and technology developers to solicit and incorporate their input as well as to ensure autonomy, equitable access, and appropriate constraints on data use and sharing.

Going forward, the continued investigation of older adults' attitudes toward in-home technology can build on existing evidence while making important new contributions. There is a paucity of studies with large samples of participants who have direct experience with the technologies of interest. While hypothetical assessments are useful in the early stages of in-home technology research, the field has progressed to where those perceptions and stated attitudes need to be tested against actual interactions with systems and devices. Although it has been established that older adults are not averse to in-home monitoring or assistance under certain circumstances and for certain purposes, there are clearly many differences in how this would translate into acceptance on an individual basis. The potential disconnect between acceptance in the abstract and willingness to use in-home technology in reality has not been adequately examined.

The engagement of other involved participants is also a crucial issue for future research. Family members, health care providers and paid caregivers will have particular points of view regarding both the utilization of in-home technology as well as the preferred avenues for transmission of collected data. Remote family members may find value in receiving continuous data describing social activity of their loved one; paid caregivers might find use in reports of changes in self-care ability; and primary care providers might seek input regarding blood pressure or other physiological parameters. The consent and cooperation of the end user of technology may vary with each intended application. Additionally, the frequency of data transmission and the format in which data are communicated are not trivial matters. As noted above, the control of technology and dissemination of information present ethical challenges for researchers and clinicians alike.

As these technologies become more readily available, the cost of implementation will be an important consideration. Expense was a prominent concern among the older adult population in the studies described above, and can be expected to be a critical variable in their acceptance and utilization of any system or device. Funding options for broad based deployment, whether in research or clinical applications, must be investigated. A key factor for potential funding sources will likely be related to the cost effectiveness of any system. Thus it is essential that there is collaboration among geriatricians, engineers, and policy makers in pursuing the goal of successful and widespread implementation of technology in the service of maintaining health and independence of older adults.

References

[1] M. Alwan, Passive in-home health and wellness monitoring: Overview, value and examples, in: *Proceeding of the Annual International Conference of the IEEE EMBS*, 2009, pp. 4307–4310.

[2] American Association of Retired Persons, Healthy @ Home, Washington, D.C., 2008.

[3] N. Andersson, E. Hanson and L. Magnusson, Views of family carers and older people of information technology, *British Journal of Nursing* **11** (2002), 827–831.

[4] K.A. Bauer, Home-based telemedicine: A survey of ethical issues, *Cambridge Quarterly of Healthcare Ethics* **10** (2001), 137–146.

[5] L. Boise et al., How older adults respond to home-based monitoring: Results of a survey from the Oregon Bio-Medical Research Partnership Study (Abstract), *Annual Meeting of the Gerontological Society of America* (2009).
[6] H. Bouma, Professional ethics in gerontechnology: A pragmatic approach, *Gerontechnology* **9** (2010), 429–431.
[7] S.J. Brownsell et al., Do community alarm users want telecare? *Journal of Telemedicine and Telecare* **6** (2000), 199–204.
[8] C. Cannuscio, J. Block and I. Kawachi, Social capital and successful aging: The role of senior housing, *Annals of Internal Medicine* **139** (2003), 395–399.
[9] M.D. Cantor, No information about me without me: Technology, privacy, and home monitoring, *Generations Summer* (2006), 49–53.
[10] M.C. Carillo, E. Dishman and T. Plowman, Everyday technologies for Alzheimer's disease care: Research findings, directions and challenges, *Alzheimer's and Dementia* **5** (2009), 479–488.
[11] M. Chan et al., Smart homes – Current features and future perspectives, *Maturitas* **64** (2009), 90–97.
[12] K. Chen and A.H. Chan, A review of technology acceptance by older adults, *Gerontechnology* **10** (2011), 1–12.
[13] J. Cohen-Mansfield et al., Electronic memory aids for community-dwelling elderly persons: Attitudes, preferences, and potential utilization, *Journal of Applied Gerontology* **24** (2003), 3–20.
[14] K.L. Courtney, Privacy and senior willingness to adopt smart home information technology in residential care facilities, *Methods of Informatics in Medicine* **47** (2008), 76–81.
[15] K.L. Courtney et al., Needing smart home technologies: The perspectives of older adults in continuing care retirement communities, *Informatics in Primary Care* **16** (2008), 195–201.
[16] S.J. Czaja et al., Factors predicting the use of technology: Findings from the Center for Research and Education on Aging and Technology Enhancement (CREATE), *Psychology and Aging* **21** (2006), 333–352.
[17] G. Demiris, Independence and shared decision making: The role of smart home technology in empowering older adults, in: *Proceeding of the Annual International Conference of the IEEE EMBS*, 2009, pp. 6432–6435.
[18] G. Demiris et al., Findings from a participatory evaluation of a smart home application for older adults, *Technology and Health Care* **16** (2008), 111–118.
[19] G. Demiris et al., Older adults' attitudes towards and perceptions of "smart home" technologies: A pilot study, *Medical Informatics* **29** (2004), 87–94.
[20] G. Demiris et al., Senior residents' perceived need of and preferences for "smart home" sensor technologies, *International Journal of Technology Assessment in Health Care* **24** (2008), 120–124.
[21] A. Dorsten et al., Ethical perspectives on emerging assistive technologies: Insights from focus groups with stakeholders in long-term care facilities, *Journal of Empirical Research and Human Research Ethics* **4** (2009), 25–36.
[22] T. Hayes et al., A study of medication-taking and unobtrusive, intelligent reminding, *Telemedicine Journal and e-Health* **15** (2009), 770–776.
[23] A. Hein et al., Monitoring systems for the support of home care, *Informatics for Health and Social Care* **35** (2010), 157–176.
[24] H.G. Kang et al., In situ monitoring of health in older adults: Technologies and issues, *Journal of the American Geriatrics Society* **58** (2010), 1579–1586.
[25] J. Kaye et al., Home-based activity changes associated with MCI, in: *Annual American Academy of Neurology Conference*, 2010.
[26] J.A. Kaye et al., Deploying wide-scale in-home assessment technology, in: *Technology and Aging: Selected Papers from the 2007 International Conference on Technology and Aging*, 2008, pp. 19–26.
[27] J.A. Kaye et al., Intelligent systems for assessing aging changes: Home-based, unobtrusive and continuous assesment of aging, *Journal of Gerontology: Psychological Sciences*, in press.
[28] E. Kimbuende et al., *U.S. Health Care Costs*, 2010.
[29] L. Magnusson and E.J. Hanson, Ethical issues arising from a research, technology and development project to support frail older people and their family carers at home, *Health and Social Care in the Community* **11** (2003), 431–439.
[30] D. Mahoney et al., In-home monitoring of persons with dementia: Ethical guidelines for technology research and development, *Alzheimer's and Dementia* **3** (2007), 217–226.
[31] W.C. Mann et al., Elder acceptance of health monitoring devices in the home, *Care Management Journals* **3** (2002), 91–98.
[32] M. Marschollek et al., People's perceptions and expectations of assistive health-enabling technologies: An empirical study in Germany, *Assistive Technology* **21** (2009), 86–93.
[33] C. McCreadie and A. Tinker, The acceptability of assistive technology to older people, *Ageing and Society* **25** (2005), 91–110.

[34] A. Melenhorst et al., Potential intrusiveness of aware home technology: Perceptions of older adults, in: *Proceedings of HFES Annual Meeting*, 2004.
[35] A. Mihailidis et al., The acceptability of home monitoring technology among community-dwelling older adults and baby boomers, *Assistive Technology* **20** (2008), 1–12.
[36] R.L. Mitzner et al., Older adults talk technology: Technology usage and attitudes, *Computers in Human Behavior* **26** (2010), 1710–1721.
[37] F. Moretti et al., A standardized approach to qualitative content analysis of focus gorup discussions from different countries, *Patient Education and Counseling* **82** (2011), 420–428.
[38] D. Morrison-Beedy, D. Cote-Arsenault and N. Feinstein, Maximizing results with focus groups: Moderator and analysis issues, *Applied Nursing Research* **14** (2001), 48–53.
[39] V. Rialle et al., What do family caregivers of Alzheimer's disease patients desire in smart home technologies? *Methods in Informatics Medicine* **47** (2008), 63–69.
[40] R.P. Ricci, L. Morichelli and M. Santini, Remote control of implanted devices through home monitoring technology improves detection and clinical management of atrial fibrillation, *Europace* **1** (2009), 54–61.
[41] A. Sixsmith and J. Sixsmith, Smart care technologies: Meeting whose needs? *Journal of Telemedicine and Telecare* **6**(Suppl. 1) (2000), 190–192.
[42] R. Steele et al., Elderly persons' perception and acceptance of using wireless sensor networks to assist healthcare, *International Journal of Medical Informatics* **78** (2009), 788–801.
[43] A. Tinker and P. Lansley, Introducing assistive technology into the existing homes of older people: Feasibility, acceptability, costs and outcomes, *Journal of Telemedicine and Telecare* **11** (2005), 1–3.
[44] V. Wibeck, M. Dahlgren and G. Oberg, Learning in focus groups: An analytical dimension for enhancing focus group research, *Qualitative Research* **7** (2007), 249–267.
[45] K.V. Wild et al., Unobtrusive in-home monitoring of cognitive and physical health: Reactions and perceptions of older adults, *Journal of Applied Gerontology* **27** (2008), 181–200.

Devices and Infrastructure to Facilitate Ambient Assisted Living

Handbook of Ambient Assisted Living
J.C. Augusto et al. (Eds.)
IOS Press, 2012

doi:10.3233/978-1-60750-837-3-115

Devices and Infrastructure to Facilitate AAL

Paul MCCULLAGH*
School of Computing and Mathematics, University of Ulster, UK

Abstract. This section explores technology used to identify an individual in their environment, promote their safety and wellness at home and beyond and support rehabilitation. All three aspects need to be addressed if AAL is to flourish.

Keywords. Biometrics, face recognition, gait monitoring, behaviour pattern, bio-signals, wellness, safety, rehabilitation

Introduction

This section of the Handbook is about technological advances and their applications to support Ambient Assisted Living (AAL) for healthcare, well-being and rehabilitation. A major focus is on identifying an individual in an AAL environment. This provides technical and computational challenges beyond normal identification scenarios, in which the individual is actively involved in the process, for example fingerprint access to an information system. Ideally such identification should be unobtrusive. For example, in a smart home assisted living application, we may wish to identify an individual in need of assistance, in a multi-person environment, whilst of course leaving other occupants unaided. This of course requires the introduction of Ambient Intelligence into the process [1]. The typical user is likely to be older or possibly more vulnerable than the general population demographics and this represents another major challenge for engagement.

Modi provides an overview of the possibilities for biometric identification, including prevalent fingerprint and iris identification. The chapter states: "Biometric technologies open up unprecedented opportunities in ambient assisted living (AAL) applications, but they also raise some unanswered questions". Future challenges and direction of use of biometric technologies in AAL applications are discussed.

Candidate identification strategies are presented in this section (face recognition, upper body behaviour, and electrocardiogram identification), with underlying research providing the evidence base. Video monitoring hardware and image processing and segmentation algorithms are key enabling technologies for the first two case studies.

Franco et al. address face recognition. Indeed as a human's primary means of person identification, it is an obvious choice, so long as the hardware and software can combine to undertake what is a complex task. The chapter cites: "The extreme variability of faces in such applications, due to continuous changes in terms of pose, illumination and subject appearance, requires very robust and fast algorithms to be developed".

---

*Corresponding Author: Dr. P.J. McCullagh. E mail: pj.mccullagh@ulster.ac.uk.

A semi-supervised video-based template approach is presented. This can account for day-to-day changes in appearance with continuously updates to the templates on the basis of new inputs.

Drosou and Tzovaras monitor a person's behaviour in the environment. Can this provide us with a biometric? Exploiting the behavioural variations between different users performs identification. The upper body limb anthropometric information is extracted for each user and an attributed body-related graph structure framework is employed for the detection of discriminative biometric features. The authors state: "Biometric monitoring can enhance the performance of the Smart Home technology, offering intelligent control over home… the user will be authenticated by the way he/she moves into the room. The system will then be able to understand who the person entering the room is, and apply his/her preferences, e.g. favourite music, TV channel, lighting scene, etc."

Less obvious biometrics are biosignals, usually electrical potentials, which can be measured using, attached electrodes, but sometimes by capacitive contact, e.g. during exercise on a treadmill in the gymnasium. Does the electrocardiogram (ECG) provide a characteristic as unique as a fingerprint? Nowadays this can be measured unobtrusively as we undertake other activities, and it is a fertile area of investigation for 'smart garments' [2]. Agrafioti et al. investigate its potential in AAL. The authors state: "ECG falls under the umbrella of medical biometrics i.e., physiological signals that are typically used for disease diagnosis, but also carry subject discriminative information. As opposed to traditional static biometric modalities like the iris, the fingerprint or the face, ECG is a time dependent signal affected both by physical and emotional activity". This provides additional technical challenge, for feature detection. The authors argue that ECG by itself may not be able to provide the required performance for typical identification applications, however the incorporation of a secondary external factor, i.e., a validation key can be beneficial. Anyone familiar with 'on-line banking' will appreciate this motivation.

However technological assistance has the potential go well beyond identification. Safety is a key concern, especially for a vulnerable person. AAL should offer benign and welcomed assistance to address wellbeing, in the form of a 'guardian angel', rather than as an authoritarian 'big brother'. Achieving this balance provides an ethical dimension, which research much address, especially as solutions become more critical and traditional support structures provide less guarantees.

Yi-Luen Do and Jones introduce the idea of a smart living environment in which the home tracks and supports 'happy healthy' living for the residents with implementations toward health, awareness and entertainment. The chapter provides a holistic solution to AAL. Home based sensors monitor and assist activities of the occupant such as cooking. Entertainment applications include a 'gesture pendant', which allows gestures to control home devices and the 'Piano Touch', a light-weight glove fitted with little vibration motors wirelessly synchronized with an iPod, or other music playing device. It can cue the musicians about which finger they need use to play the next note. This can of course have rehabilitation potential.

Of course the AAL environment is not restricted to the home, and Tan et al. explore the options for AAL support while traveling on an aircraft by providing support for good posture. In the chapter an adaptive neck support system is described. The system, which consists of sensors, actuators, database and processor, can improve the aircraft passenger's neck comfort by reducing muscle stress on the journey. This may encourage older people to continue to take holidays, visit relatives etc, and hence promote inclusion.

Gait monitoring is discussed by Hodgins. The chapter describes a range of medical conditions that affect a person's gait and how gait monitoring can be used to improve the outcomes following rehabilitation (e.g. after Stroke or a surgical implant). Hodgins provides examples where monitoring has been used to help the treatment and rehabilitation process. Technologies are becoming available that will allow us to monitor gait, using 'smart insoles' in a totally unfettered way. These depend on appropriately devised feedback (possibly through an iPod or smartphone) that can allow dysfunction to be addressed and hopefully corrected in real-time.

This takes us to the area of rehabilitation. Whilst the environment can provide support, the frailties of the body mean that illness and disease will inevitably cause us problems, especially in our later years. Rehabilitation at home is an exciting prospect. It can be cost effective for the healthcare system and promotes a 'self-management' philosophy with AAL technology as an enabler [3]. Whilst technological advances and improved software may well be the facilitators for AAL, it is probable that economic considerations and our desire for independence into our later years will be the motivational factors.

References

[1] *Ambient Intelligence and Future Trends – Proceedings of the International Symposium on Ambient Intelligence (ISAmI 2010)*, J.C. Augusto, J.M. Corchado, P. Novais and C. Analide, eds, Advances in Intelligent and Soft Computing, Vol. 72, Springer, 2010.

[2] I. Cleland, C.D. Nugent, D. Finlay and R. Armitage, Optimal placement of accelerometers within the constraints of a smart garment system, in: *10th IEEE International Conference on Information Technology and Applications in Biomedicine (ITAB)*, 2010.

[3] P.J. McCullagh, C.D. Nugent, H. Zheng, W.P. Burns, R.J. Davies and N.D. Black, Promoting behaviour change in long term conditions using a self-management platform, in: *Designing Inclusive Interactions*, Springer, 2010, pp. 229–238.

Handbook of Ambient Assisted Living
J.C. Augusto et al. (Eds.)
IOS Press, 2012

doi:10.3233/978-1-60750-837-3-118

Biometrics in Healthcare – A Research Overview

Shimon K. MODI[*]
Independent Biometric Technology Specialist

Abstract. Digitization of the healthcare sector has been a major impetus for rapid adoption of biometric technologies, ranking it only behind the financial sector in consumer facing applications. The highly critical nature of healthcare records, the legal and medical risks associated with mis-identification, and the requirement of quick access to user information makes biometrics a preferred technology. The body of research supporting the theoretical effectiveness and efficiency of biometric technologies is quite substantial but users, the deployment environment and the type of biometric technology heavily impact its actual effectiveness and efficiency. Biometric technologies open up unprecedented opportunities in ambient assisted living (AAL) applications, but they also raise some unanswered questions. The aim of this chapter is to provide its readers with a basic understanding of biometric technologies and processes, discuss research in this area, and future challenges and use of biometric technologies in the healthcare environment, and specifically AAL applications.

Keywords. Biometrics, healthcare, fingerprint recognition, iris recognition, performance evaluation

Introduction

An individual's ability to access their healthcare information is rapidly changing as digitization of healthcare records gains momentum. As the concepts of electronic healthcare records (EHR) and electronic medical records (EMR) gain a foothold in an evolving healthcare environment, the role of paper records and filing cabinets will be reduced. Undoubtedly this change will result in an increase in efficiency, convenience, and fraud control, but it also raises several identity management related issues. Who will have access to this information? How can access be regulated in reliable manner? Can proper security controls be implemented to ensure unauthorized individuals do not violate privacy, confidentiality and integrity of information? The traditional means of authentication based on secret knowledge or secure tokens are not deemed strong enough for controlling access to sensitive information for primarily the following reasons: (i) they can be misplaced or forgotten (ii) non-repudiation is impossible to ascertain (iii) susceptible to automated attacks. Biometrics, which is the automated recognition of individuals based on physiological or behavioral traits is an alternative, and stronger, method of authentication. Fingerprint recognition, face recognition, voice recognition etc. are examples of biometric technologies and their use in access control applications has increased steadily in the last decade. Biometric technologies funda-

[*]Corresponding Author: Shimon K. Modi. E-mail: shimonmodi@gmail.com.

mentally bind an identity credential to an individual, which prevents it from being stolen or lost and thus provides strong authentication. They are used in various applications like password replacement and password management for computer log-on, physical access to secure areas, national ID programs, border control, time and attendance for employees, and user access to personal data. The use of biometrics is gaining traction in the healthcare environment as preferred means of identity management and now only trails behind the financial sector in number of consumer facing deployments [16]. The body of research supporting the theoretical effectiveness and efficiency of biometric technologies is quite substantial but users, the deployment environment and the type of biometric technology heavily impact its actual effectiveness and efficiency. The potential benefits of biometrics in the healthcare environment outweigh its detriments as it moves towards an increasingly digitized infrastructure. The aim of this chapter is to provide its readers with a basic understanding of biometric technologies and processes, discuss research in this area, and future challenges and direction of use of biometric technologies in the healthcare environment, and specifically ambient assisted living (AAL) applications.

1. Biometrics Overview

The word biometrics is derived from the Greek words *bios* meaning life and *metron* meaning measurement. Although many different parts of the body are candidates for recognition purposes, biometric technologies have to fulfill the following criteria to be useful in a real world application [10]:

- Uniqueness. The technology should extract features that are relatively different among members of the population.
- Universality. The technology should use features present in the normal part of the population.
- Collectible. The technology should be able to collect data in real time using socially acceptable capture techniques.
- Permanence. The technology should use features, which do not change over the lifetime of the individual.
- Performance. The technology should be able to perform consistently and reliably in real time.

In addition there are other practical consideration like scalability of the technology, user interaction between the individual and capture system, liveness detection and throughput which should be taken into account as these will contribute to the success of the technology. The final design of the biometric system has to take all these factors into account in order to decide its feasibility in identity management.

Biometric technologies have been researched and in use for over a century, and today there are several different types of commercially available technologies, which are discussed later in this chapter. As the definition of biometrics suggests these can be categorized into two groups: *physiological* and *behavioral*. Physiological biometric technologies are based on physical characteristics like fingerprints, face, and iris patterns. Behavioral based biometric technologies are based on actions or mannerisms that are acquired or learned over time like signature, gait, and typing pattern. Generally physical characteristics provide a more consistent reading as it is minimally affected by the behavior of the individual and are considered to be more secure, but research has shown behavioral biometrics can be used effectively to improve security and convenience.

1.1. Overview of Biometric Technologies

The field of biometric technologies is extremely dynamic and new developments are occurring rapidly. The technologies described in this section are all commercially available and are in use in various consumer-facing applications.

Fingerprint recognition is the oldest and most widely deployed biometric technology. The surface of skin on each finger-tip has friction ridges with discontinuities in it. These discontinuities are called minutiae points and the patterns of minutiae points provide uniqueness to the fingerprint. These minutiae points can be described using their spatial location; their type and the angle of its orientation and these details are used by pattern matching algorithms for matching fingerprints. The flow of the friction ridges have also been analyzed at a global level for recognition purposes, but minutiae based systems are by far the most dominant.

Face recognition is something that humans use in their everyday lives and are quite adept at performing. The automated process of face recognition uses either a collection of distinct facial landmarks and their interrelationship, or the overall structure of the face. This is one of the least intrusive biometric technologies as no physical interaction is required between the subject and the biometric system.

Iris recognition uses the texture pattern formed by presence of muscle tissues and blood vessels in the iris. The iris is the colored part of the eye that surrounds the pupil. Although there is color information available, iris recognition uses infrared-illumination to capture the texture patterns in the iris as they provide a higher level of discrimination. The initial iris systems required users to stand extremely close to the camera but recent developments have made it less intrusive. Contrary to popular belief iris recognition uses only a detailed 2D image of the iris and lasers are not used for imaging the iris.

Hand recognition uses the contour of the hand, length of fingers, width of fingers, and distances between distinct points on the hand for recognition purposes. Commercial systems capture an infrared-illuminated image of the back of the hand, which is then used for feature extraction and matching. The imaging mechanism of this technology results in a larger form factor, which makes it suitable for controlling physical access.

Voice recognition uses distinct acoustic features of an individual for recognition purposes. The behavioral characteristics like accent as well as the physical makeup of vocal chords provide uniqueness to a person's voice. Standard microphones like the ones in mobile phones can be used for capturing voice samples, which makes it an easy technology to deploy.

Vascular pattern recognition uses the structure formed by the network of veins for recognition. Using infrared illumination vein patterns from the subcutaneous region can be captured and used for matching. Currently commercial technologies use three different parts of the hand fore recognition purposes: the finger, palm of the hand and back of the hand.

Dynamic signature verification uses features like the velocity, direction, number of strokes, time of each stroke, and pressure applied by the user. The use of signatures in everyday transactions makes it an appealing technology, which can be integrated easily into a variety of applications.

Keystroke dynamics uses the unique typing rhythm and pattern of a user. The accuracy and reliability of this technology is still improving and as a software only solution it holds potential as an additional layer of authentication along with passwords.

DNA identification has typically been used in forensic sciences but is now being pursued as a biometric technology. There are still technology issues like invasive nature of data capture and its inability to provide a decision in real time which need to be addressed but its high level of distinctiveness among individuals makes it an extremely promising technology.

Biometric technologies like retina recognition, gait recognition, ear lobe recognition, scent recognition, hand gesture recognition, knuckle recognition and others are being researched by the academic and scientific community but their commercial applications have not been deployed yet.

1.2. Biometric System Model

A biometric system is essentially a pattern recognition engine, which is capable of capturing and extracting physiological and behavioral characteristics of an individual. Any biometric technology can be seen as a collection of 5 subsystems, each with its own specialized function [9]. These five subsystems are:

- Data Acquisition. This subsystem is responsible for capturing the raw biometric sample from the user. Typically acquisition is done using a sensor, which could require physical interaction with the user depending on the type of technology. This is the only point of interaction between the user and the biometric system and also where all the interaction issues are introduced into the system. The errors introduced in this subsystem are propagated throughout the other subsystems and could potentially result in errors.
- Signal Processing. This subsystem is responsible for isolating the signal of interest from the biometric sample and extracting features which represent uniqueness of the sample. This module will pre-process the sample for enhancement, perform quality assessment and create a feature vector which is a compact representation of the raw signal, also called a template.
- Data Storage. This subsystem stores the feature vector produced by the signal processing subsystem which is used for subsequent transactions. Data storage can be either centralized i.e. stored on a central server, or localized i.e. stored on a smart card or some token.
- Matching. This subsystem takes two extracted features from biometric samples as input and produces a similarity score. The similarity score is the degree of confidence that the two feature vectors are from the same individual. A biometric matching subsystem is probabilistic in nature and two samples even from the same individual will never provide a perfect match. Password and cryptographic token techniques require a perfect match in order to declare it a success. Due to the human interaction with the acquisition subsystem successive samples from the same individual are never exactly the same. Instead of providing a binary response a similarity score is produced by this subsystem.
- Decision. This subsystem uses the similarity score from the matching subsystem as an input and compares it to a threshold value to generate a yes or no

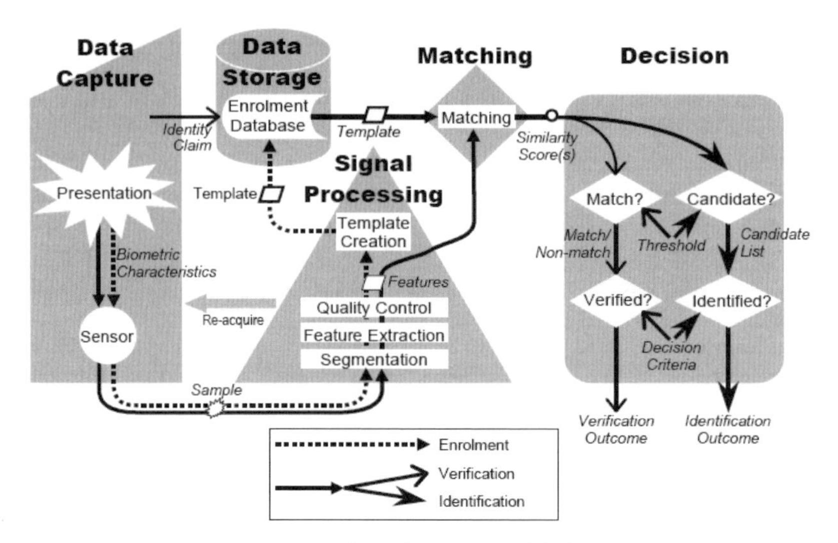

Figure 1. Biometric System Model [9].

decision. Every biometric system requires a threshold, which reflects the variability that is allowed in the biometric samples for them to be considered from the same source. The threshold value is a reflection of the risk that the owner of a biometric system is willing to accept. The threshold value plays an instrumental role in the decision errors produced by a biometric system, and these errors are discussed in later chapters. The decision about the particular threshold value should be taken after careful discussions among all business units that are affected by the biometric system.

A complete biometric system is designed and tuned with the dual goals of maximizing inter-class variance and minimizing intra-class variance. Maximizing inter-class variance ensures that the same features from different individuals are distinct. Minimizing intra-class variance ensures that the same features from same subject remain stable over time and can be captured consistently. These dual principles of distinctiveness and stability are the essential functions of any biometric system.

1.3. Biometric System Processes

A biometric system is capable of performing three main processes: *Enrolment*, *Verification* and *Identification*. During the enrolment process an individual provides their biometric sample to the system and a template is extracted and stored for future use. Verification is a type of a matching process where an individual provides a claim to an identity. Providing a user ID number along with a biometric sample is an example of verification. Verification is also referred to as 1:1 matching. Knowledge based and token based recognition techniques always work in verification mode since they require additional information like usernames or the physical token itself. Identification is a type of matching process where an individual does not make a claim to a specific identity but rather lets the biometric system decide if he or she is enrolled with the system. Identification is also referred to as 1:many matching and is used extensively in law enforcement and border control applications. Some biometric applications, which operate in identification mode, might require that the system return a list of closest matching candidates, called a candidate list. Candidate lists are popular in applications, which require human intervention, like law enforcement, but is unlikely to be seen in the healthcare environment.

For a practical application vetting the user's credentials is extremely important. During the enrolment process the user's biometric template is linked to an identity that is established based on veracity of the credentials provided by the user. Any error at this stage is perpetuated throughout the identity credential lifecycle and defeats the purpose of strong authentication.

1.4. Biometric System Errors

The accuracy and reliability of a biometric system is a function of the errors generated by the 5 subsystems and they can be categorized into acquisition errors and matching errors.

An acquisition error occurs when the data capture subsystem is unable to capture the biometric characteristics of a user or if the signal processing subsystem is unable to extract features from the sample. An acquisition error can depend on variety of factors including user training, user interface and the physical shape of the sensor, environment conditions, and sample quality threshold. A user who has not undergone proper training or is unsure about the correct way of interacting with the device may provide an incomplete sample or take longer than the system defined threshold for a time-out. In an unsupervised system interaction issues become even more important as there is no operator to guide the user on how to interact appropriately with the system. A classic example of an interaction issue is a user not knowing how long to keep their finger placed on the sensor. First time users of fingerprint recognition often remove their finger before the capture process is completed and this leads to an acquisition error. Environment conditions have a significant impact on biometric systems. Measuring sample quality ensures that biometric samples with a high ratio of noise are rejected from further processing. Each biometric system with a quality assessment component will have a quality threshold and all biometric samples, which do not pass this quality threshold, will be rejected.

The biometric matching process provides a similarity score which reflects the confidence that the two samples are from the same source. A matching system based on passwords or tokens will require the input to be exactly the same as the registration to declare a true match. Such a matching process always produces a yes or a no decision. Biometric matching and decision making, in contrast, is probabilistic and is dependent on the matching threshold value.

The capture of two biometric samples from the same individual will never be exactly the same because of the interaction between the user and the biometric sensor. For example, the orientation of the fingerprint, the amount of pressure applied on the sensor surface, the skin condition etc. will be different between successive acquisitions. This distortion and variation will never allow two fingerprint images to be exactly the same. As a result, errors can occur in the decision-making process because biometric systems must use a probabilistic matching process. This is true for any type of a biometric system because randomness and variation will always be introduced into the capture process making the two samples slightly different.

Biometric systems can make two forms of decision errors: false rejects (also known as Type I errors) and false accepts (also known as Type II errors). False rejects occur when an enroled user is incorrectly rejected as not being that user. False accepts occur when a user is incorrectly accepted as another enroled user. In statistics, a Type I error is caused by rejecting a true null hypothesis, and a Type II error is caused by failing to reject a false null hypothesis. For a biometric system, the true null hypothesis states that the two samples being compared are from the same individual. A Type I error is equivalent to a false reject error and a Type II error is equivalent to a false accept error.

The threshold and the distribution of genuine and impostor matches determine the proportion of false accepts and false rejects. Changing the threshold will result in a change in the proportion of false accepts and false rejects. So if a system administrator wants to reduce the proportions of false accepts, it is likely that the number of false rejects will increase. The type of application will determine the relative importance of these two errors. For example, a physical access control system for a nuclear power plant might be required to minimize the number of false accepts at the cost of increased false rejects. This tradeoff can also be viewed as a conflict of security versus convenience and the policies surrounding the application will determine the acceptable tradeoff cost.

Evaluation of biometric systems will typically express these errors in terms of rates. The following are the error rates most frequently used to describe acquisition, matching and decision error rates [25]:

- Failure to Enrol (FTE) Rate: An FTE occurs if a user cannot complete the enrolment process. The FTE rate is calculated as the proportion of users who are unable to complete the enrolment process.
- Failure to Acquire (FTA) Rate: The FTA rate is calculated as the proportion of users who cannot provide an adequate sample during verification or identification.
- False Accept Rate (FAR): FAR is calculated as the proportion of verification transactions from imposters that are incorrectly accepted.
- False Reject Rate (FRR): FRR is calculated as the proportion of verification transactions from genuine users that are incorrectly rejected.

1.5. Biometric System Evaluation Methodologies

There are three different methodologies for evaluating biometric systems: Technology evaluation, Scenario evaluation and Operational evaluation [9]. It is important to understand the differences between these, as they are fundamental to research discussed later in the chapter.

The goal of a technology evaluation is to evaluate multiple algorithms of the same technology. Such an evaluation is conducted on biometric data collected from a group of users on the same sensor. Technology evaluation allows separation of the different subsystems and can be evaluated separately. Technology evaluation provides several benefits. Since data collection and matching comparisons are conducted at different times a full cross comparison of all samples can be performed. This is the preferred means of laboratory testing and extremely effective at testing incremental changes in any of the subsystems.

The goal of a scenario evaluation is to determine the overall performance of a biometric system in a simulated environment that is representative of operational environment. A scenario evaluation will include the entire biometric system – from the data capture subsystem to the decision subsystem. Typically this evaluation is conducted in real time, although the data collected can be stored for later processing. A scenario evaluation does not allow a true comparison of multiple systems, as the biometric data used for evaluation is not collected from the same single sensor. Environment conditions, human interaction issues and subject demographic differences have an impact on the final performance of the system and it is difficult to replicate all of these among multiple systems. The true benefit of a scenario evaluation is the understanding it provides of the impact of real world application factors on the final performance.

The goal of an operational evaluation is to determine performance of a deployed biometric system. The results of such an evaluation are typically used for monitoring and maintenance of the system. Comparison of multiple operational systems is also unrealistic since the deployment environment and the target population using the biometric system will be different.

2. Healthcare Environment and Biometric Applications

Digitization of the healthcare sector has been a major impetus for rapid adoption of biometric technologies, ranking it only behind the financial sector in consumer facing applications. The highly critical nature of healthcare records, the legal and medical risks associated with mis-identification, and the requirement of quick access to user information makes biometrics a preferred technology. A general classification of adoption drivers is listed below.

2.1. Patient & Personnel Identification

The requirement of positive identification of patients and healthcare personnel stems from the following reasons: avoid medical errors, reduce risk of fraud and improve capability to handle medical emergencies [17]. Medical errors have a significant contribution to the number of avoidable deaths and is a drain on limited medical resources. Medical identity theft is also on the rise due to the increasing costs of healthcare. The main aim of identity theft here is to defraud insurance companies and public welfare programs. Identifying individuals during an emergency that might not have identity documents on them, or might not be in a state to provide it could have an impact on their ability to recover. Although such a process would require previous enrolment of the individual and an infrastructure to support identification of users who might be unconscious, the technical capabilities do exist for this.

2.2. EHR & Facility Access

Maintaining confidentiality and authorized access to critical digital information and physical resources is required by legislation in the US and European Union [8]. Today's healthcare infrastructure provides multiple access points to critical information, and some of these access points may not even be within the vicinity of the actual physical location of the hospital. The proliferation of mobile device use by doctors and other healthcare professionals increases the risk of inadvertent disclosure of critical information. Qualified healthcare professionals can only administer certain types of prescription drugs and physical access to these drugs has to be controlled.

2.3. Context-Aware Personalization

Context-aware applications hold the most potential in ambient assisted living environment. Context can be generally described as information that is characterized by interaction between people, applications and the surrounding environment [6]. Identification and personalization are a basic requirement for context-aware applications. The ability to recognize individuals in their environment, cross referencing the identity with their medical requirements and assisting them in their daily activities makes context-aware applications a key factor in increasing autonomy of individuals and make AAL more practical and give users a more satisfying experience.

3. Overview of Research

Although biometric technologies have experienced a rapid rate of adoption in the healthcare environment, there are several challenges, which need to be addressed for them to cross the chasm from pilot deployments to industry standard. Biometric technologies are affected by a variety of non-technology factors like user interaction, deployment environment, user physiology and technical factors like system architecture, quality and matching threshold and number of user enrolled in the system. The healthcare environment has its own set of unique challenges like strict hygiene standards, impact of medical conditions on biometric traits and privacy and legal legislation. Applied research in biometrics is an active area with a significant body of work, and although not all of it is focused on healthcare, research from other areas can be generalized to healthcare. An overview of relevant research along with a categorization of challenge areas is discussed in this section.

3.1. Hygiene

Maintaining hygiene standards is one of the biggest concerns in the healthcare environment. The fear of an infection spreading because of patients and doctors using the same biometric sensors is a valid one, and is a growing concern with the increase in use of biometrics in this area. There are several biometric technologies like face and iris recognition which do not require physical interaction with the sensor, but technologies like fingerprint recognition and vascular pattern recognition require the user to come in physical contact with the sensor. The survivability and transferability of bacteria was analyzed in a study conducted on three different biometric sensors and a doorknob used as a control surface; fingerprint recognition, hand recognition and back of the hand vein recognition [24]. Two different species of bacteria Staphylococcus Aureus and Escherichia Coli were used in this study. Survivability of the bacteria species was tested by sterilizing the sensor area and then applying the bacteria culture and analyzing samples at a time period of 5, 20, 40 and 60 minutes. Transferability of the bacteria was tested by sampling a surface which came in contact with the contaminated sensor 50 times at the rate of one touch per minute. The study found that survivability decreased to a maximum of 40% after 5 minutes and close to 0% after 20 minutes for all three sensors. The study observed that surface hardness had an impact on transferability of bacteria as the more porous surface providing a safer environment for bacteria. As would be expected, the transferability of bacteria decreased with each consecutive contact and the transfer rates for the two bacteria species was found to be similar after

10 touches. Although no statistical conclusions can be drawn about similarity of survivability and transferability between the biometric sensors and the doorknob, graphical analysis of the survival and transfer rates showed a similar trend. This is the only study of its kind which empirically tested and analyzed the hygiene impact of physically interacting with biometric sensors and several recommendations were given by the authors to further the body of knowledge in this area, including: expanding the number of bacteria species and biometric sensors, and simulating humidity and temperature conditions of a hospital.

A logical solution to the issue of hygiene issues is to develop a sterilization procedure for biometric sensors and users. The use of alcohol swabs was explored for cleaning the finger surfaces but performance analysis showed that alcohol reduces moisture content in the skin and impacts the clarity of the fingerprint image captured. Biometric sensors capable of cleaning themselves will have a huge impact on allaying hygiene concerns and represents an interesting area of research.

The strict hygiene restrictions require doctors and nurses to sanitize their hand repeatedly. The constant exposure to soap and other cleaning agents has an impact on the epidermis of the finger skin and its ability to retain moisture. This affects the skin characteristics of their hands and potentially the fingerprint image quality. There is a significant body of research in fingerprint recognition, which shows the adverse impact of fingerprint image quality on recognition performance rates [22]. A research study assessed the impact of moisture content, temperature, oiliness and elasticity of finger skin of 30 healthcare professionals on image quality and recognition rates of fingerprints collected on an optical and capacitive sensor [3]. The same data was collected from a control group consisting of 30 non-healthcare professionals labeled the general population. The study found a statistically significant difference in the fingerprint image quality between the healthcare and general population samples, with the general population providing a higher image quality score. An interesting observation of the study was that recognition rates of the two population samples were similar for fingerprints collected on optical sensor but not for the capacitance sensor. The authors noted that the sample size was too small for generalizing results to a larger population. This study illustrated the need to gain a better understanding of how the healthcare environment impacts the underlying physical characteristics used by biometric technologies. To the best knowledge of this chapter's author no study has yet explored the impact of healthcare environment on behavioral characteristics.

3.2. Medical Conditions

This is an area, which is receiving increasing attention as the biometrics community attempts to analyze the impact of individuals who might not be part of the ideal user population. The impetus for this research has stemmed from national identity programs as they have to accommodate individuals irrespective of medical conditions but the healthcare environment will come across these cases with a much higher frequency.

The technology makeup of iris recognition makes it appealing for use in the healthcare environment. Empirical studies have shown it is highly accurate [5]. It does not require any physical interaction for data capture. Current advances have led to systems capable of capturing iris images from more than a 1 meter away [13]. But most of the research in iris recognition has used data from the normal population. One of the first research studies disorders was conducted on individuals who underwent cataract surgery. From an anatomical perspective cataract surgeries affect the iris texture. Roizenblatt et al. analyzed the verification rates of 55 individuals before and after they underwent cataract surgery [19]. Their results showed that 6 individuals were falsely rejected after the surgery. Even though the similarity scores showed a lower level of confidence, it was not enough to cross the system threshold. A recommendation from the study was to re-enrol all individuals who undergo a cataract surgery to reduce the probability of a false reject.

A more comprehensive study analyzing the impact of ocular pathologies on iris recognition was conducted by Aslam et al. [1]. Their experiment involved 54 patients who suffered from one of the following: glaucoma requiring laser iridotomy, inflammation of the iris, corneal pathologies, episcleritis, scleritis and conjunctivitis. Their experiment was designed as a pre-post study that compared the similarity scores of the iris images. Their results indicated that except for inflammation of iris, the other eye pathologies had no significant impact on similarity scores.

Skin diseases are an underrepresented factor in fingerprint recognition research in spite of its potential to adversely impact the feature extraction and matching process. Drahansky et al. published a research report classifying several skin diseases into three different categories: affecting only papillary line structure, affecting skin color and affecting both papillary line structure and skin color [4]. Fingerprint acquisition technologies capture grayscale fingerprint images and skin color should have no impact on recognition rates. Although this research did not conduct performance analysis on fingerprint data, the structural changes brought about by several diseases in papillary ridges is outlined and is an excellent foray into this problem space. The research hypothesized an adverse impact on fingerprint recognition, and future research should test this hypothesis.

A recent finding indicates that the drug Xeloda used by patients during cancer treatment has a destructive influence on the papillary ridgelines of finger skin [20]. These patients cannot use fingerprint recognition systems and this represents a new challenge area in biometrics.

Voice recognition is an appealing candidate for use in ambient assisted living; it is non-invasive and requires a regular microphone to capture the voice sample. But the sheer number of different disorders or ailments, which have an impact on the voice of a person, makes it a challenge. Preliminary evidence has shown that severe cold or laryngitis has an impact on performance of voice recognition [12]. This has not been specifically analyzed within the domain of healthcare and requires feasibility studies to assess voice recognition's performance.

Vascular pattern recognition has seen a growing number of healthcare providers using it for patient and staff identification. Due to the nature of the imaging system, medical conditions which lead to excess deposit of thick fatty tissue can interfere with capture of subcutaneous vein patterns [14]. Medical conditions like superficial thrombophlebitis could change the structure of vein patterns, but its impact on recognition rates has not been analyzed yet.

There is a logical connection between various medical conditions and changes in anatomy that they bring about, and analysis of this connection with respect to biometric systems is a necessity for its success.

3.3. Environment Conditions

Although research investigating specific healthcare ambient environment conditions has not been conducted, evidence from research on general environment conditions indicates its importance. Several research studies have analyzed impact of environment conditions on different biometric technologies [21]. Research has shown that different illumination levels affect recognition rates of face recognition systems [11]. This could be of importance for an AAL application as face recognition would be a likely candidate technology, which would have to accommodate for daytime and nighttime lighting levels. The benefit of the general healthcare environment is that it is highly controllable, at least from outdoor factors and thus represents a slightly smaller challenge compared to other categories.

3.4. User Demographics

Certain external biological characteristics like skin get degraded through years of wear and tear, loss of collagen and it ability to retain moisture. The differences in fingerprint image quality and recognition rates between samples of the young and elderly population was analyzed by Modi et al. [15]. Their results showed a significant difference in image quality and recognition rates between the two age groups with the elderly population showing a high level of error rates. Considering that the ambient assisted living users will belong to the elderly population these results have a direct impact on which biometric technologies are suitable in such an environment.

Occupational impact on human anatomy is widely understood with respect to physically demanding activities like construction work, but beyond that this area remains largely unexplored. Years of repetitive occupational activities can have an impact on biometric technologies, which needs to be better understood.

3.5. User Interaction

The quality of a captured biometric sample is largely affected by how a user presents themselves to the acquisition sensor. Research in the area of human interaction has shown the significant impact it has on performance of the biometric system as well as user experience [23]. The elderly population is more likely to suffer from musculoskeletal disorders and thereby affect their ability to interact with the sensor. Arthritis makes it difficult to straighten the body joints, and technologies like fingerprint recognition and vein pattern recognition that require physical interaction with the sensor could be problematic to use. There is a growing body of research in this area and although they might not be targeting the healthcare environment, the results can be generalized to ensure a better user experience and fewer errors in a variety of conditions.

3.6. Privacy

The need to apply privacy preserving principle to biometric systems is universally accepted but extremely difficult to implement due to its subjectivity. The concept of privacy is significantly shaped by geo-cultural factors, but there is consensus that individuals should have control over release of personal information thereby controlling their own anonymity. The ability to link medical information with personal identifiers like biometrics represents a risk of unintentional disclosure. Section 3.2 discussed impact of medical conditions on biometric system performance; a corollary to that is the ability to detect certain disorders using the same biometric sensors. The application of privacy preserving techniques to biometric technologies represents a growing area. Pedraza et al. outlined the need to create social guarantees in context aware healthcare applica-

Table 1. Description of requirements that should be satisfied by the administrator [18]

Administrator	Requirement Description
Private Company	Users must be acquainted with the technology, output of the application and how the output of the application will be used
Private Company	Users consent must be sought
Private Company	Users have the right to revoke their consent
Private Company	Users must be able to exercise their rights in accordance with protection provided by legal systems
Private Company	Proper security measures should be used to protect user data
Government	General principles of proportionality of use should be respected
Government	Application should respect user's personal dignity
Government	Users can exercise their right to protect personal files owned by government

tions along with a list of requirements, which should be satisfied [18]. They identify that a private company or the government could administer ambient assisted living environment and they put a greater onus when the administrator is the government. When the government is the administrator they should satisfy the requirements placed on private companies as well.

Balancing privacy and legal requirements with identification technologies, which are non-cooperative and non-intrusive, is difficult but should remain a goal that is not overshadowed by the technical requirements alone.

The European Union, under the Seventh Framework Programme (FP7) for Research and Technology Development initiated a project name TURBINE (Trusted Revocable Biometric Identities) to enhance the protection and privacy of identity management systems which use fingerprint recognition. The overall goal of TURBINE is to create mechanisms with [7]:

- Ability to create identity credential from fingerprint such that the original fingerprint image cannot be recreated.
- Ability to create different pseudo-identities for different applications using the same fingerprint.
- Ability to revoke pseudo-identity permanently.

Since its inception TURBINE has been extremely active in this area with application domains ranging from eHealth, eGovernment, mobile transactions and physical access control. Although this work might not have a direct application to ambient assisted living, it definitely has the potential to address privacy concerns raised by the use of biometric technologies.

The Biometrics Institute in Australia published the Biometric Privacy Code report that recommended guidelines on how biometric data should be collected, used and disclosed to protect privacy of users [2]. The report outlined three specific goals of the code (1) to facilitate the protection of personal information provided by, or held by, biometric systems; (2) to facilitate the process of identity authentication in a manner consistent with the Australian Privacy Act; (3) to promote biometrics as privacy-enhancing technologies (PETs).

This particular category of research represents a crossroads of technology and policy, which will have a significant near term implications on adoption of biometrics in healthcare.

4. Biometric System Implementations

Healthcare applications which provide staff and patient identification are currently the frontrunners in adopting biometrics within the healthcare environment. The most often stated reason for using biometric is to streamline the check in process, eliminate data input errors and provide single-sign-on access to nurses across various applications. A large hospital chain in the North Carolina called Carolinas HealthCare System (CHS) has enrolled over 200,000 patients using a palm vein recognition system since they installed it in 2007. The technology is predominantly used for protecting patient's EHR and optimizing the patient check-in process.

Sutter Solano Medical Center in Vallejo, California is using fingerprint recognition to provide caregivers access to the healthcare IT systems. The original process of logging into the system using a login-password combination was proving to be cumbersome and time consuming, and fingerprint recognition was introduced to replace that process. They have deployed over 600 fingerprint scanners many of which are attached to PCs at nursing stations, along with mobile computer carts and medication cabinets. An interesting finding from their deployment was that fingers covered with non-powdered latex gloves were capable of providing fingerprint images, thereby alleviating concerns about caregivers who have to keep their gloves on. With growing acceptance of biometric technologies in traditional healthcare applications, their next logical transition will be in the field of tele-medicine and ambient assisted living applications.

5. Summary

This chapter provides an introduction to different biometric technologies, concepts for understanding system performance and an overview of research as it impacts the general healthcare environment. The existing body of research gives a fascinating insight into some fundamental issues of using biometrics in the healthcare environment, as well as solutions to some challenging problems, but this work is still in the beginning stages.

One of the biggest challenges of any biometric system evaluation is the need to collect biometric data from a representative sample of the population. This problem becomes an exponentially difficult one in the context of healthcare environment. As noted in these chapters there are several factors that have an impact on biometric systems, and collection of representative data is often difficult and sometimes impossible. Without access to appropriate data it will be impossible for researchers to provide the necessary results for solving these operational challenges. The typical user demographic of the ambient assisted living environment is be on the older side and this represents another research area widely unexplored as of yet. The ambient assisted living technology elements will be a collection of unobtrusive sensors as well as self-monitored mobile devices, and a seamless identity verification mechanism will require solving secure data storage and architecture challenges. Context-aware applications will constitute the majority of applications in AAL, and identity verification technologies, which do not disrupt a user's behavior, will be key.

Biometric technologies open up unprecedented opportunities in AAL applications, but they also raise some unanswered questions. Future research in this area will require a cross section of technologists, policy makers, users and system integrators to come together and address these research challenges.

References

[1] T.M. Aslam, S.Z. Tan and B. Dhillon, Iris recognition in the presence of ocular disease, *J.R. Soc. Interface* **6** (2009), 489–493.
[2] Biometrics Institute Privacy Code, 2009.
[3] C. Blomeke, S. Elliott, B. Senjaya and G. Hales, A comparison of fingerprint image quality and matching performance between healthcare and general populations, in: *IEEE BTAS*, 2009, pp. 1–4.
[4] E. Brezinova, M. Drahansky and F. Orsag, dermatologic diseases and fingerprint recognition, *Database Theory and Application, Bio-Science and Bio-Technology* **118** (2010), pp. 251–257.
[5] J. Daugman and I. Malhas, *Iris Recognition Border-Crossing System in the UAE*, 2004.
[6] A. Dey, D. Saber and G. Abowd, A conceptual framework and a toolkit for supporting the rapid prototyping of context-aware applications, *Human-Computer Interaction (HCI) Journal* **16** (2001), 97–166.
[7] EU, TrUsted Revocable Biometric IdeNtitiEs, 2008.
[8] Health Insurance Portability and Accountability Act (HIPAA), 1996.
[9] International Standards Organization, *ISO/IEC 19795-2: Information Technology – Biometric Performance Testing and Reporting – Part 2: Testing Methodologies for Technology and Scenario Evaluation*, ISO/IEC, Geneva, 2007.
[10] A. Jain, P. Flynn and A. Ross, *Handbook of Biometrics*, Springer, 2007.
[11] E. Kukula and S. Elliott, *Effects of Illumination Changes on the Performance of Geometrix FaceVision 3D FRS*, IEEE, Albuquerque, New Mexico, 2004, pp. 331–337.
[12] J. Markowitz, J. Markowitz Consultants.
[13] J. Matey and L. Kennell, Iris recognition – beyond one meter, in: *Handbook of Remote Biometrics*, Springer Verlag, London, 2009, p. 37.
[14] G. Michael, T. Connie, L. Hoe and A. Jin, Design and implementation of a contactless palm vein recognition system, in: *SoICT 10*, ACM, 2010, pp. 92–99.
[15] S. Modi and S. Elliott, Impact of image quality on performance: Comparison of young and elderly fingerprints, *Recent Advances in Soft Computing (RASC) 2006*, Canterbury, UK, 2006, pp. 449–454.
[16] E. Mordini, Final Scientific Report, 2007, p. 18.
[17] E. Mordini and C. Ottolini, Body identification, biometrics and medicine: Ethical and social considerations, *Ann. Ist. Super Sanità* **43** (2007), 51–60.
[18] J. Pedraza, M.A. Patricia, A. Asís and J.M. Molina, Privacy and legal requirements for developing biometric identification software in context-based applications, *International Journal of Bio-Science and Bio-Technology* **2**(2010), 13–24.
[19] R. Roizenblatt, F. Schor, P. Dante, J. Roizenblatt and R. Belfort Jr., Iris recognition as a biometric method after cataract surgery, *Biomedical Engineering Online* **3** (2004).
[20] R. Rubin, Checking fingerprints when a person has none, in: *USA Today*, 2009.
[21] R. Sanchez-Reillo, B. Fernandez-Saavedra, J. Liu-Jimenez and Y. Kwon, Changes to vascular biometric system security & performance, *Aerospace and Electronic Systems Magazine, IEEE* **24** (2009), 4–14.
[22] E. Tabassi and C. Wilson, A novel approach to fingerprint image quality, in: *IEEE International Conference on Image Processing, 2005, ICIP 2005*, Genoa, Italy, 2005, pp. 37–40.
[23] M. Theofanos, S. Orandi, R. Micheals, B. Stanton and N. Zhang, *Effects of Scanner Height on Fingerprint Capture*, National Institute of Standards and Technology, Gaithersburg, 2006.
[24] T. Walter, C. Blomeke and S. Elliott, Bacterial survivability and transferability on biometric devices, in: *41st IEEE Carnahan*, Institute of Electrical and Electronics Engineers, Ottawa, Ontario, 2007, pp. 80–84.
[25] J. Wayman and A. Mansfield, Best Practices in Testing and Reporting Performance of Biometric Devices, 2002, p. 32.

Handbook of Ambient Assisted Living
J.C. Augusto et al. (Eds.)
IOS Press, 2012

doi:10.3233/978-1-60750-837-3-133

Face Recognition in Ambient Intelligence Applications

Annalisa FRANCO[*], Dario MAIO and Davide MALTONI
C.d.L. Scienze e Tecnologie Informatiche, University of Bologna, Italy

Abstract. Face recognition is certainly the most natural approach to person recognition in smart home environments. The extreme variability of faces in such applications, due to continuous changes in terms of pose, illumination and subject appearance (hairstyle, make-up, etc.), requires very robust and fast algorithms to be developed. Moreover the variations of the subject's face cannot usually be adequately encoded in the initial user template, typically created starting from a few example images, thus making necessary to continuously update the templates on the basis on new inputs. After a review of the state of art of video-based face recognition approaches, suitable for home environments, a semi-supervised video-based template updating approach introduced by the authors is presented.

Keywords. Template updating, video-based face recognition, home environment, subspace learning

1. Introduction

The rapid development of technology and the contextual reduction of hardware costs characterizing the last decades, have made computers more and more present in everyday life; initially dedicated to very specific applications, microprocessors are now embedded in common objects and used, more or less consciously, by a wide range of the population. The challenge is now to go a step forward making these technological facilities "smart", i.e. sensitive and reactive to the presence of people. The idea is to embed technology in the environment enriching it with the capability of recognizing people and adapting itself to user specific needs and preferences. This ability is usually referred to as Ambient Intelligence (AmI), a concept with many different definitions that indeed share some common features: the AmI technologies should be extremely user-friendly, i.e. non-intrusive, ubiquitous, sensitive, adaptive, responsive and, of course, intelligent.

Four main application scenarios of AmI have been depicted by the European Commission in [16]; the document, released in 2001 by the IST Advisory Group, illustrates how Ambient Intelligence might be experienced in daily life and work around 2010 and suggests some research directions. The four scenarios hypothesized are: personal ambient communicator, connecting people and expressing identities, traffic optimization, social learning by connecting people and creating a community memory. The document specifies precise technological requirements for the development of this kind of application:

---

[*]Corresponding Author: Annalisa Franco. E-mail: annalisa.franco@unibo.it.

- very unobtrusive hardware, i.e. miniaturized devices (nanodevices) with sensors and actuators, smart surfaces, self-generating power;
- a seamless mobile/fixed web-based communications infrastructure, needed to realize interoperability between complex heterogeneous networks;
- dynamic and massively distributed device networks, since AmI applications should rely on almost uncountable interoperating devices;
- a natural feeling human interface that makes the system very intuitive to use;
- dependability and security, i.e. the AmI-world should be safe and secure against deliberate misuse. Biometric recognition plays an important role in the pursuit of this objective.

Over a decade later an analysis of the application of ambient intelligence in real world reveals that the forecasted scenarios are still far to be realized, suggesting that innovative techniques are still expected from the research community. Contributions from multiple disciplines, such as pattern recognition, artificial intelligence and hardware design, are needed.

A complete review of the state of the art of ambient intelligence is beyond the aim of this work; interested readers can refer to the recent survey in [28]. One interesting application of AmI is called Ambient Assisted Living (AAL) that refers to applications aimed at improving the quality of life in home environments; examples are home automation, entertainment, health care and household work. These applications are dedicated to different categories of users, ranging from young people requiring some "intelligent" ambient personalization appliances to older people who require support to maintain independent living at home.

Despite their different nature, AmI applications share a common issue, i.e. the need for a person identification mechanism, a basic requirement for ambient personalization. The most natural and proper approach to recognition in AMI applications is certainly based on the use of biometric systems, i.e. automated methods of identifying an individual based on his/her physiological (e.g., face, fingerprint, iris, retina, etc.) or behavioral (e.g., signature or voice) characteristics. Each biometric characteristic has peculiar attributes in terms of recognition accuracy, efficiency and ease of use. Behavioral characteristics, being more sensitive to environmental conditions and strongly influenced by user's emotions, are considered less reliable and effective with respect to physiological characteristics. Iris, retina and fingerprint analysis provide the most accurate recognition results, but unfortunately the acquisition of such characteristics is quite "invasive" and requires the user cooperation thus making these traits unsuitable for home environments. On the contrary, face acquisition can be performed continuously, discreetly, and without any supervision while users perform their daily activities; for this reason there are many fields where face recognition finds its ideal application, such as video-surveillance, anti-robbery protection systems in banks and post offices and smart home environments. Unfortunately, face recognition accuracy is generally lower with respect to that achievable with other characteristics.

This chapter will focus on face-based recognition systems in AmI applications. A typical face recognition system represents each user of the application by means of a template, created for example when the application is installed or when a new user is recorded, and then stored and exploited subsequently for continuous recognition. Unfortunately the template, initially created starting from a few example images of the user, is not able to capture the extreme variability of faces in unsupervised applications, due to continuous changes in terms of pose, illumination and subject appearance (hairstyle, make-up, etc.). This phenomenon makes it necessary to setup an updating mechanism that, exploiting the large quantity of face images continuously collected, gradually updates the user template, thus allowing to limit the negative effects of aspect variations on recognition performance. The need for performing template updating in an unsupervised and totally transparent manner makes the problem very difficult: the system in fact does not know with certainty the identity of the persons represented in the images collected and consequently has first to estimate their identity and then to decide if the acquired image is worth using for template updating. This topic will be the main focus of this chapter whose organization is as follows: an overview of the state of the art of face recognition in home environments is given in Section 2; in Section 3 the problem of template updating is described and the existing approaches are reviewed; Section 4 describes a video-based template updating approach validated by several experimental results; finally Section 5 draws some conclusions.

2. Face Recognition in Home Environments

Face recognition refers to the capability of an automatic system to identify or verify the identity of one or more subjects represented in still images or videos. It actually involves two sub-problems: *face detection*, i.e. finding the position of an unknown number of faces within a still image or a video frame, and *face recognition*, i.e. identify or verify the identity of each face detected in the previous stage. A considerable literature exists about face detection and recognition in different applications (see [1,17,41] for a comprehensive review). However, AmI applications present some peculiarities that can be summarized as follows:

- *unconstrained image acquisition* – images are recorded by an unattended system while the user performs his/her normal activities, by means of inexpensive devices, typically resulting in low quality images, with very complex background and large variations in terms of pose and lighting conditions;
- *availability of video information* – face recognition is usually performed starting from video sequences that can provide additional information for identification with respect to static images;
- *limited number of users* – differently from other applications, the number of enrolled users in this case is usually limited, thus making the recognition task relatively easier;
- *need for real time processing* – person recognition is just the first step for ambient personalization and must be performed very quickly and efficiently to avoid an overall performance degradation;
- *need for automatic updating procedures* – the system should be able to capture changes in users' aspect and to automatically update the stored template to avoid a progressive increment of recognition errors;
- "*closed set identification*" – the unidentified individual is known to be enrolled in the user database and the system only has to determine his/her identity. In such applications, in fact, the system has to recognize a predefined set of users that normally attend the house. The opposite scenario is called "open-set" and is characterized by the possibility of access attempts by unauthorized users; in this case the system has first to determine if the person is registered in the database and, successively, establish his/her identity. Most of

the AmI applications assume a closed-set scenario, while a small subset of them (e.g. access control, surveillance) operate in a open-set scenario.

Some of the above requirements make face recognition in this field a very complex task and often determine a failure of many of the approaches in the literature that usually reach good performance in the presence of images acquired with controlled illumination and pose but unfortunately fail to deal with more realistic operational conditions. Bespoke algorithms need to be designed to properly address the problem. The most recent approaches will be reviewed in the next subsection.

2.1. State of the Art

In the field of pattern recognition, face recognition is certainly one of most interesting and studied problems. In the last decades several solutions have been proposed: the earlier studies addressed the simpler problem of face recognition from controlled 2D images, but progressively more and more complex problems have been addressed by the research community, ranging from recognition based on 2D uncontrolled images (with pose and lighting variations) or 3D data to video-based face recognition that nowadays draws the attention of many researchers. Besides ambient intelligence, the latter category of approaches based on video analysis has several practical applications such as video-surveillance, video conferencing, video indexing and retrieval and entertainment. Most of the video-based algorithms are quite general purpose, only a few of them have been designed appositely for AmI applications and tested in real environments. The main contributions will be summarized in the rest of this section, starting from general video-based face recognition techniques (for which a more detailed survey can be found in [27]), followed by specific approaches designed for home environments.

2.1.1. Video-Based Face Recognition

Many video-based face recognition techniques are simple extensions of recognition approaches previously proposed for still images: the frames of a video sequence are individually processed and a final decision is obtained by combining the single decisions/scores of each image by some fusion rule (e.g. sum, average, majority vote rule, etc.). The classical subspace-based approaches have been extended to video processing in several works. In [34] the basic Eigenface approach [37] is used to compare two video sequences; the similarity between two videos is obtained by considering the smallest distance between frame pairs (one from each video), in the reduced feature space. Analogous extensions are proposed in [18] where the final decision is taken by integrating the decisions of each frame with decision fusion techniques. Other approaches use multiple subspaces to represent each user and perform recognition by comparing the test frames to the multiple subspaces, according to a distance-from-space metric [34,36]. In [36] different subspaces capture information related to different color channels, in [34] non-linear subspaces are used to better represent the data distribution. In [29,39] multiple subspaces are used to model both the user's template and the test images and a space-to-space distance is defined to obtain the similarity score. In other methods, Active Appearance Models have been used to represent users. In particular the authors of [7,8] propose to isolate the model parameters related to identity from those not related to identity (pose, expression, etc.) and to integrate identity evidence over a sequence of frames. In [22] A multi-view dynamic face model is designed to extract shape-and-pose-free facial texture patterns, successively represented by feature vectors extracted with Kernel Discriminant Analysis. In that work the shape information is used only in the normalization step and not exploited for recognition. A partitioning strategy based on pose information is implemented to compare similar views; for each predefined view the related features are approximated using a plane and the pose information is then exploited for matching testing frames with facial models of corresponding frames. Euclidean distance is used to compute the similarity between frames and the final score is obtained by simply averaging the contribution of each frame.

The previous described approaches do not exploit all the information existing in videos. The techniques exploiting the whole video information available usually perform simultaneously face tracking and recognition using a common representation. Some works propose the use of stochastic approaches in which tracking and recognition is performed on the basis of the posterior probability density function of a time series state space model (TSSSM). Tracking is formulated as a Bayesian inference problem, and it is solved as a probability density propagation problem; recognition is obtained by applying the MAP rule on the posterior probabilities. Li and Chellappa [21] implemented a simplified TSSSM with no identity variable, in which only the tracking motion vector was estimated and propagated. Face was represented either by the common intensity image or by Elastic Bunch Graph Matching (EGM) representation of the facial landmarks. Successively in [43] the approach was improved with the inclusion of identity information. A complex measure of observation likelihood is proposed where the appearance changes in videos are represented by a truncated Laplacian and the intra-personal variations are modeled using a probabilistic subspace density. A further refinement was proposed in [42] where the use of an adaptive motion model is adopted. In [20] a different model, based on probabilistic appearance manifold, is used for tracking and recognition. Bayesian inference is used to include the temporal coherence of human motion in the distance calculation. Finally some techniques propose to use face motion information as new biometric identifiers. In [5] recognition is based on optical flow: a sequence of optical flow fields are calculated for each frame and then concatenated to form a unique feature vector. Recognition is performed with nearest neighbor classifies in feature spaces calculated by Principal Component Analysis (PCA) and Linear Discriminant Analysis (LDA). Gaussian mixture modeling is used in [25] to represent the head motion information, extracted by tracking a few facial landmarks in the image. Successively in [26,33] the authors integrated the head motion information with mouth motion and facial appearance into a unified framework.

2.1.2. Face Recognition in Home Environments

Some face recognition approaches have been specifically designed for home environments. In [45] a face recognition system designed to be embedded in smart home applications is proposed. The system, named *HomeFace*, consists of three different modules for face detection, facial feature extraction and face recognition, respectively. The system operates on video and is based on the assumption that motions of faces from the same user form a smooth trajectory, and a new user can be identified by detecting a break of this trajectory. The images characterized by an excessive rotation or too low resolution are discarded, while the others are processed in the subsequent steps. As with many recent approaches, the face detection module adopts a cascade of detectors of increasing complexity: the first one is based on skin color analysis, the second one on geometry and the last one uses a neural network. The selected face candidates are successively normalized by applying an affine transform that warps an input face to a standard frame. Finally identification occurs, based on a multistage rejection-based LDA (Linear Discriminant Analysis). The authors claim that their system is able to operate near real-time and it is designed to operate in a distributed mode, where face detection and recognition are performed at different processing units, thus improving the overall efficiency. The authors of [40] propose a face analysis system, designed for AmI applications, that consists of two main agents: the former performs face recognition and is used to identify different users entering the room; the latter is designed to estimate the face orientation in order to drive the camera pan-tilt toward the user. The face recognition agent performs face detection, feature extraction and face recognition and is based on a two-layer Hidden Markov Model (HMM), whereas the orientation estimation module is based on the Wavelet transformation. A real-time video-based door monitoring system for smart environments has been recently proposed in [9]. The system, designed to identify subjects while entering a room, first detects and tracks the eyes for face registration and then exploits a local appearance-based algorithm with DCT (Discrete Cosine Transform) features for face recognition. The scores of each image are progressively combined to provide the identity estimate of the entire sequence. The algorithm has been tested on 2292 video sequences of 41 subjects recorded during 6 months, providing interesting results.

2.1.3. Open Issues

Despite of the large number of approaches proposed in the literature, the problem of face recognition in home environments is still challenging. Several aspects need to be further investigated to provide effective solutions for this specific application.

- *Evaluation benchmarks*. A comparison between the existing approaches, and of consequence a real performance assessment, is still quite difficult due to the lack of common benchmarks for performance evaluation. Most of the works proposed in the literature exploit self-acquired sequences for testing their own approaches. Moreover the data used are often not very realistic: the videos usually capture only one person at a time, and present a relatively good quality, in contrast to the characteristics of videos acquired in more realistic scenarios.
- *Performance*. The results of the existing approaches, particularly for those tested on realistic data, are quite unsatisfactory. The recognition error rate obtained on low quality data is too high and far from the one obtained in more controlled environments.
- *Long-term template validity*. Unfortunately, compared to other characteristics (e.g., fingerprint), face presents a very low permanence and a large intra-class variability: the face aspect can vary considerably, even in a very short period of time, due both to physical changes (e.g., hair style, presence of moustache or beard) or to different acquisition conditions (e.g., varying light, different poses). For these reasons the templates acquired during the enrollment session are often poorly representative of the user and can quickly become out-of-date. In relation to this problem, the home environment presents an undeniable advantage: a large quantity of unlabelled face images can be continuously collected and exploited to gradually update the user template, thus limiting the negative effects of aspect variations on recognition performance. The problem of exploiting unlabelled data is usually referred to as semi-supervised or unsupervised learning; despite of the variety of approaches proposed in the literature for general pattern recognition problems [4,19,44], a few works have been proposed to deal specifically with biometric recognition problems.

The rest of this chapter will focus on the last issue, template updating for face recognition from video sequences; a review of the state of the art will be followed by the detailed description of an approach named ITU algorithm introduced by the authors.

3. State of the Art on Template Updating for Face Recognition

In the field of face recognition only a few works in the literature address the problem of exploiting unlabelled data for template updating. Two main categories of approaches have been proposed: *supervised* and *semi-supervised* [4,6]. In both cases the user's template is initially created starting from a few labeled data and the newly acquired data are automatically labeled (i.e. an identity label is assigned), but in the supervised approaches the intervention of a human expert is finally required to validate the assignment and to correct the possible misclassifications. For instance, Argus [35] is a supervised system for automatic visitor identification. An interface agent notifies system users when visitors arrive and users can provide feedback to the system.

The main issue in semi-supervised learning is the ability to successfully exploit the unlabelled data to improve recognition accuracy; the main risk is of course to perform wrong assignments that could progressively deteriorate the template. The complexity of the task is highlighted in [6] where a theoretical analysis shows under what conditions unlabelled data can improve classification accuracy and when, on the other hand, their use can be detrimental. Most of the semi-supervised approaches proposed in the literature suggest to limit the error probability by selecting for updating only the data which can be recognized with a high confidence level. Under this assumption, an approach was proposed in [24] in which the initial template is successively enriched using available unlabeled images. The Eigenface technique is used to reduce the dimensionality of the image space and then template updating is performed by an iterative process where an ensemble of classifiers is used to classify the unlabeled data. An experimental comparison of different semi-supervised multi-classifier systems for template updating in face recognition was proposed in [10]. Even in this case only the images that can be recognized with a high confidence are used for updating. Another PCA-based technique has been proposed in [32] where the initial template is successively updated by iteratively analyzing the unlabeled images. Of course exploiting only the images that can be classified with high confidence allows a "local" optimization of templates because the data for updating are derived from the neighborhood of the enrolled templates; the most useful information actually comes from the data not adequately represented and consequently more difficult to recognize. In [31], on the basis of this observation, a "global" optimization approach to template updating based on the graph mincut algorithm is proposed. A graph is used to represent the intra-class variations by analyzing the structure of the input data and the similarity information among them. Since all the unlabelled images available for update are included in the graph, the approach deals with difficult samples and exploits them to improve the template.

In the attempt of identifying for updating the images "far" from the user template, a great contribution could come from the video information that can be extracted from a video sequence of frames which represents the natural source of information in the home environments, subject of this work. To the best of our knowledge, one of the few published works focusing on template updating for face recognition from video sequences is [2]. The approach is graph-based, but in this case the graph edges include information related to time adjacency between frames in addition to other measures re-

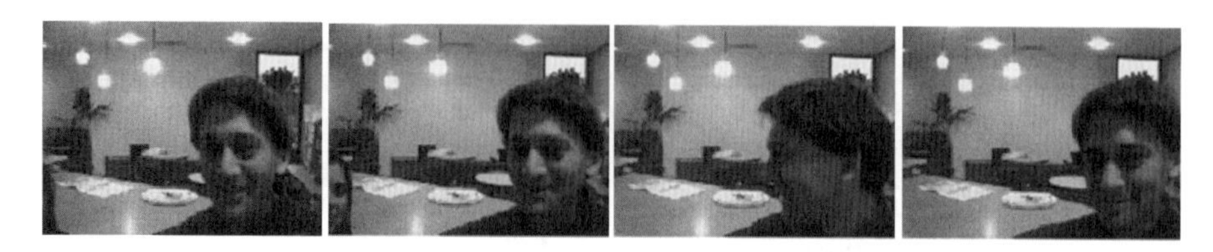

Figure 1. Four consecutive frames of the same subject: in some frames (1st, 2nd and 4th) the face is clearly visible and is selected for its similarity to the template; in the 3rd frame the image, despite the particular pose, can be selected thanks to the information extracted from the video.

lated to the visual similarity between images. The unlabelled images are assigned to a given individual by walking through the graph, according to a similarity criterion, until a labeled image is reached. The approach in [2] has been tested on an ad-hoc database, acquired with a low quality webcam. Data collection has been carried out in 7 acquisition sessions of 5–10 minutes each, distributed over a period of four months; the images have been acquired from the same camera (in a fixed position), and each image contains at most one person.

The approach described in [14], developed by the authors of this chapter, was designed to address face recognition for AmI applications in a very realistic operational scenario: both image similarity and video information are exploited for template updating. The approach will be described in detail in the following sections.

4. Incremental Template Updating

The Incremental Template Updating algorithm (ITU) operates on video sequences; it performs an analysis at "scene level" of the detected faces (a scene is intended as a sequence of continuous and related frames). The basic idea of the algorithm is that, within a scene, the position of an individual is approximately constant and his/her face should be detected in subsequent frames roughly in the same position (a relevant change in the image would determine a scene change detection). Within each scene the video information, represented by the frequency of detection of the different subjects and the related positions, is stored and exploited to select the images for updating. At the beginning of a scene, when the video information is not yet sufficiently reliable, the images are selected only according to the similarity with the existing templates. As the video information becomes more significant, the algorithm starts to exploit it to select images "far" from the current template but that can be reasonably assigned to the subject based on their spatial and temporal closeness with other images more similar to the template. An example is provided in Fig. 1 where the image in the third frame, which has probably a low similarity with the template due to the particular face pose, can nevertheless be selected thanks to its spatial and temporal proximity with the faces in the neighboring frames.

The updating technique presented in Section 4.1 has been designed without any assumption about the specific kind of template adopted, thus making the procedure suitable for different face representations. Of course the definition of specific template selection and updating procedures are representation-dependent; a possible implementation for subspace-based templates is presented in detail in Section 4.2.

```
ITU (T, V)

Initialize variables
for each frame v_j ∈ V
    F ← Detect faces in v_j
    for each face candidate cf in F
        x ← Extract features from cf
        T_i1, T_i2 ← Get the two templates closest to x
        if RecognitionConfidence(x, T_i1, T_i2) ∧ InterframeContinuity(cf, i_1, RI) then
            R_i1 ← R_i1 ∪ {x} // add the face to the set of images relevant to template T_i1
        else
            NR ← NR ∪ {cf} // add the face to the non-relevant images
        end if
        // Detection information updating
        if RecognitionConfidence(x, T_i1, T_i2) then
            Update RI with cf
        else
            if InterframeContinuity(cf, i_1, NRI) then
                // the repeated detection in the same position justifies promotion
                Move the detection info related to cf from NRI to RI
            else Update NRI with cf
            end if
        end if
        if Scene change detected between v_j and v_j+1 then
            Try assigning images in NR
            Update templates (T_i, R_i), i = 1,...,N
            Initialize variables
        end if
    end for
end for
```

Figure 2. High level pseudo-code of the ITU algorithm.

4.1. The ITU Algorithm

Given a set of templates $T = \{T_1, T_2, \dots, T_N\}$ representative of N users and a video sequence V, the Incremental Template Updating algorithm ITU (T, V), described as high level pseudo code in Fig. 2, updates the templates with the faces detected in V. The video sequence is partitioned in scenes according to relevant changes in the frame sequence: within each scene, frames are analyzed and the detected faces are evaluated and labeled either as *relevant* for one of the templates or *non-relevant*. At the end of the scene, the images that were previously considered as non-relevant are newly evaluated and possibly exploited for updating and finally template updating is carried out as a batch procedure. Then all the scene-related variables are re-initialized. Readers interested in implementing the algorithm can refer to [14] for a more detailed description of the pseudo code.

The relevance of a face relies both on its recognition confidence (similarity with template) and interframe continuity (repeated detection of the same individual across different frames of the same scene). If both conditions are fulfilled the face is considered feasible for updating and added to the set R_{i1} containing the images that will be used to update template T_{i1} (where T_{i1} is the template closest to the face), otherwise it is added to the set of non-relevant images *NR* and will be reconsidered at the end of the scene. To evaluate the interframe continuity the detection information is continuously updated. To this aim the algorithm maintains two data structures called *RI* (**R**elevant face detection **I**nformation) and *NRI* (**N**on-**R**elevant face detection **I**nformation). In particular:

- *RI* stores quadruples $RI_i = (id, v, \mathbf{p}, s)$ each denoting that a *relevant* face for a subject *id* (i.e., a face belonging with high probability to the subject *id*) was detected v times at a position close to **p** and with scale close to s.
- *NRI* maintains quadruples $NRI_i = (id, v, \mathbf{p}, s)$ denoting that a *non-relevant* face for the subject *id* (i.e., possibly belonging to the subject *id* but with low confidence), was detected at a position close to **p** and with scale close to s for v times.

In Fig. 3 the result of the application of the proposed approach to a sequence of frames (single scene) is given. Only the images of the sequence where a face was detected are reported. For each image, the face candidate is framed with different colors to indicate whether it satisfies or not the recognition confidence and the interframe continuity conditions and can consequently be considered relevant.

At the beginning of the scene some images satisfying the recognition confidence condition are detected, but since the subject is moving in the room the interframe continuity condition is not fulfilled and the images are not considered relevant; however, the detection information is stored in *RI*. After a first set of detections, several images start to satisfy both conditions and are thus labeled as relevant. The second image of the last row (dark green), initially considered non-relevant, is recovered at scene change thanks to its interframe continuity with other relevant images. On the other hand, the first faces of the sequence (light blue and violet) cannot be recovered due to the unstable position of the subject. The following subsections provide more details on the main steps of the algorithm.

4.1.1. Face Detection

The first step of the algorithm is the detection of face images in the current frame. The face detector provided by the OpenCV Library [30] is used in this work. The classifier implemented in the library was initially proposed by Viola and Jones [38] and successively improved by Lienhart in [23]; it consists of a cascade of boosted classifiers working with haar-like features. In this work one of these pre-trained classifiers made available with the library, optimized for nearly frontal faces is used. The result of face detection is a set of candidate faces $F = \{cf_1, cf_2, \dots, cf_m\}$, where $cf_i = (\mathbf{f}_i, \mathbf{p}_i, s_i)$ $i = 1, \dots, m$ is associated to a squared sub-image containing the face (**f**), the x and y coordinates of the upper-left corner of the window containing the face (**p**=[x, y]) and the window size (s).

4.1.2. Feature Extraction

A very simple feature extraction technique is adopted in this work to extract features from the detected faces: a bank of Gabor filters (with 3 scales and 8 orientations) is applied to the 2D image in correspondence of the 64 nodes of a uniform grid (8×8) superimposed to the image. The feature vector is then constituted by $3 \times 8 \times 64 = 1536$ elements, each corresponding to the module of the real and imaginary responses of a Gabor filter on a grid node.

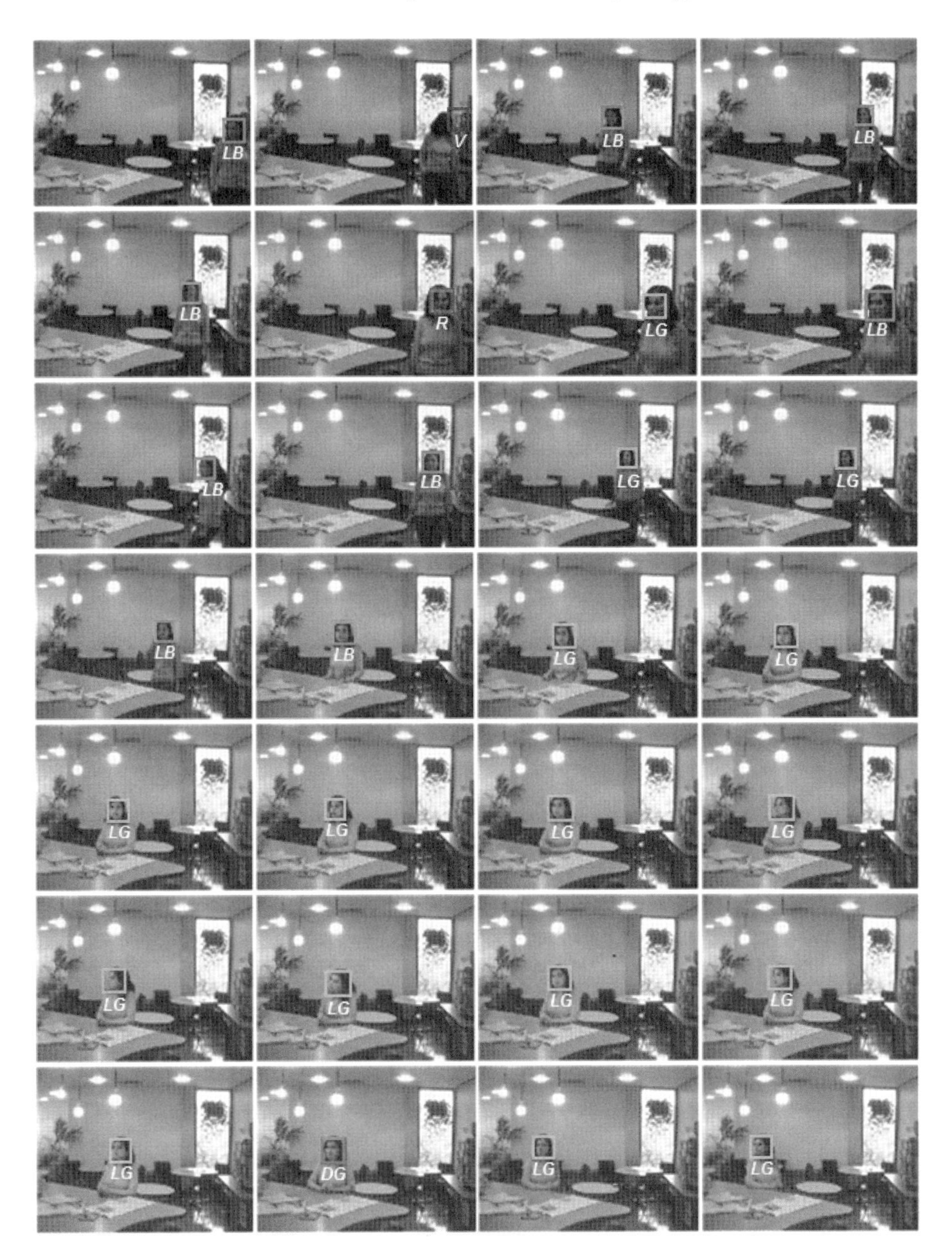

Figure 3. A sequence of images (single scene) from the FreeFoodCam database. The faces detected are framed with different colors: *light blue* (*LB*) denotes images satisfying only the *recognition confidence* condition; *violet (V)* indicates images that satisfy only the *interframe continuity* condition; *red (R)* refers to images that do not satisfy *none* of the two conditions; *light green (LG)* indicates images considered *relevant at the first stage* (they satisfy both conditions); *dark green (DG)* represents images initially labeled as non-relevant which are *re-labeled as relevant* at the scene change thanks to the video information.

4.1.3. Recognition Confidence

Given a face candidate (represented by the feature vector **x**), let T_{i1} and T_{i2} be the two templates closest to **x**, then the *Recognition Confidence* (*RC*) condition is fulfilled if the ratio $\frac{d(\mathbf{x},T_{i2})-d(\mathbf{x},T_{i1})}{d(\mathbf{x},T_{i1})}$ is greater than a predefined threshold, where $d(\mathbf{x}, T)$ is the distance (i.e., dissimilarity) between a feature vector **x** and a template T.

It was experimentally found that the use of subject-specific dynamic thresholds, rather than a single fixed one, leads to better performance. In our implementation, at the beginning of each scene the subject-specific thresholds ($\boldsymbol{RC_{Thr}}$) are set to the same prefixed value (RC_{Thr0}) for all the individuals and then gradually reduced (at steps of sRC_{Thr}) according to the frequency of detection (**df**) of the subjects. In Bayesian terms, reducing subject thresholds based on the subject frequency of detection in the current scene, corresponds to modulate their prior probabilities according to the recent history.

The *RC* condition is then expressed as follows:

$$RC(\mathbf{x}, T_{i1}, T_{i2}) = \begin{cases} 1 & if \ \dfrac{d(\mathbf{x}, T_{i2}) - d(\mathbf{x}, T_{i1})}{d(\mathbf{x}, T_{i1})} \times 100 > RC_{Thr}[T_{i1}] \\ 0 & otherwise \end{cases}$$

The threshold RC_{Thr0} and the related decrement step sRC_{Thr} are two main parameters of the algorithm and their effects on the recognition performance are evaluated in detail in the experiment section.

4.1.4. Interframe Continuity

The *Interframe Continuity* (*IC*) condition validates the assignment of a candidate face $cf = (\mathbf{f}, \mathbf{p}, s)$ to an individual i_1 according to its consistency with previous detections: the individual i_1 must have been detected at least v_{Thr} times in the previous frames of the same scene, approximately in the same position (i.e., with an Euclidean distance lower than IC_{Thr} with respect to the face size s). Given a candidate face $cf = (\mathbf{f}, \mathbf{p}, s)$, the *IC* condition is defined as:

$$IC(cf, i_1, X) = \begin{cases} 1 & if \ \exists (i_1, v', \mathbf{p}', s') \in X \mid (\|\mathbf{p} - \mathbf{p}'\| < IC_{Thr} \times s) \land (v' \geq v_{Thr}) \\ 0 & otherwise \end{cases}$$

The threshold v_{Thr} is generally higher for the set *RI* (i.e. when $X = RI$) with respect to the set *NRI* (i.e. when $X = NRI$). Of course the *IC* condition is never satisfied at the beginning of a new scene, and a temporal gap is necessary at the beginning of each scene to collect detection information before starting to update.

4.1.5. Detection Information Updating

For each face detected the sets *RI* and *NRI* containing the detection information are updated. If only the *RC* condition is verified the face image is added to set *RI*. If *RC* is not fulfilled but the *IC* condition is verified for the set *NRI* (i.e. *NRI* contains a sufficient number of previous detections indicating the presence of the individual i_1 approximately in the same position) the image is promoted to relevant face (i.e. added to the set *RI*), otherwise the detection information is simply added to the set *NRI* (see pseudo-code in Fig. 2). The choice of promoting images from *NRI* to *RI* is aimed at updating the "weak" templates that would need to be updated more than others but at the same time are not sufficiently robust to fulfill the two conditions. An example of promotion is reported in Fig. 4a, where the first images in the sequence (red and violet) are considered non-relevant and their detection information is stored in *NRI*. However, for some of these images, the closest template is the same, so that at a certain point the detection information is moved to *RI*. This is the reason why the 3rd, 4th and 5th image in the second row (violet) satisfy the *IC* condition with respect to the set *RI*.

4.1.6. Scene Change Detection

A very simple scene change detection method, based on the difference between subsequent frames, has been implemented. The absolute difference (pixel by pixel) between two frames $\mathbf{v}_i$ and $\mathbf{v}_{i+1}$ is calculated on the three channels (RGB), and if the overall difference is higher than a fixed threshold (related to the image size) a scene change is reported.

4.1.7. Possible Assignment of Non-Relevant Images

The images labeled as non-relevant in the template selection step are re-analyzed when a scene change is detected. In fact, thanks to the additional information gathered during the analysis of the successive frames, a face previously considered non-relevant could become relevant for a given template. In practice, the relevance of each face in *NR* is evaluated according to the interframe continuity with respect to the relevant images in the scene, thus potentially updating the sets of relevant images $R_i, i = 1, \dots, N$ for the different templates.

In Fig. 4a sequence of faces detected in a single scene of the FreeFoodCam database is reported to show the effect of the assignment of non-relevant images; each image is framed with a color indicating whether it satisfies or not the *IC* and the *RC* conditions, and if they are considered relevant or not. In particular Figs 4a and 4b represent, respectively, the situation before and after the attempt of assignment. Initially only a few images are considered relevant since they satisfy both the *IC* and the *RC* conditions. The other images satisfy just one of the two conditions or none; they are thus labeled as non-relevant.

At the end of the scene the non-relevant images are then re-evaluated. In particular a non-relevant image is re-labeled as relevant if it satisfies the *IC* condition with respect to the relevant images. As shown in Fig. 4b, this process is very useful; it allows to recover most of the detected faces. Some of the faces cannot be re-labeled since the (quite restrictive) *IC* condition is not fulfilled; however imposing such a restrictive condition is necessary, particularly in images containing more subjects, often close one to each other (e.g. in the Big Brother database). The experiments carried out confirm that this stage is reasonable since the percentage of incorrect assignments is negligible.

4.1.8. Template Updating

At this stage each template T_i is updated with its set of relevant images R_i. Template updating is carried out by a batch procedure, either when a scene change is detected (as in Fig. 2) or on a daily basis. In our implementation, for optimization purposes, the templates are updated once a day. After updating, the sets *NR* and R_i ($i = 1,\dots, N$) are re-initialized to $\varnothing$.

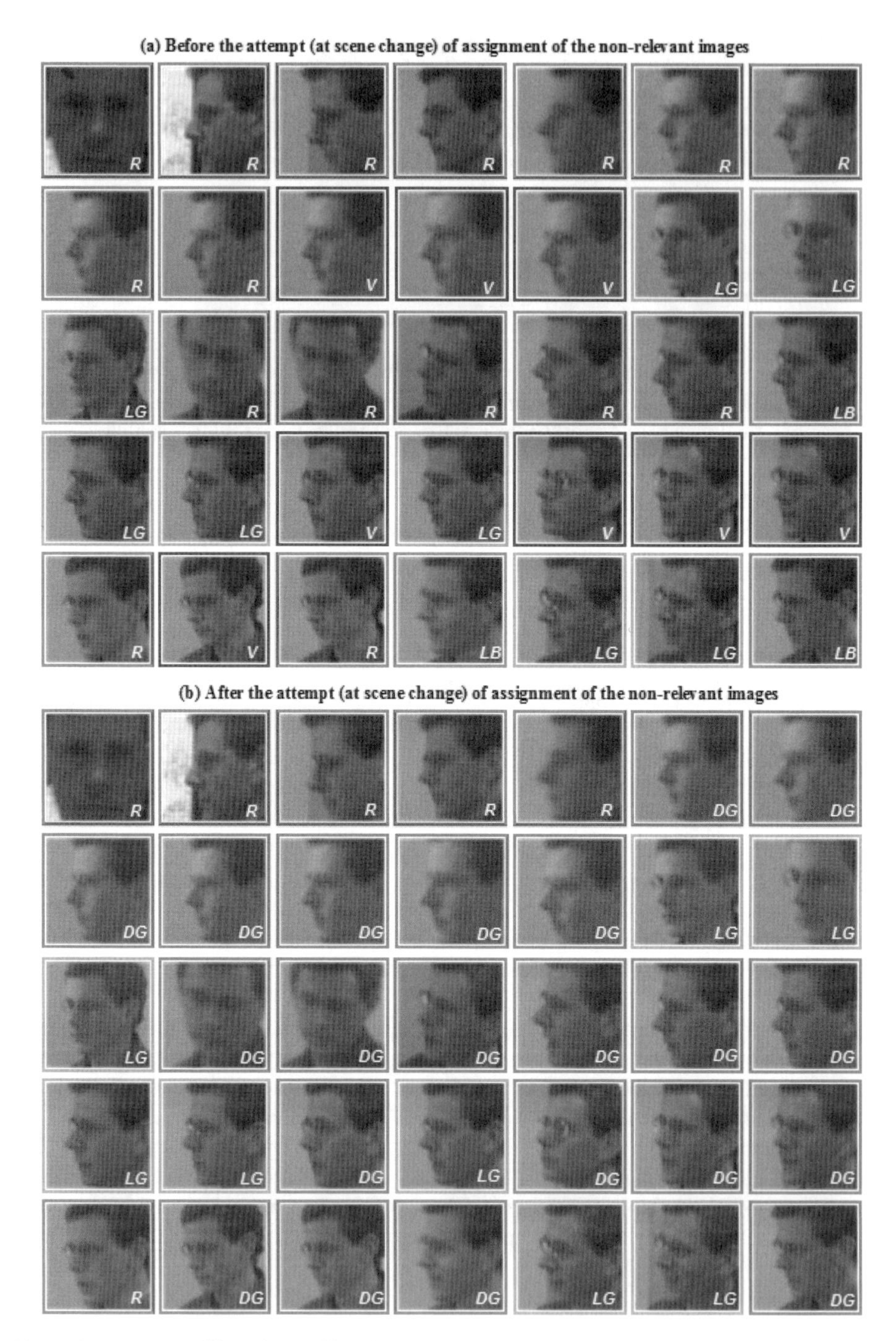

Figure 4. A sequence of faces detected in a single scene (FreeFoodCam database), before (a) and after (b) the attempt to assign the non-relevant images. *Light blue* (*LB*) denotes images satisfying only the *recognition confidence* condition; *violet (V)* indicates images that satisfy only the *interframe continuity* condition; *red (R)* refers to images that do not satisfy *none* of the two conditions; *light green (LG)* indicates images considered *relevant at the first stage*; *dark green (DG)* represents images initially labeled as non-relevant which are *re-labeled as relevant* at the scene change.

4.2. Updating Procedure for Subspace-Based Templates

In order to verify the efficacy of the proposed approach, an implementation for subspace-based templates has been proposed. Even if the procedure refers to MKL-based templates, it can be simply adapted for other subspace-based approaches.

4.2.1. Template Representation

Each template T_i is represented by a MKL space [3], i.e. a mixture of KL subspaces [15] of the original feature space. For a better understanding of the following concepts a brief review of the KL and MKL notation and operators is here reported.

Let $P = \{x_i \in \Re^n | i = 1, \ldots, m_P\}$ be a set of images constituted by n-dimensional feature vectors. A single k-dimensional KL subspace S_P can be computed [15] to represent P by selecting the first k eigenvectors from the KL transformed space of P: $S_P = [\bar{\mathbf{x}}_P, \Phi_P, \Lambda_P, m_P]$, where $\bar{x}_P$ is the mean vector over P vectors, Φ_P and Λ_P are the matrices of the first k eigenvectors and eigenvalues of the covariance matrix of P vectors. The value of k is a parameter bounded by the dimension of the feature space n and the number of available samples m_P. Given a subspace S_P, the distance of a $\mathbf{x}$ pattern from S_P, called *distance from space*, is defined as: $d_{FS}(\mathbf{x}, S_P) = \sqrt{\|\mathbf{x} - \bar{\mathbf{x}}_P\|_2^2 - \|\Phi_P^T(\mathbf{x} - \bar{\mathbf{x}}_P)\|_2^2}$. The MKL transform [3] is a generalization of the KL transform where more subspaces are used to better represent a set of patterns. A MKL space S is thus defined by a set of KL subspaces $S = \{S_{P_1}, S_{P_2}, \ldots, S_{P_s}\}$, representing a partition $\wp = \{P_1, P_2, \ldots, P_s\}$ of P, where each S_{P_i} is the KL subspace representing P_i. The definition of distance of a pattern $\mathbf{x}$ from a KL subspace $d_{FS}(\mathbf{x}, S_P)$ can be generalized to the concept of *distance from set of subspaces* $d_{FSS}(\mathbf{x}, S_P)$ as follows: $d_{FSS}(\mathbf{x}, S) = \min(d_{FS}(\mathbf{x}, S_{P_i}) | i = 1, \ldots, s)$.

4.2.2. Updating Procedure for MKL Templates

The template updating algorithm presented in Fig. 2 is very generic and can be easily adapted to different kinds of template. The only two aspects really specific to the template representation adopted are the distance metric d and the final template updating procedure, i.e. the technique used to update the templates with the selected images. As to the distance metric, for MKL-based templates the *distance from set of subspaces* (d_{FSS}) is used. As to the updating algorithm, in this case a complete recalculation of the subspaces is not a viable solution due to its high computational complexity. For this reason an incremental updating procedure is here adopted: the relevant images R_i for template T_i are used to calculate a new MKL space T_i' which is then "merged" to template T_i according to the procedure described in Appendix A of [11]; the algorithm is simply a multi-space extension of the basic subspace updating procedure [12]. Template updating is thus performed very efficiently.

4.3. Experiments

Several experiments have been performed with the aim of demonstrating the efficacy of the Incremental Template Updating (ITU) technique. In all the experiments template updating is carried out on a daily basis to simulate real operative conditions: the images considered useful for template updating are stored during the day and a batch update is performed in the evening.

The ITU approach is compared with other two techniques:

- *Similarity-based updating* (RC). To understand the relevance of video information, a typical similarity-based updating technique is implemented where images for update are selected according to the recognition confidence (RC condition) only.
- The approach described in [2].

The following indicators are considered to evaluate performance:

- *Recognition Rate (RR)*: percentage of images of the testing set correctly recognized in a closed-set identification scenario;
- *Percentage of relevant images*: percentage of images in the daily updates set selected by ITU algorithm and used for updating;
- *Percentage of correct updates*: percentage of relevant images assigned to the right user and hence used to update the correct template.

The tests have been conducted on the following databases:

- *Big Brother.* This database, whose detailed description is given in [13], has been created to evaluate the updating approaches in very realistic conditions. It consists overall of 23842 images belonging to 19 subjects. The structure of the database is different from the traditional one, where the data are simply partitioned into Training and Test sets. Here an additional set of images, intended for template updating purposes, is provided so that the database is composed by the following subsets:

  - *Training set*. Two sets of images are available for initial training (i.e., first creation of templates): 652 images extracted from the video presenting the participants' biography (taken during the everyday life of each subject, at home or work, with friends, etc., low quality) and 5950 acquired during the participants' audition. The auditions video are not available for some of the participants.
  - *Updating set*. A set of 11898 images is available to update templates as proposed in this work; images are hierarchically organized: the images are first partitioned according to the day they were recorded, and then according to the subject represented.
  - *Testing set*. Some of the videos available do not report the day of recording. The images that cannot be included in the daily updates, since the temporal information is not available, can be used as testing set. These images refer to events occurred during the 99 days and are representative of the whole stay in the house. The number of images in this set is 5342 and they are reserved to performance evaluation.

  The number of images for the 19 subjects and their distribution in training, daily updates and testing sets are given in Table 1, together with the number of days the person lived in the house. Some subjects lived in the house for a short period and too few images are thus available for an in-depth evaluation. For this reason a subset of the whole database, referred to as SETB in the following, has been defined; it includes the images of the 7 subjects (indicated with the symbol "×" in column 3 of Table 1) who lived in the house for a longer pe-

Table 1. Details of the composition of the Big Brother database. For each subject the following information is given: number of days the subject lived in the house, inclusion of the subject in SETB, number of training images (partitioned into biography and audition images), number of images for daily updates, number of testing images

ID	# days	Set B	# training		#updating	#testing
			# biography	# audition		
S0	70	×	42	341	1183	337
S1	14		49	510	237	96
S2	91	×	29	288	1158	525
S3	21		5	250	153	112
S4	47		10	489	565	230
S5	99	×	25	376	1617	499
S6	99	×	33	500	1527	616
S7	91	×	35	590	773	190
S8	15		20	0	471	442
S9	7		26	325	7	7
S10	99	×	57	396	1212	577
S11	84	×	32	349	1043	316
S12	21		31	458	114	259
S13	29		26	480	340	236
S14	50		10	0	640	453
S15	28		16	598	130	150
S16	21		82	0	247	101
S17	49		62	0	481	193
S18	0		62	0	0	3
Tot.			**652**	**5950**	**11898**	**5342**

riod; such number of users seems realistic for a home environment application. The SETB database contains: 253 images from the participants' biography and 2840 form their auditions (to be used for training), 8513 images for the updating set and 3060 testing images. The SETB database is certainly the most significant one for the evaluation of the efficacy of template updating, in fact: on the one hand it contains many images of each subject, thus allowing to appreciate the results of template updating; on the other hand, the long sequence of consecutive updates may gradually deteriorate the template and consequently determine a performance drop. It is worth noting that during updating, the information about the subjects effectively present in the house is not exploited, i.e. all the templates are evaluated for possible updating.

- *FreeFoodCam*: it consists of 5254 images (640 × 480 pixels). We used the tool described in [13] to analyze the frames, detect and label the faces and to store the video information needed by the template updating algorithm. A total of 2563 faces have been detected and, analogously to the approach used in [2], two different subsets have been extracted: in the first subset, 100 images (the first 10 images of each of the 10 subjects) have been included in the training set and the other images are used for updating and testing; in the second one 200 images (20 of each subject) are used for training and the others for updating and testing purposes.

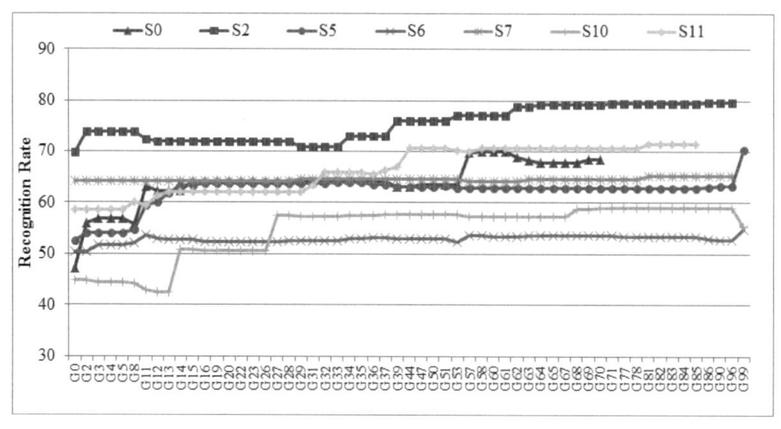

Figure 5. Recognition rate measured for each day of presence of each subject of SETB when an unsupervised template updating is carried out by the ITU algorithm (RC_{Thr}= 10%, sRC_{Thr0} = 1%).

Experimental Results on the Big Brother Database

Extensive experimentation has been initially carried out on the SETB of the Big Brother database to evaluate the algorithm sensitivity to its main parameters: the initial distance threshold RC_{Thr0} and the related decrement step sRC_{Thr} (see Section 4.1.3) are two parameters that could have a great impact on the selection of the relevant images and consequently on the probability of performing wrong updates. The main outcomes of the experiments are discussed here; interested readers can refer to [14] for detailed results. The tests carried out show that increasing the distance threshold (RC_{Thr0}) results in a more restrictive selection of relevant images as confirmed by the lower percentage of images selected for updating; on the other hand, the higher is the distance constraint, the higher is the percentage of correct updates. However, even for quite loose constraints the percentage of correct updates is satisfactory (more than 88%), with a corresponding percentage of images used for updating higher than 65%. When a sufficiently high distance threshold is considered, i.e. 10% or higher, a very high percentage of correct updates (95%–99%) is achieved. The decrement step (sRC_{Thr}) is even less critical to the performance of the method in terms of percentage of relevant images and correct updates. Furthermore some experiments aimed to evaluate the impact on the recognition rate of the parameters RC_{Thr0} and sRC_{Thr} have been conducted on SET B, and the results obtained are very encouraging: for most of the subjects the recognition rate significantly increases with respect to the initial value. In conclusion these preliminary results show that the two parameters RC_{Thr0} and sRC_{Thr} have a limited impact on the performance of the method, thus confirming the robustness of the approach.

Further experiments have been executed on the SET B of Big Brother database to measure the day by day trend of ITU recognition rate. The experiments were obtained by fixing RC_{Thr0} to 10% and sRC_{Thr} to 1%. In Fig. 5, the recognition rate measured for the subjects of SETB is reported for each day of his/her presence in the house. The graph exhibits a positive trend for most subjects, thus confirming the efficacy of the updating procedure. The increment is less evident for subject S07 for which the images in the updating set were mainly low quality (e.g. significantly blurred).

Finally, an experiment on the whole Big Brother (19 subjects) database has been conducted and the results obtained are summarized in Table 2. The following performance indicators are reported: the recognition rate measured (after updating) for each

Table 2. Summary of the results obtained on the whole Big Brother database. For each of the 19 subjects the following information is reported: days of presence, number of training, updating and testing images, recognition rate obtained using the initial template (RR_I), the final recognition rate after updating (RR_F) and the maximum recognition rate measured during the presence of the subject (RR_{Max}), the deviation of RR_F and RR_{Max} from RR_I (dev_F and dev_{Max} respectively). The last row of the column reports the average deviation weighted according to the number of testing images of each subject. The results are given for the ITU and the RC algorithms

						ITU				RC			
ID	#days	#training	#daily updates	#testing	RR_I	RR_F	RR_{Max}	dev_F	dev_{Max}	RR_F	RR_{Max}	dev_F	dev_{Max}
S0	70	383	1183	337	40.06	65.58	65.58	**63.70**	**63.70**	62.91	62.91	**57.04**	**57.04**
S1	14	559	237	96	77.08	81.25	81.25	**5.41**	**5.41**	77.08	77.08	0.00	0.00
S2	91	317	1158	525	40.38	47.81	47.81	**18.40**	**18.40**	45.14	45.14	**11.79**	**11.79**
S3	21	255	153	112	35.71	48.21	49.11	**35.00**	**37.50**	34.82	35.71	–2.50	0.00
S4	47	499	565	230	46.52	53.48	53.48	**14.95**	**14.95**	46.96	46.96	**0.93**	**0.93**
S5	99	401	1617	499	43.89	47.09	47.90	**7.31**	**9.13**	50.30	50.30	**14.61**	**14.61**
S6	99	533	1527	616	37.50	42.21	43.51	**12.55**	**16.02**	39.77	39.77	**6.06**	**6.06**
S7	91	625	773	190	45.26	47.37	47.37	**4.65**	**4.65**	46.32	46.32	**2.33**	**2.33**
S8	15	20	471	442	1.81	0.90	1.36	–50.00	–25.00	0.00	1.81	–100.00	0.00
S9	7	351	7	7	28.57	14.29	14.29	–50.00	–50.00	14.29	14.29	–50.00	–50.00
S10	99	453	1212	577	35.01	61.35	61.35	**75.25**	**75.25**	42.11	42.11	**20.30**	**20.30**
S11	84	381	1043	316	49.37	61.39	61.39	**24.36**	**24.36**	54.75	54.75	**10.90**	**10.90**
S12	21	489	114	259	47.49	46.33	47.10	–2.44	–0.81	47.49	47.49	0.00	0.00
S13	29	506	340	236	40.68	41.95	41.95	**3.12**	**3.12**	41.53	41.53	**2.08**	**2.08**
S14	50	10	640	453	1.10	0.88	0.88	–20.00	–20.00	1.10	1.10	0.00	0.00
S15	28	614	130	150	51.33	51.33	51.33	0.00	0.00	51.33	51.33	0.00	0.00
S16	21	82	247	101	14.85	19.80	19.80	**33.33**	**33.33**	14.85	14.85	0.00	0.00
S17	49	62	481	193	3.63	2.59	3.63	–28.57	0.00	3.11	3.63	–14.29	0.00
S18	0	62	0	3	0.00	0.00	0.00	0.00	0.00	0.00	0.00	0.00	0.00
				AVG	33.60	41.00	41.35	**+12.88**	**+16.69**	37.35	37.53	**+0.96**	**+9.81**

subject the last day he/she was in the house (RR_F), and the percentage deviation (bolded) with respect to the initial recognition rate (RR_I), calculated as follows: $dev_F = (RR_F - RR_I)/RR_I \times 100$. A positive value for the deviation denotes an improvement of the recognition rate, while a negative value indicates a result worsening. Since the updating is carried out on a daily basis, the recognition rate on the test set can be measured every day; the maximum daily recognition rate (RR_{Max}) (measured over the whole period of the show) is given as well.

For the subject in Set B for which a large quantity of data is available, very good results are achieved. For most of the subjects not included in SETB the ITU algorithm does not provide a noticeable performance improvement due either to the lack of training images, which determines a very poor initial template (e.g. S14), or to the limited number of images in the daily updates set, which does not allow an effective template updating to be carried out (e.g. S9, S15). Indeed the results are encouraging: the template updating, even in this very difficult scenario, exhibits an average increment of the

Table 3. Percentage of relevant images and correct updates, initial recognition rate (RR_I), final recognition rate (RR_F) and recognition rate deviation (dev_F) in the tests carried out with the ITU and the RC algorithms on the FreeFoodCam database with 100 and 200 training images

	100		200	
	ITU	**RC**	**ITU**	**RC**
Relevant images	65.95%	22.27%	68.23%	23.97%
Correct updates	93.10%	96.53%	96.40%	100.0%
RR_I	56.03%		63.22%	
RR_F	77.71%	62.40%	82.14%	69.32%
dev_F	**+38.69%**	**+11.38%**	**+29.93%**	**+9.65%**

recognition rate of about 13% with a percentage of relevant images and of correct updates equal to 38.04% and 87.38% respectively.

The comparison between the ITU and the RC algorithms clearly shows the importance of using video information for template updating. The RC algorithm, based exclusively on the similarity between images and templates, allows to obtain a very limited increment of the recognition rate (< 1%) with respect to the good result of the ITU algorithm (about 13%). The unsatisfactory behavior of the RC algorithm can be explained considering that the images more useful for template updating are those more "distant" from the template; such images cannot be selected without the contribution of the video information.

Results on the FreeFoodCam Database

Experiments analogous to those presented in the previous section have been performed on the FreeFoodCam database. In these experiments the algorithm parameters have been fixed to RC_{Thr0} = 10% and sRC_{Thr} = 1%. The results obtained with 100 and 200 training images are summarized in Table 3; in particular, the table reports for the ITU and the RC algorithms: the percentage of images effectively exploited for template updating and the percentage of correct updates performed, the initial recognition rate, the final recognition rate and the percentage deviation with respect to the initial recognition rate. The results confirm the efficacy of the approach obtained on the Big Brother database: the percentage of correct updates and the resulting performance improvement are quite relevant. The results obtained with the FreeFoodCam dataset are generally better than those obtained on the Big Brother database, certainly due to the lower complexity of this dataset. We believe that the performance measured are very encouraging, considering the very limited number of images available for training (10 or 20 for each subject) which are not sufficient to create robust subspaces. The superiority of the ITU algorithm with respect to the RC approach is confirmed in this test as well.

The final recognition rate obtained with the proposed updating technique (RR_F) is higher than that measured for analogous experiments in [2], (from the graphs it can be estimated around 74% with 100 training images and 78% with 200 images); this result is interesting, even considering that the method in [2] exploits color information not considered in the current implementation of the proposed approach. Moreover, the updating technique presented in this work confirmed its ability to deal with a very large quantity of data, whereas the method in [2] could present some scalability problems: in fact, each new image corresponds to a node in the graph and its labeling requires walking through the graph according to a similarity criterion until a labeled image is reached. Of course increasing the graph size makes this procedure more complex.

5. Conclusions

This work is framed into the context of face recognition in home environments where the images acquired are usually low quality, often significantly blurred or partial occluded, with large variations in terms of pose of the subject and illumination conditions. Traditional recognition algorithms cannot be applied to this difficult recognition problem for which specific techniques need to be developed. A review of the state of the art reveals that the problem is not yet solved: the performance of many existing algorithms are quite poor with respect to the results reached in other fields; moreover a fair comparison between different algorithms is not yet possible due to the lack of a common benchmark for these specific applications. The chapter also highlighted the importance of template updating since it represents the only mechanism that allows to gradually capture the inevitable changes occurring in face aspect. In relation to this issue, a semi-supervised updating algorithm has been presented. An analysis of the results obtained shows that templates can be successfully updated exploiting unlabeled images with a very limited error rate and that the video information is crucial to this aim.

References

[1] A.F. Abate, M. Nappi, D. Riccio and G. Sabatino, 2D and 3D face recognition: A survey, *Pattern Recognition Letters* **28** (2007), 1885–1906.

[2] M.F. Balcan, A. Blum, P.P. Choi, J. Lafferty, B. Pantano, M.R. Rwebangira and X. Zhu, Person identification in webcam images: An application of semi-supervised learning, in: *ICML Workshop on Learning with Partially Classified Training Data*, 2005, pp. 1–9.

[3] R. Cappelli, D. Maio and D. Maltoni, Multi-space KL for pattern representation and classification, *IEEE Transactions on Pattern Analysis and Machine Intelligence* **23**(9) (2001), 977–996.

[4] O. Chapelle, B. Scholkopf and A. Zien, The Semi-Supervised Learning Book, MIT Press, 2006.

[5] L.-F. Chen, H.-Y.M. Liao and J.-C. Lin, Person identification using facial motion, in: *Int. Conf. on Image Processing*, 2001, pp. 677–680.

[6] I. Cohen, F.G. Cozman, N. Sebe, M.C. Cirelo and T. Huang, Semi-supervised learning of classifiers: Theory, algorithms and their applications to human-computer interaction, *IEEE Transactions on Pattern Analysis and Machine Intelligence* **26**(12) (2004), 1553–1567.

[7] G.J. Edwards, C.J. Taylor and T.F. Cootes, Improving identification performance by integrating evidence from sequences, in: *IEEE Proceedings on Computer Vision and Pattern Recognition*, 1999, pp. 486–491.

[8] G.J. Edwards, C.J. Taylor and T.F. Cootes, Learning to identify and track faces in image sequences, in: *IEEE Proceedings on Automatic Face and Gesture Recognition*, 1998, pp. 260–265.

[9] H.K. Ekenel, J. Stallkamp and R. Stiefelhagen, A video-based door monitoring system using local appearance-based face models, *Computer Vision and Image Understanding* **114** (2010), 596–608.

[10] N. El Gayar, S.A. Shaban and S. Hamdy, Face recognition with semi-supervised learning and multiple classifiers, in: *Int. Conf. on Computational Intell., Machine Systems and Cybernetics*, 2006, pp. 296–301.

[11] A. Franco and A. Lumini, Mixture of KL subspaces for relevance feedback, *Multimedia Tools and Applications* **37**(2) (2008), 189–209.

[12] A. Franco, A. Lumini and D. Maio, Eigenspace merging for model updating, in: *International Conference on Pattern Recognition*, Vol. 2, 2002, pp. 156–159.

[13] A. Franco, D. Maio and D. Maltoni, The Big Brother database: Evaluating face recognition in smart home environments, in: *International Conference on Biometrics*, 2009, pp. 142–150.

[14] A. Franco, D. Maio and D. Maltoni, Incremental template updating for face recognition in home environments, *Pattern Recognition* **43**(8) (2010), 2891–2903.

[15] K. Fukunaga, *Statistical Pattern Recognition*, Academic Press, San Diego, 1990.

[16] I.A. Group, Scenarios for ambient intelligence in 2010, 2001.

[17] E. Hjelmåsa and B.K. Low, Face detection: A survey, *Computer Vision and Image Understanding* **83** (2001), 236–274.

[18] S.K. Huang and M.M. Trivedi, Streaming face recognition using multi-camera video arrays, in: *Proceedings of Pattern Recognition*, Vol. 4, 2002, pp. 213–216.
[19] T.M. Huang, V. Kecman and I. Kopriva, Kernel Based Algorithms for Mining Huge Data Sets, Supervised, Semisupervised and Unsupervised Learning, Springer-Verlag, Berlin, Heidelberg, 2006.
[20] K.-C. Lee, J. Ho, M.-H. Yang and D. Kriegman, Visual tracking and recognition using probabilistic appearance manifolds, *Computer Vision and Image Understanding* **99**(3) (2005), 303–331.
[21] B. Li and R. Chellappa, A generic approach to simultaneous tracking and verification in video, *IEEE Transactions on Image Processing* **11**(5) (2002), 530–544.
[22] Y. Li, S. Gong and H. Liddell, Recognising trajectories of facial identities using kernel discriminant analysis, *Image and Video Computing* **21**(3–4) (2003), 1077–1086.
[23] R. Lienhart and J. Maydt, An extended set of Haar-like features for rapid object detection, in: *IEEE International Conference on Image Processing*, Vol. 1, 2002, pp. 900–903.
[24] C. Martinez and O. Fuentes, Face recognition using unlabeled data, *Computacion y Sistems, Iberoamerica Journal of Computer Science Research* **7**(2) (2003), 123–129.
[25] F. Matta and J.-L. Dugelay, Person recognition using human head motion information, in: *International Conference on Articulated Motion and Deformable Objects*, 2006, pp. 326–335.
[26] F. Matta and J.-L. Dugelay, Video face recognition: A physiological and behavioural multimodal approach, in: *IEEE Proceedings on Image Processing*, 2007, pp. 497–500.
[27] F. Matta and J.L. Dugelay, Person recognition using facial video information: A state of the art, *Journal of Visual Languages and Computing* **20** (2009), 180–187.
[28] H. Nakashima, H. Aghajan and J. Augusto, eds, *Handbook on Ambient Intelligence and Smart Environment*, Springer Verlag, 2009.
[29] M. Nishiyama, O. Yamaguchi and K. Fukui, Face recognition with multiple constrained mutual subspace method, in: *Proceedings of Audio- and Video-Based Biometric Person Authentication*, 2005, pp. 71–80.
[30] OpenCV, http://sourceforge.net/projects/opencvlibrary/.
[31] A. Rattani, G.L. Marcialis and F. Roli, Biometric template update using the graph mincut algorithm: A case study in face verification, in: *Biometric Symposium*, 2008, pp. 23–28.
[32] F. Roli and G.L. Marcialis, Semi-supervised PCA-based face recognition using self-training, in: *International Workshop on Structural and Syntactical Pattern Recognition and Statistical Techniques in Pattern Recognition*, 2006, pp. 560–568.
[33] U. Saeed, F. Matta and J.-L. Dugelay, Person recognition based on head and mouth dynamics, in: *IEEE Proceedings on Multimedia Signal Processing*, 2006, pp. 29–32.
[34] S. Satoh, Comparative evaluation of face sequence matching for content-based video access, in: *IEEE Proceedings on Automatic Face and Gesture Recognition*, 2000, pp. 163–168.
[35] R. Sukthankar and R. Stockton, Argus: The digital doorman, *IEEE Intelligent systems* **16**(2) (2001), 14–19.
[36] L. Torres and J. Vila, Automatic face recognition for video indexing applications, *Pattern Recognition* **35**(3) (2002), 615–625.
[37] M.A. Turk and A.P. Pentland, Face recognition using eigenfaces, in: *IEEE Proceedings on Computer Vision and Pattern Recognition*, 1991, pp. 586–591.
[38] P. Viola and M.J. Jones, Rapid object detection using a boosted cascade of simple features, in: *IEEE International Conference on Computer Vision and Pattern Recognition*, Vol. 1, 2001, pp. 511–518.
[39] O. Yamaguchi, K. Fukui and K.I. Maeda, Face recognition using temporal image sequence, in: *IEEE Proceedings on Automatic Face and Gesture Recognition*, 1998, pp. 318–323.
[40] Z. Yong, L. Yuliang, Z. Ying, X. Guo, H. Jian, H. Yibin and H. Zhangqin, Novel interactive mode based on face-recognition and facial orientation-estimation applied to AmI, in: *International Conference on Bioinformatics and Biomedical Engineering*, 2008, pp. 1996–1999.
[41] W. Zhao, R. Chellappa, P.J. Phillips and A. Rosenfeld, Face recognition: A literature survey, *ACM Computing Surveys* **35** (2003), 399–458.
[42] S. Zhou, R. Chellappa and B. Moghaddam, Visual tracking and recognition using appearance-adaptive models in particle filters, *IEEE Transactions on Image Processing* **13**(11) (2004), 1491–1506.
[43] S. Zhou, V. Krueger and R. Chellappa, Probabilistic recognition of human faces from video, *Computer Vision and Image Understanding* **91**(1–2) (2003), 214–245.
[44] X. Zhu and A.B. Goldberg, Introduction to Semi-Supervised Learning (Synthesis Lectures on Artificial Intelligence and Machine Learning, Morgan & Claypool Publishers, 2009.
[45] F. Zuo and P.H.N. de With, Real-time embedded face recognition for smart home, *IEEE Transactions on Consumer Electronics* **51** (2005), 183–190.

Handbook of Ambient Assisted Living
J.C. Augusto et al. (Eds.)
IOS Press, 2012

doi:10.3233/978-1-60750-837-3-155

Biometric Monitoring of Behaviour

Anastasios DROSOU [a,*] and Dr. Dimitrios TZOVARAS [b]
[a] *Department of Electrical Engineering, Imperial College London, SW7 2AZ, London, UK*
[b] *Informatics and Telematics Institute (Ce.R.T.H.), P.O. Box 361, 57001 Thermi-Thessaloniki, Greece*

Abstract. This chapter presents a novel framework for dynamic biometric monitoring of behaviour towards user authentication, utilizing dynamic and static anthropometric information. The recognition of the performed activity is based on Generalized Radon transforms that are applied on spatiotemporal motion templates. User authentication is performed exploiting the behavioural variations between different users, regardless of small variations in the interaction setting. The upper body limb anthropometric information is extracted for each user and an attributed body-related graph structure framework is employed for the detection of static biometric features of important discrimination power. Finally, a quality factor based on ergonomic criteria evaluates the recognition capacity of each activity. Experimental validation illustrates that the proposed approach for integrating static anthropometric features and activity-related recognition, advances significantly the authentication performance. In this concept, a series of possible applications of the proposed system is also presented.

Keywords. Biometrics, biometric monitoring, activity recognition, behavioural biometrics, biometric authentication, activity related recognition, motion analysis, body tracking, HMM, anthropometric profile, attributed graph matching, applications of biometrics

1. Introduction

Monitoring of activities has been extensively researched during the last decades, mainly for identifying ongoing activities [36], detecting anomalies in their execution [7], providing access control to restricted areas [14], etc. The results of this research field can be directly applied to surveillance [9], identity verification and medical applications [10].

Extending this, biometric monitoring of behaviour, exploits the inborn tendency of humans to develop their own unique motion patterns for performing activities, or for reacting to specific environmental stimuli, in order to identify both the performed activity, but also the person that performs it. In the current chapter, an unobtrusive, privacy-enabled, framework for real-time user authentication, is presented, where applicability of dynamic behavioural biometric traits is enhanced by static biometric information.

Specifically, the rest of the current chapter is organized as follows: In Section 2 the concept of activity detection is introduced. In Section 3 a short review of existing biometric recognition research his presented, while activities with high authentication

*Corresponding Author: Anastasios Drosou. E-mail: a.drosou09@imperial.ac.uk.

potential are suggested. The methodology followed towards accurate activity detection and the classification of the latter to normal/abnormal ones is elaborated in Section 4. The core of the current work, which includes the dynamic behavioural feature extraction, the compensation for small variations in the interaction setting, the exploitation of soft, static anthropometric information and the evaluation of the measurements, is thoroughly discussed in Section 5. Last, the performance of the proposed system is illustrated in Section 7, followed by a series of possible applications for the proposed framework (Section 8).

2. Activity Recognition – Background

A crucial issue in biometric monitoring of behaviour is the recognition of the ongoing activity. Activity detection can be either performed as a pre-processing step in behavioural analysis or as a stand-alone application for triggering several types of alarms in areas under surveillance (i.e. identifying ongoing activities, detecting anomalies in the execution of activities, and performing actions to help achieve the goal of the activities). In both cases, the main challenge lies in the segmentation of the activity of interest in a given frame sequence [19]. In other words, it is in some sense necessary to identify the portion of the sequence supposedly corresponding to an action, in order to recognize each action that appears in a given sequence.

The interest in human activity recognition stems from a number of applications that rely on accurate inference of activities that a person is performing. These include, context aware computing to support for cognitively impaired people [24], health monitoring and fitness, and seamless services provisioning based on the location and activity of people. Applications enabling activity recognition methods may range from directly medical and healthcare issues [25] to Ambient Assisted Living [30,35] and to surveillance of secured areas [27]. In general, activity recognition methods can be categorized in two main approaches: methods based on various sensors placed on the subject to extract meaningful features and methods based on video analysis to detect human activity.

In [3], multiple accelerometers were used placed on the subject's body to estimate activities such as standing, walking or running. One of the drawbacks of the methods based on multiple sensors and measurements taken all over the body is that they often lead to unwieldy systems with large battery packs. Lester et al. [22] tries to overcome this problem by enabling a small low-power sensor board that is mounted on a single location on the user's body. However, the relationship between the extracted features and the corresponding activities still remains an open problem.

On the other hand, Zouba et al. presented a video-based, less obtrusive, multimodal approach for the automatic monitoring of everyday activities of elderly people in [36]. Specifically, video analysis from a set of video cameras installed in an apartment was combined with information from contact sensors installed on the doors and the windows and from pressure sensors installed on the chairs. The system was able to detect a set of activities such as dish washing, cupboard opening, walking into a room etc. Moreover, a real-time video understanding system, which automatically recognizes activities occurring in environments observed through video surveillance cameras, was presented in [9]. Similarly, a system for recognizing activities in the home setting using a set of small and simple state-change sensors was introduced in [32].

3. Behavioural Biometrics – Background

Behavioural biometrics refer to the unique way a person performs certain activities, such as gait, interaction with environmental objects, keystroke pattern, signature and voice. If processed correctly, all these features possess significant discrimination power, since they indicate unique characteristics of each person. Additionally, emerging biometrics can potentially allow the non-stop (on-the-move) authentication or even identification in an unobtrusive and transparent manner to the subject and become part of an ambient intelligence environment.

Typical physiological biometric [16] technologies for recognition like fingerprints, palm geometry, retina and/or iris, and facial characteristics demonstrate among others, a very restricted applicability to controlled environments. More than being obtrusive and uncomfortable for the user, static physical characteristics can be digitally duplicated, i.e. the face could be copied using a photograph, a voice print using a voice recording and the fingerprint using various forging methods. In addition, static biometrics could be intolerant of changes in physiology such as daily voice changes or appearance changes.

These drawbacks in the person recognition problem could be overcome with the mobilization of behavioural biometric characteristics [16], using shape based activity signals (gestures, gait, full body and limb motion, etc.) of individuals as a means to recognize or authenticate their identity. Behavioural and physiological dynamic indicators (as a response to specific stimuli) could address these issues and enhance the reliability and robustness of biometric authentication systems when used in conjunction with the usual biometric techniques. The nature of these physiological features allows the continuous authentication of a person (in the controlled environment), thus presenting a greater challenge to the potential attacker. Further they could potentially allow the non-stop (on-the-move) authentication or even identification [6,18] which is unobtrusive and transparent to the subject and become part of an ambient intelligence environment.

Previous work on human identification using activity-related (behavioural) signals can be mainly divided in two main categories. a) sensor-based recognition [17] and b) vision-based recognition. Recently, research trends have been moving towards the second category, due to the obtrusiveness of sensor-based recognition approaches. Additionally, recent work and efforts on human recognition have shown that the human behavior (e.g. extraction of facial dynamics features [13]), motion exploiting human body shape dynamics during gait [11,14] or motion trajectory [8], provide the potential of continuous authentication for discriminating people, when considering behavioural signals.

Moreover, shape identification using behavioral activity signals has recently started to attract the attention of the research community. Behavioral biometrics are related to specific actions and the way that each person executes them. The most known example of behavioural biometrics is gait recognition [6]. However, earlier, in [4,18] person recognition has been carried out using shape-based activity signals, while in [5], a method for human identification using static, activity-specific parameters was presented.

Prehension biometrics also belong to the general category of behavioral biometrics and can also been thought as a specialization of activity related biometrics [8,18]. In this concept, an interesting biometric characteristic can be the user's response to specific stimuli within the setting of an ambient intelligence (AmI) environment.

Table 1. Table with activities with high authentication potential.

Activities for driver pilot	Authentication Potential
Pull fasten seat belt	HIGH
Regulate radio/CD player	Potential identifier
Regulate air conditioning	Potential identifier
Check and adjust the Radio	Potential identifier
Put on / off glasses	HIGH
Handle steering wheel	Potential identifier
Handle the gear	Potential identifier
Unfasten seat belt	HIGH
Abnormal activities for driver pilot	Authentication Potential
Rapid move of the head and keep it there for a while	HIGH
Activities for office pilot (Fixed Seat User) & Activities for fixed work place pilot	Authentication Potential
Walking in the room	HIGH
Wearing protective clothes, e.g. gloves	Potential identifier
Using keyboard	Potential identifier
Writing (e.g. notes)	HIGH
Phone Conversation	HIGH
Throw away objects in the waste bin	HIGH
Drinking from glass	HIGH
Stretching (head, arms, shoulder, trunk)	Potential identifier
Getting up	Potential identifier
Abnormal activities for office pilot (Fixed Seat User) & Abnormal activities for fixed work place pilot	Authentication Potential
Hands up	HIGH
Pressing buttons too often	Potential identifier
Rapid, explosive action	HIGH
Sudden stand up	Potential identifier

3.1. Classification of Activities

The variations, that are exhibited by different users in the execution of the same activity [20,28], comprise the main difficulty for an activity detection system. However, this significant problem for activity recognition systems turns into a fundamental advantage when dealing with behavioural biometrics that try to exploit these variations to identify/authenticate individuals [8,28].

In this concept, various activities that can be adequate for authentication purposes in safety and security environments can be selected on the basis of their frequency, reproducibility, distinctiveness and rituality. According to the experiments performed in [1], there is quite a number of common, everyday activities taking place in work environments, which demonstrate high authentication capacity as shown in Table 1.

4. Detection of the Activities

Activity recognition is an important task of a biometric monitoring system not only for the segmentation of the activity from the full captured frame sequence, but also for the

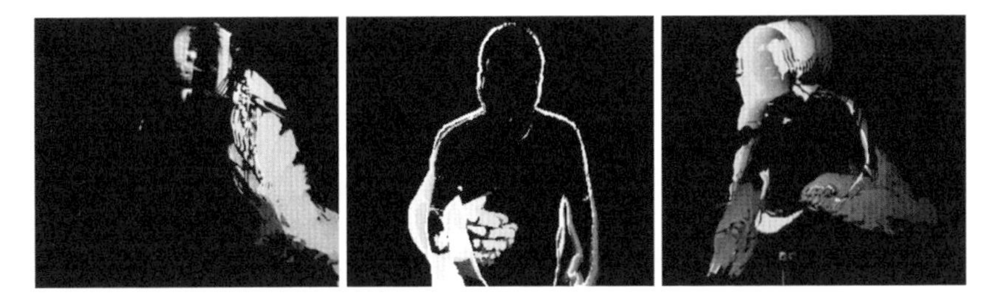

Figure 1. MHI samples: a) Phone conversation – b) Typing pin on a wall-keyboard – c) Talking to microphone.

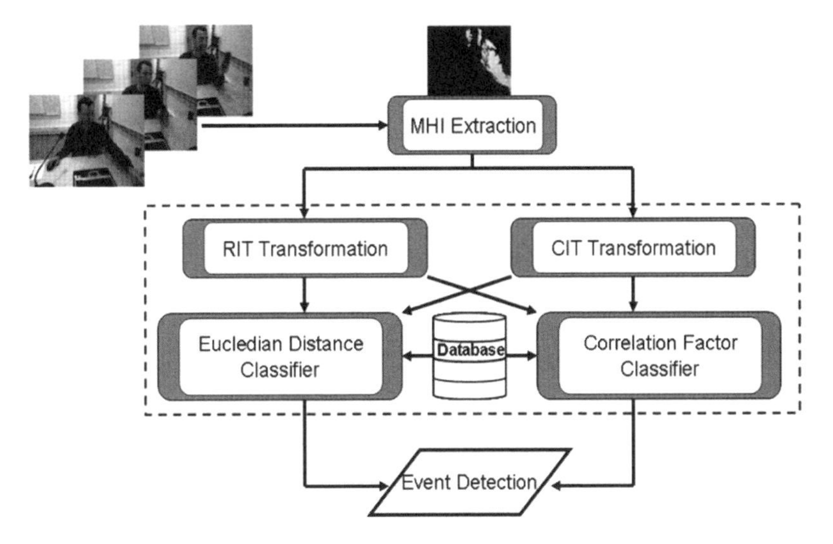

Figure 2. Proposed system for the event detection.

classification of the activities to Normal or Abnormal ones, in order to trigger specific alarms.

In the current framework activity recognition is performed utilizing utilizing the concept of Motion History Images (MHI) [4]. Specifically, a MHI is a temporal template, where the intensity value at each point is a function of the motion properties at the corresponding spatial location in an image sequence according to Eq. (1).

$$\mathrm{MHI}_T(x, y, t) = \begin{cases} \tau, & \text{if } D(x, y, t) = 1 \\ \max(0, \mathrm{MHI}_T(x, y, t-1) - 1), & \text{otherwise} \end{cases} \quad (1)$$

where the $D(x, y, t)$ equals 1 if there is a difference in the intensity of a pixel between two successive frames $I_{t-1}(x, y)$; $I_t(x, y)$ and τ is the number of frames contributing to the MHI generation (i.e. $\tau = 15$). The older a change is, the darker its depiction on the MHI will be, while changes older than 15 frames faint completely out (Fig. 1).

The proposed system for activity recognition through event recognition is presented in Fig. 2.

An MHI is extracted for each frame, using the last τ frames. The MHI is then transformed according to the Radial Integration Transform (RIT) and the Circular Integration

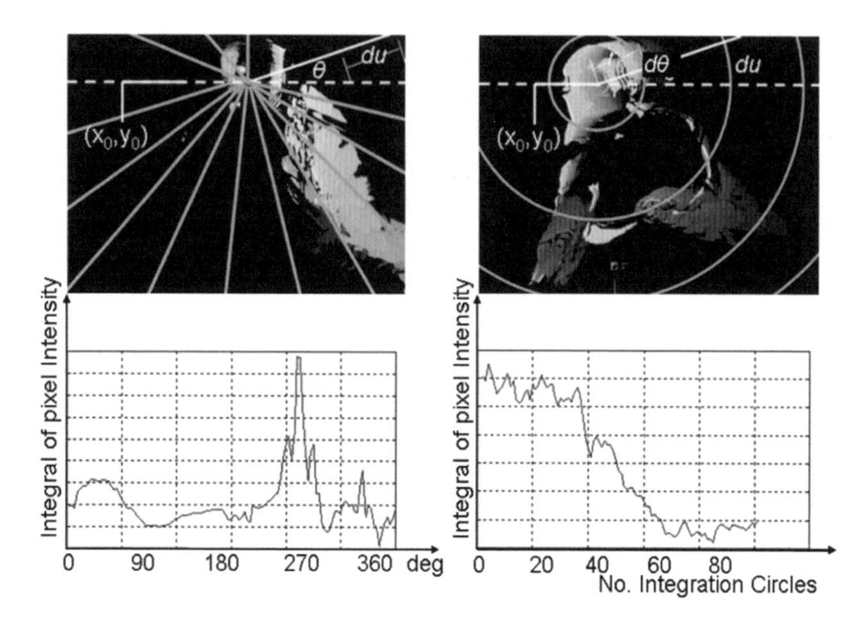

Figure 3. Visual description of RIT (left) & CIT (right) for the activity "Phone Conversation" and "Talking to Mic. Panel" respectively.

Transform (CIT) [31], which are used due to their aptitude to represent meaningful shape characteristics. The location of the head (x_0, y_0) is detected following the approach in [33] and is used as the center of integration for both transformations.

In particular, the RIT transform of a function $f(.., ..)$ is defined as the integral of $f(.., ..)$ along a line starting from the center of the image (x_0, y_0), which forms angle θ with the horizontal axis (Fig. 3 (left)). In our feature extraction method, the discrete form of the RIT transform is used, which computes the transform in steps of $\Delta\theta$ and is given by Eq. (2).

$$\mathrm{RIT}(t\Delta\theta) = \frac{1}{J}\sum_{j=1}^{J}\mathrm{MHI}(r_0 + j\Delta u \cdot \cos(t\Delta\theta), y_0 + j\Delta u \cdot \sin(t\Delta\theta)) \tag{2}$$

$$\text{for } t = 1, \ldots, T \text{ with } T = 360^\circ/\Delta\theta$$

where $\Delta\theta$ and Δu are the constant step sizes of the distance u and angle θ and J is the number of the pixels that coincide with the line that has orientation R and are positioned between the center of the head and the end of the MHI in that direction.

In a similar manner, the CIT is defined as the integral of a function along a circle curve with center (x_0, y_0) and radius ρ. Similar to the RIT transform, the discrete form of the CIT transform is used, as illustrated in Fig. 3 (right), which is given by Eq. (3)

$$\mathrm{CIT}(t\Delta\rho) = \frac{1}{T}\sum_{t=1}^{T}\mathrm{MHI}(x_0 + k\Delta\rho \cdot \cos(t\Delta\theta), y_0 + k\Delta\rho \cdot \sin(t\Delta\theta)) \tag{3}$$

$$\text{for } k = 1, \ldots, K \text{ with } T = 360^\circ/\Delta\theta$$

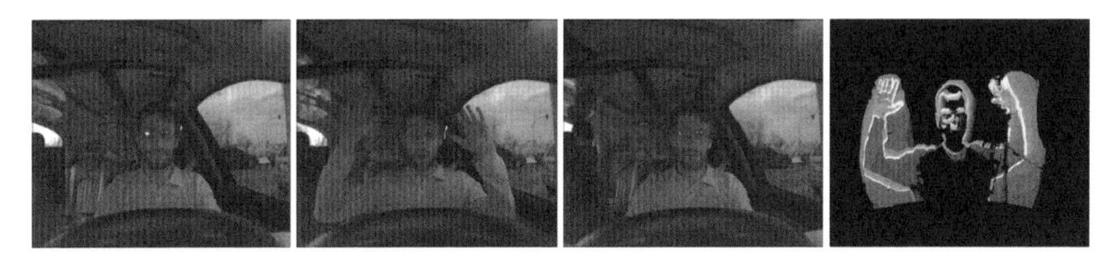

Figure 4. IR vision in driver pilot.

where $\Delta\rho$, and $\Delta\theta$ are the constant step sizes of the radius and angle variables and finally $K\,\Delta\rho$ is the radius of the smallest circle that encloses the grayscaled MHI (Fig. 3 (right)).

Similarly, the database consists of several sets of MHIs transformed according to RIT and CIT methods for each activity. Thus, an incoming transformed signal **x** is compared to a stored one **y** according to two separate classifiers; namely an Euclidian distance classifier, Eq. (4) and a correlation factor distant curves, Eq. (5).

$$D_E = \sqrt{\mathbf{x} - \mathbf{y}^2} = \sqrt{\sum_{i=1}^{n} (x_i - y_i)^2} \tag{4}$$

$$corr(x, y) = \rho_{\mathbf{x},\mathbf{y}} = \frac{\mathrm{cov}(\mathbf{x}, \mathbf{y})}{\sigma_{\mathbf{x}}\sigma_{\mathbf{y}}} = \frac{\mathrm{E}((\mathbf{x} - \mu_{\mathbf{x}})(\mathbf{y} - \mu_{\mathbf{y}}))}{\sigma_{\mathbf{x}}\sigma_{\mathbf{y}}} \tag{5}$$

The detected event is the one that has the most matches with the prototype MHIs from several subjects, stored in the database, according to the *majority voting* method. Accordingly, an activity is considered to be performed within the time period of two corresponding events. It has to be noted, an event is only then detected, when the returned scores from both classifiers exceed the experimentally selected thresholds, so as to deminish the false positives.

The same methodology can be exploited in settings with no light at all (i.e. driving a car in the night) via the use of a near infrared (nIR) camera as illustrated in Fig. 4.

5. "Measuring" the Behaviour

The novel concept discussed in the current chapter, suggests analyzing the response of the user to specific stimuli generated by the environment, while the user is performing everyday tasks, without following a specific protocol. An illuminating example of such an activity is a phone conversation, held in an office environment, while the user is seated at his/her desk. The expected response of the user to the ringing of the phone (stimuli) is to raise the latter and bring it to his/her ear before starting talking. Similarly, at the end of the discussion, the user is expected to place the earphone back on its base. Similarly, the typing of the personal pin on a keyboard panel reveals behavioural information (Fig. 5). Both of these activities are considered to contain biometric information, since each human is used to answer the phone in a different behavioral way (e.g. using different hands, moving the head towards the phone, etc.).

In the same respect, there can be found plenty, event triggered, activities in everyday life (Section 3.1), which can be very revelational about human behavioral biometric characteristics. Generally speaking, any activity could be revealing about the users' behaviour biometry. This information can be useful if we only manage to detect the starting and ending of the certain activity (Section 4).

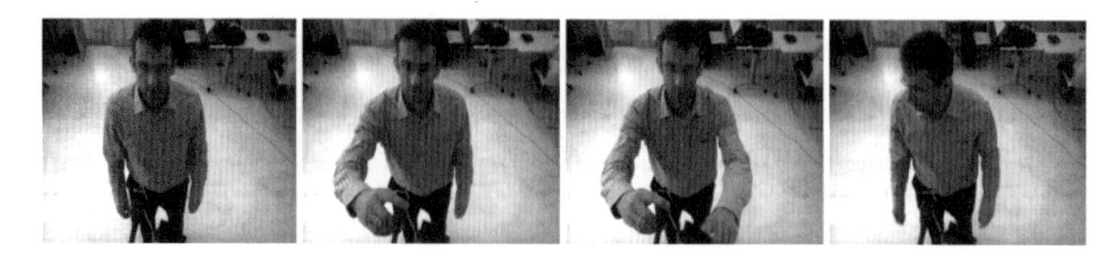

Figure 5. User typing his pin on a keyboard panel.

Initially, the event detection module identifies and extracts the image sequence that corresponds to a specific activity. This sequence is then processed so as to extract the user's static anthropometric profile that refers to the an upperbody skeleton model and the activity related dynamic features, which correspond to the motion trajectories of the head and the hands. Once small changes in the interaction setting have been handled via spatial warping of the trajectories, the full signature for claimed used ID is restored from the database and the actual extracted features are used to classify the user as a client or an impostor to the system via a Hidden Markov Model (HMM) classifier and an Attributed Graph Matcher (AGM). Finally, a score level fusion of both classifiers is performed by a Support Vector Machine (SVM) algorithm implemented on a Gaussian kernel and the validity of the final score is then verified by a quality factor based on ergonomic restrictions.

The novelty of this approach lies in the fact that the measurements that will be used for authentication will correspond to the response of the person to specific events being however, fully unobtrusive, comfortable and also fully integrated in an Ambient Intelligence infrastructure. The objective of our study is the description of a biometric system, able to authenticate a subject without the latter noticing any sensor and without having to wait or stand in any pre-defined posture. This concept is called "on-the-move biometry" [23].

5.1. Tracking

5.1.1. Face Tracking

The constant tracking of the face (Fig. 7a) is achieved via the combination of two different algorithms. Specifically, the algorithm is based on the use of haar-like features and their classification by the cascade architecture boosting algorithm AdaBoost [33]. This algorithm is extended with an object tracking method, which exploits the mean-shift algorithm [26]. The mean-shift algorithm comes into play, only when the face detection algorithm fails to detect the face on a given frame. As a last verification step for the correct tracking of the head, the skin color proportion in the detected head rectangle is calculated. If this proportion exceeds a certain threshold the detected face rectangle is considered as valid.

5.1.2. Skin Color Filtering

The skin color classification of the pixels on each frame I is implemented by setting constraints on the normalized values of both RGB and HSV color spaces according to [12]. This way, a skin-mask image $S(I)$ is acquired (Fig. 7b).

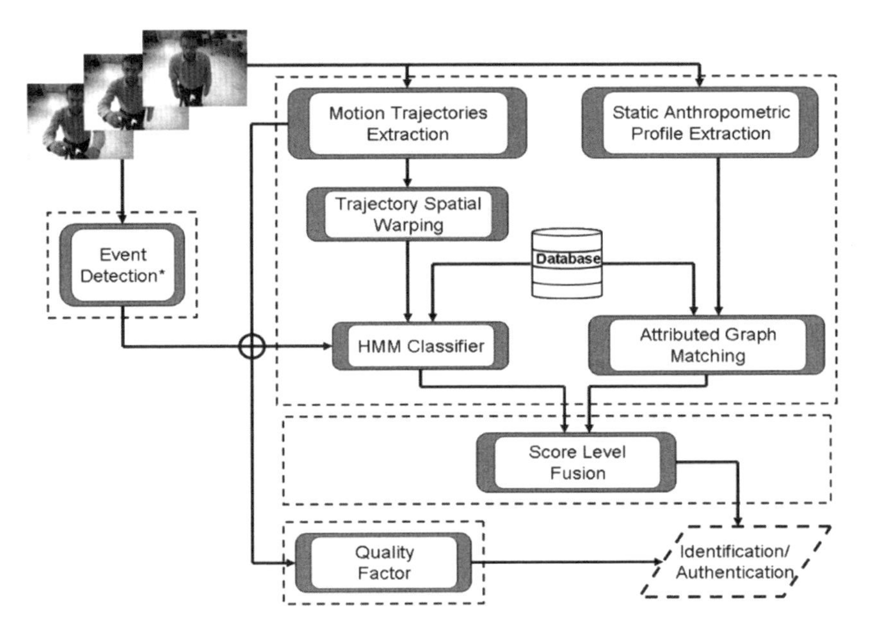

Figure 6. Proposed system overview.

5.1.3. Background Removal

In the current approach, all pixels that depict objects or humans with a bigger disparity value than the mean disparity value of the head rectangle are considered as background and are discarded as shown in Fig. 7d, including persons that lie behind the user's head. Thus, a second mask image $B(I)$ is obtained that corresponds to the active foreground.

The binary masks $S(I)$ and $B(I)$ are used to extract the active skin-coloured foreground (Eq. (6)).

$$D(I) = S(I) \cap B(I) \tag{6}$$

5.1.4. Motion Detection

Although the mask image *D(I)* has filtered out most of the unwanted information of the initial image *I*, it still contains a lot of noise (Fig. 7d), which deteriorate the accuracy of the tracking. Specifically, skin-coloured foreground objects, shadows, illumination variances, etc. could be removed, if the moving objects on *D(I)* would be detected. The final step towards the detection of the exact position of the two palms on each frame is performed by a motion detection algorithm. Therefore, the concept of Motion History Images (MHI) [4] is employed. An MHI is a static image template, where pixel intensity is a function of the recency of motion in a sequence (recently moving pixels are brighter) In our case, an MHI M can be derived for each pair of two sequential filtered frames $D(I)$ according to Eq. (7), as shown in Fig. 7c.

$$M_t(x, y) = \begin{cases} 2, & \text{if } D(I(x, y)) = 1 \\ \max(0, M_{t-1}(x, y) - 1), & \text{otherwise} \end{cases} \tag{7}$$

where by $t = 1, \ldots, N$.

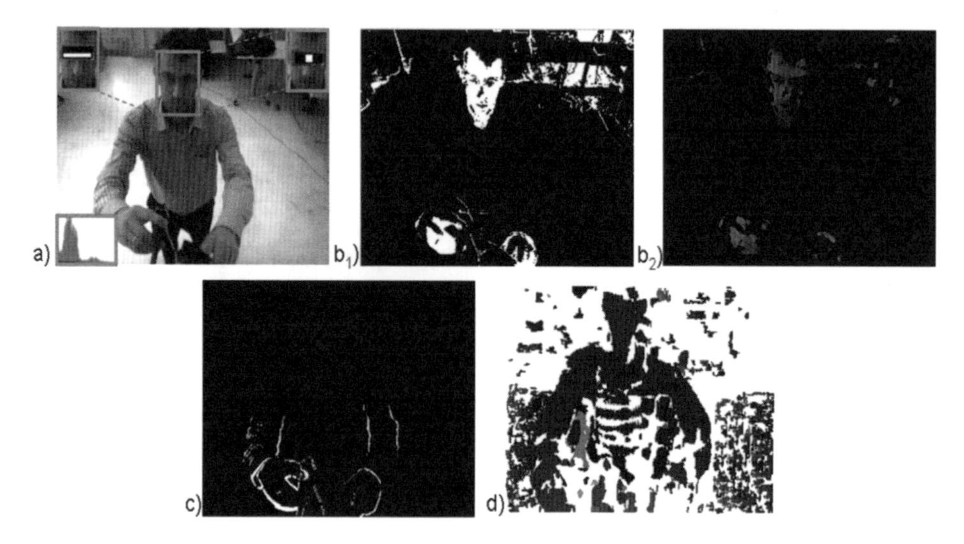

Figure 7. Applied filtering masks towards head and palms tracking.

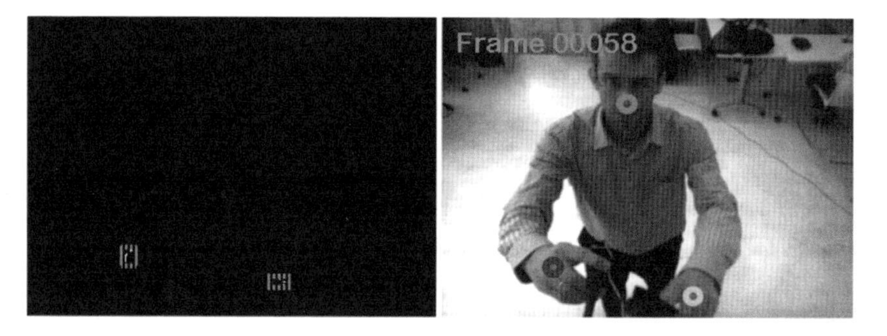

Figure 8. a) Remaining valid blobs after filtering. b) Estimated head and hand positions on the raw, initially captured frame.

The remaining active pixel-blobs (Fig. 8a) on each frame M_t indicate the users' palms with high accuracy. Accordingly, the head's and palms location are marked on the initially captured coloured frame as illustrated in (Fig. 8b).

5.1.5. Trajectory Extraction

Just like the approach suggested in [8], the estimated positions of the head and the palms on each frame are used to describe the movement performed by the user. Before the actual feature extraction, a series of normalization operations are applied to the trajectories. The trimming performed on these signals is a 4-step procedure, as shown in Fig. 9. Additionally, the transition from the 2D image to a 2.5D state and then to the real world 3D coordinates can be easily achieved via the depth information provided by the the disparity image (see Section 5.1.3).

The motion pattern for a given movement is considered consistent from trial to trial and independent of the movement speed assumption [20]. Based on this, it can be claimed that the trajectories of each body part for a given activity can be seen as a biometric

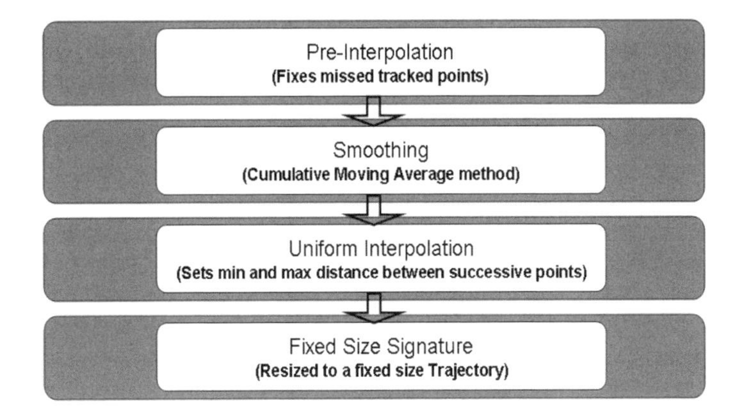

Figure 9. Processing of the raw trajectories.

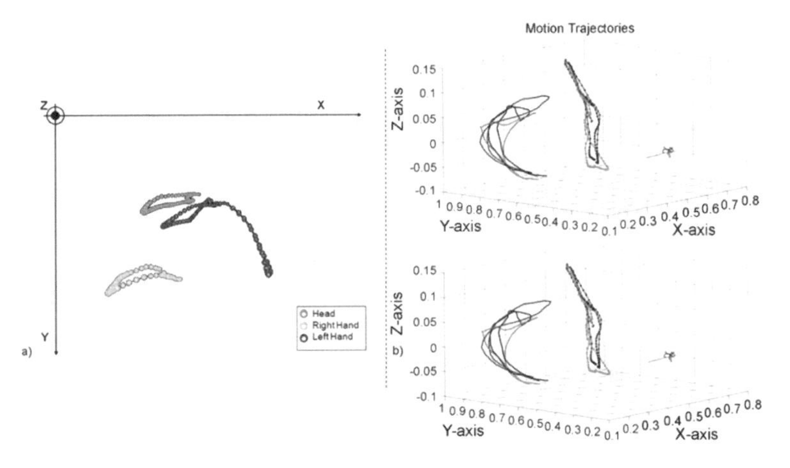

Figure 10. Motion trajectories illustrating the hand movement during a combined activity: a) "Interaction with an office Panel during a phone conversation", b) "Inserting a card before typing the personal PIN".

pattern. Thus, this motion patterns are going to form the main activity-related feature. Trajectory smoothing and homogenization is subsequently performed as described in [8]. Additionally, homogenization of the extracted trajectories is further improved by resizing them to a fixed, a priori set vector length.

The acquired set of smooth trajectories (head & two palms) is shown in Fig. 10. These trajectories represent with high accuracy the movement of the corresponding body parts. In Fig. 10a, depth is represented by the diameter of the circles.

5.2. Handling the Variances in Interaction Setting

The invariance of the extracted trajectories in slightly different interaction settings between separate trials (different positions of the interaction objects) is of high importance. Normally, an increased False Rejection Rate (FRR) would appear, due to variances in the interaction setting (object's positions, etc.) and not because the user is not a genuine client for the system. In order to provide enhanced invariability to the extracted trajectories, the concept of spatial warping is introduced, inspired from the Dynamic Time

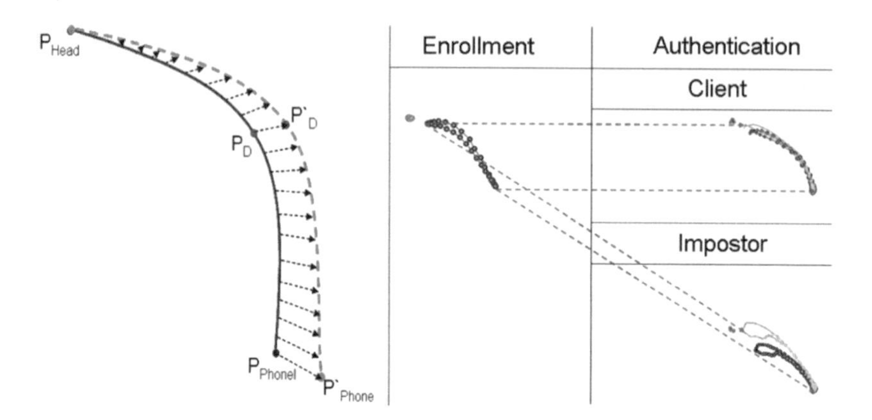

Figure 11. a) Visual explanation of warping method. b) Warping of trajectories.

Warping (DTW) method [29]. Without loss of generality regarding the environmental object, the case of a user answering a phone will be studied. In the sequel, the relative distance between the initial hand position and the phone is not expected to remain fixed, either due to a shift of the user's body or due to small displacements of the panel.

In a similar "Phone Conversation" scenario, where the user is asked to pick up the phone, there are two "extreme" positions of the hand that types the code. Specifically, these can be seen in Fig. 11b at point P_{Phone}, when the user has just touched the phone just before he starts picking it up and at point P_{Hand}, when the phone has reached the user's ear. The distance between these two "extreme" spots may vary even between the same user from trial to trial, since it depends on the slight variations of the environmental setting. Nevertheless, since we are mainly interested in the motion pattern of the trajectories and not its size, we apply the warping method on the hand trajectories.

Specifically, the exact location of these two points in the 3D space is automatically stored in the database for each user during the enrollment procedure. Accordingly in the authentication process, the trajectory is warped to the environmental characteristics of the enrollment moment.

In other words, the head-to-phone distance d is used for the warping (stretching/compression) of an incoming set of trajectories, according to the claimed ID. Specifically, the blue line in Fig. 11a indicates the actual extracted trajectory in the authentication stage. P_{Phone} and P_{Head} are the stored locations of the user's head and the phone respectively obtained in the enrollment phase. The suggested method indicates that P_{Phone} and P'_{Phone} as well as P_{Head} and P'_{Head} are mapped onto each other, while all other points P_D of the XYZ signature in between are linearly transformed to the new point P'_D as indicated by Eq. (8).

$$P_{D'} = qP(D),$$
$$\text{where } q = \frac{||P_{Head} - P_{Phone}||}{||P_{Head} - P'_{Phone}||}. \quad (8)$$

5.3. Confidence Metrics

Due to restrictions set by the structure of the human body, it is easy to understand that there are regions around the human, where the movement of the hands is more convenient

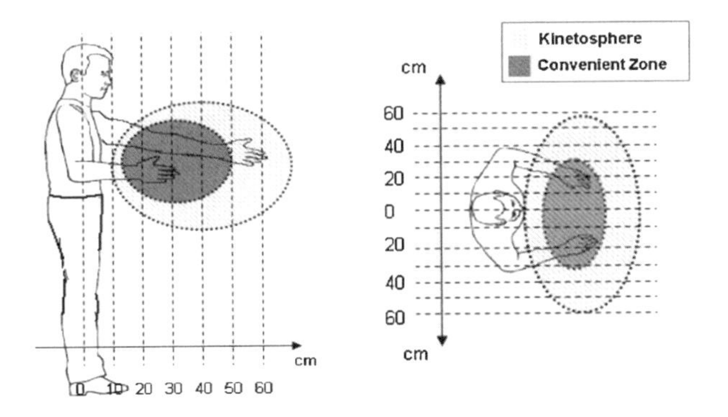

Figure 12. Convenience zones for a human.

than in other regions. These assumptions have been scientifically formulated in [21]. Specifically, it has been proven that the area in front of a seated human can be divided in three different spheres, according to the easiness with which the user can reach an object within certain regions (Fig. 12). It is suggested that the dark grey area is the one where the user moves most convenient and is thus called the "convenient zone". On the contrary, the light grey area indicates the "kinetosphere", whereby the user has to stretch or to bend his body in order to reach something. The white areas on Fig. 12 are out of reach for the user.

Consequently, it can be assumed that the user performs more relaxed movements within the "convenient zone" than in the "kinetosphere". Accordingly, it can be claimed that the movements within the "convenient zone" reveal more information about the user's behavioral response, since they are performed under no pressure or with force. On the other hand, the movements within the "kinetosphere" can be considered as forced movements. Thus, the ergonomic zones taken into account are dependent on the distance between the user's torso and the interaction objects.

As a result, an important metric about the quality and the evaluation of the extracted signature is proposed and is defined in Eq. (9) as the product of the tracking quality factor f_q (Eq. (10)), enhanced by a user-object distance factor b ($0 \leq b \leq 1$), which changes over the human ergonomic spheres (Eq. (11)).

$$f_{q,final} = b \cdot f_q \tag{9}$$

$$f_q = \frac{N_{missHead} + N_{missRHand} + N_{missLHand}}{3N_{frames}} \tag{10}$$

where $N_{missHead}$, $N_{missRHand}$, $N_{missLHand}$ are the amount of frames in which the Head, the right and the left Hand were not detected, respectively. N_{frames} is the total number of frames of the sequence.

$$b = \begin{cases} 0.1 \cdot d_{torso,object} + 0.5, & \text{if } d_{torso,object} \leq 5 \text{ cm} \\ 1, & \text{if } 5 \text{ cm} \leq d_{torso,object} \leq 35 \text{ cm} \\ -0.02 \cdot d_{torso,object} + 1.7, & \text{if } d_{torso,object} \geq 35 \text{ cm} \end{cases} \tag{11}$$

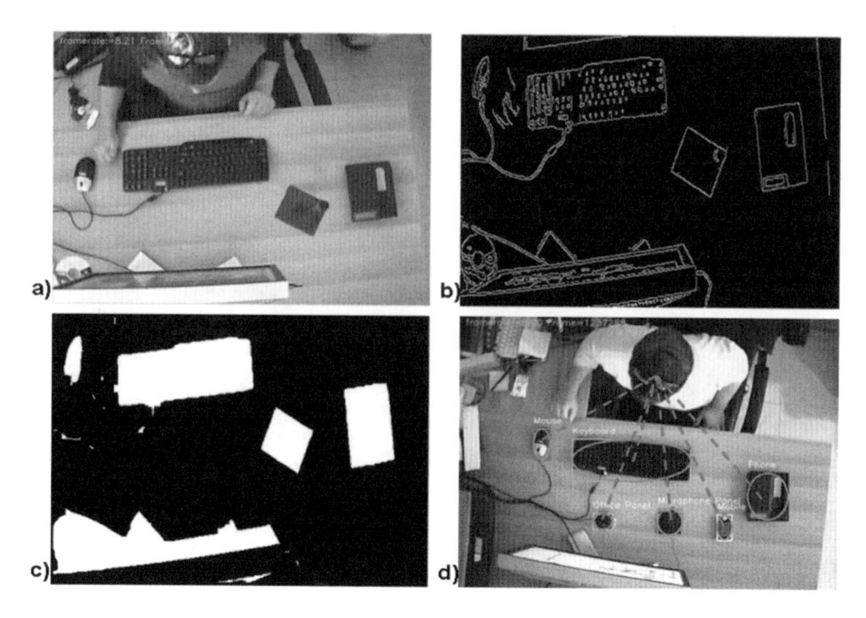

Figure 13. Object detection from top camera.

The lowest the quality factor the less probable the extracted dynamic features to contain valuable biometric information for authentication. Accordingly, if $f_{q,final} \leq 0.5$ the extracted features are discarded and no authentication process takes place.

5.3.1. Torso – Object Distance Estimation

In order the distance $d_{torso,object}$ to be calculated, both the torso and each object have to be first detected on the recording setting. Given that the head rectangle is detected as described in Section 5.1.1, the rectangle area below it refers to the user's torso. On the other hand, each object can be detected from the top camera as shown in Fig. 13. Generally, objects are coarsely described in a rotation-invariant way based on their contours. Specifically, each object is described by its aspect ratio, the area it occupies and its colour.

Since the two cameras are calibrated with each other, the distance $d_{torso,object}$ can be easily calculated, as illustrated by the red dotted lines shown in Fig. 13d.

6. Augmenting with Static Anthropometric Information

The robustness and the performance of a solely behavioural biometric system can be significantly improved by the fusion of soft biometrics (i.e. gender, height, age, weight, etc.) recognition capacity [15]. Specifically, soft biometrics can be implanted in any existing biometric system in the market and enhance its authentication performance, providing auxiliary information to the primary authentication module. For example the information about height can augment the information obtained by the primary biometric system. This approach has great potential when dealing with extreme database cases (i.e. the user is very tall or very short, the user has very long/short limbs, etc.) since in this case these characteristics are quite representative for the user.

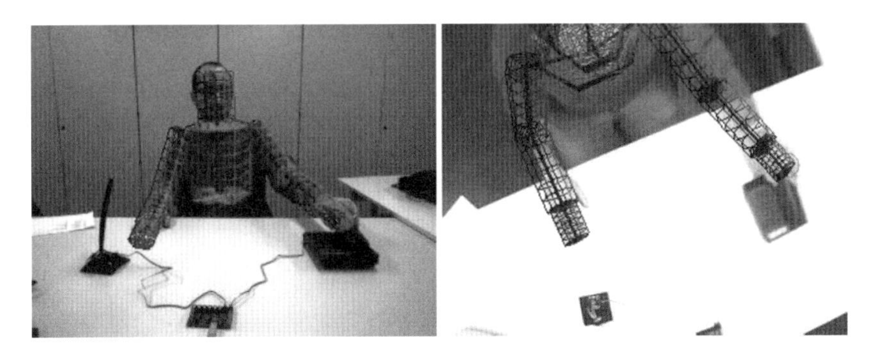

Figure 14. Adjusted skeleton model (frontal – top view).

Such a soft biometrics feature can also be considered the static anthropometric information about the user's body, which can be a significant enhancement to the authentication performance of the system described in Section 5. Thus, the architecture of the soft biometrics module is included in Fig. 6, whereby it is utilized in parallel to the proposed dynamic authentication system. The initial frame of the sequence sequence is processed so as to extract some soft biometric features of the user.

In the current approach, the static anthropometric profile for a subject can be estimated according to [2], which utilizes hierarchical particle filtering towards the accurate shape adjustment of the virtual model to the user's body (Figs 14a and 14b).

The proposed multicamera environmental setting (Fig. 14) consists of two calibrated cameras (i.e. a frontal stereo-camera and a top monocular camera). Furthermore, the skeleton model of the user is extracted and represented through an Attributed Relational Graph (ARG) $G = \{V, E, \{\mathrm{A}\}, \{\mathrm{B}\}\}$ [34], whereby V are the nodes, E the edges, and A and B the corresponding attributes, respectively. The nodes and the edges stand for the joints and the limbs of the actual body, respectively, as shown in Fig. 15. Attribute matrix **A** is not used, since no attributes for the joints are utilized in the current framework, while attribute matrix **B** corresponds to the lengths of the limbs.

6.1. Attributed Graph Matching

In some difficult cases, such as partial occlusions of the hands from other foreground objects or incomplete tracking due to bad illumination, etc., partially connected anthropometric graphs may be generated. Thus, the Attributed Graph Matcher (AGM) based on Kronecker Graphs [34] has been utilized, whereby comparison between fully and partially connected graph is possible.

Let us assume two random anthropometric Graphs G and G' as shown in Eq. (12)

$$
\begin{aligned}
G &= \{V, E, \{\mathrm{B}\}_{i=1}^{n}\}, \quad \text{where } n := |V| \\
G' &= \{V', E', \{\mathrm{B}'\}_{i=1}^{n'}\}, \quad \text{where } n' := |V'|
\end{aligned} \tag{12}
$$

where B_k carries the lengths of the user's upper body limbs.

The case of $n \neq n'$ indicates a Sub-Graph Matching (SGM), while $n = n'$ a Full-Graph Matching (FGM). In any case, Graph **G** is claimed to match to a sub-graph of $\mathbf{G}'$, if there exists an $n \times n'$ permutation sub-matrix **P** so that Eq. (13) are fulfilled.

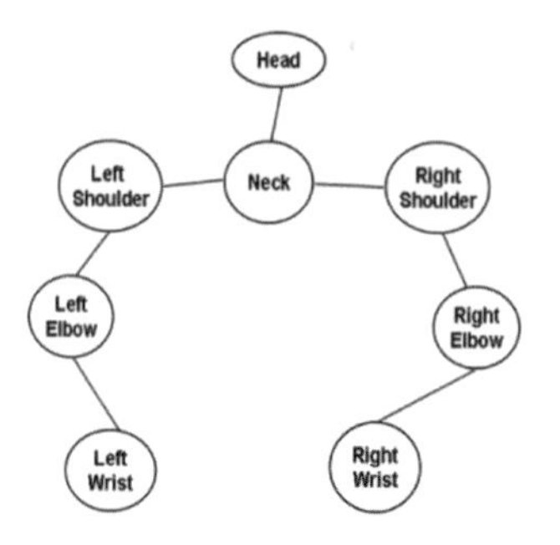

Figure 15. Adjusted skeleton model (frontal/top view) – Anthropometric graph.

$$\mathbf{B_j} = \mathbf{P_0 B'_j P_0^T} + (\varepsilon \mathbf{M_j}), \text{ where } j = 1, \ldots, s \tag{13}$$

where $\mathbf{M_j}$ is an $n \times 1$ noise vector and ε is related to the noise power and is assumed to be independent of the indices i and j.

To accommodate inexactness in the modelling process due to noise, the AGM problem can be expressed as the combinatorial optimization problem of Eq. (14).

$$\min_{p} \left(\sum_{j=1}^{s} \mathbf{W_{j+r}} ||\mathbf{B_j} - \mathbf{P B'_j}||^{\mathbf{q}} \right) \tag{14}$$

where $||\cdot||$ represents some norm $\mathbf{P} \epsilon Per(n, n_0)$ denotes the set of all $n \times n_0$ permutation submatrices and $\{\mathbf{W_i}\}_{k=1}^{r+s}\}$ is a set of weights satisfying $0 \leq \mathbf{W_k} \leq 1, k = 1, \ldots, r+s$ and $\sum_{k=1}^{r+s} \mathbf{W_k} = 1$.

7. Experimental Results

7.1. Database

The presented system has been evaluated on the proprietary ACTIBIO-dataset. This database was captured in an ambient intelligence indoor environment and is extensively described in [8]. More precisely, the current, annotated database consists of 29 subjects, performing a series of everyday office activities (i.e. a phone conversation, typing, talking to a microphone panel, drinking water, etc.) with no special protocol. Each subject has performed 8 repetitions in total, equally split in two sessions. Among the five cameras which have been recording each user from different angles, only the recordings from a frontal stereo camera and the top USB-camera have been used for the current work.

7.2. Activity Recognition

The performance of the proposed activity detection framework (Section 4) exhibited high accuracy, as illustrated in Table 2. The experiment that has been carried out on the 29 subjects of the database, forced a simultaneous search for the detection of four different activities. Namely, the phone conversation, the interaction with an office panel, the talking to the microphone and the drinking from a glass, have been looked for simultaneously at each frame.

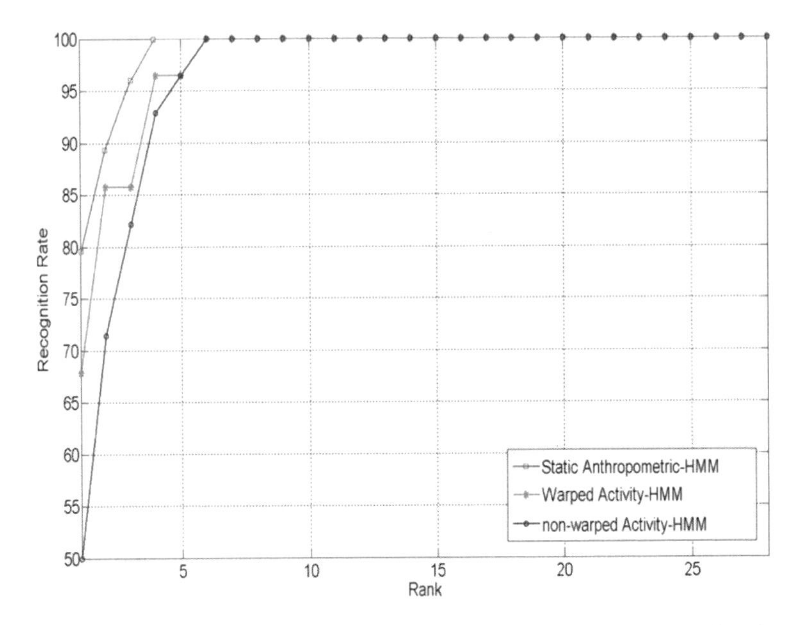

Figure 16. Improvements in recognition performance of the system due to the warping/static anthropometric method, respectively.

Table 2. Frequency of Special Characters.

Events	Phone	Panel	Microphone	Drink
Phone	93.1%	0%	0%	6.9%
Panel	0%	89.7%	10.3%	0%
Microphone	0%	10.3%	86.2%	3.44%
Drink	0%	3.44%	3.44%	93.1%

Activities, which gather a lot of (motion) energy in the same areas of the frame (i.e. glass and phone are on the same side of the user and are both brought towards his head), are most likely to be mismatched. On the other hand, activities performed on distinctive areas on the image (i.e. the users picks the phone with the left hand but leans to the microphone on his right side) are more likely to be distinguished.

7.3. Behavioural Recognition

In Fig. 16, one can notice the recognition capacity of the proposed system and the improvements performed, when applying the warping method (Section 5.2) and the static anthropometric information (Section 6) to the simple dynamic information.

7.4. Behavioural Authentication

Similarly, in Fig. 17 the authentication capacity of the proposed system is exhibited. Specifically, the Equal Error Rate of the two different activities is presented, when only the dynamic information is extracted. The score level fusion score from these two activities is illustrated with the red line in Fig. 17.

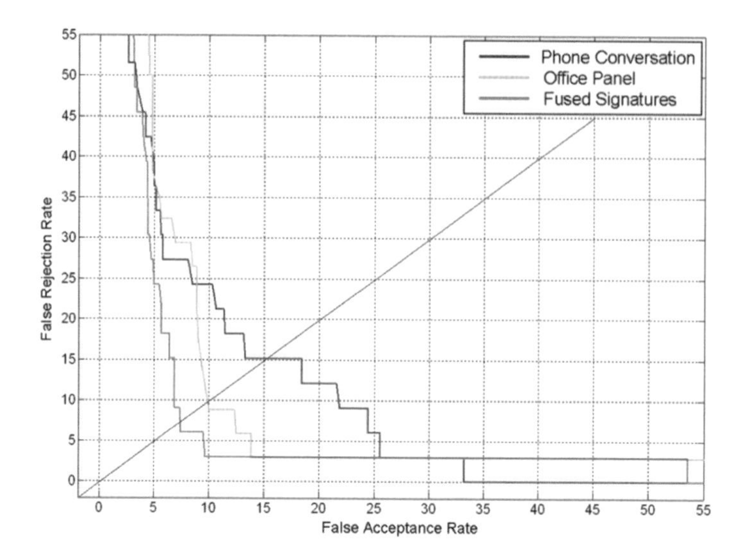

Figure 17. Authentication performance of the initial system.

The improvements succeeded in similar experiments, when applying the the warping method (Section 5.2) and when augmenting the algorithm with the user's static anthropometric profile (Section 6), are exhibited in Figs 18 and 19, respectively.

Of course, it is expected that for larger datasets, the authentication capacity of the static part to fall, due to increased number of similar bodytypes of the users. However, secured areas are not expected to have big amounts of registered users. Moreover, the static information is expected to be used auxiliary to the dynamic authentication method.

8. Discussion on Applications of Biometric Monitoring of Behaviour

There is little doubt that biometrics technology is very sophisticated and can be utilized in a number of ways, depending on the nature of the application. Fertile ground for applications regarding the biometric monitoring of behaviour can be found in the field of Ambient Intelligence (AmI) environments or Infrastructures (AmII), which are characterized by significant commercial growth nowadays.

8.1. Comfort-Oriented Applications

Specifically, AmI environments have the following characteristics:

1. unobtrusiveness – the devices embedded in the environment should not aggravate the users life or intrude into his/her consciousness,
2. personalization (i.e. it can recognize the user, and its behaviour can be tailored to the user's needs),
3. adaptiveness (i.e. its behaviour can change in response to a person's actions and environment),
4. anticipation (i.e. it anticipates a person's desires and environment as much as possible without the need for mediation).

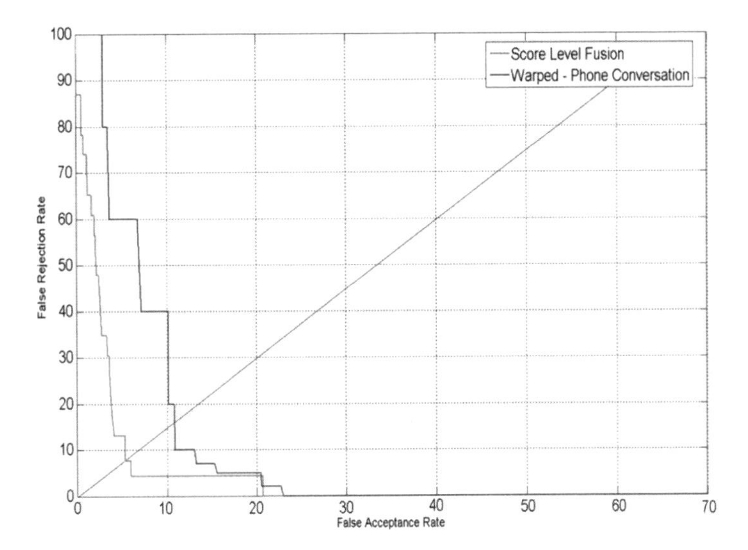

Figure 18. Improvements in authentication performance of the system due to the warping method (phone coversation).

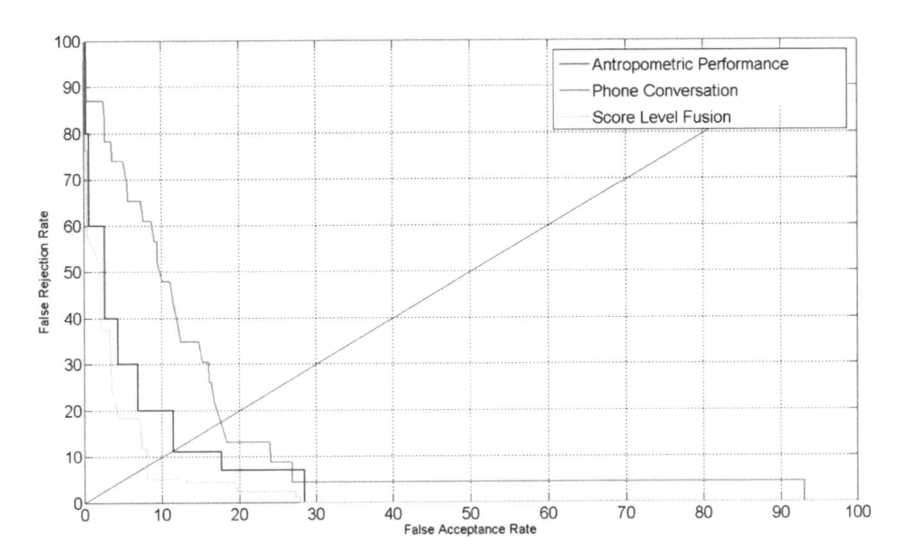

Figure 19. Improvements in authentication performance of the system due to the static (anthropometric) biometrics enhancement.

A smart home is a very popular example of an AmI environment, since it is a house that has highly advanced automatic systems for, lighting, temperature control, multimedia (e.g. control of home entertainment systems), window and door operations, security and many other functions. It appears "intelligent" because its computer systems can monitor so many aspects of daily living.

Biometric monitoring can enhance the performance of the Smart Home technology, offering intelligently control over home. Applying the unobtrusive biometric monitoring method, proposed in Section 5, the user will be authenticated by the way he/she moves into the room. The system will then be able to understand who the person entering the room is, and apply his/her preferences, e.g. favourite music, TV channel, lighting scene, etc.

A further application of the Ambient Intelligence is in the Ambient Assisted Living, which can be utilized in order to extend the time people can live in their preferred environment by increasing their autonomy, self-confidence and mobility (and thus, to improve their quality of life). Thereby, AAL can greatly help Europe to face the social change, which is brought about by the unprecedented demographic change: the share of elderly people to the entire population is steadily growing, while the share of the youngest (esp. the working population) is shrinking. Therefore, healthcare has nowadays a new aim, namely to increase independence, mobility, safety and social contact of elderly and disabled persons' through increased communication, inclusion and participation using available technologies.

Such infrastructures include new medical devices for health monitoring, home care and telediagnostics, which create large amount of health related information, usually from sensors organized into body sensor networks (BSNs). In this concept it is possible that the user does not accept that people other than his/her doctor (e.g. family members) have access to his/her medical record. A behavioural monitoring system undertakes the protection of these important and private data. Only authorized persons will be allowed to login to the computer or to the medical device. The user will be authenticated and will accept or deny the access, respectively.

In the same framework the development of systems, which automatically register and analyze the purchasing preferences of customers in real time, according to their daily transactions, is of great interest for commercial applications (e.g. supermarkets and shops) towards redesigning the shelves, forming the advertising policy, etc. Thus, the development of a customer profile system can be enhanced.

8.2. Security-Oriented Applications

Nevertheless, interest in biometrics was kick-started by the new wave of security threats, terrorist attacks and identity theft in the early years of this decade. With this as driving force, a biometrics-based technology (including identification and verification using human characteristics and behavioural traits) can be provided that will play an increasingly important role in securing information systems and physical assets.

Biometric technology for high secure access is important to both commercial and military community. Currently, biometrics is being investigated around the world as a means to manage borders and combat identity fraud. The proposed biometric monitoring methods (i.e. activity recognition and event detection) can greatly enhance the border control application and provide with the necessary unobtrusiveness such system requires. In such a surveillance application, the proposed behavioural biometric system provide a) enhanced security against trespassing and b) fully automated border control processing of pre-enrolled, trusted or frequent travellers.

In the same concept, the already well-established biometric access control applications for critical security areas will soon proliferate into many other areas where controlled access is required. The proposed framework is able to provide with the much desired continuous authentication that the safety critical infrastructures require.

Similarly, the field of forensics can benefit as well. The areas of both biometrics and forensics focus on concepts related to identity and are an integral to growing part of the security and law enforcement landscape. Thus, biometric monitoring of behaviour is possible to assist crime solving or at least be auxiliary for such purposes. The use of advanced behavioural biometrics that can be recorded on video, trajectories and gestures has the potential to dramatically impact the accuracy of making correlations in forensics at a stand-off distance.

Regarding the field of surveillance, the presented system can contribute with novel data analytics methods and information visualization to an unsupervised approach to abnormal event detection (Section 4). The detection of anomalous or abnormal events is extremely useful for surveillance operators located at airport waiting areas, metro stations, stadiums or even at supermarkets, because it is precisely this category of events that characterizes a situation in which action may need to be taken.

Last, the safety and security of hazardous materials transportation (i.e. off-route or stolen vehicles, drivers' attacks, lost or stolen dangerous goods, etc.) can be enhanced as well. In that extent, the current framework can significantly contribute to such a "biologin in the track/vehicle" and shipping application.

However, the issue of "big brother" feeling is arising when talking about behavioural tracking in AmI environments. The user should not have the impression that he/she is under control. Within the proposed concept all raw data from the cameras are treated in order to extract the characteristics traits that will be used either for authentication or specific event detection. Consequently, only the information required for the extraction of behavioural information is processed and stored, while all other information, such as pictures from third persons or timestamps are destroyed on-the-fly.

9. Conclusions

In this chapter the concept of biometric monitoring of behaviour has been extensively discussed and a novel behavioural, unobtrusive authentication method augmented by static anthropometric information has been presented, that is related to behavioural biometrics and that effectively handles small environmental variations in the interaction setting when performing everyday activities. The system is triggered by a robust event detection algorithm, while the quality of the extracted features is verified with respect to both, the accuracy of the tracking algorithm and the ergonomy of the setting. The proposed framework is seen experimentally to provide very promising verification rates. Although state-of-the-art solutions show inferior performance compared to static biometrics (fingerprints, iris, etc.), this drawback could be eliminated by the inferential integration of different independent activities and different modalities. Moreover, taking also into account that no hard constraints have been forced during the capture of the input signals, the proposed approach makes a step forward in the context of the very challenging problem of unobtrusive on-the-move-biometry. Moreover, the current framework is fully privacy enabled, since no obtrusive information about the user's privacy is being stored. Last, a series of modern and interesting possible applications for the presented system towards both Ambient Assisted Living (AAL) and highly secured environments have been presented.

Acknowledgements

This work was supported by the EU funded ACTIBIO ICT STREP (FP7-215372).

References

[1] ACTIBIO ICT STREP (FP7-215372), http://www.actibio.eu:8080/actibio.
[2] M. Alcoverro, J.R. Casas and M. Pardas, Skeleton and shape adjustment and tracking in multicamera environments (to be published), in: *VI Conference on Articulated Motion and Deformable Objects (AMDO)*, Mallorca, 2010.
[3] L. Bao and S.S. Intille, Activity recognition from user-annotated acceleration data, in: *Proc. of the Int. Conference on Pervasive Computing and Communications (PerCom)*, A. Ferscha and F. Mattern, eds, 2004, pp. 1–17.
[4] A. Bobick and J. Davis, The recognition of human movement using temporal templates, *IEEE Trans. Pattern Anal. Mach. Intell.* **23**(3) (2001), 257–267.
[5] A.F. Bobick and A.Y. Johnson, Gait recognition using static, activity-specific parameters, in: *IEEE Proc. Computer Society Conference on Computer Vision and Pattern Recognition (CVPR)*, Vol. 1, 2001, pp. 423–430.
[6] N. Boulgouris and Z. Chi, Gait recognition using radon transform and linear discriminant analysis, *IEEE Trans. Image Process* **16**(3) (2007), 731–740.
[7] Q. Dong, Y. Wu and Z. Hu, Pointwise motion image (PMI): A novel motion representation and its applications to abnormality detection and behavior recognition, *IEEE Transactions on Circuits and Systems for Video Technology* **19** (Mar. 2009), 407–416.
[8] A. Drosou, K. Moustakas, D. Ioannidis and D. Tzovaras, On the potential of activity-related recognition, in: *The International Joint Conference on Computer Vision, Imaging and Computer Graphics Theory and Applications (VISAPP 2010)*, 2010.
[9] F. Fusier, V. Valentin, F. Brémond, M. Thonnat, M. Borg, D. Thirde and J. Ferryman, Video understanding for complex activity recognition, *Mach. Vision Appl.* **18** (Aug. 2007), 167–188.
[10] A.P. Glascock and D.M. Kutzik, Behavioral telemedicine: A new approach to the continuous nonintrusive monitoring of activities of daily living, *Telemedicine Journal* **6**(1) (2004), 33–44.
[11] M. Goffredo, I. Bouchrika, J.N. Carter and M.S. Nixon, Performance analysis for automated gait extraction and recognition in multi-camera surveillance, *Multimedia Tools and Applications* (Oct. 2009).
[12] G. Gomez and E.F. Morales, Automatic feature construction and a simple rule induction algorithm for skin detection, in: *Proc. of the ICML Workshop on Machine Learning in Computer Vision (MLCV)*, 2002, pp. 31–38.
[13] A. Hadid, M. Pietikäinen and S.Z. Li2, *Learning Personal Specific Facial Dynamics for Face Recognition from Videos*, Springer, Berlin / Heidelberg, 2007, pp. 1–15.
[14] D. Ioannidis, D. Tzovaras, I. G. Damousis, S. Argyropoulos and K. Moustakas, Gait recognition using compact feature extraction transforms and depth information, *IEEE Trans. Inf. Forensics Security* **2**(3) (2007), 623–630.
[15] A.K. Jain, S.C. Dass and K. Nandakumar, Soft biometric traits for personal recognition systems, in: *Proc. of International Conference on Biometric Authentication (ICBA)*, 2004, pp. 731–738.
[16] A.K. Jain, A. Ross and S. Prabhakar, An introduction to biometric recognition, *IEEE Trans. Circuits Syst. Video Technol.* **14**(1) (2004), 4–20.
[17] H. Junker, J. Ward, P. Lukowicz and G. Tröster, User activity related data sets for context recognition, in: *Proc. Workshop on 'Benchmarks and a Database for Context Recognition'*, 2004.
[18] A. Kale, N. Cuntoor and R. Chellappa, A framework for activity-specific human identification, in: *IEEE Proc. International Conference on Acoustics, Speech, and Signal Processing (ICASSP)*, Vol. 4, 2002, pp. 3660–3663.
[19] D. Kawanaka, T. Okatani and K. Deguchi, HHMM based recognition of human activity, *IEICE Trans. Inf. Syst. (Inst. Electron. Inf. Commun. Eng.)* **7** (2006), 2180–2185.
[20] F. Lacquaniti and J.F. Soechting, Coordination of arm and wrist motion during a reaching task, *The Journal of Neuroscience: The Official Journal of the Society for Neuroscience* **2** (Apr. 1982), 399–408.
[21] L. Laios, $\Sigma \acute{\upsilon} \gamma \chi \rho o \nu o \eta$ $\epsilon \rho \gamma o \nu o \mu \acute{\iota} \alpha$ (Modern Ergonomy), Papasotiriou, Athens, 2003.

[22] J. Lester, T. Choudhury, N. Kern, G. Borriello and B. Hannaford, A hybrid discriminative/generative approach for modeling human activities, in: *Proc. of the International Joint Conference on Artificial Intelligence (IJCAI)*, 2005, pp. 766–772.

[23] J. Matey, O. Naroditsky, K. Hanna, R. Kolczynski, D. LoIacono, S. Mangru, M. Tinker, T. Zappia and W. Zhao, Iris on the move: Acquisition of images for iris recognition in less constrained environments, in: *Proc. of the IEEE*, Vol. 94, 2006, pp. 1936–1947.

[24] D.J. Patterson, L. Liao, K. Gajos, M. Collier, N. Livic, K. Olson, S. Wang, D. Fox, and H. Kautz, Opportunity knocks: A system to provide cognitive assistance with transportation services, in: *Proc. of International Conference on Ubiquitous Computing (UbiComp)*, Springer, 2004, pp. 433–450.

[25] T. Pawar, S. Chaudhuri and P. Siddhartha Duttagupta, Body movement activity recognition for ambulatory cardiac monitoring, *IEEE Transactions on Biomedical Engineering* **54**(5) (2007), 874–882.

[26] D.C.V. Ramesh and P. Meer, Real-time tracking of non-rigid objects using mean shift, in: *IEEE Proc. Computer Vision and Pattern Recognition 2007 (CVPR)*, Vol. 2, 2000, pp. 142–149.

[27] P. Remagnino, A.I. Shihab and G.A. Jones, Distributed intelligence for multi-camera visual surveillance, *Pattern Recognition* **37**(4) (2004), 675–689.

[28] D.A. Rosenbaum, R.J. Meulenbroek, J. Vaughan and C. Jansen, Posture-based motion planning: Applications to grasping, *Psychological Review* **108**(4) (2001), 709–734.

[29] H. Sakoe and S. Chiba, Dynamic programming algorithm optimization for spoken word recognition, *Readings in Speech Recognition*, 1990.

[30] D. Sánchez, M. Tentori and J. Favela, Activity recognition for the smart hospital, *Intelligent Systems, IEEE* **23**(2) (2008), 50–57.

[31] D. Simitopoulos, D.E. Koutsonanos and M.G. Strintzis, Robust image watermarking based on generalized Radon transformations, *IEEE Trans. Circuits Syst. Video Technol.* **13** (8) (2003), 732–745.

[32] E. Tapia, S.S. Intille and K. Larson, Activity recognition in the home using simple and ubiquitous sensors, in: *Proc. of PERVASIVE*, A. Ferscha and F. Mattern, eds, Springer, Berlin, Heidelberg, 2004, pp. 158–175.

[33] P. Viola and M. Jones, Rapid object detection using a boosted cascade of simple, in: *IEEE Proc. Computer Society Conference on Computer Vision and Pattern Recognition (CVPR)*, Vol. 1, 2001, pp. 511–518.

[34] B.V. Wyk and M.V. Wyk, Kronecker product graph matching, *Pattern Recognition* **36**(9) (2003), 2019–2030.

[35] J. Yang, B.N. Schilit and D.W. McDonald, Activity recognition for the digital home, *Computer, IEEE* **41**(4) (2008), 102–104.

[36] N. Zouba, F. Bremond, M. Thonnat and V.T. Vu, Multi-sensors analysis for everyday activity monitoring, in: *4th International Conference: Sciences of Electronic, Technologies of Information and Telecommunications (SETIT2007)*, 2007.

Handbook of Ambient Assisted Living
J.C. Augusto et al. (Eds.)
IOS Press, 2012

doi:10.3233/978-1-60750-837-3-178

Medical Information Management with ECG Biometrics: A Secure and Effective Framework

Foteini AGRAFIOTI *, Francis M. BUI and Dimitrios HATZINAKOS
The Edward S. Rogers SR. Department of Electrical and Computer Engineering, University of Toronto, 10 King's College Road, Toronto, ON, Canada, M5S 3G4

Abstract. This chapter discusses the feasibility of using the Electrocardiogram (ECG) for human identification. ECG falls under the umbrella of medical biometrics, i.e., physiological signals that are typically used for disease diagnosis, but also carry subject discriminative information. As opposed to traditional static biometric modalities like the iris, the fingerprint or the face, ECG is a time dependent signal affected both by physical and emotional activities. Therefore, one of the challenges that are studied in this work is the design of permanent and, at the same time discriminative features, which are robust to heart rate changes.

A feature extraction methodology based on the autocorrelation of ECG recordings is presented and evaluated on a public database. In addition, the advantages of using the standard 12 lead ECG system in the recognition process are discussed, and various fusion strategies are presented. Experimental results indicate increased recognition accuracy for the fused case (100% for 14 subjects).

Furthermore, this chapter advocates ECG biometrics as a natural choice for handling medical information. Given the medical origin of the signal and the fact that in a clinical setting this measurement is collected irrespective of the recognition task, an ECG based biometric signature can be used to manage the patient's information. A body area network (BAN) is described as the application environment, while the findings can be generalized for a wide range of clinical settings.

Keywords. Electrocardiogram, autocorrelation, linear discriminant analysis, biometric recognition

Introduction

As identity verification is becoming increasingly critical in our every day lives, the need for automatic and effective recognition solutions is prominent. Traditional strategies for human recognition rely on something that the user must remember or possess (for example ID cards, PIN numbers or passwords). Despite the wide deployment of token-based authentication, these entities can be easily lost, stolen or forgotten. The resulting security gap has been filled by biometrics.

Biometric characteristics comprise physiological or behavioral features of the human body, which can be used to identify individuals. With biometrics, the authentication modality is directly linked to the subjects and as such it bypasses the above mentioned

*Corresponding Author: Foteini Agrafioti. E-mail: foteini@comm.utoronto.ca.

shortcomings. Examples of widely deployed physiological features are the fingerprint, the iris and the face. Similarly, behavioral biometrics may include features such as the keystroke or the gait.

Every biometric feature has unique properties which make it appropriate for particular applications. For example, a face can be captured from a distance, thus this feature can be used in surveillance. Furthermore, some biometrics are more robust to attacks than others, or more publicly acceptable. However, for a feature to be used as a biometric characteristic, criteria such as the *universality*, *permanence* and *uniqueness* need to be met. In addition, it is of great importance for the biometric to be robust against attacks. Given this set of standards, it is difficult, if not impossible, to choose one feature that satisfies all criteria simultaneously. Every feature has its own strengths and weaknesses, and deployment choices are made based on the characteristics of the envisioned application.

This chapter proposes the use of the electrocardiogram (ECG) signal for biometric recognition. The ECG falls under the category of *medical biometrics* which is relatively new. This chapter is organized as follows: Section 1 introduces the ECG as a biometric characteristic and describes the motivation for this deployment. Section 2, discusses the proposed pattern recognition algorithm for ECG biometric signal processing. The same section reports the performance of this algorithm when tested over ECG signals from 14 individuals. Section 3 introduces the envisioned medical information management environment and extends the previously presented algorithm to the application settings. The reported performance of the enhanced recognition algorithm, for the purpose of handling medical records, is evaluated over ECG signals from 52 subjects.

1. Medical Biometrics

The medical biometrics technology has been developed to address security concerns with respect to falsification and replay attacks, i.e., attacks for which the actual biometric was stolen and presented to the system by an adversary. This set of physiological traits includes signals that are traditionally used for diagnostic purposes, such as the electrocardiogram (ECG), phonocardiogram (PCG), electroencephalogram (EEG) or blood pressure (BVP). The essence of medical biometrics is that, by definition, they constitute life indicators, thus decreasing the possibility of a replay attack. Furthermore, medical biometrics, being internal to human body, cannot be copied or falsified by third parties easily.

This chapter discusses the problem of cardiac biometric recognition, with emphasis on ECG signals. The following sections provide an overview of the advantages and disadvantages of this biometric feature, as well as the challenges of using it for subject identification and authentication.

1.1. ECG Biometric Recognition

ECG describes the electrical activity of the heart over time. It is recorded at the surface of the body with electrodes attached to specific locations. One can record a variety of ECG signals depending on the electrode placement.

The fact that ECG can be collected from any living human subject, directly establishes its *universality* as a biometric feature. *Permanence* is also satisfied among healthy people. Even though certain localized characteristics of the pulses might get distorted with time, the overall diacritical waves are still observable. Permanence will be demonstrated experimentally in the subsequent sections.

The *uniqueness* of a biometric feature is directly related to the underlying inter-individual variability in a population. In the ECG case, this is a result of several parameters of the cardiac function that controls the waveforms. Electrophysiological variations of the myocardium such as the heart mass orientation and exact position, or the timing of depolarization and repolarization add to the idiosyncratic properties of every subject's ECG waveforms [14,19]. What is more, the medical research community has long been focusing on diminishing this variability for the establishment of universal diagnostic standards. For instance in [12], where the objective is to determine the normal ranges of particular ECG waves, the inter-individual variability is treated with appropriate normalization.

Among the strengths of ECG in biometric recognition is its continuous property. This credential is suitable for long term monitoring and authentication of individuals, since a new reading can be acquired every couple of seconds to be used for recognition. Standard biometric modalities are static identifiable signatures, which lack this property. Continuous authentication can be vital in monitoring applications, e.g., for security in field operations of soldiers, fire fighters and policemen. In health care, ECG is usually collected for diagnostics irrespective of the recognition task. Thus, utilizing the same information to authenticate individuals and not requiring extra credentials, is conducive to data minimization.

On the other hand, ECG biometrics comes with enormous privacy concerns. Having been traditionally linked with medical activities that only physicians and authorized personnel have access to, it is considered as sensitive and highly personal information. When compromised, privacy is directly intruded, as not only medical information can be revealed, but also the current psychological status of the subject [13,23].

1.2. Signal Morphology and Acquisition

For the electrocardiogram to be recorded, electrodes are attached on the surface of the body in multiple configurations that provide representation of typical aspects of the heart cycle. Up to now, ECG has been under analysis mostly for clinical applications, as it can provide a first indication for a cardiac irregularity. However, ECG has only recently been suggested for biometric recognition [2–5,7,8,10,11,14–16,19,20,22,24,25,29].

From a signal processing point of view, ECG is a non-periodic but highly repetitive signal that is mainly composed of three waves. Figure 1 shows the most significant components of an ECG signal i.e., the P wave, QRS complex and the T wave.

The P wave has usually positive polarity and a duration of approximately 120 ms [26]. This wave mainly reflects the depolarization of the right and left atria. The QRS complex describes the depolarization of right and left ventricles. In normal sinus rhythms, its duration varies between 70–110 ms. Finally, the T wave reflects a repolarization of the ventricles and is usually observed about 300 ms after the QRS complex. However, its exact position depends on the heart rate and appears closer to the QRS complex at rapid rhythms [26].

The spectral characteristics of ECG waves are central to the application of signal processing algorithms. A healthy P wave is considered to contribute to the low frequency

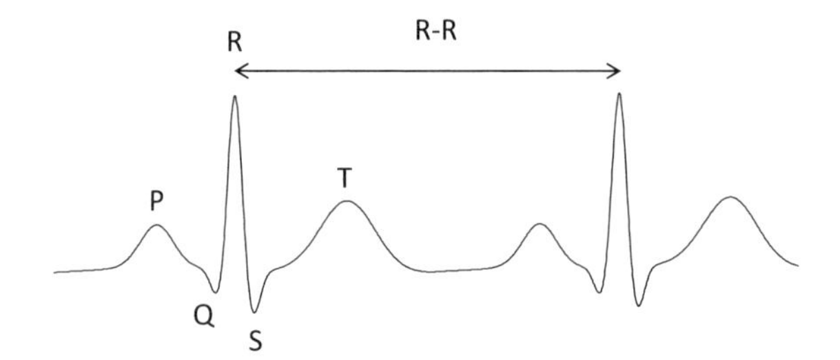

Figure 1. Major fiducial points on a heart beat.

components at about 10–15 Hz. On the other hand, a QRS complex has a spectrum of comparably high frequencies due to its steep slopes. The spectral content of this complex is usually found in the 10–40 Hz band.

There is more than one approach to ECG recording, such as the orthogonal leads and synthesized leads [26]. However, the most widely applied system is the *standard 12-lead ECG* where there are three main sets of lead orientations. The *bipolar limb leads* are usually denoted as I,II, and III and they track the electrical potential of the heart when three electrodes are attached at the right and left wrist and left ankle [26].

By convention, lead I measures the potential difference between the two arms. In lead II, one electrode is attached on the left leg and the other one on the right hand as depicted in Fig. 2. Finally, in lead III configuration, the measured potential is between the left leg and right hand.

Following the electrode position as pictured in Fig. 2, the limb leads are measured in the following combinations:

$$I = V_{LH} - V_{RH} \tag{1}$$

$$II = V_{LL} - V_{RH} \tag{2}$$

$$III = V_{LL} - V_{LH} \tag{3}$$

The preceding equations suggest that, having recorded any two of the bipolar limb lead signals, the third one can be directly derived.

The *augmented unipolar limb leads* fill the 60° gaps in the directions of the bipolar limb leads. Using the same electrodes, the augmented unipolar leads are measured as:

$$aVR = V_{RH} - \frac{V_{LH} + V_{LL}}{2} \tag{4}$$

$$aVL = V_{LH} - \frac{V_{RH} + V_{LL}}{2} \tag{5}$$

$$aVF = V_{LL} - \frac{V_{LH} + V_{RH}}{2} \tag{6}$$

The third category of lead orientation involved in the conventional 12-lead system comprises the *precordial leads* (V1, V2, V3, V4, V5, V6). These signals are recorded with 6 electrodes attached successively on the left side of the chest, thus capturing more detailed information in the electrocardiogram [26].

For identity verification one lead ECG is usually sufficient. It is however expected, and herein experimentally justified, that when more than one leads are used in the pro-

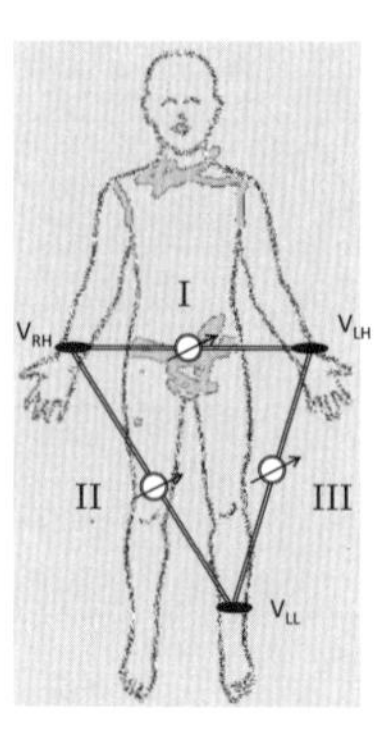

Figure 2. Configuration of leads I, II and III.

cess, the identification decision is strengthened. This property is similar to the multi modal biometrics idea, where individuals are recognized using multiple biometric modalities, to increase the probability of positive recognition.

2. ECG Pattern Recognition

The application of ECG biometrics fundamentally involves a pattern recognition problem, where the objective is to find unique waveform patterns relative to particular individuals. A standard recognition framework has usually three steps, i.e., *preprocessing*, *feature extraction* and *classification*.

In preprocessing, the acquired signal is subjected to filtering and artifact removal. ECG is vulnerable to both high (powerline interference) and low (baseline wander) frequency noise. This step cleans and prepares the signal for further processing. Feature extraction follows with the goal of determining features of high discriminative power, using machine learning algorithms. Classification is the process of matching the designed feature vector against the respective ones that have been previously (during enrollment) saved in the gallery set.

This section describes the Autocorrelation – Linear Discriminant Analysis (AC/LDA) method [6] which can be used for one lead ECG recognition. As opposed to other approaches [8,10,15,29], the AC/LDA does not require detection of fiducial points, which makes it appealing for real time implementation. Subsequently, a decision level fusion is presented, that strategically merges information from the 12 lead ECG system, to increase the overall accuracy of the recognizer.

2.1. The AC/LDA Method

First, to eliminate the effects of noise, ECG is filtered with a Butterworth band-pass filter of order 4. The cutoff frequencies of this filter are set to 0.5 Hz–40 Hz since the expected maximum frequency content of a heart beat is at 40 Hz (*QRS* complex) [26]. The AC/LDA method relies on the autocorrelation (AC) of an ECG segment for feature extraction. Since AC captures the repetitive property of the signal, the ECG segment should be long enough (approximately 5 sec) for a number of pulses to be included.

Utilizing the AC for feature extraction essentially eliminates the need for fiducial points detection, since a segment is allowed to cut the signal even in the middle of a

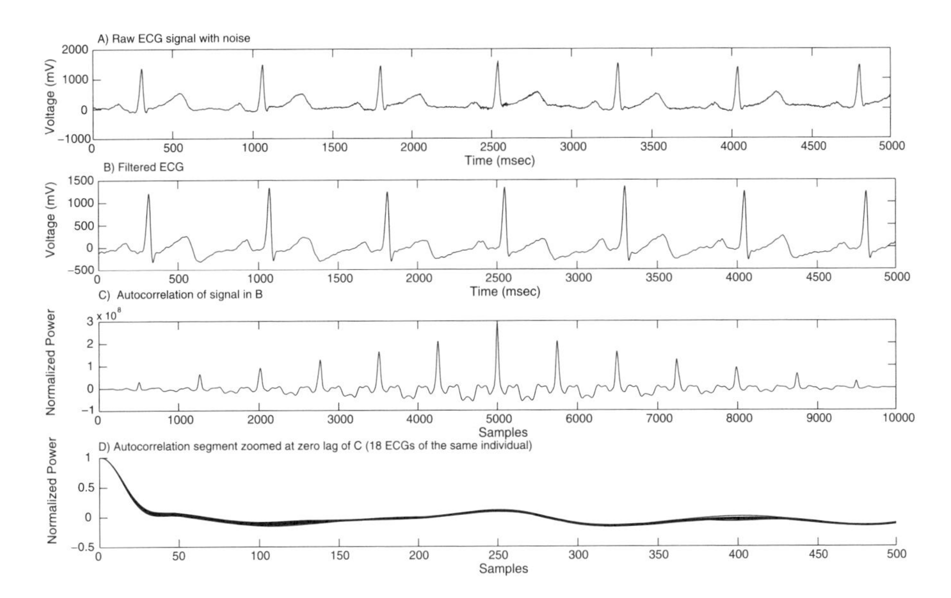

Figure 3. The AC/LDA method for ECG feature extraction.

pulse. Avoiding fiducial points detection reduces the complexity of the system and at the same time bypasses the risk of poor detection results. The autocorrelation of a repetitive signal, such as the ECG, captures the finest characteristics of the ECG's main waves that are repeated at every pulse. Artifacts or transient effects that appear at isolated pulses are not conveyed by the autocorrelation function.

Following filtering, the normalized autocorrelation (AC) is computed for every 5 sec ECG using:

$$\widehat{R}_{xx}[m] = \frac{\sum_{i=0}^{N-|m|-1} x[i]x[i+m]}{\widehat{R}_{xx}[0]} \tag{7}$$

where $x[i]$ is the windowed ECG for $i = 0, 1...(N - |m| - 1)$, $x[i+m]$ is the time shifted version of the windowed ECG with a time lag of $m = 0, 1, ...(M - 1)$; $M << N$, N is the length of the windowed signal and $\widehat{R}_{xx}[0]$ is the magnitude of the autocorrelation at zero lag. Out of $\widehat{R}_{xx}$ only a segment, defined by the zero lag instance and extending to approximately the length of a *QRS* complex, is used for further processing. Figure 3 graphically depicts the ECG signal after every step.

The autocorrelation is chosen for feature extraction because it explores the quasi periodic nature of the ECG. This is particularly important because typical cardiac disorders do not necessarily affect the ECG waveform in total, therefore the recognizer can be robust to them. In other words, only acute events detrimentally affect the recognition precision (atria fibrillation, premature ventricular contraction etc.). Isolated incidents, such as atria premature contractions that are very common among all age groups, are tolerated by the recognizer. More information regarding the robustness of the AC/LDA algorithm to cardiac disorders can be found in [4].

The Linear Discriminant Analysis (LDA) is subsequently applied on the AC segment. LDA is a well known machine learning technique, which reduces the dimensionality of the feature space. Given a training set $\mathcal{Z} = \{\mathcal{Z}_i\}_{i=1}^{U}$, containing U classes with each class $\mathcal{Z}_i = \{\mathbf{z}_{ij}\}_{j=1}^{U_i}$ containing a number of windows $\mathbf{z_{ij}}$ a set of K feature basis vectors $\{\psi_m\}_{m=1}^{K}$ is estimated by maximizing Fisher's ratio. This ratio is defined as the between-class to within-class scatter matrix. The maximization is equivalent to the solution of the following eigenvalue problem:

$$\psi = \arg\max_{\psi} \frac{|\psi^T \mathbf{S}_b \psi|}{|\psi^T \mathbf{S}_w \psi|} \tag{8}$$

where $\psi = [\psi_{\mathbf{1}}, ..., \psi_{\mathbf{K}}]$, and $\mathbf{S_b}$ and $\mathbf{S_w}$ are the between and within class scatter matrices respectively. Linear Discriminant Analysis finds ψ as the K most significant eigenvectors of $(\mathbf{S}_W)^{-1}\mathbf{S}_b$ that correspond to the first K largest eigenvalues. Having obtained the basis vectors, any test input window $\mathbf{z}$ is subjected to the linear projection $\mathbf{y} = \psi^T \mathbf{z}$ space by maximizing the between-subject variability and accordingly minimizing the within-subject one. In essence, this process outputs biometric signatures that are optimally differentiated from one subject to another.

2.2. Lead Fusion

The motivation for lead fusion is that ECG signals recorded simultaneously from different electrode orientations, can be combined to increase the distinctive information for every subject. Although using more than one leads is optional, the larger the amount of identifying information the better the chances of correct identification [5].

Fusion can be roughly performed in three different levels: the raw-data level, the feature level and the decision level.

Combining raw information suggests direct fusion of various sources for the same trait. In the ECG case for instance, one could average the signals from different leads. However there is no practical reason why such a process would offer more substantial information for subject recognition.

For feature level fusion, the data are concatenated in one feature vector with higher dimensionality, provided that the respective features are in the same type of measurement scale.

The third type of fusion is decision based. Different classifiers make identifying decisions on specific feature vectors; and the final decision is a result of a structured synthesis (such as majority voting). An extensive description of methods for combining the outcomes of different classifiers can be found in [30].

In this work, the AC/LDA features of different ECG leads are combined at the decision level, based on variants of the voting principle. More specifically, 12 classifiers are trained each on signals recorded from the standard 12 lead ECG system. We denote a classifier k is tested on an input x as $cl(x)^k$. The final decision is denoted as $CL(x)$. If the system has N enrolled subjects who can be identified, then every classifier would make a decision from the set $\Omega = 1, 2, \ldots,$ N. The following characteristic function is introduced to simplify the description on the fusion methodology:

$$\Phi_k(x \in C_i) = \begin{cases} 1, & \text{if } i \in \Omega \text{ and } cl(x)^k = i \\ 0, & \text{otherwise} \end{cases} \tag{9}$$

We introduce here four rules that guide the decision fusion of different classifiers.

- *Case 1*:
  This rule is used to make conservative decisions. Voting takes place, but the system rejects (*R*) the input unless all classifiers agree on the same cluster. The final decision $CL(x)$ is given from:

$$CL(x) = \begin{cases} j, & \text{if } j \in \Omega \text{ and } \sum_{k=1}^{12} \Phi_k(x \in C_j) = 12 \\ R, & \text{otherwise} \end{cases} \tag{10}$$

- *Case 2*:
  A less conservative rule for decision synthesis can be given from:

$$CL(x) = \begin{cases} j, & \text{if } \Psi(x,j) = \max_i \Psi(x,i) > 6 \\ & \text{and } j, i \in \Omega \\ R, & \text{otherwise} \end{cases} \tag{11}$$

  where $\Psi(x,j) = \sum_{k=1}^{12} \Phi_k(x \in C_j)$. Here an input *x* is identified as subject *j* if more than half of the classifiers agree on that (majority voting).
- *Case 3*:
  This case is a generalization of case 2, to accommodate more or less conservative decision fusions, based on the parameter α which takes values in (0,1]. The final identity of the subject is given from:

$$CL(x) = \begin{cases} j, & \text{if } \Psi(x,j) = \max_i \Psi(x,i) > 12\alpha \\ & \text{and } j, i \in \Omega \\ R, & \text{otherwise} \end{cases} \tag{12}$$

  For $\alpha = 0.5$ cases 2 and 3 are equivalent, so this rule can be regarded as a generalization of majority voting.
- *Case 4*:
  To account for situations of equal votes for two or more subjects, or cases where the final subject is chosen with votes which are not considerably higher than the second maximal, the final decision can be made using:

$$CL(x) = \begin{cases} j, & \text{if } \Psi(x,j) = \max_1 \\ & \text{and } (\max_1 - \max_2) \geq 12\alpha \\ R, & \text{otherwise} \end{cases} \tag{13}$$

  where

$$\max_1 = \max_i \Psi(x,i) \tag{14}$$

$$\max_2 = \max_{i-j} \Psi(x,i) \tag{15}$$

  When α is large, this rule becomes very conservative, since in order to assign an input to an identity, it needs to be supported by many classifiers and not to have opponents [30].

Table 1. Experimental results from classification of the PTB data from different leads

Lead	ECG Recognition Rate
I	97.2%
II	97.9%
III	97.58%
αVR	97.58%
αVL	97.88%
αVF	97.88%
V1	82.47%
V2	97.88%
V3	92.74%
V4	84.29%
V5	98.48%
V6	99.39%

2.3. Experimental Performance

2.3.1. ECG Signals

The performance of the proposed ECG recognition system, for the one-lead and multi-lead cases, was evaluated on the PTB [28] database. This database is offered for public use from the National Metrology Institute of Germany and the signals were collected at the Department of Cardiology of University Clinic Benjamin Franklin in Berlin. Each record contains the conventional 12-lead and 3-Frank-leads ECGs. The signals were sampled at 1000 Hz, with a resolution of 16 bit over a range of 16.384 mV. For the purposes of the current experiment, only healthy subjects were considered. Therefore, a subset of the PTB dataset containing 14 subjects for which two recordings were available (collected a few years apart) was composed. The older recording of a subject was included in the gallery set, and the newer one was reserved for testing.

2.3.2. One-Lead Performance

The normalized autocorrelation is computed using Eq. (7) on a 5 sec ECG segment, and the linear discriminant analysis is applied for dimensionality reduction of an AC window. The length of this window corresponds approximately to the length of a *QRS* complex. This is because this wave is less affected by varying heart rates [21], as opposed to the rest of the pulse. With this treatment, the performance of the recognizer will not be affected in cases of anxiety, stress and exercise, all of which may increase the heart rate.

The Euclidean distance is used as a similarity measure, and the nearest neighbor for classification. Given the 5 sec segmentation on the input, there are a number of ECG testing recordings available for every subject. The reader should note, however, that longer ECG windows are expected to increase further the recognition rates, at the expense of longer recording times.

Table 1 lists the recognition performance for individual leads. All lead signals have discriminative power and it is expected that the integration of this information in the right framework (multi-lead) can enhance the overall identification procedure.

Table 2. Rejection and identification rates under fusion cases 1 and 2

Case	ECG Rejection Rate	ECG Identification Rate
1	32.32%	100%
2	0.9%	100%

2.3.3. Multi Lead Performance

In order to combine the 12 leads at a decision level, 12 classifiers are trained, each on the corresponding source.The output of every classifier can be viewed as a binary decision for every class, given an input x. The four cases described earlier introduce rules which guide the fusion of the 12 decisions.

Decision level fusion may cause rejections (R), when the classifier is unable to a finalize a decision. Rejection can take place either because the system is too conservative, or the input is ambiguous. Essentially, rejection might be unacceptable for biometric identification systems, since the subject will need to be recognized with a different module or provide again his/her signal. On the other hand, it reduces significantly the possibility of illegal penetration. When the system is not absolutely confident about a person's identity, it sets off the alarm rather than assigns someone to a false identity. However, it is useful to configure a fusion framework, which would be conservative enough to detect intruders, and at the same time have as low rejection rates as possible.

The identification rates presented in this section are computed among the subjects that were not rejected by the system. The first rule is conservative enough, since a subject is identified upon agreement of all classifiers. As expected, this rule leads to high rejection rates, as reported in Table 2. However, in this scenario, the identification performance is 100%.

Since the second rule operates on majority voting, it is less conservative than the first and is thus expected to have less rejection cases. Table 2 shows that the window rejection rate is reduced to 0.9% while still being able to identify correctly all the subjects.

Cases three and four introduce rejection as well. In these cases, the degree of rejection is controlled by parameter α. This measure expresses the order of confidence about formed decision. Naturally, there is a tradeoff between highly confident decisions and rejection rates. The greater the number of the classifiers that participate in the voting process, the higher the probability of successful identification. Given that α lies in the interval (0,1], several values have been tested, offering 100% recognition rates. Accordingly, Fig. 4 shows the rejection rates for different values of α.

Even though the proposed framework was tested on 14 healthy subjects, the analysis was carried out for multiple ECG windows of every individual. The *training* set consists of 331 ECG segments, while *testing* was done using 324 windows. However, the feasibility of using ECG for human identification, as well as the benefits of fusing information from different sources are clear with the current experimental setup.

3. Managing Medical Information

Focusing on one lead ECG identification, this section discusses an application of ECG biometrics in managing health care information. The monitoring environment considered here, employs a Body Area Network (BAN), i.e., a wearable network of sensors which

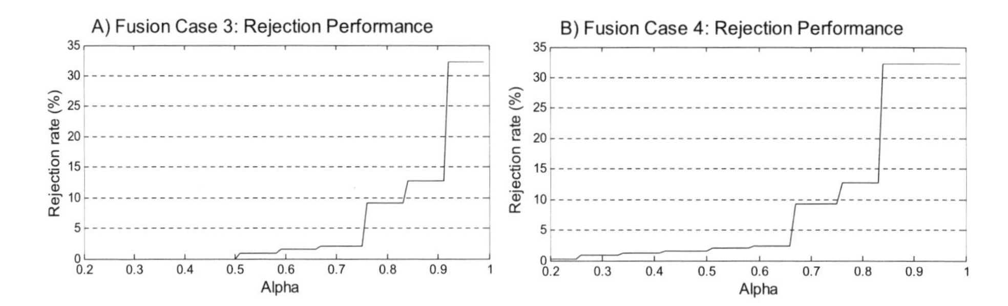

Figure 4. Rejection rate as a function of α for fusion cases 3 and 4.

collects various physiological signals and transmits this information to the monitoring authority (health care provider, nurse's desk and so on). However, the essence of ECG biometrics in handling information can be extended to other environments as well.

BANs offer a promising solution to subject monitoring. Their portable nature allows for unobstructed aggregation of medical information over a long period of time. A variety of signals such as BVP, PPG, ECG, temperature and so on can be collected simultaneously, to continuously assess the subject's well being. In such a setting, where ECG is naturally collected, irrespective of the recognition task, using it to manage the collected information instead of requiring extra credentials, works in favor of privacy and data minimization.

Medical information is very sensitive, and traditionally only designated personnel have access to it. With ECG being the focus of the current technology, it should be noted that a variety of cardiac irregularities can be observed, thus confidentiality must be guaranteed for any recognizer to become socially acceptable and trusted.

There are two ways to address this problem. One option is to use encryption techniques for any transmitted or stored information [27]. However, the purpose of this work is to design an architecture for information mapping which is unlinkable to a specific identity. Biometric data which cannot be linked to identities effectively limit their usability by unauthorized third parties. The proposed monitoring and recognition scheme is driven essentially by the privacy concerns of this technology. The two main norms of the system are:

- Any information received by the server is stored *automatically* to the respective personal file.
- Apart from the medical data, there is *no subject specific information* transmitted or used at any point.

To deal with these requirements, the proposed framework encompasses two modules (Fig. 5): 1) Data aggregation and transmission, and 2) Information allocation in personal folders. The first module runs within the BAN environment, while the second one at the server.

Module I: The BAN Environment Module I describes the internal functionalities of the BAN. Note that the physiological measurements depicted in Fig. 5 are only examples of vital signals that can be collected. This information can vary according to the requirements of a specific application. The BAN essentially consists of a number of peripheral nodes and one central node.

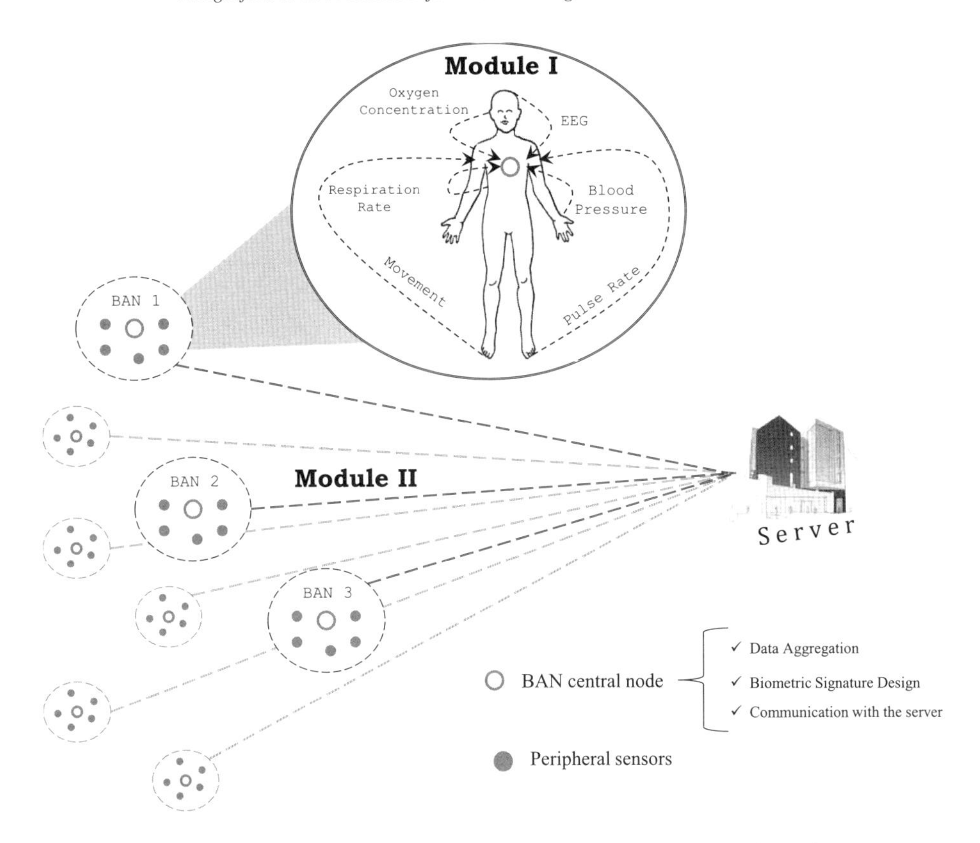

Figure 5. An ECG biometrics enabled system for handling health care information.

The peripheral nodes are transmission enabled sensors, which can have a cardiovascular origin or not. The essence of the network is that these nodes will simultaneously collect vitals and transmit them to the central node of the network. The central node is responsible for the centralization and transmission of the data to the server. This node is located on the chest, to easily acquire an ECG signature, that will also be transmitted. The ECG signature is based on the AC/LDA feature extractor that was discussed previously. Given the limited number of computations that are required for this process, feature extraction can be done with a micro-controller on the central node, without significant power consumption.

Module II: Information Handling Architecture Given a number of BANs that are simultaneously transmitting biometric signatures and medical data to the servers of the monitoring authority, the challenge is to automatically allocate this information to the respective personal folders. ECG biometrics are used in this regard, to match an incoming signature against the respective signatures of all previously enrolled subject that are subjected to monitoring. Matching is a two step process (Fig. 6), as follows:

1. **Identification**. This step performs a *one to many* match based on a distance measure. There is no a priori knowledge on possible identities. The output is a *ranked list of candidates*. However, identification itself is a very difficult problem, and the matching is usually not adequate for safe decisions.

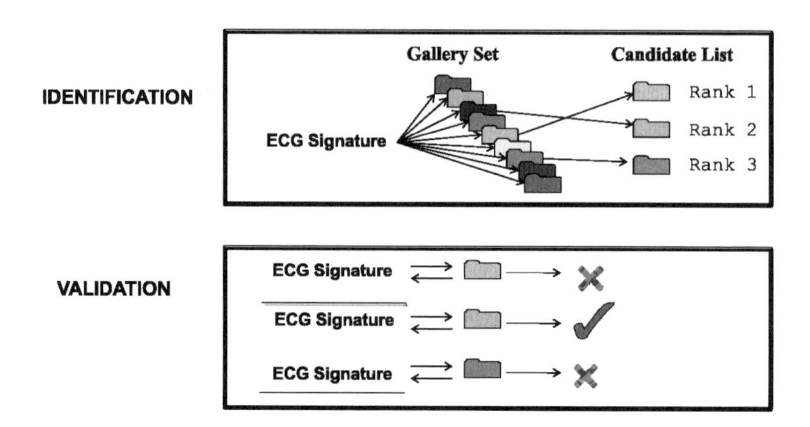

Figure 6. The two steps of Module II.

2. **Validation**. The ranked list of candidates serves as input for validation. The problem is transformed into a *one to one* match. Bound keys which are already stored in the personal files are used to authenticate one of the identified candidates.

This hierarchical fusion of the two techniques is expected to increase the confidence of the final recognition decision. Identification pre-screens the subjects and validations looks among a pruned space to find the possible match. More precisely, while the sole application of identification leads to misclassification rates that may be deemed unsuitable for practical applications, the secondary validation step reinforces the quality of identification. However, for validation, an extra modality is required to effectively strengthen the identification decision.

To this end, a scheme is employed based on the fuzzy commitment principle [9,17], which excels at addressing one-to-one verification problems. Since this comparison is based on a stricter and a more controlled criteria, the quality of the previous identification can be reinforced. On the other hand, the fuzzy commitment principle is unsuitable for pure identification applications, since the output is intended for a binary-type decision. As such, the described two-stage combination offers synergistic advantages derived from the two blocks in achieving a practical overall framework. The technical details of fuzzy commitment with ECG biometrics are beyond the scope of this chapter. The interested reader can find more information in [2] and [1].

3.1. Experimental Performance

3.1.1. ECG Signals

Two ECG recording sessions took place at the BioSec.Lab[1] of the University of Toronto, scheduled approximately a month apart, in order to test the signal's stability with time. Lead I ECG recordings from 52 healthy volunteers of ages between 21–40 years old, were acquired using a Vernier ECG Sensor[2] (1mV body potential / 1V sensor output). Each recording lasted for 3 minutes and the sampling frequency was set to 200 Hz.

[1]http://www.comm.utoronto.ca/~biometrics/
[2]http://www.vernier.com/

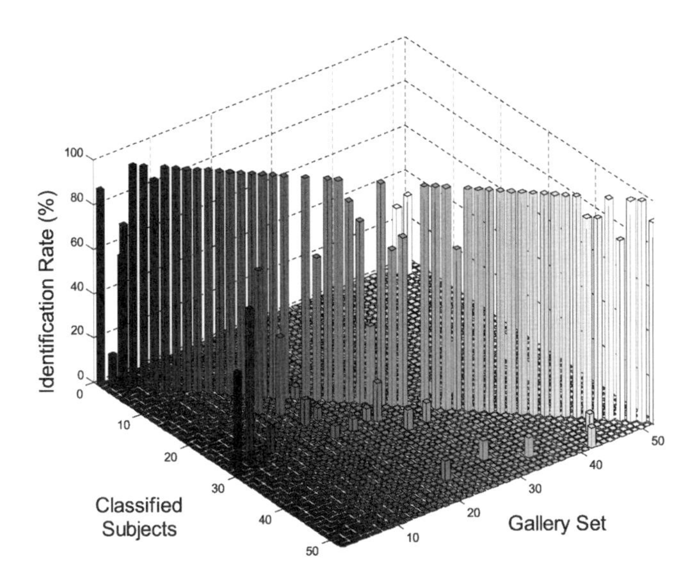

Figure 7. The contingency table for the identification step. 85.3% of the ECG windows are correctly identified.

During the experiments, all volunteers signed consent forms prior to connection to the sensor. Two electrodes were attached conveniently on the subjects' wrists to record one lead ECG. During the collection, the subjects were given no special instructions, in order to allow for mental state variability to be captured in the data. The signals which were collected during the first session were used for training the proposed algorithm, and accordingly the second's session readings were reserved for testing.

3.1.2. ID Management Performance

Every signal was segmented into windows, each of 5-second length. A Butterworth bandpass filter of order 4 was applied, with cutoffs at 0.5 Hz and 40 Hz, to suppress noise. Subsequently, the autocorrelation of every ECG window was computed, and normalized based on the zero lag magnitude as in Eq. (7). The LDA was trained on the first set of recordings, which constitutes the training set. Accordingly, every recording in the testing set was projected in lower dimensions using the trained LDA. The projected feature vector constitutes the signature that is transmitted to the server for matching.

At the server, for the *identification* step, classification was performed using the nearest neighbor classifier, and using Euclidean distance as the similarity measure. The output of this step is a ranked list of identities, i.e., file indices for every input ECG to be recognized. Due to the nature of biometrics, the first ranked result, i.e., the best match, is not always the correct class, because of the inherent intra-class variability and the stochastic nature of the signal.

The identification performance is graphically depicted in Fig. 7 which is a bar plot of the contingency matrix. In a perfect system, the diagonal is expected to show 100% recognition for all subjects. Up to this point, the average identification performance is 85.3%. Nevertheless, this step manages to accurately prune the search space as reported in Table 3. There are however cases of lower ranking for the correct class (6.29% was ranked second and 2.54% third) which suggests that if recognition depended entirely on first ranked results, ID management would be compromised.

Table 3. Identification performance based on ranking of the true class

Rank of correct class	Percentage of ECG windows
1	85.3%
2	6.29%
3	2.54%
4	0.3%
5	0.75%
6	1.05%
7	0.15%
8	0%
9	0.15%
10	3.4%

Table 4. Verification performance for two triplet cases

BCH triplet	FAR	FRR	Verification Rate
(31,6,7)	7.6%	11.2%	92.4%
(31,11,5)	5.1%	17.8%	94.9%

An information management application typically does not tolerate such incorrectly classified data, and for this reason, the validation step is applied to reduce the possibility of false acceptance. In this subsequent step, the Bose-Chaudhuri-Hocquenghem (BCH) family is employed as the error-correcting code scheme. Details regarding the code construction and properties can be found in [18]. In essence, this code is governed by three parameters i.e., code dimension, information dimension, error-correction capability. Tuning these parameters can make the code more or less stringent, which will directly affect the authentication rate, the false acceptance (FAR) and rejection (FRR) rates, defined as follows:

- **Authentication Rate** Percentage of ECG windows for which the true class was ranked first, and the system accepted the pair.
- **FAR** Percentage of ECG windows for which the correct class was not ranked first, and the system accepted the pair.
- **FRR** Percentage of ECG windows for which the correct class was ranked first, but the system rejected the pair.

In biometric systems, there is an inherent tradeoff between authentication, false acceptance and false rejection i.e., the more the subjects that are correctly authenticated the higher the chances of authenticating an intruder as well. Table 4 lists the verification rate along with the corresponding FAR and FRR for two BCH triplet cases. In both scenarios the verification rate increases significantly, to ensure a better overall recognition performance.

4. Conclusion

As the technology for falsification advances, accurate, robust and reliable identification of individuals becomes increasingly critical. Conventional strategies for identity authentication rely on entities or passwords that the user must remember or possess (ID cards,

PIN numbers, tokens etc.). Although the security gap is nowadays filled by typical biometric modalities such the fingerprint or the iris, there is still a high risk of systems being fooled with falsified credentials.

In this chapter, a human identification system based on the electrocardiogram signal is reported. The AC/LDA method for feature extraction is presented, to provide a means of analyzing ECG without fiducial points detection, suitable for the design of highly discriminative features in a population. In addition, the benefits of using the 12-lead ECG system for subject recognition are discussed. A multi-modal framework is presented, to fuse the information from the 12 sources at a decision level. The employment of all lead signals in the recognition process increases significantly the accuracy of the recognizer, at the expense of increased intrusiveness to the user.

Furthermore, a privacy-oriented BAN topology is explored in a health monitoring setting. Since it has been previously established that medical biometrics will play an important role in realizing security in BAN, the dual goal is to investigate the use of the ECG biometric in the topology. It is argued that ECG identification itself may not be able to provide sufficient performance for typical applications, however the incorporation of a secondary external factor, i.e., a validation key can be beneficial.

A two-stage framework is envisioned, in which the ECG identification block first performs an *one to many* match in order to find possible candidates from the database, and then validation takes over with *one to one* searches between the input and the identified candidates. This secondary step is shown to offer more flexibility in achieving improved classification rates. Subsequently, ECG can be strategically employed in medical environments for the distribution of incoming information to the appropriate medical files and can provide a sound alternative to patient authentication.

Acknowledgements

This work has been supported by the Natural Sciences and Engineering Research Council of Canada (NSERC).

References

[1] F. Agrafioti, F. M. Bui and D. Hatzinakos, Medical biometrics in mobile health monitoring, *Security and Communication Networks* (July 2010), 10.1002/sec.227.

[2] F. Agrafioti, F.M. Bui and D. Hatzinakos, On supporting anonymity in a BAN biometric framework, in: *16th International Conference on Digital Signal Processing*, July 2009, pp. 1–6.

[3] F. Agrafioti, F.M. Bui and D. Hatzinakos, Medical biometrics: The perils of ignoring time dependency, in: *IEEE 3rd International Conference on Biometrics: Theory, Applications, and Systems, 2009. BTAS'09*, Sept. 2009, pp. 1–6.

[4] F. Agrafioti and D. Hatzinakos, ECG biometric analysis in cardiac irregularity conditions, *Signal, Image and Video Processing* (2008), 1863–1703.

[5] F. Agrafioti and D. Hatzinakos, Fusion of ECG sources for human identification, in: *Third International Symposium on Communications, Control and Signal Processing (ISCCSP)*, Malta, March 2008.

[6] F. Agrafioti and D. Hatzinakos, Ecg based recognition using second order statistics, in: *6th Annual Communication Networks and Services Research Conference*, May 2008, pp. 82–87.

[7] F. Agrafioti and D. Hatzinakos, Signal validation for cardiac biometrics, in: *IEEE International Conference on Acoustics Speech and Signal Processing (ICASSP)*, Mar. 2010, pp. 1734–1737.

[8] L. Biel, O. Pettersson, L. Philipson and P. Wide, ECG analysis: A new approach in human identification, *IEEE Trans. on Instrumentation and Measurement* **50**(3) (2001) 808–812.
[9] F.M. Bui and D. Hatzinakos, Biometric methods for secure communications in body sensor networks: Resource-efficient key management and signal-level data scrambling, *EURASIP Journal on Advances in Signal Processing* (2008), 1–16.
[10] A.D.C. Chan, M.M. Hamdy, A. Badre and V. Badee, Wavelet distance measure for person identification using electrocardiograms, *IEEE Transactions on Instrumentation and Measurement* **57**(2) (Feb. 2008).
[11] D.P. Coutinho, A.L.N. Fred and M.A.T. Figueiredo, One-lead ECG-based personal identification using ziv-merhav cross parsing, in: *20th International Conference on Pattern Recognition (ICPR)*, Aug. 2010, pp. 3858–3861.
[12] H. Draper, C. Peffer, F. Stallmann, D. Littmann and H. Pipberger, The corrected orthogonal electrocardiogram and vectorcardiogram in 510 normal men (frank lead system), *Circulation* **30** (1964), 853–864.
[13] A.F. Folino, G. Buja, P. Turrini, L. Oselladore and A. Nava, The effects of sympathetic stimulation induced by mental stress on signal averages electrocardiogram, *International Journal of Cardiology* **48** (1995), 279–285.
[14] R. Hoekema, G.Uijen and A. van Oosterom, Geometrical aspect of the interindividual variaility of multilead ECG recordings, *IEEE Trans. Biomed. Eng.* **48** (2001), 551–559.
[15] S.A. Israel, J.M. Irvine, A. Cheng, M.D. Wiederhold and B.K. Wiederhold, ECG to identify individuals, *Pattern Recognition* **38**(1) (2005), 133–142.
[16] S.A. Israel, W.T. Scruggs, W.J. Worek and J.M. Irvine, Fusing face and ecg for personal identification, in: *Proc. of 32nd Applied Imagery Pattern Recognition Workshop*, 2003, pp. 226–231.
[17] A. Juels and M. Wattenberg, A fuzzy commitment scheme, in: *Proc. 6th ACM Conf. Comp. and Commun. Sec.*, 1999, pp. 28–36.
[18] G. Kabatiansky, E. Krouk and S. Semenov, *Error Correcting Coding and Security for Data Networks: Analysis of the Superchannel Concept*, John Wiley and Sons, 2005.
[19] G. Kozmann, R.L. Lux and L.S. Green, Geometrical factors affecting the interindividual variability of the ECG and the VCG, *J. Electrocardiology* **33** (2000), 219–227.
[20] M. Li and S.S. Narayanan, Robust ECG biometrics by fusing temporal and cepstral information, in: *Proceedings of 20th International Conference on Pattern Recognition (ICPR)*, Aug. 2010.
[21] D. Mucke, *Elektrokardiographie Systematisch*, UniMed Verlag, 1996.
[22] K.N. Plataniotis, D. Hatzinakos and J.K.M. Lee, ECG biometric recognition without fiducial detection, in: *Proc. of Biometrics Symposiums (BSYM)*, Baltimore, Maryland, USA, Sept. 2006.
[23] J. Scheirer, R. Fernandez, J. Klein and R.W. Picard, Frustrating the user on purpose: A step toward building an affective computer, *Interacting with Computers* **14**(2) (February 2002) 93–118.
[24] T.W. Shen, Biometric identity verification based on electrocardiogram (ECG), PhD thesis, University of Wisconsin, Madison, 2005.
[25] T.W. Shen, W.J. Tompkins and Y.H. Hu, One-lead ECG for identity verification, in: *Proc. of the 2nd Conf. of the IEEE Eng. in Med. and Bio. Society and the Biomed. Eng. Society*, Vol. 1, 2002, pp. 62–63.
[26] L. Sornmo and P. Laguna, *Bioelectrical Signal Processing in Cardiac and Neurological Applications*, Elsevier, 2005.
[27] F. Sufi, S. Mahmoud and I. Khalil, A wavelet based secured ECG distribution technique for patient centric approach, in: *Medical Devices and Biosensors, 2008. ISSS-MDBS 2008. 5th International Summer School and Symposium on*, June 2008, pp. 301–304.
[28] The PTB diagnostic ECG database, national metrology institute of Germany, http://www.physionet.org/physiobank/database/ptbdb/.
[29] G. Wübbeler, M. Stavridis, D. Kreiseler, R.D. Bousseljot and C. Elster, Verification of humans using the electrocardiogram, *Pattern Recogn. Lett.* **28**(10) (2007), 1172–1175.
[30] L. Xu, A. Krzyzak and C.Y. Suen, Methods of combining multiple classifiers and their applications to handwriting recognition, *IEEE Transactions on Systems, Man and Cybernetics* **22**(3) (May 1992), 418–435.

Handbook of Ambient Assisted Living
J.C. Augusto et al. (Eds.)
IOS Press, 2012

doi:10.3233/978-1-60750-837-3-195

Happy Healthy Home

Ellen Yi-Luen DO[a,*] and Brian D. JONES[b]
[a]*College of Architecture and School of Interactive Computing, Health Systems Institute*
[b]*Interactive Media Technology Center, Aware Home Research Initiative*
Georgia Institute of Technology, USA

Abstract. This chapter introduces the idea of a smart living environment in which the home tracks and supports happy healthy living for the residents. We start with the introduction of the concepts of wellness and the Aware Home Research Initiative at Georgia Institute of Technology. We then present several interesting projects to illustrate the approaches and implementations toward health, awareness and entertainment and conclude with some reflections and discuss possible future research directions.

Keywords. Ubiquitous computing, ambient intelligence, aware home research initiative

1. Introduction – Toward a Smart Living Environment

It's a spring day in the year 2050. As you finish your breakfast your table displays a picture of the medicine and vitamin to take after the meal. When you go to the kitchen to get yourself a glass of water, you notice the handle of the kettle is red to remind you that the water is hot and ready for tea. Glancing out the window, you see fresh snow accumulated on the ground overnight and feel thankful that the heat was automatically turned up while you were asleep. Meanwhile the living room starts playing the music for your exercise routine. You may be sixty, eighty or a hundred years old now. You are happy and healthy. You are aging gracefully and living alone with your life style partner, the Aware Home.

We have entered the age of ubiquitous/pervasive/ambient computing. Increasingly we are seeing computing and information processing diffused into everyday life, and become invisible. The question is, can our homes help us stay active, alive and vital?

This vision is already becoming a reality. Nowadays there is a wide variety of network sensors and computers that can be installed in a home. A computer is no longer a desktop machine, instead, it is becoming part of the room, part of the building, and constantly present. Can we imagine the world with things that think, spaces that sense, and places that play? Can we employ computing creatively to enhance our lives? Can we use technological innovation to unlock and augment human potential? Design and Human-Computer Interaction are crucial components of information technologies in daily life and they color our experience of computation and communication. Computing that is aware of what people are doing and what they want would significantly impact our life.

At Georgia Tech, the Aware Home Research Initiative (AHRI), an interdisciplinary group of researchers, is exploring emerging technologies and services based in the

*Corresponding Author: Ellen Yi-Luen Do, Georgia Institute of Technology, Atlanta, GA 30332, USA. E-mail: ellendo@gatech.edu.

home. Since 1998, faculty and students involved in the initiative have focused their efforts on solving problems of significant social and economic impact, particularly in the areas of wellness and health. Core to this research and teaching is an understanding of individual needs; how individuals perceive and interact with different devices; and how differently individuals accept these technologies and devices in their homes and everyday lives. One of the facilities used in this research effort is "The Aware Home," a two-story single-family house that serves as a living laboratory for ubiquitous computing research, built with sensing infrastructure that is capable of knowing information about itself and the whereabouts and activities of its inhabitants [16]. In this chapter, we focus on the idea of ambient assistive living, discuss and reflect on the development and deployment of these technologies in the context of a Happy Healthy Home.

2. Be Well – Happy Healthy Living at Home

The idea of wellness is related to human potential. What is wellness? Wellness is the presence of wellbeing. Wellness is about being active, alive and vital. It concerns individuals, communities and our environments. Wellness has multiple dimensions. A popular notion of the six dimensions of wellness consists of: physical, emotional, occupational, social, intellectual and spiritual [11]. The physical dimension concerns diet, nutrition and physical activities. The emotional dimension recognizes awareness and acceptance of feelings and behaviors. The occupational dimension realizes achievement and enrichment through work. The social dimension encourages contribution to the environment, community and the world. The intellectual dimension seeks creative and stimulating activities. The spiritual dimension recognizes the search for values, meaning and purpose in life.

Achieving wellness is a Grand Challenge. We are concerned about the quality of life for ourselves and for our society. As human beings we want to develop and cultivate our untapped potential for a happy, healthy, creative and fulfilling life. Technological innovation may be just the key to unlock human potential for the Holy Grail of wellness.

The Georgia Institute of Technology aspires to the commitment to improving the human condition through advanced science and technology. As a top technological university with genuine concerns about human conditions, Georgia Tech has created a culture of possibilities fostering the growth of interdisciplinary research centers such as the Aware Home Research Initiative, GVU Center, the Health Systems Institute and the Center for Music Technology.

The research and innovating projects produced by these centers are too numerous to list them all. To briefly demonstrate the spirit and the scope of the types of the research efforts, the rest of this chapter will focus on three areas of interest – health, awareness, and entertainment, each illustrated by a couple projects, to form part of the picture of the theme of "happy, healthy living at home with ambient intelligence."

3. Health: For the Old and the Young, with Capturing, Recording and Notification

Besides supporting healthcare services and capabilities ranging from surgery planning to diagnosing and treating chronic disease, many opportunities exist to help people live a more carefree and independent life.

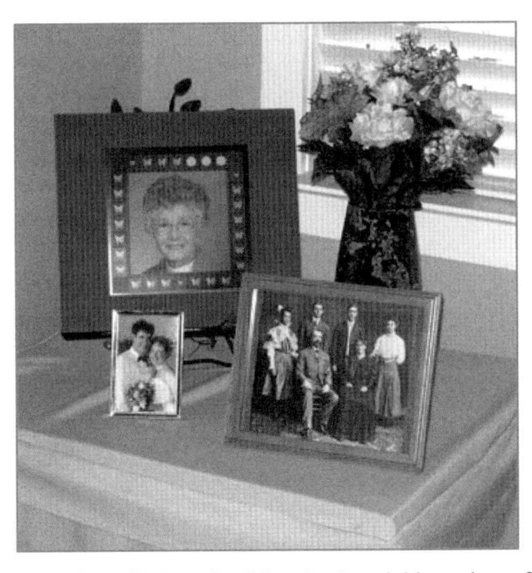

Figure 1. Digital Family Portrait of Grandma's activities as butterfly icons.

3.1. Digital Family Portrait

The Digital Family Portrait [19,24] helps family members at a distance to "keep an eye" out for their family members in a casual, lightweight manner. Figure 1 shows a picture of Grandma displayed together with other family portraits. Displayed on a LCD monitor, the picture is surrounded by the images of the butterflies that change daily, reflecting some portion of Grandma's activities recorded by the non-obtrusive sensors installed in the house. In the Aware Home, the Digital Family Portrait uses motion sensors to collect the activity data on the first floor of the home, while other installations have used strain sensors on the joists of the house to get activity information. A server in the home collects the information and serves it up as a portal from which the client systems retrieve the data.

An earlier version of the picture frame provides many icons for users to understand the activity level of the individual in the sensed home. Study participants found the interface too complex to understand what was going on. Thus, as a result, four levels of information (two representing low and high average activity, one low activity and one high activity) were portrayed in the size of the butterflies, based on the typical activity level of the individual on that day of the week over the last month. Multiple days were included on the screen as this feature helped users to be able to compare different days (e.g., today vs. the past days) on the frame. A touchscreen option allows the user to "scrub" or replay the days' activity for a better understanding of when and where the activity occurred in the home.

3.2. Cook's Collage

Although for privacy reasons, one may appreciate not being constantly under the surveillance camera, there are times that a recording and monitoring service may come in handy. Take Cook's Collage [26] for example, a capture system installed under the kitchen cabinets, that provides a visual summary of recent cooking activity can serve as a memory aid. Imagine you are in the middle of making a cake and you stop to answer

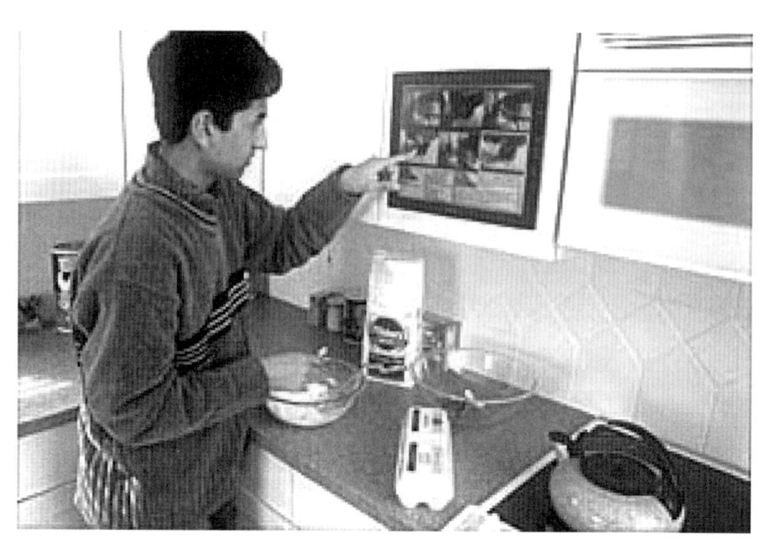

Figure 2. Cook's Collage captures cooking activities for later review.

the phone. When you get back, you wonder if you have already put in either three or four cups of flour in your mixing bowl. The display shows visual snapshots (from two or three mounted webcams under the cabinets providing different perspectives) arranged as a series of comic strip panels for you to touch and review past events. Figure 2 shows a person touching Cook's Collage display to check to see how many cups of flour he already put into the bowl.

The system as shown in Fig. 2 was part of a user study conducted in the Aware Home. The researcher used a Wizard of Oz approach, with an application created to simulate a computer vision system that can quickly pick out images (e.g., when an object being touched or moved) that would best indicate the latest steps in the recipe and display those on the kitchen display.

3.3. Pervasive Remote Asthma Monitoring

Living well at home is a concern for people of all ages. Children with asthma enjoy playing outdoors as much as others. Parents are concerned about their children's well-being even when they are out of sight. With the Pervasive Remote Asthma Monitoring [4] added to a cell phone or a cute animal pendant worn on their necks, children's coughing and wheezing can be recorded no matter where they are located. This monitoring could alert caregivers remotely and enable them to quickly supply medical attention in the event of an emergency. Figure 3 shows a diagram of the system. With embedded electronics and software, the voice can be processed through digital signal processing, sent through the network and incorporated into patients' electronic medical records.

3.4. Personal Robotic Assistant

If you are disabled or confined to a wheelchair at home, Personal Robotic Assistant [15] can turn your world into a clickable interface with a laser pointer. If you want your robotic assistant to pick up a toy or a remote control on the floor and deliver it to your

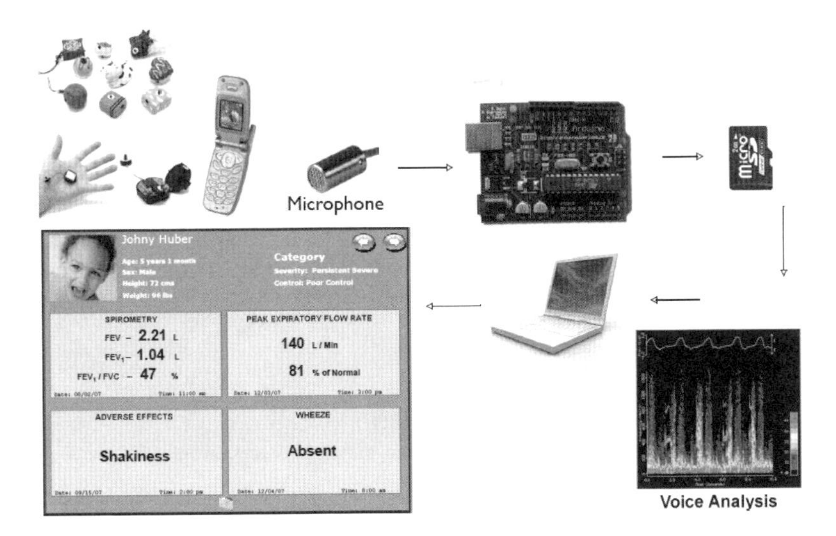

Figure 3. Pervasive Asthma Monitoring helps detect patients' coughing and wheezing patterns.

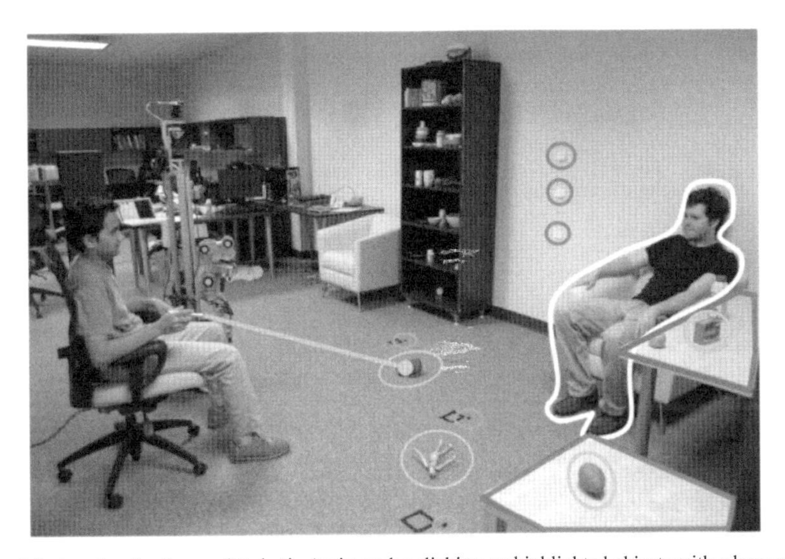

Figure 4. Instructing the Personal Robotic Assistant by clicking on highlighted objects with a laser pointer.

friend on the other side of the room, all you need to do is to point the green laser at the object first, and then at the person. Your robotic helping hand will then follow your command and deliver the object. Figure 4 illustrates how the robot would perceive objects and a person, instructed using a green laser pointer.

In order to complete this task, the robot must perform a number of computations in parallel. It must be capable of detecting the laser pointer when positioned in any orientation. This was accomplished with a camera oriented vertically and monitoring a 360-degree mirror, allowing it to see the laser pointer at any location. Then, the robot must determine the path to reach the object safely and identify the object in order to determine the best manner to retrieve that object (where to grip it, how much force to

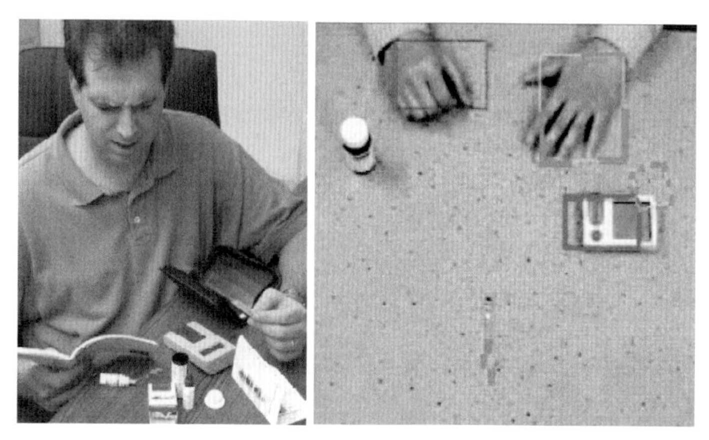

Figure 5. Technology Coach "watches" user actions to provide feedback on home medical device operation.

apply, etc.). Once the object is retrieved, it will turn toward the individual (a social expectation by participants) and wait for a location to which it should deliver the object (human or table top). While the price tag for a full-scale robot is quite hefty, this research has lead to smaller, more affordable versions that can really make a difference in the independence of people who are limited in their mobility.

3.5. Technology Coach

The in-home personal assistant does not have to look like a robot. It could be an invisible fairy or a guardian angel that watches over your shoulder and guides you through unfamiliar or difficult tasks. For example, the Technology Coach [22] provides feedback to assist older adults in using medical devices (such as a blood glucose meter) for the first time, or when the system detects the user did not follow the procedure for using the device. Figure 5 shows that the Technology Coach using a computer vision system to recognize user actions and to recognize potential errors and provide appropriate guidance.

3.6. ClockReader

Worried about your memory and cognitive function but don't want to (or can not) get an appointment with the doctors? Want to self-administer cognitive impairment test at home just like how you could monitor weight with a scale or blood sugar level with a glucose meter? The Clock Drawing Test is one of the simplest, but most commonly used screening tools to detect Alzheimer's disease and related disorders [8]. The task is to draw a clock with a pencil on a given sheet of paper and set a specific time (e.g., 11:10, 1:45). Neurologists or neuropsychologists then spend hours analyzing and scoring the test for diagnosis and treatment. The ClockReader system [17] provides automatic recording and scoring of the Clock Drawing Test on a tablet PC so you could perform the test at the comfort of your own home without the need for the visit of a specialist or a trip to the hospital. Figure 6 left shows the screen of the ClockReader system with the result of the recognition shown in small window. Figure 6 right shows the interaction of drawing a clock using a stylus on a tablet PC.

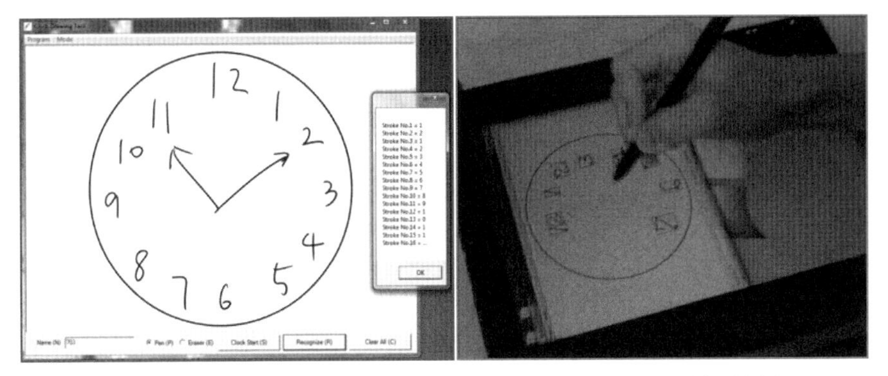

Figure 6. ClockReader interface and scoring (left) with a stylus-and-tablet (right).

There are many scoring systems with differing emphases on visual-spatial, executive, quantitative, and qualitative issues [8,14]. Missing or extra numbers, reversal of the minute and clock hand proportion or misplaced clock hands often appear in clock drawings from people with cognitive impairment. The ClockReader system has three main components: data collection, sketch recognition, and data analysis. Each stroke drawn on a Tablet PC is given a bounding box. Every coordinate of the cusps and intersections of each stroke are stored in the memory for character recognition processing. The recognition engine takes into consideration that some characters have more than one stroke and consequently more than one bounding box. The system then automatically analyzes the drawing and reports the result based on the scoring criteria.

4. Awareness: of Self & the Environment, for Physical, Emotional, Social & Spiritual Wellness

Information technology can serve as a medium to help us connect with ourselves, with other people, and with our environment. Applications in a hospital setting may be designed to help relieve anxiety of the patients and their family members. Applications in a household that inform people about energy consumption patterns may help residents monitor their energy use and modify their behavior patterns. Application in a prayer practice may even help people connect with their spiritual needs. Custom home sensor networks using multiple cameras or existing residential power line could provide location and event detections to support a variety of applications in our daily activities. Let's look at some examples here.

4.1. Patient Interactive Communication & Learning System

Being sick is no fun. It is uncomfortable and stressful. While confined in a hospital bed, a patient may feel overwhelmed and alone. Being able to learn about one's own illness and medical procedures, or to communicate with clinicians, friends and families may help alleviate the stress. The Patient Interactive Communication and Learning System (PILS) simplifies the patient's hospital communication experience by combining communication tools into one easy-to-use system mounted on the patient bed [7]. As shown in Fig. 7, PILS has a one-touch call button that connects to nurse's videophone. Family video conferencing, educational video, entertainment media, and vital signs informa-

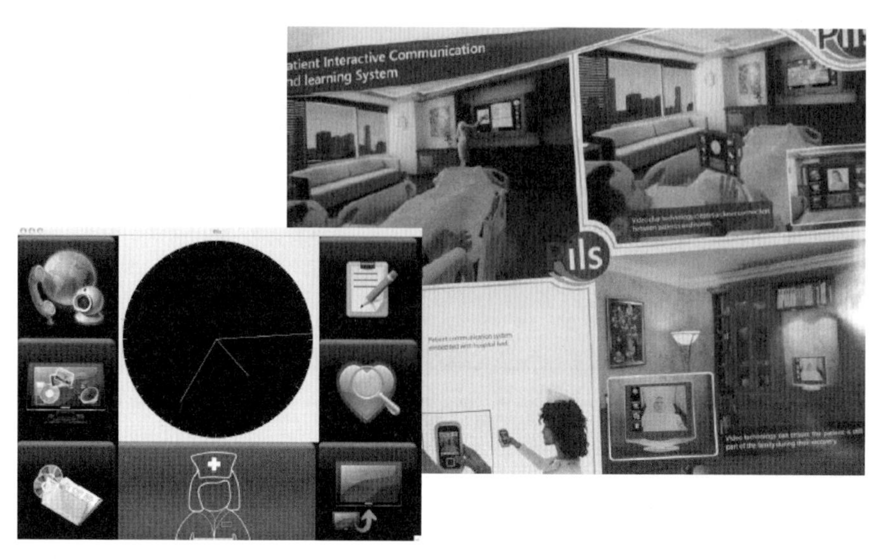

Figure 7. Patient Interactive Communication & Learning System mounted on the bedside connects patients, care givers & family members at home, monitors vital signs and provides learning opportunities.

tion are all just "one-touch away." The entertainment system also doubles as a display for medical records so that the clinicians could use it to explain medical conditions and treatment options to the patients and concerned family members.

4.2. Energy Puppet

Or consider energy awareness – we are all concerned about climate change and our impact on the environment and the world. Would you like to be aware of the energy consumption at your home and change how you use energy? Would you adopt an electronic pet for this purpose? The Energy Puppet [1] is an ambient display device that provides peripheral awareness of energy consumption for individual home appliances. The display produces different "petlike" behavioral reactions according to energy use patterns of the appliances to give homeowners an indication of their energy consumption. The puppet would raise its "arms" in victory to display normal consumption rate (see Fig. 8), or its "eyes" would change color to red and "roar" to warn the homeowners when the specific appliance reaches high consumption rates.

4.3. Power Line Positioning

Besides energy monitoring, many home automation, entertainment and healthcare applications with activity sensing require large numbers of sensors or extensive installation procedures. Wouldn't it be nice if we could have low-cost and easy-to-deploy location and sensing technologies at home by simply leveraging the existing infrastructure? Power Line Positioning [21] is an inexpensive technique that uses fingerprinting of multiple tones transmitted along the power line for location detection within the home space, offering an lower-cost alternative to location aware systems.

The system is based on a popular wire-finding technique used by electricians to locate or trace hidden wires behind a wall or underground. The diagram in Fig. 9 illu-

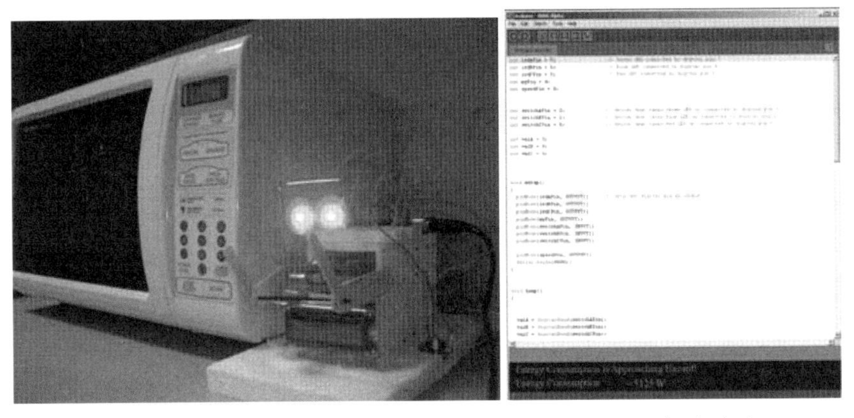

Figure 8. Energy Puppet raises its arm to celebrate low energy consumption in the home.

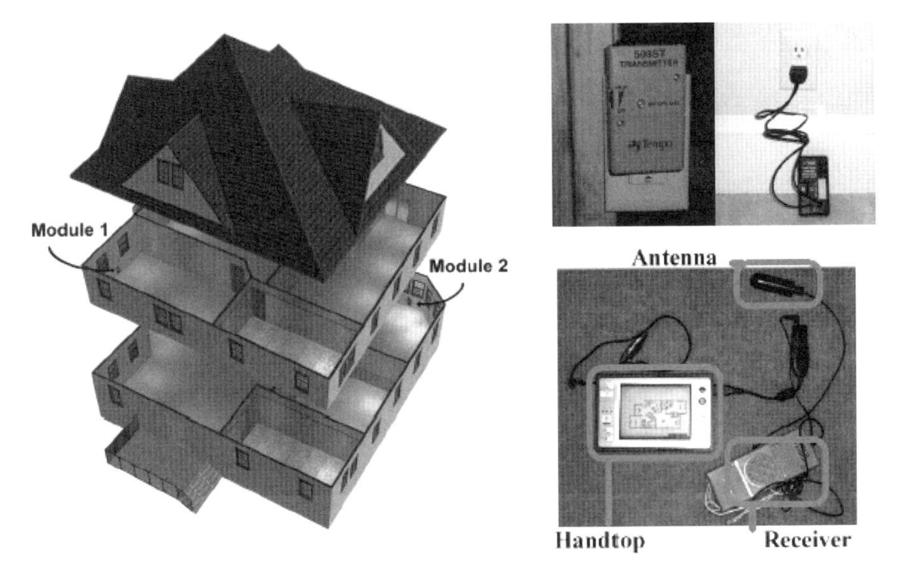

Figure 9. Power Line Positioning system: two signal-generating modules (top right) at extreme ends of a house (left), the location tag with a receiver and antenna connected to a handheld computer (bottom right).

strates the components of the positioning system. A custom wireless tag can detect signals generated by plugging in two signal generator modules into electrical outlets at extreme ends of a house. The power lines essentially act like antennas, but since the signal attenuates over the length of all the power lines in the home, the strength of the signal at every point in the home is the contribution of all the power lines in the vicinity. Thus, after a look up list of signal signatures is generated for the home, the sensor tag is able to sense and transmit the values to determine its location within the home. The detection was able to determine location at better than a 1 meter × 1 meter resolution. With this resolution, the system can be used for many applications like "where are my keys?" or assist in determining the location of an individual in the home to help in understanding the context of their needs.

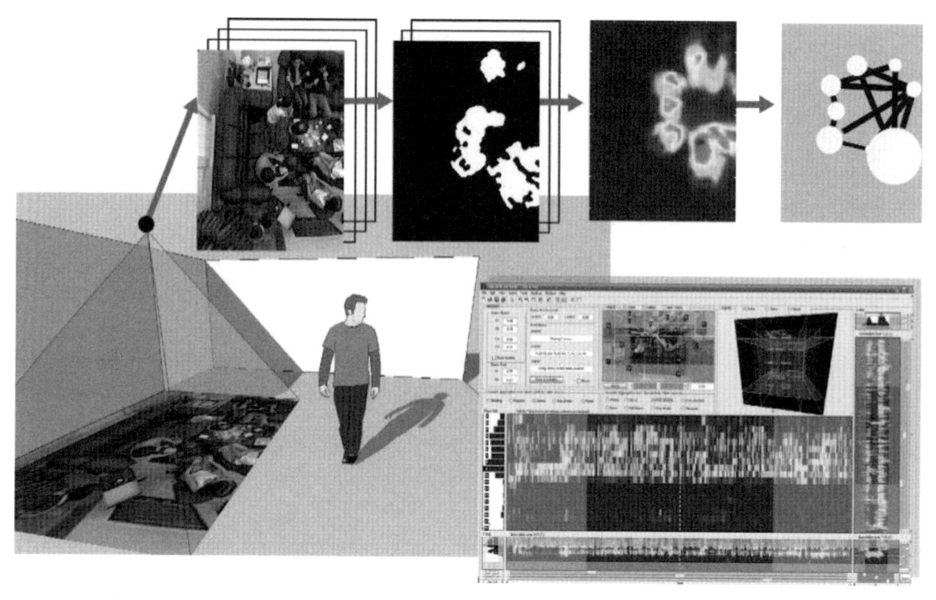

Figure 10. Vis-a-Viz system processes data from overhead camera and turns it into blobs, activity data and activity map for further analysis.

A sister project called Power Line Event Detection uses a single plug-in sensor to detect a variety of electrical events throughout the home using machine learning techniques to recognize electrically noisy events, such as switching on or off a particular light switch, a television set, or an electric stove and classify various electrical events with accuracies ranging from 85–90% [20]. This technology would be very helpful for low-cost monitoring of activity in the home that may have health implications. Further research is being conducted into the use of water line sensing [10] using a pressure sensor to determine which water tap or appliance is currently using water. This too could be used to monitor certain aspects of health or activities of daily living.

4.4. Vis-a-Viz

An approach to understand human activity in natural environments over long periods of time is to use camera and visualization tools to facilitate longitudinal in-situ behavioral analysis. Vis-a-Viz is a visualization tool (see Fig. 10) that interprets data from the overhead cameras, computes motion and blob tracking, aggregates over space and time and provides interactive navigation of the results [23]. By having interpretation and visualization in a spatial or geographical information system, where the floor plan of the inhabited space serves as the geography and time is stacked as layers on top of the plane, the tool helps contextualize video analysis in the space and time to facilitate rapid overview, filtering and zooming, and details on demand of large volumes of video data, that helps identify potentially sparse target behaviors.

Built in Google Sketchup, the system allows the researcher to interactively manipulate the 3D volume (2D floorplan on x and y axis and time on z) to find video of interest. Being able to monitor and analyze behaviors in space could contribute to understanding of the wellness of the inhabitants. For example, Vis-a-Viz data and analysis could be the back end for Grandma's Digital Family Portrait.

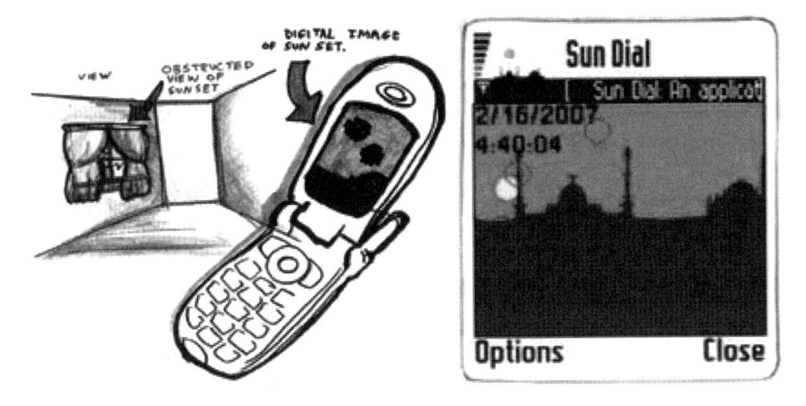

Figure 11. Sun Dial provides environmental cues on a cell phone for prayer opportunities.

4.5. Sun Dial

Sun Dial [28] is an application that supports Muslims' prayer practices by showing the natural environmental cues of the movement of the sun through the sky pictorially in the screen of a mobile phone. The ritual involves several cycles and prayer takes place during a "window of opportunity," instead of an exact time. Therefore, an alarm clock function is not appropriate. With a simulated sun movement through the sky on a cell phone, even people in an interior space with no view to the sky can perceive the different phases of the day for prayer opportunities. This project provides an example of how prayer as an activity can be supported with technology. Figure 11 shows the sketch used in the study with the Muslim community and the resulting screen shot for Sun Dial showing a mosque in profile and the sun locations in the blue sky background.

5. Entertainment – Video, Music and Technology

Watching TV or listening to stereo is a favorite passtime for many people. Finding the remote control can be a chore. You can't quite remember where you put it. You want to change the channel or turn the volume up but you just can't find the remote. Some remotes may be too complicated and difficult to use. Or you may be listening to music when the phone rang and you just wanted to wave at your music player to turn it off.

5.1. Gesture Pendant

The Gesture Pendant project [25] allows control of ordinary household devices, literally, with the wave of a hand (see Fig. 12). Acting as an input device, the pendant enables a number of applications that can use a gesture in place of the remote control. By making gestures in front of the pendant you could control anything from a home theater system, to lighting, to the kitchen sink. In order to detect gestures, a wireless camera is embedded in the small pendant you wear and infrared LEDs illuminate objects (hands) in front. Researchers also investigated the use of the system to analyze user movements and detect loss of motor skill or tremors in the hand that might indicate an illness or problems with medication. Other applications include monitoring of regular eating or activity patterns for detection of health conditions or enabling elderly and disabled people in achieving greater independence in their homes.

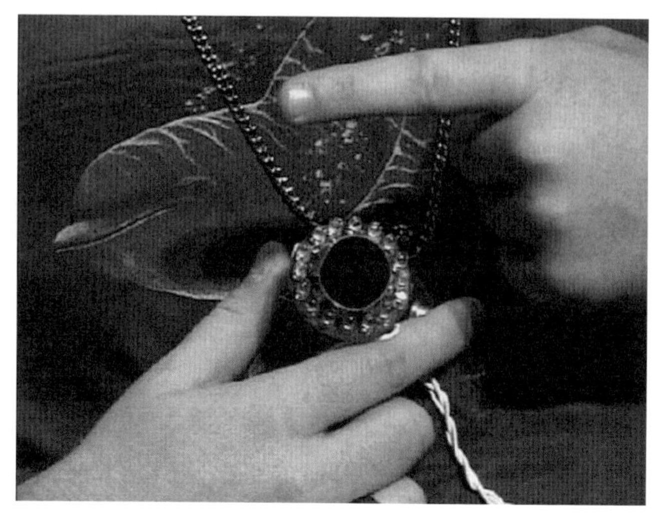

Figure 12. Waving a finger in front of the Gesture Pendant could control a device at home.

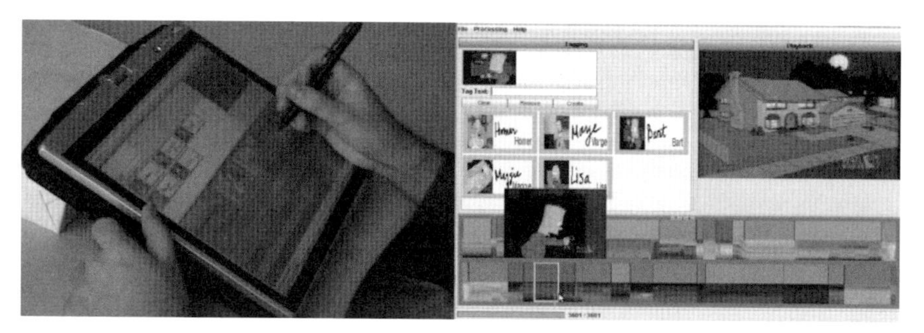

Figure 13. Videotater supports video segmentation and tagging with a pen-based interface.

5.2. Videotator

Interested in editing and annotating video for personal diary or to send a commentary along with a video program to your friends? With Videotater you can play, cut segments of digital video and tag them by using a pen on a Tablet PC [6]. The tool provides efficient and intuitive navigation, selection, segmentation, and tagging of digital video. It automatically segments the video into meaningful categories (i.e., by characters or events) and signals to the user where appropriate segment boundaries should be placed. It also allows rapid review and refinement of manually or automatically generated segments, all with simple pen gestures. Figure 13 shows the editing interface of videotater.

5.3. Music

Music is an important part of life. We hear it everywhere: in elevators, vehicles, concert halls and shopping malls. Music is an art form that helps us express ourselves, and our feelings. Music is fun. An upbeat happy tune can cheer you up. A soft melody can soothe you. Appreciation of music is more than just entertainment. It also has social,

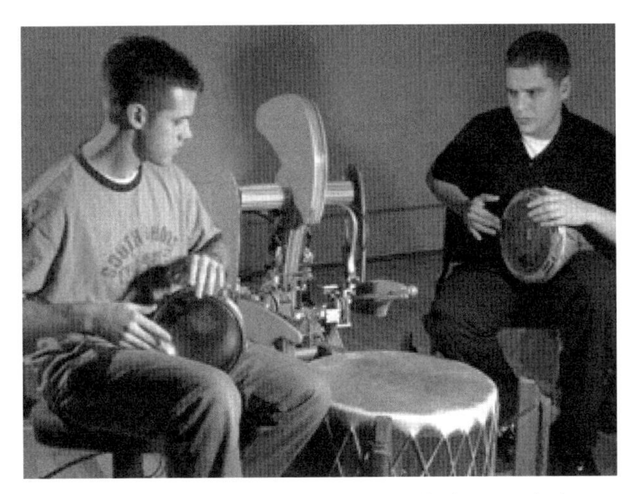

Figure 14. Drumming with an interactive robotic percussionist.

cultural, and emotional implications. Music helps promote wellness, manage stress, alleviate pain, express feelings and improve communication [2,3]. Hand drums have been used to help Alzheimer's patients improve their short-term memory and increase social interaction, help autistic children increase their attention spans, and to aid Parkinson's patients and stroke victims to regain their movement control of or increase their gaits [5,9].

5.4. Haile the Robotic Percussionist

Imagine finding a musician who can jam with a group of players and produce inspiring rhythms in various varying speed and intensity that go beyond human player's ability? Haile is an interactive robotic percussionist that can listen to live players, analyze their music in real-time, and use the results of the analysis to play back in an improvisational manner [27]. Besides being able to imitate human musicians, Haile can sense, analyze, and react to perform with acoustic diversity and dynamic range, and with varying velocities between the two arms that are difficult for human players. The experience of playing with an interactive robotic percussionist may facilitate a musical experience that is inspiring and encourages novel expressions and interactions or serves as effective music therapy [2,3,5,9]. Figure 14 shows a drumming session with the interactive robotic percussionist.

5.5. Piano Touch

Too busy and can't find time to practice piano? How about wearing a glove that can help you learn to play music while you're at your desk or on the move. The Piano Touch [12] project provides a new way for people to learn to play the piano. Wirelessly synchronized with an iPod, cell phone or other music playing device, the Piano Touch is a light-weight glove outfitted with little vibration motors to cue the musicians about which finger they need to use to play the next note. Figure 15 shows a converted golf glove with vibration electronics playing on a lighted keyboard. A pilot study shows that students learned the songs that they were practicing with the Piano Touch glove with

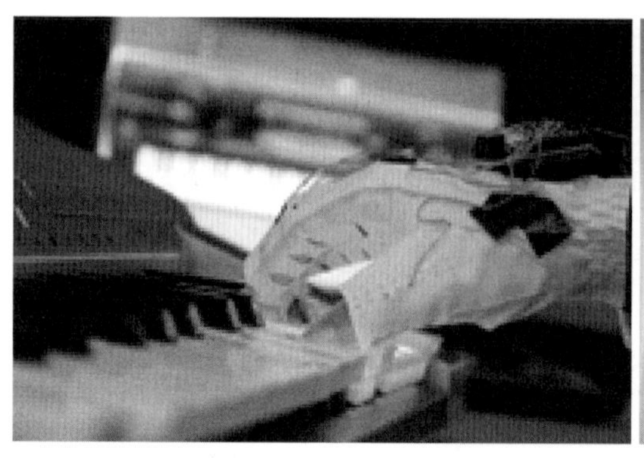

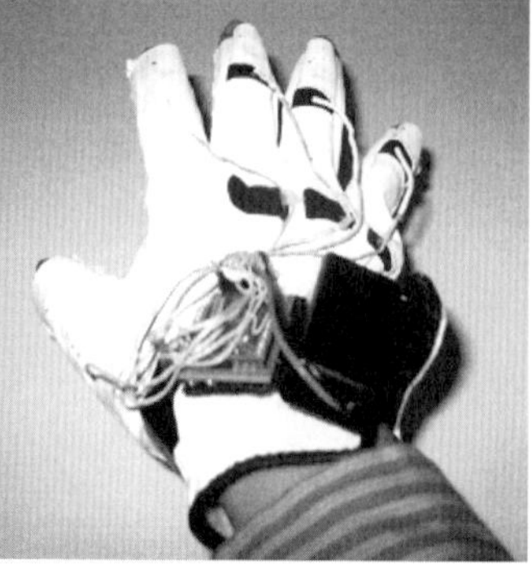

Figure 15. Piano Touch is a lightweight glove that cues which fingers to play.

fewer fingering mistakes than the songs that they were practicing without the glove. Extending Piano Touch's passive haptic learning, we are currently working on making Mobile Music Touch an engaging, pervasive hand rehabilitation aid for patients who suffer loss of functionality of their hands [13,18].

6. May You be Happy and Healthy at Home!

In this chapter we have covered topics of human potential and the dimensions of wellness and presented a holistic view of ambient assistive living. We have seen technological innovation projects addressing different aspects of wellbeing in our everyday lives – about health, awareness and entertainment. Researchers in these projects came from the disciplines of computer science, electrical engineering, human-computer interaction, health systems, industrial engineering, digital media, architecture, industrial design, and music. These projects would not have been possible without the culture of interdisciplinary collaboration, the synthesis of research across many domains, and the aspiration to support fundamental human needs.

To quote from an old Irish Blessing here: "May the road rise up to meet you, may the wind be always at your back. May the sun shine warm upon your face and the rain fall softly on your fields." Extending ambient assistive technologies to understand and support human needs, our home, and the larger built environment could make happy healthy living a reality.

References

[1] S.M. Abdelmohsen and E.Y.-L. Do, Energy puppet: An ambient awareness interface for home energy consumption, in: *SID 08, 7th International Workshop on Social Intelligence Design, Designing Socially Aware Interactions, Dec. 3–5*, Universidad de Puerto Rico, San Juan, PR, 2008, http://cdr.uprrp.edu/SID2008/default.htm.

[2] AMTA, American Music Therapy Association, 2008, http://www.musictherapy.org/.

[3] D. Campbell, *The Mozart Effect for Children: Awakening Your Child's Mind, Health and Creativity With Music*, William Morrow Publishing, 2000.

[4] J. Chhabra, A. Asmi and L. Ragavan, Pervasive asthma monitoring, in: *Pediatric Center of the Future Class, Taught*, E.Y.L. Do, C. Zimring, D. Cowan, G. Lamb, J. Lindgren and J. Jones, eds, 2007, http://www.hsi.gatech.edu/pedcenter.

[5] M.M. Chiang, Research on Music and Healing in Ethnomusicology and Music Therapy, Master Thesis, University of Maryland, College Park, 2008.
[6] N. Diakopoulos and I. Essa, *Videotater: An Approach for Pen-Based Digital Video Segmentation and Tagging, Symposium on User Interface Software and Technology (UIST)*, 2006, pp. 221–224.
[7] T. Fischer, T. Davis and C. Vargas, Patient interactive communication and learning system, in: *The Patient Room of the Future Class at Georgia Tech, Taught*, E.Y.L. Do, C. Zimring, D. Cowan, G. Lamb, S. Kahn, A. Mullick and C. Winegardend, eds, 2006, http://cool.coa.gatech.edu/patientroom.
[8] M. Freedman, L. Leach, E. Kaplan, G. Winocur, K. Shulman and D.C. Delis, *Clock Drawing: A Neuropsychological Analysis*, Oxford University Press, USA, 2004.
[9] R.L. Friedman, *The Healing Power of the Drum*, White Cliffs Media, Inc., 2000.
[10] J.E. Froehlich, E. Larson, T. Campbell, C. Haggerty, J. Fogarty and S.N. Patel, HydroSense: Infrastructure-mediated single-point sensing of whole-home water activity, in: *Proceedings of the 11th International Conference on Ubiquitous Computing (Ubicomp'09)*, ACM, 2009, pp. 235–244, doi:10.1145/1620545.1620581, http://doi.acm.org/10.1145/1620545.1620581.
[11] B. Hettler, *Six Dimensions of Wellness*, National Wellness Institute, 1976, www.nwi.org, and http://www.hettler.com/sixdimen.htm.
[12] K. Huang, E.Y.-L. Do and T. Starner, PianoTouch: A wearable haptic piano instruction system for passive learning of piano skills, in: *ISWC 2008, 12th IEEE International Symposium on Wearable Computers*, Pittsburgh, Pennsylavania, Sep. 28–Oct. 1, 2008, pp. 41–44, http://www.iswc.net/.
[13] K. Huang, T. Starner, E. Do, G. Weiberg, D. Kohlsdorf, C. Ahlrichs and R. Leibrandt, Mobile music touch: Mobile tactile stimulation for passive learning, in: *Proceedings of the 28th International Conference on Human Factors in Computing Systems (CHI'10)*, ACM, New York, NY, USA, 2010, pp. 791–800, doi:10.1145/1753326.1753443, http://doi.acm.org/10.1145/1753326.1753443.
[14] E. Kaplan, The process approach to neuropsychological assessment of psychiatric patients, *Journal of Neuropsychiatry* 2 (1990), 72–97.
[15] C.C. Kemp, A. Cressel, H. Nguyen, A. Trevor and Z. Xu, A point-and-click interface for the real World: Laser designation of objects for mobile manipulation, in: *3rd ACM/IEEE International Conference on Human-Robot Interaction (HRI)*, 2008, pp. 241–248.
[16] C.D. Kidd, R.J. Orr, G.D. Abowd, C.G. Atkeson, I.A. Essa, B. MacIntyre, E. Mynatt, T.E. Starner and W. Newstetter, The aware home: A living laboratory for ubiquitous computing research, in: *Proceedings of the Second International Workshop on Cooperative Buildings – CoBuild'99*, Position Paper, October 1999, http://awarehome.imtc.gatech.edu/publications.
[17] H. Kim, Y.S. Cho and E.Y.-L. Do, Computational clock drawing analysis for cognitive impairment screening, in: *TEI'11 Proceedings of the Fifth International Conference on Tangible, Embedded, and Embodied Interaction*, 2011, pp. 297–300, doi:10.1145/1935701.1935768.
[18] T. Markow, N. Ramakrishnan, K. Huang, T. Starner, M. Eicholtz, S. Garrett, H. Profita, A. Scarlata, C. Schooler, A. Tarun and D. Backus, Mobile music touch: Vibration stimulus as a possible hand rehabilitation method, in: *Proceedings of the 4th International Pervasive Health Conference*, Munich, Germany, March 2010.
[19] E.D. Mynatt, J. Rowan, S. Craighill and A. Jacobs, Digital family portraits: Providing peace of mind for extended family members, in: *Proceedings of the ACM Conference on Human Factors in Computing Systems (CHI 2001)*, ACM Press, Seattle, Washington, 2001, pp. 333–340.
[20] S.N. Patel, T. Robertson, J.A. Kientz, M.S. Reynolds and G.D. Abowd, At the Flick of a switch: Detecting and classifying unique electrical events on the residential power line, in: *Proceedings of Ubicomp*, 2007, pp. 271–288.
[21] S.N. Patel, K.N. Truong and G.D. Abowd, PowerLine positioning: A practical sub-room-level indoor location system for domestic use, in: *Proceedings of Ubicomp*, 2006, pp. 441–458.
[22] W.A. Rogers, I. Essa and A.D. Fisk, Designing a technology coach, in: *Ergonomics in Design: A Publication of the Human Factors and Ergonomics Society*, 2007, pp. 17–23.
[23] M. Romero, J. Summet, J. Stasko and G. Abowd, Viz-A-Vis: Toward visualizing video through computer vision, *IEEE Transactions on Visualization and Computer Graphics* 14(6) (Nov./Dec. 2008), pp. 1261–1268, doi:10.1109/TVCG.2008.185.
[24] J.T. Rowan, Digital family portraits: Support for aging in place, PhD Dissertation, Georgia Institute of Technology Atlanta, GA, USA, 2005, ISBN:0-542-43423-7.
[25] T. Starner, J. Auxier, D. Ashbrook and M. Gandy, The gesture pendant: A self-illuminating, wearable, infrared computer vision system for home automation control and medical monitoring, in: *ISWC 2000*, 2000, pp. 87–94.
[26] Q. Tran, G. Calcaterra and E. Mynatt, Using memory aid to build memory independence, in: *Proceedings of HCII, Human Computer Interaction International*, 2007, pp. 959–965.

[27] G. Weinberg and S. Driscoll, The interactive robotic percussionist: New developments in form, mechanics, perception and interaction design, in: *Proceedings of the ACM/IEEE International Conference on Human-Robot Interaction*, Arlington, Virginia, USA, 2007, pp. 97–104.
[28] S. Wyche, K.E. Caine, B. Davison, M. Arteaga and R.E. Grinter, Sun Dial: Exploring Techno-Spiritual Design Through a Mobile Islamic Call to Prayer Application, CHI Extended Abstract, 2008, pp. 3411–3416.

Handbook of Ambient Assisted Living
J.C. Augusto et al. (Eds.)
IOS Press, 2012

doi:10.3233/978-1-60750-837-3-211

Adaptive Neck Support for Wellbeing During Air Travel

CheeFai TAN[a,b,*], Wei CHEN[b] and Matthias RAUTERBERG[b]
[a] *Universiti Teknikal Malaysia Melaka, Melaka, Malaysia*
[b] *Department of Industrial Design, Eindhoven University of Technology, Netherlands*

Abstract. Air travel is becoming increasingly more accessible to people both through the availability of low cost flights. Health problems may arise due to anxiety and unfamiliarity with airport departure procedures prior to flying, whilst during the air travel, problems may arise as a result of the food served on board, differences in the environmental conditions inside the cabin, the risk of cross-infection from fellow passengers, seat position, posture adopted and duration of the flight. These can be further compounded by changes in time zones and meal times, which may continue to affect an individual's health long after arrival at the final destination. The aircraft passenger comfort depends on different features and the environment during air travel. Seat comfort is a subjective issue because it is the customer who makes the final determination and customer evaluations are based on their opinions having experienced the seat. The aircraft passenger seat has an important role to play in fulfilling the passenger comfort expectations. The seat is one of the important features in the passenger aircraft and is the place where the passenger spends most of time during air travel. This chapter describes the development of adaptive neck support system to improve the wellbeing experience during air travel for economy class aircraft passenger. Design concept, prototyping, system implementation, experimental testing and design evaluation in an aircraft cabin simulator developed at Eindhoven University of Technology will be presented in the chapter.

Keywords. Adaptive, air travel, neck support

Introduction

Travel by air, especially long distance, is not a natural activity for human. Many people experience some degree of physiological and psychological discomfort and even stress during flying. Excessive stress may cause the passenger to become aggressive, overreaction, and even endanger the passenger's health [2,6,24]. A number of health problems can affect flying passengers. Seat comfort is an attribute that demand by today's passenger. The results of seating comfort and discomfort survey [13,14,18] indicated that the neck is one of the most discomfort body parts after one hour and after five hours travel for truck drivers as well as economy class aircraft passengers. In the survey, the neck support is one of the top ranking comfort descriptors for economy class aircraft seat. The observation in the economy class aircraft cabin also indicates that most observed passengers preferred sitting posture with head facing forward. The head

*Corresponding Author: CheeFai Tan, Senior Lecturer, Department of Design and Innovation, Faculty of Mechanical Engineering, Universiti Teknikal Malaysia Melaka, Melaka, Malaysia. E-mail: cheefai@utem.edu.my.

facing forward is the most comfortable head position [21]. Therefore, an adaptive support system prototype was developed that focuses on neck. The objective of an adaptive system is to reduce the neck muscle stress of the economy class passengers during air travel. This chapter describes the development of an adaptive neck support system for aircraft passenger wellbeing during air travel.

1. Current Neck Support for Vehicle Seat

In this subsection, the study on the neck support for long haul travel and vehicle seat e.g. aircraft, bus and train are described.

1.1. Travel Type Neck Support

From the product search using web services, several neck supports related products were found. There are different types of neck supports that are used during air travel such as inflatable neck pillow [9], polyester filled pillow [9], memory foam pillow [9], feather filled pillow [12] and the aircraft seat with mechanical neck support [3,7,16].

Inflatable Neck Pillow

The inflatable neck pillow is low in price and can be found in the travel shop. The air pressure in the inflatable air pillow is proportional to the aircraft flying altitude. When the aircraft flies in the higher altitude, the air pillow will expand and it will contract in the lower altitude. The aircraft passenger will be disturbed by the air pillow when the flying altitude changes. The air pillow holds the passenger's head in one position and the passenger is unable to change the head posture freely. Most of the inflatable air pillows are made from vinyl material that will cause the user to feel hot and sticky. The advantages of the inflatable pillow are that it is easy to store and light-weight [9].

Memory Foam Travel Pillow

The memory foam travel pillow provides good and comfortable support during travel. The memory foam is able to respond to the passenger's body shape and to hold the passenger's head firmly. The memory foam pillow can be compressed into smaller size for storage purpose. The memory foam pillow is light-weight and durable. On the other hand, the memory foam pillow is the most expensive in comparison with commercially available neck support pillows [9].

Polyester Travel Pillow

The polyester travel pillow does not provide good support for aircraft passenger. The polyester pillow will become flat after it is used for some time. Some people also have polyester allergy because the polyester pillow is made from synthetic material. Some airlines such as Air France-KLM Airlines, Malaysia Airlines and China Southern Airlines do supply polyester pillows in the cabin. The advantage of polyester travel pillow is its very low cost [9].

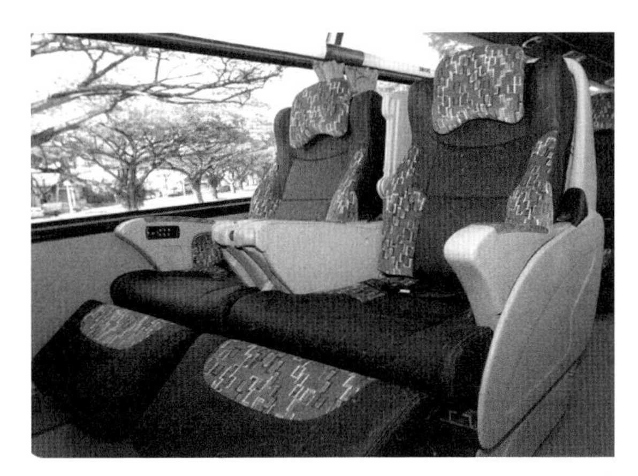

Figure 1. The luxury coach passenger seat with neck support (Photograph reprinted from [5]).

Feather Filled Pillow

The feather filled pillow is soft and easy to mold around the passenger's head for better support. The feather filled pillow is light in weight and can be scrunched. On the other hand, the feather filled pillow will sink into some degree when it is used for some time. The passenger needs to adjust the feather filled pillow to its preferred loft from time to time. The feather filled pillow creates noise when passenger moves their head during resting condition [12].

1.2. Long Distance Commercial Vehicle Passenger Seat with Neck Support

The Coach Passenger Seat with Neck Support

Long-distance coach services, e.g. express buses, are transporting passengers from city to city and serve as main commuter for towns without any railway service [22]. The coach passenger seat is one of the important features to ensure the comfort of the passenger for long distance travel. For example, an express coach that travels from Singapore to Thailand as shown in Fig. 1 was equipped with neck, side and leg support for their passenger's comfort during long distance bus travel.

The Train Passenger Seat with Neck Support

Long distance high speed railway companies, such as ICE, Thalys and Eurostar offer luxury passenger seat to ensure the seating comfort of passengers during train travel. German ICE offers a passenger seat with the neck support as shown in Fig. 2. The neck support is a soft cushion attached to the seat with two strings.

1.3. The Aircraft Passenger Seat with Neck Support

The economy class seat of major airlines such as KLM, Malaysia Airlines, Qantas Airlines and Cathay Pacific Airlines are equipped with adjustable head rest to improve the head and neck comfort during air travel. The headrest of an economy class seat is a mechanical device that supports head and neck. The device needs to be adjusted manually by the passenger for comfort improvement. The headrest (Fig. 3) available in the

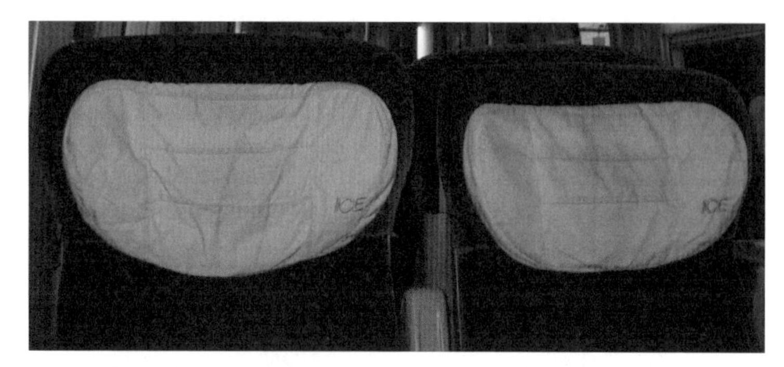

Figure 2. The German train ICE passenger seat with neck support.

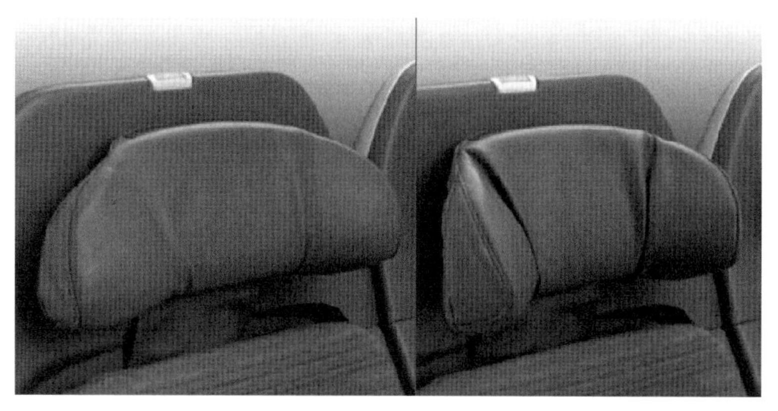

Figure 3. The Cathay Pacific Airlines economy class aircraft seat with built-in neck suppor (Photograph reprinted from [3]).

economy class aircraft seat of Cathay Pacific Airlines can be adjusted in four ways – up, down and sideways (with the adjustable ears). The headrest aims to maximize comfort and support for the passenger's head and neck [3]. Most of the headrests available in current aircrafts [3,7,11] are a mechanical system where the passenger needs to adjust the head rest manually to the required position.

2. Survey of Body Discomfort for Economy Class Aircraft Passenger

Long haul economy class aircraft passengers are at risk of discomfort for long sitting and experience significant discomfort at different body parts. This study was set out to examine the relationship between body discomfort and travel time for economy class aircraft passengers. There were 104 anonymous questionnaires completed at Schiphol International Airport, the Netherlands, from October through November 2008.

2.1. Methods

The objective of the questionnaire is to investigate the seating discomfort for economy class aircraft passengers over travel time. The questionnaire consists of three sections: (1) questions about the respondents' air travel frequency per year, common flight dura-

Table 1. Body map and scales for body discomfort evaluation

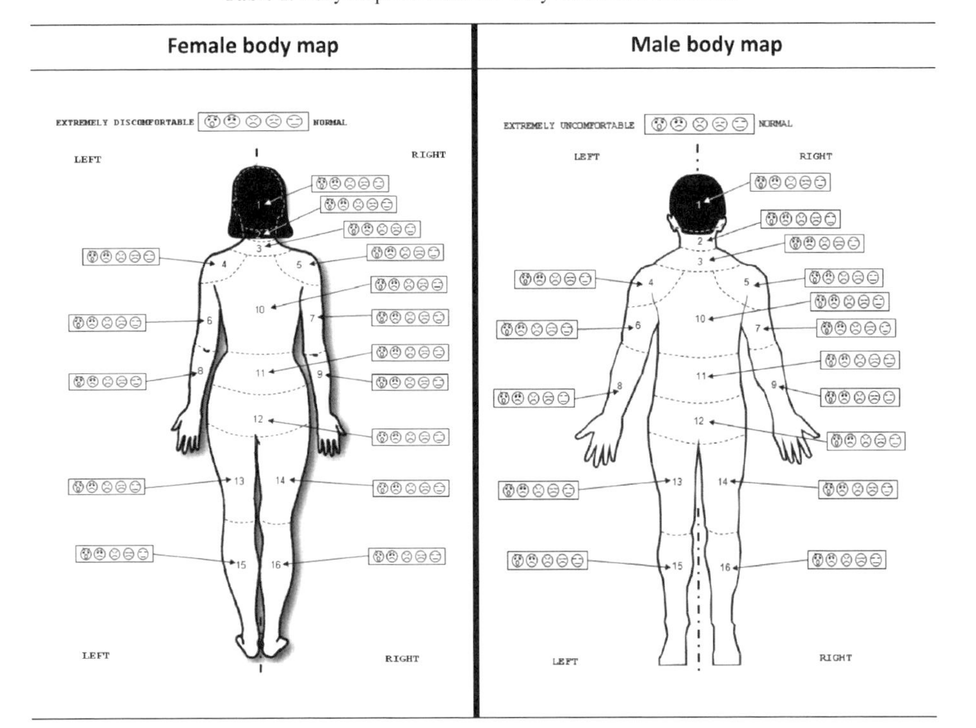

tion and the travel class; (2) questions about their discomfort level for each body part after one hour and five hours flight; (3) questions about demographic background of respondents.

The questionnaire begins with a short, self-explanatory introduction in which the purpose and background of the survey are explained; it is also emphasized that data will be treated with confidentiality and analyzed in an anonymous manner.

The respondents were asked to report on travel frequency in a four point scale (1 = 1 time, 2 = 2–5 times, 3 = 6–10 time, 4 = 11 times or more), common flight duration in a four point scale (1 = less than one hour, 2 = 2–5 hours, 3 = 6–10 hours, 4 = 11 hours or more) and the travel class in a three point scale (1 = economy class, 2 = business class, 3 = first class). The questionnaire was devised to identify the body part discomfort, to indicate the discomfort level for each defined body part after one hour and after five hours travel. In order to identify the body part discomfort level, a body mapping method is used. The body map and scales were used for discomfort assessment. In this method, the perception of discomfort is referred to a defined part of the body. The subject is asked for the discomfort experiences during flight for each defined body part. The scales are graded from 'extremely discomfort' to 'normal'. The body map and scales of body discomfort evaluation for economy class aircraft seat is shown in Table 1.

The questionnaire was completed by 104 aircraft passengers who were randomly sampled at Schiphol International Airport in the Netherlands. The investigator was present on each occasion, during which aircraft passengers were approached and the aims of the investigation were briefly outlined. The questionnaire with female body

Table 2. Body discomfort ranking of aircraft passengers after one hour and after five hours of travel

Ranking	Body discomfort after 1 hour travel	Body discomfort after 5 hours travel
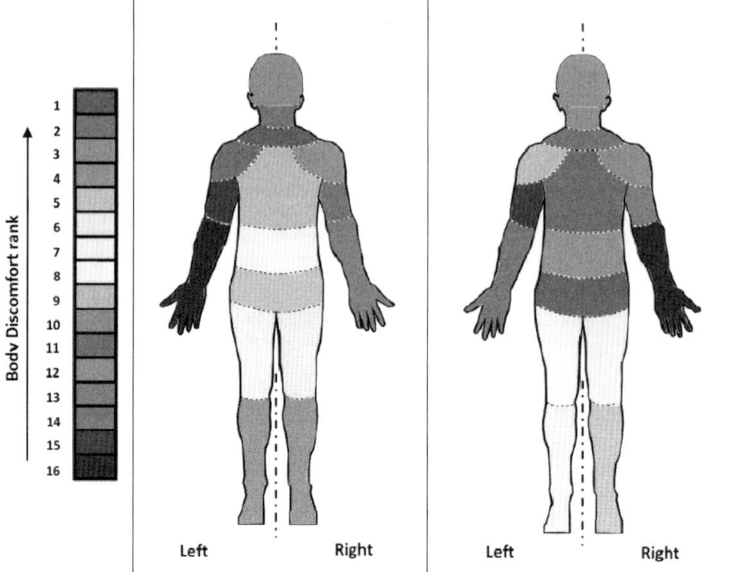 Body Discomfort rank 1 2 3 4 5 6 7 8 9 10 11 12 13 14 15 16	Left Right	Left Right

map was distributed to female respondents and the questionnaire with male body map was distributed to male respondents. Approximately 90% of those approached accepted to participate. The questionnaire took between three to five minutes for self-completion.

2.2. Results

The nonparametric Friedman test was used to test the mean rank of the sixteen body parts. For each body part, the sixteen body parts were ranked from 1 to 16 based on body discomfort rating score. The test statistic is based on these ranks. From the result of body discomfort after one hour travel, it showed that shoulder (MR = 10.57) exhibited the highest discomfort ranking. It was followed by neck (MR = 10.37) and right lower leg (MR = 10.29). The difference in medians among 16 body discomfort after one hour travel, is significant χ^2 (15, N = 104) = 286.27, $p < 0.001$. For the body discomfort level after five hours travel, the result showed that buttocks (MR = 10.74) was ranked as the highest discomfort level after five hours travel. It was followed by shoulder (MR = 10.24) and neck (MR = 10.15). The difference in medians among 16 body discomfort after one hour travel, is significant χ^2 (15, N = 104) = 312.93, $p < 0.001$. Univariate analysis of variance was conducted to find the differences of body discomfort level between after one hour travel and after five hours travel. The results showed the body discomfort level after five hours travel was higher than after one hour travel. The detailed comparison between body discomfort ranking after one hour travel and after five hours travel is shown in Table 2.

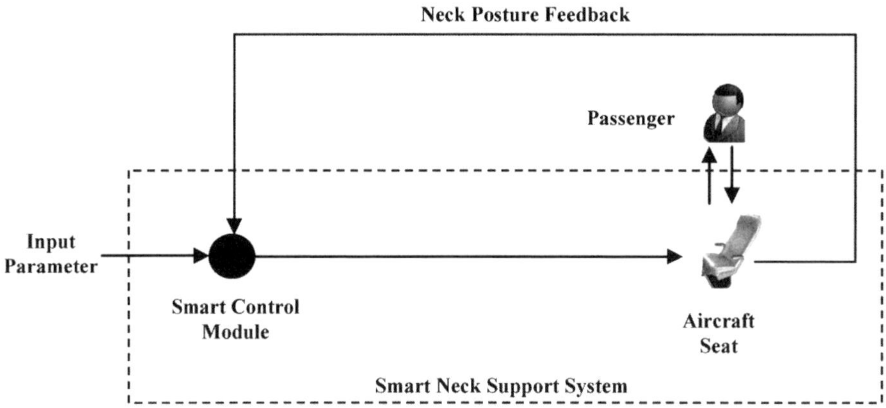

Figure 4. Feedback loop for smart neck support system.

2.3. Discussion and Conclusion

There were 104 respondents who filled up the questionnaire about body discomfort after one hour and after five hours travel. In line with the survey hypothesis, findings confirmed that the body discomfort of aircraft passenger after five hours travel is higher than after one hour travel. The body discomfort of economy class aircraft passengers was associated with flight duration. The finding also showed that the neck is one of the top three most discomfort body part after one hour and after five hours of travel. The result of the study on body discomfort of economy class aircraft passenger demonstrates the need for the development of a neck support system.

3. Adaptive Neck Support System

An adaptive neck support system is developed to reduce neck muscle stress during air travel for economy class aircraft passenger seat. Feedback loop for adaptive neck support system is illustrated in Fig. 4. The system commences by detecting the passenger's head posture. Two air pressure sensors are embedded in the seat body to detect the head posture of the passenger. Subsequently, the information of the head posture is sent to a smart control module which performs the following functions:

- Providing support to the passenger's head based on his or her current head posture.
- Changing the head rotation angle of the passenger to reduce neck muscle stress in an adaptive and autonomous way. When the smart control module detects that the passenger is in low activity and the passenger has been in contact with the airbag for some time, the smart control module will be activated to provide neck support to the passenger. The passenger's head will be moved towards front facing position, as this would reduce the neck muscle stress and it is known that the head facing front position is the most comfortable position [21].

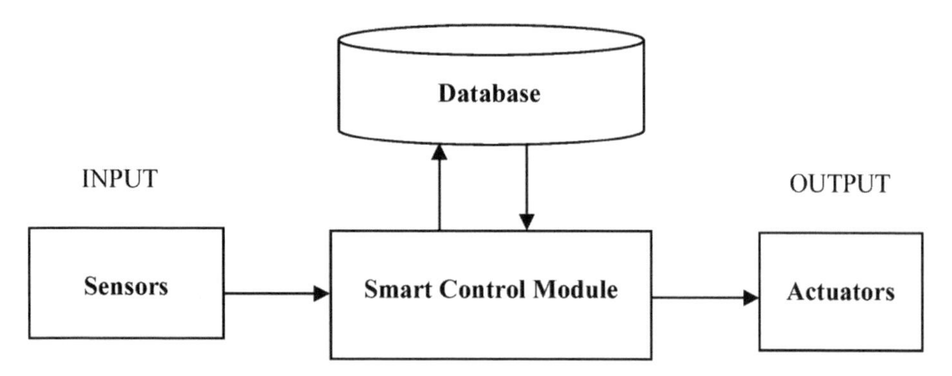

Figure 5. The simplified architecture of an adaptive neck support system.

3.1. The Architecture of Adaptive Neck Support System

The architecture of an adaptive neck support system is shown in Fig. 5. Both sides of the upper part of the aircraft passenger seat are embedded with air pressure sensors. The sensors are used to detect the passenger's head posture. The input parameter to the smart control module is the analog value from the air pressure sensor and the potentiometer. The air pressure sensor is used to measure the air pressure in the airbag and the potentiometer detects the presence of passenger. The output parameter is the analog value from the smart control module used to control the proportional solenoid valve. The proportional solenoid valve is used to control the air flow to and from the airbag. The smart control module is the core component of the system where it is used to mediate between sensors and actuators. The air pressure detection model is the main component in the smart control module. The algorithm for the system is to support the aircraft passenger's neck adaptively. The database is used to record the airbag pressure as well as to provide input to the smart control module. The output from the system is the actuators. The actuators will change the airbag condition such as inflate and deflate.

3.2. System Design

State Transition Diagram

The state transition diagram (Fig. 6) is used to describe the behavior of an adaptive neck support system. The state transition diagram describes the possible states of the airbags as events occur. Each circle represents a state. All states are inter-related to each other. When the passenger is not in touch with adaptive neck support system, the adaptive neck support system is in the initial airbag pressure condition (C1). For example, when the passenger head is in contact with the head cushion (Fig. 9) and the system senses the presence of the passenger (C2), the system will move from 'Stand-by State' to 'Passenger Presence State'. If the passenger's head turns to the right and is in contact with the right airbag for *t* time (p3), the system will move from 'Passenger Presence State' to 'Right Support State'. Similarly, if the passenger's head turns to the left and is in contact with the left airbag for *t* time (C4), the system will move from 'Passenger Presence State' to 'Left Support State'. When the passenger leaves the system, all states will transit to 'Standby State' and become condition one (C1).

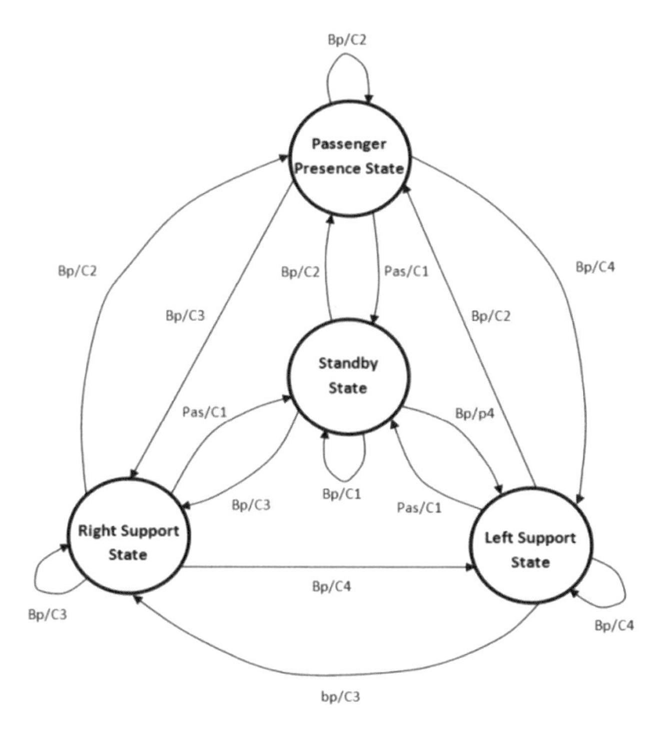

Legend:

Input Stimuli:
Bp: airbag pressure increase/decrease
Pas: passenger is move away from SnS[2]

Conditions:
C1: initial airbag pressure
C2: the passenger is presence
C3: the passenger is in touch with the right airbag for t time
C4: the passenger is in touch with the left airbag for t time

States:
Standby state
Passenger presence state
Right support state
Left support state

Figure 6. State transition of an adaptive neck support system.

State Transition Description for Smart Neck Support System

State transition is used to describe the behavior of an adaptive neck support system. There are four transition states of an adaptive neck support system. The description of the state transition for an adaptive neck support system is as follows.

Standby State

In 'Standby State', the right airbag (RA) and the left airbag (LA) are filled with air based on a pre-set air pressure. The arrangement of the head cushion, right airbag and left airbag is shown in Fig. 7. Each airbag is equipped with an air pressure sensor and a potentiometer. The adaptive neck support system is in stand-by mode.

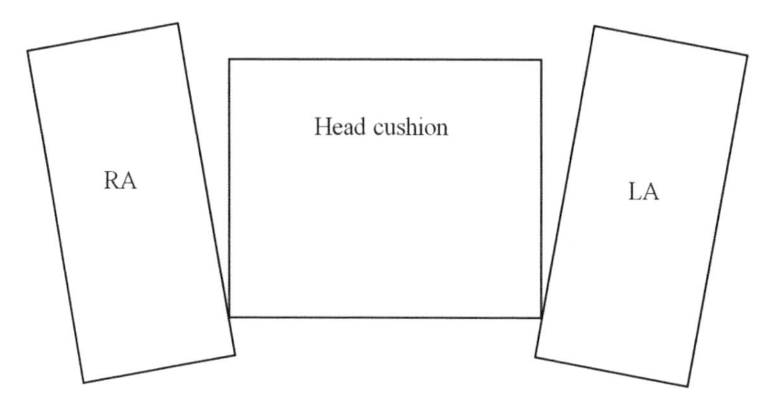

Figure 7. Schematic of 'Standby State'.

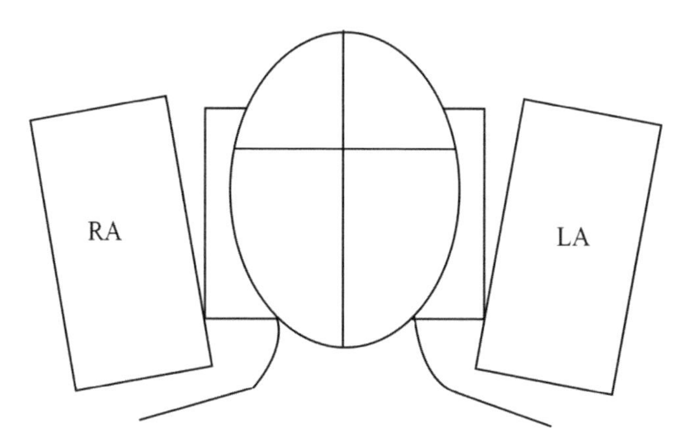

Figure 8. Schematic of 'Passenger Presence State'.

Passenger Presence State

The head cushion detects the presence of the passenger. As shown in Fig. 8, the passenger's head is perpendicular to the head support and it is not in touch with the right and left airbag.

Right Support State

In the 'Right Support State' (Fig. 9), the passenger's head moves to the right and is in touch with the right airbag. After one minute, when the system detects low activity of the passenger, the system is activated. Low activity is defined as the change of the air bag pressure during a time window to be within a predefined upper threshold and lower threshold. If the passenger stays in position for some time, the neck support system is activated to give support to the passenger's head. The rotation angle of the right airbag for the initial position and the supported position is shown in Fig. 10. When the system is activated, the airbag will be inflated from the initial position (45°) to the supported position (15°).

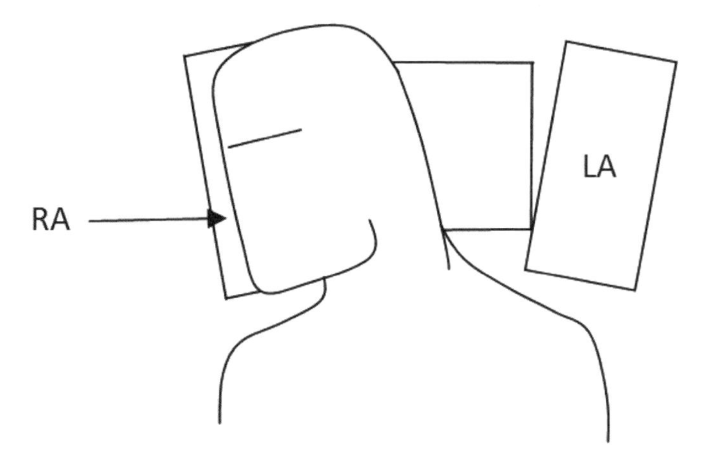

Figure 9. Schematic of 'Right Support State'.

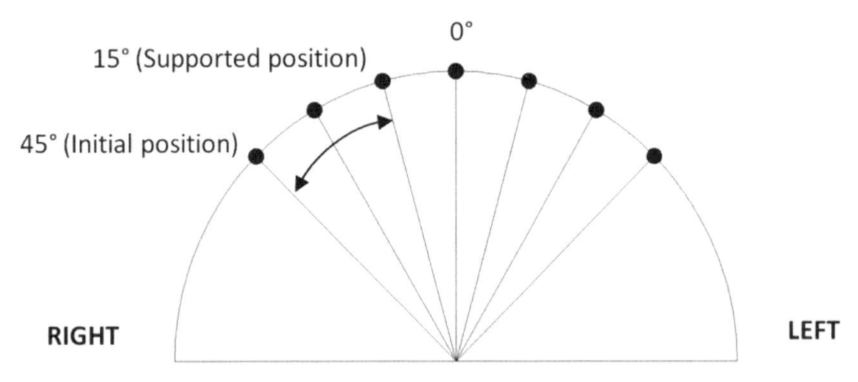

Figure 10. The schematic of example initial position and supported position for right airbag.

Left Support State

In 'Left Support State', the passenger's head is in touch with the left airbag (Fig. 11). The right airbag will be reset to initial state mode. If the passenger's head is in touch with left airbag and in low activity mode for one minute, the neck support system is activated to give support on the left side of the passenger's head. The rotation angle of the left airbag for the initial position and the supported position is shown in Fig. 12. During the activation of the system, the airbag will be inflated from initial position (45°) to supported position (15°).

Air Pressure Detection Model

An air pressure detection model was developed. The objective of the developed air pressure detection model is to detect the passenger's head position by using an airbag system. The developed model takes into account the passenger's head posture while computing the air pressure differences in the airbag. The air pressure detection model is used for the right airbag and the left airbag. The proposed model records the increase and decrease of air pressure in the airbags. The actuator is not activated when the re-

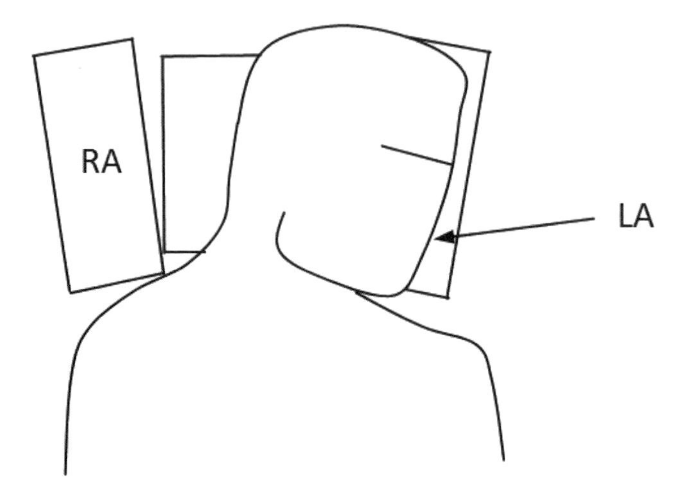

Figure 11. Schematic of 'Left Support State'.

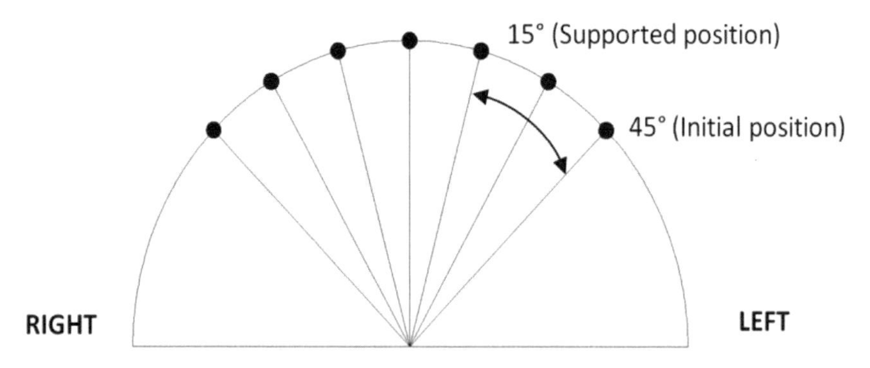

Figure 12. The schematic of example initial position and supported position for left airbag.

cording of air pressure takes place. This because the air that flows into the airbag or exhaust from the airbag will be interfering with the current air pressure value. The model can be easily modified to take into account any variation in the air pressure during implementation. For example, if the passenger's head is away from the supported airbag, the current air pressure in the airbag will change.

Let,

$P_{current}$ = current air pressure in the airbag
$P_{recorded}$ = recorded air pressure when passenger is in touch with the airbag
n_1 = value for upper threshold
n_2 = value for lower threshold

P_{airbag} is the difference between the recorded air pressure and the current air pressure. P_{airbag} is defined as

$$P_{airbag} = P_{recorded} - P_{current} \tag{1}$$

P_{airbag} is used for data logging purpose.

Mathematically,

When passenger is in touch with the airbag,

$$P_{current} < P_{recorded} + n_1 \ \&\& \ P_{current} > P_{recorded} - n_2 \qquad \text{comparing the airbag pressure}$$

If the current air pressure in the airbag is within the defined upper threshold and the lower threshold, the SnS^2 is activated.

When passenger is away from the airbag that supports the neck,

$$P_{current} < P_{recorded} \qquad \text{comparing the airbag pressure}$$

The current air pressure in the airbag will decrease to a value that is less than the recorded air pressure when the head is not in touch with airbag. Hence the system can infer that passenger's head has left the airbag and deactivate the SnS^2. The algorithm of air pressure detection model for the right airbag and the left airbag is shown in Fig. 13.

4. Prototype

The final prototype setup is an adaptive neck support system that contains a head cushion, a neck cushion, two side airbags, a microcontroller with sensors and actuators connected. The installation of an adaptive neck support system to the economy class aircraft seat in aircraft cabin simulator is shown in Fig. 14. The aircraft cabin simulator is a testbed used for experimental purposes as well as product evaluation purposes.

4.1. Hardware

Arduino Mega [1], transformer, air pressure sensor and proportional solenoid valve were used to build the control system for SnS^2. The Arduino MEGA is a microcontroller board based on the ATmega1280. It has 54 digital input/output pins (of which 14 can be used as pulse with modular outputs), 16 analog inputs, 4 UARTs (hardware serial ports), a 16 MHz crystal oscillator, a USB connection, a power jack, an ICSP header and a reset button. Arduino is an open-source electronic device that used for prototyping purpose. The Arduino receives input from sensors and controls the output such as actuator and valve. The communication between the Arduino Mega and the computer is using 9600 baud via USB cable.

The air pressure sensor is a Phidget 1115 [8] type sensor that is used to measure the air pressure inside the airbag. It measures absolute gas pressure from 20 to 250 kPa with a maximum error of ±1.5%. The air pressure sensor is a ratiometric sensor. The membrane potentiometer is a sensor embedded in the head cushion and used to detect the presence of the passenger. The resistance of the membrane potentiometer can be changed linearly from 100 Ohms to 10,000 Ohms [4].

4.2. Software

The software is an integral part of an adaptive neck support system. It enables different components to be controlled and integrated in the way best suited to the functions of the smart neck support system, ensuring data flow and information flow throughout the

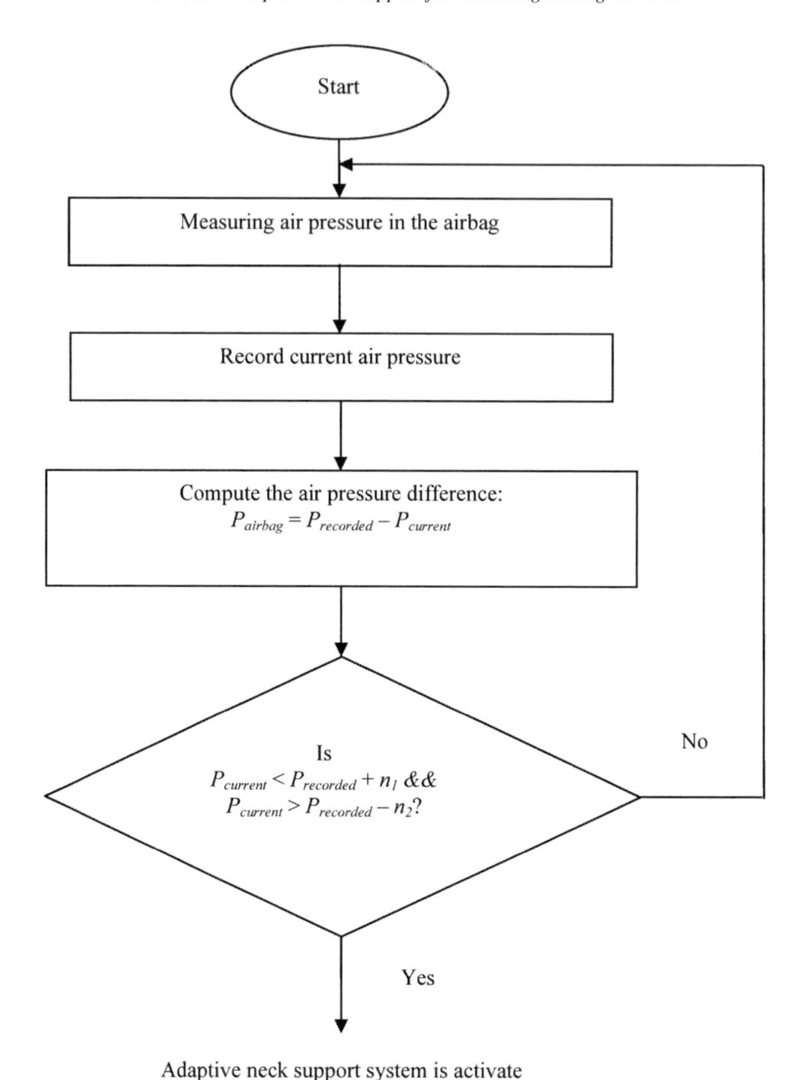

Figure 13. Flowchart for the neck support state transitions when the passenger is touching the airbag.

system. The aims of the developed program are to control the right and the left airbag of an adaptive neck support system.

In term of programming implementation, two programming languages were used in the adaptive neck support system prototype. Arduino programming language [1] was used to program the Arduino microcontroller. The Arduino programming language is based on *Wiring* [23] and the Arduino development environment was based on Processing [10]. The Arduino programming language is an open-source program and the environment is written in Java. For the database development, we used *Processing* to write the code. Processing [10] is an open source programming language and environment for prototyping purposes. Processing was used to log the sensors and actuators data.

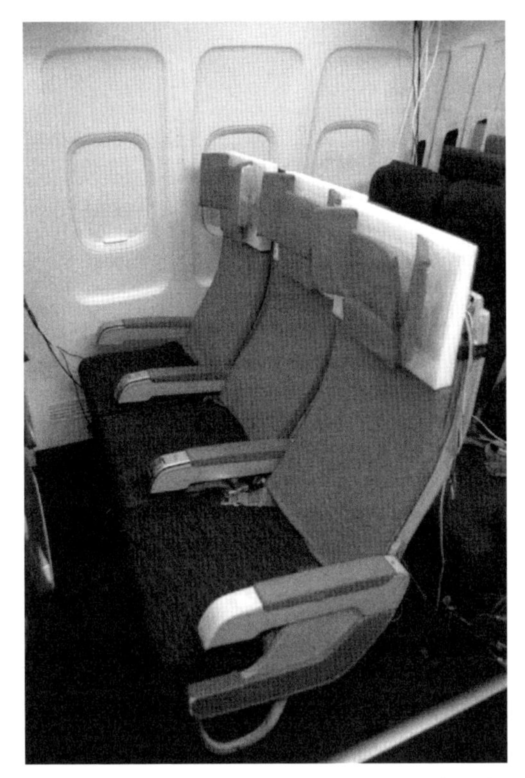

Figure 14. An adaptive neck support system on economy class aircraft seat.

5. The Validation of Adaptive Neck Support System

The proposed adaptive neck support system was evaluated in an aircraft cabin simulator [15,17,20] as shown in Fig. 14 developed at Department of Industrial Design, Eindhoven University of Technology. Calibration experiments and evaluation experiments were carried out. The purpose of the calibration experiment [16,19] was to provide input such as the neck support condition, time factor and the neck rotation angle to validate the adaptive neck support system. In this section, details of the validation experiment are reported.

5.1. Participant

Four participants (2 females and 2 males) with no neck pain from the last three months were recruited. They were informed regarding the procedure of experiment such as sitting inside the aircraft cabin simulator for one hour, video recording and attachment of EMG electrodes on their sternocleidomastoid (SCM) muscle.

5.2. Experimental Setup

Two validation experiments were conducted in the aircraft cabin simulator. The location of experiment is in the simulation lab in the main building of Eindhoven University of Technology. The first experiment was the aircraft seat without smart system and the second experiment was the aircraft seat with smart system. Both experiments recruited same participant. The observation cameras used to monitor the activity of each participant.

5.3. Apparatus and Data Recording

The hardware used in experiment was MP150 Biopac Systems with (electromyography) EMG module, aircraft cabin simulator, a adaptive neck support system, computer and observation camera.

Two EMG module of MP150 Biopac system were used for each participant. The aircraft cabin simulator is a test bed was designed and built to simulate the average economy class cabin. Three adaptive neck support systems were installed in each aircraft seat. The computer was used for data logging and video recording. The cameras were installed at the front as well as above the participant. The acquisition of EMG signal and procedure are same as calibration experiment.

5.4. Experimental Procedure

We started the experiment with 30 minutes of briefing to participants and attachment of electrodes on SCM muscles. The participant was performed maximal voluntary contraction of the SCM by rotate the head to left hand side and right hand side for 10 seconds. After that, we positioned the participant on the economy class aircraft seat. The aircraft seat sitting position was classified as aisle seat, center seat and window seat. Next, light in the aircraft cabin was dimmed and the participant was advised to rest during the one hour experiment. The EMG signals for participants were monitored and recorded in parallel with system log and video recording.

5.5. Data Analysis

For each experiment, the average normalized EMG value was used for statistical analysis. A descriptive statistical method was used to analyze the questionnaire. A one-way analysis of variance with repeated measures was used.

5.6. Results

After the experiment, the results from EMG measurements were selected and analyzed. From the statistical result, the mean scores of normalized EMG value for after supported by adaptive neck support system ($M = 2.817$, $SD = 2.130$) is lower than the mean scores of normalized EMG value for before supported by adaptive neck support system ($M = 3.029$, $SD = 2.312$). The mean scores of normalized EMG value for the participant in relation with neck support activity are shown in Fig. 15.

6. Summary

This chapter presents the development of an adaptive neck support system to improve the neck comfort during air travel. The architecture of an adaptive neck support system described the structure of the system which consists of sensor, actuator, database and central processor. The framework showed that the behavior of the developed system

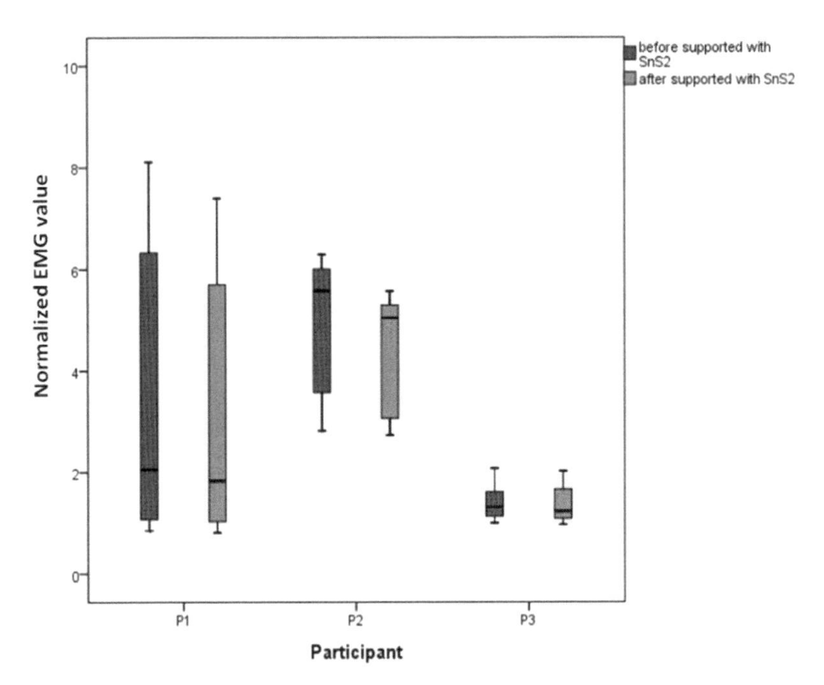

Figure 15. The mean scores of normalized EMG value for the participant in relation to neck support activity.

can improve the aircraft passenger neck comfort. The state transition diagram was used to describe the behavior of an adaptive neck support system. Four transition states were designed and implemented. The air pressure detection model was related to the airbag system. The air pressure detection model is used for the implementation of an adaptive neck support system, the airbag is capable to detect the passenger's posture and support the passenger's neck adaptively. The final setup of an adaptive smart neck support system contains a head cushion, a neck cushion, two side airbags, an Arduino microcontroller with air pressure sensors and a proportional solenoid valve connected. The open-source programming language, namely Arduino and Processing, were used for programming implementation in the adaptive neck support system. For the experiment to validate the adaptive neck support system, the results showed that the developed system is able to provide the necessary neck support to reduce the SCM muscle stress.

References

[1] Arduino, Arduino Mega, http://arduino.cc, accessed on 20 February 2010.

[2] G. Brundrett, Comfort and health in commercial aircraft: A literature review, *The Journal of the Royal Society for the Promotion of Health* **121**(1) (2001), 29–37.

[3] Cathay Pacific, Your Guide to the Economy Class Seat, http://downloads.cathaypacific.com/cx/new_seat/seatguide/Olympus_y.pdf, accessed on 15 February 2010.

[4] Eztronics, Air Pressure Sensor, http://www.eztronics.nl, accessed on 20 February 2010.

[5] Five Star Tours, http://www.fivestarsonline.com/?q=en/coach, accessed on 17 June 2010.

[6] S. Kalogeropoulos, Sky rage, *Flight Safety Australia* (1998), 36–37.

[7] Malaysia Airlines, Economy Class, http://www.malaysiaairlines.com/hq/en/flymh/cabin/eclass/economy-class.aspx, accessed on 10 February 2010.

[8] Phidgets, http://www.phidgets.com, accessed on 20 February 2010.

[9] Pilot Paul, It's A Shame For You Not To Use A Travel Neck Pillow To Help You Sleep While Traveling – When Other People Do It So Easily, http://www.pilot-pauls-travel-accessories.com/travel-neck-pillow.html, accessed on 15 February 2010.
[10] Processing, http://processing.org/, accessed on 20 February 2010.
[11] Qantas, Qantas A380 Awards, http://www.qantas.com.au/travel/airlines/economy-seat-award/global/en, accessed on 15 February 2010.
[12] N. Robinson, Feather Pillows – Advantages and Disadvantages You Should Know, http://ezinearticles.com/?Feather-Pillows---Advantages-and-Disadvantages-You-Should-Know&id=1122787, accessed on 15 February 2010.
[13] C.F. Tan, Smart System for Aircraft Passenger Neck Support, PhD Thesis, Eindhoven University of Technology, 2010.
[14] C.F. Tan, W. Chen and M. Rauterberg, An approach to study the sitting position and neck discomfort of economy class aircraft passenger during air travel, in: *Proceedings of International Conference on Applied Human Factors and Ergonomics*, Miami, Florida, USA, Chapter 40, 2010, pp. 376–382.
[15] C.F. Tan, W. Chen and M. Rauterberg, Design of aircraft cabin testbed for stress free air travel experiment, in: *5th International Conference on Planning and Design*, Tainan City, Taiwan, 2009, p. 157.
[16] C.F. Tan, W. Chen and M. Rauterberg, Experimental design for sternocleidomastoid muscle stress measurement, in: *7th International Conference on Methods and Techniques in Behavioral research*, Eindhoven, The Netherlands, 2010, pp. 44–47.
[17] C.F. Tan, W. Chen and M. Rauterberg, Interactive aircraft cabin testbed for stress-free air travel system experiment: An innovative concurrent design approach. In: *Proceedings of International Conference on Advances in Mechanical Engineering 2009*, Shah Alam, Malaysia, 2009, p. 137.
[18] C.F. Tan, W. Chen and M. Rauterberg, Self-reported seat discomfort amongst Dutch commercial truck driver, in: *Proceedings of FISITA 2010*, Budapest, Hungary, paper code: FISITA2010/FISITA2010-SC-P-36 (2010).
[19] C.F. Tan, W. Chen and M. Rauterberg, The relationship of head rotation angle and SCM EMG value for the development of AnS2, in: *Proceedings of World Congress on Engineering 2010*, London, UK, Vol. 3, 2010, pp. 2082–2085.
[20] C.F. Tan, W. Chen and M. Rauterberg, Total design of low cost aircraft cabin simulator, in: *Proceedings of Design 2010*, Cavtat, Croatia, 2010, pp. 1721–17280.
[21] A.R. Tilley and H. Dreyfuss, The *Measure of Man And Woman: Human Factors in Design*, John Wiley & Sons Inc., New York, 2002.
[22] D. van de Velde, Long Distance Bus Services in Europe: Concession or Free Market, Discussion Paper no. 2009-21, Joint Transport Research Centre, 2009.
[23] Wiring, http://wiring.org.co, accessed on 20 February 2010.
[24] World Health Organization, Travel by Air: Health Considerations, http://whqlibdoc.who.int/publications/2005/9241580364_chap2.pdf, accessed on March 2007.

Handbook of Ambient Assisted Living
J.C. Augusto et al. (Eds.)
IOS Press, 2012

doi:10.3233/978-1-60750-837-3-229

Gait Profile – A Biometric that Defines Our Mobility

Diana HODGINS*
European Technology for Business Ltd.

Abstract. This chapter discusses gait monitoring and why it is important to the health and wellbeing of individual, at any time of their life. It then describes a range of medical conditions which affect a person's gait and gait monitoring could be used to improve the outcomes following rehabilitation. Different techniques for monitor gait are also discussed, together with their relative merits and limitations. Finally, examples where monitoring has been used to help the treatment and rehabilitation processes have been provided.

Keywords. Gait monitoring, mobility, health and wellbeing, gait disorders

Introduction

It can be said that the way a person walks, or their gait, is one of their biometrics [1,3]. The gait profile can be defined through a number of different parameters, all which can be measured, and hence a person's 'gait' biometric can be defined. The gait parameters include a description of the way the trunk, arms, left and right lower limbs move through a stride cycle; specifically the trunk, thigh, shank and foot segments and the shoulder, hip, knee and ankle joints. The biomechanics of movement have been well documented and there are books which cover the topic in detail [9].

There are a number of reasons why it is important to measure a person's gait profile, including personal identification for security purposes and identification of potential health problems or deterioration in body movement. It is the latter that is the focus of this chapter, where maintaining health and well-being are of interest, as gait is a biometric that can change significantly with age, illness and injury. People learn to walk at a very early age and their gait characteristics develop. However, if a person grows up with a poor gait then compensatory gait deficits may introduce musculoskeletal pain in different parts of the body, or osteoarthritis later in life. There are many books and papers that describe the normal function of the gait cycle, which provide the reference from which deviations can be identified.

Identifying the precise abnormality within the gait profile is essential if it is to be corrected, either by training or surgical intervention. If it is identified early enough training can be sufficient and should alleviate pain and reduce injury and surgical intervention later in life. An unstable or uneven gait can result in a worsening in a medical condition, for example uneven wear on a knee joint, or in the elderly it may result in a fall. Gait profiling as part of a medical diagnosis makes it possible to quantify the real situation for each individual and prescribe the best course of treatment. For example,

*Corresponding Author: Diana Hodgins. E-mail: DMH@etb.co.uk.

for a damaged knee the person may be offered a partial rather than complete knee replacement. For an elderly person they may be offered a set of exercises to strengthen particular muscles. Changes of gait over time monitored over time would identify whether rehabilitation exercises are suitable and adapted where necessary. These are some examples which are discussed in some detail.

Gait profiling can be performed by a skilled practitioner, either visually or using equipment designed for this application. In this chapter different methods of gait profiling are discussed that could be applied to the different age groups and medical conditions.

1. The Need

Mobility is key to living a healthy life and to keep mobile we need to retain a normal gait. If we become sedentary then our muscles weaken and ultimately we lose the ability to walk. Mobility is recognized as one of the key aspects of keeping the population healthy and with a good quality of life [12] and with the percentage population above 70 increasing every year it is becoming more important to address this. A poor gait can occur at any time in a person's life, as a result of accident, injury, illness, or change in lifestyle. Specific examples are discussed in the following sections.

1.1. Falls in the Elderly

Injuries due to falls claim over 235,000 lives of EU citizens annually and represent the fourth leading cause of death within the European Union. Many of these falls are related to gait disorders. After a fall, 48% of older people report a fear of falling and 25% have a functional decline, which often leads to long-term care.

Elderly people fall for a variety of reasons, including a poor gait, which is currently identified by a range of subjective tests or a visual Gait Assessment [7]. For people who have fallen a Gait Assessment would provide a clear starting point and identify progress towards that of a healthy elderly person. There are many reasons why this approach is adopted including:

- Elderly people, particularly those with a known gait disorder are frail, unable to stand for any length of time.
- They do not like to have to prepare for a test e.g. change their clothes, have markers on, walk along a set route etc.
- They would not be able to negotiate a treadmill.

Optical, video and force plate systems all include one or more of these aspects. Recent sensor based systems overcome these problems and have been used on the elderly.

1.2. Orthopedics and Osteoarthritis

There are approximately 2.3 million knee and hip replacements carried out in Europe every year [8]. These are performed because the knee or hip joint has failed, causing pain and an abnormal gait. In most cases the person suffers extreme pain and in this case surgery is seen as the only solution. In addition, there are a number of knee injuries, for example a meniscus tear, or a problem with the anterior cruciate ligament. Whilst these also require surgical intervention, they are far less invasive that a total knee replacement and hence recovery time is shorter and the risk is less. Gait profiling can be used in the clinical assessment to help identify the problem. For example, hip abduction in stair climbing has been shown to be a key indicator to identify recovery levels after different types of surgery for total knee arthroplasty [11].

Once the type of operation has been chosen and the patient has undergone the surgery, they should undergo physiotherapy. Their gait profile should be assessed soon after the operation (1–2 weeks) either visually by a trained practitioner or with the assistance of technology based systems. Either way a target outcome of their gait profile can be set, to help ensure that the patient makes a full recovery. Clinical evidence suggests that a return to normal activity after surgery is important [6].

Osteoarthritis in later life causes an asymmetric gait [5]. A routine gait assessment would identify any asymmetries and then physiotherapy could be used to correct these. Objective measurements would help to identify exactly when symmetry has been achieved, whereas a visual assessment by a skilled practitioner can identify noticeable asymmetries in different parts of the anatomy. If this is left untreated then surgical intervention is normally the only solution. However, if it is identified early enough, alternative treatment strategies can be adopted, for example a hyaluronan injection could be sufficient to delay the further deterioration of the knee joint and help the person resume a normal gait profile.

1.3. Spina Bifida and Cerebral Palsy

Cerebral Palsy is caused by damage to the motor control centres of the developing brain and can occur during pregnancy, during childbirth or up to about age three. The person has limited movement which affects their gait. Spina Bifida is a developmental birth defect to the spinal cord and this causes nerve damage which affects their gait.

For both of these conditions, where it is considered that surgery can improve their movement a full gait analysis is carried out to assess the situation prior to surgery. This may be done either using complex 3D optical systems or observational kinematics [4].

1.4. Foot Disorders

Orthotics are often prescribed for people with foot problems, to correct their abnormal gait identified from pressure profiles on foot loading in stance.

1.5. Prosthesis

Accidents, or medical conditions which affect blood circulation in the lower limbs, can result in a partial or full lower limb prosthesis. Learning how to walk with the prosthesis, with attention to symmetry of movement, is recognised as important for the person's long term health and wellbeing.

There has been extensive technological advancements made in prosthesis design and now there are a wide range of active devices which alter their dynamics depending upon the terrain and speed that the person is moving. These devices have been designed using the latest modeling methods, manufactured using high strength, low density materials and enable people with lower limb prosthesis not only to carry out day to day activities but also compete is sports which were previously inaccessible to them. However, even with the very latest technology, the person may not attain the full potential from their prosthesis because it is incorrectly set. Skilled practitioners are used to fit and set the prosthesis. To do this they visually assess the person, generally in an indoor environment and adjust setting until the person feels most comfortable and noticeable asymmetries are minimized. Recent advances in measuring techniques means that dynamic measurements on a variety of terrains can be taken and adjustments then made to optimize the performance and minimize asymmetries under the variety of conditions they will experience in everyday use.

1.6. Neurological Disorders

Parkinson's disease and dementia are two examples of medical conditions that can affect a person's gait. Parkinson's disease (PD) is a common neurodegenerative disorder with prevalence rates in western countries estimated at 0.3% of the entire population and about 1% in people over 60 years of age. PD is believed to be due to substantial dopaminergic neuron reduction in a brain region. The symptoms include rigidity on passive movement and slowness of movement (bradykinesia), often referred to as a shuffling gait. Drugs, like levodopa, are the most common form of treatment, often combined with physiotherapy. However, measurable metrics that quantify the improvements in gait due to these interventions are difficult using current technologies as gait parameters change during the day.

Dementia is another neurological condition which is associated with changes in gait patterns through the day. Gait profiling would identify the changes in gait with treatment but would need to be available over the entire 24 hour cycle. For this reason, this approach is not currently followed, except for research. However, with the development of wireless, sensor based system, simple gait parameters, for example when strides occur over a 24 hour period, could soon be in commercial use.

2. The Gait Cycle

The gait cycle is the continuous, repetitive pattern of walking or running. The locomotion is primarily concerned with the lower limb movement, although there is also some movement in the trunk and the upper limbs. For the purpose of this chapter, only the lower limb movement will be analysed.

The complete gait cycle is the motion from any time in the cycle to the same time in the next cycle. The combination of the motion of the different limb segments over a gait cycle and the phase information of these provides a comprehensive understanding of the kinematic features of the gait cycle.

A gait cycle is repetitive and can therefore any analysis can start at any point in the cycle, for example initial placement of the supporting heel on the ground to when the same heel contacts the ground for a second time. The phase data is normally separated out as two main sectors: stance and swing phase, where a complete gait cycle includes both a stance (shown in Fig. 1) and a swing phase (shown in Fig. 2) on both limbs. By evaluating each individual phase of the gait cycle, in terms of both the amplitude of movement, the orientation and the timing of the movement, a skilled practitioner, e.g. a physical therapist obtains important information into specific muscular weaknesses and joint problems. Addressing these issues in a rehabilitation programme will lead to a more efficient gait pattern, resulting in decreased risk of injury, less energy expenditure,

Stance Phase

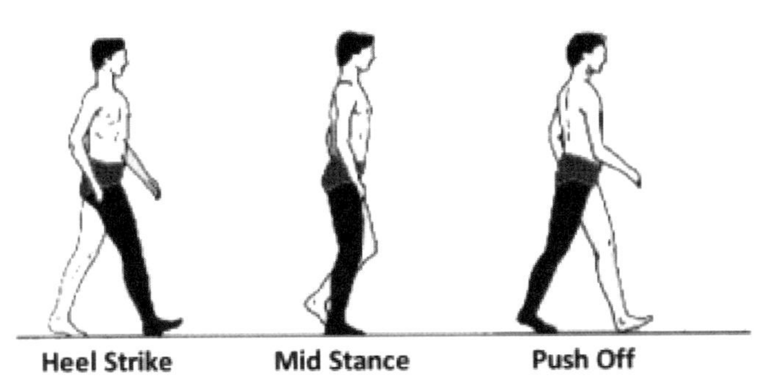

Figure 1. Stance phase through the gait cycle on the right leg.

Swing Phase

Acceleration
Swing Through
Deceleration

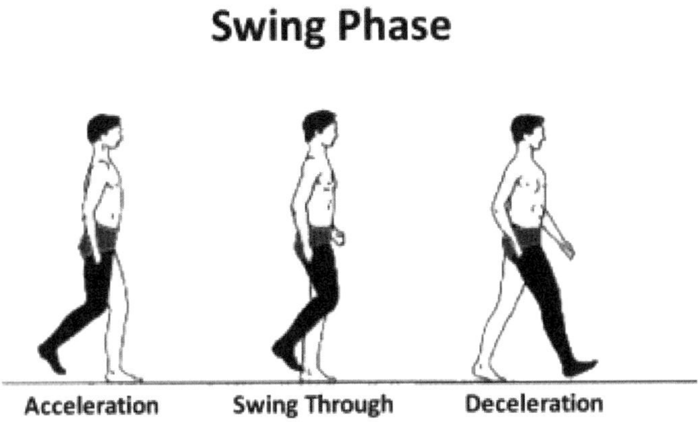

Figure 2. Swing phase through the gait cycle on the right leg.

greater functional independence, and improved muscular balance. Monitoring the progress, either visually, or using technology designed for gait monitoring, identifies when the problems have been rectified and a normal gait cycle has been resumed.

The stance phase is the element where the foot is in contact with the ground and equates to approximately 60% of the cycle when walking. The swing phase takes up the remaining 40%. During walk there is a period called double stance. This is where both feet are in contact with the ground. The swing and stance phases can be further broken down into the following elements:

- Heel strike – The point when the heel hits the floor.
- Foot flat – The point where the whole of the foot comes into contact with the floor.
- Mid stance – Where weight is transferred from the back of the foot to the front of the foot.
- Toe off – Using the toes to push off thereby propelling us forwards.
- Acceleration – The period from toe off to maximum knee flexion in order for the foot to clear the ground.

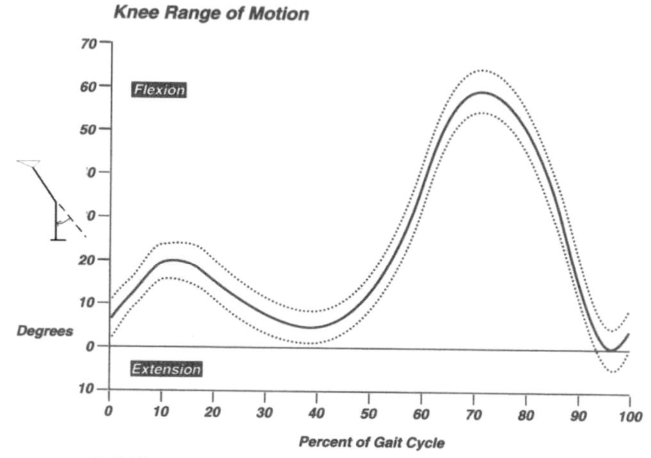

Solid line –Average value, Dotted line – Standard deviation

Figure 3. Knee flexion profile for a typical healthy adult.

- Mid-swing – The period between maximum knee flexion and the forward movement of the tibia (shin bone) to a vertical position.
- Deceleration – The end of the swing phase before heel strike.

Human visualization, plus optical measurement systems are suitable for identifying events, like those listed above and optical systems can also provide information on the range of motion, temporal information and a complete profile, with events identified on them if required. Force and pressure systems can identify the start and end of the stance phase and the pressure characteristics of the foot during this part of the gait cycle but cannot provide any information on the swing phase when there is no load.

The lower limb movement can be presented and summarized as the knee flexion profile over an entire stride. For a healthy person this should be the same for both knees and should look like the curve shown in Fig. 3 [12]. This shows a high flexion of around 60°, which occurs in the swing phase, and a lower flexion of around 20°, which occurs as the body weight goes over the foot in stance. Deviations from this profile, particularly if it deviates just on one leg, would be an indication of a problem in the gait cycle. The temporal phase information of this movement is also important.

In order to examine the movement in more detail, the lower limb movement can be further broken down into the thigh and calf segments. In a healthy subject the hip, knee and ankle joints are optimized for movement thigh, shank and foot movement in the sagittal plane. Any coronal movement (abduction or adduction) introduces out of balance movement and should be avoided. This more involved analysis of lower limb movement can only be carried out using true 3D optical systems or the more recently available sensor based systems and therefore only limited published data is available.

3. Methods and Technologies used to Obtain a Gait Profile

Gait information can be obtained using a skilled practitioner alone, a technological approach, or a combination, where a skilled practitioner enhances their assessment by using one or more technologies. Where the analysis relies entirely on a skilled practitioner the following points must be considered:

- the skilled practitioner's availability;
- the limitations of the skilled practitioner to quantify parameters.

If a technology based solution is chosen, then a decision must be made on what method to choose. This will be based on the amount of information and the accuracy required, which is directly related to the medical application. For example, for Cerebral Palsy and Spina Bifida sufferers, the information will be used to identify the surgical intervention, and must therefore be 3-dimensional and provide information on the legs, feet and trunk. At the other extreme, people with dementia may just require a simple stride counter. Cost, availability and applicability for the different medical applications are all important criteria when choosing the most suitable technology.

4. High Cost, Low Availability, High Accuracy Optical Systems

The optical Gait Laboratory is the most extensive system available today. People who attend these laboratories normally have a serious medical condition that requires a detailed analysis.

The analysis is usually performed on a level walking surface. The surface may have force measurement built into the surface and there would be optical camera capability. Markers would be placed on the patient and optical data will be obtained from a number of angles, using cameras suitably positioned around the laboratory. The optical data can be input into a bespoke software application for more detailed review by the Gait Laboratory specialist.

The trial can be quite involved and take up to 3 hours. The data is then analysed by the specialist and presented in a report for the doctor or surgeon treating the person. The time required to run the trial and analyze the results makes this an expensive solution. The availability of facilities, time for analysis and cost make this approach unsuitable for integration into daily healthcare services.

However, this is the most comprehensive and accurate gait analysis tool available to date and therefore it is the most commonly used system for academic studies on all of the clinical applications described previously and many more besides. The data obtained provides the basis for defining the gait abnormalities that are present and the magnitudes of these for the different conditions. Unfortunately, these studies normally only have a small sample set, due to the cost and complexity of the trials. Therefore, this approach has been used for defining conditions but not for determining typical values and spreads in a large population. For example, only a very small percentage all people who have undergone total knee arthroplasty have been monitored after surgery and then 1 year later.

5. Low Cost, Minimal Information, Low Accuracy Video Solutions

The use of low cost video systems is becoming far more widespread, with the availability of high speed cameras and motion analysis software. It is often available in physiotherapy clinics, where it is used to identify certain gait abnormalities and more recently in high performance sports shops, where it is used to look at foot loading with different shoes.

This analysis is often done on a treadmill to maintain the person in a steady position in the view of the video. The benefit of using a treadmill is the speed variable is removed and a large number of strides can be examined. The most common use is the camera behind the person under test, to obtain the rear view of the customer walking or running. The foot and calf position during stance is used to ascertain whether there is over-pronation or under-pronation of the foot. It is also possible to gather elements of data on problems like fallen or collapsed arches and leg length issues. Recommendations on footwear are normally made after a test. Stride duration, stride length and step time can also be determined, by manually identifying events in each cycle.

Other information that can be obtained if more than one camera is used is the range of motion of the thigh, calf and knee joint. This requires a camera each side of the person and the analysis of the data requires identifying specific events, e.g. maximum protraction and maximum retraction of each segment. Most of the information is obtained from freezing specific frames and drawing lines through key anatomical features. The accuracy of such a system is therefore dependent upon the positioning of the camera and the accuracy of identifying the anatomical features.

6. Basic Foot Pressure Systems

The pressure system provides information on the foot loading during stance. From this information, certain aspects of gait are calculated and the rest are inferred. The force distribution throughout the stance phase from initial foot contact is examined. This may be through pressure pads placed in the sole of the person's shoes or the treadmill or floor may have force measurement capabilities built into the walking surface. This will provide a force measurement, normally as a number of discrete frames. This type of analysis is particularly suitable for providing footwear recommendation, or as part of the information in a full gait analysis. The limitations, particularly with the internal pressure pads are accuracy [13]. For this reason, this type of system is generally used to provide a pressure distribution profile rather than absolute values of pressure.

Stride duration can be determined from the time between consecutive events e.g. initial foot contact on the left foot. Symmetry of load can be determined (left to right) and the loading over the foot through the stance phase. From this over-pronation or supernation are inferred. No information on the knee, thigh or shank range of motion can be determined.

7. Low Cost, High Accuracy, Sensor Based Gait Monitoring System

Over the last decade there has been significant development in the area of sensor systems for monitoring motion. The evolution of this type of system has been rapid due to the advancement in solid state accelerometers and gyroscopes. Around 2005 the first 3-axis accelerometers became available, followed in 2010 by the first 3-axis gyroscopes and 3-axis magnetometers. These sensors, which have the range, accuracy and resolution to be able to monitor human body motion, have meant that sensor modules can be mounted onto limb segments, without affecting the movement of that limb. Combined with the advancement in wireless technology and storage capabilities, complete motion sensing systems have started to appear on the market.

Sensor based solutions are an effective, validated method of quickly and easily assessing key parameters of a gait profile, either in a clinical or home environment. This means that they can easily be used as part of the initial assessment in the hospital and in the follow up assessments in a clinic or at home in large scale programmes.

The main advantages that these systems offer over those previously mentioned are:

- Quantifiable data to the accuracy of a full optical gait laboratory.
- Ability to monitor a large population in their environment.
- Suitability of use on people of all ages and disabilities.
- Automatic analysis of digital data.

The systems could be used as a gait assessment tool, to provide quantifiable data throughout the treatment and rehabilitation cycle for all people undergoing a certain clinical procedure, for example a total knee arthroplasty (TKA). Thus, it will provide a more robust assessment of the intervention process than has been possible previously. In the longer term systems like this could become widely available in general practitioners, or walk in clinics, in a similar way to other medical diagnostic equipment. This would then help pick up early signs of gait abnormalities before they cause medical problems.

8. Typical Data That Can be Obtained from Sensor Based Systems

With this type of system it is possible to measure segments by placing a sensor along that segment, so in theory any body segment can be analysed, either in isolation, or with respect to other body segments. If a multiple of sensors are to be used, for example, to monitor lower limb movement, then these need to be synchronized, in order that temporal phase information can also be captured.

In research applications, sensors have been placed on different segments and the information relevant to the study calculated. This would be classed as a universal research tool, where individual Inertial Measurement Units (IMUs) are arranged by the research group and custom analysis software developed for their application. There are many research papers which cover clinical investigations using these tools [2].

For commercial applications, a system needs to be defined and the user and analysis software prepared for ease of use, if the full benefits of this type of system are to be realized. For example, if every person undergoing TKA is tested after surgery and then through rehabilitation, a system needs to be in place which can be attached to the patient, a short test carried out, the results obtained and a report prepared for the clinician, all within 10 minutes. The person carrying out the test would typically be a trained technician or nurse, and should not require any specific system knowledge.

9. The Gait Trainer, a Sensor Based Product

The ‘Gait Trainer’ system, developed by European Technology for Business (ETB) Ltd under the Technology Strategy Board (TSB) Assistive Living Innovation Platform (ALIP1) and an earlier EC Framework 6 Integrated Project ‘Healthy Aims’, is an inno-

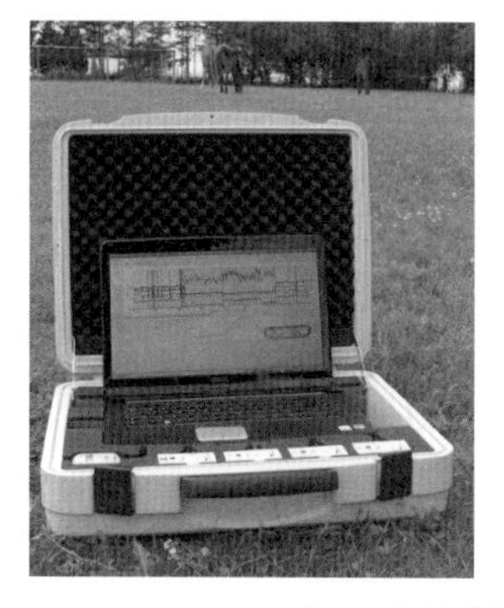

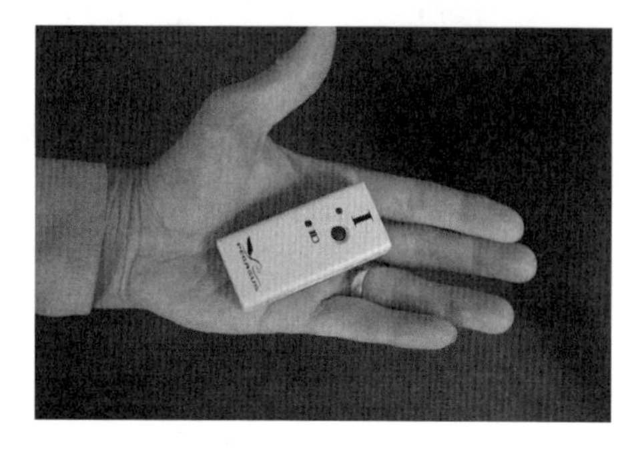

Figure 4. Gait Trainer system and the sensor.

vative new solution, designed to provide gait assessment in a person's natural environment. It is designed to form an integral part of medical procedures used in hospitals, outpatients and day centres.

The system shown in Fig. 4 provides the user with information on the lower limb movement at walk, either on level ground, slopes or stairs, making it suitable for the wide variety of medical conditions described previously. The Gait Trainer produces easy, quick, relevant output analysis reports, providing critical information to consultants to assist them in diagnostic evaluations in the specific medical sectors described previously. The tests are non-invasive and the equipment is completely portable, allowing gait measurement in the users' natural environments without being observed, as shown in Fig. 4. The user follows a protocol related to their particular market area. The gait trainer allows healthcare workers to 'assess', 'treat' and 'monitor'.

The product uses 4 inertial motion sensors (IMS), shown in Fig. 4. Each IMS, total weight 54 grams and measuring 73 × 36 × 19 mm, contains a tri-axial 5g accelerometer and three single axis, 1200 deg/s gyroscopes. The sensor data is filtered by anti-aliasing filters with a cut-off frequency of approximately 50 Hz, the outputs of which are sampled with a 12 bit analogue-to-digital converter at a frequency of 102.4 Hz. Each IMS is factory set to within 1 ppm (equivalent to 3.6 ms per hour) of a reference time traceable to national standards, with the aim of achieving less than 10 ms per hour relative drift between units after synchronization. The IMS sample interval is 1/102.4 or 9.77 ms, which is greater than the relative drift between two units in one hour. Before every test the four IMS units were synchronized with a computer clock, using custom software. Each IMS unit is time synchronized at the start of each trial, by a simultaneous pulse sent to the respective units.

These sensors are fitted to the calf and thigh of both legs using simple straps, as shown in Fig. 5. The straps, with the sensors, need to be light enough not to influence the limb segment movement and yet retain the sensor in place. For the thigh sensor straps an additional tie support it attached between the thigh strap and a belt, to stop any slippage whilst walking. The sensor alignment along the segment is important if absolute values are required, but if an offset is acceptable then it is only necessary to retain the sensor in position. If the sensor is misplaced around the leg, then there will be some difference between the sensor result and the movement in the sagittal plane.

A simple test would be a short walk along a level surface. Different protocols can be used depending on the application, such as stairs or uneven surfaces (grass, stones,

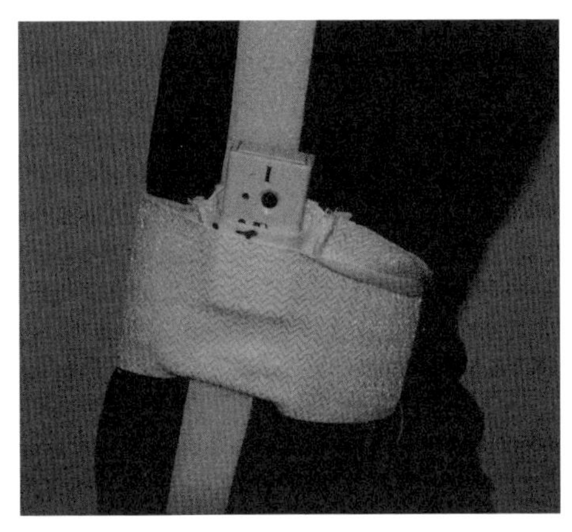
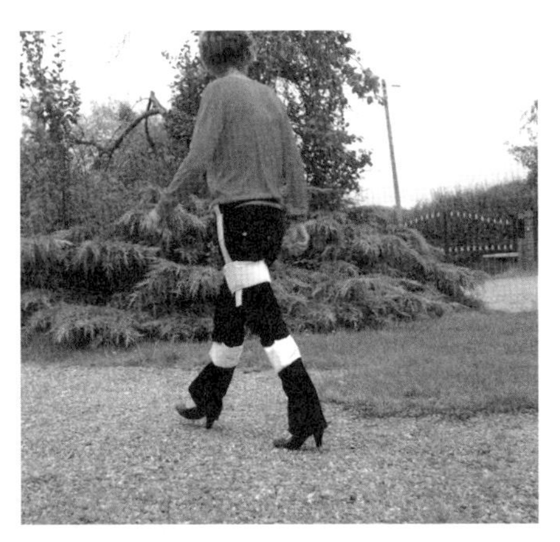

Figure 5. Left thigh strap with tie with sensor partially mounted and all four straps.

slopes, steps). Currently the output of the Gait Trainer is a report giving the required information for the specific market. This can be a simple one line report informing the patient that their gait is say 40% symmetric, to a full detailed analysis of how each limb is moving relative to the other for each and every stride.

Because sensor based systems can record data continuously and the analysis is done automatically, it is logical to analyse the entire trial and then extract the results from the most relevant sections. This is different to optical or video based systems, where data is normally only collected over a short period within the trial, typically around 10 seconds.

The data that is output for the user is system dependent. For a system with sensors on the thigh and calf of each leg, the following information can be obtained and is available from the Gait Trainer system.

- Stride duration.
- Knee angle – left and right for the entire trial.
- Phasing between the left and right leg within a gait cycle.
- Sagittal and coronal angle profile for both the thigh and calf segments.

From this, sections can be chosen and the following values can be calculated

- Typical profile for the knee, thigh and calf in the region (left and right).
- Phasing between the left and right for the typical stride.
- Range of motion (ROM) for knee, thigh and calf.
- Asymmetry between the left and right knee flexion, thigh or calf segments.

Profile plots can be provided, plus a table with the ROM values, stride duration and phasing data.

10. Segment Angle Measurement

The analysis of the movement of a segment enables users to measure the angle of any limb segment during normal activity, for example walking on a level surface or up or down stairs. Sensor based systems and optical systems with 3D capability can provide

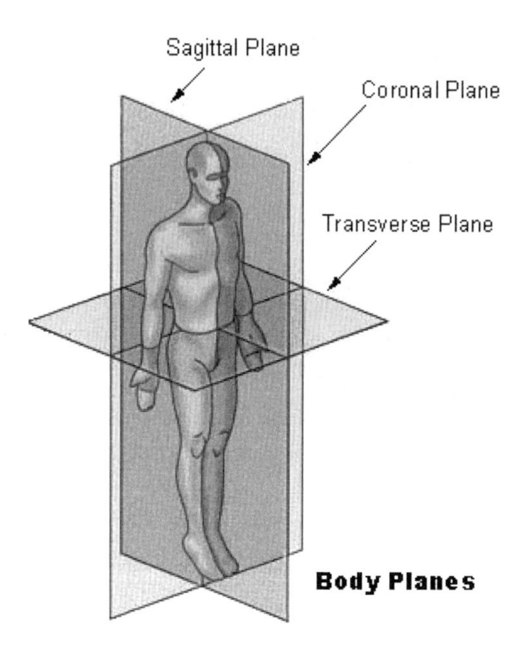

Figure 6. Definition of body planes used in gait analysis.

measurements of angle over time in the sagittal (cranial caudal) and coronal (mediolateral) planes for both the thigh and calf segments. For the sensor based systems the sensors would typically be mounted with their axes along the sagittal, coronal and transverse planes shown in Fig. 6. For the optical systems the markers are normally mounted on the joints, in both the sagittal and coronal planes.

This approach enables the stride parameters to be analysed in detail and any anomalies can be directly related to a specific limb segment. Video and pressure or force plate systems are not able to provide this level of information.

10.1. Characteristics of a Normal Stride

When a person walks they swing both the thigh and calf in the sagittal plane. In a healthy subject the calf segment typically swings through 70 degrees and a shorter percentage of the stride occurs from retraction to protraction than from protraction to retraction. The thigh segment typically swings through 37 degrees and is only negative for 35% of the stride. The calf and thigh are out of phase with each other producing a variable knee flexion angle through the stride. These values have been taken from a study on over 100 healthy adults using the Gait Trainer system.

The angle for both legs in both the sagittal and coronal planes for the calf and thigh provides an indication of the degree of symmetry between the left and right leg and also the amount of flexion that the person is producing when walking. In addition, it provides information on whether the leg is swinging out of plane, which can cause imbalance in the stride and asymmetric loadings on joints and the back.

The thigh segment provides the momentum to move the leg forward and the flexion angle provides precise information on how well this is achieved on both legs. The

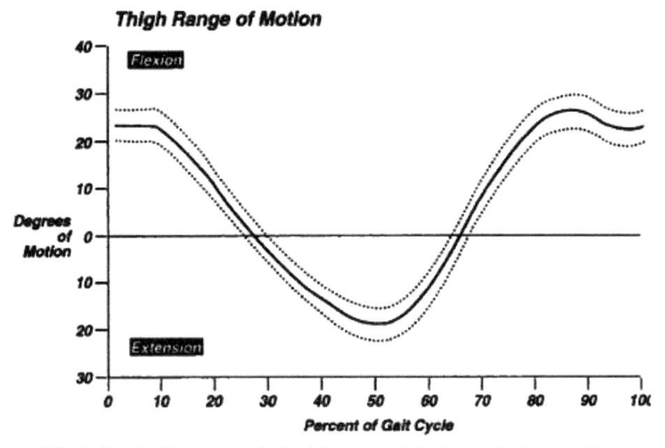

Black line is the mean, dotted lines are +/– 1 standard deviation

Figure 7. Typical profile for a thigh through a gait cycle.

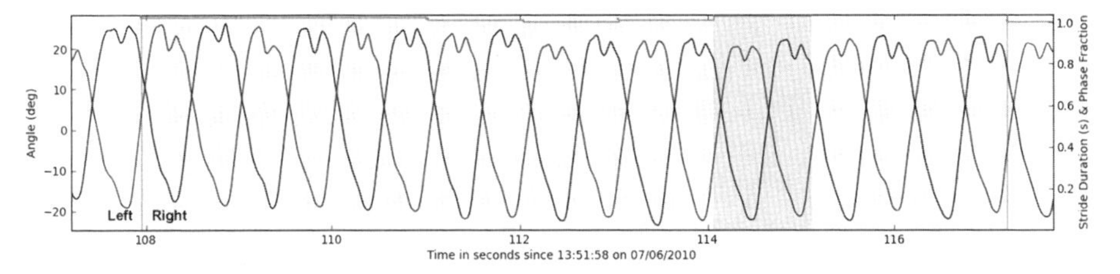

Figure 8. Sagittal angles with time for the left and right thigh.

plot below shows the thigh range of motion for a healthy person walking. A typical profile is shown in Fig. 7, obtained using an optical based system.

10.2. Example from the Gait trainer System – Thigh Segments

Data are processed automatically using the Poseidon software [10]. The sagittal and coronal angles, stride duration and temporal phasing between the left and right segments are calculated. The angle is taken from the vertical, where vertical is zero. In the sagittal plane retraction is negative and protraction is positive. In the coronal plane a swing inwards is negative and outwards is positive. The data are presented as a plot and from this, sections can be chosen for review.

The thigh segments are calculated in the same way as the calf segments and the plot of the entire test provided. In the example shown in Fig. 8, the highlighted section is the sagittal angle for the left and right thigh when the person is walking. The dark stride is the one that has been identified as the typical stride, i.e least error when compared to all the other strides.

From this the left and right thigh typical stride is plotted in Fig. 9, together with the standard deviation (dotted lines). The sagittal and coronal angles are shown on one plot for the left thigh and a second plot for the right thigh.

The left and right thigh profile has two peaks on protraction, which relates to the initial contact and load on the limb. The left to right comparison shows that the profiles are almost identical. There were nine strides in the region and the average stride duration was 1.03 s.

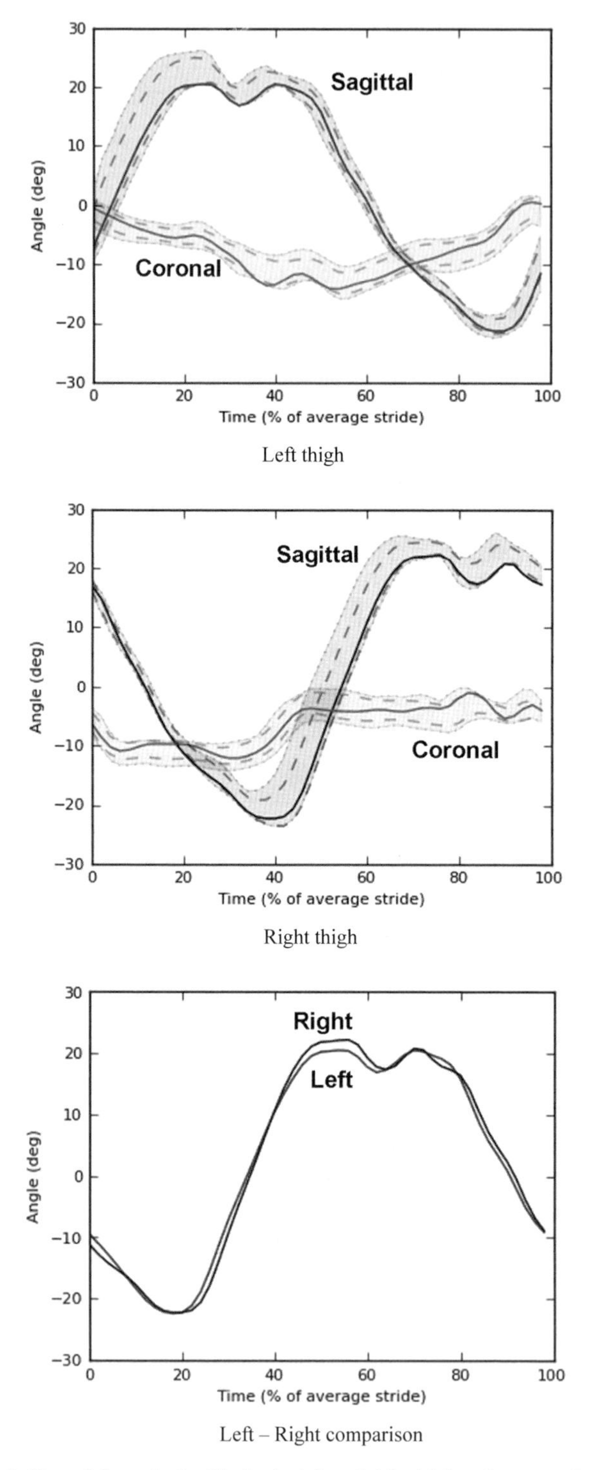

Figure 9. Plots of the typical stride for the left and right thigh and a comparison plot.

Table 1. Summary data for the left and right thigh

	Left S Angle	Left C Angle	Right S Angle	Right C Angle
Typ Peak to Peak (°)	43.8	13.2	45.1	10.0
Min Peak to Peak (°)	41.8	11.9	43.8	9.0
Max Peak to Peak (°)	46.2	14.8	46.5	11.3

Note: S – Sagittal, C – Coronal

Table 1 summarises the data from the same strides as the calf segments and therefore the typical stride duration and the variation is the same as for the calf segments at 1.03 s. The variation in thigh flexion angle is low, as for the calf segments, further supporting the earlier statement that the stride profile is steady and symmetric.

10.3. Example from the Gait Trainer System – Calf Segments

In this example the highlighted section of normal walking has been selected for analysis and the dark stride identified as the typical stride as shown in Fig. 10.

For this section the typical stride is then plotted in Fig. 11, together with the standard deviation (dotted line). The sagittal and coronal angles are shown on one plot for the left calf, and a second plot for the right calf.

The plots show that the flexion angle profile in the sagittal plane on the left calf is slightly different from that of the right, whilst the total flexion angle is comparable. There is minimal coronal movement in both the left and right calves, which means that there is minimal out of plane swing of the calf on either leg. The comparison shows very quickly that the profiles are similar.

The statistics are also provided for each region in tabular form (Table 2), where total flexion angle, stride duration and temporal phasing, are quoted for the 8 strides, the highlighted section. The average stride duration was 1.03 s.

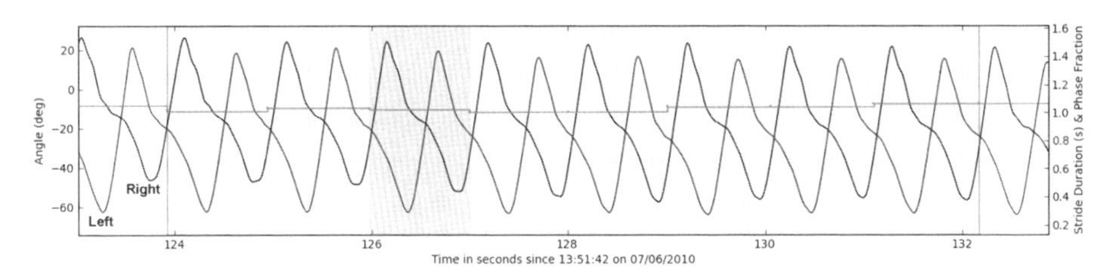

Figure 10. Sagittal angles with time for the left and right calf.

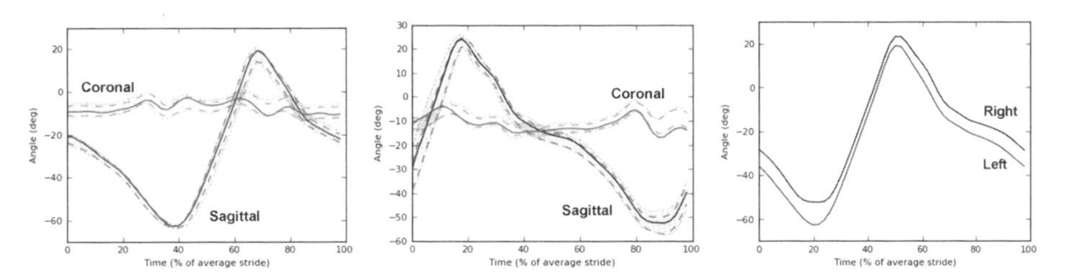

Figure 11. Plots of the typical stride for the left and right calf and a comparison plot.

Table 2. Summary data for the left and right calf

	Left S Angle	Left C Angle	Right S Angle	Right C Angle
Typ Peak to Peak (°)	80.2	9.6	76.9	11.1
Min Peak to Peak (°)	78.7	7.1	72.6	10.1
Max Peak to Peak (°)	83.4	12.0	80.2	12.9

Note: S – Sagittal, C – Coronal

The variation in calf flexion angle over the 8 strides is low, providing evidence of steadiness. The asymmetry between the left and right is also very low.

11. Knee Flexion Angle Measurement

In Section 3 the gait cycle was described and the knee flexion angle profile for a typical healthy adult plotted. This is one parameter that is frequently quoted in clinical papers as it provides a good summary of both the thigh and calf motion through both the swing and stance phase of the gait cycle. The sensor based systems and the 3-D optical systems can provide this information accurately. Video based systems can only provide knee flexion on both limbs if cameras are placed each side of the person, which is not common practice. Force and pressure based systems cannot provide this data.

In sensor based systems the knee angle analysis software measures the angle between two segments, where sensor units are mounted on the calf and thigh of each leg. In the Gait trainer system the angle over time is defined as the minimum angle to rotate one sensor onto the other as shown in Fig. 12. It measures the knee joint angle of both legs simultaneously, providing additional information on the relative phasing of the joint angle, as well as the profile for each joint. It does this during normal activity, for example walking on a level surface, or on slopes and stairs and does so with minimal hindrance and with no practical range limit.

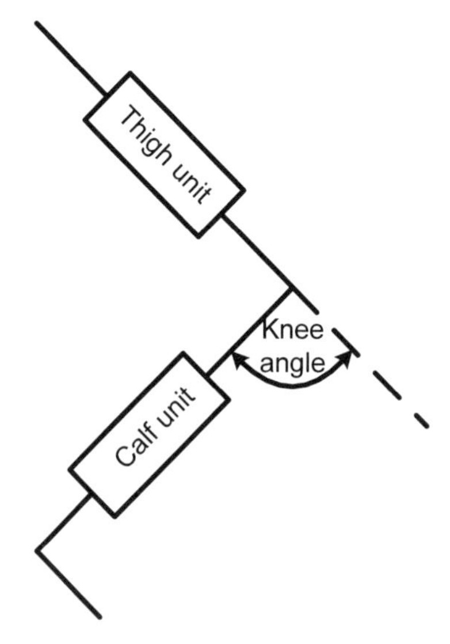

Figure 12. Definition of the knee joint angle.

11.1. Knee Flexion in a Person with a Normal Gait

When a person walks the calf motion is out of phase with respect to the thigh motion through the stride cycle, thus producing a knee flexion angle that changes through the stride.

11.2. The Results of a Knee Flexion Analysis Using the Gait Trainer System

The data are processed automatically and the knee flexion angles, stride duration and temporal phasing between the left and right calf calculated for the entire trial. From this, sections can be analysed. This plot shown in Fig. 13 shows the left and right knee flexion angle for a steady period of walking. The left and right knee are shown. The angle in degrees is the scale on the left hand axis. The top straight line is the stride duration in seconds and the bottom straight line the phasing between the left and right calf, quoted as a fraction of a complete stride, where 1 is a complete stride. Both of these have the scale on the right hand axis. This plot provides an overview of the stability and uniformity of the knee flexion angle for both the left and right leg. In this example the left and right leg knee flexion is comparable.

From the shaded section the left and right flexion angles for a typical stride (highlighted as darker shaded region) is calculated as well as the standard deviation over the strides chosen (dotted lines). This is plotted as shown below in Fig. 14, with the phase between the left and right knee as a percentage of the complete stride (a) and then with the phase information removed (b).

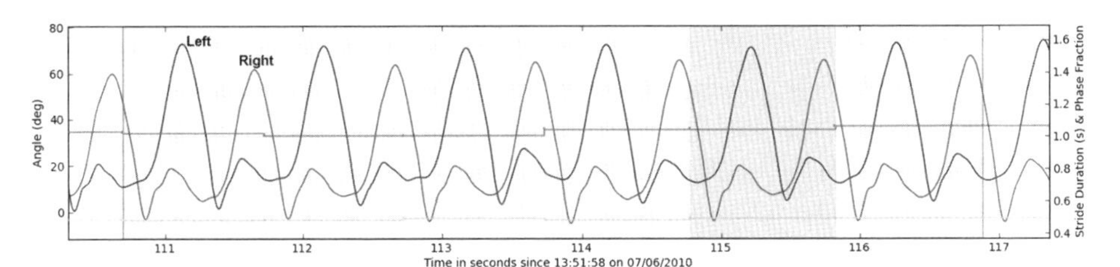

Figure 13. Knee flexion plot for a healthy person at walk.

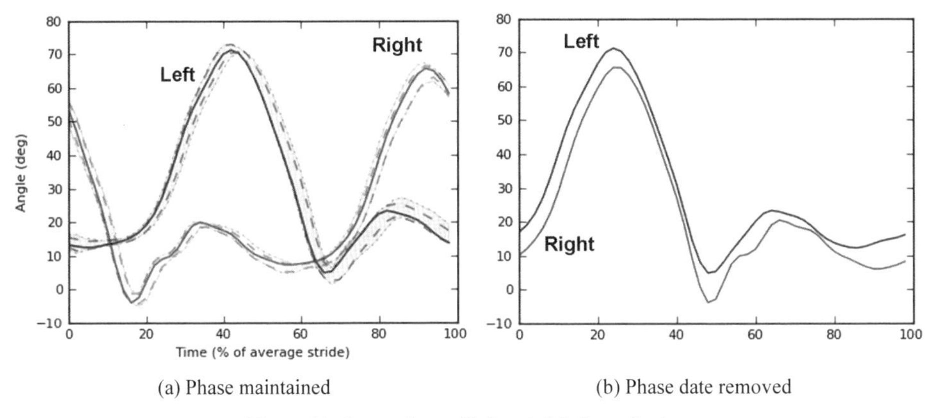

(a) Phase maintained (b) Phase date removed

Figure 14. Comparison of left and right knee flexion.

Table 3. Summary data for the left and right knee

	Left knee	Right knee
Typ Peak to Peak (°)	68.5	68.3
Min Peak to Peak (°)	66.2	64.8
Max Peak to Peak (°)	71.5	71.5

The final piece of information that is provided for the chosen section is a summary (Table 3). This shows that 6 strides were chosen with an average stride duration of 1.03 s and a variation of 0.05 s, or 5%. The typical knee flexion angle was 68 degrees on the left and right leg, showing excellent symmetry of movement.

12. Case Studies

The benefit to monitoring a person's gait profile has already been discussed. In this section some examples of people being monitored through rehabilitation following treatment, using the Gait Trainer system, are presented.

12.1. Case Study 1. Pre and Post Exercise on an Elderly Person

An elderly lady who was mobile with the use of a roller frame had a fall on her left side. Her gait was monitored and the major asymmetry of her left to right was quantified in terms of difference in knee flexion. She then started to attend balance classes, and one month later her gait was re-assessed.

She continued to attend the Balance Class and also do some exercises at home for a further month. She regained sufficient strength that she could walk unaided and she was measured again. The results shown in Fig. 15 show that there is a marked improvement in her gait profile over the 8 weeks when she has been attending the balance classes. Immediately after her fall, the motion of her left leg was considerably less than the right leg. By week 4 her left leg now had almost the same range of motion as the right leg, making the gait pattern far more symmetric. By week 8 she was walking unaided with a symmetric gait pattern. Her stride duration had also reduced from 1.7 s to 1.5 s, which is closer to the 1.1 s value for a person over 60.

12.2. Case Study 2. Patient with Osteoarthritis

This patient had previously had a right total knee replacement and recently had been having a problem with his left (normal) knee. X-rays of the left knee showed that it was now affected by osteoarthritis, and the patient had significant discomfort on walking. Gait analysis was carried out and revealed a near normal pattern in the right knee that had previously been replaced and a significant deficit in the left knee. An injection of hyaluronan was recommended and a single dose of 6ml was inserted under local anaesthesia. One month later the patient was reviewed. At this stage he had complete relief of pain. Gait analysis was repeated and revealed that a symmetrical gait had now been restored as shown in Fig. 16.

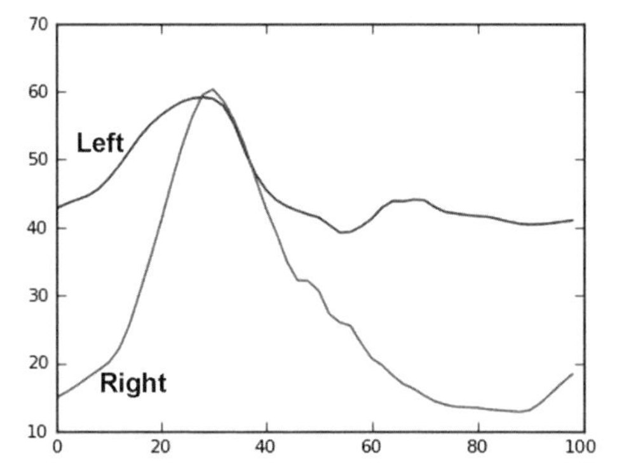

Immediately after the fall, with Roller frame. Left knee 24°, right knee 45°

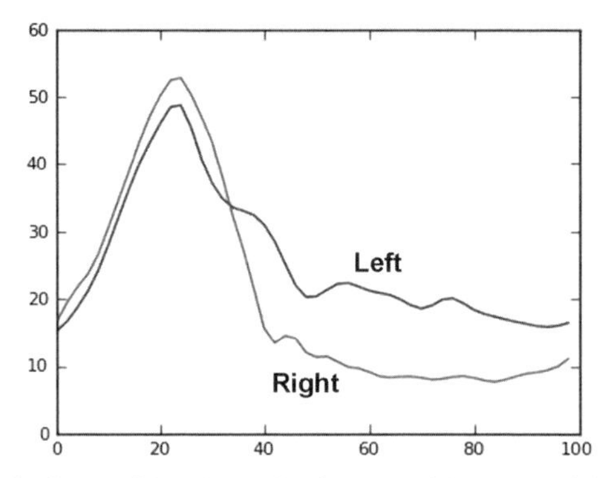

One month after the fall, with Roller frame. Left knee 38°, right knee 45°

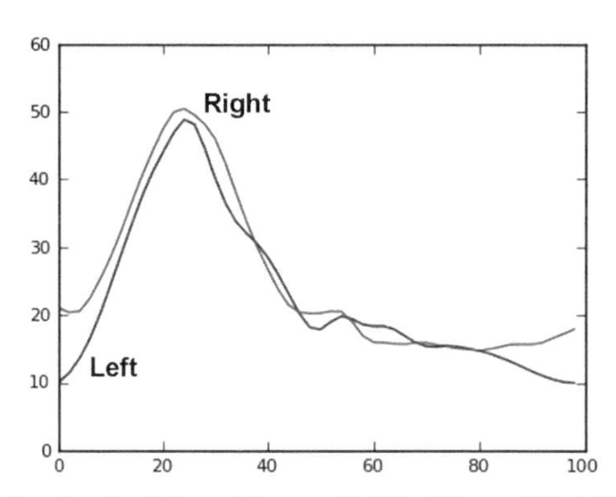

Two months after the fall, walking unaided. Left knee 42°, right knee 35°

Figure 15. Knee flexion profiles and stride data for an elderly person.

Knee flexion and stride duration were measured at the first examination. The left leg had a lower flexion in the swing phase compared to the right knee, but the difference was only 6° (48° left, 54° right). The time of swing was also slightly less on the left compared to the right. The stride duration was slow at 1.38 s, suggesting some reluctance to walk. The right knee flexion at 54° is within 1 standard deviation for a healthy person.

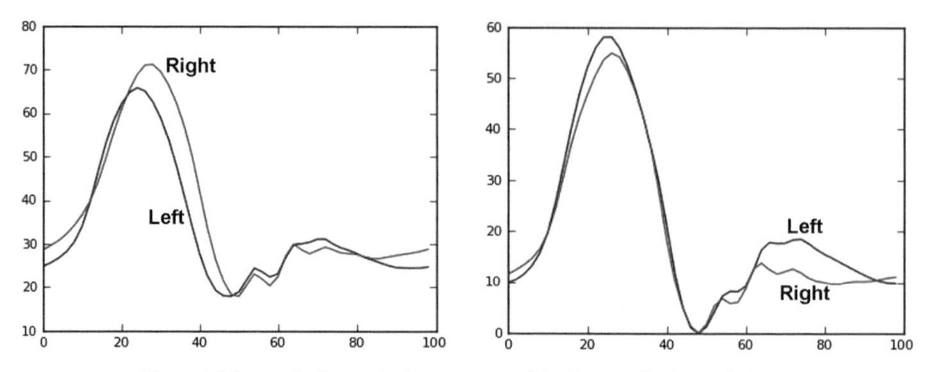

Figure 16. Person before and after treatment of hyaluronan (before and after).

One month after the injection the patient was brought back for a second gait test. This showed that the left leg had improved with the knee flexion now symmetrical with comparable amplitude (56° left, 55° right) and the time in the swing phase almost identical. The stride duration has also reduced significantly from 1.38 s to 1.24 s, which is further indication that a normal gait has been resumed.

In many cases where a patient has already had one total knee replacement with a good result and the second knee starts to deteriorate the first thought of both patient and surgeon is to consider a second joint replacement. However, even when there is moderately severe osteoarthritis hyaluronan injections may be sufficient to restore normal knee function as least in the short term. The availability of gait analysis in this patient as part of the consultation meant that it was possible to demonstrate objective improvement and return of symmetry.

12.3. Case Study 3. Patient Treated for a Meniscus Tear

This 59 year old patient underwent surgery on his left knee to repair a meniscus tear. A gait analysis was performed every week from week 1 to week 6. At the end of week 6 he completed his physiotherapy.

The recovery process of this patient who has undergone surgery to repair a torn meniscus in the left knee has shown that close to a normal gait profile has been obtained 6 weeks after surgery. From week 3 to 4 the patient suffered a recurrence of pain, which resulted in a reduction in knee movement. The doctor associated this with too much physiotherapy and this was reduced to massage and hot/cold treatment in week 5. So the increase in knee flexion from week 1 to week 3 was more than should be expected for a normal slow painless recovery.

The asymmetry in knee flexure at the end of treatment by week 6 was minimal as shown in Fig. 17, with the subject reducing the flexion on the healthy leg to bring it in line with the leg that had been operated on. However, one noticeable difference with this patients gait and a typical healthy gait profile is that there is no straightening of the knee after flexion on load. This is true for both knees, not just the treated one.

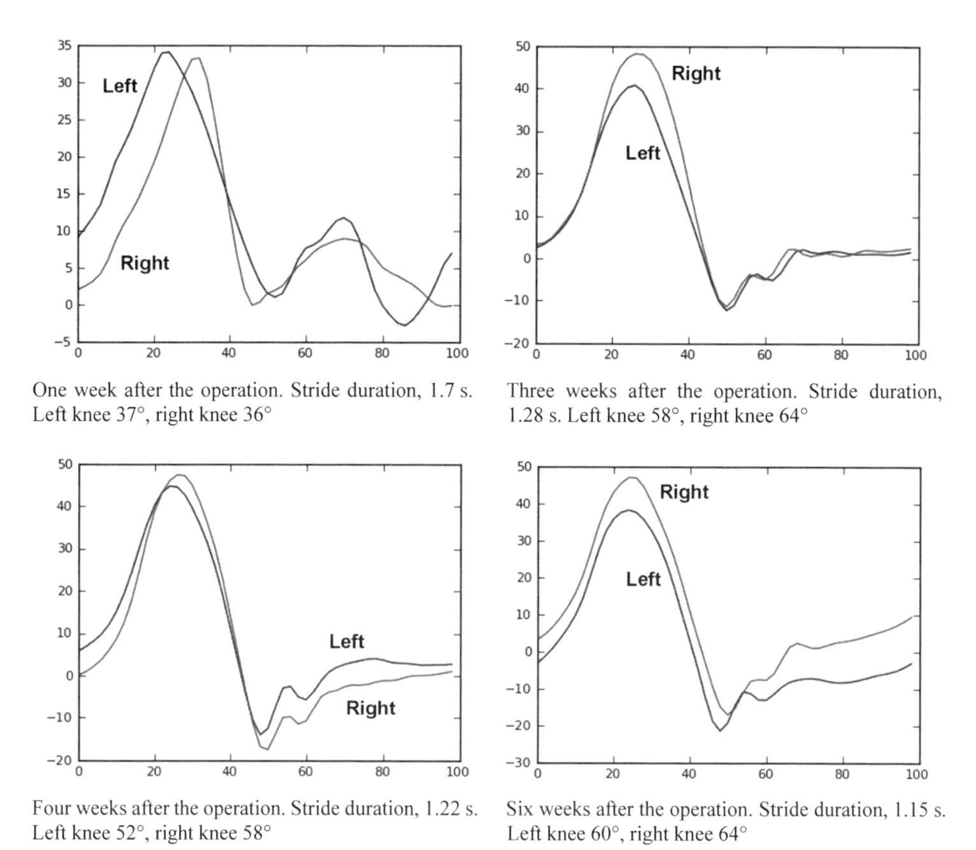

One week after the operation. Stride duration, 1.7 s. Left knee 37°, right knee 36°

Three weeks after the operation. Stride duration, 1.28 s. Left knee 58°, right knee 64°

Four weeks after the operation. Stride duration, 1.22 s. Left knee 52°, right knee 58°

Six weeks after the operation. Stride duration, 1.15 s. Left knee 60°, right knee 64°

Figure 17. Changes in gait through rehabilitation for a patient treated for a meniscus tear.

13. Conclusion

Gait is recognized as one of a person's biometric, yet to date little attention has been given to monitoring it. The reasons why monitoring a person's gait profile is so important to the long term health and well being have been discussed, with a particular focus on medical conditions that will affect a person's mobility. Different methods of measuring gait have been discussed, and the limitations of each presented. These limitations are largely technology dependent, which has restricted their use to primarily research activities for medical conditions where accuracy is required. However, with the latest technology advancements in motion sensor technology, new systems are now appearing which can be used in the clinical as well as the research environment. Some examples have been provided, showing how treatment and rehabilitation can be improved by knowing the gait abnormality at the start and providing goals for the individual.

It is believed that over the next decade there will be further advancements in gait systems, primarily based on sensor technology and this will lead to gait analysis being integrated into the diagnosis and rehabilitation process. It will also, it is believed, form part of the assessment of elderly people as they lose mobility, providing achievable goals linked to exercises.

References

[1] J.E. Boyd and J.J. Little, Biometric gait recognition, *Advanced Studies in Biometrics* (2005), 19–42.
[2] G. Cooper et al., Inertial sensor-based knee flexion/extension angle estimation, *Journal of Biomechanics* (2009).
[3] A.A. Kale, N.P. Cuntoor, B. Yegnanarayana, A.N. Rajagopalan and R. Chellappa, Gait analysis for human identification, in: *AVBPA*, 2003, pp. 706–714.
[4] D. Krebs, Reliability of observational kinematic gait analysis, *Physical Therapy* **65**(7) (1985).
[5] V. Lugade, Gait asymmetry following an anterior and anterolateral approach to total hip arthroplasty. *Clinical Biomechanics* **25**(7) (2010), 675–680.
[6] R.G. Marx, T.J. Stump, E. Jones, T.L. Wiskiewicz and R.F Warren, Development and evaluation of an activity rating scale for disorders of the knee, *Am. J. Sports Med.* **29** (2001), 213–218.
[7] National Institute for Clinical Excellence, FALLS, The assessment and prevention of falls in older people NICE, Nov. 2004.
[8] Organisation for Economic and Cultural Development, Health at a Glance 2010: OECD EU Edition, 2010.
[9] J. Perry, *Gait Analysis Normal and Pathological Function*, SLACK Incorporated, 1992.
[10] Poseidon software written by European Technology for Business Ltd.
[11] M. Varnell, Surgical approach results in different strategies at the hip and knee during the performance of stair negotiation at 2 years following TKA, ORS 2011 Annual Meeting.
[12] World Health Organization, Diet, nutrition, and the prevention of chronic diseases, WHO Technical Report Series 916, World Health Organization, Geneva, 2003.
[13] G.V. Zammit, H.B. Menz and S.E. Munteanu, Reliability of the TekScan MatScan® system for the measurement of plantar forces and pressures during barefoot level walking in healthy adults, *Journal of Foot and Ankle Research* **3** (2010), 11.

Ambient Assisted Living in Gerontology

Handbook of Ambient Assisted Living
J.C. Augusto et al. (Eds.)
IOS Press, 2012

doi:10.3233/978-1-60750-837-3-253

Gerontological Perspectives on Ambient Assisted Living

Andrew SIXSMITH*
Gerontology Research Centre, Simon Fraser University, Canada

Abstract. This section explores AAL from a gerontological perspective, both in terms of the types of AAL systems and applications that have been developed for older users and the contributions that technology can make to their health, independence and quality of life. The six chapters are representative of the range of research and development activities focusing on meeting the needs of older people and are organized in three themes: monitoring activity and health; AAL and dementia; market and policy issues.

Keywords. Gerontology, older people, activity monitoring, dementia, markets, policy

Introduction

Population aging is a global phenomenon. Today almost 1 in 10 people are over 60 years old, but by 2050 the figure will be higher than 1 in 5 and people aged over 60 will outnumber children aged 0–14. Globally the 60–79 and 80 plus age groups are growing the fastest with the number of people over 80 is growing at 4% per annum, whereas the population as a whole is growing at 1% per annum [1]. Illustrating these trends at a more local level, such as the province of British Columbia in Canada [2], out of a total population of around 4.5 million some 679 thousand or 15.3% are currently aged 65 and over. This figure will rise to about 1.3 million by 2031 (25.4%). Moreover, BC currently has 96 thousand people aged 85 and over, which is set to rise to 166 thousand by 2031. What are the implications of population aging for the health, independence and quality of life of seniors? Around 214 thousand people aged 65 and over in BC (43.2%) will have some kind of disability, rising to 54% for the over 75s, of which about 40% will have "severe" or "very severe" disabilities. Around 22 thousand over 65s in BC have disabilities due to memory impairment. 143 thousand BC seniors live alone, or about 27%, rising to 34% of the over 75s. The incidence of falls amongst persons aged over 65 is at least 30% and are the most common cause of injury for the very old (85+).

Clearly, population aging presents many challenges: How to improve the health status of older people who are living with the everyday realities of chronic disease? How to respond to people's desire to "age-in-place"? How to improve services and enhance people's independence and quality of life? How to respond to these challenges in the context of limited resources? It is in this context that advances in the area of

*Corresponding Author: Andrew Sixsmith, PhD, Gerontology Research Centre, SFU Harbour Centre, Vancouver BC V6B 5K3, Canada. E-mail: sixsmith@sfu.ca.

AAL may play a crucial role. The aim of this section of the Handbook is to explore AAL from a gerontological perspective, both in terms of the types of AAL systems and applications that have been developed for older users and the contributions that technology can make to their health, independence and quality of life. While it would be impossible to cover all aspects of AAL for older people, this section comprises six chapters that are representative of the wide range of research and development activities focusing on meeting the needs of older people.

1. Monitoring Activity and Health

A major component of AAL systems is "activity monitoring", which uses data collected from environmental sensors installed in the home and wearable biomedical sensors to build a profile of the dweller's typical pattern of living and health status, such as when the person gets up and goes to bed, level and location of movement, etc. Any variation from the typical pattern of activity may be a source of concern, for example a reduced level of activity during the day may be indicative of a decline in health status. Activity monitoring may be useful in generating health or emergency alerts in the short term, possibly requiring immediate intervention and also for monitoring changes in the health and independence of people in the longer-term.

Two chapters in this section have a specific focus on activity monitoring. Floeck and colleagues provide an overview of the state-of-the-art of activity monitoring and describe the results of an AAL system that was installed in Kaiserslautern in Germany. The AAL system was seen to have potential benefits for monitoring a range of alert situations, for example critical events requiring immediate intervention (e.g. heart attack) to non-critical situations requiring longer-term preventative interventions (e.g. exacerbations of a chronic illness). The chapter looks at technical issues (e.g. problems of merging different types of sensor data) and user issues (e.g. acceptability of the technology) as well as discussing some of the problems relating to the interpretation of activity data. A solution to many of these problems is to focus on patterns of inactivity and the benefits of this approach are illustrated in examples from the Kaiserslautern project. One of the major concerns that many people have is the loss of privacy and the "big brother" effect of monitoring people in the private space of their homes. Some people are very uncomfortable with this kind of surveillance, while others can be sceptical about its usefulness. However, many older people appreciate the value of the additional peace of mind afforded by this kind of system, which may contribute to their ability to continue living in their familiar home and neighbourhood.

Bhachu and colleagues describe a field trial of an AAL system that was implemented to support the health care professionals caring for people living with chronic illness in a community setting. A key idea behind the project is that any technology cannot work in isolation and always needs to be part of integrated care solution that enhances the formal and informal networks that are already in place. To this end, the field trial was aimed at using activity monitoring and bio-medical sensoring to provide information to aid "community matrons" in the management of people with diseases such as chronic obstructive pulmonary disease (COPD). The role of community matrons in the UK health system focuses on the case management of very vulnerable people with an aim to coordinate care, to manage the condition and to avoid unnecessary hospital admissions. The field trail provides strong evidence for the effectiveness of the system in supporting the delivery of care to patients, for example by aiding patients in the self-management of their conditions by providing them with easily accessible health and well-being data.

2. AAL and Dementia

Dementia is an age-related condition that effects around 5% of all people aged 65 and over and, while it should not be seen as part of the "normal" ageing process, dementia is a highly debilitating condition for many seniors. Although most of the applications within the area of AAL are likely to be relevant to this group, a specific focus on dementia has emerged because of the very significant challenge it presents in terms of the kinds of problems that people with dementia and their carers encounter and the challenges and costs in providing effective care and support. Dementia is a condition where mental faculties, such as memory, orientation in time and space and the ability to communicate decline significantly due to degeneration of the brain and consequent decline in cognitive function. Early symptoms may include forgetfulness and disorientation, progressing to very severe problems of communication, mental functioning and the ability to carry out everyday tasks of living in later stages.

There are many underlying diseases that give rise to dementia, with the most common one being Alzheimer's disease (AD). Currently, drugs are not effective in curing or significantly affecting the progress of AD and care interventions focus on managing the symptoms and providing help and support to informal carers. Typically, the application of technology for people with dementia has addressed issues of safety and security. For example, wandering is seen as a major problem for both people living in the community and in nursing homes and there are commercially available systems to trigger an alert if a person leaves their dwelling place. Another common problem concerns household safety and AAL systems often have in-home sensors and actuators to detect and control a range of potentially dangerous situations, such as flooding, extreme temperatures, fire and gas leaks. These are clearly important areas, but emerging AAL technologies also have the potential to develop interventions that can positively enhance independence and quality of life.

Two chapters have a specific focus on applying AAL to people with dementia. The chapter by Mihailidis and associates examines how technology can help people to perform everyday tasks of living that are important to continued independence. While tasks such as dressing, washing and preparing food are straightforward to cognitively intact people, they often become significant problems for people with dementia. The chapter highlights some of the key challenges facing people with dementia and their carers and outline key technological features and design principles for the development of AAL solutions. A major principle in the design of these kinds of systems is that they should foster and support the completion of tasks rather than autonomously performing the task for the person. By adopting this approach, the aim is to take into account the limitations of the person, encourage and facilitate task completion by the person themselves and thus help to maintain remaining skills and abilities and foster a sense of control and independence. The chapter illustrates these ideas in a review of various systems to support activities of daily living. For example, the COACH system was developed to assist with hand washing. COACH uses computer vision and artificial intelligence to track and interpret the user's performance of the various components of hand washing. An audio-visual interface gives appropriate prompts to aid completion if these are identified as necessary.

The chapter by Kearns and Fozard also focuses on dementia, but examines the potential of AAL in the assessment of cognitive status, by examining the relationship between ambulatory movement within the dwelling space and the level of cognitive function. Their research involves the monitoring of "path tortuosity", or the extent to which a person's movement path deviates from a straight line, using a wrist-worn tagging device that can accurately determine a person's location. Their research with residents in an assistive living facility found a significant negative association between path tortuousity and the cognitive status as measured by the Mini Mental State Exam (MMSE). Put simply, the more erratic the pattern of movement, the lower the cognitive function of the person. This kind of assessment is particularly useful because it generates objective data from within the natural home environment, rather than in artificial contexts such as a clinic. Moreover, such a system has the capacity to monitor a large number of people in a location such as a nursing home and provide frequent measures over time that may be helpful in the early detection of changes in cognitive status.

3. Market and Policy Issues

It is interesting to note that some of the key ideas within AAL have been around for many years. For example, push-button alarms to send an emergency alert to a call centre or carer has been around since at least the 1960s. The idea of smart housing, where the home environment adapts to the needs and preferences of the dweller has also been around for many decades, while the idea of activity monitoring has been around since the 1980s. However, many of these ideas have failed to get beyond the prototype stage. Care and support for older people living at home remains overwhelmingly based on direct face to face contact and markets for commercially available products and services remain patchy.

Two chapters in this section address these issues from market and policy perspectives. Meyer and colleagues look at the international market situation for AAL, where uptake of systems remains low despite the considerable benefits that they can potentially provide. The chapter provides an overview of international markets for the different generations of systems and highlights international differences in penetration. The barriers to the development of AAL markets remain considerable, reflecting factors such as funding and reimbursement systems, organisation of care services, cultural differences and ethical/legal concerns. Despite these barriers, the case for incorporating ICT within the spectrum of care is increasingly compelling. Following their market analysis, Meyer and colleagues argue that a holistic approach is needed for AAL deployment that includes three key activities: user requirement analysis; care process design; business case modelling. This approach aims to ensure that AAL solutions are aligned with the all the key actors involved in the consumption and delivery of AAL-based services.

In the final chapter in this section, Martin and Mulvenna look at technology policy initiatives, with a particular focus on the UK, one of the world leaders in integrating ICT-based solutions within the spectrum of care. Contemporary health and social care exists within a complex economic, social and political context and is increasingly technologically mediated and geographically dispersed. End-user and cost factors are driving the delivery of care away from traditional settings, such as hospitals, into the community and emerging AAL solutions will play a significant role in this process. The policy analysis looks at global, cross-national (EU) and national (UK) level policy and assesses the significance of policy initiatives in realizing technological innovation. In the UK, a range of initiatives have been demonstrated to have significant cost savings and improved delivery of services. A key component in the effective implementation of technological solutions is a research and development cycle that is closely aligned to policy objectives, is evidence-based and is driven by end-user involvement. The chapter provides two case studies of how this approach has been effective in practice, for example the TRAIL network of living labs.

References

[1] http://www.helpage.org/resources/ageing-data/.
[2] A. Wister, A. Sixsmith, R. Adams and D. Sinden, *Fact Book on Aging in British Columbia*, Gerontology Research Centre Simon Fraser University, Vancouver, 2010.

Handbook of Ambient Assisted Living
J.C. Augusto et al. (Eds.)
IOS Press, 2012

doi:10.3233/978-1-60750-837-3-258

Monitoring Patterns of Inactivity in the Home with Domotics Networks[1]

Martin FLOECK[a], Lothar LITZ[a,*] and Annette SPELLERBERG[b]
[a] *Institute of Automatic Control, Faculty of Electrical and Computer Engineering, University of Kaiserslautern, Kaiserslautern, Germany*
[b] *Institute of Urban Sociology, Faculty of Architecture, Regional and Environmental Planning, Civil Engineering, University of Kaiserslautern, Kaiserslautern, Germany*

Abstract. This chapter describes a state of the art AAL project in Kaiserslautern, Germany, which aims at monitoring inactivity patterns under real-world-conditions. Twenty flats have been inhabited by approximately 26 individuals since the end of 2007. The flats are equipped with several home automation sensors and actuators, thus allowing the collection of extensive data sets representing the typical user behaviour over long periods of time. Inactivity is the focus of the presented approach since it is assumed that inactivity and not activity is indicative of potential emergencies. The ultimate goal of the system is supporting senior citizens with modern home automation technology and thus helping them to maintain their independence and self-determination. In addition, illnesses and medical emergencies are to be detected by analysing and interpreting the captured sensor data. Based on this automated reasoning, appropriate help is administered to the persons affected. It is important to note that the development procedure of the Kaiserslautern AAL environment had been implemented from the onset as an evolutionary, user-centred design process to ensure user feedback and to allow easy identification of potential shortcomings or flaws of the developed solutions. Choosing such a user-centred design process facilitated meeting one of the paramount objectives of the AAL project, *viz.*, that the AAL technology satisfies the users' needs and wants.

Keywords. Ambient assisted living, home automation, assistive technology, alarm management, activity and inactivity recognition, acceptance evaluation

1. Introduction and State of the Art

Ambient Assisted Living (AAL) is a comparatively new term. Numerous technologies, however, can be associated with it, either as technological predecessors or as more advanced visions currently being under development. Artificial Intelligence (AI), Ubiquitous Computing (UC), and Ambient Intelligence (AmI) paved the way for AAL, whereas Cyber-Physical Systems (CPS's) are the next evolutionary step towards truly ambient, autonomous, and intelligent systems.

---

[*]Corresponding Author: Prof. Dr.-Ing. habil. Lothar Litz, Faculty of Electrical and Computer Engineering, University of Kaiserslautern, P.O. Box 3049, 67653 Kaiserslautern, Germany. E-mail: litz@eit.uni-kl.de.

[1]This chapter is a digest of the dissertation 'Activity Monitoring and Automatic Alarm Generation in AAL-enabled Homes' by Martin Floeck (ISBN 978-3-8325-2722-8) with permission from Logos-Verlag, Berlin. It has been extended with the most recent results and was complemented with outcomes of sociological research by A. Spellerberg. All images/tables taken from/based on the above dissertation (except for Table 2).

The idea of Artificial Intelligence had first been discussed by ALAN M. TURING in 1950 ("can a machine think?") [14]. In this groundbreaking paper, the idea of intelligent machines had been introduced. In 1991, MARK WEISER presented his vision of Ubiquitous Computing (UC) [15]. In this seminal paper, the idea of technologies that "weave themselves into the fabric of everyday life until they are indistinguishable from it" is first expressed. WEISER believes that our current computers are only a transitional step towards their disappearance into the background of everyday life. The next step towards the concept of AAL was the EU's announcement of their Ambient Intelligence (AmI) programme [3]. A world comprising a large number of easy-to-use interfaces, seamlessly embedded into everyday objects, is envisaged. This AmI-enabled environment is to recognise and respond to individuals in an unobtrusive way, thus assisting them in living, working, and relaxing (together). Hence, AmI systems need to be *context-sensitive*, *personalised*, *able to reconfigure themselves dynamically* to unforeseen conditions, *able to adapt to varying needs* of the user, *compatible* to neighbouring AmI systems, *failsafe*, even if parts of the network malfunction, and *trustworthy*, i.e., safeguarding the privacy, security, and safety of the user. Cyber-Physical Systems are the most recent step forward in the development of ambient, smart, and autonomous computing [16]. This novel concept was first envisioned by the U.S. National Science Foundation in 2006 [9]. The genuine novelty of this technology is the fusion of computation and physical processes: The fundamental principle of a CPS is that embedded systems monitor and control physical processes and physical processes affect the computations executed by the embedded systems [6]. There is, however, a significant overlap with the above existing approaches in the projected applications: health care, assisted living, bionics, and wearable devices are expressly listed as potential application domains [9].

With regard to the theme of the present book – AAL technologies –, numerous research groups are conducting research. The large scope of AAL research topics, however, makes it impossible to give an exhaustive overview of all AAL projects worldwide. In the following, only a brief synopsis of four realms of AAL research relevant to the work presented in this chapter will be provided. The attempt to give a comprehensive account of all research endeavours the authors are aware of would go far beyond the scope of this section.

1.1. Telecare and Monitoring Chronic Illnesses/Vital Functions

Medical conditions and vital functions can be observed for multiple reasons. First, telecare solutions can help users to cope with already existing illnesses. Second, vital functions can be monitored in order to assist medical staff in caring for the affected individual. Third, long-term trends may be identified to allow early intervention in case of a deteriorating health state.

In [10], an approach is presented that illustrates how individual users can be supported in handling their illnesses independently. The work aims at integrating and standardising the management of personal medication into the OSGi framework, a technology widely used in a huge variety of applications, building and home automation being one thereof.

Numerous works also tackle the collection of vital signs for evaluation by medical staff. In [17], a miniaturised, wearable sensor for the collection of heart and respiratory rates was developed. In [2], a wrist-worn device for the collection of multiple vital signs and their wireless transmission using a cellular link to a medical centre was implemented. These two works try to give (high-risk) patients the greatest possible degree of independence and freedom while at the same time guaranteeing that their vital functions are being monitored continuously. Hence, emergencies can be detected instantly.

1.2. Emergency Avoidance and Detection

In [8], a visionary model of human vitality is introduced. Human vitality is divided into three regions, i.e., healthy, non-critical, and critical. Furthermore, this model hypothesises that even with the most advanced technology, the vitality of an individual can only be approximated. Hence, emergencies can only be detected with a certain delay in time. In order to anticipate and detect emergencies as early as possible, vital signs and activities need to be monitored continuously. Moreover, one particular field of research, especially targeted at seniors living single, is fall detection. Considerable effort is devoted to this problem by various research groups in order to detect this class of emergency and to counteract the implications it can have, i.e., early formal care in nursing homes or even hospitalisation.

1.3. Maintaining Independence and Increasing Quality of Life

Many AAL research groups strive to enable seniors to live in their accustomed homes as long as possible. This aspect of AAL research is particularly important since it contributes to maintaining independence and thus quality of life and at the same time helps to reduce expenditures of public health schemes. Numerous projects are currently under way, however, most of them have not yet reached a state that would allow the deployment to the end user. Further research needs to be carried out to reach viable solutions that do indeed meet the users' needs and wants without being intrusive and that fulfil the expectations of health professionals and family members.

1.4. Acceptance of Monitoring Technologies by and Their Impact on Seniors

The Kaiserslautern AAL project described in this chapter has previously been evaluated, e.g., [5,12]. One pivotal finding of the acceptance evaluations was that the inhabitants of the AAL-enabled block of flats do not perceive the developed AAL solution as intrusive, privacy-violating, or interfering with their self-determination. On the contrary, when prompted for their opinion regarding the collection of activity data for monitoring their health status, only positive feedback was given by the users. In [1], similar findings obtained in a study conducted with 22 individuals requiring formal care are reported. The perceived quality of life of the participating individuals increased during the first three month of the project. This study concludes that activity monitoring and sharing the data with healthcare professionals were acceptable to older adults when in return an increased sense of safety and timely intervention in case of an emergency were to be anticipated.

As mentioned above, a detailed overview of related works relevant to the AAL approach presented here cannot be provided within this chapter. However, such an overview along with in-depth considerations about ethical and privacy implications of AAL developments is presented in [4].

Table 1. Severity levels of domestic emergencies or medical conditions for AAL.

Severity level	Life-threatening	Description	Examples	Action required
A – high	Yes	Sudden, genuine emergency	Heart attack Stroke	Immediately (within few minutes)
B – medium	No	Sudden, genuine emergency	Fall Unconsciousness	As soon as possible (within minutes to few hours)
C – low	No	Onset or exacerbation of a chronic illness	Hypertension Dementia Decrease of activity	Subject should see a doctor (within days to weeks)

2. Experimental Foundation: The Kaiserslautern AAL Approach[2]

2.1. Preliminary Considerations

The principal aim of the presented AAL solution is detecting medical emergencies arising among senior citizens. As illustrated in Table 1, three different classes of emergencies need to be distinguished. Since the approach followed here is genuinely ambient, i.e., not involving any sensors worn on the body, class A emergencies requiring immediate attention cannot be addressed. Instead, the AAL solution discussed here is ideally suited for detecting incidences of class B. Since some delay is inherently attached to this approach, class B emergencies can, however, only be noticed with a certain delay. Examples for class B emergencies are falls, faints, and the like. To a degree, behavioural changes associated to class C (i.e., potentially pointing at the deterioration of the user's state of health slowly manifesting itself) may be detected as well but are not the focus of this chapter.

2.2. A Real-World AAL Installation in 20 Flats

The Kaiserslautern project emerged from a cooperation of the University of Kaiserslautern and a local housing society, Gemeinnützige Baugesellschaft Kaiserslautern AG (BauAG). BauAG administers, maintains, and rents out 5300 flats. In the 1990s and 2000s, BauAG went to great lengths to modernise large parts of their housing stock. One of the buildings that had been modernised is the one shown in Fig. 1. After a renovation phase of one year, the building now accommodates 16 two-room flats, 3 three-room flats, and one single-family home attached to the block of flats. The flats can be accessed from a shared walkway ("access balcony"). The block of flats consists of three storeys and is equipped with a lift to facilitate access to the upper storeys and to ensure handicapped accessibility.

The 26 tenants living in these flats constitute a representative cross-section of the population of Kaiserslautern (as in February 2008): former skilled and unskilled labourers, housewives, as well as two university graduates. Of them, five are 60 years or younger and four are 80 years or older. The majority of tenants are 60 to 80 years old. Their mean age is 69 years [12].

[2]The project was funded by the *Ministry of Treasury* of Rhineland-Palatinate (Ministerium der Finanzen) and *Stiftung Rheinland-Pfalz für Innovation* (Foundation for Innovation RLP) and kindly supported by BauAG Kaiserslautern.

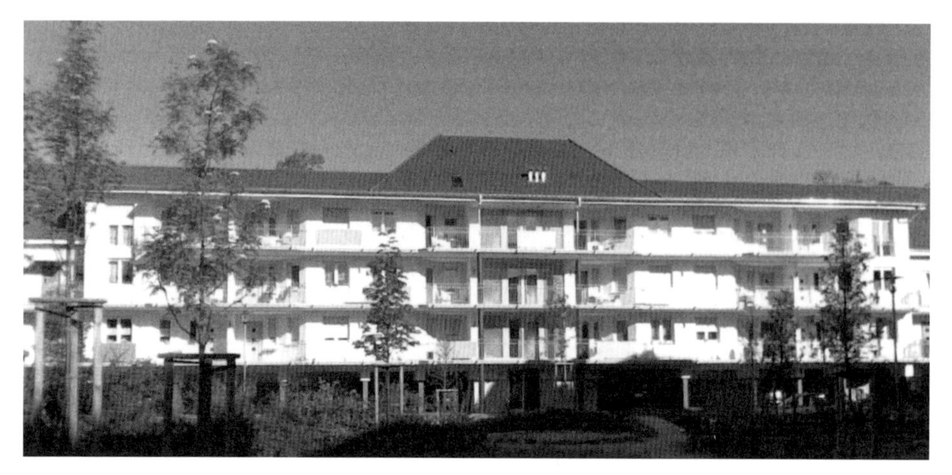

Figure 1. Block of flats of the Kaiserslautern AAL project.

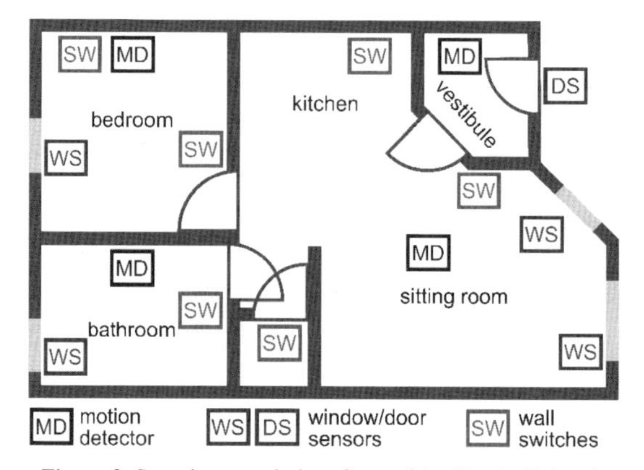

Figure 2. Sample ground plot of one of the flats in Kaiserslautern.

2.3. Home Automation Technology and the Personal Assistive Unit for Living

Figure 2 shows a ground plot of a typical two-room flat. All of the flats are extensively equipped with KNX home automation technology (KNX was formerly known as EIB, the European Installation Bus). Today, most major manufacturers of home automation equipment, white goods (domestic appliances), HVAC (heating, ventilation, and air conditioning) equipment, and related trades offer KNX-compliant products. The sensors used for gathering information about the activity of the tenants are marked in Fig. 2 and listed in Fig. 4.

The advantage of a building automation bus system is that all nodes can exchange data. Hence, by programming the nodes (which essentially are microcontrollers) *inherent intelligence* can be added (e.g., regarding power saving, lighting scenarios, or combined HVAC schemes). Moreover, all components are easily re-programmable so that changing requirements regarding the function of sensors (e.g., light switches) or actuators (e.g., relays) can be accommodated. Finally, the telegrams exchanged by the bus nodes can be tapped for further processing, e.g., with an Ethernet gateway. If a gateway

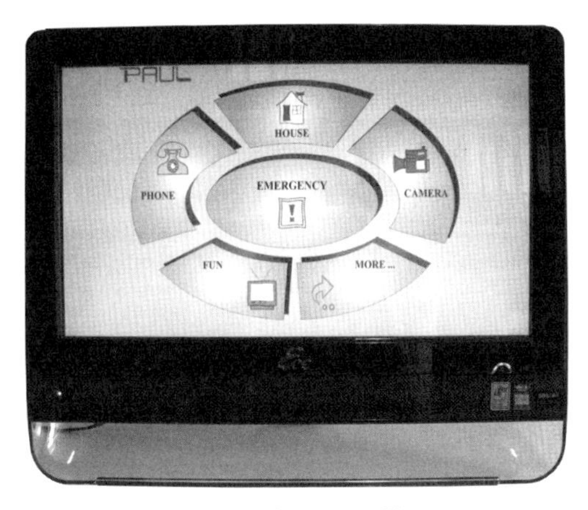

Figure 3. PAUL, the Personal Assistive Unit for Living. Icons: *House, camera, more, fun, phone, emergency.*

supports bidirectional communication, sophisticated control algorithms can be implemented on external controllers and be fed back onto the bus system [11].

In the Kaiserslautern project, this control unit is called *PAUL*, the *p*ersonal *a*ssistive *u*nit for *l*iving (Fig. 3). PAUL is based on a tablet PC featuring a touch screen. Having such a computer in each flat offers numerous advantages.

First, an individual computer in each flat allows storing all personal sensor data of the user locally. Thus, no sensitive data are disclosed to anyone unless the tenant wishes to participate in a *monitoring and alarming programme* (see Section 5). Taking part in an alarming programme is by choice and not compulsory. At the time of writing, the alarming programme is in its test phase and is expected to be available to every tenant at the end of 2011.

Second, the algorithms required for activity and health monitoring can be executed locally on PAUL. This greatly contributes to the protection of the users' privacy as well.

Third, having a computer at one's disposal in each flat is very convenient in order to give the user the opportunity to control and interact with the AAL system: For instance, visualising the inactivity history along with the inactivity graph of the current day enables the user to monitor their behaviour very easily and to identify possible mismatches between their real activity/inactivity pattern as perceived by the user and the one observed by the AAL system. In addition, being able to review the captured data is believed to improve both acceptance and grasp of the AAL system.

Fourth but not least, the AAL system may in no way stigmatise the users on the basis of their age-related needs or incapabilities. On the contrary, if an AAL solution is to be successful, it must provide real benefits for the users which are useful in everyday life without too obviously revealing that age-related deficiencies are existent. These requirements can be met by setting up a sleek computer that is likely to be perceived rather as a cutting-edge gadget than as a clumsy contraption for elderly people. In order to further boost the acceptance and prestige of PAUL and to give the users extra incentives to use it on a daily basis, PAUL has been equipped with additional functionalities: It will assist the user in their everyday life with some of their chores (e.g., rolling up shutters), provide entertainment and means of communication (e.g., Internet access, electronic bulletin forum functionality, web radio), and safety (e.g., video entry phone). These features are believed to be of pivotal importance to motivate users – no matter

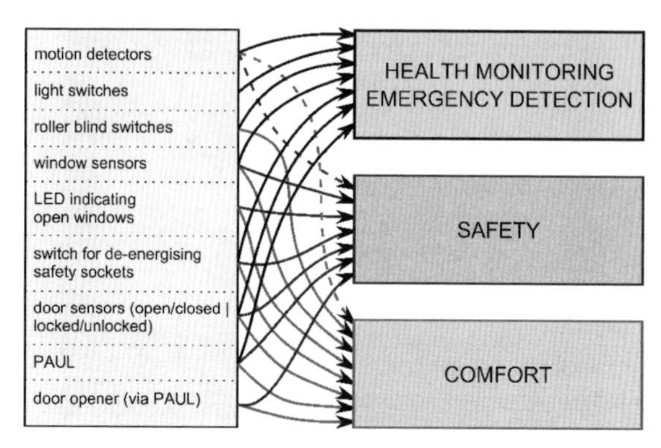

Figure 4. Multiple uses of domotics components for AAL functionalities.

whether they need health monitoring or not – to use PAUL regularly and thus become acquainted with PAUL, its functionalities, and how to operate it at an age at which doing so does not pose a problem. If PAUL is only installed when prospective users *ultimately need* it, learning how to operate it may form an insurmountable hindrance to the users.

In conclusion, it can be stated that all home automation components – sensors as well as actuators – contribute to more than just health and emergency monitoring (see Fig. 4). The home automation technology provides safety and comfort as well.

2.4. Acceptance Evaluation

The aim of the project is to not only promote technical assistance but also social integration through an active community and integration in the neighbourhood. Therefore, emphasis is placed on community building in addition to the technical concept of the project. At monthly tenants meetings, the residents arrange joint activities in the recreation room and come up with ideas how the technical concept may be developed further. The iterative, human-centred development process is based on these meetings, observations of usage, round table discussions as well as interviews of tenants.

A first evaluation of PAUL which mainly focussed on its usability took place in May 2007 when a model apartment was completed. However, the results have restricted validity only as all test persons (7, between 60 and 76 years of age) were "normally aging" persons without any specific health impairments and had an above-average technical competence for their age, too.

Two months after implementing the technical devices in all apartments (February 2008) and again eight months later (October 2008) the residents were questioned about their experiences and usage of the PAUL and the other home automation devices. The initial face-to-face interview was supplemented by a participant observation. Nineteen people were interviewed. The latest survey was carried out nearly two years after the tenant's having moved in (October 2009). Eighteen of 19 households (21 of 25 people) were reached.

This latest survey focussed on the evaluation whether and to which extent the acceptance and daily use of AAL technology changed after two years, and also how the tenants value the technological devices, the apartment itself, the living environment, and the neighbourhood. The survey was conducted using guideline-based interviews. In addition, 16 people were observed and filmed while using PAUL.

Here we mainly present the results of the third survey and focus on the usage and acceptance of the technology in the apartments. Comparisons with the survey in February 2008 can only be made to a limited extent, as not all tenants participated in both surveys: Two tenants only participated in the survey in February 2008, five only participated in the one in October 2009.

2.4.1. Usability and Location of PAUL

The majority of residents got accustomed to operating PAUL. Except for two interviewees, all observed manage to operate PAUL without any problems. Fourteen out of 16 residents quickly find the options on the menu bar and handle the tasks with ease. One senior woman, most likely suffering from incipient dementia, is not able to operate any functions of PAUL by herself – even though she was able to do so during the first survey one and a half year earlier. The fact that PAUL is operated with ease by most of the tenants also corresponds to the statements of some interviewees that PAUL would not react quickly enough to their commands:

> *"Ich komme damit gut zurecht, doch. Wirklich. Ich bin manchmal ein bisschen zu schnell."*
> *(I'm getting along with it well. Really. I'm sometimes a bit too fast.)*

In general, PAUL is highly accepted and after almost two years of using, PAUL is integrated in most of the tenants' everyday life. However, the interviews and the observations showed that the tenants use PAUL in different ways. In the majority of visited households (13 out of 18) PAUL is installed in the sitting room, the place where the tenants spend most of their time during the day. The number of households having PAUL in the sitting room has even increased since the last survey. In only one sixth of the households PAUL is situated permanently in the bedroom. Two thirds of the surveyed tenants (14 out of 20) use PAUL daily, whereas the intensity of use varies.

The process of adoption was not homogeneous. Concerning the degree of interest in new technology, the number of used options, and the frequency of utilisation, the tenants can be assigned to three different types of use: creative adoption, pragmatically use, and disuse.

Tenants belonging to the "creative type" are especially technophile. For acquisition they apply the trial-and-error method in an independent and creative manner. They use the majority of the offered functions including the internet feature. Furthermore they propose additional options for use. For this group, PAUL is a valuable contribution to their everyday life, as it offers diversion, it is convenient, and new actions can be learned. Nine out of 21 users are assigned to this type, six women and three men.

The tenants matching the "type of pragmatic use" apply only some selected features which they judge to the best advantage, such as the door camera or the remote-controlled blinds. These persons do not use the other functions regularly. This group also judges PAUL as a surplus but the enthusiasm is considerably lower than in the first group. Ten out of 21 users are assigned to this type, six women and two men.

Tenants who can be described as "disusers" do not use PAUL at all or solely to show it to visitors. So PAUL is of little importance to this group. Two female tenants match this group.

The results of the surveys show that for the tenants the implemented technical devices do not represent "technology", as they would think of technology being compli-

Table 2. Use of selected devices over the course of time (total times mentioned).

	February 2008 used (mentioned)	October 2009 used (mentioned)	Change of use
Door camera	15 (17)	16 (19)	+1
Internet	12 (18)	11 (21)	–1
Electric roller blinds	11 (16)	14 (18)	+3
Light control	1 (5)	6 (18)	+5
Radio	6 (13)	8 (20)	+2

cated and only understandable using a manual. Instead, the features are inconspicuously integrated into their everyday life and adopted playfully.

2.4.2. Comparison: Use of PAUL in the Course of Time

A detailed comparison of the number of users in the October 2009 survey to the first one in February 2008 is not possible, as for some functions there are only a small number of statements. As not all features were implemented in the first survey, an evaluation of the change of use was not possible for the TV and the picture gallery. A comparison of the users of the light control is not possible, due to the small number of users in February 2008. In addition, some tenants were not able to use all functions in February 2008 because they were malfunctioning but operated well during the recent survey (e.g., radio and door camera).

There are statements on the general use of PAUL for all three survey periods (February 2008, October 2008, and October 2009) of 14 tenants. Of these, twelve used PAUL in all survey periods. Within this group of 14 there were no significant changes in usage. Altogether, the number of statements of actual users of the light control (+5), the electric blinds (+3), the radio (+2), and the door camera (+1) have increased. This might also be due to a greater number of respondents in the recent survey and the fact that the tenants were explicitly asked about the functions more often. The total numbers of users of the alarm clock (–2) and Internet users (–1) have decreased. Although the total number of users of the internet has only decreased by one from February 2008 until October 2009 (12 to 11 users), there has been a further change, not visible in Table 2, as four former users no longer use PAUL's Internet feature partly because they bought a PC or laptop.

The electric shutters and light control, the automatic door opener, and "security" were mentioned as important factors for a good feeling in the apartment. For some tenants the devices are on one hand some kind of compensation for age-related physical limitations and on the other hand they promote a sense of security. Nevertheless, the decisive factors for feeling at home are primarily the community and the fact of not being alone (anymore), respectively, and the matter of fact that the tenants feel comfortable in the building which again is predominantly due to the barrier-free design and the good building quality of the apartments.

Overall it can be concluded that PAUL and the other home automation devices certainly contribute to the tenants' coping in everyday life and to the positive feeling of living. To what extent the implemented automation components can actually contribute to a longer, self-determined life in an own home cannot yet be answered. Whether they contribute effectively and independently compared to a conventionally equipped home designed according to senior persons' requirements to enable a longer life in their own homes still remains questionable since the contribution for the physical impaired is

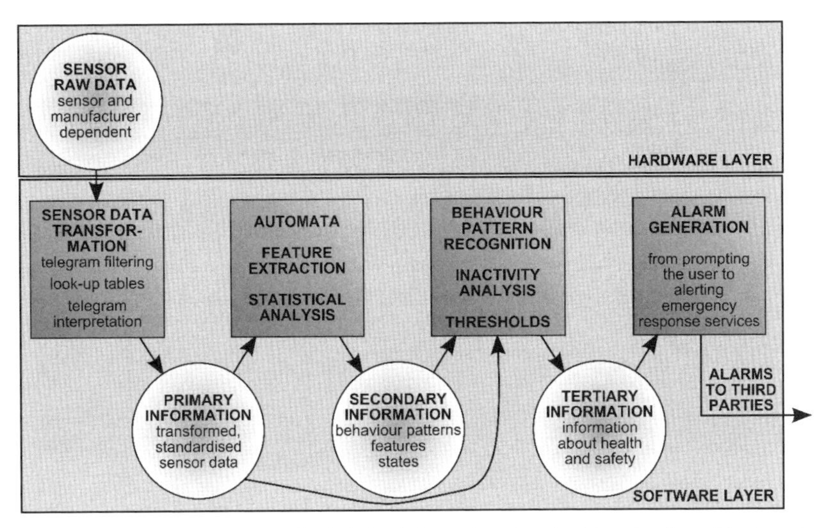

Figure 5. Data processing steps for deriving information about health and safety of the tenant.

small. The facilitation of everyday life as well as safety, entertainment, and information aspects might allow for a quality enhancement rather than a temporal extension of independent living. The automatic generation of alarms using inactivity patterns marks a milestone as it increases the sense of security both for seniors and their relatives.

3. Activity vs. Inactivity Approach

3.1. Sensor Data Collection, Storage, and Processing

It is important to understand that the activity signals captured by the various sensors in the home are processed in several steps (see Fig. 5). The signals provided directly by the sensors are referred to as *sensor raw data*. Two fundamentally different types of sensors exist: First, there are genuine sensors of various kinds whose only function is capturing data and, second, quasi-sensors whose primary use is not gathering information but being used for controlling the home environment. Examples for quasi-sensors are, for instance, wall switches that are connected the KNX bus so that information about when they are actuated can be retrieved. Thus, normal interaction of the user with their environment also generates information about their location and activity level. Sensor raw data is highly unstructured and must be standardised before being processed in subsequent steps.

After having decoded and transformed the telegrams sent by the sensors, primary data can be passed on to further data processing algorithms. This way, it is ensured that the monitoring and alarming algorithms can handle the primary information, no matter which type of sensor captured the original data or which sensor technology (i.e., technology standard) is being used. All algorithms operating on primary, secondary, or tertiary data that were implemented in this work require generic, unambiguous, well-defined strings that are *not* specific to a particular flat or AAL installation.

Secondary information is the first type of information that consists of aggregate, condensed information based on data from previous processing steps. In order to obtain

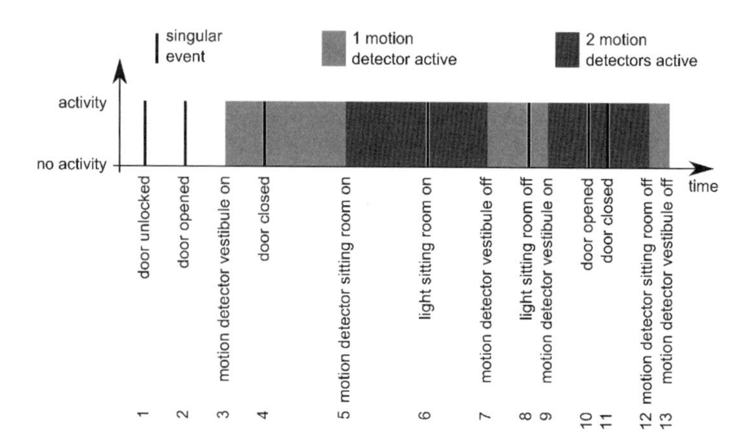

Figure 6. Singular events vs. continuous activity.

secondary information, primary data has to undergo multiple steps of further refinement, the first step being running finite state machines (FSMs) on the data. The FSMs are used to model the states of the individual sensors, e.g., the information about doors (open/closed), windows (open/closed), lights (on/off), and roller blinds (up/down). More importantly, FSMs are suitable for deducing knowledge that is not immediately obvious from raw or primary data. Two FSMs for obtaining specific knowledge are particularly important: First, the *activity FSM* for determining whether or not there is any activity inside the flat and second, the *presence FSM* for reasoning whether or not the flat is occupied by a human.

The techniques for obtaining tertiary information are the main focus of this chapter and revolve round behaviour pattern recognition, inactivity analysis, and threshold application. In these steps, high-level information about health and safety of the tenant is deduced. These techniques are elucidated in full detail below.

3.2. Singular (Transient) Events and Continuous (Non-Transient) Activity

Two different basic types of human actions encountered in AAL settings need to be distinguished: singular transient events and continuous activity. Most sensors detect singular events, lasting only an instant, e.g., wall switches, door sensors, etc. Motion detectors, however, signal continuous activity, representing a time span rather than a discrete event, and remain in their active state for a certain period of time (12 seconds in case of the sensors used in the Kaiserslautern project) after the last activity was observed. Figure 6 represents these two different types of activity by means of an example in which a person returns to their home, opens the front door and enters the flat (telegrams 1–4), resides in the sitting room (telegram 5–8), and finally leaves the flat again (telegrams 9–11).

As a rule, all interactions of the user with their environment raise singular events – pressing buttons, opening doors, etc. rarely have a duration. In contrast, activity observed by motion detectors (marked grey in Fig. 6) is not transient but continuous and lasts as long as a person is moving plus the switch-off delay, i.e., an arbitrary period of time.

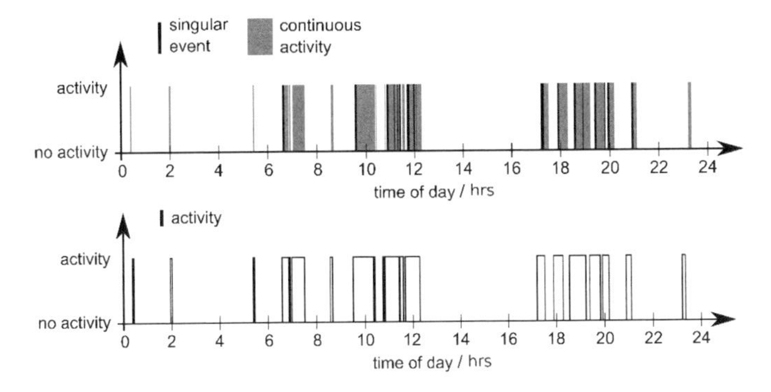

Figure 7. Merging continuous activity and singular events (top) into general activity (bottom).

The inherently different natures of those two types of activity render it very difficult to merge them. Figure 6 shows that while at least one motion detector is active (grey areas), all information about singular events becomes redundant. On top of that, singular events should rarely be received outside periods of continuous activity since motion detectors are expected to detect human presence even without relying on singular events being raised. However, singular events can become very important on one condition: They contribute to the redundancy of the sensor array and can still provide some information about the user if one of the motion detectors fails or the tenant is out of range of the sensor so that the sensor cannot "see" him.

3.3. Composite Singular/Continuous and Condensed Activity Patterns

As outlined above, merging singular events and continuous activity is not straightforward. The main issue regarding merging singular events and continuous activity is that the "cardinality" of the observed activity has to be constant – either there is activity or there is none. Thus, overlapping activity signals from multiple motion detectors and singular events must be condensed into a single parameter, i.e., general activity (Fig. 7).

This can be achieved by constructing the envelope of all activity signals, regardless of their source. By dividing each day into 24 h × 3600 s/h = 86 400 s and assigning timeslots to each thereof, activity patterns accurate to the second can be created.

Looking at Fig. 7, one may be inclined to think that such activity patterns constitute a possible approach for tackling the recognition of emergencies. Visualising and interpreting the recorded activity data in such a way, however, illustrates the two main drawbacks of this rather simple activity evaluation method: First of all, interpreting activity data in the above way hardly allows the detection of emergencies because – as a preliminary assumption – no emergency should have occurred as long as activity can be observed. I.e., in case of a genuine emergency, e.g., a faint or unconsciousness, all activity is expected to cease entirely. Thus, employing activity patterns of the above type for detecting emergencies is not very promising since focussing on activity is counterproductive if inexplicable or unanticipated *inactivity* periods indicate potential emergencies. This consideration leads to the approach of instead exploiting inactivity as a criterion for detecting emergencies: If extended periods of inactivity cause any suspicion – be it because they are extremely long or at unexpected times – alarms can be triggered. In Fig. 7, several examples of such inactivity periods are visible, notably

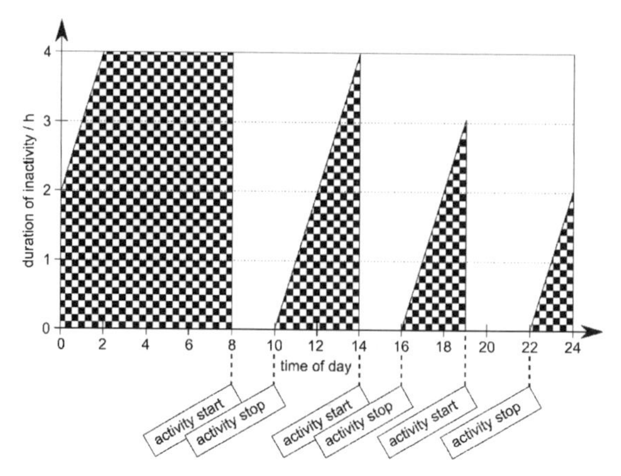

Figure 8. The inactivity principle.

before 0630[3], between 1200 and 1700, and between 2000 and 2400. Yet, the knowledge about these inactivity periods cannot be utilised directly for identifying dangerous situations and triggering alarms because of the second drawback: This data representation does not include any information about the user being at home or the flat being empty. Without that knowledge, any attempts of reliable emergency detection will be futile because the AAL system cannot decide whether an actual extended period of inactivity was caused by a genuine emergency or the user having left their flat.

Thus, a sophisticated model for representing the users' inactivity is needed, taking into account whether or not the tenant is at home. Detecting presence and absence of the user is possible using finite state machines. For details on their functional principle and how they are implemented, please refer to [4].

3.4. Inactivity Patterns

In contrast to the *activity* patterns introduced in the previous section, *inactivity* patterns focus on the time *between* activity periods. This approach has several advantages over activity patterns. First, merging multiple sources of activity data is no longer necessary – inactivity is the case if *no sensor* whatsoever signals activity. Second, inactivity data interpretation as shown in Fig. 8 provides additional knowledge – other than in case of the activity envelope in Fig. 7 that only shows whether or not there is activity at any given time, the inactivity representation also contains information on how long a person had been inactive at a given time. Third but not least, monitoring inactivity protects the users' privacy. No activities of daily living or other information potentially giving rise to privacy concerns need to be processed or generated.

In the schematic sample diagram in Fig. 8, four inactivity periods (chequered spikes) occurred throughout the day: Before 0800, 1000–1400, 1600–1900, and after 2200. Between each of them, activity periods were observed: 0800–1000 and so forth, i.e., each inactivity period commenced after activity ceased entirely and ended upon the reception of an arbitrary activity telegram.

[3]In order to avoid any ambiguity when referring to the time of the day, all times are given as "railway time" rather than using the 12-hour clock notation, i.e., 5:35 p.m. will be written as 1735.

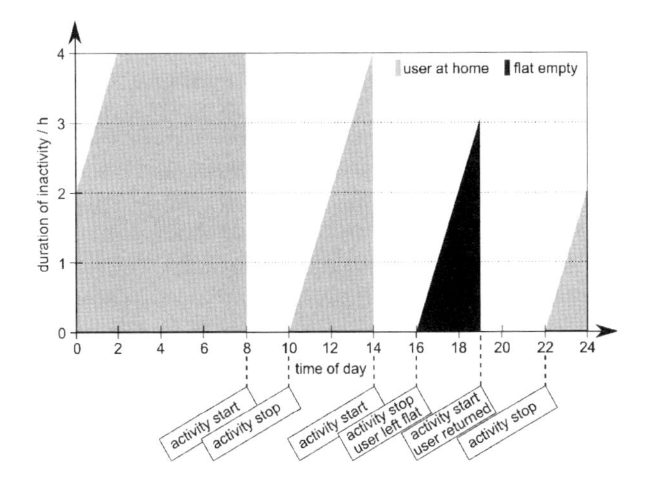

Figure 9. Enhanced inactivity principle distinguishing presence and absence.

When an inactivity period begins, a spike starts rising linearly from the abscissa. The height of a spike indicates the duration of the inactivity period, e.g., the duration of the inactivity period between 1000 and 1400 is four hours which is reflected by the height of the corresponding spike. Upon reception of an activity telegram, the inactivity period is terminated and the spike plummets back to zero.

A formal expression for the duration of inactivity *DI* is given in Eq. (1).

$$DI(t,d) := \text{elapsed time after last observed activity} \\ t \in (0\,\text{h},\ 24\,\text{h}),\ \ d \in \mathbb{N} \tag{1}$$

where *DI* is a non-negative function, *t* is the time of the day, and *d* is the day considered.

The third advantage of inactivity patterns over activity patterns becomes apparent if the inactivity monitoring procedure is expanded in such a way that presence and absence of the tenants can be accommodated in the inactivity representation which cannot be accomplished by the activity approach. The activity graphs (Fig. 7) do not inherently include knowledge about the user being at home or not and may thus lead to faulty reasoning. In contrast, statistical analyses of inactivity data as in Fig. 9 will not be distorted because the impact of absence can be quantified and can thus be compensated for.

In Fig. 9, grey spikes indicate inactivity while the tenant is at home whereas black spikes denote periods of inactivity due to the flat being empty. In the above example, the tenant left their flat at 1600 and returned at 1900. Using the knowledge about the tenant being at home or away, Eq. (1) can be modified to only represent inactivity while the tenant is present (see Eq. (2)). Periods during which the tenant is not at home do not need to be considered for detecting emergencies or building long-time inactivity patterns.

$$DI_{\mathrm{p}}(t,d) := \begin{cases} DI(t,d), & \text{if tenant present} \\ 0, & \text{elsewhere} \end{cases} \tag{2}$$

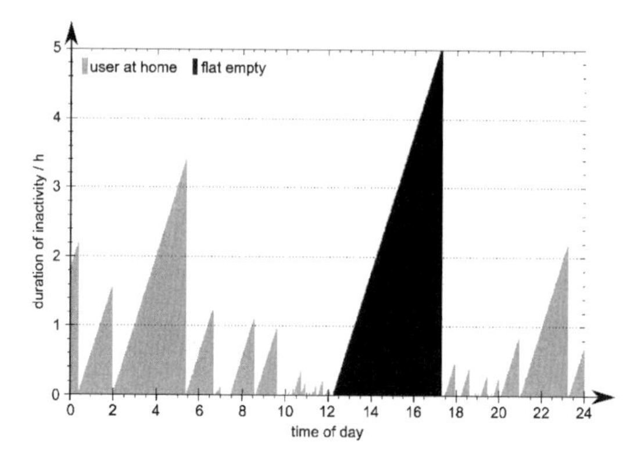

Figure 10. Inactivity graph of real-world data shown in Fig. 7.

Applying the above considerations to the real-world data shown in Fig. 7 yields the inactivity diagram in Fig. 10. This diagram illustrates that the tenant was not at home during the long period of inactivity between 1200 and 1700. All other phases of inactivity can be put down to the tenant being rather passive, i.e., only moving little and not interacting with any buttons or sensor-equipped objects in their surroundings. Possible reasons for this include taking a nap or sitting on the sofa and reading a newspaper – if only little physical action is exercised, the presence sensors may not detect it.

A detailed discussion on how inactivity patterns can be further interpreted and which conclusions can be drawn from them follows in Section 4.

4. Multi-Day Patterns and Alarm Generation

4.1. General Considerations

Based on the above inactivity graphs, extensive analyses of the personal long-term inactivity patterns of a user can be performed. A sample inactivity pattern of a single day, however, will not suffice as reference, no matter what kind of emergency is to be identified. Thus, statistically more significant inactivity reference data sets need to be generated that well reflect the typical daily routine of a person. Long-term graphs created by combining inactivity patterns of multiple days, thus representing the average long-term behaviour of a user, are believed to be a suitable representation of the daily routine. Based on these multi-day patterns, alarm thresholds will be deduced that can serve as alarm criteria for emergencies of type B.

4.2. Multi-Day Inactivity Patterns

Two methods for condensing sets of single-day profiles are presented here: First and most straightforwardly, overlaying multiple single-day patterns and removing inactivity periods during which the user was not at home ("black spikes"), thus eventually representing maximum inactivity, generates multi-day patterns. Second, long-term inactivity graphs with statistical outliers being removed will be introduced.

Equation (3) represents the calculation rule for determining the maximum value-based multi-day patterns:

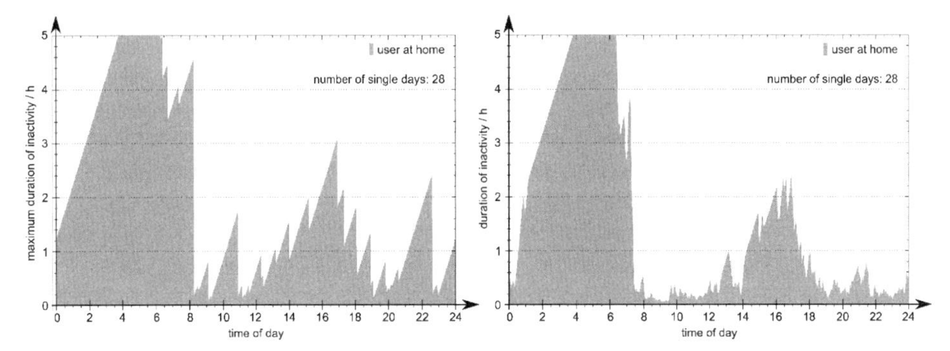

Figure 11. Left: Maximum value-based multi-day pattern of 28 days. Right: Outlier-free multi-day pattern of 28 days.

$$MDI_{\mathrm{p}}(t,S_{\mathrm{i}}^{\mathrm{A}}) := \max_{\forall d \in S_{\mathrm{i}}^{\mathrm{A}}} DI_{\mathrm{p}}(t,d) \tag{3}$$

where $MDI_{\mathrm{p}}(\cdot)$ is the maximum duration of inactivity, S_{i} is the set of i days from which the maximum-based inactivity pattern is calculated, and A is an arbitrary identifier for the set under consideration.

Equations (4) and (5) show how to compute the outlier-free multi-day pattern:

$$DIE_{\mathrm{p}}(t,S_{\mathrm{i}}^{\mathrm{A}}) := \begin{cases} MDI_{\mathrm{p}}(t,S_{\mathrm{i}}^{\mathrm{A}}), & \text{if } MDI_{\mathrm{p}}(\cdot) < Q3 + 3.0 \times IQR \\ Q3 + 3.0 \times IQR, & \text{elsewhere} \end{cases} \tag{4}$$

$$DIE_{\mathrm{p}}^{*}(t,\, S_{\mathrm{i}}^{\mathrm{A}}) := \alpha \times DIE_{\mathrm{p}}(t,\, S_{\mathrm{i}}^{\mathrm{A}}) + (1-\alpha) \times DIE_{\mathrm{p}}^{*}(t-1\mathrm{s},\, S_{\mathrm{i}}^{\mathrm{A}}) \tag{5}$$

where $DIE_{\mathrm{p}}(\cdot)$ is the duration of inactivity with outliers eliminated, $DIE^{*}_{\mathrm{p}}(\cdot)$ is the smoothed $DIE_{\mathrm{p}}(\cdot)$, Qn is the nth quartile, α is the smoothing factor, and $(1 - \alpha)$ is the discount factor. *IQR* stands for *interquartile range*, a term used in descriptive statistics. An in-depth explanation on this outlier-removal procedure and the *IQR* in particular can be found in [4,7,13].

Figure 11 shows multi-day patterns based on 28 days of inactivity observed in a flat: On the left, the maximum value-based pattern is displayed whereas the outlier-free pattern is shown on the right.

In the following, multi-day patterns of the above types will be used for both deriving and establishing alarm thresholds as well as verifying the chosen thresholds.

4.3. Alarm Stages

In order to enable the use of alarm thresholds of whatever kind for monitoring the health state or detecting potential emergencies in a flat, first of all the concept of alarm stages (AS) needs to be introduced. In the following, three basic AS's will be defined:

OK: *no alarm* whatsoever

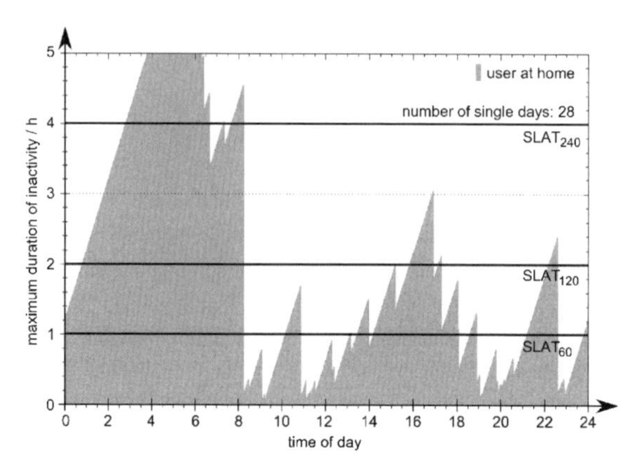

Figure 12. Three sample SLATs of 60, 120, and 240 minutes.

PA: *potential alarm* – user triggered alarm manually or PAUL assumes alarm but neither is confirmed

CA: *confirmed alarm* – alarm not cancelled by user within specified period of time OR confirmed by third party (emergency call centre).

The nature of OK and CA should be immediately clear. PA had been introduced to reduce the number of false alarms: procedures are implemented that allow cancelling spurious alarms triggered unintentionally before they become CAs actually being forwarded to an emergency call centre. This alarming plan will be discussed in detail in Section 5.1.

4.4. Static Linear Alarm Threshold

Alarm thresholds, derived from the multi-day patterns introduced above, are the principal instruments for identifying potentially dangerous situations. Based on such thresholds, alarms are triggered if any inactivity longer than allowed by the threshold is observed. The simplest threshold one can use for generating inactivity alarms is a static linear alarm threshold $SLAT_x = x$ minutes. Once that static, linear threshold is exceeded by the current inactivity duration at any given time, an alarm will be triggered (Def. 1).

Definition 1. Alarm principle of SLATs

IF	inactivity $DI_p(t, d) > SLAT_x$
THEN	alarm stage $AS \leftarrow$ potential alarm PA

Figure 12 shows three sample SLATs being applied to the 28-day-pattern discussed above. This example illustrates the most striking disadvantage of a plain SLAT: Since SLATs are active 24/7, long nightly periods of inactivity which do not constitute abnormal behaviour will inevitably trigger numerous false alarms. It needs to be noted in addition that low SLATs in the range of 60 or 120 minutes will cause false alarms during day-time as well. However, SLATs of 180 minutes or more are unlikely to trigger unacceptably many false alarms during the day. On the contrary, occasional false alarms play an important role in the monitoring approach presented here and will be addressed in Section 5.

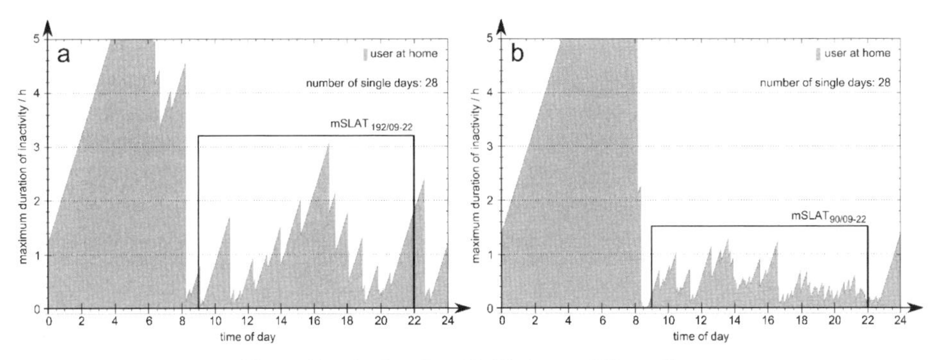

Figure 13. a, b: Sample mSLATs in two different flats.

In order to circumvent the detrimental effect the nightly periods of inactivity can have on rate of false alarms, masked SLATs are only active during certain times of the day, the so-called period of operation *PO* (Def. 2).

Definition 2. Alarm principle of mSLATs.

IF	time of day $t \in PO$
	AND
	inactivity $DI_p(t, d) > mSLAT_x$
THEN	alarm stage $AS \leftarrow$ potential alarm PA

Figure 13 illustrates how mSLATs can be used for inactivity monitoring without triggering an overabundance of false alarms at night. By setting $PO = [0900, 2200]$, sleeping phases cannot set off alarms. Moreover, Figs 13(a) and 13(b) exemplify that multiple users' behaviours in different flats can vary considerably: In case (a), significant inactivity peaks of up to three hours were observed in the early afternoon whereas in case (b) inactivity was generally lower and distributed more evenly. The following Section 4.7 "Long-Term Trends" addresses the issue of temporal constancy and user-dependence of the inactivity patterns more in detail.

As illustrated by Fig. 13, the response time, i.e., the time that has to elapse before PAUL can detect a potential health threat or emergency, typically ranges from 1.5 up to 4 hours. Whilst several hours still may be considered long if, e.g., one has fallen and has to wait for help to arrive, it must to be noted that being able to detect states of distress based on automated reasoning and administer help within reasonable periods of time is a major advancement that is well capable of preventing emergencies from not being noticed at all.

4.5. Multi-Day Inactivity-Derived Threshold

In order to shorten the response time before an alarm is raised, another kind of alarm threshold can be employed: the multi-day inactivity-derived threshold (*MIT)*. The MIT is based on the smoothed, outlier-free multi-day pattern. In contrast to mSLATs, the PO of an MIT can be 24 hours. Twenty-four hour monitoring, however, is only feasible if false alarms are tolerated as they are inevitable in the long run. The *mean time between false alarms* (MTFA) is a concept to handle these inevitable false alarms: The user is given the possibility to set the MTFA according to their wishes, i.e., a personal

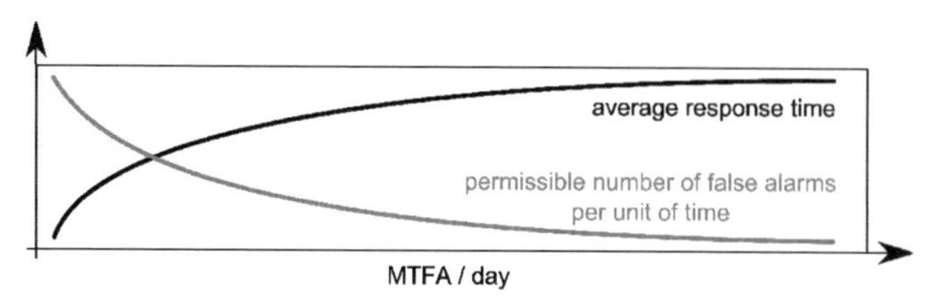

Figure 14. Qualitative dependence of permissible number of false alarms/avg. response time on MTFA.

trade-off between quick response times on the one hand and low number of false alarms on the other hand has to be made (Fig. 14). The multi-day inactivity patterns assist the users in setting their personal MTFA by letting them estimate when false alarms are most likely to occur, i.e., at peak inactivity durations.

Since false alarms are explicitly tolerated in case of the MIT, Eq. (6) gives the respective calculation rule.

$$\forall t \in [0000,\ 2400]: MIT(t, S_i^A, \tau) = DIE_p^*(\cdot) + \tau$$

$$\tau = \min \left\{ T \mid MTFA_{\text{specified}} = MTFA(MIT(t, S_i^A, \tau = T)) \right\} \tag{6}$$

The alarm principle of MITs is very similar to that of mSLATs (Def. 3).

Definition 3. Alarm principle of MITs.

IF	inactivity $DI_p(t, d) > MIT(\cdot)$
THEN	alarm stage $AS \leftarrow$ potential alarm PA

In the following example, an MTFA of 10 days was chosen, i.e., on average one false alarm in ten days is tolerated. This means that within a period of twenty-eight days roughly three false alarms may occur.

In Fig. 15, MITs are shown for the same multi-day patterns as in Fig. 13. The most notable difference to Fig. 13 is that that the MITs well reflect the typical user behaviour: Inactivity peaks observed during the training period are incorporated in the alarm threshold. Along with the acceptance of false alarms, the MITs can be as low as approximately two hours both in Figs 15(a) and (b). In (a), two out of three false alarms are expected at night and one during day-time. In (b), false alarms are mainly anticipated around 0800 since the sleep period is very constant and thus slight deviations can lead to a false alarm.

4.6. Conclusions with Regard to Alarm Thresholds

The three alarm principles introduced above can be summarised as shown in Table 3. The table illustrates that the transparency of the system is inversely correlated with the adaptation to the users' behavioural profile and quick response times.

Since the users only have to set the MTFA and the central control unit PAUL takes all necessary measures to achieve the desired MTFA, all of the alarm principles can be implemented. However, thorough understanding on the side of the users is advisable because informed consent from the users can only be ensured if they fully understand how assistive technologies in their surroundings work.

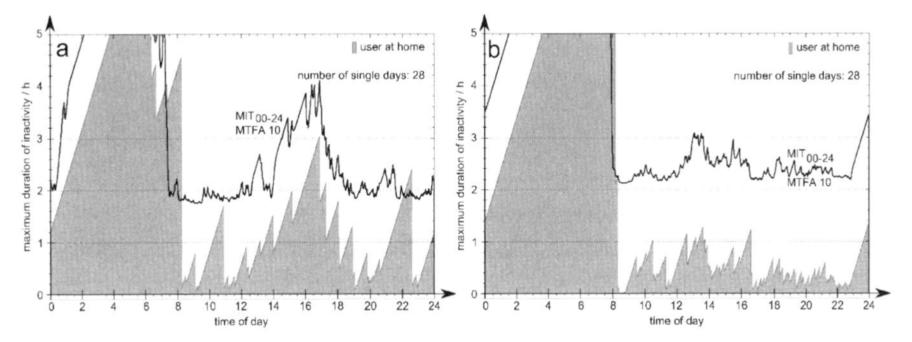

Figure 15. a, b: Sample MITs in two different flats.

Table 3. Overview of the three alarm principles introduced above.

Alarm principle	Period of operation	Transparency/under-standability for seniors		Impact on alarm generation
Singular linear alarm threshold **SLAT**	24 hours	++	Very easy to understand	Very coarse, no adaptation to specific user's profile
Masked singular linear alarm threshold **mSLAT**	Any	+	Easy to understand	Medium coarse, some adaptation to user's profile possible
Multi-day inactivity-derived threshold **MIT**	24 hours	–	Difficult to understand	Fine-grained, excellent adaptation to user's profile

4.7. Long-Term Inactivity Trends

Processing and interpreting sensor data from various flats over several years proved that behavioural patterns in a particular flat are both quite constant and unique to a user whereas other tenants in other flats may have entirely different behaviours.

As a result, conclusions or alarm thresholds generated in one flat cannot easily be generalised and be transferred to another one. Within a particular flat, however, the inactivity level remains fairly constant throughout the year, i.e., only a slight seasonal impact is found. However, it needs to be pointed out that the seasonal change in the patterns is not uniform – in some flats, inactivity is higher in winter than in summer and in some flats the opposite observation can be made. Light switch utilisation is the sole feature that varies significantly and rather concordantly in several flats between summer and winter but it does not have any measurable influence on the overall inactivity level. In conclusion, it needs to be stated that no easily and immediately identifiable correlation of inactivity level and time of the year can be extracted.

The constancy of the inactivity patterns renders it unnecessary to update the alarm threshold permanently in order to adapt to changing user behaviour over time. This finding is corroborated by the fact that the number of false alarms per month using alarm thresholds based on four weeks' training data are very constant over extended periods of time, i.e., the false alarm rate did neither increase nor decrease significantly. Moreover, this result illustrates that long-term behaviour changes cannot easily be detected using only a limited array of ambient sensors. Further research, incorporating both a larger total number and a greater variety of sensors, will be needed to provide a deeper understanding of which features of long-term behaviour are indicative of the onset, course, or worsening of chronic illnesses, e.g., dementia, diabetes, or heart diseases. Notwithstanding the above, it must be noted there is good reason to assume that evaluating user behaviour does indeed allow detecting and monitoring chronic medical conditions.

However, behaviour and inactivity monitoring need to be seen from two perspectives: One conceivable scenario is that the long-term data of a tenant exhibit inexplicable patterns that cannot easily be explained by the lifestyle of the respective person. In such a case, these observations may either point in the right direction or may be misleading, but eventually no compelling conclusions can be drawn as to what exactly caused those unexpected patterns. In another scenario, a health professional or other person might suspect a potential health problem based on observations or medical statements not linked to the AAL environment. In such a case, looking at the inactivity pattern of the respective person may support or refute a hypothesis regarding the suspected health issue and thus form a valuable additional source of information for doctors and caregivers.

Last but not least, it is noteworthy that the absolute inactivity durations vary substantially when comparing the inactivity patterns from several flats. In the Kaiserslautern AAL project, the lowest peak inactivity duration within one month observed in one flat was 35 minutes whereas –in another flat– peak inactivity amounted to almost 200 minutes. Similarly, the absolute tripping rates of the sensors, i.e., the number of sensor activations per unit of time, also vary greatly. For example, the smallest average number of light switch actuations per day observed in one flat was 15 whereas 175 were recorded elsewhere. On the one hand, this observation partly explains the varying inactivity levels mentioned above. On the other hand, it underscores that the daily routine is very unique to the respective user due to individual circumstances such as personal habits, working hours, hobbies, and so on. The inactivity patterns of individual sensor groups (e.g., light switches) and the overall inactivity, however, showed a good degree of correlation in a given flat.

5. Alarm Management

5.1. Necessity of False Alarms

False alarms are not only deemed to be unavoidable but the authors believe that they are downright indispensable. In chemical industries or process engineering, however, false alarms (i.e., spurious trips) are undesired because they can cause a plant to go from the normal productive state to a safe state in which the plant is halted. Nevertheless, spurious trips form an integral part of any safety equipment used in process engineering. Thus, procedures must be put in place to handle spurious trips appropriately. Moreover, all safety loops in industrial settings must periodically undergo routine proof tests to ensure that the safety equipment will indeed be capable of fulfilling its task upon a demand, i.e., initiating the transition into a safe state or shutting down the plant. With regard to AAL applications, false alarms may act as proof tests but it needs to be ensured that there will not be an overabundance of false alarms that might ultimately turn into an annoyance for the user. To avoid this from happening, the average number of false alarms per month that is acceptable can be limited by the user setting the mean time between false alarms (MTFA), as introduced above. Employing false alarms to verify that the AAL monitoring system does work properly has a number of plausible advantages.

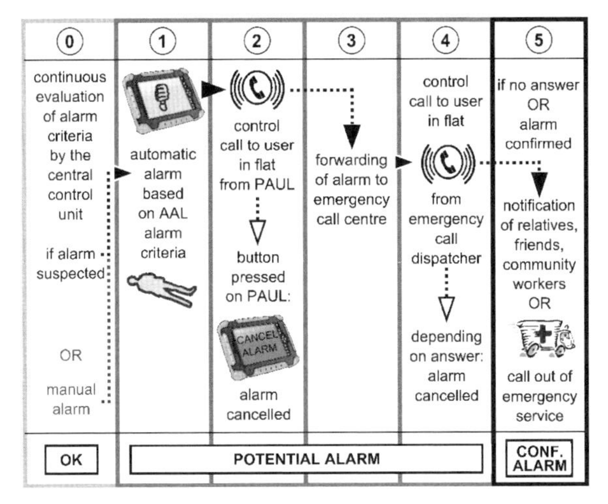

Figure 16. Alarm levels and forwarding plan.

First, false alarms test the entire alarming system: By means of a regular proof test, PAUL (the central unit), the software, and the communication line to the emergency call centre can be tested. The operability and availability of the sensors, however, cannot be tested since they work fully automatically. In contrast to that, in case of a false alarm the AAL system does what it is made for – observe an inactivity pattern that is outside the normal range and initiate an alarm sequence. Thus, malfunctions of the system would become apparent if any of its components had failed. Second, moderate numbers of false alarms that do not annoy the user instead train him how to deal with (false) alarms. This contributes to the user feeling confident about the AAL system so that the user knows how to handle and react to the system and alarms in particular. Third, false alarms will typically occur much more often than regular proof tests. Thus, the operability of the AAL system will be monitored more closely than in case of normal proof tests. As a result, the requirements towards the individual components constituting the AAL system can be lower than in case of safety equipment tested only once a year. This in turn allows the use of reasonably priced standard components that might otherwise have to be ruled out.

5.2. Alarm Handling and Forwarding

From the authors' point of view, an AAL alarming plan should comprise several stages (Fig. 16).

Alarm stage 0 means that the user is okay and that no potentially dangerous situation in the flat is detected by PAUL.

Stage 1 is entered if PAUL detects a potential case of emergency. This can have multiple causes: First, the automatic inactivity data processing algorithms running on PAUL may have reasoned that a potential emergency is present. Second, the user may have initiated a manual alarm via the emergency switch. It is, however, inherently impossible for PAUL to differentiate genuine alarms from false alarms: An automatic alarm may be caused by both a genuine emergency involving unconsciousness of the user or a false alert due to an exceptionally long inactivity phase which is, however, owed to normal user behaviour and not indicative of an emergency. Manual alarms can be raised either because the user did so intentionally or because the emergency button was pressed inadvertently, e.g., during cleaning or by a visitor who is not familiar with the alarming mechanisms.

In order to intercept as many of these spurious alarms, the alarming plan comprises stage 2: To avoid an overabundance of false alarms being forwarded to the emergency call centre, the user is given the chance to cancel the alarm before that. For this reason, PAUL rings the user on his (mobile) phone. If the user answers the call, a voice message will be played back, notifying the user of the impending alarm. The message will also prompt the user to interact with PAUL within a given short period of time by touching a cancel button displayed on the touch screen. The alarm forwarding time delay is typically only a few minutes, giving the user enough time to realise and react to the alarm but not unduly delaying contacting help in case of a real situation of distress. If the alarm does turn out to be a false alarm and the user presses the cancel button displayed on PAUL, the AAL system will switch back to the normal state and continue monitoring the user passively. The interaction with PAUL in order to cancel the false alarm is interpreted as activity so that all inactivity counters are thus reset to zero.

Once stage 3 is reached, PAUL assumes that the current alarm is genuine. PAUL now contacts the emergency call centre and transmits all necessary information to the dispatcher, e.g., in which flat the alarm originated, who might be affected, what criterion triggered the alarm, etc. It is important to note, though, that the privacy of the user is ensured to the greatest possible extent since no details regarding the collected raw activity data is transmitted but only the condensed information that at least one alarm criterion went out of the normal range and that assistance may be required immediately.

In stage 4, the emergency call dispatcher tries to verify the alarm by calling the user in their flat again. If the user answers the call and informs the dispatcher that a false alarm slipped through, no further actions will be taken, i.e., the alarm is cancelled by the call dispatcher. Stage 5 will not be entered.

In all other cases, the dispatcher proceeds to stage 5. There are two conceivable scenarios: First, the user answers and confirms the emergency, e.g., by telling the dispatcher that he fell and now requires help. Second, the call is not answered at all. In the former case, the operator tries to work out what kind of support is required and dispatches appropriate help. Possible options range from relatives or community workers to medical professionals and emergency medical services (EMS). If the control call is not answered by the user at all or the situation cannot be assessed properly, an EMS will as well be dispatched right away.

Even this multi-stage alarm handling plan, however, will not prevent a certain number of false alarms being reported to the call centre. However, German emergency call centre operators are prepared to handle these false alarms.

5.3. Acceptance of Automatic Alarming

During the interviews in October 2009 a total of 17 respondents (out of 18) indicated that the inactivity-based alarm generation was a good system. Even without being asked, two tenants mentioned the alarm generation to be an important function which should be implemented as soon as possible. Eight of the supporters, including two couples, indicated, however, that they do not see the system as useful for themselves but for other people living single. Only one younger tenant was afraid of surveillance and thus was against the alarm generation. The other tenants did not mention fears because of surveillance or heteronomy. Nevertheless, some of the tenants questioned whether the system will work. During the interviews the concept of the inactivity detection had to be explained to four residents.

Although one respondent was sceptical about whether and how the inactivity-based alarm generation works exactly, she sees advantages over other emergency detection systems if the emergency transmission goes to the neighbours who have access to the apartment. For most of those interviewed, the advantage of alarm generation lies in the fact that the person in need does not have to actively call for help but the call is sent automatically.

6. Summary

In this chapter, an AAL approach to enable senior citizens to live independently in their own homes using a *p*ersonal *a*ssistive *u*nit for *l*iving (PAUL) was introduced. The primary methods for supporting and assisting the seniors are pattern monitoring techniques that were developed in the course of an AAL project in Kaiserslautern, Germany. Inactivity proved to be a suitable means of assessing potential risks or emergencies in a flat. By monitoring user behaviour over a period of four weeks, the typical behavioural patterns were learned by the AAL system and inactivity profiles of each of the participating tenants could be established.

Based on these long-term inactivity patterns, alarming principles were developed. Both linear alarm thresholds (i.e., constant throughout the day) and tenant-specific thresholds (i.e., derived from the typical long-term inactivity profile) are used to generate automatic alarms if the current inactivity level in a flat exceeded the respective thresholds. It needs to be noted, however, that medical emergencies requiring immediate action (e.g., strokes or heart attacks) cannot be detected by the current monitoring system. Instead, it is most suitable for detecting emergencies in which help needs to be administered within a period of time of minutes to a few hours rather than immediately.

It is further assumed that in any such system false alarms cannot be avoided. Thus, procedures are defined and implemented that are capable of handling false alarms. In the presented work, false alarms are not seen as something to be avoided or penalised but rather as an important and valuable tool for giving the user the opportunity to adjust selectivity and response time of the monitoring system. By allowing a small mean time between false alarms (MTFA), the system will swiftly report potential emergencies whereas it will react more conservatively if a large MTFA is set. Since false alarms are anticipated in any real-world application of the monitoring system, a multi-stage alarming plan, involving the users and an emergency response call centre, is introduced and described in detail as well.

Regarding the acceptance of the introduced AAL concept, it can be stated that the system offers many useful features which can be controlled by a single device called PAUL. After two years of usage it became evident that the tenants do not have any problems with using PAUL. Most of them have well integrated PAUL and the other technological features in the apartment in daily life, they judge them as important for enhancing quality of life. The usage of the functions door camera, electric blinds, and internet became normal for the residents. Overall, the tenants in Kaiserslautern are very satisfied with their living conditions. The main reasons are the suitable apartments that guarantee mobility and access to inner city infrastructure. Another important reason is the lively neighbourhood with good personal relationships, high level of engagement, and leisure activities. Living in the social community with neighbours and preserving this integration are as well considered crucial factors for a high standard of living, regardless of the health situation. PAUL is seen by most tenants as a convenient amenity but not a necessity. Nevertheless, the advanced technology and PAUL are main topics in neighbourhood talks. In this sense AAL is more than technology: It is an important and positive factor for a newly composed neighbourhood that grows together.

References

[1] M. Alwan, S. Dalal, D. Mack, S.W. Kell, B. Turner, J. Leachtenauer and R. Felder, Impact of monitoring technology in assisted living: Outcome pilot, *IEEE Trans. Inf. Technol. Biomed.* **10**(1) (2006), 192–198.
[2] U. Anliker, J.A. Ward, P. Lukowicz, G. Troester, F. Dolveck, M. Baer, F. Keita, E.B. Schenker, F. Catarsi, L. Coluccini, A. Belardinelli, D. Shklarski, M. Alon, E. Hirt, R. Schmid and M. Vuskovic, AMON: A wearable multiparameter medical monitoring and alert system, *IEEE Trans. Inf. Technol. Biomed.* **8**(4) (2004), 415–427.
[3] EU, *Ambient Intelligence,* 2004. Online. http://ec.europa.eu/information_society/tl/policy/ambienti/index_en.htm (retrieved 2 Nov 2009).
[4] M. Floeck, *Activity Monitoring and Automatic Alarm Generation in AAL-Enabled Homes*, Logos-Verlag, Berlin, 2010, ISBN 978-3-8325-2722-8.
[5] J. Grauel and A. Spellerberg, *Attitudes and Requirements of Elderly People Towards Assisted Living Solutions*, Springer, Heidelberg, 2008.
[6] E.A. Lee, Cyber physical systems: Design challenges, in: *Proc. 11th IEEE International Symposium on Object Oriented Real-Time Distributed Computing (ISORC)*, 2008, pp. 363–369.
[7] R. McGill, J.W. Tukey and W.A. Larsen, Variations of box plots, *The American Statistician* **32**(1) (1978), 12–16.
[8] J. Nehmer, Elektronische Notfallüberwachung für Alleinlebende, *Notfall & Rettungsmedizin* **12** (2009), 19–24.
[9] NSF, National Science Foundation, in: *NSF Workshop on Cyber-Physical Systems – Research Motivation, Techniques and Roadmap*, 2006, Online: http://varma.ece.cmu.edu/CPS/, (retrieved 12 Nov. 2009).
[10] J.M. Reyes Alamo, J. Wong, R. Babbitt, H.-I. Yang and C.K. Chang, Using web services for medication management in a smart home environment, in: *ICOST '09: Proc. of the 7th International Conference on Smart Homes and Health Telematics*, Springer-Verlag, Berlin, Heidelberg, 2009, pp. 265–268.
[11] M. Rose, *Gebäudesystemtechnik in Wohn- und Zweckbau mit dem EIB*, 2. bearb. Aufl., Huethig Heidelberg, 1995.
[12] A. Spellerberg, J. Grauel and L. Schelisch, Ambient assisted living – Ein erster Schritt in Richtung eines technisch-sozialen Assistenzsystems für ältere Menschen, *Hallesche Beiträge zu den Gesundheits- und Pflegewissenschaften* **8**(39) (2009).
[13] J.W. Tukey, Data-based graphics: Visual display in the decades to come, *Statistical Science* **5**(3) (1990), 327–339.
[14] A.M. Turing, Computing machinery and intelligence, *Mind* **59** (1950), 433–460.
[15] M. Weiser, The computer for the 21st century, *Scientific American* **265**(3) (1991), 66–75.
[16] W. Wolf, Cyber-physical systems, *Computer* **42**(3) (2009), 88–89.
[17] D. Zito, D. Pepe, B. Neri, D. De Rossi, A. Lanata, A. Tognetti and E.P. Scilingo, Wearable system-on-a-chip UWB radar for health care and its application to the safety improvement of emergency operators, in: *Proc. 29th Annual International Conference of the IEEE Engineering in Medicine and Biology Society EMBS 2007*, 2007, pp. 2651–2654.

Handbook of Ambient Assisted Living
J.C. Augusto et al. (Eds.)
IOS Press, 2012

doi:10.3233/978-1-60750-837-3-283

The Role of Assistive Technology in Supporting Formal Carers

Amritpal S. BHACHU[a,*], Nicholas HINE[a] and Ryan WOOLRYCH[b]
[a] *University of Dundee*
[b] *Manchester Metropolitan University*

Abstract. In an increasingly ageing population, solutions are being sought to enable older people to live independently in their own homes. Assistive technology has the potential to develop supportive environments for older people through "ambient assisted living". This chapter is based on results from the implementation of an assistive technology project designed to provide formal carers with patient information to support them in their case management. The study followed the trial use of a telecare system, capturing the experiences of formal carers and documenting the impact of assistive technology. The findings identify that assisted living devices have the potential, once trust is established, to support formal carers to undertake their role more effectively. However, in accepting assistive technology as part of an integrated care solution, there are implications on the role and responsibilities of the formal carer, existing mechanisms for delivering community care and the quality of the relationship between the carer and the cared for. The paper concludes by considering the challenges for assistive technology if it is to be directly supportive of formal care-givers.

Keywords. Telecare, patient management, older adults, chronic conditions

1. Ambient Assisted Living, the Home and Formal Care

Global population ageing is pervasive, representing a significant health and social care burden to society [34] as increasingly more people require high intensity care and support to undertake activities of daily living [13]. An ageing population has raised pertinent questions about how we can best meet the needs of older people, through providing care and assistance that supports their independence, choice and quality of life. Effectively addressing these challenges has spawned a plethora of policy initatives, frameworks, and declarations emphasising the role of Information and Communcation Technologies (ICT) in helping to care for older people [14,15]. The challenge is to support older people to 'live independently', 'in a secure environment' with 'peace of mind', priorities identified in The Ambient Assistive Living Road Map [2]. This road map defined the need for a solution which supports ageing in the home, as "enjoying a healthier and higher quality of life for a longer time, assisted by technology, whilst maintaining a high degree of independence, autonomy and dignity" [2]. However, in delivering on these aims, assistive technology needs to be considered within the context of existing delivery mechanisms, and its potential impact upon formal methods of delivering care in the community.

*Corresponding Author: Amritpal S. Bhachu. E-mail: abhachu@computing.dundee.ac.uk.

This overarching objective is supported by aging-in-place literature, which has identified the home as the preferred living environment for older people [41]. In a survey of 2000 people undertaken by Bayer and Harper [6], amongst those aged 45 and over, over 80 percent of respondents felt 'somewhat strongly' or 'very strongly' that they wish to remain in their own home as long as possible. Furthermore, when asked about where respondents would prefer to receive care, 82 percent stated that they would prefer to receive care at home, rather than move to a care facility. Other literature has established reasons for the home as a valued place in the lives of older people, identifying the importance of the home as a source of shared memories for the older person, constituting an important factor in sense of belonging and identity [38,39]. The home has been articulated as being central to the independence and autonomy of older people, representing an environment where notions of freedom and choice are exercised [42]. Moreover, research on restorative environments suggests that the home is a place of security, to recover from stressful life events and to maintain a well-being equilibrium between positive and negative effect [19]. The importance of the home has also been situated with the context of service delivery. Research examining the impact of health and social care provision has evidence that services delivered within the home environment can enable older people to retain higher perceived levels of independence and quality of life [9], whilst moving to a care facility brings about feelings of dependence and represents a downward trajectory in old age [3].

Given the importance of the home as a place to deliver care, a key priority is creating a domestic environment, and ICT solutions, that encourage and support health aging. In the areas of falls prevention, lifestyle and activity monitoring and alarm response systems, assistive technologies have been designed to support people living at home [10,16]. Here, research suggests that assistive technology can play a significant role in sustaining or enhancing levels of perceived safety, encouraging freedom of movement around the home and in the completion of activities of daily living [25,26]. Technology for older people has been considered as 'freeing' and a protection of individual privacy, as it enables older people to stay in their home longer, encouraging independent living and preventing the need for institutional care [8,12]. Whilst technology might be considered supportive, other research has identified barriers to the long-term acceptability of assistive technology in the homes of older people, identifying ethical issues related to privacy, confidentiality and obtrusiveness [23,35], which can potentially compromise or undermine personal identity [17].

In delivering care to older people within the home, existing evidence suggests that technology cannot work in isolation and must be part of a more integrated care solution [27]. This requires that the development of ICT solutions for independent and assisted living are designed to support and enhance the care delivered through existing informal (friends, family members, neighbours) and formal (doctors, nurses, healthcare professionals) pathways. Research suggests that formal carers can develop close relationships with older people, establishing a strong sense of trust and reciprocity in the process; such that formal carers assume an active role in the decision-making process concerning access and take-up of services [21,37]. Given the central role of the formal carer in delivering care, they have a fundamental role to play in the ways in which older people interrelate with assistive technology and therefore in the overall acceptability and usability of healthcare technologies within the home. Moreover, as assistive technology is likely to be delivered through formal service mechanisms and providers, it needs to be supportive of the working practices of care providers and empower them to make better-informed decisions about care.

Assistive technology has the potential to support care providers, whilst delivering high quality care. Research has evidenced improvements in the effectiveness and efficiency of care delivery through providing formal carers with health and care information [1,24]. Remote monitoring facilitates the possibility that clinical decision-making can be undertaken by formal carers away from the home, or can be combined with home care visits, to better assess health and social conditions and deliver high quality care. The monitoring and interpretation of patient information can be reactive (action to a change in specific data) or proactive (to monitor long term trends and determine intervention) [16], enabling the prioritisation of care and better care management thus improving efficiency (better use of carers time and resources) and thereby reducing costs [20]. Assistive technology thus becomes an 'enabler' of care, acting as the interface between older person and formal carer and delaying the need for acute intervention.

Prioritising case management has prompted concerns regarding the quality of care, where technology is perceived as a replacement of patient-centred care, leading to the loss of the 'human factor' in care delivery [18]. Access to patient information is also an area of concern, ensuring that the caregiver has accurate, reliable and readable information to make better informed care decisions regarding the patient. Importantly, in introducing remote monitoring, such solutions potential redefine the role of the formal carer, thereby introducing cultural barriers associated with changes to working practices. Here, technology which is to be acceptable and usable in making decisions about the delivery of care, needs to be predicated upon an experiential understanding of the impact of ambient assisted living technology on the working practices of the formal carer and their relationship with the older person.

2. Formal Carers as Community Matrons

In this study we explored the impact of telecare technology in supporting the role of Community Matrons (CMs) in delivering care to older people. By definition, CMs are experienced and skilled nurses who deliver a personalized, case management approach to supporting older people within their homes. The emphasis of their role is upon addressing problems before they escalate and require high intensity, and more costly, service interventions. CMs are responsible for: reviewing and prescribing medication; needs assessment; providing health and social care interventions; co-ordinating input from other health and social care agencies and teaching and educating patients about their condition [32]. The Community Matron acts as the single point of contact for the provision and procurement of care for the older person, developing a relationship founded upon a degree of trust and reciprocity. CMs are required to monitor individuals care, providing one-to-one support to a caseload of vulnerable patients with long-term conditions. Appropriate interventions can be widespread and are based upon an in-depth knowledge of the client, but may include dietary, behavioural, lifestyle, medication aspects of health and well-being.

The role of the Community Matron emerged from the NHS Improvement plan [33], a key UK policy objective of which is to promote independence, well-being and choice amongst older people. This plan recommended a new clinical role for nurses, predicated upon the holistic management of individual cases i.e. case management. Case management is an extension of 'care in the community', adopted in the Community Care Act [31], which encourages the delivery of health and social care within people's homes, providing people with services that meet their individual needs [5]. With case management there is an emphasis on the Community Matron to co-ordinate the delivery of the care, whilst encouraging the patient to self manage their condition, ensuring that older people are able to remain at home longer and preventing unplanned admission to hospital. The objective of the Community Matron is to increase choice, prevent unnecessary hospital admissions and improve outcomes, thereby enabling patients to live in their own homes independently. Research assessing the success of the case management approach, reveals mixed results regarding its impact on reducing unplanned hospital admissions and in alleviating the costs of care [30]. Others have highlighted the complexity of the role, identifying skills gaps, training requirements and the need for closer working with other healthcare professionals [28].

Whilst community care is well grounded in UK policy, the approach of providing services to older people within their own homes, through a healthcare professional, is widespread [4]. In the US, this operates within a framework of managed care aimed at frail older people with multiple problems. It is therefore intended that the results from this study have relevance across different domains.

3. The Project

This project evaluated the impact of assistive technology in helping to support CMs, as formal carers, to undertake their role more effectively. Assistive technology was trialed in the homes of older people, technology that integrated unobtrusive pervasive sensing in the homes of older people and linked to physiological/metabolic parameters and lifestyle patterns. Ambient sensing was used to capture information including activity monitoring, sleeping pattern, room occupancy, and gait and posture changes. The technology used a variety of non-invasive sensors throughout the home to provide continual activity and environmental monitoring of the individual.

The objective of the technology was to ensure CMs were provided with patient health and well-being information in a readable form, potentially providing a tool for improved well-being monitoring and early detection of changes in disease state. The data collected from the homes of patients, via ambient and body worn sensors, was transmitted via a home hub to a secure network platform, to the care provider systems for access by the formal carer. This raised the possibility of accessing patient information remotely or when stationed within their place of work, providing the means to make decisions regarding patients without the need to undertake a home visit. In addition to interpretation by CMs, the system provides the opportunity for older people themselves to access the information, through a specific television channel presenting their information. Here, the technology has the potential to empower older people themselves, through the ability to interpret and act upon any changes to their own condition.

The aim of this study was to examine the role of assistive technology in helping to support the role of the Community Matron in making informed decisions about the care of their patients. By presenting collected sensor data in a meaningful way for healthcare professionals, it was hoped that this would help them better manage their patient loads and make patient care more efficient.

The project aim was underpinned by a number of research questions:

1. To what extent can assistive technology better support the role of the formal carer in the decision-making process?

2. In what ways does assistive technology impact on the relationship between the carer and cared for?
3. What factors contribute to the acceptability and usability of assistive technology by formal carers?
4. What are the key factors influencing the acceptability and usability of assistive technology amongst formal carers?

In undertaking this role, CMs were recruited via the local NHS trust. CMs attended a number of recruitment days where the system was explained to them and they had the opportunity to ask any questions. CMs were asked to recruit patients to the trial, based upon who they felt would be most appropriate for the trial. Following recruitment, and the consent of the patients themselves, the equipment was installed in the home environment. A total number of eleven patients and four CMs were involved during the course of the trial.

4. Methods

For assistive technology to be directly supportive of the workload of the CMs, it was necessary to establish their expectations and requirements from the system, and to capture an understanding of the ways in which the system impacted on the ways in which they currently deliver care to their patients. The experiences of CMs and older people themselves were captured through a variety of methods. These included: An Older Adults Workshop, Live Forum Theatre, Trial and Case Conferences, Exit Interviews and a Dissemination session. Mixed methods were important for determining the requirements and expectations of the Community Matron pre-trial, to ensure ongoing issues were identified during the trial and to determine the overall impact and recommendations for the future post-trial. Older adults were involved at an early stage to ensure that the project was grounded in an experiential understanding of the needs of those receiving care.

This mixed methods approach was necessary to incorporate the views of both older people and CMs and to develop an in-depth understanding of the working practices, care delivery mechanisms and the development of the carer-cared for relationships. Given that the trial was six months and overall project length forty-two months, creative methods were used alongside more traditional research approaches in order to elicit a breadth and depth of information that a single method research could not achieve. Moreover, more creative approaches were perceived as an opportunity to alleviate participant fatigue, ensuring that they were engaged in varied ways across the course of the project. The application and development of the methods was underpinned by a participatory approach, ensuring that comments and feedback from each of the methods was incorporated into system re-design where possible. Incorporating the views of stakeholders in this way results in product development which is more reflective of the experiences of end users themselves; an inclusive approach advocated in the design and development of assistive technology for older people [22,40].

4.1. Older Adults Workshop

An Older Adults Workshop was undertaken at an early stage of the work to determine the applicability of the technology within the lives of older people. It was felt important to elicit the feedback of older participants, and determine if the proposed ICT was fit for purpose within the home environment, before capturing the views of CMs. The workshop method was chosen as, if conducted effectively, it represents a participatory and inclusive way for older people to have their say in the design and development of technology [11].

A group of 13 older adults were invited to attend a workshop in the School of Computing at the University of Dundee. Members of the group had varying degrees of computing skills, some with little experience of using computers and some with everyday experience. They were of pensionable age, between the ages of 60–80 years old. The group all came from different educational and working backgrounds. There were three who had experience of working in a professional office environment, two who had worked in education, four manual workers and one ex-nurse. There were also several who hadn't worked. This gave the study a wide range of people from the target group. The health conditions of group members were not considered in the scope of this workshop, although many of the group referred to their health during discussions.

The workshop outlined the aims and objectives of the project, and presented the key features and specific aspects of the technology as the stimulus for discussion. The session incorporated both hands-on activities (interacting with system components) and information presentation (the visual representation of the information). Older people were asked for the comments on the system, identifying aspects of current care delivery, levels of acceptability concerning individual components of the system and likelihood of use within the home environment. All discussions were facilitated by a member of the research team with audio and video recorded for transcription.

4.2. Live Forum Theatre

After capturing the feedback of older people, it was necessary to elicit the opinions of the CMs themselves regarding the supportive role that the technology could play in their everyday working practices. To ensure that the technology was fit-for-purpose it was necessary to understand the working practices of healthcare professionals including the specific ways in which they delivered care to the older person and how technology can best support them. Live Forum Theatre is a method through which storytelling and the presentation of typical scenarios can be acted out to enable participants to reflect upon and engage with key aspects of the research [29].

Use case scenarios were developed as a result of earlier work conducted with CMs. These scenarios presented typical work examples confronting the matrons on a regular basis, incorporating the use of the technology. During the forum theatre event, scenarios were scripted and acted out by professional actors. The audience was given the opportunity to comment on what they have seen after each scene as a prompt for further discussion. This method was used as it gave the audience a chance to see how a telecare system could be used to support CMs in the delivery of care, and provided the platform for them to contribute their opinions. The Live Forum Theatre provided the opportunity to bring together the formal carers, technicians and academics, establishing a common ground, which is often difficult to establish when engaging end uses in research [36].

Two Live Forum Theatre sessions were conducted focused on working through typical care delivery scenarios and discussing the way in which the technology could support them. Each Live Forum Theatre event lasted for between two and three hours with a rich level of discussion being produced during this time. In both sessions, the audience comprised healthcare professionals including CMs, telecare developers, technicians and academics. In line with the ethical submission of the project, potential service users could not take part in the Live Forum Theatre. However, on discussion with the formal carers prior to the events taking place, the research team was happy that the CMs and other healthcare professionals could represent the opinions and feelings of their patients.

The scenarios and discussions provided knowledge of the working practices of CMs and the specifics of delivering care within the home. The feedback also enabled a better understanding of the relationships that CMs have with their patients and the informal aspects of care delivery which technology needs to support. The Live Forum Theatre sessions were audio and video recorded and made available for analysis.

Seven healthcare professionals and six developers/technicians attended the first live forum theatre. This session introduced the notion of assistive technology to the audience and detailed the aims and objectives of the technology. The individual scenarios were scripted after detailed discussions with the script-writer and local community nurses. Each scenario was based upon typical situations confronting the CM when they are delivering care to the patient. Following presentation of the scenarios, CMs were asked about the processes for delivering care, their response to the needs of the situation and any additional support which could be provided to the formal carers to help them manage the delivery of care more effectively.

Having developed an understanding of the working practices of CMs, a further Live forum Theatre event was conducted. This event presented scenarios which included on 'A Day in the Life of a Community Matron Using a telecare system' and depicted the possible course of events and situations that may be encountered by CMs during a typical day using a telecare system. Responses were elicited from CMs, identifying the positive ways in which the technology could better support their decision-making without acting as a hindrance or barrier to the delivery of care. Eight healthcare professionals and twelve developers/technicians attended this event.

By re-enacting familiar scenarios, and asking CMs to respond to them, the control of the discussion was transferred to the formal carers themselves. This provided them with an environment where they felt more able to share their opinions, thoughts and feelings concerning the system. The Live Forum Theatre enabled deeper understandings to emerge of the issues impacting on the acceptability of assistive technology amongst CMs. Establishing their responses prior to the commencement of the trial, provided the opportunity to monitor these attitudinal changes as the trial commenced, monitoring expectations and identifying previously unconsidered benefits.

4.3. Trial and Case Conferences

CMs recruited to the project recommended a number of patients who they felt would benefit most from continuous monitoring in the home environment. Patients were approached in the first instance by CMs to determine their likelihood of being involved. The research team then contacted the older participants to explain the aims and objectives of the project, to introduce the key features of the system and to outline the anticipated benefits of their involvement. Where the older participant felt it was desirable, informal carers were involved in the discussions. After acquiring informed consent, the equipment was installed in the homes of the participant for a duration of six months. Altogether, four CMs and eleven patients took part in the trial. During the trial, the CMs had access to the data produced from the sensors and devices of their patient's system through a secure online Community Ward website.

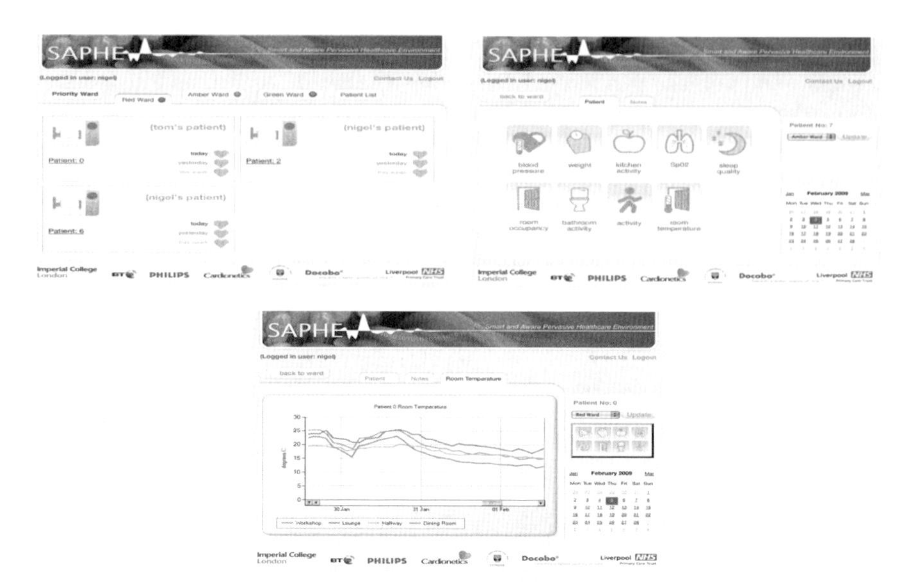

Figure 1. Community ward screenshots.

The Community Ward website gave the CM a three level display of the patients collected data. The top level displayed all of the patients that a single CM cared for. From here, the CM could choose to view the data of an individual patient. The next screen gave an overview of the statistics being collected for the selected patient. The third level of data gave a more detailed breakdown of a selected statistic in the form of a graph. The Community Ward website allowed the CM to view patient data at a level that was appropriate to the patient and the specific information that the CM required at the time of viewing. Screenshots of the Community Ward website can be seen in Fig. 1.

At monthly intervals during the trial, case conferences were facilitated with the CMs as a group. Altogether, six case conferences were conducted. Each case conference lasted for between 2 and 3 hours in duration, were facilitated by two members of the research team and were recorded for purposes of transcribing. A group format was deemed most appropriate to facilitate shared dialogue and active discussion between CMs.

The aim of the case conferences was to determine the impact of the technology on the working practices of CMs, identifying any aspects of the system that were/were not working well, any perceived changes in the relationship between the carer and cared for as a result of using the technology and issues relating to the usability and acceptability of the system over time. Capturing their perceptions over the duration of the trial, enabled the development of their attitudes towards the technology to be monitored over the course of the trial. Patients were discussed on a case-by-case basis, identifying examples of where technology had positively/negatively impacted on supporting/delivering care to the patient. It also provided the opportunity for CMs to relay any comments from their patients or informal carers about the system.

4.4. Exit Interviews

After completion of the 6 month trial, the equipment was removed from the homes of the older person. This was immediately followed by one-to-one exit interviews conducted with each of the CMs. All interview were conducted at a date, time and venue convenient to the Community Matron, lasted for between 45 and 90 minutes and were recorded for purposes of transcribing.

The aim of the exit interviews was to establish the overall impact of the technology in the context of their initial expectations. Both anticipated outcomes and unanticipated benefits and drawbacks of the technology were discussed and their implications for the adoption of monitoring technology commented on. The exit interviews provided the opportunity for CMs to evaluate their own experience of being involved in the trial, as well as the perceived advantages and disadvantages of assisted technology for the older participants themselves. Additionally, they proposed recommendations for the successful integration of such technology in the future, and identified potential practical and political barriers to adoption.

4.5. Dissemination Session

A final dissemination session was held 4 weeks after the trial was completed. The aim of the dissemination session was to engage CMs in workshop to feedback on the key findings from the trial and to determine if the findings were an accurate portrayal of their experiences. The emerging results provided the stimulus for further discussion with CMs and retrospective reflection on their engagement in the trial. Importantly, it identified any instances and examples of where the system may have been useful in supporting them to deliver care, and progress of the individual patients during the trial.

All CMs attended the dissemination session, alongside 5 members of the research team. This was a further opportunity to bring together formal carers, technicians and academics within a process of shared working to further refine the issues raised in the project. The dissemination session lasted for a duration of 3 hours and was tape recorded for transcription purposes.

4.6. Analysis

Throughout each of the activities outlined above, researcher field notes and audio and/or visual recordings were taken.

Thematic analysis [7] was applied to this content and the main themes were extracted. The thematic analysis followed the key principles outlined by Braun (i) familiarisation with the data (ii) generating initial codes (iii) searching for themes (iv) reviewing themes (v) defining and naming themes (vi) producing the reports.

Key themes and findings were mapped across the course of the work and synthesized across the Adult Workshops, Live Forum Theatre, Case Conferences, Exit Interviews and Dissemination Event.

5. Key Findings

The CMs (CMs), as providers of health and social care to the older person, identified a number of key issues in the application and development of assistive technology with the homes of older people. They relate to the acceptability of the technology within the homes of the patients, the impact of the technology on the relationship that they have with their patients and also identify ways in which assistive technology needs to be supportive of the everyday needs of CMs. These issues emerged and developed in different ways throughout the project, as CMs and patients became more familiar with the technology.

5.1. Role of the Formal Carer in Integrating Assistive Technology

Research into patient privacy has revealed that assistive technology within the home can lead to perceptions of being monitored, heightening levels of anxiety and feelings of being watched [3,16]. The findings from this project suggested that CMs, by placing them in a position of control, can alleviate concerns related to monitoring and privacy, thereby increasing levels of acceptability of technology amongst older people.

Issues relating to patient privacy were first reported by CMs during the forum theatre sessions, and was a theme raised in the early discussions with older people. The older adults in the workshop session were the first to question how telecare systems, through being visible within the older person's home, would compromise an individual's privacy. They felt that having telecare devices visible to family members, friends and other visitors could increase the stigma associated with having a telecare system in the home i.e. visitors would know the patient is being monitored and would perceive them as being 'ill' or in need of assistance.

Similarly, the CMs felt that privacy would be a significant issue if the system and its features were not adequately explained to the patient, thereby increasing levels of anxiety and concern if the older person does not understand the purpose of the individual sensors. CMs felt that there was the potential of some sensors to be intrusive as they closely resembled a camera, for example, particularly the Passive Infra Red (PIR) sensors which had integrated flashing lights when activated. During the initial theatre session, the CMs commented that with the introduction of a telecare system, the patient may feel like:

> "*everyone is watching their every move*" [CM FT1]

CMs felt issues relating to privacy and monitoring could have a specific impact on the adoption and acceptability of the technology amongst older people. The CMs felt that patients would feel as if they are being watched, potentially restricting their behaviours within the home and increasing anxiety levels/tension as a result of having the system within the home. In the early case conferences, the issue of privacy and intrusiveness was again raised by CMs, within the context of informal carers acceptability of the system. A Community Matron relayed the story of the wife of one patient who felt that the system was watching her movements and activities within different rooms and actively intervened to turn the sensors off.

However, the Community Matron, being responsible for making care-related decisions, played an active role in minimizing concerns over privacy and increasing levels of acceptability. CMs revealed that they were often in a position of trust; patients relying upon the formal carer to make the most appropriate decisions to benefit them. CMs therefore acted as the mediator, allaying the everyday concerns of older people and informal carers regarding privacy and behavioral monitoring. The Community Matron were also available to explain and regularly reinforce the potential benefits of the system to the patient, resulting in increased levels of acceptability amongst patients. However, this requires that CMs understand how the technology operates and that they 'buy-in' to the anticipated benefits of the system. Given this, the Community Matron may still feel uncomfortable promoting a system that has not yet become an integral part of their care provision.

In empowering CMs, it was important they felt a sense of ownership in accessing the data. Here, CMs were asked to make the decisions concerning how and when they chose to act upon the data and also had the freedom to halt the trial and ask for a removal of the system if they felt it was not working. Moreover, through the regular case conferences they were provided with the forum for voicing their concerns which where possible resulted in changes to the equipment. Transferring control to the CMs provided participants with feelings of safety, as they were aware that the formal carer themselves were representing the needs and wants of the patient. Older people felt more secure in the knowledge that CMs were the individuals monitoring their data and responding to changes. The fact that the CM were the ones undertaking the 'watching' and being in control of the technology was seen as fundamental to patients accepting being monitored:

> "*there was nobody [in the end] that felt threatened or paranoid in any way that we were watching at all... but I think that's to do with your relationship with the patient... they were very very happy that they knew that I was watching and that I was proactive in it all and I think that's what gave them a bit more confidence really knowing that I was watching.*" [CM1 End of Trial Interview]

CMs, in acting as the mediator to the system, provided the everyday support to older people to become familiar with the system, minimising any concerns or worries and educating the patient about the system to minimise perceptions of 'being watched' and suspicions about what the system is designed to achieve. Here, CMs can play a significant role in smoothing the integration of technology within people's home. Additionally, the CMs were in the best position (as the main point of contact with the older person) to relay any issues with operability and reliability of the equipment. As well as feedback through the case conferences, CMs were encouraged to provide daily or weekly feedback on their experiences via e-mail or telephone. This provided formal carers with a channel for raising and discussing queries and issues, and was beneficial to the development of the technology as it allowed for re-design.

5.2. Assistive Technology and Impact Upon Role of the Formal Carer

CMs identified the importance of trust and reciprocity in the relationship that they developed with their patients and often spoke about a 'partnership approach to care'. This was a theme that was evident from a very early point in the research from the first forum theatre session. The CMs felt that such trust took a considerable time to develop with the client, predicated upon a continuity of care with the client and maintained by regular personal contact and communication. Indeed, this close relationship gave rise to early suspicions regarding the intention of the technology. CMs reported that patients felt that the system was designed to replace the role of the Community Matron:

> "*one patient thought the system was a replacement for me.*" [CM 2 CC4]

The CMs felt that maintaining this trust was fundamental to patients talking openly about their condition, ensuring their compliance with recommended treatments and their concordance with decisions made by the CMs. Prior to the trial, CMs reported that the involvement of the patients in the trial was dependent on the involvement of the CMs:

> "*they know that you have made a difference in the past, if they can see the difference before where you've improved things then they're more willing to have a go at something new.*" [CM FT1]

This was evidenced in later case conferences where CMs explained how a number of the trial participants were engaging in the study as they thought that it might 'help out' the CM and therefore accepting the system as it supported their own health and well-being.

Indeed, CMs reported the continued involvement of the participants being dependent on the relationship with the older person. During the second forum theatre session, and the first case conference, CMs stressed the importance that any system should not compromise this relationship and the levels of trust that they had developed with their patients. In particular, it was highlighted that any false positives that led to the CM questioning the patient based on the data could result in the patient not wanting to be as open to discuss issues with the CM.

During the trial, the issue of trust continued to be raised on a number of occasions. In some instances the system was used by CMs to directly challenge the perceptions of the patient. For example, on one occasion the patient informed the CM that they had not been the toilet but the system suggested otherwise. Assistive technology thus provided the source of tension, challenging the CM/patient relationship. The CM was keen to ensure that they system did not compromise the CM/patient relationship and the knowledge of the client and the monitoring of the CM were prioritised over reliance upon the system. CMs consistently reported that they did not substitute patient visits as a result of what they interpreted from the system data, although the data was often used as a prompt for a visit or telephone call, but was not seen as a replacement.

The issue of trust was again raised in the post-trial interview stage with CMs. They felt that being involved in the trial brought additional responsibilities, through increased patient expectations (that the CM were continuously monitoring and interpreting the data). If such a system was to be adopted in the long-term, CMs felt that this would bring a mental burden (stress and worry) in meeting patient expectations:

> "*if you'd been on annual leave it worried me that nobody had been monitoring... when you're away for two weeks holiday, what's happening in the meantime... how do you reassure the patients... I'm going on holiday now, who's looking at the data?*" [CM1 End of Trial Interview]

This raises the question that if CMs are to be seen as mediators in the implementation and management of such a system, how can this be best facilitated without compromising the CM/patient relationship. CMs recommended the possibility of an alternative person monitoring and identifying patterns in the data, a person with clinical experience who could raise any concerns with the CM. They felt that this would alleviate the resource burden of interpreting such technology, whilst ensuring continuous monitoring of the data.

5.3. Assistive Technology as a Supportive Tool in Delivering Care

In the discussions held during the first Live Forum Theatre, the CMs expressed concerns in relying on technology for making care-related decisions. The CMs felt that they needed to develop trust in the system, through ensuring (i) that the equipment was consistently reliable and (ii) that the data generated was timely and accurate.

During the first forum theatre session, CMs were asked about the potential of the technology to increase efficiency through more effective case management. This might include using assistive technology and the patient information to better prioritise visits or to reduce the number of unnecessary calls. CMs were wary of replacing or re-prioritising visits based upon what the assistive technology was telling them. This was partly attributable to their lack of trust in the system but also to their uncertainty of the role of the technology in replacing established working practices. One CM reported:

> "*I wouldn't particularly think about swapping appointments just by judging what's on the screen.*" [CM FT2]

At this point, CMs revealed that their patients typically experienced multiple problems and that making a decision based on the datasets within the system would be problematic. CMs often combined their intimate knowledge of the client, with specific medical information, and observed behaviours to arrive at a decision. The assistive technology itself could not combine the tacit knowledge which the CM possesses. In the initial stages, CMs felt that the system would actually decrease levels of efficiency, as it represented another responsibility i.e. monitoring the data, which they would need to undertake in addition to a patient visit:

> "*if the patient says they aren't feeling well then we have to visit no matter what the data says.*" [CM FT2]

Additionally, CMs felt that there was a limit to the intelligence that the system could possess. Whilst the sensors yielded information around the home, it did not provide the CMs with in-depth knowledge of the patient within the home. Everyday patterns and intentions for patients movement around the home were more complex and could not be integrated into the system. For example, door sensors provided them with data relating to room usage, but provided little contextual information about the activities of the person within the room. For example, "entering the toilet does not tell us that they used the toilet", "opening the fridge, does not provide us with evidence that they have consumed solids and liquids". In being supportive of the role of the CMs, there was a requirement for data that expressed a finer level of granularity.

However, there was a notable change in CM attitudes and perceptions during the second Live Forum Theatre session, as they began to perceive the system in a supportive role, as opposed to something designed to replace the care they were received. Here CMs began to articulate assistive technology as part of an integrated care solution, where the information generated by the assistive technology might provide the prompt or the stimulus for action on behalf of the carer. At this stage, benefits in terms of patient management, were still not being articulated, yet the potential assistive role of the technology was being expressed:

> "*If the system wasn't showing things, I wouldn't take it as definitive, but if it was showing things, it would prompt me to make a visit.*" [CM FT2]

Evidence of improved case management were further hampered with reliability issues with the equipment. Here, there was some disparity in the readings taken by the CM and those relayed by the system. This difference caused some early anxiety for CMs, prompting unnecessary visits to corroborate the data and undermining trust in the system. This had the effect of decreasing frequency of use in the early stages of the trial. Moreover, by placing CMs in control of the system, the CM becomes the conduit for reporting problems with the reliability of the equipment. This represented an extra burden for the Community Matron, who had to manage the integration of the system with their own everyday workload, directing time and efforts away from caring towards the integration of the technology.

However, CM feedback was used constructively to facilitate the re-design of the technology. Comments were fedback into the technicians who made subsequent improvements to the technology and to the presentation and readability of the data. Alterations mainly focused on the graphs to allow a CM to view exact data at a particular point as well as removing any outliers that were clearly not part of the patient data to make the graph easier to view. Also, changes were made to the design and implementation of the sensors used in the system to better fit the way in which the patients were using them. As the trial progressed, CMs re-engaged with the system, as they began to see that the changes that they had proposed were used for meaningful system change and development.

5.4. Assistive Technology as a Tool for Improved Case Management

As the trial progressed, CMs began to identify specific examples of where the technology helped support the CMs to undertake their role i.e. patient management. Here, the data from the system assisted the CMs in making specific interventions that may not have arisen without the trial equipment. It was when the CMs shared these benefits that a change in perception towards the technology was noted and the CMs began talking about the system as assistive and supportive technology for them rather than as a direct replacement of what they do. A movement from using the system reflectively, as noted in early case conferences, to using it proactively for early intervention was seen during the later case conferences. The CMs began to see the system as enabling them to monitor long-term trends in the condition of their patients. Here, CMs began to make changes to lifestyle and diet as a result of trends in the data. This prevented crisis situations from occurring through making necessary interventions based upon patterns in the data. Importantly, where there were inconsistencies in the data, CMs through their knowledge of the client, felt able to establish that they were outliers and removed them from the interpretation of the data in some cases where automated monitoring of the data or a third person analyzing the information may have yielded false alarms or incorrect inferences, the Community Matron was able to interpret the results within the context and circumstance of the individual, for example, where changes in medication resulted in higher or lower rates of blood pressure or where room activity could be linked to friends of relative visiting.

> "*I did most of the time, I didn't initially because there were a few blood pressure checks that I had to make that didn't seem to ring true and there was a bit of a difference in the beginning but over the month it ironed out, could see that a few different readings didn't matter over the long term.*" [CM 2 End of Trial Interview]

Moreover, CMs were in the best position to interpret the multiple problems of the patient and bring about an intervention that would best support the older person. Whereas the data itself might have suggested one intervention, the knowledge of the CM, and there ability to undertake a visit when necessary resulted in the optimum intervention. CMs cited examples where they needed to synthesis a number of datasets for a particular patient in order to make a recommendation i.e. a patient living with high blood pressure, low weight, and abnormal sleeping patterns. Whilst the system presented this data to the Community Matron, this needed to be interpreted meaningfully for an appropriate intervention to be initiated:

"*it [the system] picked up that she'd had no sleep, she hadn't gone to bed at all and it picked up that her blood pressure was low and picked up that she hadn't eaten, that she'd lost weight... it actually helped her pain control because she wasn't taking her long acting pain relief in the right way... it also it got her back into a routine basically, it made her put her alarm on and not spend all day in bed at the weekends.*" [CM2 CC 3]

The requirement of assistive technology if it is to function as an efficient clinical decision-making tool is to be supportive to the formal carers, supplying information for the appropriate decision to be made. It is unlikely to function successfully in isolation, as technology cannot incorporate the knowledge that the Community Matron possesses. The CM has knowledge of: personal histories, backgrounds, family situations, home and environmental circumstances, daily routines which are all drawn upon to arrive at an accurate clinical decision. Whilst technology may not be able to incorporate these facets of individual well-being, there is a need to ensure that assistive technologies are tailored to the requirements of the individual. Moreover, that there is a recognition of the 'softer' elements of care delivered by the formal carer.

In the early stages of the study, CMs were initially skeptical about the impact of the technology on their roles and work responsibilities. CMs raised early concerns about the aims and objectives of the system, frequently discussing the technology versus person debate. The CMs defined their role more broadly than the delivery of task-oriented, health-based care, and identified components of social, psychological and emotional well-being, as well as mediating with other carers and healthcare professionals. The CMs identified a limitation in the assistive technology which presented information to the carer through monitoring and sensor information.

The CMs felt that their role constituted more of what was described as the 'softer' elements of care, such as prompting, encouraging and supporting. This form of care was seen as important for assisting patients to self manage their own condition and thus fundamental to their independence. These 'softer' elements of care operated *alongside* the collection of diagnostic information.

5.5. Patients Viewing their Healthcare Data and Self-Management of Health

The system provided the opportunity for older people to visualize their own data through their television. Patient data could be relayed to the older person through a series of graphs available through a television channel. From the outset of the project, this was seen as important in ensuring that users had a sense of control over the system. Moreover, a key responsibility of the role of the CM is to encourage self management amongst patients and patients viewing their own data was seen as a potential tool to support the self-identification of health and well-being issues.

When this aspect of the system was raised in the early workshops, older people felt that this could be empowering, enabling older people to be more directly involved in analyzing their own condition and promoting self management:

"*A patient would feel confident using such visualisations to help with the self-management of health.*" [OA2 during OA Workshop]

In enabling older people to have control of their data, it placed the older person more central to the decision-making process, shifting from their role as the 'passive recipient' of care:

> "*They share information with the carer rather than just listen and be dictated to.*" [OA5 during OA Workshop]

Others felt that viewing their own data might be alarming for the older person. Here, there was the possibility that the patients could become obsessed with the readings generated by the system, leading to stress, worry and hyper-tension:

> "*Maybe the user/patient is better not to know because they might get obsessive about whether they slept or not and this would mean that they suffer a greater lack of sleep as they worry more about the readings.*" [OA2 during OA Workshop]

These concerns were echoed by CMs themselves. When the CMs were asked during the second forum theatre session about patients viewing their own data, the initial response was that it could be potentially inappropriate. They felt that some patients may not want to be confronted by information regarding their own health:

> "*Any new information will be alarming to a patient and could cause them concern.*" [CM during FT2]

CMs felt that there was an assumption that older people would know how to interpret the data. Whilst a key responsibility for CMs is educating patients about their own condition, they still had patients who were less confident when interpreting their own health and well-being data. This resulted in increased workload for the CM:

> "*...half the time I was going out for reassurance, they had been looking at particular data such as blood pressure rather than looking at the whole thing and saying about how they felt in* themselves *so yes it was a downfall from that point of view... you would be there for ages because there is always something else they remember.*" [CM4 End of Trial Interview]

At the end of trial interview, one CM commented on the example of a patient whose anxiety levels (as a result of reading the system data) led to an unnecessary hospital admission:

> "*Think it [the system] was more of a hindrance than a help in some ways though because it just gave him hyper vigilance, he went off to hospital because he was telling me he was* nauseating *and vomiting and he had a fast pulse and when he got to the hospital he told them he'd seen it on the monitor.... It [the system] was not good for him... it raises the stress levels.*" [CM1 End of Trial Interview]

A consistent theme through the case conferences and reiterated at the exit interviews with the CMs was that such a system would only work if it is has the compliance of patients. The CMs also felt that this compliance would be more complex to develop amongst those that are 'more ill' as they would have greater difficulty when self monitoring etc. due to their condition. This would also be true of those that were less educated about their own condition.

> "*a lot more* education *needs to go on so that if you do get raised blood pressure that this could be this and not to worry.*" [CM2 during CC5]

However, patients viewing their own data was potentially beneficial when a telephone call flagged up an issue that needed to be addressed and this occurred with patients who were more knowledgeable about their own condition. This demonstrated that assistive technology can play a role in self management provided that CMs have established the conditions (awareness and education) for the data to be interpreted and acted upon sensibly.

CMs did however report during the last three case conferences that a number of their participants were using the system to self-manage. Here, patients who were actively using the system were using the readings from the system to self-manage their condition. On one such occasion, a patient identified that they were putting on weight. After calling the CM to let them know about this, the CM was able to diagnose that the patient had been retaining water, and so was able to prescribe water tablets. On this occasion the CM felt that the system being used in this way by the patient almost certainly prevented a hospital admission. This improved communication levels between patient and CM, where the information and awareness of the patient was used to empower patients in the care delivery process' no longer just the CM going in and taking measurements and recommending a course of treatment (one way communication) but rather the patient being in control of their own data:

> "*... it did empower them a little bit more because they were looking at there own data and* able *to gauge things.*" [CM1 during CC4]

CMs felt that this improved communication strengthened the relationships between the carer and the care door:

> "*the* system *has reinforced the partnership between CM and patient.*" [CM1 End of Trial Interview]

This partnership was strengthened as a direct result of the patient undertaking care decisions which the Community Matron felt responsible for. In the following example, this led directly to the prevention of an hospital admission:

> "*...it [the system] has worked when it stopped an inappropriate admission with one of the patients, I think it was one where they would've rang 999 normally and because they were able to see the data themselves.*" [CM 1 End of Trial Interview]

At the last forum theatre and in the exit interviews, CMs also talked about the improved quality of patient visits as a direct result of information generated by the system. Patients, prompted by the data, would engage in discussion with the CMs about their progression since the last visit. This conversation provided the opportunity for CMs to further educate their patient, on the reasons for fluctuations in the data and to recommend potential interventions.

Other CMs felt that there was little appetite for self-management amongst patients. Whilst choice and control were perceived as beneficial, not all patients wanted to be in a position to self manage. CMs felt that a number of patients were content to transfer decision-making to the formal carer:

> "*It's difficult to know how people are going to react, some people do not want to take responsibility for anything and they're the ones that say oh I'll do it for you love, they want you to make all the decisions for them. They want you, you're the professional, they trust your judgment, they just want you to do what needs to be done.*" [CM3 End of Trial Interview]

These findings suggest that for some patients the system brings about a sense of control and independence as a result of viewing, interpreting and acting upon the data, yet for others (who do not wish to have this level of choice and independence) CMs need to be in the position to make that decision. Here, assistive technology is potentially problematic if it takes an element of the decision-making away from the CM.

6. Conclusions

Formal care providers have a key role in ensuring that older people are able to live independently in their own homes whilst receiving high standards of care. Within the context of care in the community and a case management approach, the formal carer is fundamental to ensuring that older people have the support which enables them to stay at home as they become increasingly frail and vulnerable. In this study we have explored the impact of assistive technology in helping to support formal carers to make care-related decisions with the home.

The results of the project indicate that technology can play a supportive role in helping CMs to monitor patients, enabling earlier detection of problems (proactive use) and assisting in delivering care (reactive user). Here, assistive technology can provide information which results in changes to patient lifestyle, diet and behavior. However, in delivering these benefits, assistive technology has the potential to impact upon the mechanisms for delivering care and thus the roles and responsibilities of the formal carer. Initially, the integration of technology can represent a tension, as CMs perceive its role as a threat to their own traditional forms of face-to-face delivery. As the trial progressed this perceived threat minimized, as CMs become familiar with the system, and shaped the system as a 'supportive tool' rather than using technology as the sole mechanism for delivering care. Moreover, as the assistive technology began to yield benefits for case management, they began to see it as the opportunity to increase efficiency and prioritise care. Here, issues relating to privacy and intrusions became less well cited by CMs and patients as the technology became a more familiar and accepted.

The application of technology can also have implications on the relationship between the carer and cared for. Being the main carer for the older person places them in a position of trust and responsibility; care-related decisions thus need to be predicated on timely, reliable and accurate information. It is therefore perhaps understandable that CMs are initially apprehensive in trusting assistive technology to help them make decisions that impact on the health and well-being of the older person. Moreover, CMs did not wish to compromise the close, person-centred relationship which they developed with their patients, and so were reticent to use the assistive technology to either question the older person or to make a change to the way in which they delivered care. Over time, as CMs began to trust the system, the information delivered through the technology was relied upon to make care-related decisions.

A key aspect of the role of the Community Matron is to better educate patients (as expert patients) to self manage their condition. This study demonstrated that assistive technology can support older people, by providing them with health and well-being data in a readable format in order for them to make their own decisions regarding medication, diet and lifestyle. However, this needs to work alongside concerted efforts by the Community Matron to appropriately educate their own patients about their condition. In those older people who were not appropproiately aware of their condition, accessing their own data could produce increased anxiety and tension, as they did not have the knowledge to make decisions which would benefit them. However, those that were more informed about their own condition were able to respon to changes in their own data in order to bring about changes in their life. Thus technology can assist in working alongside CMs to fill a key responsibility of their work.

Overall, the experiences of the healthcarers during the research indicate that assistive technology implemented in this way has the potential to have a positive impact on the way that they work. Continuous monitoring of patient information allows the carer to ascertain an understanding of the patient's condition outside of normal visits. When combined with the knowledge of the care giver, this enables care to be managed more efficiently. However,feedback from CMs suggests that technology cannot work in isolation; it needs to be combined with the tacit and situated knowledge of the Community Matron to arrive at a decision regarding the care of the patient. Importantly, the Community Matron is fundamental to the acceptability of assistive technology within the home, in encouraging patients to adopt the technology and accept it as part of their everyday environment. For many patients, the inclination to have it in the home is that it is of purpose and assistance to the person making the decisions about their care, thus maintaining their health and well-being status. Thus, assistive technology needs to be seen a part of an integrated care solution, at the interface between the formal carer and the cared for.

Acknowledgements

This study would not have been possible without the contribution of the participants, in particular the CMs from Liverpool Primary Care Trust and their patients. Additionally, the support provided by all partners in the project, including Oliver Wells from Imperial College, David Walker from Philips and Nigel Barnes from BT.

References

[1] E. Agree, Incorporating assistive devices into community-based long-term care, *Journal of Aging and Health* **12** (2000), 426–450.
[2] ALIP, Ambient assisted living road map, Available at http://www.aaliance.eu/public/documents/aaliance-roadmap/aaliance-aal-roadmap.pdf, 2009.
[3] F. Aminzadeh, W.B. Dalziel, F.J. Molnar and L.J. Garcia, Symbolic meaning of relocation to a residential care facility for persons with dementia, *Aging & Mental Health* **13** (2009), 487–496.
[4] R. Applebaum, J. Straker and S.M. Geron, *Assessing Satisfaction in Health and Long-term Care: Practical Approaches to Hearing the Voices of Consumers*, Springer Publishing Co., New York, 2000.
[5] M. Barnes, *Care, Communities and Citizens*, Longman, London, 1997.
[6] A.-H. Bayer and L. Harper, Fixing to stay: A national survey of housing and home modification issues, *AARP* (2000), 1–82. Washington, DC.
[7] V. Braun and V. Clarke, Thematic analysis, *Qualitative Research in Psychology* **3** (2006), 77–101.
[8] S. Brownsell, D. Bradley and J. Porteus, *Assistive Technology and Telecare: Forging Solutions for Independent Living*, Policy, Bristol, Avon, 2003.
[9] V. Burnholt and G. Windle, Literature review for the strategy of older people in Wales social inclusion for older people, Available at http://www.wales.gov.uk/subisocialpolicy/content/ssg/LR3.pdf, 2001.
[10] K. Doughty, R. Lewis and A. McIntosh, The design of a practical and reliable fall detector for community and institutional telecare, *Journal of Telemedicine and Telecare* **6** (2000), 150–154.
[11] R. Eisma, A. Dickinson, J. Goodman, A. Syme, L. Tiwari and A.F. Newell, Early user involvement in the development of information technology-related products for older people, *Universal Access in the Information Society* **3** (2004), 131–140.
[12] A. Essen, The two facets of electronic care surveillance: An exploration of the views of older people who live with monitoring devices, *Social Science and Medicine* **67** (2008), 128–36.
[13] EU, E-europe 2005: An information society for all: An action plan, Available at http://ec.europa.eu/information_society/eeurope/i2010/archive/eeurope/index_en.htm, 2005.

[14] EU, i2010 eGovernment action plan: Accelerating eGovernment in Europe for the benefit of all, Available at http://ec.europa.eu/information_society/activities/egovernment/docs/action_plan/comm_pdf_com_2006_0173_f_en_acte.pdf, 2006.
[15] EU, ICT and Ageing: European study on users, markets and technologies, Available at http://www.ict-ageing.eu/ict-ageing-website/wp-content/uploads/2008/11/ictageing_vienna_handout_final2.pdf, 2008.
[16] M.J. Fisk, *Social Alarms to Telecare: Older People's Services in Transition*, Policy Press, Bristol, 2003.
[17] L.N. Gitlin, M.R. Luborsky and R.L. Schemm, Emerging concerns of older stroke patients about assistive devices, *The Gerontologist* **38** (1998), 169–80.
[18] J. Glasby and R. Littlechild, *The Health and Social Care Divide*, Policy Press, Bristol, 2004.
[19] T. Hartig and H. Staats, Guest editors' introduction, *Journal of Environmental Psychology* **23** (2003), 103–107.
[20] H. Hoenig, D. Taylor and F. Sloan, Does assistive technology substitute for personal assistance among the disabled elderly?, *American Journal of Public Health Information* **93** (2003), 330–337.
[21] G. Huby, J. Stewart, A. Tierney and W. Rogers, Planning older people's discharge from acute hospital care: linking risk management and patient participation in decision-making, *Health Risk and Society* **6** (2004), 115–132.
[22] Lacey et al., User involvement in the design and evaluation of a smart mobility aid, *Journal of Rehabilitation Research and Development* **37**(6) (2000), 709–723.
[23] L. Magnusson and E. Hanson, Ethical issues arising from a research, technology and development project to support frail older people and their family carers at home, *Health and Social Care in the Community* **11** (2003), 431–439.
[24] W. Mann, K. Ottenbacher and L. Fraas, Effectiveness of assistive technology and environmental interventions in maintaining independence and reducing home care costs for the frail elderly: A randomized controlled trial, *Archives of Family Medicine* **8** (1999), 210–217.
[25] A. Melander-Wikma, Y. Faltholm and G. Gard, Safety vs. privacy: Elderly persons' experiences of a mobile safety alarm, *Health and Social Care in the Community* **16** (2008), 337–346.
[26] F.G. Miskelly, Assistive technology in elderly care, *Age Ageing* **30** (2001), 455–458.
[27] S. Müller, P. Quinones, I. Meyer, D.M. Rueda and C. García Cazalilla, Process and IT innovation: Experiences from the CommonWell project, *Gerontechnology* **9**(2) (2010), 135. Paper presented at the International Society for Gerontechnology's 7th World Conference, 27–30 May 2010, Vancouver, Canada.
[28] E. Murphy, Case management and community matrons for long term conditions, *British Medical Journal* **329** (2004), 1251–1252.
[29] A.F. Newell, M. Morgan, P. Gregor and A. Carmichael, Theatre as an intermediary between users and CHI designers, CHI 2006 Experience Report, April 22–26, Montreal, Quebec, Canada, 2006.
[30] NHS, Modernisation Agency, CCIT update, http://www.wise.nhs.uk/sites/workforce/retainingand-developingstaff/Consultant%20Contract%20Document%20Library/1/CCIT%20Update/CCIT%20Update%2014.pdf, 2004.
[31] NHS, Community care act, Available at http://www.legislation.gov.uk/ukpga/1990/19/contents, 1990.
[32] NHS, Community matrons, Available at http://www.dh.gov.uk/en/Healthcare/Longtermconditions/DH_4134132, 2007.
[33] NHS, The NHS improvement plan: Putting people at the heart of public services, Available at http://www.dh.gov.uk/en/Publicationsandstatistics/Publications/PublicationsPolicyAndGuidance/DH_4084476, 2004.
[34] NIA, Why population aging matters – A global perspective, Available at http://www.nia.nih.gov/researchinformation/extramuralprograms/behavioralandsocialresearch/globalaging.htm, 2009.
[35] J. Percival and J. Hanson, Big brother or brave new world? Telecare and its implications for older people's independence and social inclusion, *Critical Social Policy* **26** (2006), 888–909.
[36] M. Rice, A.F. Newell and M. Morgan, Forum theatre as a requirements gathering methodology in the design of a home telecommunication system for older adults, *Behaviour and Information Technology* **26** (2007), 323–331.
[37] K. Roberts, Exploring participation: Older people on discharge from hospital, *Journal of Advanced Nursing* **40** (2002), 413–420.
[38] R.L. Rubinstein, J.C. Kilbride and S. Nagy, *Elders Living Alone: Frailty and the Perception of Choice*, Aldine de Gruyter, New York, 1992.
[39] J. Sabia, There's no place like home: A hazard model analysis of aging in place among older homeowners in the PSID, *Research on Aging* **30**(1) (2008), 3–35.

[40] J. Seale, C. McCreadieb, A. Turner-Smitha and A. Tinkerb, Older people as partners in assistive technology research: The use of focus groups in the design process, *Technology and Disability* **14** (2002), 21–29. IOS Press.
[41] A. Sixsmith and J. Sixsmith, Ageing in place in the United Kingdom, *Ageing International* **32** (2008), 219–235.
[42] J. Sixsmith and S. Sixsmith, Places in transition: The impact of life events on the experience of home, in: *Household Choice*, T. Putnam and C. Newton, eds, Futura, London, 1990.

Handbook of Ambient Assisted Living
J.C. Augusto et al. (Eds.)
IOS Press, 2012

doi:10.3233/978-1-60750-837-3-304

Ambient Assisted Living Technology to Support Older Adults with Dementia with Activities of Daily Living: Key Concepts and the State of the Art

Alex MIHAILIDIS [a,*], Jennifer BOGER [a], Stephen CZARNUCH [a], Tizneem JIANCARO [a] and Jesse HOEY [b]
[a] *Intelligent Assistive Technology & Systems Lab, University of Toronto and Toronto Rehabilitation Institute*
[b] *David R. Cheriton School of Computer Science, University of Waterloo*

1. Introduction to the Chapter

This chapter provides an overview of research that has been completed in the field of Ambient Assistive Living (AAL) for older adults with dementia. Information will be presented through a discussion of key concepts from within this field, as well concepts from other fields, such as engineering, design, social sciences, and computer science, that have informed the design and development of these types of technologies. In the first part of this chapter, the authors present findings from their own research and the experiences of others in this field with respect to best practices related to designing AAL technologies for older adults with dementia. This includes a discussion of the application of new approaches such as artificial intelligence that the authors, and others, have found useful in the development of new AAL technologies. In the following sections, the authors present a summary of key projects and their findings, focusing on projects that have applied the concepts presented in this chapter, such as AI. The chapter concludes with a discussion of the possible future of this field and new areas of research that need to be explored. Throughout this chapter key concepts are presented and will include 1) potential design approaches and philosophies that may be useful in the design of AAL technologies; 2) the effects and importance of considering other potential users of these technologies, such as family members and caregivers; 3) how to measure the success of these technologies; and 4) ethical considerations.

2. Older Adults with Dementia

Before presenting AAL technologies for older adults with dementia and discussing key design concepts, it is important for the reader to have an understanding of the popula-

[*] Corresponding Author: Dr. Alex Mihailidis, Barbara G. Stymiest Research Chair in Rehabilitation Technology & Associate Professor, Department of Occupational Science & Occupational Therapy, University of Toronto, 160-500 University Avenue, Toronto, Canada, M5G 1V7, 416-946-8565. E-mail: alex.mihailidis@utoronto.ca.

tion and to explore the unique characteristics of this population that will affect the development and use of AAL technologies. Therefore one must understand demographics, disease etiology, and current practices in providing care.

As life expectancies around the world increase, so too does the prevalence of dementia. In 2010, there were 36 million people globally with dementia and this figure is expected to reach 115 million by 2050, which will equate to one person in 85 [6,13].

The personal implications of dementia can be devastating. Cognitive decline, such as impairments in memory, attention, judgment, and decision making, often profoundly affect a person's ability to perform everyday activities, and thus significantly reduces his or her quality of life [36]. On an everyday level, these changes may hamper activities related to safety, hygiene, meal preparation, and mobility. A person may no longer be able to make breakfast or remember to turn the stove off; she may forget how to operate a phone or, should help be needed, not know whom to call. At the more advanced stages, a person may not be able to complete self-care activities and may become completely reliant on a caregiver.

As independent living becomes more challenging, informal caregivers often fill the gap, though not without consequences. While caring for a person with dementia can be rewarding, many informal caregivers, who are usually family members, also experience considerable physical and psychological stress. Caregivers under stress possess weakened immune systems, 15 to 32% present symptoms of clinical depression, and 40 to 75% experience significant mental illness [5].

The financial costs of dementia are formidable too. The costs to support people with dementia in 2010 were estimated to be US $604 billion, which is equivalent to 1% of the world's GDP [6]. To place this into perspective, this figure exceeded the yearly revenue of corporations such as WalMart (US $414 billion) and Exxon Mobil (US $311 billion) and if dementia care represented a country's GDP, it would be the 18th largest in the world [6]. Of the total, 42% (US $252 billion) of the costs were assumed by informal care, namely the care given by unpaid (informal) caregivers such as family members [6]. Professional residential care in the community accounted for another 42%, while the direct medical costs associated with treatment and care of dementia accounted for only 16% of the total cost.

2.1. Living with Dementia

The symptoms exhibited by people with dementia vary considerably, not only from person to person, but also from day to day. Memory loss is often the first sign of the disease, though in time, virtually all cognitive processes will be touched, from judgment and decision making to personality and sleep patterns [4].

The most common type of dementia is Alzheimer's Disease, which is classified as a cortical type of dementia because the primary pathology of Alzheimer's occurs at the cortex of the brain. Other cortical dementias include frontotemporal dementia and Creutzfeldt-Jakob Disease. Subcortical dementias include Huntington's and Parkinson's Diseases, while mixed-variety dementias (affecting both cortical and subcortical regions) include vascular dementia and AIDS dementia [7]. As they have different pathologies, it is possible for a person to concurrently have more than one type of dementia.

These degenerative and diffuse neurological diseases all involve losses in memory, although an additional impairment is necessary for a specific diagnosis. This secondary impairment might involve one or more of the following: object recognition; motor function; language production; language comprehension; planning; judgment; and decision making [4]. Currently, diagnosis of most dementias can only be implied based on a person's behaviour, ability to perform everyday activities, and neuropsychological tests.

Dementia is typically divided into three stages, though the boundaries between the stages blur over the course of the disease. At the mild stage, people may experience problems with memory and decision making. Their capacity to travel to new places or handle money diminishes and they may experience mood changes. Instrumental activities of daily living (IADL), such as preparing meals, doing light housework, shopping, managing money, and using the phone, become challenging and the person with dementia may need assistance with activity completion from a caregiver [67]. Temporal and spatial disorientation can make IADLs that occur in the community especially challenging [35,57]. At the moderate stages, people need progressively more assistance to live independently. IADLs are usually assumed by a caregiver and people begin to have trouble with basic activities of daily living (ADL), such as bathing, dressing, eating, toileting and transferring (between seated and standing positions). In the moderate stage, people become even more disoriented in time and place, and can easily become lost or experience hallucinations. Various emotional and personality changes may occur, ranging from apathy and depression to bouts of anger or feelings of euphoria. In the severe stages, people lose motor and toileting skills, rely mostly or completely on a caregiver for IADL and ADL completion, and usually have great difficulties comprehending events and recognizing people [5,55].

While many abilities change or become impaired, there are some which remain relatively intact. In the case of Alzheimer's Disease, emotional processing can be present well into the course of the disease and therefore can potentially be supported indefinitely [14]. Therapeutic strategies and assistive technologies, targeting emotional facial expression and emotional prosody via singing and music, for instance, are being developed to take advantage of these remaining skills and enhance quality of life [21,65].

2.2. Caring for People with Dementia

Being able to plan and sequence events is crucial to independent living as this ability is central to performing everyday activities [53]. For most people with mild dementia, a caregiver, who is often a family member, helps with IADL, which includes providing indirect support by encouraging a person's participation and engagement with IADLs [61]. Three caregiver strategies to offer this kind of indirect support include reducing the demands asked of someone with dementia by re-structuring activities to support cognitive strengths; issuing reminders and instructions throughout the execution of an activity to support completion; and keeping a person company in a social and supportive manner throughout a wide variety of activities [46]. At the moderate stage of dementia, the person is usually no longer able to complete IADL and has trouble completing ADL. This dependence on a caregiver to complete ADL and IADL increases as the disease progresses and causes related increases in caregiver burden.

Letting people choose where they wish to age (i.e., aging in place or aging with choice) is increasingly becoming recognized as an important avenue for future healthcare development. One reason for this shift is that aging in place is considered to have more positive health outcomes compared to long-term care placement [39]. The high costs of formal (institutional) care is another driving force, especially considering that most current healthcare systems are already overloaded. Finally, like anyone else, people with dementia and their families want to be able to make the care decisions that best suit their particular needs and resources. Placement of a person with dementia into long-term care is usually out of necessity, rather than choice, and is can be devastating for both the person who is moved and his or her family.

These arguments for enabling a person with dementia to remain at home must be carefully weighed against the physical and psychological realities of caregiver burden. One study with over 1500 participants that was conducted in the United States compared caregivers of people with and without dementia found that personal time, employment issues, and family conflict are all compromised more for people who were caring for someone with dementia than for those who were not [45].

One way of balancing the needs of people with dementia, the burden placed upon caregivers, and both the financial and physical limitations of overextended healthcare systems may lie in the application of intelligent technologies to help support older adults with dementia.

2.3. The Potential of Ambient Assisted Living (AAL) Technologies

There are many potential areas where AAL technologies could be used to provide support for people with dementia. By assuming or supporting tasks that are traditionally completed by a formal or informal caregiver, the application of well-designed AAL technologies would simultaneously reduce caregiver burden. As such, AAL technologies have the potential to support functional limitations directly, which would, in turn, indirectly support financial ones as these technologies would cut down their users' needs for (potentially costly) formal care. The following section begins the discussion of using AAL technologies to support older adults with dementia through an initial discussion of how to design these types of technology and the key aspects that need to be taken into consideration.

3. Designing Ambient Assisted Living Technologies for Older Adults with Dementia

Technologies are only as useful as their designers make them. There are many factors that developers of AAL technologies must consider to build devices that are appropriate and, therefore, useful. As such, the first key theme in this chapter is how best to design AAL technologies for older adults with dementia. This section presents key concepts of AAL technologies for older adults with dementia, while specific examples of these technologies are presented in Section 4.

3.1. Key Features of AAL Technologies for Older Adults with Dementia

AAL technologies for older adults with dementia must reflect the needs and capabilities of the demographic to be accepted and used. Research shows that encouraging a person with dementia to interact in his environment can slow cognitive decline and foster feelings of control and independence [68,72]. As such, AAL technologies should support task completion rather than autonomously doing tasks for a person with dementia. By taking into account possible user limitations and facilitating active user involvement, AALs leverage what a person is able to do and compensate for what they cannot, helping a person to maintain his or her residual skills by encouraging participation in the world around him or her as much as possible. This includes supporting not only ADL but also enabling social and communication activities, which are necessary for positive mental health and feelings of connectedness. The following is a detailed list of key features that AAL technologies should incorporate, based on evidence and experiences collected by the authors and others in this field.

3.1.1. Dynamic and Customised Support

Dementia generally causes a progressive degradation in several cognitive and physical abilities. The abilities of a person with dementia can also change dramatically from day to day and even from hour to hour. AAL technologies must be able to support the dynamic and complex nature of dementia either by responding appropriately across a great range of abilities or by detecting changes in ability and adapting accordingly. In particular, memory impairments can make it difficult for people with dementia to deviate from routines or remember how to use new objects. Thus AAL technologies that can accommodate the preferences that have been accumulated through a lifetime of habit are more likely to be successful [44].

3.1.2. Simple, Clear, Unobtrusive, and Intuitive Interfaces

In addition to the challenges posed by dementia, older adults often have co-morbidities that occur as a result of the aging process, such as impairments in mobility, fine motor control, eyesight, and hearing. Large displays, loud and clear audio cues, simple layouts, and high contrasting colours are examples of appropriate interface features for older adults with dementia. If an AAL technology requires users to interact with it, employing objects and operation techniques that are familiar to the user are likely to be more intuitive and therefore make the device more usable [44]. Embedded ambient technologies (i.e., technologies that are seamlessly incorporated into an environment) are particularly appropriate as they free the user from having to remember to wear a device, maximise communication connectivity, and minimise maintenance.

3.1.3. Include the Caregivers' Needs

Caring for an older adult with dementia requires enormous physical and emotional efforts that often cause high levels of caregiver burden, which can translate into high levels of stress, depression, and even an increased risk of mortality [60,70]. As most caregivers are stretched to their limits, devices designed to support people with dementia *must* also support their caregivers. Additionally, many caregivers are the spouses of the care recipient and have morbidities of their own to manage, which places restrictions on interaction modalities with the technology. AAL technologies for people with dementia should require as little explicit input from the caregiver as possible and, when it cannot be circumvented, input should be intuitive and minimal. This requirement dictates that technology developers carefully weigh the benefits of direct device configuration by the user with the demands of requiring explicit input. It must be acknowledged that some caregivers appreciate the sense of control and candid personalisation that user-driven device customisability provides; therefore, this design feature should not be discarded altogether, but should be an option rather than a requirement.

3.1.4. Expandability

AAL technologies should be able to operate as stand-alone devices or in tandem with other AAL technologies and assistive devices. This capability allows consumers to pick which AAL technologies are appropriate for their particular needs and addresses the practical challenges associated with developing a single technology that can support multiple daily activities. Moreover, combining data from multiple AAL technologies allows the creation of a richer and more holistic representation of the people they are supporting. This information can be used to provide targeted and tailored care to match the individual's needs.

3.2. User Centred Design

There are many approaches employed by AAL technology developers to ensure that the devices they create incorporate the features described in Section 2.1, and that they are appropriate and useful to the people they are intended to support. As people with dementia are the ultimate consumers of the product, their needs, preferences, and abilities should be the primary consideration throughout the design process. However, it is important to remember that professional and informal caregivers are also primary consumers of AAL technologies by virtue of their relationships to the person (or people) they care for. Caregivers are usually involved in the initial device procurement, as well as any daily operational and maintenance requirements; if the technology is rejected by the caregiver, then it will not be available for use by the person with dementia. Therefore, anticipating and incorporating the needs and preferences of caregivers is as important as those of people with dementia.

To capture these requirements, researchers are starting to employ a *user centred design* approach, where users are included in a three stage design process to increase the likelihood of device acceptance [10,51]. The first stage determines user needs; specifically device characteristics, the target environment, and relevant daily tasks in need of intervention. The second stage involves the synthesis of user goals into formal design criteria and development of functional prototypes. The third stage is the evaluation of the prototypes in real-world settings. These three stages are then repeated as necessary until an acceptable device has been created. In the case of AAL technologies designed for people with dementia, user centred design also includes caregivers for their own experiences and as proxies for the people they care for.

Caregivers' extensive experience with people who have dementia allows them to provide design guidance and give critical feedback on technology feasibility. Including caregivers throughout the design process allows relatively easy access to expert information (compared to clinical trials) and allows access to caregivers' own preferences as well. While caregivers can provide valuable information, it is the people with dementia who are the true experts regarding being a person with dementia. Reliable and specific opinions can be difficult to obtain from this population; however, when approached by skilled practitioners (such as occupational therapists or mental health professionals) many people with dementia are able to provide definite opinions regarding products [1]. Direct feedback from people with dementia themselves constitutes invaluable design information as the behaviours and preferences of people with dementia can be extremely hard to predict, particularly when creating novel products. Therefore, it should not be assumed that people with dementia are unable to contribute to an evolutionary design process, but rather should be included at the core of development efforts.

3.3. AAL Technology Development Techniques for Older Adults with Dementia

The device development process, guided by methods just described (e.g. user centred design), is iterative in nature, becoming more involved as a product evolves. Depending on the resources available, the stage of development, and the nature of the technique, designers may use the following techniques sequentially or throughout the device development process.

3.3.1. In Silico Testing

In silico testing consists of debugging and optimising a new technology in a virtual environment on a computer. In this technique, developers use button presses (e.g., using a keyboard or buttons) or scripted code to simulate input the device could receive if it were operating in the real world and to estimate device responses to them. As *in silico* testing has explicit and known inputs; it is a powerful and effective method for creating the initial version of a device, adding new functionalities, targeting problem areas for debugging and optimisation, and investigating specific scenarios.

3.3.2. Benchtop Trials

In benchtop trials, developers interact with a physical version of the device in a controlled environment. Interacting with the device and its components adds a layer of complexity as the device's hardware and software are physically present, integrated, and usually running in real-time. Benchtop trials allow the developers to identify and address numerous physical design requirements, such as the selection of hardware that will be used, the assembly and installation of the device, and communication between device components and external services. Parts of the device can be developed, integrated, and optimised sequentially or in parallel, resulting in a functional prototype. Benchtop trials can range from assembly at a workstation to testing in mock-ups of real environments.

3.3.3. Actor Simulations

While experienced developers may have a good understanding of the general behaviours and attitudes of people with dementia, these traits are quite difficult to replicate authentically. Actors have trained extensively to take specified emotions and attitudes to play specific roles. Actors can use role-playing to simulate conditions or situations of interest and have commonly been used for teaching and assessments in medicine [8,31]. More recently, actors have been used to optimise devices for people with disabilities [12,32]. In a recent set of trials with an AAL technology, actors were able to emulate older adults with dementia in a manner that was considered to be believable by professional caregivers and elicited reactions from the technology that were comparable to older adults with dementia [12].

3.3.4. Clinical Trials

Conducting clinical trials with people with dementia and caregivers is the most direct method of gauging how a device will react to real-world applications. Clinical trials can range from pilot studies in controlled environments to large-scale, long-term installations in peoples' homes. While clinical trials are a crucial step in the development process, they are also the most complex and costly. Older adults with dementia are a frail and vulnerable population; therefore, trials involving people from this group generally require special considerations and extra resources. The technology to be tested needs to be optimised prior to trials, methodologies carefully planned, and resources available to complete the trials and analyse the data. However, these trials are the most conclusive and informative, and are the only way to truly evaluate a device. Although they are more appropriate for later stages in the development process, the benefits of gaining a good understanding of how the device operates negate logistical difficulties of clinical trials.

3.4. Including Privacy in Design

Elements to ensure the privacy and security of users and data being used by the technology must be maintained throughout the design process and approaches described. It is important to recognize people have different levels of comfort regarding the sharing of personal information. With respect to healthcare related AAL technologies, these preferences change over time and depend on factors such as the person's health status, care requirements, and confidence in the data collection method. End user education (e.g., knowing what data are being collected, why sharing the collected information may be beneficial, and what safeguards to privacy and dignity are in place) are key ways of making the person who is being monitored more likely to accept the technology, share information, and to feel more comfortable when doing so [16]. As such, AAL technologies need to be transparent about the information they gather and what happens to this data afterwards. Stakeholders (e.g., the primary user, his or her caregiver, family members, health practitioner, etc.) should have some degree of control over what is being collected, stored, and transmitted and be able to change these preferences to match their comfort level and needs. Apart from respecting people's rights concerning their own data, transparency enables device users to evaluate the efficacy of a device and make better decisions regarding device use.

Healthcare is becoming increasingly more ubiquitous, automated, and electronic-based. In response to this trend, experts and governments are creating guidelines and regulations to ensure data are handled in an appropriate manner, such as those described in [28,56,71]. These guidelines highlight the need for privacy by design: that the highest possible levels of privacy and security should be the default setting of any data collecting devices and should be changed to more permissive settings only when the owner unequivocally wishes to do so, thus ensuring privacy is respected. The inclusion of appropriate privacy and security measures that handle data in an ethical manner is a critical design requirement.

Privacy by design may appear to be at odds with the fundamental concept of AAL technologies, particularly those that collect and disseminate health-related data. However, privacy by design does not maintain that sensitive data should not be collected or shared, but rather that whatever data is used should be appropriate for the application, that the stakeholders be aware of what is being collected and why, and that people have control over who the information is shared with. As such, privacy by design not only ensures privacy is respected, but encourages device users to become educated about what the device does, assume a level of responsibility and control over data, and participate in the process of what happens to their own information.

3.5. Zero-Effort Technologies

A final critical design consideration in the development of AAL technologies is to minimize the interactions and effort required from the user. This is especially important when designing these technologies for users such as older adults with dementia, who are often unable to initiate the use of these technologies and do not possess the procedural memory required to operate them. Zero-effort technologies (ZETs) are a class of technologies that employ techniques such as artificial intelligence and unobtrusive sensors to support the collection, analysis, and application of data about the user and their context autonomously. ZETs operate with minimal or no explicit feedback, which translates into minimal or no learning or behaviour modification requirements for the users. This emphasis on little to no demands from the devices' users makes ZETs an excellent fit for people with dementia and their (often overburdened) caregivers.

Artificial intelligence and other computer algorithms are able to manipulate and interpret the incoming data making it possible for ZETs to respond to situations or trends of interest in an appropriate fashion. ZETs are able to perform autonomous data manipulation, which allows the targeted and customisable presentation of data in formats that are tailored to the interests of different stakeholders, such as clinicians, professional and informal caregivers, and, importantly, the person being monitored. The "hands off" functionality of ZETs can encourage device acceptance and use as it places little or no demands on the users, thereby providing support with virtually no human effort. The following section provides an overview of artificial intelligence, including sensors and issues related to using these approaches in the design of AAL technologies. Examples of ZETs are presented in Section 5.

4. Overview of Key Technical Concepts and Artificial Intelligence (AI)

A primary sub-theme in this chapter has been the recognition and support of the dynamic and diverse needs of older adults with dementia and their caregivers. The characteristics of dementia make it such that one solution cannot fit all users. As described in Section 3.2, a user-centred design approach needs to be used to ensure that this type of technology is able to meet the various needs of each individual user. However, manually applying this approach can be extremely costly and time consuming. In response, there has been an increase in the number of AAL projects that are applying more sophisticated paradigms and approaches, such as artificial intelligence (AI). AI allows for technologies to be developed that can autonomously sense, learn, and adapt to individual users, lending itself well to tasks that involve learning and decision-making (two of the primary limitations resulting from dementia). This concept helps researchers to design AAL technologies with a universal design approach in mind, while the resulting technology operates within a user-centred design framework.

Specifically within the field of AI, *sensing* and *machine learning* have proven to be especially useful AI techniques that can help new AAL technologies to be more autonomous and usable by a variety of populations. This section will focus on an overview of how sensing and machine learning can be applied in the development of AAL technologies within the context of older adults with dementia.

4.1. Commonly Used Sensing Techniques

A critical feature of any system is the ability to sense the environment to determine what a user is trying to do, and how he or she is interacting with the environment. In the AAL field there has been a variety of different types of sensors that have been used. These sensors can be classified according to different criteria, such as whether they are active or passive (i.e., require power or not), worn on the person or installed within the environment, and wired or wireless communication. Within these broad categories there have been several specific sensor types that have been used in the development of AAL technologies, the most common with respect to older adults with dementia being 1) environmental sensors; 2) radiofrequency transmitters; and 3) computer-vision.

4.1.1. Environmental Sensors

This class of sensors consists of a wide variety of low-cost sensors that are commercially available and are often meant to measure a single factor only. One of the most commonly used environmental sensors in AAL technologies is an electronic motion detector that simply detects the presence of motion within a specific room. There are several versions of this type of technology including motion sensors that measure movement based on optical or acoustical changes in the field of view, as well as the inclusion of an occupancy sensor that integrates a timing device to measure how long a person may be within the view of the sensor. More advanced motion sensors also use a passive infrared sensor (PIR), which detects body heat from occupants in the room.

In addition to motion sensors, other commonly used environmental sensors include devices that can measure specific events such as mechanical devices that measure water usage, thermostats to measure environmental temperature and humidity, and micro-switches that can detect if a person is lying on a bed, sitting on a chair or has opened a door.

4.1.2. Radiofrequency Transmitters

The use of radiofrequency-based sensors has been steadily increasing in the development of AAL technologies. A common type of this sensor is Radio Frequency Identification (RFID), which consists of 'readers' that are able to sense the presence of 'tags' and a communication protocol that allows the sensed tag to transmit any data stored in its memory back to the main system for processing. This data is often a unique identification number assigned to the tag but can be a more descriptive label such as the name or location of an object. These tags, or responders, can be placed onto different objects or as bracelets that may be worn by a user. Similar form factors can also be used for the readers that are used to collect the required data. Typically there are three types of RF-ID tags: passive, active, and battery assisted passive (BAP). A passive tag does not have a battery, but requires an external source to initiate and perform signal transmission, such as an external reader that is powered and thus also powers the passive tag. An active tag requires a battery and can transmit signals to an external source. Similar to a beacon, active systems can be used for real-time locating systems by actively emitting a signal to a reader at pre-set intervals, and typically have transmission ranges of up to 300 feet. Finally, a BAP tag contains a battery that eliminates the need for the tag to gather energy from the reader, resulting in performance levels that are much greater than a normal passive system. In addition, BAP tags can often incorporate other sensors such as temperature, humidity, and illumination.

4.1.3. Computer Vision

The use of visual-based sensors, such as web cameras, in AAL technologies is becoming increasingly popular as a result of the decreasing hardware costs, vast improvements in image processing algorithms with respect to computational costs and robustness, and the recognition by AAL researchers that the rich data set that can be collected via cameras has many potential benefits. The latter includes reducing the need for the use of several environmental based sensors to monitor a specific activity. Computer vision uses a camera and various image processing techniques to extract information from an image that is necessary to solve some kind of task, such as image recognition, motion analysis, scene reconstruction, or image restoration. For recognition, image processing techniques are used to determine if the image data contain some specific object, feature, or activity. This is achieved by the system learning what a specific object or activity looks like based on training data that consist of various features and poses that describe the desired target. Within motion analysis, tracking a target object, such as a person, is typically used in AAL systems in order to determine the actions and intentions of a person. This is achieved by algorithms that analyse sequential video frames and outputs the movement of the object between each frame. A key aspect of these algorithms is the ability to differentiate the object being tracked from the background and other irrelevant features in the environment.

4.2. Commonly Used Machine Learning Approaches

Machine learning (ML) is an area of AI concerned with the study of computer algorithms that improve automatically through experience. There are a variety of different ML techniques that have been used in AAL applications. In all cases, the basic idea is to learn a function that maps between some inputs (e.g. sensor readings in a smart home or database query results) and some outputs (e.g. categories of human behaviour or actions that a system must take). This learning is done based on a set of training examples and is evaluated on a separate set of test examples. The metric for success is the performance on the test examples, and a ML algorithm is considered successful if it is able to generalise from the training data to the test data. An unsuccessful ML algorithm often performs very well on the training data, but very poorly on test data, a phenomenon known as overfitting.

Machine learning algorithms can be grouped into three categories that describe how the approach learns about the application for which it is being used: 1) supervised learning; 2) unsupervised learning; and 3) reinforcement learning. A review of the AAL literature shows that there are a growing number of different ML techniques in each of these three learning categories that are being used in the development of new AAL technologies. This subsection will provide an overview of each of these three different categories, and examples of specific ML algorithms for each. A discussion of generalization and overfitting can be found in Section 4.4.

Details on the ML concepts introduced in this section can be found in texts on machine learning [11,38,54,63] and artificial intelligence [49,58].

4.2.1. Supervised Learning

Supervised learning (i.e., when the training data are labelled) is one of the most common ML approaches. Supervised algorithms are presented with training data, which consist of examples that include both the inputs and their desired outputs. From these data, the algorithm can learn a relationship between the two sets of data so that it is able to map, or classify, new inputs into appropriate outputs. The simplest supervised learning technique is linear regression, where inputs and outputs are assumed to be related by a linear function, the parameters of which can be estimated from the training data (by fitting a linear function to the data). A generalisation is to non-linear fitting, in which a variety of methods are used to fit a (usually parameterized) curve to a dataset. If the target labels are binary (e.g. disease/no-disease), then a logistic regression is often successful, in which the non-linear fit is done to a logistic (sigmoid) function.

Typically, data for a supervised learning approach take the form of a number of discrete or real-valued input *attributes* and a single output target attribute. For example, in an AAL application, the input attributes may be the values of a number of sensors in an older adult's home, while the target attribute may be a category of human activity. The input attributes may be discrete-valued (e.g. a switch that is on/off) or may be continuous-valued (e.g. a temperature value), and there may be a mixture of the two different types. The output attribute is typically discrete-valued (e.g. an activity label), but could also be continuous-valued (e.g. a probability that a fall is imminent).

The most well-used supervised learning technique for a discrete-valued target attribute is a decision tree, in which input attributes are used to divide the data into sets, each of which is better able to predict the target attribute. The learned decision tree consists of a set of nodes arranged in a tree structure, each of which is associated with a *test* of a particular input attribute. The possible results of the test are then *branches* emanating from the node, leading to other, similar nodes, or to *leaves* of the tree. The leaves are labelled with a target attribute value. Classification of a data sample proceeds from the root of the tree by applying the test at that node, and then following the branch that corresponds to the output of the test. This process is repeated until a leaf is reached, at which point the predicted target attribute is read off. A decision tree can be learned using a simple greedy approach. In the greedy approach, each input attribute is evaluated as per its ability to divide the input data into sets that have similar output attribute values and the best performing input attribute and test is chosen as the root node. This process is repeated recursively for each test result and associated training data. The choices of how to choose attributes, how to split data based on those attributes, and how to choose when to stop splitting data and creating new branches are settings that bias the final decision tree results. Care in assigning these settings is key to learning an effective decision tree (i.e. one that generalises and does not overfit). The standard text on decision tree learning is described in [52].

Another very popular supervised learning approach is the neural network. The neural network was one of the early attempts to emulate human intelligence on a machine by replicating neuron-like processing units. In this case, each input attribute is assigned to an input node in a network of neuron-like processing units. Each artificial neuron takes values from a set of these input nodes and compares a weighted sum of these values to a threshold, firing an output *pulse* if the threshold is crossed. A second layer of neurons then combines the outputs from the first layer in a similar way. The outputs of the second layer are the predictors of the target attribute. The neural network is trained by repeated presentations of inputs and outputs and a simple update rule is used at each node to bring the predictions closer to the true outputs. Often this training procedure can be time consuming.

4.2.2. Unsupervised Learning

In many situations, it is difficult or undesirable to assign output labels to a set of training data. For example, one may be interested in detecting changes in a person's behaviour in a smart home. In order to detect change, a model must be built of the person's normal routines. New data can be tested for novelty by comparison to this normality model. In this case, it is not desirable to assign categories of human behaviours to a training set, but rather is important to learn what types of patterns are normally present [40]. Unsupervised learning tackles this problem.

Probably the most common unsupervised approaches are statistical in nature. A statistical model is hypothesised and its parameters are learned by a computer from a set of data. The simplest example is the mixture model, where we define a probability distribution over the input attributes given a set of (unknown but of fixed size) labels. The expectation-maximization (EM) algorithm can then be used to learn the parameters of this probability distribution such that the likelihood of the data given the parameters is maximized. Mixture models can handle multi-dimensional, mixed continuous and discrete inputs, and can learn output attributes with many values [11]. A generalisation is to allow the model to also learn the number of output values or labels, by placing hierarchical Bayesian priors over the mixture categories. Such methods have been used recently in many text categorisation and machine translation problems [64].

Unsupervised learning can be seen as a form of clustering, in which patterns are sought in the data. The *clustering objective* is to find a set of subsets of the input data such that the data within each subset are all very similar (small intra-class distance), and all data in different subsets are very dissimilar (large inter-class distance). Many clustering approaches exist, the simplest based on computing the ordered eigenvectors of the input data (also known as principal components analysis or PCA). The principal (first) eigenvector is a vector in the high-dimensional space of input attributes along which the data vary the most. Splitting the input data into two sets at the mid-point of this vector is often an effective method for finding sets which satisfy the clustering goal. A recursive application of this method is sometimes referred to as *vector quantization.*

Neural networks are also used for clustering. The self-organising map (SOM) is a classic example of a neural network with an unsupervised training rule [30]. In a similar fashion to the supervised case, they are trained by slowly adjusting the weights of each neuron. However, in this case, the adjustments cannot be made to bring the predictions in line with the true outputs, and some other measures of success must be used. Maximizing the entropy of the target labels given the inputs is one approach that is attempting to satisfy an objective similar to the one defined above for clustering.

4.2.3. Reinforcement Learning

In this approach, an agent (i.e., something that perceives and acts), explores the environment and receives a reward, which may be either positive or negative. Reinforcement learning (RL) can be seen as a form of supervised learning in which the output (target) labels are the reward values. The difficulty in RL is that the reward is often delayed, and the agent has a blame attribution problem to solve. For example, a personal assistant robot may only learn that it has done a good job at the end of the day when its performance is evaluated. It will not know which specific actions led to that reward signal. The agent therefore needs to learn how to act so that, in the long run, it achieves the maximum cumulative reward. The function that tells an agent what to do in any situation is known as a *policy* [63].

There are two major types of RL algorithms: model-based and model-free. In a model-based approach, the agent assumes some parameterized model of the dynamics of the environment (and of its actions in it) and of the rewards. The agent then gathers evidence about these parameters while acting in the world. Once the model has been learned, a policy can be computed (using e.g. dynamic programming) that optimises the (learned) reward function. Model-free approaches, however, do not assume a model and attempt to learn the policy directly from the data. The most commonly used model-based approach uses the Markov decision process (MDP) as a simple Markovian model of the environment. Dynamic programming is a classical search algorithm that can be used in an MDP to guide the agent towards the goal (or towards optimal long-term reward) [9]. Q-learning is the simplest model-free approach, and many variants of it have been proposed, mostly focussed on efficiency gains. The advantages of a model-based approach are that it is easily interpretable and prior knowledge about the domain is relatively easy to incorporate. The advantage of the model-free approaches is that there is less bias imposed on the structure of the environment (e.g. a Markovian assumption) and more complex dynamics can be learned given enough data.

Central to the problem of RL is the exploration/exploitation tradeoff. An RL agent can either exploit its current knowledge of reward (e.g. it may know of a particular action that will yield a good outcome), or it can try something new by exploring a new action that it has not yet tried. While the first option is safe, the second carries some risk, but may potentially yield higher overall return. Many RL agents use heuristic methods to trade-off exploration and exploitation. For example, an RL agent may try a random action some percentage of the time, slowly decreasing this percentage as it learns more and more about the environment. Another alternative is *optimism in the face of uncertainty* in which an agent always assumes an untested action is best. This second approach is often very effective (fast) for RL. Bayesian reinforcement learning (BRL) explicitly quantifies uncertainty over this tradeoff and is the optimal method for RL, but carries a significant computational overhead [18]. Efficient methods for BRL are a topic of much current research [17].

4.3. Modelling Interactions Between Users and AAL Technologies

When designing new AAL technologies it is important to first understand the types of interactions that may occur between the system and the user(s). In addition, the system needs to take into account the various aspects of these interactions and other aspects of the context within which the system will be used. These aspects are critical in that they will determine how best to model the variables that are related to the user, activity, and the environment, and direct the choices of sensing and ML approaches that are needed to deal with them. The following is an overview of some of the key variables that should be considered in the design of the chosen sensing and ML algorithms when developing AAL technologies for older adults with dementia.

4.3.1. Uncertainty

The world is full of uncertainty, and AAL contexts are no exception. This becomes an even larger issue when deploying these technologies into the homes of older adults, which are typically highly unconstrained, dynamic, and unpredictable. Sources of uncertainty include noise from sensors, unobservability of events and states, and uncertain effects of actions. The latter is particularly important when working with older adults with dementia, whose behaviours are difficult to predict. For example, when assisting a user during a self-care task, such as handwashing, an assistive system may need to sense what the user is doing using a variety of sensors (such as those described previously). These sensors carry with them explicit uncertainty, sometimes providing false readings. Further, the technology cannot directly measure various "hidden" states such as a user's awareness, level of frustration, or affect. Finally, a user may not always have predictable behaviours, even though completing the same task, within the same environment. This uncertainty about the future state of the user can be reduced by increasing the complexity of the model (thereby taking into account more factors). ML can play a significant role in helping to better model these various factors.

4.3.2. Time

An older adult with dementia often does not need help just once, but rather will need it repeatedly, through different tasks, and at different times of the day. As such, any assistance provided by an AAL technology needs to be an ongoing interaction, requiring the system to build and maintain an explicit model of time. In AI-based approaches there are typically two ways of modelling time: event-based and clock-based. Event-based approaches use events as delineations of time. For example a person entering the kitchen denotes the start of a kitchen event that lasts until the person leaves the kitchen. These events may have even finer resolution, such as the person touching the water faucet, indicating the start of that specific sub-step of handwashing. Event-based modelling is very intuitive and powerful, as it allows for hierarchical modelling of nested events, and corresponds to human perceptions of time. Clock-based approaches are event-based in which the only events that denote time are (regular) ticks on a real clock. The advantage of a clock-based approach is it removes the need to specify what an event is, at the expense of having possibly far too many (or even too few) events for a particular task.

4.3.3. Adaptivity

One of the primary reasons for using AI in the design of AAL technologies is to make these systems adaptable in their operations. Humans are individuals and behave in different ways in similar situations. Humans are also dynamic, and change over time. This is especially true for older adults with dementia, which is a progressive disease and causes significant changes in a person's cognition and abilities over time (both in the short and long term). Therefore, AAL systems must have the ability to adapt to a user over time.

There are two ways to approach adaptivity: learning and inference. The learning approach considers that the model being used has some parameters that govern how the model works, and that these parameters change over time. For example, the system may learn the probability that a user needs help washing his/her hands. This is a single number that may be close to zero for a non-cognitively disabled person, while it may be much higher for an older adult with dementia. A learning algorithm can track this change, learning how the parameter changes over time, thus adjusting its responses to the user accordingly.

In the inference approach, the system estimates some underlying factors that govern the change in how the model operates. In the previous handwashing example, a factor that affects the probability of needing assistance could be dementia level (e.g. mild, moderate, or severe), or dementia type (e.g. cortical vs. sub-cortical). Some fixed parameters then govern how the user's need for assistance during handwashing depends on these variables. The model can then be used to infer the person's level or type of dementia and use this to change its response characteristics.

4.3.4. Abstraction

A common thread in AAL technologies is the ability to sense real world events using the various sensor types presented previously, where the result is often a large quantity of data. For example, a video stream of a person using the soap during handwashing might contain large volumes of raw data describing the user's hand positions, interactions with the soap, and extraneous data that are irrelevant to the task at hand. Furthermore, these data points are often collected with high frequency (typically around 10 to 30 frames per second). Even with a simpler type of sensor, such as a switch, the raw data emanating from it will be a continuous signal through time, sampled at a rate that could provide a large amount of data over a period of hours, days, weeks, or years. As such, AAL technologies need to be able to sift through all of these data, and create appropriate abstractions of it, both in time and in space, and over a range of sensors. These abstractions (classes or categories) are critical in order to allow for simple and fast decision making for actions by the system.

In ML there are two primary techniques that are for creating and learning appropriate abstractions: generative and discriminative. Generative techniques attempt to model the complete distribution over all the sensor data by learning a function that maps between the abstract categories or classes and the raw sensor data. This function typically is very large and complex and can be quite difficult to learn. Discriminative techniques, meanwhile, attempt only to find a method for classifying the data into the necessary categories, without worrying about the complete distribution of the data. A simple example is a water flow impeller in a pipe, used to detect if a person has turned on the water during handwashing. A generative approach will build a function describing the distribution of sensor readings for each situation: water on or off. The distribution might take some parametric form, such as a Gaussian, or might be described by a non-parametric form, such as a histogram of values the sensor reading normally takes on for each of the states of the water flow. A discriminative approach will find the threshold for the sensor's output that will be the best predictor of the water being on or off. It should be noted that in theory, a generative modeling approach will always outperform a discriminative one if it is a correct model (if it is expressive enough) and if enough training data are available to learn the model. In practice, discriminative techniques offer better performance in terms of classification, when only limited training data are available. However, for decision-making, it is very important to maintain some generative model of the raw sensor noise.

4.3.5. Preferences

An important aspect is developing AAL technologies for older adults with dementia is to ensure that the system incorporates the preferences and needs of the user in order to ensure that the technology maximizes the abilities of the person. These preferences may be as simple as a list of things that a person likes or does not like (e.g. doesn't like audio prompts in a male voice), or may be more complex conditional preferences (e.g. likes audio prompts when in the kitchen, but not in the bathroom), or may be relational (e.g. likes audio prompts better than video prompts, but not as much as tangible prompts).

While it is important for designers of AAL technologies to elicit these preferences during the design phase, it is also critical for the technology itself to be able to extract this information during the operation of the system to ensure that the changing needs of the user are met. In machine learning, this can be achieved through the concept of *utility*, which can be used to map a user's preferences onto a numerical utility function. These concepts originate in the study of game theory, operations research, and decision theory. Essentially, game theoretic theorems guarantee that a rational human's preferences can be mapped onto a numeric scale of utility, and that decisions made according to this numeric scale will be the best, or optimal, for that person.

4.4. Experimental Performance

The final topic in the building of effective ML algorithms is a consideration of data. All the techniques presented rely on some training data. However, the actual aim of the learning process is to provide accurate classifications on future, unseen, test data. That is, our classifiers are not generally useful for the training data, as we already know how to classify this data (what the labels are, for example).

A recurrent problem in machine learning is that of overfitting, in which a classifier is trained on some training data, and learns to perform very well (e.g. predict the labels) very well on this data, but then fails to perform well on the test data. The model in such a case is too complex, in the sense that it is able to model the training data too closely and, therefore, does not generalise well to real-world applications.

The avoidance of overfitting is an art in itself and requires the model designer to carefully select the parameters to be learned in relation to the complexity of the classification problem. However, a simple technique for dealing with overfitting involves simply separating the training data into two sets: a training set and a validation set. The validation set is essentially a stand-in for eventual test data. The machine learning algorithm is then applied to the training set, but performance is evaluated on the validation set. The best performing classifier on the validation set is the one that is chosen as having the best ability to generalise. In practice, one only has to select a fraction (e.g. 10%) of the data that is to be reserved for validation.

5. Examples of AAL Technologies

As discussed in the previous sections, AAL technologies come in many forms and are targeted to support different needs. Growing pressures to support an aging population combined with significant advances in computer science have resulted in an increasingly rapid growth in the research and development of AAL technologies for people with dementia, both in academia and industry. While intelligent or adaptive AAL technologies are just beginning to appear in the marketplace, the current pace of development will likely result in the increased use of these technologies in the near future. It is beyond the scope of this chapter to list all the advances in AAL technologies for dementia; therefore, the following examples are intended to provide an illustration of possible AAL technology applications.

5.1. Examples of AAL Technologies Being Developed by the Research Community

Being able to complete ADLs, such as toileting, bathing, and dressing, is a key component to maintaining independence and dignity. It is also one of the most difficult forms of support for a caregiver to provide because of the amount of care involved and the highly personal/private nature of most ADLs. A person's inability to complete ADLs independently results in high levels of burden, depression, and other difficulties for both the caregiver and care recipient, which can become overwhelming and often results in the care recipient's placement into long-term care. As a result, much research has focused on the creation of AAL technologies that can support ADL completion.

One example of such a technology is the COACH, which is prototyped to assist with handwashing [27,42]. COACH consists of a video camera mounted over the sink, a computer, speakers, and a flat-screen monitor. Using computer vision, COACH tracks the user's hands, the towel, and the soap as he or she interacts with the sink area. As described in Section 4, this is achieved by using image processing techniques that learn the different characteristics of the user's hand (e.g. skin colour), and the other relevant objects (e.g. location). This information is passed to a planning module, which employs machine learning and inference techniques to determine autonomously where in the task the user is and to estimate parameters such as the user's overall level of dementia, current responsiveness, and preferred ordering of steps. The planning module then uses this information to decide the best course of action to take; namely, to continue to observe the user, give the user an audio or video prompt to guide him or her to the next step in the activity, or to summon the caregiver should the user require assistance. COACH is also able to select different levels of prompting autonomously to match the user's abilities and current context, with prompts ranging from simplistic (e.g., an audio prompt that says "Turn the water on") to specific (e.g., an audio prompt "John, push the silver handle to turn the water on" with an accompanying demonstrative video). COACH is an example of a ZET as it does not require any explicit input from the user with dementia or the caregiver to make decisions and provide support autonomously. COACH is also able to learn about the user's preferences and is able to change its short- and long-term strategies to complement the dynamic nature of dementia. In pilot trials with COACH participants with moderate to severe dementia were significantly more independent, requiring little or no human assistance. Improvements are being made to the tracking and planning modules of COACH with the intention of deploying the device into people's homes for further evaluation. In addition, the system is currently being developed for other ADLs, including toothbrushing, nutrition, and work-related tasks.

Autominder is an AAL technology that has been developed to provide flexible and context-sensitive reminders to people who have trouble with memory tasks through the application of many of the AI techniques and sensors described in Section 4 [47,48]. For example, this particular system uses probabilistic approaches that use supervised machine learning algorithms to model what the person is doing, and what the person should be doing. Autominder is not intended to give detailed instructions on how to complete a task (as COACH does), rather it is meant as a high-level reminder system. When a new task is scheduled with Autominder, the person inputting the task not only specifies when the task should happen, but can also specify a temporal tolerance for the task (i.e., an acceptable "window" for the task to be initiated, such as +/- 30 minutes from the scheduled time). Autominder employs environmental sensors and machine learning to learn about the user and his or her context (i.e., the user's preferences, what the user is doing, and the state of his or her environment) and combines this with the temporal tolerance of the task to deliver prompts at times when he or she may be the most effective. For example, if a person is scheduled to take medication every day at 1 PM, but Autominder knows his or her favourite TV show is on at 1 PM on Wednesdays, on Wednesday Autominder may prompt the person to take his or her medication at 12:55 rather than delivering the prompt during the show, when it may be ignored or forgotten. Unlike a conventional reminder system, Autominder's context awareness means it will not provide a prompt to the user for a task he or she has already completed. This is important in supporting independence and minimising confusing messages (e.g., if a non-context aware system reminds a person to take medication they have just taken, it could result in a double-dose). Preliminary field tests with older adults and people who have traumatic brain injury have shown promising results, although an in-depth evaluation has yet to be completed. Autominder was "...developed with four sometimes competing goals in mind: 1) user awareness of planned activities; 2) a high level of user and caregiver satisfaction; 3) avoiding introduction of inefficiency into the user's activities; and 4) avoiding over-reliance on the reminder system – that is, reliance to the extent that use of the system actually decreases rather than increase [the] user's independence" [47, p. 69]. These goals are an excellent and succinct example of design criteria for an AAL technology for people with dementia.

At the mild stages of dementia, people are often able to still function independently outside of the home, but may easily forget their destination, how to get there, or why they were going there. The Assisted Cognition project was initiated in an effort to create a portable reminder and guidance system for people in the mild stages of dementia and other forms of cognitive impairments [33,34]. The resulting handheld system uses a mobile phone with WiFi and employs artificial intelligence to learn about the user's normal wayfinding behaviours and to customise directions according to the user's preferences for how they best recognise directions. For example, using GPS and street-view images of the area the user is in, the device is able to display images of the nearby area with an overlaid directional arrow indicating the direction the user should be going. The device is also able to provide directions by showing landmarks (e.g., building, sculptures, etc.) that are downloaded from a Graphical Information System (GIS) databases or the internet. Two sets of pilot trials with the device have shown promising results. From these trials, researchers have highlighted that users' needs are very different and that directions must not only be given to the user in a way that he or she can interpret them, but also must be able to support changes in a user's abilities.

AAL technologies can also be used directly and indirectly to detect changes in health. For example, research being done by Hayes and colleagues has shown that slower walking speeds may be indicative of an increased risk for conditions such as disability, cognitive impairment, institutionalisation, falls, mortality, and complications following surgery [2,23,25,26,29,62,66]. Hayes et al. are using infrared sensors to measure both variability in daily activities and changes in walking speed over extended periods of time continuously. In a year-long study of seven older adults with mild cognitive impairment (MCI) and seven healthy aged-matched controls, it was found that the variability in daily activity was significantly higher in subjects with MCI [24].

Alwan et al. have developed a home monitoring system to identify changes in normal patterns of living that uses motion detectors, a stovetop monitor, and an instrumented mattress [3,69]. Data are autonomously analysed to develop models of a person's usual behaviour, detect if an abnormal situation has occurred, and raise alerts that reflect the probable level of the event's severity. In pilot trials with 22 older adults (some who had dementia) living in an assisted living facility, the system correctly detected two serious changes in health and four falls before clinicians were aware of them. Clinicians felt the system also helped them gain a better understanding of some of the participants' chronic conditions as well as a more complete picture of participants' overall health, enabling better treatment and health management. Feedback from study participants and their families found that people were generally accepting of the technology, willing to share their data with caregivers, and reported significantly higher quality of life after three months of monitoring.

AAL technologies are also starting to be developed for non-traditional applications in improving the quality of life of older adults with dementia. For example, leisure activities and expressive creation are important ways to counter depression and stress and foster communication with others. Hoey et al. are developing a device to assist older adults with dementia perform arts therapy [41]. The device consists of a large multi-touch screen acting as a canvas, a computer, and a camera. Prior to a therapy session, an arts therapist is able to select and customise the virtual tools their client will use (e.g., paintbrush, shapes, colours, and effects) and add themes and pictures that they feel might interest their client. The device employs artificial intelligence to gauge a person's engagement by monitoring their interactions with the canvas and tracking where they are looking using the video camera. The device can encourage engagement by adding items for the person to interact with the canvas and by providing audio prompts, all of which are customisable by the therapist. Artwork is saved for review by the therapist and can be printed and shared with caregivers and family members. The device also logs each session, allowing therapists to quantitatively analyse their clients' use of the device. While the prototype is intended to be used during sessions with arts therapists, future versions may be appropriate for individuals to use with their informal caregivers, thereby providing a tool to encourage meaningful communication and expression.

The intelligent AAL technologies presented above are able to perform a multitude of autonomous functions and could be integrated to provide a detailed, subtle, and highly-personalised support as well as being able to diagnose conditions (possibly before a human could) and provide quantifiable rates of change in health. Intelligent AAL technologies have the potential to give clinicians, family, and the individuals themselves a deeper understanding of a person's health and represent invaluable tools in the current trend towards a preventative, rather than reactionary, approach to healthcare.

5.2. Examples of Commercially Available AAL Technologies

While truly intelligent AAL technologies are not yet commercially available, there are many AAL technologies available in the marketplace to support people with dementia. These products are usually targeted toward specific areas or conditions, require a good deal of effort from the caregiver and cooperation from the care recipient to operate. The following examples highlight the wide variety of commercially available technologies that support limitations and challenges faced by people with dementia and their caregiver.

Wandering is a prevalent behaviour with dementia and can be very stressful for both the caregiver and care recipient as the confusion caused by dementia often results in the person with dementia becoming lost. There is a multitude of devices intended to detect and prevent wandering, such as EmFinders (EmFinders), Quest Guard (Quest Guard Alliance), and Wherify Wireless (Wherify Wireless Inc.). These systems are about the size of a wristwatch, are worn by the person with dementia, and use GPS or cellular towers to locate the care recipient. With Quest Guard, the caregiver is able to set safety zones and is notified if the care recipient moves outside of these while Wherify can store up to 10 contact numbers that the user can page with a simple button press. These technologies have been helpful for people with mild dementia who are still able to function outside of the home but are prone to bouts of confusion. With more severe levels of dementia, technologies such as the SafeDoor and SafetyBed (Emfit Ltd.) may be more appropriate. SafeDoor is a wireless device that can raise an alarm if a person walks out a door, but not when they open it, which can be especially helpful in managing people who are prone to night-time wandering. The SafetyBed is a sensor that is able to alert the caregiver when a person has gotten out of bed. The caregiver can choose to set a delay on the alarm (from 10 seconds to 90 minutes) which allows the bed's occupant to get out of bed and return (e.g., going to the washroom) without disturbing the caregiver.

There are several home health monitoring devices now on the market such as Health Buddy (Bosch), Telestation (Phillips), Genesis DM (Honeywell), Health Guide (Intel), LifeView (American TeleCare), Ideal LIFE Pod (Ideal Life), and Healthanywhere (Healthanywhere Inc.). These systems are able to take physiological readings (e.g., blood pressure, heart rate, temperature, glucose levels, etc.) using conventional measurement devices (e.g., blood pressure cuff, thermometer, blood glucose meter, etc.) and shares them remotely with clinicians. Many of these devices allow the person being monitored to interact with clinicians over video screens, enabling more personal communication. Some also have access to online, multimedia educational materials, caregiver networks, and other resources that can help people to manage conditions. While these devices are not designed for older adults with dementia in particular, they can be valuable tools for caregivers and clinicians who are managing the health of older adults with dementia living at home.

Although they do not yet possess the level of autonomy that intelligent AAL technologies currently being researched do, commercially available AAL technologies can provide a great deal of assistance and peace of mind for both the caregiver and care recipient. It is only a matter of time before intelligence will be readily available in AAL technologies in the marketplace enabling significantly greater levels of convenience and support.

6. Measuring the Success of AAL Technologies for Older Adults with Dementia

The final sub-theme that is important to discuss is how to measure the successfulness of an AAL technology. For intelligent AAL technologies to make inroads within the established healthcare system and marketplace, their value may need to be proven further in the research domain. Typically, healthcare research involves rigorous testing protocols that can range from descriptive case studies to randomized controlled trials [50]. The research-based technologies described in Section 4.1 are a good representation of the general state of the field of intelligent AAL technologies; most projects are in the initial stages of research and, while many have a working prototype, only some have been pilot tested, few have been tested in true real-world applications, and very few have been involved in longitudinal studies. In the context of evidence-based testing, these projects are at early phases of development along the continuum of proof, which is a fitting stage that reflects the recent and rapid growth of intelligent technologies themselves.

Intelligent AAL technologies lie within the broader domain of assistive technologies (ATs), which have been increasingly evaluated in recent years with respect to their research protocols. For instance, in their evaluations, reviewers studying ATs for dementia as well as for other cognitive impairments have suggested researchers 1) ground their work in solid theoretical frameworks [37]; 2) incorporate mixed methods that combine qualitative and quantitative studies [65]; 3) investigate the many factors that influence AT use in greater depth [59,65]; 4) develop designs that shift from demonstrations of 'efficacy' in controlled clinical environments to 'effectiveness' in 'real-world' environments [37,59]; and 5) perform follow up studies that can assess outcome measures of AT use over the long term [65].

Notably, these considerations are all discussed in a framework that is intended to help plan complex research protocols for interventions that involve multiple interacting variables [15]. The framework proposed by Campbell et al. [15] involves an iterative, phased approach that combines qualitative research with quantitative analysis. Phases proceed from a preclinical phase (descriptive theory), to Phase I (modeling and preliminary testing), to Phase II (exploratory trials), with the protocol becoming increasingly specified within each phase. Activities in the preclinical phase of the framework include selecting an intervention and proposing a basic research proposal. In Phase I, the factors are increasingly specified by simulating the intervention. Descriptive and qualitative studies, such as focus groups, can contribute to this phase of research, identifying both barriers and facilitators to the outcomes of interest. By the time Phase II testing is reached, technical feasibility has been proven, preliminary testing has been completed, relevant mediating factors have been identified, a suitable comparison test (possibly a standard or no-treatment trial) has been selected, and outcome measures have been defined. Subsequent Phase II activities then involve further refinement of the intervention and the protocol based on Phase I activities as well as implementation of the controlled trial itself.

The framework described above is relevant because AT research has been identified as complex [19,59]. The phased progression within the framework is mirrored in Fuhrer's work [19], for instance, which recommends AT protocols that shift from 'small theory' studies to efficacy trials under controlled conditions and effectiveness trials under externally valid conditions. Similarly, Scherer et al. [59] refer to both the importance of identifying the complex series of factors at play and of real-world testing, which they cite as particularly relevant to the high rate of AT abandonment estimated at 90%. The reasons for abandonment can vary widely depending on the type of technology and user. It has been speculated that abandonment issues include users not accepting their own disabilities and thus being resistant to using an assistive technology, technologies being too complex and costly for users to use and acquire, and caregivers and family members rejecting the technology because it actually increases their own workload and burden (e.g. by having to set-up the technology, install it, etc.). This final issue is further testament to this chapter's sub-theme on the importance of including caregivers in the design and testing of AAL technologies.

The ENABLE project, a large European effort involving development of several assistive devices for people with dementia, followed a structured protocol, functioning at a Phase II level of research [22]. Besides employing a phased protocol, researchers on this project recognized that various outcomes, in addition to functional effectiveness, were important. So besides functional outcomes, they selected the Dementia Quality of Life instrument to consider outcomes for the care recipient and the Relative's Stress Scale to measure caregiver stress. Similarly, in an aggregated analysis that was conducted over several studies, Nygård [43] found functional outcomes to be eclipsed by other outcomes relevant to people with dementia, particularly by perceived control and mastery. In both of these series of studies, one element that becomes clear is the importance of assessing a variety of outcomes that are relevant to the multiple stakeholders involved.

In work on AT outcomes, Fuhrer et al. [20] not only specified different kinds of outcomes, including usability, psychological impacts and subjective wellbeing, but also noted that different stakeholders possess different values and, in turn, particular outcomes would be more relevant for some than for others. In addition, they recommended narrowing the list to examine only a few outcomes in a research study, considering weighting these outcomes relative to their importance, and using both objective and subjective measures in assessment.

In summary, work in iterative phased research coupled with implementation of appropriate outcome measures may shift development of research-based AAL technologies further along the evidence-based continuum and, in turn, prove their value within the broader healthcare community.

7. The Future of AAL Technologies for Older Adults with Dementia

The future of AAL technologies will continue to become more important as the older adult population grows and the number of people who have dementia increases. As described in this chapter, in order to be effective these technologies need to be easily adaptable to these users' needs. The requirement for this adaptability to be automatically performed by the technology will become even more important as the trend towards providing care to older adults with dementia in their own homes becomes more prevalent. In response, advanced sensing, machine learning, and other applications from the field of artificial intelligence will continue to play a large role in the development of future AAL technologies. This will be true not only for those technologies related to cognition, but also to those needed for mobility and sensory impairments. It is becoming apparent that AAL technologies can no longer just focus on the single dimension of cognition, but must also take into account the other co-morbidities that older adults face. For example, there is growing literature in the area of intelligent powered wheelchairs that can help older adults with dementia navigate their environments more safely. There has also been work to add intelligence and complex sensing to more "traditional" assistive technologies such as walkers and canes to help users to maintain their balance and to help with wayfinding. In addition, there are several new "frontiers" that are starting to be explored that can have a significant impact on the lives of older adults with dementia. One potential area is the use of advanced robotics to help care for older adults with a variety of disabilities. For example, it could be imagined that personal robotics can play a significant role in supporting older adults in their own homes. Robots can be developed that can help older adults complete a variety of activities, such as meal preparation or house work, and could also play a role in the monitoring and assessment of a person's overall health and well-being. Within the area of AAL technologies to help monitor the health and well-being of older adults, researchers (e.g., at the University of Toronto) are developing ways of placing sensors into building materials. Dubbed *brick computing*, this incorporation of sensors into floor, wall, and ceiling materials allows for continuous and autonomous ambient readings, without any kind of manual interactions from the user. For example, a floor tile is under development that will be able to measure a person's physiological parameters (e.g. heart rate and blood pressure) simply by the person standing on the tile in bare feet.

The future of the AAL field for older adults with dementia will also require more work to be completed on the development and use of new design paradigms that will allow for data to be collected with respect to user needs. While traditional approaches, such as user-centred design, are proving to be somewhat useful, it is still difficult to include this population in the design process. The dynamic nature of dementia is forcing this field to begin to incorporate design and evaluation strategies that are as equally dynamic. However, issues around how to instill these new approaches while still being able to complete the required work effectively, in a timely manner, and without increasing the end costs of the resulting technology, are still significant barriers that need to be addressed.

Finally, as AAL technologies become more ubiquitous in the care of older adults with dementia, more research on the social and ethical implications of these types of technologies needs to be completed. This population is not similar to other typical AAL users, such as those who have physical or sensory disabilities. Special considerations need to be taken in the design and use of these technologies when a cognitive impairment exists. In practice, older adults with dementia are unable to provide their own consent for the use of these various technologies. This issue becomes even more problematic as more AAL technologies are developed for private and personal activities, and are being installed in sensitive locations within a person's home (e.g., in the bathroom). Careful consideration needs to be taken in determining how consent will be obtained to use these new technologies, and how users will be educated about the potential benefits and limitations of these systems in a fashion that is consistent with their cognitive abilities. These issues have not been fully addressed within the field of AAL technologies and hold the potential for a new and fruitful area of research.

References

[1] T. Adlam, R. Faulkner, R. Orpwood, K. Jones, J. Macijauskiene and A. Budraitiene, The installation and support of internationally distributed equipment for people with dementia, *IEEE Transactions on Information Technology in Biomedicine (TITB), Special Issue on Pervasive Healthcare* **8** (2004), 253–257.

[2] J. Afilalo, M.J. Eisenberg, J.-F. Morin, H. Bergman, J. Monette, N. Noiseux, L.P. Perrault, K.P. Alexander, Y. Langlois, M. Gharacholou, P. Chamoun, G. Kasparian, S. Robichaud and J.-F. Boivin, Gait speed as a predictor of mortality and major morbidity in older adults undergoing cardiac surgery: Preliminary results from the FRAILTY ABC'S study, *Circulation* **120** (2009), S988–S989.

[3] M. Alwan, S. Dalal, D. Mack, S.W. Kell, B. Turner, J. Leachtenauer and R. Felder, Impact of monitoring technology in assisted living: Outcome pilot, *IEEE Transactions Information Technology in Biomedicine* **10** (2006), 192–198.

[4] Alzheimer's Association, 2009 Alzheimer's disease facts and figures, *Alzheimer's and Dementia* **5** (2009), 234–270.

[5] Alzheimer's Disease International, World Alzheimer Report 2009, London, UK, 2009.

[6] Alzheimer's Disease International, World Alzheimer Report 2010: The Global Economic Impact of Dementia, Alzheimer's Disease International, London, UK, 2010.

[7] M.T. Banich, *Cognitive Neuroscience and Neuropsychology*, Houghton Mifflin College Div, 2004.

[8] H.S. Barrows, An overview of the uses of standardized patients for teaching and evaluating clinical skills, *Academic Medicine* **68** (1993), 443–451.

[9] R.E. Bellman, *Dynamic Programming*, Princeton University Press, Princeton, 1957.

[10] A.J. Bharucha, V. Anand, J. Forlizzi, M.A. Dew, C.F. Reynolds III, S. Stevens and H. Wactlar, Intelligent assistive technology applications to dementia care: Current capabilities, limitations, and future challenges, *American Journal of Geriatric Psychiatry* **17** (2009), 88–104.

[11] C.M. Bishop, *Pattern Recognition and Machine Learning*, Springer, 2006.

[12] J. Boger, J. Hoey, K. Fenton, T. Craig and A. Mihailidis, Using actors to develop technologies for older adults with dementia: A pilot study, *Gerontechnology* **9** (2010), 431–444.

[13] R. Brookmeyer, E. Johnson, K. Ziegler-Graham and H.M. Arrighi, Forecasting the global burden of Alzheimer's disease, Johns Hopkins University, Dept. of Biostatistics Working Papers, 2007.
[14] R.S. Bucks and S.A. Radford, Emotion processing in Alzheimer's disease, *Aging & Mental Health* **8** (2004), 222–232.
[15] M. Campbell, R. Fitzpatrick, A. Haines, A.L. Kinmonth, P. Sandercock, D. Spiegelhalter and P. Tyrer, Framework for design and evaluation of complex interventions to improve health, *British medical journal* **321** (2000), 694.
[16] A.-M. Dorsten, K.S. Sifford, A.J. Bharucha, L. Person Mecca and H. Wactlar, Ethical perspectives on emerging assistive technologies: Insights from focus groups with stakeholders in long-term care facilities, *Journal of Empirical Research on Human Research Ethics* **4** (2009), 25–36.
[17] F. Doshi-Velez, The infinite partially observable markov decision process, in: *Proc. Neural Information Processing Systems (NIPS)*, 2009.
[18] M.O. Duff, *Optimal Learning: Computational Procedures for Bayes-Adaptive Markov Decision Processes*, University of Massassachusetts Amherst, 2002.
[19] M.J. Fuhrer, Assessing the efficacy, effectiveness, and cost-effectiveness of assistive technology interventions for enhancing mobility, *Disability & Rehabilitation: Assistive Technology* **2** (2007), 149–158.
[20] M.J. Fuhrer, J.W. Jutai, M.J. Scherer and F. DeRuyter, A framework for the conceptual modelling of assistive technology device outcomes, *Disability & Rehabilitation* **25** (2003), 1243–1251.
[21] E.S.B. Gotell and S.-L. Ekman, Influence of caregiver singing and background music on posture, movement, and sensory awareness in dementia care, *International Psychogeriatrics* **15** (Dec. 2003), 411–430.
[22] I. Hagen, T. Holthe, J. Gilliard, P. Topo, S. Cahill, E. Begley, K. Jones, P. Duff, J. Macijauskiene, A. Budraitiene, S. Bjørneby and K. Engedal, in: *Development of a Protocol for the Assessment of Assistive Aids for People with Dementia*, Vol. 3, 2004, pp. 281–296.
[23] S. Hagler, D. Austin, T.L. Hayes, J. Kaye and M. Pavel, Unobtrusive and ubiquitous in-home monitoring: a methodology for continuous assessment of gait velocity in elders, *IEEE Transactions on Biomedical Engineering*, 2010 (in press).
[24] T.L. Hayes, F. Abendroth, A. Adami, M. Pavel, T.A. Zitzelberger and J.A. Kaye, Unobtrusive assessment of activity patterns associated with mild cognitive impairment, *Alzheimer's & Dementia* **4** (2008), 395–405.
[25] T.L. Hayes, M. Pavel and J. Kaye, An approach for deriving continuous health assessment indicators from in-home sensor data, in: *Technology and Aging*, A. Mihailidis, J. Boger, H. Kautz and L. Normie, eds, Assistive Technology Research Series, Vol. 21, IOS Press, 2008, pp. 130–137.
[26] T.L. Hayes, T. Riley, M. Pavel and J.A. Kaye, A method for estimating rest-activity patterns using simple pyroelectric motion sensors, in: *32nd Annual International Conference of the IEEE Engineering in Medicine and Biology Society*, Buenos Aires, Argentina, 2010.
[27] J. Hoey, P. Poupart, A. von Bertoldi, T. Craig, C. Boutilier and A. Mihailidis, Automated handwashing assistance for persons with dementia using video and a partially observable Markov decision process, *Computer Vision and Image Understanding – Special Issue on Computer Vision Systems* **114** (2010), 503–519.
[28] Information and Privacy Commissioner of Ontario (Canada), *Sensors and In-Home Collection of Health Data: A Privacy by Design Approach*, Information and Privacy Commissioner, 2010.
[29] J.A. Kaye, S.A. Maxwell, N. Mattek, T.L. Hayes, H. Dodge, M. Pavel, H. Jimison, K. Wild, L. Boise and T. Zitzelberger, Intelligent systems for assessing aging changes: Home-based, unobtrusive and continuous assessment of aging, *Journal of Gerontology; Series B: Psychological Sciences*, 2010 (in press).
[30] T. Kohonen, *Self-Organization and Associative Memory*, Springer-Verlag, Berlin, 1989.
[31] S.M. Kurtz, J. Silverman and J. Draper, *Teaching and Learning Communication Skills in Medicine*, 2nd edn, Radcliffe Publishing, Oxon, UK, 2005.
[32] J.A. Lenker, M.F. Nasarwanji, V. Paquet and D. Feathers, A tool for rapid assessment of product usability and universal design: Development and preliminary psychometric testing, *Work: A Journal of Prevention, Assessment, and Rehabilitation*, 2010 (in press).
[33] A.L. Liu, G. Borriello, H. Kautz, P.A. Brown, M. Harniss and K. Johnson, Learning user models to improve wayfinding assistance for individuals with cognitive impairment, in: *Workshop on Interactive Systems in Healthcare Atlanta, GA*, 2010.
[34] A.L. Liu, H. Hile, G. Borriello, H. Kautz, P.A. Brown, M. Harniss and K. Johnson, Informing the design of an automated wayfinding system for individuals with cognitive impairments, in: *3rd International Conference on Pervasive Computing Technologies for Healthcare (PervasiveHealth)*, London, UK, 2009, pp. 1–8.
[35] K.P.Y. Liu, C.C.H. Chan, M.M.L. Chu, T.Y.L. Ng, L.W. Chu, F.S.L. Hui, H.K. Yuen and A.G. Fisher, Activities of daily living performance in dementia, *Acta Neurologica Scandinavica* **116** (2007), 91–95.

[36] R. Logsdon, S.M. McCurry and L. Teri, Evidence-based interventions to improve quality of life for individuals with dementia, *Alzheimers Care Today* **8** (2007), 309–318.
[37] E.F. Lopresti, A. Mihailidis and N. Kirsch, Assistive technology for cognitive rehabilitation: State of the art, *Neuropsychological Rehabilitation* **14** (2004), 5–39.
[38] D.J. MacKay, *Information Theory, Inference, and Learning Algorithms*, Cambridge University Press, Cambridge, 2003.
[39] K.D. Marek and M.J. Rantz, Aging in place: A new model for long-term care, *Nursing Administration Quarterly* **24** (2000), 1–11.
[40] M. Markou and S. Singh, Novelty detection: A review – part 1: Statistical approaches, *Signal Processing* **83** (2003), 2481–2497.
[41] A. Mihailidis, S. Blunsden, J. Boger, B. Richards, K. Zutis, L. Young and J. Hoey, Towards the development of a technology for art therapy and dementia: Definition of needs and design constraints, *The Arts in Psychotherapy* (2010), 4, (in press).
[42] A. Mihailidis, J. Boger, T. Craig and J. Hoey, The COACH prompting system to assist older adults with dementia through handwashing: An efficacy study, *BMC Geriatrics* **8** (2008).
[43] L. Nygard, Responses of persons with dementia to challenges in daily activities: A synthesis of findings from empirical studies, in: *International Congress, 13th, Jun 2002, Stockholm, Sweden, Earlier Preliminary Results of this Study Were Presented at the Aforementioned Conference*, Vol. 58, Jul.-Aug. 2004, pp. 435–445.
[44] R. Orpwood, C. Gibbs, T. Adlam, R. Faulkner and D. Meegahawatte, The design of smart homes for people with dementia – User-interface aspects, *Universal Access in the Information Society* **4** (2005), 156–164.
[45] M.G. Ory, R.R. Hoffman, J.L. Yee, S. Tennstedt and R. Schulz, Prevalence and impact of caregiving: A detailed comparison between dementia and nondementia caregivers, *The Gerontologist* **39** (1999), 177–186.
[46] A. Phinney, Family strategies for supporting involvement in meaningful activity by persons with dementia, *Journal of Family Nursing* **12** (2006), 80–101.
[47] M.E. Pollack, Autominder: A case study of assistive technology for elders with cognitive impairments, *Generations: The Journal of the American Society on Aging* **30** (2006), 67–69.
[48] M.E. Pollack, Intelligent technology for an aging population: The use of AI to assist elders with cognitive impairment, *AI Magazine* **26** (2005), 9–24.
[49] D. Poole and A. Mackworth, *Artificial Intelligence: Foundations of Computational Agents*, Cambridge University Press, 2010.
[50] L.G. Portney and M.P. Watkins, Multiple comparison tests, *Foundations of clinical research: Applications to practice* (2009), 479-501.
[51] D. Poulson and S. Richardson, USERfit – A framework for user centred design in assistive technology, *Technology and Disability* **9** (1998), 163–171.
[52] J. Quinlan, *C4.5: Programs for Machine Learning*, Morgan Kaufmann, San Mateo, CA, 1993.
[53] C. Rainville, H. Amieva, S. Lafont, J.F. Dartigues, J.M. Orgogozo and C. Fabrigoule, Executive function deficits in patients with dementia of the Alzheimer's type: A study with a Tower of London task, *Archives of Clinical Neuropsychology* **17** (2002), 513–530.
[54] C.E. Rasmussen and C.K. Williams, *Gaussian Processes for Machine Learning*, MIT Press, 2006.
[55] B. Reisberg, E.H. Franssen, M. Bobinski and S. Auer, Overview of methodologic issues for pharmacologic trials in mild, moderate and severe Alzheimer's disease, *International Psychogeriatrics* **8** (Sum. 1996), 159–193.
[56] S. Rogerson, *Ethics and e-Inclusion*, European Commission (Information Society and Media), Brussels, Belgium, Sept. 2008.
[57] L. Rosenberg, Navigating through tecnological landscapes: Views of people with dementia or MCI and their significant others, in: *Department of Neurobiology, Care Sciences and Society*, Vol. PhD, Karolinska Institutet, Stockholm, Sweden, 2009, p. 97.
[58] S. Russell and P. Norvig, *Artificial Intelligence*, A Modern Approach, Prentice Hall, 2010.
[59] M.J. Scherer, T. Hart, N. Kirsch and M. Schulthesis, Assistive technologies for cognitive disabilities, *Critical Reviews in Physical and Rehabilitation Medicine* **17** (2005), 195.
[60] R. Schulz and S. Beach, Caregiving as a risk factor for mortality: The caregiver health effects study, *Journal of the American Medical Association* **282** (1999), 2215–2219.
[61] M. Smith, L.A. Gerdner, G.R. Hall and K.C. Buckwalter, History, development, and future of the progressively lowered stress threshold: A conceptual model for dementia care, *Journal of the American Geriatrics Society* **52** (2004), 1755–1760.
[62] F.A. Sorond, A. Galica, J.M. Serrador, D.K. Kiely, I. Iloputaife, L.A. Cupples and L.A. Lipsitz, Cerebrovascular hemodynamics, gait, and falls in an elderly population: MOBILIZE Boston study, *Neurology* **74** (2010), 1627–1633.

[63] R. Sutton and A.G. Barto, *Reinforcement Learning: An Introduction*, MIT Press, 1998.
[64] Y.W. Teh, M.I. Jordan, M.J. Beal and D.M. Blei, Hierarchical Dirichlet processes, *Journal of the American Statistical Association* **101** (2006), 1566–1581.
[65] P. Topo, Technology studies to meet the needs of people with dementia and their caregivers, *Journal of Applied Gerontology* **28** (2009), 5–37.
[66] G.A. van Kan, Y. Rolland, S. Andrieu, P. Anthony, J. Bauer, O. Beauchet, M. Bonnefoy, M. Cesari, L.M. Donini, S. Gillette-Guyonnet, M. Inzitari, I. Jurk, F. Nourhashemi, E. Offord-Cavin, G. Onder, P. Ritz, A. Salva, M. Visser and B. Vellas, Gait speed at usual pace as a predictor of adverse outcomes in community-dwelling older people, *Journal of Nutrition, Health and Aging* **13** (2009), 881–889.
[67] L.M. Verbrugge and A.M. Jette, The disablement process, *Social science & medicine* **38** (1994), 1–14.
[68] J. Verghese, R.B. Lipton, M.J. Katz, C.B. Hall, C.A. Derby, G. Kuslansky, A.F. Ambrose, M. Sliwinski and H. Buschke, Leisure activities and the risk of dementia in the elderly, *New England Journal of Medicine* **348** (2003), 2508–2516.
[69] G. Virone, M. Alwan, S. Dalal, S.W. Kell, B. Turner, J.A. Stankovic and R. Felder, Behavioral patterns of older adults in assisted living, *IEEE Transactions Information Technology in Biomedicine* **12** (2008).
[70] L.C. Watson, C.L. Lewis, C.G. Moore and D.V. Jeste, Perceptions of depression among dementia caregivers: findings from the CATIE-AD trial, *International Journal of Geriatric Psychiatry*, 2010, (online, pre-print).
[71] S. Wey, *The Ethical Use of Assistive Technology*, 2007.
[72] R.S. Wilson, L.L. Barnes, N.T. Aggarwal, P.A. Boyle, L.E. Hebert, C.F. Mendes de Leon and D.A. Evans, Cognitive activity and the cognitive morbidity of Alzheimer disease, *Neurology* **75** (2010), 990–996.

Handbook of Ambient Assisted Living
J.C. Augusto et al. (Eds.)
IOS Press, 2012

doi:10.3233/978-1-60750-837-3-331

Tracking Natural Human Movements Identifies Differences in Cognition and Health

William KEARNS, PhD[a,*] and James L. FOZARD, PhD[b]
[a] *Department of Rehabilitation and Mental Health Counseling, University of South Florida, Tampa, Florida USA 33612*
[b] *Department of Aging Studies, University of South Florida, Tampa, Florida USA 33612*

Abstract. In this chapter we discuss efforts to measure natural human movement and describe a novel location aware technology to study the relationship of movement to health changes. Several syndromes whose understanding may be increased by a more thorough analysis of movement are identified. We conclude with a discussion of how location aware technologies can play a role in identifying problems and solutions in the design of living spaces for the elderly.

Keywords. Movement path tortuosity, chronic diseases, fractal dimension, dementia, gerontechnology goals

Location Aware and Health Surveillance Technology in Health Care

The estimated number of countries with two million persons 65 years of age and older is 26, 38 and 72 respectively for 1990, 2008, and 2040 [33]. The 2000 figure for the US is 12.4% due largely to sustained immigration of younger persons and their families. The swelling healthcare budget associated with older populations has forced governments to consider innovative technological approaches to mitigate rising healthcare costs. One innovation under study is to implement "smart house" technologies in the homes of persons who may be at risk of developing expensive chronic disorders or suffering the effects of their sequelae [47]. This strategy includes monitoring and evaluating behavioral changes [20] including the early detection of potentially expensive or lethal disorders, the delineation of high fall risk areas in the home through the study of resident traffic patterns [61], or detecting falls and injuries rapidly and summoning prompt assistance in order to minimize recovery costs [19].

In each case the intent is to improve care through improved surveillance and significantly reduce the likelihood that the resident will transit into an expensive formal care environment before it is absolutely necessary. A considerable body of mental and physical health evidence supports the practice of maintaining persons in their own homes vs. transferring them to formal care settings where they may be cut off from their social support networks [11,38,43,54].

*Corresponding Author: William Kearns, PhD, Department of Rehabilitation and Mental Health Counseling, University of South Florida, Tampa, Florida 33612. E-mail: kearns@usf.edu.

1. Space Provides the Context for Movements, Memories and Goals

The movement ecology paradigm provides a theoretical framework for studying human path tortuosity (the degree to which an person's movement path deviates from a straight line); it is a transactional analysis that links three features of an individual – their internal state, their navigational capacity and their motion capacity – with features of their external environment [42, p. 10954]. Each change in the location of the individual, termed a "movement path", brings about a change in the person-environment dynamic that potentially alters any or all of the three components of the moving individual. The internal state, or "why move", is defined by the goal of traversing a space for a meal, getting to a sleeping area, or to engage in recreation. Navigational capacity, having the ability to execute "where to move", is differentially affected by the presence of dementia and by differences in the individual's cognitive abilities. Motion capacity, or knowing "how to move", applies to both persons who walk independently, with the aid of a walker, or who use a wheelchair.

The movement ecology paradigm informs our understanding of dementia's effect on navigational capacity, as reflected in the shape of the movement paths elders make while traveling. Luis and Brown (2007) argue that dementia may affect navigational capacity either by changing orientation [10,21,55] or by difficulty shifting attention – an executive function – [8,46,52]. At present no convincing evidence exists to refute either hypothesis, partly because researchers have included persons at different stages of dementia.

Another way dementia might affect path tortuosity is through motion capacity or "how to move". Stride to stride gait speed variability and length, measured when elders walk on prescribed paths, correlates negatively with cognitive performance measures, including the MMSE, in both normal aged and in persons with clinical diagnoses of dementia [7,60]. Standardized gait and balance assessments (SGB) include stride length, step length, support base, step time, swing time, stance time, single support time, double support time and average velocity measures [25,51]. Static balance assessment includes body sway measures recorded when standing on one or two legs with eyes open or closed; dynamic balance assessments are made while walking and performing an additional task such as talking on a cell phone. Recently researchers [7,59] have employed fractal analytic techniques to SGB thereby unveiling gait and balance variability information leading to improved fall prediction. Hausdorff and colleagues [7] have found that increased stride time variability predicted heightened fall risk in community dwelling elders; stride time variability in this study also correlated negatively (–.47) with participants' MMSE scores. To summarize, in dementia, all three movement ecology paradigm hypotheses (why move, where to move and how to move) predict dementia will increase movement path tortuosity through its degenerative neurological effects on structures controlling motivation, navigational abilities, and skeletal muscle activity.

When applied to the study of animal models of movement path tortuosity, the movement ecology paradigm has focused on four main factors; the ability or strength to orient towards a specific goal in space [6], the distance at which an animal orients towards that goal [16], the tendency for the animal to continue travelling in the direction it has been going (i.e. angular momentum) [36] and speed of travel [9]. An animal travels with a more tortuous path when any of orientation strength, orientation distance, angular momentum or speed decreases. Both disordered spatial orientation and shifting attention would affect the ability to consistently orient towards a spatial goal. Increased gait variability would decrease angular momentum. All of these factors individually or combined would result in more tortuous movement paths. Obtaining accurate spatial data requires accurate mapping of movement paths over long intervals in natural environments using sensor networks.

2. Normal Aging and Chronic Diseases Affect Gait, Balance and Falls

Normal aging itself, depression and vascular dementia, diabetes, cardiovascular disease, Parkinson's disease and iatrogenesis – a result of drugs used to treat some of the others – are age associated diseases with consequences for gait, balance and falls. An abbreviated summary [30], of the varied consequences of these diseases on gait, balance and falls is given below.

2.1. Normal Physical Changes With Age

- Slower reaction times, gait changes, decreased muscle strength, endurance, and sensory perception often resulting in falls and fractures Falls related to these physical changes are associated with high mortality and morbidity rates in the elderly population.

2.2. Mental Status, e.g., Depression and Dementia Is Affected By Chronic Diseases

- Fall risks for cognitively impaired older persons are double those for normal elders [32, p. 131].
- Limited activities result in isolation of the individual and
- Increased risk for cardiac disease and "metabolic syndrome" that may cause vascular dementia.

2.3. Diabetes Mellitus

- Disease characterized by impaired output of the Islet cells of the pancreas, and/or resistance of end-organ receptors to the utilization of insulin. This results in muscle strength loss and atrophy, weakness of cardiac muscle, inability to metabolize lipids, and changed endothelial artery lining throughout the body.
- Alterations in cerebral, renal, cardiac, and peripheral vasculature occur resulting in impaired mental functioning, inability to walk, lethargy and visual deficits [35]. During hypoglycemic episodes insulin is suppressed decreasing glucose uptake and utilization in peripheral tissues resulting in neuroglycopenic symptoms that include confusion, dizziness, convulsions and loss of consciousness. Diabetics may also exhibit tremors, palpitations, and loss of coordination and these symptoms may produce impaired mental functioning and gait disturbances.

2.4. Coronary Artery Diseases

- Arteriosclerosis, atherosclerosis, and arteritis of the coronary arteries [44, p. 1159] often cause peripheral vascular diseases such as stroke and arterial venous malformations.
- Strokes may result in the loss of physical ability to speak, ambulate and/or do self care thus producing limitations of activities [22, p. 757].

- Iatrogenesis often results from the side-effects of the anti-hypertensive drugs; patients often become lethargic, dizzy, hypotensive, and often experience diuresis. Iatrogenic patients may experience the loss of proprioception producing impaired coordination and an inability to ambulate. Neurological changes affecting gait and balance in hypertensives may begin long before treatment starts and may thus be evaluated using gait detection algorithms [34].

2.5. Metabolic Syndrome

- Metabolic syndrome is a cluster of cardiovascular risk factors including the major components of dyslipidemia, hypertension, and insulin resistance [49, p. 58]. These physiological changes cause generalized weakness, altered gait, and decreased sensory perception.

2.6. Parkinson's Disease

- A movement disorder characterized by stiffness, rigidity, resting tremor and postural instability; a progressive neurodegenerative disorder occurring when neurons in the substatia nigra die or become impaired. Movement disorder measurement related to fatigue and autonomic nervous system alterations may provide early diagnosis and intervention with neuroprotective therapies.
- Impaired ambulation and instability is highly correlated with injury in this population. They may also exhibit "freezing", being stuck in place when attempting to walk. Retropulsion, a tendency to fall backwards, is also experienced when the elders are ambulating [23]. These physical impairments alter the ability to ambulate in a direct pathway, thus technological supervision of movement may assist in the prevention of falls and accidents. Considerable effort has been placed on early diagnosis of Parkinson's Disease through the evaluation of stride time variability measures [7].

2.7. Iatrogenesis

- May result from medications that may precipitate confusion, psychosis, and behavioral changes. Polypharmacy may result in pseudo-dementia as well as physical complications and individuals may exhibit changed gait, and an inability to control body functions which may result in injury. Studies of movement and changes in gait offer early recognition of instability leading to catastrophic physical events.

3. Location Aware Technology Tracks a Person's Location and Movement in Space

Gerontechnology [13] identifies four health related goals of technology, three of which correspond closely to the major goals of public health – primary, secondary, and tertiary prevention. Location aware technology plays a role at all three levels.

Prevention and engagement refers to technology that delays or prevents age-associated physiological and behavioral changes that restrict functioning. In housing, this includes long term support of health through creation and monitoring of safe environments, technology that facilitates the performance of ADLs and IADLs, and adaptability of housing to support the changing needs of people as they age. Active location aware technology can be used to evaluate the safety and use of furniture and appliances in a monitored living space. In congregate living situations it provides information about how residents use space and furnishings for social activities, hobbies, and interactions with fellow residents and staff.

Compensation and assistance refers to technology that compensates for common age associated losses in strength and mobility, sensory and perceptual function, and cognitive function. In living settings, interventions are designed to alter intensity and placement of sources of light or sound, reduce visual glare and masking noise and provide alternative sources of environmental information and the means to respond to it. The goals for persons with cognitive limitations relate to safety, communication, use of environmental information to compensate for memory loss, and assistance to caregivers. The roles of location aware technology include triggering lights, thermostats, alarm systems, controls on doors, etc.

Care support and organization refers to the use of technology either for self-care by elderly persons with existing functional limitations or for care provided by nonprofessional or professional caregivers. Examples include devices that lift and move physically disabled persons, machines that monitor and administer oral and injectable medications, and technology that provides behavioral and physiological information to remote – usually professional – caregivers. Location aware technology supports the monitoring of movements by persons with disabilities, the deployment and monitoring of robots and other devices that serve as surrogates to human caregivers.

Cutting across the other three is technology for *enhancement and satisfaction* – interactive communication, self adapting equipment, and simpler devices – that expand the range and depth of human activities related to comfort, vitality and productivity. Location aware technology facilitates communication with equipment and other people.

3.1. Inexpensive Sensor Technology Monitors Movement in Homes and Formal Care Settings

These technologies are low cost, have wide availability and there is a considerable body of private sector expertise in their use. They are found in home security systems and at least one commercial smart home surveillance system employs a modified home security system and sensor technologies to keep an eye on the residents [50]. They provide key information about general health, e.g., a simple switch attached to the flush control of a standard toilet may provide information about daily elimination. Passive infrared sensors located near bedroom entrances provide information on when an individual arises and retires, but also about disturbances in sleep patterns which may affect general cognitive functioning [1]. Changes in sleep patterns may presage other health problems and may result in increased sedative and/or alcohol consumption; sleep deprivation is associated with an increased risk of traffic fatalities in the general population. Inexpensive sensors include passive infrared devices (PIR) [57] which detect the presence of infrared energy emitted by the human body during normal thermogenesis. PIR systems yield binary (on/off) data similar to contact closures. These sensors can be "tuned" to admit IR from a specific direction thereby enabling detection of the presence of persons in a small region of a room or within a wide area. This feature enables multiple devices to be used in conjunction to get rudimentary data on direction and speed of travel as one sensor "hands off" to the next sensor in the path of the resident as they pass by. A shortcoming of the PIR sensor is that detectable IR emissions do not differ reliably by individual making it impossible to differentiate among persons living in the same environments. Attempts have been made using PIR and mathematical models to study individuals based on patterns of sensor firings [48]. However these approaches have shown only modest success and depend on a consistent census in the dwelling being monitored. The introduction of a new resident renders the process of accurate differentiation impossible using only PIR based systems.

Radio frequency identification devices (RFID) in conjunction with PIR and contact switch closures offer a method to improve differentiation of individuals [47] and improve localization. RFID is widely used in the commercial sector to manage inventory, prevent theft and to speed checkout lines. A miniaturized RFID "tag" includes a transponder which echoes an identification number whenever it is struck by radio waves of a specific frequency. Some versions of the tag are implantable in humans (Verichip) and have a 10 year lifespan inside the body but have raised ethical and security concerns [18]. The most commonly used RFID tags, termed "passive RFID", derive their power from a stationary reader less than a few meters from an individual which emits radio waves and listens for the echoed tag number. When used in conjunction with a network of PIR sensors it is possible to obtain data on an individual's location, rate and direction of travel. Using this approach Pavel, Hayes and colleagues have successfully studied movement variability in persons with Parkinson's syndrome [47].

A second more capable but also more expensive form is "active RFID" which is used to manage wandering behavior in persons with dementia in assisted living facilities and nursing homes. Active RFID systems employ a powered electrical circuit in the tag which allows readers to be far more sensitive to the presence of the tag [62]. This approach has distinct advantages over passive RFID which can operate only at short ranges. A person wandering and intending to elope may deliberately charge an exit door, giving very short notice of their intentions to leave. A passive RFID system might not have sufficient time to respond to a rapid approach since it activates when the tag is very close to the reader and may fail to lock the door in time, prohibiting their departure. Active tags readable at hundreds of meters can be precisely programmed to lock an exit door when an individual is several meters away from it. Unfortunately, active tags must be worn on the wrist, ankle or as a pendant and cannot be implanted. Implantation of powered RFID devices results in significant attenuation of the RFID radio signal, shortening their range from a few hundred meters to just a few meters. There are also teratogenicity issues related to long term exposure to strong radio waves generated from the internal device and the possible interference of active implanted RFID with implanted pacemakers and other devices; experience with external low power active RFID devices has found them to be safe, however [63]. Most active RFID systems improve upon passive RFID through extended transmission range [62]. In general, however they do not provide information about their location unless readers are placed in strategic locations, and the received signal strength (RSSI) from the active RFID tag is used as an indicator of the position of the tag relative to the readers (where greater signal strength equates to proximity to the reader). This strategy works provided the tag's signal strength remains constant over time, which cannot be guaranteed since signal strength varies with battery power level, and battery life decreases the more frequently the tag is probed for its position by the reader. A tag receiving infrequent probes may have its battery last 2 years, while a tag probed multiple times per second may exhaust its battery in just a few hours. An additional problem associated with attempting to triangulate tag position based on signal strength alone is the "multipath" problem which confronts RFID use in indoor environments. Multipath refers to the phenomenon of multiple radio reflections which originate from a source confounding the reliable location of the source of the radio signal [12]. Multipath problems loom large in buildings and vary as a function of the amount of reflective materials in the building's structure, the number of steel items such as desks and filing cabinets, stoves, tables and refrigerators.

3.2. Use of Active Location Aware Technology to Study Movement Patterns Related to Dementia and Cognitive Decline

The authors' work relates the measurement of people's movement inside structures to their health and cognitive function including the early detection of dementia. Dementia affects 6 million Americans [4] for Europeans the 2010 estimate is also 6 million, which will grow to over 14 million by 2050 [39]. There is no known cure for dementia although early detection coupled with medications such as Aricept has shown some effectiveness in slowing the rate of decline [15]. Blood tests for dementia do not exist and differential diagnosis of Alzheimer's dementia from other varieties (vascular dementia and others) must be obtained postmortem. Behavioral symptoms such as memory loss, confusion, inability to perform common activities such as adding up a column of numbers typically eventuate in a neurological assessment being performed and a diagnosis rendered by a qualified professional.

A characteristic of 40–60% of persons with dementia is a tendency to wander, which is defined here as aimless locomotion coupled with confusion resulting in becoming lost in familiar locales [3]. At last count there were in excess of 20 different definitions of wandering which included among other elements the determining of the intent of the wanderer, i.e. to go to unrealistic places such as to visit a dead relative [2], making comprehensive study of the phenomenon rather difficult. Our studies focus on aimless movement as a key component of dementia and we assert that, when correctly measured, all walking, including that of normal individuals, contains a certain amount of "aimlessness" which increases proportionately with the severity of the dementia.

The measurement of aimless movement presupposes the existence of two elements: The first is a system capable of providing accurate positioning of an individual's location over extended observation intervals and, second, a means to quantify "aimlessness" in the movement pattern. Fortunately the first element exists in a specialized variant of active RFID known as Ultra Wideband RFID or UWB [26,28]. UWB is designed for indoor operation in environments which produce multipath interference and gives tag locations to better than +/– 20 cm. Tag dimensions and weight makes it acceptable as a "wristwatch" for most elders and in practice observed battery life is about 2 months. Positional data can be rendered at up to 10/sec; however, we have determined that one update per 0.43 seconds is adequate to obtain accurate tracking information from our freely moving research participants.

Our research environment is an assisted living facility (ALF), which offers hotel services but no professional medical care to individuals needing assistance with one or more activities of daily living. The proportion of residents with diagnoses of dementia at our ALF partners' sites ranges up to 70%. To detect aimless movement we employ four UWB RFID "readers", one each at four corners of an atrium connecting dormitory areas to a dining area and front porch [27,31]. Because the area is a conduit to important locations, research participants pass through the area frequently and provide a sample of their walking behavior. Hence our subjects generate thousands of paths for evaluation in the span of a single month.

The extraction of the aimless component (tortuosity) from the path data is performed using fractal mathematics, specifically "Fractal Dimension" (or Fractal D)

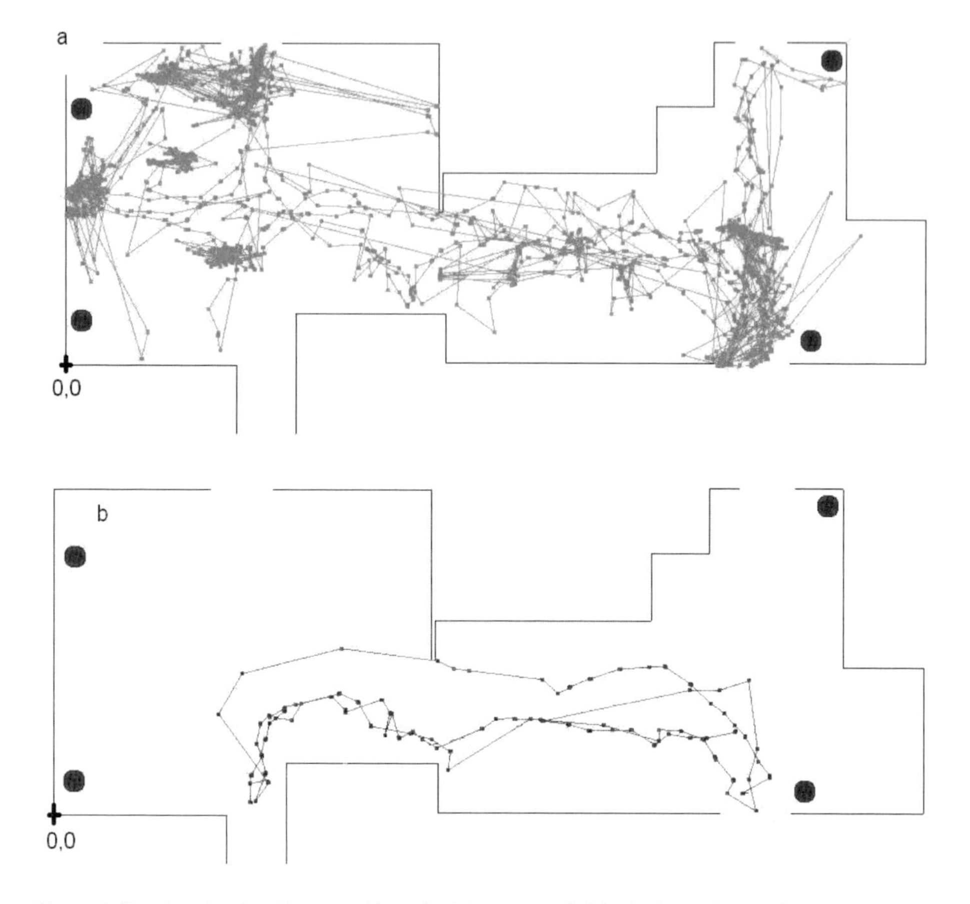

Figure 1. Raw location data for two subjects for 2 hours recorded beginning at 9 a.m. The top panel (a) reveals a subject (#10) with a highly variable paths resulting in a mean Fractal D of 1.62. The lower panel (b) shows a subject who followed relatively straighter paths (#13) and who had a mean Fractal D of 1.24. The subject in the upper frame had the 4th highest fractal D value of any subject and suffered a hip fracture from a fall which occurred after the study's completion. Ovals denote the locations of sensors in the room.

[40,41] which is a method for estimating the tortuosity of a path composed of X and Y coordinates. In its simplest form, Fractal D can vary from a value of 1 for a perfectly straight path requiring only 1 dimension (length) to describe it to a value of 2 which describes a path which is so chaotic that it covers the entirety of a 2 dimensional plane (i.e. Brownian motion). Hence Fractal D may vary continuously from a value of 1.0 to 2.0 according to the amount of the second dimension (width) that is required to describe the path. Using Fractal D we were able to obtain measures of path tortuosity for all subjects taking part in our study.

In a recently completed investigation of 25 elders monitored using UWB over a one month period, a significant negative association ($r = -0.44$ $p = 0.02$) was found between Fractal D path tortuosity and subjects' MMSE scores [29] supporting our working hypothesis that disordered movement predicted cognitive decline in elders. Figure 1 presents data from the tracks of two elders recorded for two hours at approximately the same time one with a diagnosis of dementia (top) and the other without (bottom). The differences in their paths are readily apparent. Further investigations will determine whether Fractal D calculations can be used as a proxy for conventional cognitive measures and allow the near realtime detection of dementia in its nascent stages.

While the application of Fractal D to the study of movement variability has shown promise for the early detection of dementia, it is likely that other physical and mental disorders may have unique movement characteristics which make them amenable to study using the technology described above.

3.3. Home Modifications and Health Surveillance Technologies to Maintain Independent Living by Seniors

The well documented desire of older persons to maintain their independence in their own home [14] is complemented by policy makers' interest in using technology to reduce the costs of health care services provided in institutional settings. The relevant technologies address modification of the home and health and safety surveillance of the occupants of the home. One role of location aware technology in these efforts is to facilitate the evaluation of the effectiveness of the home modifications and surveillance technologies by gathering information about ordinary movement patterns in the areas affected by the interventions.

"Independence" requires the ability to move or be moved safely and effectively throughout different living spaces and to manipulate and operate the products and appliances that support the multiple activities carried out in the home. Both the common age-related changes in gait and those associated with strokes as well as progressive diseases that affect gait can create challenges to maintaining independence – challenges involving one or more of the three dimensions of movement, why, where and how to move. For example, the normal age-related changes in gait relate most clearly to the 'how' dimension – relatively shorter strides taken in a wider stance – both adaptations in gait that result in greater stability while walking [56]. Those associated with chronic and progressive diseases that involve gait vary with the disease as described earlier in the chapter.

The modal pattern of aging occurs and will continue to occur in existing individual homes with multiple occupants – homes not designed to be user-friendly for persons who have or who are developing limitations in personal mobility. Determining what 'user-friendly' means for individuals in specific homes is an idiosyncratic and complex process; the starting point for many planners are the building codes used for congregate living settings for elderly and wheel-chair bound persons. They do not apply to individual homes although Great Britain has introduced such a code for new private home construction. With some variations, such building codes typically include: a level entry to the principal entrance; an entrance door wide enough to allow wheelchair access; wide hallways; a bathroom on the entrance level or first habitable story; and a level or gently sloping approach from the parking space to the dwelling [24]. These architectural features may be supplemented by additional modifications in working and living spaces that support independent functioning for wheelchair-bound persons. Modifying existing individual housing stock along the lines of the building codes described is impractical, expensive and for most elderly persons, unnecessary.

Systematic efforts to customize specific modifications to existing homes to the unique individual needs of its aging occupants have been made in Europe and the United States mostly by occupational therapists. The most sophisticated of these grew out of a six-country study of housing used by elderly persons in Europe [45]. Data from this study, called ENABLE-AGE, included descriptions of the house, the health and functional capacities of its elderly occupants and observations of the occupants carrying out daily tasks. Iwarsson [24, p. 98, Fig. 4.3] lists 15 functional limitations including interpreting information, limitations in vision, hearing, balance, reaching, use of mobility aids, extremes of weight, etc, and relates them to necessary modifications in the interior and exterior of the house. The instrument used by the expert observer is called the Housing Enabler; a self-administering version for use by the resident is called "Usability in my home." Iwarsson recommends that both versions be used in planning home modifications, partly to engage the interest and cooperation of the resident. A similar instrument, "Comprehensive Assessment and Solution Process for Aging Residents" (CASPAR) [53] has been developed in the United States; it is specifically designed to actively involve the resident in decisions about home modifications.

The home adaptations can take many forms depending on the structure of the home and the specific needs of the occupants. Grayson [17] identifies three levels of complexity: I – no modification of existing physical, mechanical or electrical systems; II – replacing and adding to existing elements – widening doorways, installing grab bars, installing emergency alerting systems; and III – major time consuming alterations, e.g., replacing kitchen and bathroom fixtures, adjustable height cabinets and work surfaces.

Location aware technology can supplement and broaden the observations and recommendations made by the expert observer and it provides a longer time frame for establishing patterns of movement and use of these new resources, as well as changes in those patterns after modifications are made. When coupled with other technologies that identify hand and arm movements, information about approaches to and leaving sites where daily activities are performed can be made using machine based information to supplement information gained by expert observers.

4. Uses of Active Location Aware Technology in Intervention Studies

In home-based studies of persons with dementia and their caregivers we have recorded up to two months of daily readings using active tag UWB RFID (Kearns et al. unpublished observations). The array, which costs $7,000, collects data from a room of interest in the home, but nowhere else, with the objective of studying exiting in persons with dementia who wander. Behavioral interventions are then introduced and their impact on exiting evaluated for effectiveness in reducing exiting frequency; the intent in this study is *not* to provide realtime monitoring of behaviors nor consequate exiting but to evaluate the impact of relatively inexpensive behavioral interventions on wandering. Simple behavior management technologies for reducing exiting in persons with dementia include alarms, warning signs and visual illusions which deter approaches to the doorway. Because the system can track approaches to the door and selectively detect those which successfully egress it provides a more thorough description of the exiting process than would be attainable using passive RFID.

The main advantage of active location aware technology over passive devices is its ability to uniquely relate location information of objects or persons wearing the transponders. The UWB RFID technology was developed for tracking location of physical assets, e.g., the location of mobile equipment in a hospital, or the location of parts used in construction of complex pieces machines such as airplanes or cars. The technology is also used in military training exercises showing the precise movements of soldiers in house to house combat simulations.

One feature of Ubisense's active location aware ultra-wideband technology is the wide range of sensitivity of the transponders. In earlier research using this equipment

[31] the location of the tag was determined approximately every 0.43 sec. However, it is possible to estimate tag location more than ten times per sec, thereby making it possible to track movements more precisely. Accordingly, we are currently comparing this technology against other conventional methods and equipment used to assess gait and balance. If comparable results can be obtained, the equipment used to monitor everyday movements of residents in congregate living settings might also perform the standard gait and balance assessments.

Using ultra-wideband RFID technology it is possible to monitor the movements of large numbers of people simultaneously. This creates opportunities to study the locations and time course of interactions among residents in congregate living situations. If staff in the congregate living settings also wear transponders, further opportunities are created for studying the location and time course of interactions between staff and residents, something of considerable interest to managers of Assisted Living Facilities. By the same token, it is possible to evaluate the use of furniture, and appliances placed in common spaces of congregate living settings. Analyses of hourly activity levels in two assisted living facilities [31] have shown that activity increases around scheduled events such as meals and administration of medications by staff to residents (Zeitgebers), and decreases during other times of the day. Altering the arrangement and type of furniture and appliances in the common spaces may increase social interactions and amount of individual movement by residents, thereby potentially improving their mental health. Additional readers would make it possible to remotely and unobtrusively monitor residents' movements in their bedrooms and baths, thereby alerting staff of possible falls or accidents. At least one team of investigators have coupled sensing technologies with guidance algorithms [5] which are designed to encourage good sleeping habits in elders by systematically manipulating light and music levels in their bedrooms.

4.1. Limitations on the Usefulness of Home Modification and Monitoring Technologies

There are two broad categories of limitations on the usefulness of home modification and monitoring technologies. The first concerns the technological devices themselves – reliability, expense, failures and system problems. The second concerns the users of the technologies. One class of limitations include problems of the user interface with the technology e.g., ease and accuracy of linking the device with the person being monitored, difficulty in setting thresholds for triggering the devices and deciding to whom and when to route data. The second class of limitations concern a broad range of issues involved with using the technologies, e.g., the training and background of the users of the data generated by the technologies, coordination of the efforts of multiple players involved in implementing and maintaining the technologies, and the responsibility for payment for services, etc. The following paragraphs mostly address the second class of limitations.

Sensor technologies provide unprecedented opportunities for gathering large amounts of information on elders living in home and community settings. Simply having access to data, however, is not sufficient to ensure improved care. Data is not information until it is interpreted and made sensible to an individual capable of effecting change in the person's living environment or at a higher policy level. Errors in data interpretation may occur at the "living environment" level; for example, a home health worker may interpret changes in bathroom use data to indicate an elder may have a possible urinary tract infection, indicating significant declines in future health are to be expected. A home safety engineer might view the same increased bathroom use as a reason to upgrade the lighting and install bathroom safety features to lessen the likelihood of falls in that area, known to be a high risk area for falls in the elderly. A nutrition and fitness expert might take a contrary view; the increased ambulation through the house (measured in total distance travelled) might be interpreted as a positive indicator that the elder is getting more exercise and should be healthy.

In these hypothetical scenarios having data alone clearly is not sufficient to render a correct assessment of the home situation; but the presence of unexpected data values may serve as a trigger event for a more thorough investigation of the home environment. However, this does not guarantee that the care worker who performs the home assessment will immediately recognize an emerging healthcare issue (such as a nascent UTI) if their particular bias is to interpret the information according to their specialization's frame of reference (e.g. "…if all one knows how to use is a hammer, one tends to treat everything as if it were a nail."). It is the interpretation of the data by the professionals involved that will result in diminished or improved healthcare service delivery. Indeed, it is more likely that an incorrect interpretation of movement data will result in *increased* healthcare expenditures if the home safety engineer installs expensive bathroom upgrades prematurely when antibiotics were indicated, and diagnosis of a UTI is missed. Likewise the nutrition expert who through his own lens sees improved ambulation in the elder's data may literally kill the patient by assuming no visit is needed and all is well, which would prove to be a very expensive outcome indeed.

The correct interpretation of data and its conversion to useful information guiding care and policy decisions is at the heart of good science, and is the crux of creating new reliable and useful technologies that improve health care delivery. Aligning new sources of data with existing healthcare structures can produce confusion for providers who may not know how to interpret the information, and who may choose to ignore the information in favor of tried and true methods such as scheduling routine home visits, and relying on caregiver judgment as to when to visit the doctor. While securing buy-in by professionals is essential, clinicians have a duty to their patients to be skeptical since a failure to do so invites disaster.

A considerable body of research has been sponsored by the DHHS Agency for Healthcare Research and Quality which seeks to identify and remove barriers to the adoption of electronic health records (EHR) by physicians. EHR integrates data from conventional (paper) sources with information electronically produced by automated medical devices, which is then theoretically available to all specialists and physicians treating a given patient irrespective of their location. However the adoption of electronic records by physicians has been a slow process. Part of the reason for the slow rate of adoption has been the substantial initial investment, maintenance and support costs involved, although increased efficiencies and decreased medical errors are anticipated to offset these expenditures over time.

The technical aspects of integrating home tracking systems into an EHR have been mostly addressed. Standardized networked telemedicine applications such as home blood pressure monitors, electronic scales and blood glucose monitors routinely feed data into EHR for remote monitoring by specialists and physicians. However whereas increases in body weight may be easily flagged by an EHR for follow-up, it may be more challenging to draw accurate conclusions from movement tracking information. Intelligent algorithms for detecting and interpreting movement have been created using optical systems [61] as well as passive infrared and inexpensive sensors [37,47] and smart house) which can detect falls when they occur but with few exceptions these systems remain in the prototype stage. The problems associated with the human users of technology are illustrated by the discussion of Tinetti and colleagues [58, p. 720, Table 1] of fall risk evaluation and prevention practices. Although there are accepted practices to reduce the risk of falls in the elderly, their implementation is not easy. Medically oriented providers are not accustomed to dealing simultaneously with the multiple causes of falls; instead they focus on acute and chronic medical care. The potential payers for services, e.g., Medicare, which would reduce fall risk, are concerned about costs, the potential for abuse and fraud and the difficulties of paying multiple providers who might include non-medical personnel and not fit conventional models of reimbursement.

Conclusion

We have seen in this chapter how movement information can provide valuable insights into disorders and can broaden our understanding of their pathogenesis. We have focused not so much upon the gross amount of movement as we have the structure of the movement itself. By differentiating random from well ordered movement components we find significant relationships between spatial variability and disease that complement relationships observed between temporal variability and disease by other researchers such as Hausdorff and Verghese. The study of movement variability using sensor networks may provide fertile ground for the study of Diabetes Mellitus and other disorders which have movement changes as part of their symptomatology.

The study of movement variability can provide direct benefits to elders who seek to remain independent by permitting close study of their home environment's impact on their behavior and could facilitate the systematic restructuring of it to create a more well adapted home with fewer risks and more beneficial features.

Several limitations of both location aware and health surveillance technologies were discussed. The main one is limitation of machines to provide the context for interpreting the data produced.

References

[1] A.M. Adami, T.L. Hayes, M. Pavel and C.M. Singer, Detection and classification of movements in bed using load cells: Engineering in medicine and biology society, in: *27th Annual International Conference of the IEEE-EMBS 2005*, 2005.

[2] D. Algase, D. Moore, D. Gavin-Dreschnack and C. VandeWeerd, Wandering definitions and terms, in: *Evidence-Based Protocols for Managing Wandering Behaviors*, A. Nelson and D.L. Algase, eds, Springer Publishing Company, New York, 2007.

[3] D. Algase, D. Moore, C. Vandeweerd and D.J. Gavin-Dreschnack, Mapping the maze of terms and definitions in dementia-related wandering, *Aging & Mental Health* **11** (2007), 686–698.

[4] Alzheimer's Association, 2009 Alzheimer's disease facts and figures, *Alzheimers Dement* **5** (2009), 234–270.

[5] J.C. Augusto, S. Martin, M.D. Mulvenna, W. Carswell and H. Zheng, Holistic night-time care, in: *Proceedings of the 7th World Conference of the International Society for Gerontechnology*, Vancouver, Canada.

[6] S. Benhamou and P. Bovet, Distinguishing between elementary orientation mechanisms by means of path analysis, *Animal Behaviour* **43** (1992), 371–377.

[7] N. Bernstein, *The Coordination and Regulation of Movements*, Pergamon, London, 1967.

[8] Y.C. Chiu et al., Getting lost: Directed attention and executive functions in early Alzheimer's disease patients, *Dement Geriatr Cogn Disord* **17** (2004), 174–180.

[9] E.A. Codling, M.J. Plank and S. Benhamou, Random walk models in biology, *J. R. Soc. Interface* **5** (2008), 813–834.

[10] M.J. de Leon, M. Potegal and B. Gurland, Wandering and parietal signs in senile dementia of Alzheimer's type, *Neuropsychobiology* **11** (1984), 155–157.

[11] G. Demiris, M.J. Rantz, M.A. Aud, K.D. Marek, H.W. Tyrer, M. Skubic and A.A. Hussam, Older adults' attitudes towards and perceptions of smart home technologies: A pilot study, *Informatics for Health and Social Care* **29** (2004), 87–94.

[12] R.J. Fontana and S.J. Gunderson, Ultra-wideband precision asset location system, in: *IEEE Conference on Ultra Wideband Systems and Technologies, 2002*, Digest of Papers, 2002.

[13] J. Fozard, Impacts of technology on health and self esteem, *Gerontechnology* **4** (2005), 63–76.

[14] J. Fozard and W. Kearns, Persuasive GERONtechnology: Reaping technology's coaching benefits at older age, in: *Persuasive Technology*, W. Ijsselsteijn, Y. de Kort, C. Midden, B. Eggen and E. van den Hoven, eds, LNCS, Vol. 3962, Springer-Verlag, Berlin/Heidelberg, 2006.

[15] D.S. Geldmacher, Donepezil (Aricept) for treatment of Alzheimer's disease and other dementing conditions, *Expert Rev Neurother* **4** (2004), 5–16.

[16] B.J. Goodwin, D.J. Bender, T.A. Contreras, L. Fahrig and J.F. Wegner, Testing for habitat detection distances using orientation data, *Oikos* **84** (1999), 160–163.

[17] J. Grayson, Technology and home adaptations, in: *Staying put: Adapting the places instead of the people*, S. Landspery and J. Hyde, eds, Baywood, Amityville NY, 1997.

[18] J. Halamka, A. Juels, A. Stubblefield and J. Westhues, The security implications of VeriChip cloning, *Journal of the American Medical Informatics Association* **13** (2006), 601–607.

[19] M. Hamill, V. Young, J. Boger and A. Mihailidis, Development of an automated speech recognition interface for Personal Emergency Response Systems, *J. Neuroeng. Rehabil.* **6** (2009), 26.

[20] N. Harvey, Z. Zhou, J.M. Keller, M. Rantz and Z. He, Automated estimation of elder activity levels from anonymized video data, *Conf Proc IEEE Eng Med Biol Soc* **1** (2009), 7236–7239.

[21] V.W. Henderson, W. Mack and B.W. Williams, Spatial disorientation in Alzheimer's disease, *Arch. Neurol.* **46** (1989), 391–394.

[22] J. Hickey, Caring for the patient with cerebrovascular disorders, in: *Medical Surgical Nursing*, K. Osborn, C. Wraa and A. Watson, eds, Pearson, Boston, 2010.

[23] D. Houghton, H. Hurtig and M. Brandabur, *Parkinson's Disease: Medications*, Parkinson's Disease Foundation, Miami, Florida, 2008.

[24] S. Iwarsson, Assessing the fit between older people and their physical home environments: An occupational therapy research perspective, in: *Annual Review of Gerontology and Geriatrics. Focus on aging in context: Socio-physical environments*, W.E. Wahl, R.J. Scheidt and P.G. Windley, eds, Vol. 23, Springer, New York, 2003.

[25] J. Jensen, L. Nyberg, Y. Gustafson and L. Lundin-Olsson, Fall and injury prevention in residential care – effects in residents with higher and lower levels of cognition, *J. Am. Geriatr. Soc.* **51** (2003), 627–635.

[26] W. Kearns, D. Algase, D. Moore and S. Ahmed, Ultra wideband radio: A novel method for measuring wandering in persons with dementia, *Gerontechnology* **7** (2008), 48–57.

[27] W. Kearns and J.L. Fozard, Evaluation of wandering by residents in an assisted living facility (ALF) using ultra wideband radio RTLS, *The Journal of Nutrition, Health & Aging* **13** (2009), S54.

[28] W. Kearns and D. Moore, RFID: A tool for measuring wandering in persons with dementia, in: *Technology and Aging: Selected Papers from the 2007 International Conference on Technology and Aging*, A. Mihailidis, J. Boger, H. Kautz and L. Normie, eds, Vol. 21, IOS Press, Amsterdam, NL, 2008.

[29] W. Kearns, V. Nams, J. Fozard, J. Craighead, Wireless telesurveillance system for detecting dementia, *Gerontechnology* **10** (2011), 90–102.

[30] W.D. Kearns, J.L. Fozard and R.S. Lamm, How knowing who where and when can change healthcare delivery, in: *E-Health, Assistive Technologies and Applications for Assisted Living: Challenges and Solutions*, C. Röcker and M. Ziefle, eds, IGI Global, Hershey, PA, 2011.

[31] W. Kearns, V. Nams and J. Fozard, Wireless fractal estimation of tortuosity in movement paths related to cognitive impairment in assisted living facility residents, *Methods of Information in Medicine* **49** (2010), 592–598.

[32] J.M. Kinney, Nutritional frailty, sarcopenia and falls in the elderly, *Current Opinion in Clinical Nutrition and Metabolic Care* **7** (2004), 15–20.

[33] K. Kinsella and W. He, *An aging world: 2008. International population reports (P95/09-1)*, National Institute on Aging, Washington, DC.

[34] D. Krotish, P. Mitchell, V. Hirth and Y. J. Shin, The use of time-frequency analysis using electromyography and foot pressure distribution for the determination of gait disorders, in: *Proceedings of the 3rd International Congress on Gait & Mental Functions: The Interplay Between Walking, Behavior and Cognition*, 2010.

[35] R. Lamm and E. Lamm, Aging and technology, in: *Dagstuhl Seminar on Assisted Living Systems,* Kaiserslautern, DE.
[36] C.E. McCulloch and M.L. Cain, Analyzing discrete movement data as a correlated random walk, *Ecology* **70** (1989), 383–388.
[37] J.R. Merory, J.E. Wittwer, C.C. Rowe and K.E. Webster, Quantitative gait analysis in patients with dementia with lewy bodies and Alzheimer's disease, *Gait & Posture* **26** (2007), 414–419.
[38] A. Mihailidis, A. Cockburn, C. Longley and J. Boger, The acceptability of home monitoring technology among community-dwelling older adults and baby boomers, *Assist. Technol.* **20** (2008), 1–12.
[39] T. Mura, J.F. Dartigues, C. Berr, How many dementia cases in France and Europe? Alternative projections and scenarios 2010–2050, *Eur. J. Neurol.* (2009).
[40] V.O. Nams, Using animal movement paths to measure response to spatial scale, *Oecologia* **143** (2005), 179–188.
[41] V.O. Nams, Fractal computer program, v3.16, Nova Scotia Agricultural College.
[42] R. Nathan, W.M. Getz, E. Revilla, M. Holyoak, R. Kadmon, D. Saltz and P.E. Smouse, A movement ecology paradigm for unifying organismal movement research, *Proceedings of the National Academy of Sciences* **105** (2008), 19052–19059.
[43] C. Ni Scanaill et al., A review of approaches to mobility telemonitoring of the elderly in their living environment, *Ann. Biomed. Eng.* **34** (2006), 547–63.
[44] K. Osborn, C. Wraa and A. Watson, *Medical Surgical Nursing,* Pearson, Boston, 2010.
[45] F. Oswald et al., Relationships between housing and healthy aging in very old age, *Gerontologist* **47** (2007), 96–107.
[46] R. Passini, C. Rainville, N. Marchand and Y. Joanette, Wayfinding in dementia of the Alzheimer type: Planning abilities, *J Clin Exp Neuropsychol* **17** (1995), 820–832.
[47] M. Pavel, T. Hayes, I. Tsay, D. Erdogmus, A. Paul, N. Larimer, H. Jimison and J. Nutt, Continuous assessment of gait velocity in Parkinson's disease from unobtrusive measurements: CNE'07, in: *3rd International IEEE/EMBS Conference on Neural Engineering, 2007, 5/2/2007-5/5/2007*, Hawaii, USA, 2007, pp. 700–703.
[48] M. Pavel, T.L. Hayes, A. Adami, H. Jimison and J. Kaye, Unobtrusive assessment of mobility, *Conf. Proc. IEEE Eng. Med. Biol. Soc.* **1** (2006), 6277–6280.
[49] E. Roth and D. Laurent-Bopp, Challenges of treating dyslipidemia in patients with the metabolic syndrome, *American Journal for Nurse Practitioners* **8** (2004), 58–66.
[50] M. Rowe, S. Lane and C. Phipps, CareWatch: A home monitoring system for use in homes of persons with cognitive impairment, *Topics in Geriatric Rehabilitation* **23** (2007), 3.
[51] L.Z. Rubenstein, Falls in older people: Epidemiology, risk factors and strategies for prevention, *Age Ageing* **35**(Suppl 2) (2006), ii37–ii41.
[52] J.P. Ryan et al., Graphomotor perseveration and wandering in Alzheimer's disease, *J. Geriatr. Psychiatry Neurol.* **8** (1995), 209–212.
[53] J.A. Sanford, J. Pynoos, A. Tejral and A. Browne, Development of a comprehensive assessment for delivery of home modifications, *Physical & Occupational Therapy in Geriatrics* **20** (2001), 43–55.
[54] A.J. Sixsmith, An evaluation of an intelligent home monitoring system, *J. Telemed Telecare* **6** (2000), 63–72.
[55] L. Snyder, P. Rupprecht, J. Pyrek, S. Brekhus and T. Moss, Wandering, *The Gerontologist* **18** (78), 272.
[56] W.W. Spirduso, Balance, posture and locomotion, in: *Physical Dimensions of Aging*, W.W. Spirduso, ed., Human Kinetics, Champaign, Illinois, 1995.
[57] T. Suzuki, S. Murase, T. Tanaka and T. Okazawa, New approach for the early detection of dementia by recording in-house activities, *Telemedicine Journal E Health* **13** (2007), 41–44.
[58] M.E. Tinetti, C. Gordon, E. Sogolow, P. Lapin and E.H. Bradley, Fall-risk evaluation and management: Challenges in adopting geriatric care practices, *Gerontologist* **46** (2006), 717–725.
[59] J. Verghese, R. Holtzer, R.B. Lipton and C. Wang, Quantitative gait markers and incident fall risk in older adults, *J. Gerontol. A Biol. Sci. Med. Sci.* **64A** (2009), 896–901.
[60] J. Verghese, R. Lipton, C. Hall, G. Kuslansky, M. Katz and H. Buschke, Abnormality of gait as a predictor of non-Alzheimer's dementia, *N. Eng. J. Med.* **347** (2002), 1761–1768.
[61] S. Wang, M. Skubic and Y. Zhu, Activity density map dis-similarity comparison for eldercare monitoring, in: *Conf. Proc. IEEE Eng. Med. Biol. Soc.*, Vol. 1, 2009, pp. 7232–7235.
[62] R. Weinstein, RFID: A technical overview and its application to the enterprise, *IT Professional* **7** (2005), 27–33.
[63] D. Wyld, RFID 101: The next big thing for management, *Management Research News* **29** (2006), 154–173.

Handbook of Ambient Assisted Living
J.C. Augusto et al. (Eds.)
IOS Press, 2012

doi:10.3233/978-1-60750-837-3-346

AAL Markets – Knowing Them, Reaching Them. Evidence from European Research

Ingo MEYER[*], Sonja MÜLLER and Lutz KUBITSCHKE
empirica Gesellschaft für Kommunikations- und Technologieforschung mbH, Bonn, Germany

Abstract. Ambient-assisted living services are slowly but surely making their way into daily practice and life. At the same time, levels of uptake both in Europe and North America remain low and the deployment of services that are fit for this complex market remains a challenge and often fails. The present chapter provides an overview of the market for AAL services in the world and gives some guidance from practice on how these markets can be reached.

Keywords. AAL, markets, telecare, telehealth, deployment, Europe

Introduction

While there is widespread consent that information and communication technology (ICT) can be beneficial to older people and while there is also increasing evidence that ICTs are making their way into daily practice and life, developing ambient-assisted living (AAL) services that are fit for the market remains a challenging task. As far as statistics on the actual usage of AAL services are available, these show rather low levels of uptake in terms of older people actually using them. Uptake also differs widely when comparing different countries in- and outside the European Union with each other.

Factors that contribute to the situation being as it is include the perception of the role, place and value of services such as telecare and telehealth in overall care service provision, limited provision of services alongside a lack of public funding or fragmentation between different bodies with reimbursement responsibility, disparities in geographical provision, technological factors such as the update to new digital telecommunication networks or infrastructural readiness in general, the challenge of transition from pilot activities to mainstream service provision and many more.

Depending on situation and perspective, these factors can be regarded as market barriers or as characteristics of the underlying service provision systems. Regardless of what they are called it seems to be certain that these factors must be taken into account and be actively addressed in order to be able to achieve the successful deployment of AAL services and to fulfil the promises of improved quality of life for older people, people with chronic conditions and family carers, of better quality of care services, and of increased efficiency of service provision that come with them.

[*] Corresponding Author: Ingo Meyer, Research Consultant, empirica, Oxfordstr. 2, 53111 Bonn, Germany. E-mail: ingo.meyer@empirica.com.

Against this background, the present chapter wants to give an overview of the situation of the market for AAL services in the world and to provide some guidance – or food for thought – from practice on how this market can be reached. The chapter is based on research findings and practical experience stemming from our work in various European research studies, RTD and deployment projects and is divided into two main parts: The first gives an overview of today's market for AAL in key economies. The second presents an approach to support the deployment of AAL services that takes into account market characteristics and brings them to bear on different aspects of the service deployment cycle. What links the two parts is our experience that a thorough understanding of (national) deployment environments ("markets") and their framework conditions is necessary to successfully develop and implement AAL services. This understanding has to go beyond figures on potential demand or cost savings and beyond a purely technical understanding of functionalities provided by AAL devices into the area of knowing how older people organize their day-to-day life and where there is a need for outside support, how different types of services are being delivered, how provider and reimbursement structures work, and what impacts new services have on the different actors involved.

Among the first challenges confronting our task are the lack of an agreed definition of what the term "ambient assisted living" encompasses in terms of concepts, services and technologies and also the necessity to separate what is possible today or in the near future from what may become a reality in the longer run. We start by providing such a – working – definition in the first part of this chapter. In general, we decided to adopt a service-centred point of view rather than a product- or application-centred one since this seems to us to best reflect the fact that ambient-assisted living is usually part of a wider scheme, a service.

This chapter should be considered a practical guide and fresh entry-point into the topic of market-oriented development and deployment of AAL services. It aims to encourage readers to re-think the way they have done these things before. It is also a place where they will find both new things and things they have done before. It is – unfortunately – not a complete reference to all topics touched and it is certainly not the final word on the matter and we will be happy to hear our readers' comments, corrections and additions to it.

We are indebted to a number of colleagues at empirica and to former and current project partners, especially from the ICT & Ageing study [11] and the SOPRANO [29], CommonWell [8] and INDEPENDENT [12] projects for many fruitful discussions and contributions around the topics that we write about in this chapter. We would like to thank them for their direct and indirect contributions to our work.

1. The Global AAL Market – An Overview

1.1. The AAL Market – Hype or Reality?

The rise of the AAL concept has largely been driven by the interactions between two major forces of socio-economic change – demographic ageing and the increasing pervasiveness of Information and Communication Technologies (ICTs). Over recent years, the significant social and economic challenges connected with this demographic development have received attention in many countries around the world [14]. In particular, the increasing burden of long term conditions has widely been recognized as a key challenge that welfare and health systems will face during the 21st century in Europe and elsewhere [34]. At the same time, it has been frequently highlighted that current welfare and health systems tend to be rather ill-equipped when it comes to meeting the requirements of care recipients with increasingly complex needs, especially those with chronic conditions, because they are largely built around episodic models of care and support (see for instance [25,33]). Not at least, policy-makers and care planners are challenged by insufficient human and capital capacity to meet increasing demand for services, and the need to prioritize finite budgets [17].

Against this background, the use of ICT-based products and services to provide care in the community has often been proposed as a solution to mitigate the considerable strain faced by national welfare and health systems [17]. The potential offered by technology also extends into other domains. These include, for instance, more general, everyday social inclusion of older people and support for active ageing in the employment context. At least potentially, there is thus a broad range of ICT-based products and services that can be subsumed under the AAL heading.[1] In many countries, AAL is now seen to present "an opportunity for a 'win-win-win' outcome, whereby needs of older people are met in a high quality manner, the costs of providing care and support are maintained at manageable levels for society, and new market opportunities open up for ICT-based products and services" [14].

Despite the many hopes that are connected with a more widespread use of AAL solutions, it has become evident that, up till now, market forces by themselves have been insufficient to ensure the realization of the full potential in this field.[2] Part of the challenge is to separate the 'hype' from the reality. "On the surface, at least, many of the innovations in this field appear, 'self-evidently', to have a high utility value for meeting the needs of older people and of the ageing society. This can sometimes lead to a tendency to see the problem as one of relying solely on spreading the message in order for widespread deployment and market development to take-off. The reality, in fact, seems quite different – even in countries where there has long been awareness of what ICTs can offer and a high receptiveness towards ICTs, full embedding and mainstreaming of existing products and services has often been slow" [14].

When it comes to mainstreaming of AAL solutions, i.e. their routine application beyond a merely experimental or pilot stage, the recent ICT & Ageing study revealed that most market development can today be observed in three main 'market' segments that typically structure the service delivery landscape in many countries in Europe and elsewhere – social care, health care and housing.[3] These are graphically summarized in Fig. 1.

[1] In Europe, for instance the AAL Joint Program – a R&D funding program for innovative ICT-based solutions (products, services, and systems) – has been launched with a view to improving the quality of life, autonomy, participation in social life, skills, and employability of older people [34].

[2] The European Commission has for instance highlighted in its Action Plan on Information and Communications Technology for Ageing that "the market of ICT for ageing well in the information society is still in its nascent phase, and does not yet fully ensure the availability and take-up of the necessary ICT-enabled solutions" (COM((2007)) 332 final, p. 3). Although a considerable range of promising devices and systems has emerged from RTD efforts pursued in Europe and beyond for more than a decade, wider mainstreaming of ICT-enabled solutions within real world service settings has to a large extent yet to occur. Some of the underlying reasons identified in the Commission's action plan include insufficient understanding of user needs, an underdeveloped marketplace and lack of visibility of relevant solutions to potential deployer organizations and end users, as well as technical, infrastructural and regulatory barriers.

[3] This research included inter alia a benchmarking exercise in relation to the level of mainstreaming of ICT-based services across 16 countries, 14 from the EU and 2 from relevant third countries, namely US and Japan. The EU countries were selected to give a good coverage in terms of 'old' and 'new' Member States,

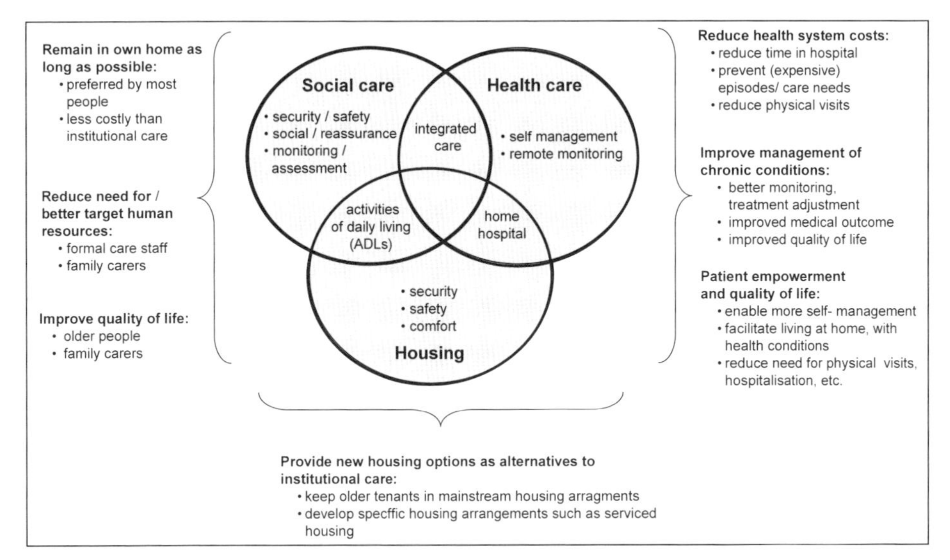

Figure 1. Today's key AAL deployment domains, functionalities and basic rationales. Source: Adapted from ICT & Ageing, 2010 [14].

In the following, we briefly discuss the evidence that has become available from this research in relation to current levels of mainstreaming of AAL solutions across these market segments (for a detailed presentation see [14]).

1.2. The Current Deployment Situation

In the social care domain, the term 'telecare' is now commonly used as a synonym for community alarm services. Increasingly, such services include a range of enhancements to the basic social alarm service concept. Here, telecare is concerned with the provision of social care (i.e. non-medical services) in the home. Typical examples include the provision of various sensors in the home (e.g. fall detectors, bed/chair occupancy sensors, smoke, gas and flood detectors, and so on) that alert social care services in the event of a problem arising in the home. Often, but not always, such telecare services are developed as add-ons to the basic social alarm services and are implemented over the social alarm infrastructure. In addition, videophone-based or other remote social care for the home can also be considered forms of telecare. At present, the most mature market in the social care domain concerns social alarms – frequently called "first generation telecare". This form of telecare can be considered mainstream in the majority of countries covered in the benchmarking exercise, in the sense that social alarms are available across the country and are provided on a regular basis. However, estimated levels of utilization vary considerably, from below 1% to more than 15% of older people, as can be seen in Fig. 2. Although basic push button alarms have been around for more than 20 years, overall levels of actual utilization have remained quite modest even in countries where they are widely available and publicly provided or at least subsi-

large and small countries, different health and social care systems, and countries that would be expected to vary in their current level of advancement as regards the use of ICTs in care and support for older people. The EU countries covered were: BG, DE, DK, ES, FI, FR, HU, IE, IT, NL, PL, SE, SI, and UK. For further details see [11].

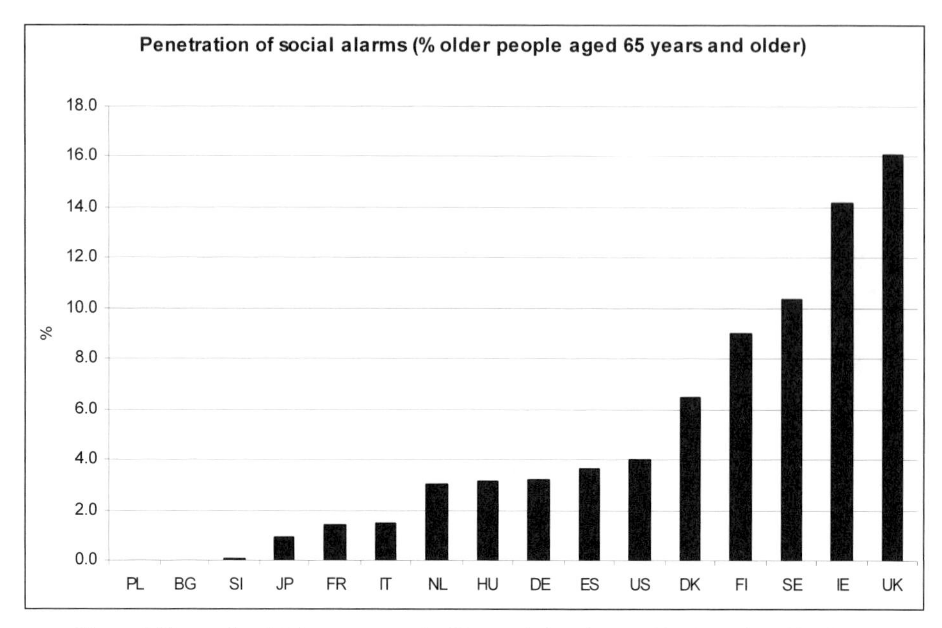

Figure 2. Usage of social alarms among the 65+ population. Source: ICT & Ageing, 2010 [14].

Table 1. Main providers of telecare services.

Mainly provided directly by (or through outsourcing by) social care and/or housing services	Mainly private provider market
DE, DK, ES, FI, FR, HU, IT, NL, SE, SI, HU, (JP), (US)	IE, PL, (US), (JP)

Source: ICT & Ageing Study, 2010.

Table 2. Who provides the physical response?

Formal care staff	Family/informal carers	Mixture
FI, SE, DK, HU	ES, IE, IT, FR, PL	SI, DE, US, NL, JP, UK

Source: ICT & Ageing study, 2010 [14].

dized, e.g. in Denmark and Germany. This finding points to the fact that – beyond the inherent functionalities of the technology – contextual factors seem to exert a major influence on the extent to which the service is taken up by the population.

Social alarm services are commonly provided by social care and/or housing organizations, either directly through alarm/response centres run by the social care (or housing) services themselves or through various forms of outsourcing to or reimbursement of private sector providers (Table 1). However, there are some countries where the main provision for older people living in their own homes is by the private sector exclusively, i.e. with little or no direct linkage to mainstream social care services.

A particular question as regards integration into the social service landscape of a given country – not least when it comes to the 'business case' – relates to how the response is delivered once the call centre has been alerted of an alarm event. The core dimension here is whether the response is expected to be made informally, e.g. by the family, or by paid social care staff (Table 2).

Table 3. Current maturity of home telehealth.

Considerable mainstreaming	Some (localized) mainstream implementations and/or extensive trials	Some pilot/trial activity	Little or no activity
US, JP	DE, DK, ES, FI, FR, IT, NL, SE, UK	HU, PL	IE, SI, BG

Source: ICT & Ageing study, 2010 [14].

More advanced telecare – frequently called "second generation telecare" – involving provision of additional sensors to enhance basic social alarm services, is only reaching a state close to mainstream in the UK. For the most advanced ("third generation") telecare, involving extensive activity monitoring, data gathering and lifestyle analysis, implementation to date has mostly been in pilots/trials, although a few examples of mainstreamed services can already be identified.

The concept of home telehealth refers to the use of ICTs in the delivery of medically-oriented care services to older people in their homes. It can include a variety of different services or applications, including telemonitoring (e.g. blood pressure, blood glucose, ECG, etc.), teleconsultation (e.g. online, by videophone, by telephone) and telerehabilitation (e.g. by videophone), as well as self-care devices to be used by people in their own homes to help them monitor and manage their health themselves. Some home telehealth applications/services may be developed as add-ons to the basic social alarm services. However, they are often developed and implemented independent of this, in part because of the traditionally separate organization of and demarcation between medical care and social care. Overall, home telehealth is less mainstreamed than telecare at present, at least in comparison to basic first generation telecare in the form of social alarms. No country has 'full' mainstreaming in the sense that all of the relevant healthcare providers, in all parts of the country, include such services within their repertoire (cf. Table 3).

Overall, the US and Japan appear to show most development, with many instances of mainstream services, including extensive home telehealth services for older clients provided by the Veterans Administration in the US and provision of a variety of services by quite a number of prefectures across Japan since as far back as the early 2000s. Some European countries do have examples, at least, of mainstream implementation of varying scope/scale, although in many cases these are quite localised initiatives involving just one provider or cluster of local providers. There are currently (and have been) a variety of relatively large-scale trials as well. In EU countries, the main providers of home telehealth services have been hospitals and, less commonly, other healthcare facilities, in some cases in collaboration with other players such as clinics or general practitioners. In the US various public and private healthcare facilities and providers have been involved. The main applications that can be found in mainstream services are the use of home telehealth to support chronic disease management and there is also some activity in relation to early discharge from hospital (hospital-at-home). In terms of chronic conditions, the main attention has been focused on conditions such as heart disease, chronic respiratory disease and diabetes, which are especially common amongst older people. To a large extent, existing approaches are generally not age-specific as such, even if many of the users are, in fact, older people.

When it comes to combined approaches that include both telecare and telehealth dimensions there seems little indication that the traditional demarcations between health and social care have been overcome. Whilst quite a number of RTD projects, pilots and trials take a more integrated, holistic approach, in reality the majority of mainstreamed services focus on one or the other dimension and to be firmly located within either the social or health care domains.

In the housing domain, the term 'smart homes' is widely used to describe a range of environmental control, home automation and home network systems that can help older people to remain living independently in their own homes. These do not necessarily rely upon a service that is delivered into the people's homes with help of ICT. In addition to such 'systems', there are also a variety of more standalone ICT-based assistive technologies that can help older people to remain independent. Examples include computer-based or other electronic communication aids, object locators, reminder systems and so on. The available evidence suggests that the extent of provision and take-up of such technologies for varies considerably across countries, with the Nordic countries generally seen as more advanced in this regard [15]. At the smart home end of the spectrum, the evidence from the 16 countries suggests that there are a lot of RTD projects, trials and demonstrators but no well-advanced mainstreaming. Only in very few countries did the smart homes 'market' seem to have become established, e.g. Netherlands where there is a dedicated policy effort towards mainstreaming 'domotics' in newly developed serviced housing for older people and Finland were a lot of serviced housing and/or residential accommodation for older people seems to incorporate some degree of intelligence.

Finally, although most observed market development seems to be in relation to ICT-based services that are implemented by or supported by social care, healthcare or housing organizations, it is also important to recognize the potential for a substantial consumer market in this field. In the social care field, there is already an emerging mixed market for telecare and other ICT-products – in some countries such services are privately purchased. As more useful devices appear it is likely that in many cases they will be purchased as consumer goods by older people or their families (e.g. medication reminders, object locators and so on). Another relevant trend is the increasing interest in the application of more general purpose consumer goods (such as the Nintendo WII) to support activation of older people. There is also a growing consumer industry focusing on 'brain trainer' type devices (or online services) that purport to help maintain cognitive capacities as they grow older. In the housing market, a number of countries have seen growing provision and demand for private retirement-village type schemes. Already some of these are beginning to include telecare, home telehealth and various smart home facilities and this can be expected to grow in the future. In the healthcare arena, there is considerable interest in the consumer health device/system market, including devices for self-monitoring and diagnosis. This may become a considerable market in the future as large electronics and other companies begin to address it. Already some of the home telehealth systems/devices that are targeted at healthcare providers are beginning to be marketed as self-help devices for private consumer purchase.

1.3. Key Factors That Impact on Further Market Maturing

Although instances of routine applications have emerged in Europe and elsewhere, the mainstreaming of ICT-based solutions still remains a challenge. Additionally, the benchmarking exercise conducted in the framework of the aforementioned ICT & Ageing study suggests that different aspects deserve attention when it comes to the further maturing of the AAL market.

To begin with, uncertainty about the role and relative value of ICT-based solutions in meeting the needs of older people is perhaps the biggest barrier at present. The benchmarking exercise revealed that there may be considerable variability across countries – at least when it comes to the implementation level – in perceptions of the role and importance that should be given to ICT-based solutions within the overall response to meeting the needs of an ageing population. More generally, there is a growing, but loosely organized, body of evaluation results emerging in this field, but much of the evidence comes from circumscribed trials and pilots. Clearly, there is a lack of evidence of the longer-term contribution and value of more advanced systems under real life conditions.

Further to this, various complexities and differences that affect the economic/business case arise across countries, linked to the ways that social/health care services are conceived, provided and funded/reimbursed and many factors can make this difficult to achieve in practice. These include disincentives built into provider and practitioner reimbursement systems, and boundaries and responsibility structures within established social and health care systems. Nevertheless, the emerging evidence-base overall is beginning to suggest a strong potential business or economic case for both telecare and home telehealth, at least at the level of the overall 'system' or public purse.[4]

The ethical perspective is central to the linking and balancing of the 'value' and 'business' cases. Issues of 'distributive' ethics come to the fore when adopting a macro-perspective, such as ensuring that technology-push and/or over-zealous search for cost savings do not result in the withdrawal of necessary and desirable human services; providing as much equality as possible across the population in regard to access to services; and transparency and fairness in the use of technology-based innovations and thus of the costs and benefits, between the state and family. Another level concerns a more micro-ethical perspective which brings attention to particular aspects of the technologies, such as in relation to surveillance in the home, lifestyle monitoring and so on. Both levels deserve careful attention in order to support wider acceptance and appropriate deployment of AAL solutions to support independent living.

Finally, changing organizational structures and cultures, work processes and behaviours are among the most difficult tasks to accomplish in making any improvement to any services delivery, not at least in the AAL domain. Professional resistance to change as well as lack of organizational willingness and capacity to change has been noted as key barriers here. Measures to help promote and enable active change management at all system levels would help facilitate better implementation of AAL solutions.

2. Supporting the Deployment of AAL Services

Following the overview of the AAL market and particularly based on the factors influencing the development of the market that we presented in Section 1.3, this second part of the chapter contains an approach for supporting the deployment of AAL services. The influencing factors – or market characteristics – are of key importance for this since the deployment approach is based on our experience that due consideration of them, at all stages of the service deployment cycle, creates the prerequisites for a successful and sustainable deployment of services on the market.

[4] In Scotland for instance, a country-wide Telecare Development programme (TTD) was put in place in 2006. Just over 7900 people were in receipt of telecare packages funded through the programme by March 2008. It was estimated in 2007/08 that costs avoided amounted to more than £11 million. See [14].

To demonstrate this, we constructed a simple deployment cycle for AAL services that is divided into different steps. These steps can, for instance, be found in research or deployment projects, but also in deployment activities outside the formal framework of (funded) projects. Following the steps of this cycle, we present a series of supporting activities that aim to ensure a close linkage of market characteristics and deployment activities.

2.1. A Deployment Cycle for AAL Services

Numerous approaches exist which describe and structure the process of product, process or system development and deployment with the objective of making it more efficient and improving the likelihood of achieving successful and sustainable results. These results take the form of products or services that will sell on the market and be stronger than the competition. Commonly, these approaches divide the overall process into a series of subsequent steps, starting from the early development of ideas and ending with the introduction of the new product or service into the market. Each step comprises a number of activities that aim to further develop the new product or service in answer to different requirements from different sides including the customer side, the technical side and the business side.

Over the course of several RTD and deployment projects we have developed our own approach to service development and deployment in AAL on the basis of generic models that already existed, our own experiences and those of the partners that we work with. We conceive this approach as being a cycle rather than a chain of steps, emphasizing that development and deployment is a continuous rather than a finite activity and also that it is iterative and relies on information flowing back and forth between the different steps. In a similar way, the steps are also not finite within the cycle but ongoing or rather recurring with varying intensity and overlapping to various degrees. While the use of iterations and also the concept of interdependencies and overlapping steps are not new aspects of product or service development, we consider it important to put a special emphasis on them in the present context of AAL. The main reason for this is that the complexity of AAL service development goes beyond what is commonly encountered in other markets, such as that for consumer electronics, in that the number of requirements imposed from different sides is exceedingly high. As outlined in Section 1.3 above, this includes requirements raised by the different actor groups:

- from clients or patients and their family members (for instance in terms of meeting demand, data security and protection, informed consent but also ease-of-use and affordability),
- from health and social care professionals (regarding integration into existing work processes, staff training, ease-of-use and others),
- from care provider organizations (regarding the role of ICT in care provision, relation of costs and benefits, more efficient service provision etc.),
- from reimbursing organizations (for instance in terms of the role of ICT in care provision, evidence on cost-effectiveness, and the inclusion into reimbursement schemes),
- and from policy makers (among other things regarding evidence on cost and benefits, alignment with existing health and social policies etc.).

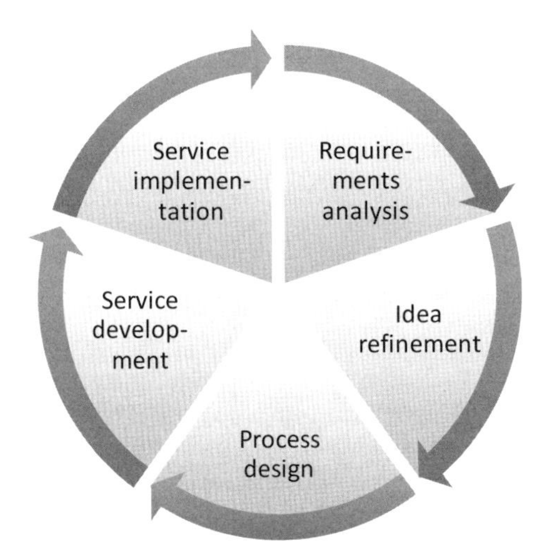

Figure 3. A deployment cycle for AAL services.

We consider that meeting these requirements, or rather balancing them between the actors, is an important, maybe even the single most important, success factor for sustainable service deployment.

Our deployment cycle for AAL services was developed with the aim to achieve this balancing act or at least to facilitate it. It is graphically depicted in Fig. 3 and starts with a first analysis of the requirements that the new service shall fulfil, commonly on the basis of a first service idea formulated by care professionals or provider organizations. On the basis of the requirements, the initial idea undergoes a first feasibility check and is refined accordingly. The feasibility check will usually take the form of a meeting, involving the technology provider and the service provider. On the basis of the refined service idea, a service process model is designed that breaks down the service into single tasks and decision points. On the basis of this model, a first prototype of the actual service is than developed and implemented for testing. The test will not only show how the service works and where there is need for improvement but also how far the requirements set in the beginning are met by it. Depending on the nature of the service, this cycle will be repeated one or several times and will finally lead to the implementation of the service in a real-life environment (either as a pilot or as a full-scale service). After this, the cycle will usually stop and only be employed at larger intervals to see if the service can be further refined to meet changed framework conditions. It should be noted that in practical implementation this circle will not necessarily run in exactly the way described. Rather, there will be a number of external influencing factors that may result in steps being skipped or repetitions being run in smaller circles, e.g. if a feasibility check shows that a certain service idea cannot be put into practice. In a similar manner, other checks like one for economic viability may halt the cycle at all stages and lead to substantial redesigning or even to the abortion of the whole strand of development.

The key characteristics of this deployment cycle can be described as follows:

- It is **conceptual** in that it provides guidance to the planning and management of deployment, rather than to the technical work in a narrower sense.
- It is **iterative** both in its overall approach and in each step, consisting of analysis, development, implementation and starting over.

- It is **open** in so far as the steps are based on information/data coming in from previous steps and on actions for further analysis, development and implementation going out to subsequent steps.
- It is **evaluative** since each step, its alignment with the previous ones (summative perspective) and its anticipated impacts on following steps (formative perspective) are evaluated empirically.
- Finally, it is **actor-centred** in that each step consists of the actions of individual or collective entities (persons or organizations) and is described, enacted and analyzed in that perspective.

In the following we will look at the main steps of the cycle in more detail and describe a set of methods and approaches to support it. To illustrate them, we refer to practical examples from our own development and implementation work in three projects: SOPRANO – Service-oriented Programmable Smart Environments for Older Europeans, CommonWell – Common Platform Services for Ageing Well in Europe and INDEPENDENT – ICT Enabled Service Integration for Independent Living. SOPRANO is an Integrated Project in the European Commission's 6th Framework Programme (IST Priority 6th Call on Ambient Assisted Living – AAL) and develops ICT-based assisted living services with interfaces specifically designed for use by older people in their home environment (see [29]). CommonWell and INDEPENDENT are both co-funded by the European Commission within the CIP ICT Policy Support Programme. CommonWell develops ICT-supported services for the integrated provision of social and health care that are being piloted in four European regions: Andalucía in Spain, Bielefeld in Germany, Veldhoven in the Netherlands and Milton Keynes in the UK (see [8]). INDEPENDENT delivers and pilots a digital infrastructure supporting coordinated cross-sector delivery of support to older people, bringing together telehealth and telecare and empowering informal carers and the voluntary/third sector to participate in delivery of support (see [12]).

2.2. Requirements Analysis and Idea Refinement

Usually, the deployment cycle starts with the formulation of a new service idea by care professionals or a provider organization, sometimes also by older end users. As a first step, requirements of the new service to be developed and later implemented need to be gathered in a comprehensive and systematic way. It is quite likely that requirements from different target groups who will later be using the new service significantly differ from each other. Thus, the process of requirements analysis needs to involve all target groups addressed. Only in this way is it possible to design a successful service that is satisfactory and usable for all actors involved. Representatives reflecting the characteristics, capabilities and experience of future users should be involved at several stages of design and development of the new service, because they have valuable knowledge about the context of use and are thus crucial to both requirement elicitation and service process design. Appropriate representatives ensure that user requirements can be identified for inclusion in service development. Iteration is necessary in order to minimize the risk that the new service fails to meet the user requirements.

The literature recommends several methods for the requirements analysis together with potential service end users. Interviews and questionnaire are, for example, well-established methods to learn more about requirements [20,24]. Both methods involve asking a set of questions to potential end users in order to capture issues such as users' subjective satisfaction, needs and possible anxieties [24]. In addition to this, interviews and questionnaires are also useful for studying how the users will potentially use the new service and what functionalities they would like to be included and, vice versa, what functionalities they dislike. The advantage of conducting face-to-face interviews is that the personal contact allows a very deep understanding of the person's life, routines and needs. The disadvantages of interviews are that they tend to be case studies that can hardly be generalized except when a high number of interviews is conducted.

Focus groups allow the involvement of a higher number of potential end users but at the same time also allow an in-depth investigation of user needs and requirements. They present another important method [5,10] that has proven to be quite successful for requirements elicitation. Focus groups are usually run by a moderator and normally involve about six to nine users who, following a pre-set schedule, identify issues over a period of about two hours. Focus groups often bring out users' spontaneous reactions and ideas through the interaction between the participants.

Another central method is the creation of scenarios of use or use cases [20,24,32]. The idea is to cut down on the complexity by describing possible uses of envisioned future services according to the characteristics of an individual user under specified circumstances [6]. Use cases include a strong reference to the social world within which the person lives or works. This is crucial as the key to creating useful and acceptable technology-based services is to understand how it is embedded in the person's everyday life. Use cases are developed by experts together with service providers.

Both focus groups and use case development were employed in some of our deployment and research projects such as SOPRANO or CommonWell. Contextual Analysis [2] is most appropriate when a set of functions is identified and methods of presenting problems and needs in the natural environment need to be understood.

The selection of methods to be applied during the requirements elicitation process of course depends on the future target group of the service under development. Addressing the target group of older people for example requires methods that perfectly suit this group. Standard tests can, for example, be too tedious, standard questionnaires might not be understood by everyone or expecting new ideas to be understood might be too challenging. In this context, the SOPRANO project used an 'ecological' model as a framework for guiding the user research and requirements elicitation [28]. This model focuses on practical aspects of everyday activities of the person, highlighting opportunities for technology and design solutions to support these activities. The model draws on the work of researchers such as Lawton and Kitwood [13,18]. The underlying idea of the model is that the activities that comprise a person's everyday life are shaped by a range of different factors such as attributes of the person (functional ability, cognitive ability, psychological factors etc.) and attributes of the immediate environment (formal support network, social network, physical environment) and wider socio-cultural contexts. These personal and situational factors operate together in a functional, 'ecological' relationship to facilitate or constrain a person's activities. The ecological model is useful in looking at the independence and quality of life of older people, because it highlights the impact and experience of age-related dependency (e.g. cognitive impairment) within its context and allows us to explore how this affects everyday life and well-being. How a person derives meaning from their everyday activities and environment is central to their well-being. Technological and design interventions can potentially play an important part by ameliorating some of the personal and contextual problems faced by a person. We argue here that a person's well-being will be enhanced if the intervention facilitates activities that are meaningful and valued by the person and takes into account the contextual factors within which the person lives [28].

The initial use cases then undergo a first feasibility check and are refined accordingly. The feasibility check will usually take the form of a meeting, involving the technology provider and the service provider.

Once technical feasibility is ensured, idea refinements will be developed, again involving all potential target groups. Depending on the maturity of the original idea, this can be done by another round of semi-structured focus groups, or, in projects with highly innovative and complex ideas and use cases, be more extensive. SOPRANO for example used two approaches for the first cycle of use case validation and idea refinement, both variants of Scenario Based Design [19,27]: a) "Design idea generation methods": refers to eliciting design ideas from end users and b) "Design idea evaluation methods": involves users in refining design decisions taken in previous activities.

One approach that we applied for the idea refinement process with good success was a theatre method. Scenario Based Dramas or Theatre methods are able to portray a situation (use case) in a very naturalistic and more immediate manner which makes it easier to imagine and remember the scene. Plays are very suitable for activating memories and emotions of spectators [3], an aspect that is particularly relevant in work with older people. Scenario-based dramas offer the possibility to enact a kind of play between users and experts and to also include first prototypes into the play. In addition, dramas give a good basis for semi-structured interviewing. As researched by Newell and colleagues in several papers [21,23], forum theatres can be promisingly applied in pre-prototype stages. The papers conclude that forum theatres can:

- encourage people with little or no technical knowledge to take part in realistic and useful discussions concerning a new technological solution; crosses boundaries of technical language and knowledge,
- encourage a creative approach to design, involving users as well as designers which is not possible in traditional focus groups and usability tests where only the opinions of the users are in focus,
- encourage real time discussion among several user groups, i.e. among the users, among the designers or among actors and the audience (users and/or designers.

In SOPRANO, theatre methods were applied in order to refine and complement service ideas developed by older people and professional carers during the requirements elicitation process. Certain use cases were transcribed into a script by a professional scriptwriter. Following the script, the use case was enacted by a theatre group, followed by discussions with the users. Participants were invited to give feedback and compare the presented solution for the ideas they had come up with themselves. The results were analyzed in order to refine/detail the original use cases. Theatre groups were a very successful approach to involve older end users in the idea refinement process and participants were actively engaged in the process and showed a lot of interest in what was going on. The ability to act scenarios out reduced confusion and meant that researchers did not have to attempt to describe abstract and complex concepts.

Once the process of idea refinement is completed, results are incorporated into the existing use cases. The refined use cases serve as a solid basis for the subsequent steps in the deployment cycle.

2.3. Process Design

However, use cases and new technologies do not exist in isolation. The identification and examination of existing care processes and how the new solution can be fitted into these processes is thus a crucial part of the whole way to go. ICT must be implemented in direct response to identified information and communication needs as expressed by the professionals rather than technology driven (see e.g. [4,7,30]). Otherwise new technologies can, for instance, increase workloads, e.g. when staff maintains a computer-based system alongside a parallel system that is paper-based. With a view to the due consideration of care processes in ICT implementation, a recent WHO policy brief [31] highlighted the need to pursue process-led innovation if telehealth is to be implemented more widely than it is today, confirming findings from research and practice [22].

Research among nurse practitioners in the UK, for example, found that nurses see a lack of effective integration of e-systems and care pathways across health and social care organizations as well as for ready access to portable, reliable hardware and 24/7 ICT support [1].

In particular when it comes to the delivery of integrated social care and healthcare services a thorough understanding of the care delivery processes and knowledge about where the developing solution needs to be fitted in is needed. This is essential not only during the development process of technical systems but also during the implementation period of these systems. This does, however, not mean that processes are completely fixed and cannot be changed. Even the most promising technical solution will very likely fail if the underlying existing care processes needed to be turned upside down. Thus, technical solutions and processes have to be carefully synchronised in order to provide successful services that support independent living. This is of particular importance since the market environment for AAL products and services is extremely complex. A large variety of different actors are involved in the service delivery process ranging from the patients and clients, their family carers to social and health care providers and reimbursing organizations and policy makers. Having said this, one inevitable step of the overall process design is to ensure that all actors involved in the service process are adequately trained and familiarised with the new technology and the adapted steps in the process of service provision. Thus, the investigation of existing care delivery processes and, in the next step, the thorough design of a service process model, need to include the identification of training needs of all actors involved. Hereby, a break-down of the service into single tasks and decision points clearly facilitates a detailed identification of these training needs, the conceptual design of adequate training concepts and the conduction of training of the actors involved. This also facilitates the acceptance of the new technology and the motivation to adopt changes in the overall process on the side of the care provider staff and has, as a consequence, the potential to overcome sometimes existing resistance at an organisational level.

Within the framework of the CommonWell project, the investigation of existing service processes, integration of the new service to be developed into existing care service delivery processes and the conceptualisation and provision of staff training was an important step. Care service providers who are well aware of the service processes thoroughly investigated the existing processes in parallel to requirements elicitation work and use case development. This ensured that the envisaged new technology-supported service was smoothly integrated into the existing processes, instead of having to completely revolutionise it. This was done with the help of focus groups involving care service providers and other relevant stakeholders in the care delivery chain.

The early identification and involvement of the service providers and other potential users in the stage of requirements elicitation and service process development also supports the business care modelling as described further below.

For the development of an integrated service supporting COPD patients in CommonWell, current processes of the social care and healthcare provision in Milton Keynes were investigated. In a second step, models (flow-charts) were drawn up showing how the envisaged new technology-supported service could fit into the whole process of service delivery (cf. Fig. 4). Key questions for the development of the flow charts were amongst others:

- What processes are performed?
- What are the work-flows?
- When is the process performed?
- How is it performed?
- Where is the process performed?
- By whom is the process performed?

Figure 4 shows the service process model developed for the new service in Milton Keynes. The aim of the Community Alarm, Telecare and Telehealth Service is to provide a comprehensive way of managing the risks to a person's health and well being within their own home environment. These are to run 24 hours a day, 365 days a year and using preventative technology to assist the individual to continue live independently for as long as possible. The Community and Telecare service receives around 700 calls from its service users per day. There are several methods of referral to telecare or community alarm. Milton Keynes has already introduced first generation monitoring systems with collaboration between the Community Alarm service and Primary Care Trust. Early results are very encouraging, but the systems are completely separate from Telecare delivered to the same patients and the data from the telehealth monitoring are not shared across any other systems – it is only received on a standalone system. Patients who are referred to telehealth have a chronic long term condition such as COPD and require daily vital sign monitoring to help manage their condition and to help them to be more involved in self-management.

Within CommonWell vital signs and telehealth equipment to test effectiveness for the management and monitoring of patients with COPD and other long term conditions will be developed and piloted. How the information can be shared within the patient pathway to ensure the opportunities to maximise the benefit to the patient and the people supporting that person is a key concern.

In the next step of service development prototypes of different levels of detail are the objects of user assessment. For example, in the early stages of a mock-up of the new ICT-based service interaction could be simulated. Later in the development, more developed prototypes can be used to assess whether usability objectives have been met.

2.4. Business Case Modelling and Cost-Benefit Analysis

The third supporting activity we are looking at is a horizontal one that cannot be assigned to one of the steps of the deployment cycle but is conceived as a process going on throughout its entire duration. The main purpose of business case modelling, as it is understood here, is to inform the deployment cycle as far as requirements from the business side are concerned and to ensure that these requirements are met to the great-

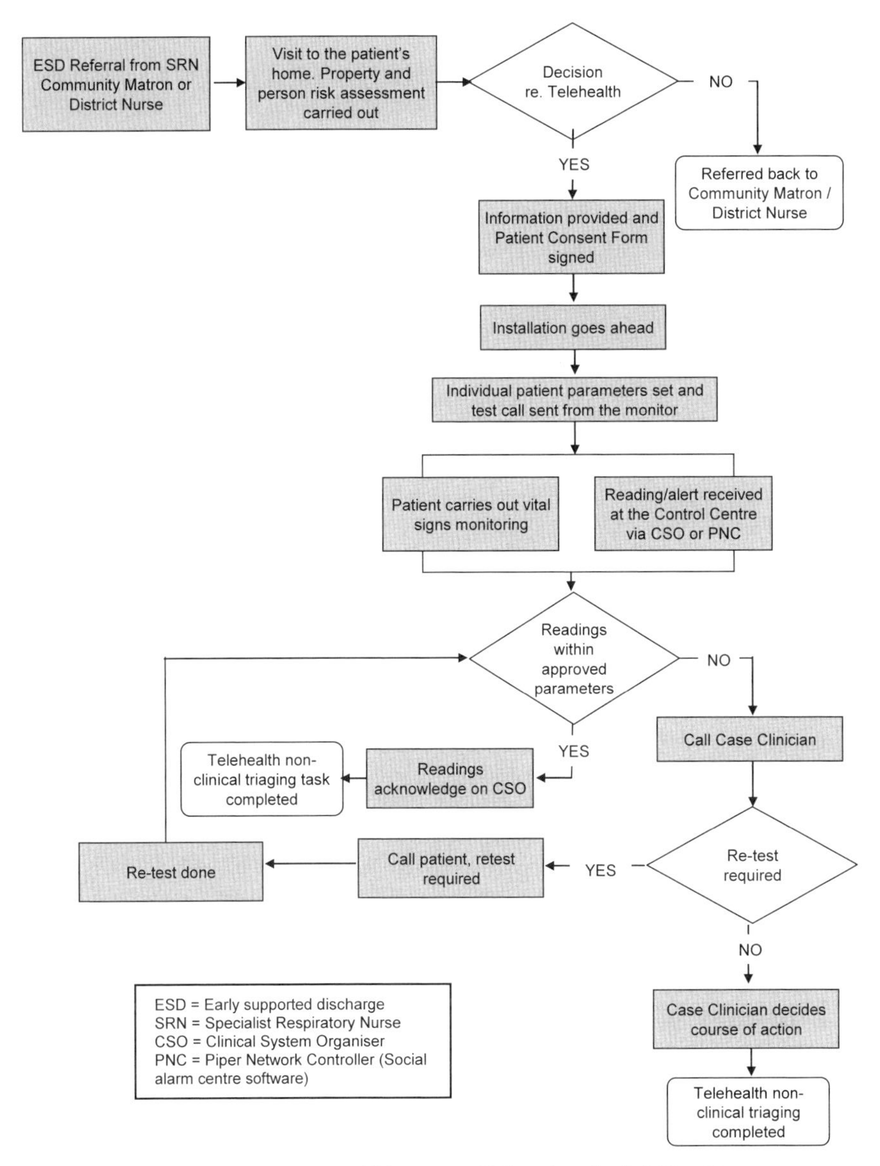

Figure 4. Service process model for a new ICT-based service in Milton Keynes.

est possible extent. This includes the analysis of service costs and benefits to different actors, the due consideration of financing means and the re-modelling of the service concept to ensure economic viability.

The overall aim of the activity is to build a business model for the developing AAL service. In this, the business case modelling approach presented here follows key characteristics of the overall development cycle. It is

- open to outcomes of all steps of the cycle and feeding back to all of them,
- an iterative approach starting from an early, basic model that is refined and expanded as the service is developed,

- based on empirical data,
- modelled around the multitude of actors usually found in AAL services and designed to optimize the cost-benefit ratio for all.

Business case modelling is here conceived as an analytic process. It is by no means a light-weight task. The integration of ICT into existing, well-established processes, such as can for instance be found in care provision, means more than introducing technical applications but usually touches deeply on each actor's way of providing a service and doing business more generally. It also, usually, necessitates substantial investments in terms of costs for hard- and software and for process adaptation. Through an analysis of eHealth services, Stroetmann et al. [31] found that investment costs can range from about 400,000€ for a service to as high as 725,000,000€! Although investments for AAL services can, of course, be considerably below these levels, even the lower boundary seems to justify solid business modelling to ensure an appropriate return.

Conceptually, a business model is a tool that contains a set of elements and their relationships and allows expression of the business logic of a specific firm, organization or group. The term was first mentioned in the accounting literature of the 1960s, but only gained widespread use in the 1990s [26]. In the most basic sense, a business model is the method of doing business by which a company or organization can sustain itself – that is, generate revenue to cover expenditure – or fulfil certain objectives – such as the provision of public services. Essentially, a business model consists of a product/service to be sold to a customer, using an infrastructure creating costs and revenue streams.

Figure 5 shows four pillars of a business model and breaks them down into nine building blocks:

- A value proposition is an overall view of a company's bundle of products and/or services that are of value to the customer. The value proposition answers the question 'Why should a customer buy the product or service?'
- The target customer is a segment of customers a company wants to offer value to.
- A distribution channel is a means of getting in touch with, and handing the product/service over to the customer.
- The customer relationship describes the kind of link a company establishes between itself and the customer.
- The value configuration describes the arrangement of activities and resources that are necessary to create value for the customer.
- A capability is the ability to execute a repeatable pattern of actions that is necessary in order to create value for the customer.
- A partnership is a voluntarily initiated cooperative agreement between two or more companies in order to create value for the customer.
- The cost structure is the representation in money of all the resources employed by the business.
- The revenue model describes the way a company secures liquidity through money inflow, usually from selling its products and services.

In the context of AAL services, this breakdown of a business model in building blocks is basically useful, yet needs to be made more precise and adapted to the characteristics of the market. In particular three important questions can help to do this.

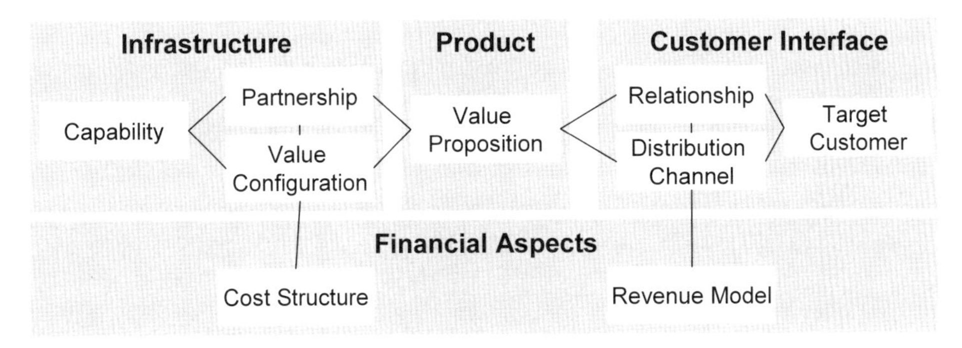

Figure 5. Pillars of a business model. Source: empirica, based on [26].

Who are the providers? In the first step the answer to this question can be as simple as a list of those actors that are currently involved in service provision. According to the ICT & Ageing study [16] the most common provider organisations for telecare are social care providers, followed by housing providers. For home telehealth, they are public/non-profit healthcare providers, although some examples of provision by private/for-profit providers were also found. Involvement of public/non-profit social care providers was also quite common, especially where combined telecare/home telehealth implementations were concerned. Hospitals and to a lesser extent primary care centres/polyclinics were by far the most common type of establishments involved. Apart from the more traditional types of providers, a certain emergence of new players can be observed, including private call/response service providers and traditionally more security-oriented service providers. Especially due to these more recent trends it may be profitable when designing a business model to look beyond traditional provider "configurations" for new partners to identify those combinations that make most sense from a service process and business point of view.

What is the service? There is quite a wide spectrum of technologies that can support the provision of AAL services and there are various ways that the technology components used for this can be conceptualised and structured. One practical approach is to distinguish between devices/systems in the older person's home, the connecting systems, and the systems at the service provider end. As described in more detail in the section on process design above, a main criterion for the choice of technology is its fit with the underlying service that is to be supported, e.g. social and health care services for people with chronic conditions. Usually, a wide array of technical solutions will be theoretically possible, but practical choice will be limited due to technical feasibility, organisational or economic constraints. More room for manoeuvre may be found in allocating the technical components of the service to the different suppliers. For example, a monitoring centre may be better placed at an existing call centre of a social alarms provider than at a hospital that currently has no call centre infrastructure at all. Same as for the provider configurations above, different choices may lead to quite different results in terms of the business model and the economic viability of the service.

What is the value chain or Who pays? This question tends to lend an additional level of complexity to building business models in the AAL domain as it is different from other IT markets, such as for consumer IT. AAL services usually do not reach the customer (e.g. a care recipient) directly but via service providers (e.g. social or health care provider). In return, payment usually takes a detour via a funding or reimbursing organisation. As the ICT & Ageing study found (see above) reimbursement regimes and their associated incentives/disincentives are among the key factors influencing – often in a negative way – the wider deployment of AAL services. Accordingly, consideration of the value chain for a given service can be considered key for successful deployment. This means more than knowing who is responsible for the payment of different types of services or knowing what is eligible under a given reimbursement scheme. It also includes knowing the flow of costs and benefits between the different actors that are involved in order to identify the quality and quantity of the impacts the service will cause.

With the knowledge about providers, technologies and value chains – that is about the framework conditions of the service – it is now possible to turn to the task of business case modelling itself. As already said above, business case modelling is here understood as an analytic and formative process, carried out on the streams of costs and benefits between the actors in the service over time and under given framework conditions.

A wide range of methods exist that analyze and model service impacts and can be used for this purpose, including wider concepts such as health technology assessment (HTA) or more specific approaches such as cost-effectiveness analysis (CEA), cost-utility analysis (CUA) and cost-benefit analysis (CBA). A good overview of different methods can, for instance, be found in Drummond [9]. We choose the approach of cost-benefit analysis as it seemed to best meet our requirements for business case modelling. In this context, its main advantages are the possibilities to adopt a multi-stakeholder perspective (i.e. costs and benefits can be analysed separately for different actors), to correct for optimism bias in cost and benefit estimates, to analyse in a time perspective and to include sensitivity analysis.

For the purposes of the cost-benefit analysis, flows of costs and benefits between the service actors – partly determined by the service model and partly by framework conditions such as the reimbursement scheme – are identified and data on the flows are collected. In doing so, three different types of costs and benefits are discerned:

1. financial costs/benefits (direct flows of money),
2. resource costs/benefits (committed resources, including redeployed resources) and
3. intangible costs/benefits (that are not immediately quantifiable as money or resources).

All three types are then included into the analysis. To this end, intangible costs and benefits are quantified and – together with resources – transformed into monetary values.

The quantification of things that are not per se of a quantitative nature, presents a major challenge for a cost-benefit analysis for AAL. From a methodological point of view there is, for instance, the problem of quantifying public goods such as social welfare, since these are usually consumed collectively and do not carry a price tag for the individual "customer" or user[5]. In practical terms this means that neither the public's evaluation of the good nor the individual's preference for a certain service are available. Further to this, there is often considerable resentment towards the quantification of quality in a social or health care setting, since this is deemed inappropriate or even

[5] For more information on this and on the issue of quantification of non-financial costs and benefits cf. for example [16].

de-humanizing. Some of the reasons for this resentment cannot be gainsaid, which is why any such attempt must be carried out carefully and with a view to the circumstances met with in a specific service. At the same time, a cost-benefit analysis necessitates this careful quantification of all factors in the same way as building a business model necessitates the analysis of costs and benefits.

On the basis of a full set of cost and benefit data, the overall model is calculated showing for each actor aggregates of different cost/benefit categories such as

- equipment cost,
- setup cost,
- costs for service provision,
- efficiency of service benefits,
- quality of service benefits,
- quality of life benefits.

Further to this, key performance measures such as overall socio-economic return, cumulative net outcomes or return on investment are calculated for the whole service. Calculating these measures for alternative models of service provision allows both to find the model that best fits the service and also to identify adaptations to the service that may be necessary from a business point of view. Also, the cost-benefit analysis can help in weighing tangible against intangible impacts, show benefit shifts where one actor bears the costs for an intervention and another profits from it without this being counterbalanced by reciprocal flows, and highlight unexpected impacts that do not necessarily come to the fore in other stages of the development cycle.

To illustrate this analytic process, we return to the example of the development of an integrated, ICT-supported social and health care service for COPD patients in Milton Keynes in the UK that is currently being piloted in the CommonWell project. Similar to the situation described for the creation of the process model, business case modelling is strongly influenced in this context by the novelty of integrating social and health care provision alongside the use of ICT. As a consequence it was not possible to start from an existing business model rather a new one had to be developed.

The main actors involved in the service are the Milton Keynes council as providers of social care services in the area. This includes the operation of a community alarm centre providing both telecare (social alarm) and telehealth (remote patient data monitoring) services. A technology provider is responsible both for the delivery of hard- and software and for technical maintenance and support. On the health care side there are several service providers acting under the roof of the National Health Service, including a district nurse and community matron (responsible for the delivery of health care services to the patient's home), the general practitioner and the hospital. The integrated services are being provided to older people diagnosed with COPD. Also involved are the patient's family members taking over a carer role.

Figure 6 shows all expected cost and benefit flows between the actors, which can be summarized as follows:

- Equipment cost for telecare and telehealth equipment and the integrated alarm centre.
- Setup cost for the development of new processes and protocols, the installation of the equipment and the training of clinicians and end-users.
- Operation costs in terms of staff effort at the alarm centre and the different health service providers, IT maintenance and end-user support.

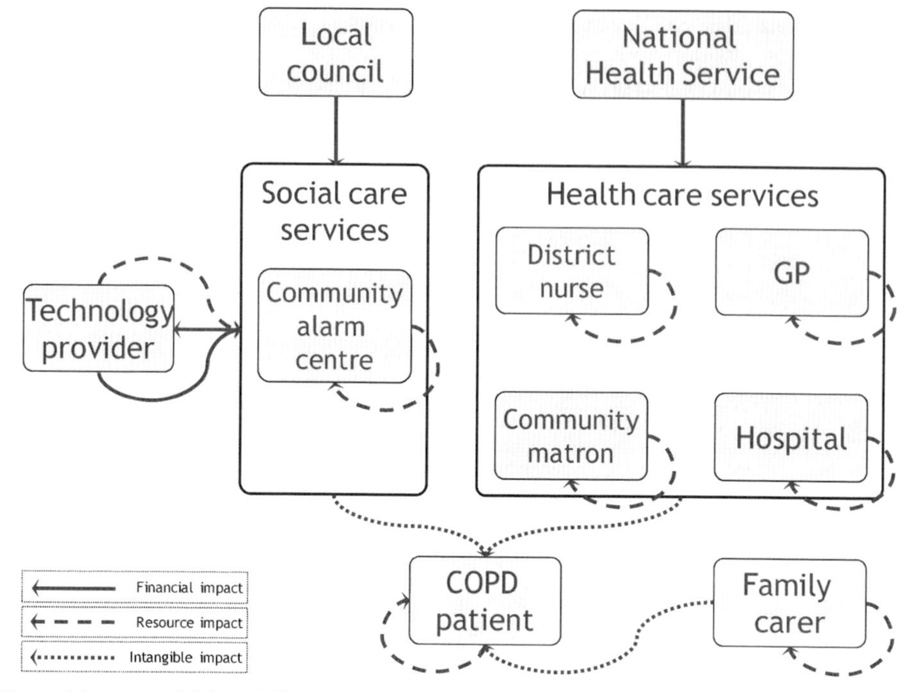

Figure 6. Impact model for an ICT-supported, integrated social and health care service in Milton Keynes in the UK.

- Quality of life benefits in terms of hospital admission avoidance, better informed patients, better support in critical situations and support for families and carers.
- Quality of service benefits in terms of a faster and more targeted response to client requests, complete access to telecare and telehealth data in one system and the availability of this data to clinicians.
- Efficiency of service benefits in terms of a decreased number of face-to-face visits to clients for health and social care staff, reduced hospital admissions costs, opportunities for early discharge from hospital and reduction in call outs to GPs and urgent care facilities.

A first modelling of the costs and benefits done before the start of the pilot test – and therefore partly based on assumptions – showed the possible effects of the new service. Included in this was an increase of effort on the side of the community matron and the district nurse due to more intensive telemonitoring and shorter reaction times to telehealth readings outside preset thresholds. At the same time, treatment efforts on the side of institutional healthcare (hospital) and general practice are envisaged to decrease due to a lower number of re-admissions and more treatment provided to the home. The COPD patients and their family carers are expected to benefit from decreased disease management efforts and increased treatment health outcomes. On the basis of the service development work that followed the approach described in this chapter, the clear expectation is that after the initial investment the Milton Keynes council and the NHS can offer better quality services to COPD patients at levels of effort comparable to those of today.

3. Some Conclusions

The last few years have shown ever increasing activity in the development and deployment of AAL services. At the same time, available evidence shows that actual deployment levels are low and widespread mainstreaming of services across Europe has not yet occurred. The factors explaining the status-quo are manifold and there relative importance can be – and often is – argued. From the knowledge about AAL markets that is available to us and from our experience in service development and deployment we come to the conclusion that only a holistic approach will eventually lead to long-term success and a possible way to achieve it has been presented. We consider the general characteristics of this approach to be as important as the more concrete work steps that we describe. While the first are open enough to be widely applicable, the latter can provide useful guidance to practitioners. More practical experience, more empirical evidence and the reflection on both will help to further elaborate it in the future.

References

[1] B. Baker et al., An investigation of the emergent professional issues experienced by nurses when working in an e-health environment, in: *Qualitative Research in Health and Social Care*, Bournemouth University, Bournemouth, 2007, available from: http://www.bournemouth.ac.uk/cfpd/pdf/prdiepien.pdf.
[2] H. Beyer and K. Holtzblatt, *Contextual Design: Defining Customer-Centered Systems*, Morgan Kaufmann, San Franciso, 1998.
[3] J. Bortz and N. Döring, *Forschungsmethoden und Evaluation*, Springer, Berlin, 1995.
[4] U. Brucker and G. Ziegler, *Grundsatzstellungsnahme Pflegeprozess und Dokumentation. Handlungsempfehlungen zur Professionalisierung und Qaulitätssicherung in der Pflege*, Medizinischer Dienst der Spitzenverbände der Krankenkassen e.V., Essen, 2005.
[5] S. Caplan, Using focus groups methodology for economic design, *Ergonomics* **33** (1990), 527–533.
[6] J.M. Carroll and M.B. Rosson, Getting around the task-artifact cycle: How to make claims and design by scenario, *ACM Transactions on Informations Systems* **10** (1992), 181–212.
[7] E. Coiera, Recent advances: Medical informatics, *British Medical Journal* **310** (1995).
[8] CommonWell consortium, CommonWell – Common platform services for ageing well in Europe, [cited 19.01.2010], available from: http://www.commonwell.eu/.
[9] M.F. Drummond, *Methods for the Economic Evaluation of Health Care Programmes*, 3rd edn, Oxford University Press, Oxford, 2005, xv, 379 s.
[10] T.L. Greenbaum, *The Practical Handbook and Guide to Focus Group Research*, D.C. Heath & Co., Lexington, MA, 1998.
[11] ICT & Ageing study team, ICT & ageing – European study on users, markets and technologies, [cited 3.3.2011], available from: http://www.ict-ageing.eu/.
[12] INDEPENDENT consortium, INDEPENDENT – ICT enabled service integration for independent living, [cited 02.11.2010], available from: http://www.independent-project.eu/.
[13] T. Kitwood, Towards a theory of dementia care: The interpersonal process, *Ageing & Society* **13** (1993), 51–67.
[14] L. Kubitschke and K. Cullen, ICT & ageing European study on users, technologies & markets – Final report, 2010, European Commission, DG Information Society and Media, available from: http://www.ict-ageing.eu/ict-ageing-website/wp-content/uploads/2010/D18_final_report.pdf.
[15] L. Kubitschke and K. Cullen, Various studies on policy implications of demographic changes in national and community policies – LOT7: The demographic change – Impacts of new technologies and information society, Final Report, 2005, available from: http://ec.europa.eu/employment_social/social_situation/docs/lot7_ict_finalreport_en.pdf.
[16] L. Kubitschke, K. Cullen and M. Rauhala, ICT & ageing European study on users, technologies & markets – Preliminary findings, 2008, European Commission, DG Information Society and Media, available from: http://www.ict-ageing.eu/ict-ageing-website/wp-content/uploads/2008/11/ictageing_vienna_handout_final2.pdf.

[17] L. Kubitschke et al., How can telehealth help in the provision of integrated care?, in: *Health Systems and Policy Analysis*, G. Permanand, ed., WHO Regional Office for Europe and European Observatory on Health Systems and Policies, Copenhagen, 2010, available from: http://www.euro.who.int/__data/assets/pdf_file/0011/120998/E94265.pdf.
[18] M.P. Lawton, Aging and performance of home tasks, *Human factors* **32**(5) (1990), 527–536.
[19] J. Machate, Von der Idee zum Produkt- mit Benutzern Gestalten, in: *User Interface Tuning. Benutzungsschnittstellen Menschlich Gestalten*, J. Machate and M. Burmester, eds, Software & Support Verlag GmbH, Frankfurt, 2003, pp. 83–96.
[20] D.J. Mayhew, *The Usability Engineering Lifecycle*, Morgan Kaufmann, 1999.
[21] S.J. McKenna et al., Requirements gathering using drama for computer vision based monitoring in supportive home environments, *International Society for Gerontechnology* **1**(5) (2006), 29–45.
[22] S. Müller, Process and IT innovation in telecare. Experiences from the CommonWell project, *Gerontechnology* **2**(9) (2010).
[23] A.F. Newell et al., The use of theatre in requirements gathering and usability studies, *Interacting with Computers* **18** (2006), 996–1011.
[24] J. Nielsen, *Usability Engineering*, Academic Press, 1993.
[25] E. Nolte and M. McKee, Caring for people with chronic conditions – A health system perspective, in: *European Observatory on Health Systems and Policies Series*, European Observatory on Health Systems and Policies, Berkshire, 2008, p. 290.
[26] A. Osterwalder, The business model ontology. A proposition in a design science approach, in: *Ecole des Hautes Etudes Commerciales*, Université de Lausanne, Lausanne, 2004.
[27] M.B. Rosson and J.M. Carroll, *Usability Engineering. Scenario-Based Development of Human-Computer Interaction*, Morgan Kaufmann Publishers, San Francisco, 2002.
[28] A. Sixsmith and J. Sixsmith, Smart care technologies: Meeting whose needs?, *Journal of Telemedicine and Telecare* **6** (2000), 190–192.
[29] SOPRANO consortium, SOPRANO – Service-oriented programmable smart environments for older europeans, [cited 19.01.2010], available from: http://www.soprano-ip.org/.
[30] M. Stefanelli, The role of methodologies to improve efficiency and effectiveness of care delivery processes for the year 2013, *Int. J. Med. Inform.* **66**(1–3) (2002), 39–44.
[31] K. Stroetmann et al., eHealth is worth it – The economic benefits of implemented eHealth solutions at ten European sites, Luxembourg, 2006, available from: http://www.ehealth-impact.org/download/documents/ehealthimpactsept2006.pdf.
[32] K. Vredenburg, S. Isensee and C. Righi, *User-Centred Design*, Prentice Hall, 2002.
[33] World Health Organisation, *Home Care in Europe*, R. Taricone and A.D. Tdouros, eds, WHO Regional Office Europe, 2008.
[34] World Health Organisation, *Innovative Care for Chronic Conditions: Building Blocks for Action*, World Health Organisation, Geneva, 2002.

Handbook of Ambient Assisted Living
J.C. Augusto et al. (Eds.)
IOS Press, 2012

doi:10.3233/978-1-60750-837-3-369

Delivering Technology Enriched Health and Social Care: Policy Context for User Focused Research

Suzanne MARTIN[a,*] and Maurice MULVENNA[b]
[a]School of Health Sciences University of Ulster
[b]School of Computing and Mathematics University of Ulster

Abstract. Implementation of ICT within Health and Social Care requires an aligned blend of strategic policy alongside research to promote innovation and creativity within services. This chapter explores the strategic context of developments within Europe, with a focus on the United Kingdom. In addition the value and opportunity for service orientated research as a mode to achieve high impact and sustainable implementation is proposed, thereby supporting evidence-based healthcare in this domain.

Keywords. ICT policy, user centred research

Introduction

The rationale supporting research into innovative use of information and communication technology (ICT) within Health and Social care is articulated well throughout this book for example changing population demographics and increased chronic disease prevalence. Building on that, this chapter will focus on two important areas that will determine to a large extent how implementation within services emerges and furthermore, how research can develop closely aligned to the needs of services and services users aiming to support successful, sustainable implementation. Initially the policy context within Europe and the United Kingdom (UK) supporting the utilization of ICT within Health and Social Care will be presented followed by an outline of the approach adopted within the Translational Research and Innovation Lab (TRAIL) Living Lab to engage with service users in a participatory user centered approach to research.

Contemporary health and social care is delivered within the context of a dynamic social, cultural and political environment. At strategic policy level within government and non-government agencies awareness prevails of meeting the healthcare needs of current populations and developing services fit for the challenges of future populations. Coyte (2007) [7] suggests that healthcare in the 21st Century is technologically mediated and geographically dispersed. Healthcare is no longer delivered solely in traditional settings for example hospitals, but in places designed for other purposes, i.e. the home.

Reviewing the literature in this area reveals a wide variation in the types of devices used within Healthcare and a great variety of applications [40] from those with a focus

*Corresponding Author: Suzanne Martin. E-mail: s.martin@ulster.ac.uk.

on the individual service user [51,53,55] to service developments over wide geographical regions [50] and in some instances national programmes of implementation are evident [42,48]. A vast array of services have been delivered for example supporting family caregivers, [43] providing rehabilitation to the elderly [52] speech and language therapy provision to children with learning difficulties [41] and interventions for chronic disease management [2,36] to cite but a few examples.

User driven research alongside open innovation is core to the work of Living Labs [32] and are considered to be most effective mode to bridge the gap between research and development and supporting commerce to enter new technologies and services onto the market place, supporting a better and faster uptake of research results.

1. Policy Context

1.1. Global

The European commission promotes the concept of eHealth for a technology facilitated health system and describes this as the

"application of ICT across the whole range of functions that affect the health sector, from doctor to hospital manager,via nurses, data processing specialists, social security administrators and – of course- patients." [30].

This definition followed on from the "Connecting for Health" [61] Strategic report published by the World Health Organization (WHO) during 2005 within which 5 eHealth paradigms are described to include the citizen, the professional, hospitals and academia, health related businesses, Governments and International Agencies. Also in that year, the WHO adopted Resolution WHA58.28 [64] establishing an eHealth Strategy which urged member states to plan for appropriate eHealth services in their countries [59]. Additionally WHO have suggested 5 strategic directions should be pursued to advance eHealth. These include:

- Strengthening health systems.
- Fostering public private partnerships in ICT research and development for health.
- Supporting capacity building for eHealth application in member states.
- Development and use of norms and standards.
- Investigating, documenting and analysing the impact of eHealth and promoting better understanding by dissemination.

Table 1 below outlines the main policy activity by the WHO to support the advancement of eHealth Globally [57,62,65].

1.2. European Context

The European Commission started to introduce public health policy as recently as 1992, when the Maastricht Treaty included an article on cooperation in public health [25]. Within Europe key policy messages are located within strategies advocating social inclusion for excluded groups and promoting aging in place.

Table 1. WHO policy activity.

Activity	Descriptor
eHealth Legal and ethics committee	Promotes respect for privacy and human rights as ehealth services develop. Provides practical guidance to member states.
Global observatory for eHealth	Network of National Nodes analyzing and reporting on eHealth activity in member states. Will provide support for development of eHealth strategy and policy.
Public-private partnerships in eHealth	Governance of eHealth partnerships which facilitate national cooperation and international exchange in eHealth.
ICT for Health education and promotion	Reach individuals at home, school and workplace. To provide education and information.
eHealth for health-care services	Improving quality and safety of access to healthcare. A set of minimum requirements for responsible use of eHealth within health systems will be produced. • Technical factors • Human factors • Financial resources All considered in relation to the operational, managerial and political levels of the health system

Examples include:

- Amsterdam Treaty; all EU citizens have a right to participate fully and without discrimination in society [21].
- 2000 and 2005 Lisbon Strategy; eradiation of poverty and social exclusion by 2010, developing a social pillar designed to modernise the European Social Model. From 2006 accessible, high quality and sustainable health are long term care is a priority policy area [22].
- eHealth 2004. eHealth-making healthcare better for European citizens: An action plan for European eHealth Areas [26].
- eEurope 2005 Action Plan aiming to stimulate secure services, applications and content based on a widely available broadband infrastructure . By 2005 Europe should have e-Health services [24].
- i2010 – A European information society for growth and employment. This policy recognises that ICT is having an increasing impact on society and aims to ensure that it all citizens of Europe will have:
    - Improves quality of life.
    - Benefits all citizens.
    - Improves public services.
    - Improves cost effectiveness.
    - Increases accessibility.
- European Parliament resolution of 23rd May 2007 (2006/2275(INI)) on the impact and consequences of the exclusion of health services from the directive on services in the internal market. This resolution states that patients should have access to medical treatment as close as possible to their own homes.

The Commission Communications, “Towards a Europe for All Ages” (COM (1999)0221) (European Commission 1999) and later paper “Europe’s response to world ageing" (COM (2002)143) (European Commission 2002) outlined a number of key challenges to inclusion and the aging population. These included:

- Managing the economic implications of ageing in order to maintain growth and sound public finances;
- Adjusting well to an ageing and shrinking workforce;
- Ensuring adequate, sustainable and adaptable pensions; and
- Achieving access to high quality health care for all while ensuring the financial viability of health care systems.

More recently eHealth priorities and strategic development throughout Europe has been presented in the following report; eHealth priorities and strategies in European countries. The European Commission places high value on the potential of ICT within Health and has made significant recurrent research funding available through Framework Programmes of activity [27,28,30]. Within the Framework 7 Research Programme the Ambient Assisted Living [1]. The objective of the AAL Joint Programme is to enhance the quality of life of older people and strengthen the industrial base in Europe through the use of Information and Communication Technologies (ICT).

1.3. United Kingdom

Within the United Kingdom Department of Health (Department of Health (DOH) 2007) is responsible for overall eHealth policy of England. Strategic Health Authorities coordinate implementation regionally within the service based local National Health Service (NHS) bodies. The DOH in England states that *"Telecare offers the promise of enabling thousands of older people to live independently, in control and with dignity for longer."* Health policy for Northern Ireland, Scotland and Wales is devolved from National Government to local administrations. Generally innovation from England will be replicated throughout the regions. Health policy generally promotes; continuing to improve the quality and capacity of services; building a service responsive to service user needs; improving value for money; preventing ill health [18].

Key policy documents from the Department of Health England are:

- Our Health, our care, our say: a new direction for community services [15].
- NHS Improvement plan 2004: putting people at the heart of public services – sets out priorities between 2004 and 2008 [1].
- Choosing Health: Making healthy choices easier recommends better use of ICT [13].
- National Standards, Local Action; Health and Social Care Standards and Planning Framework [14].
- Building the information core implementing the NHS plan. [13] Information for Social Care: A framework for improving quality in social care through better use of information and information technology [10].
- Working together with health information: a partnership strategy for education, training and development [12].
- Information for health: an information strategy for the modern NHS 1998–2005 [19].

- Building Telecare in England (Department of Health 2005) [11] providing local authorities in England and their partners with guidance to develop telecare services, and making provision for a preventative technology grant to support local implementation.

The White Paper, "Our Health, Our Care, Our Say" stated that the Governments would set up a National Demonstrator Program to prove the benefits of assistive technology. This materialized as the Whole systems Demonstrator Programme (WSD): a randomized control trial of telecare and telehealth with participant sites at Kent, Cornwall and Newham England during May 2007. The main focus of the interventions are for frail elderly and people with long terms conditions. The WSD Programme had been driven by the need to understand the true benefit of integrated health and social care supported by advanced assistive technology (telehealth and telecare). Aiming to provide the business case for implementation a robust evaluation has formed a major part of the research [56].

This work within the WSD is the largest randomized control trial of its kind ever undertaken. The results of the trial were expected by Spring 2011 however there have been delays in the public reporting of the findings.

It is hoped that the WSD will provide a better understanding of how new assistive technologies:

- promote people's long term health and independence and safety,
- improve quality of life for people and their carers,
- improve the working lives of health and social care professionals,
- improve integrated working between health and social care sectors,
- provide an evidence base for more cost effective and clinically effective ways of managing LTCs,
- inform future policy,
- determine how effectively the equipment works [39].

Within Scotland the National Telecare Development Programme (2006–2010) was established to support the development and enhancement of Telecare Services in Scotland. Led by the Joint Improvement Team (JIT2010) [38] a section of the Partnership Improvement and Outcomes Division of the Scottish Governments Health Directorates.

Key policy documents from Scotland.

- National eHealth/IM&T Strategy (NHS Scotland 2004).
- eHealth Scotland [47].

(N.B. policy documents for Wales are not available)
Key policy documents from Northern Ireland.

- Information and Communications Technology Strategy [16].
- A healthier future; A twenty year vision for health and wellbeing in Northern Ireland [17].
- Department of Health Priorities for action 2007–2008 inline with the above strategy – Priority 5; Fully Integrated Care and Support in the community. 1 million dedicated to primary care management of respiratory conditions and diabetes.
- DOH then announced 1 million for Telehealth pump-priming in Northern Ireland primarily for chronic disease management [9].

1.4. Reflections on Policy

Policy response to support the implementation of ICT within Health and Social Care has been at Global, European, National and Regional Level. The European Commission (2002) considers that Europe was one of the first Global areas to be affected by ageing and has developed a range of policy responses.

The World Health Organization (2006) states that *"income, health and social integration are the cornerstones of people wellbeing, regardless of age ... thus at policy level, multi-sectoral responses are needed"* [58,63,65].

This literature review of policy was wide however the results show that to date, the majority of policy and strategic development is occurring within the domain of Health. Further high-level collaborations and strategic output would be advantageous if bringing together the key actors required to support implementation for example housing agencies, health providers ,and non-government agencies.

Within the UK implementation of ICT into services is aligned to Health policy which currently promotes strong involvement of both patients and public in services, supporting self management along side greater choice and control of Health Services (Department of Health 2010). UK based Research Councils support a range of research themes to promote innovation and development in ICT within healthcare for example Engineering and Physical Sciences Research Council (EPSRSC) provides a range of themes in this domain one being "Towards next-generation healthcare programme" [20]. In addition Research Council collaborations bring together multidisciplinary consortia to address factors across the life course that influence healthy ageing and wellbeing in later life. The lifelong Health and Wellbeing is a case in point funded by five of the Research councils[1] this programme aims to research factors across the life course that influence healthy ageing and wellbeing in later life. This includes identifying and developing effective interventions that lead to improved health and quality of life in later life alongside informing policy and practice including the development of services and technologies to support independent living.

A recent review the Scotland National Telecare Development Program implementation of Telecare in Scotland (2006–2010) [4] highlighted the impact of the Telecare Development Programme (TDP) which allocated a spend of 16.35 million pounds sterling to drive the adoption of telecare within the region. Of the allocated funds, 2.55 million pounds was used to fund an innovation programme and meet research and administration costs, while £13.8 million was allocated directly to care partnerships to drive service expansion. Table 2 below outlines the Key findings of the telecare implementation programme achieved as a direct result of strategic and policy implementation within the region.

This significant review on the impact of Telecare also outlines the following actual benefits:

- 346,000 care home bed days (against an expected 188,000).
- 65,000 hospital bed days through facilitated discharges and unplanned admissions avoided (against an expected 80,000).
- 35,000, nights of sleepover/wakened night care (against an expected 55,000).
- 411,000 home check visits savings were less than anticipated (against an expected 615,000).

[1] Arts and Humanities Research Council, Biotechnology and Biological Sciences Research Council, Economic and Social Research Council, EPSRC and Medical Research Council.

Table 2. Key findings of Telecare implementation programme in Scotland UK [50].

Key area	Finding
Growth of Telecare Through TDP Funding	Over 29,000 people began a telecare service through TDP funding over the period 2006–2010. Over the whole period around 7,300 subsequently stopped receiving a service. Over 2,000 people that received a TDP funded service are known to have been diagnosed with dementia, but the true figure is likely to be significantly higher.
Assessment of Progress Against Business Plan Expectations	By 31st March 2010, approximately £10.4 million of TDP funding had been spent by local partnerships, and another £2.6 million as match funding. 1Around 1,500 hospital discharges were expedited as a result of TDP funding 2006–2010 against a business plan expectation of about 1,800. At the same time around 6,600 unplanned hospital admissions were avoided against an expectation of around 3,800. Over 2,650 care home admissions were also avoided against an expectation of 3,025.
Progress Against the Wider Telecare Strategy 'Seizing the Opportunity'	Much of the focus of the national telecare strategy 2008–2010 was about providing guidance and support to care partnerships, and developing the 'infrastructure' necessary to deliver effective telecare services. Some of the key elements of the broader 2008–2010 telecare strategy – targeted (non financial) support to individual partnerships, promotion of the standards agenda, and aspects of the innovation programme – were delivered. However, important aspects of the vision for 2010 have still to be achieved.
The extent to which mainstreaming of telecare has been achieved	The evidence from a self assessment survey suggests that 22% of Scottish partnerships (or 7 partnerships in absolute terms) are now there or almost there in terms of mainstreaming. The bulk of partnerships (63%, or 20 partnerships in total) may be considered to be to a greater or lesser degree solidly on their way. This leaves some 15% (5 partnerships) over which there may still be said to be a serious question mark.

Alongside this it is highlighted that overall, the gross value of TDP funded efficiencies over the period 2006–2010 is approximately £48.4 million at current prices; the financial value of gross benefits achieved was fairly close to expectations, given the uncertainties necessarily involved in business planning.

2. ICT Research for Healthcare Scenarios

An important consequence of the policies outlined above, in tandem with changing public attitudes to healthcare translates into the need for healthcare providers to justify interventions to those funding the service and most importantly those receiving services. Commonly referred to as 'evidence based practice' the onus is on clinicians to ensure they are familiar with the most recent evidence about the effectiveness of interventions and use this in parallel to clinical judgment. Muir Gray [45] stated that

'Evidence based clinical practice is an approach to decision making in which the clinician uses the best evidence available in consultation with the patient to decide upon the options which suits that patient best.'

Initially the ambition was to develop a strong flow of research findings from academia into the clinical setting. Success of this approach has been reliant on a range of fluctuating variables for example dependence on researchers disseminating in journals that are accessible and familiar to clinicians, whilst the driver in academia is for impact factors of the chosen journal which may not be a natural choice for the clinician. Furthermore there is the requirement for the clinicians to be motivated to keep up to date with the vast amount of literature produced on a daily basis and understand how to transfer the knowledge into practice.

The nature of the relationships required also suggest that researchers will instinctively be well motivated to work on pertinent practice based questions. In addition to this, consensus was sought and achieved to construe a hierarchy of research methods deemed acceptable. Hence the emergence of the randomized control trial (RCT) as the 'gold standard' of evidence because of its potential to give a conclusive answer to the basic question of treatment effects.

There are several major challenges when researching ICT within healthcare. In terms of delivering the evidence adoption of the RCT methodology would fall short of acknowledging the multidimensional nature of the phenomena being explored. The development of ICT devices for healthcare, implementation and utilization within services is extremely complex with numerous interconnect parts and as such should be considered as 'complex intervention' [6].

The Medical Research Council in the UK proposes that a phased approach to the development and evaluation on a complex intervention is best. This phased approach enables the researchers to maintain and understanding of where they are with the research and to develop and utilize a range of both qualitative and quantitative methods relevant to the various phases of the research. The research can be designed in a linear mode as in Fig. 1 moving towards long term implementation.

However an iterative approach to the research is also possible integrating both qualitative and quantitative methods.

Most recently the move for strong Patient and Public Involvement (PPI) in Health Service design and delivery is also influencing health related research and has motivated the research funding bodies to give cognizance to PPI as a core requirement within study design. Many now require patients and the public to be involved in determining research priorities, contributing to developing study and reviewing outcomes. Furthermore, a new system for assessing the quality of research from Higher Education Institutes (HEI's) in the UK known as the Research Excellence Framework (REF) [37] will be undertaken by the funding bodies of higher education by 2014. Within this scenario institutions will be assessed not only on the quality of research output but also on the wider impact and vitality of the research environment.

Add to the complex situation the recognition by policy makers and governments that future health services can only achieve success with the innovation and diffusion of healthcare technologies if partnerships are developed that includes the health service providers, academia and business partnerships. The Information Society and Media Directorate-General of the European Commission is promoting user-driven open innovation methodologies in its research, development and innovation programmes [33]. These are presented in Fig. 2.

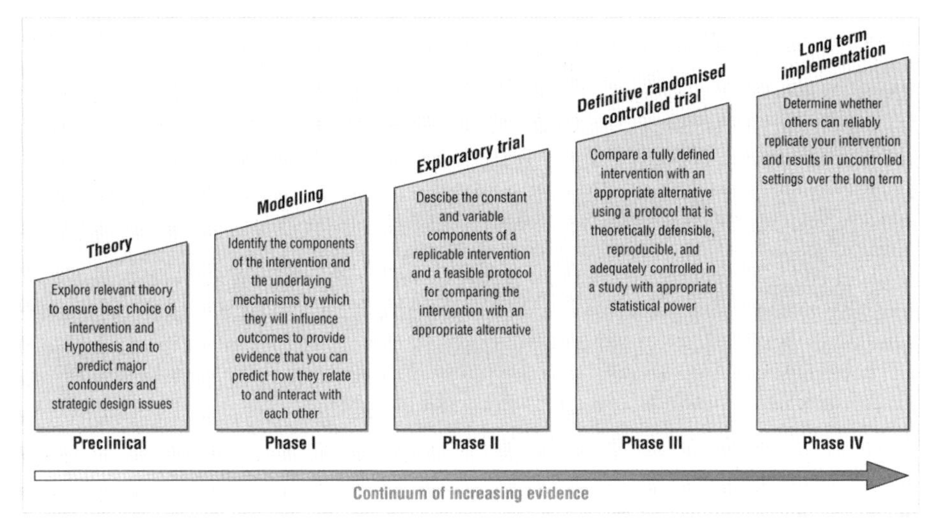

Figure 1. Sequential phases of developing randomised controlled trials of complex interventions [52].

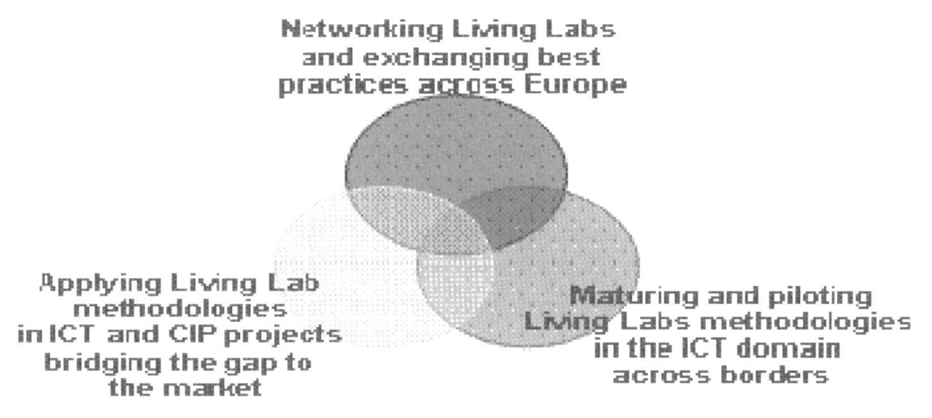

Figure 2.

The Living lab approach places the user at the centre of the innovation lifecycle, and this in real life settings.

2.1. TRAIL Living Lab

The TRAIL living lab aims to develop research methods for emerging ICT in healthcare which are user centric, promoting participation of end users and service providers whilst delivering research outputs that will impact directly into practice. TRAIL is a member of the European network of Living labs which now has approximately 212 living labs with the network. The architect and academic, William J. Mitchell, created the concept of living labs. Mitchell, based at MIT, was interested in how city dwellers could be involved more actively in urban planning and city design [44]. The ideas of citizen involvement in the design process was subsequently taken up and developed further in Europe by various research communities. A small number of living labs, created across Europe in 2005, primarily from the Computer Supported Cooperative Working (CSCW) research community, formed the European Network of Living Labs (ENOLL) in 2006. Successive waves of new living labs have since been created and, in 2010, there are, for example, 15 living labs in the UK and over 250 living labs across Europe and beyond.

Living labs are "collaborations of public-private-civic partnerships in which stakeholders co-create new products, services, businesses and technologies in real life environments and virtual networks in multi-contextual spheres" [35]. A simpler definition is "a collection of people, equipment, services and technology to provide a test platform for research and experiments" [34]. Essentially, Living Labs are community-facilitated, open and user-driven interventions.

The TRAIL living lab [54] brings a public-private-partnership approach to the research methods adopted where companies, public authorities and communities work together creating, prototyping, validating and testing new services, businesses, markets and technologies in real-life contexts in the regions, rural areas and virtual spaces between public and private players in the region of the North of Ireland. The objective of TRAIL is to conduct community-facilitated and user-driven methodologies that create service and product innovations that will enable ageing citizens to live independently in the heart of their communities.

TRAIL aims to develop pilot products and services for this sector of the community, with the added benefit of validating and fine-tuning the innovation methods. Importantly, TRAIL will support a fusion of innovation models, technology and integrated community care-based approaches. This will be achieved through executing on the following development strategy components:

- Identification and prioritization of user needs;
- Developing integrated demonstration models;
- Building capability through development, innovation, awareness and continuous process improvement;
- Growing the laboratory's reach and impact through geographic expansion, service intensification, advocacy and innovation based on evidence;
- Developing a sustainable business model for continued growth; and
- Conducting exploratory, evaluative and comparative empirical innovation studies that aim to understand better the Living Lab best practices, benchmarks, value chains, multi-level challenges and facilitators, and to understand better the core processes.

In the context of the European innovation system, the TRAIL model of open and user innovation links directly with the ambition of ENOLL, namely, to progress towards connecting the Lisbon Strategy (Lisbon Agenda, 2000) to a new and more user-driven European Innovation System. Moreover, TRAIL is equally in line with both the Lisbon Agenda and Northern Ireland regional development policy. For example, a key construct of Lisbon is "encouraging knowledge and innovation, by promoting more investment in research and development, by facilitating innovation, the take-up of information and communication technologies (ICT) and the sustainable use of resources, and by helping to create a strong European industrial base" – this is intrinsically linked to the social inclusion and economic growth in Northern Ireland. Examples of two research projects are provided below to highlight the contribution of the TRAIL lab to this research area [29].

2.2. Case Study Two: myHealth@age

The MyHealth@Age [46] project was a three year (2008–2010) research- and development initiative within the Northern Periphery Program with partners from Northern-Ireland, Norway and Sweden. The overall objectives of MyHealth@Age project where to improve health, safety and well being for elderly people in the Northern peripheral region of Europe through the use of new products and services based on mobile technologies.

The project followed Appreciative Action Research (PAAR) [3] as an umbrella methodology for the analysis, design, and test activities. PAAR embeds values such as empowerment, appreciation, ethics, and participation, as agreed overall norms and values for the project. These values were further strengthened by the Living Lab approach. The importance of starting the design and development work from the perspective of the potential users, to create as realistic situations for the work as possible, and to create traceability between needs, requirements, and prototype, as well as including continuous feedback lops throughout the project was highlighted throughout the work.

Within Northern Ireland the work focused on the needs of rural dwelling fit older people who were utilizing the community based senior citizens forum. The local healthcare trust, Southern Trust, worked in partnership on the project and supported recruitment and user engagement throughout the project. A range of qualitative tools were used to enable the voice of the older person to be heard for example face-2-face interviews, focus groups, daily diaries, photograph scrap books and regular participant meetings. In the initial phase of the project the participants attended a user workshop outlining the broad aims of our work. They were then provided with a disposable camera, scap book, diary and paper. During the following the two weeks they were asked to try to convey to us what it was like to live in a remote rural area. As general prompts they were asked to keep a daily record about their day, when they felt safe, or anxious or at risk. In addition they could make suggestions about what they considered would be really useful to them as they grew older. An iterative process of engagement with end users allowed them to significantly influence prototype device development and the associated service model. We would meet regularly in the local town where they lived and discuss rural health related issues and there views on the devices we were developing. Participants were given the devices to take home and try in a mock up situation for approximately 6 months. They give feedback to the researcher and got technical support via weekly meetings. The group of older people remained faithful to the research project through out its duration making a significant contribution and really finding a strong voice as the project developed.

2.3. Discussion of User Participation in Research

Currently within the research community discussion is taking place on individual participation in research and how to involve the wider public within research. The main drivers for this have already been presented. However legislation and policy to promote participation go back up to 35 years [8]. In fact the World Health Organization (1978) stated within the Declaration of Alma Ata (Health for all by the year 2000) [60] that:

"The people have the right and duty to participate individually and collectively in the planning and implementation of their healthcare."

It should follow in a world of evidence-based healthcare that participation in research to provide the evidence is a basic requirement. Brett 2010 [5] has stated that, "Empowering individuals and communities in order that they play a greater role in shaping health and social care research … aiming to democratise … research ensuring its maximum health and social benefit." Is a key function of patient and public participation in health service research.

However within the world of ICT enriched health and social care achieving this vision brings with it numerous challenges. By its very nature research consortiums in this domain bring together multidisciplinary groups from diverse backgrounds with differing perspectives for example engineering, healthcare and business. And whilst this brings a richness of understanding and vision to the work it can also create the circumstances for challenges and misunderstanding to emerge. For example to hold tight to the value of honouring true user participation and avoiding technological determination can at times place tensions within the consortium.

In addition to this contemporary research must only be undertaken within the framework of local ethical governance. With consortia that include academia and public healthcare providers it is often standard procedure for ethical review and approval to be sought from 3 ethical review agencies. Currently within the UK this will include the academic institution, the NHS body and the independent body for ethical review.

The administrative burden of engaging in this process must be accepted however the greater challenge in researching new and emerging technologies within healthcare can be balancing the absolute requirement of the ethical bodies to know what intervention will be developed and tested with each group against the desire for the researchers to allow the participation of itself to inform what will emerge.

Furthermore researchers need to consider the impact and expectations of participants involved in the research process. Given that most research projects will last between 2–3 years how can the research team sustain engagement with the recruited participants? This may become quite a critical issue especially if following a period of intense focus on user needs and aspirations the team retreat into the University to engage on a episode of development work.

3. Conclusion

This chapter has focused on the policy context for ICT enriched health and social care from a European and UK perspective. An example of one living lab, TRAIL is presented as a working exemplar of a single research groups attempts deliver user driven research on this complex intervention that because it has a strong user focus within its methods it may be more likely to achieve a strong impact. A recent report by OFCOM [49] identified that the opportunities and potential of next generation services for older and disabled people to achieve greater social and economic inclusion and engagement are manifold. However it is also highlighted that there are significant risks challenges and barriers to be overcome if this vision is to be realized this includes engaging with the future users of devices and services. Credible research work in this area will include multidisciplinary groups of researchers, with participants and the heart of innovation and development.

References

[1] Ambient Assisted living programme, [online] available at: http://www.aal-europe.eu/calls/aal-2008-1 [accessed on 03.02.11].

[2] J. Barlow, D. Singh, S. Bayer and R. Curry, A systematic review of the benefits of home telecare for frail elderly people and those with long-term conditions, *Journal of Telemedicine and Telecare* **13**(4) (2007), 172–179.

[3] F. Baum, C. MacDougall and D. Smith, Participatory action research, *Journal of Epidemiology Community Health* **60** (2006), 854–857.

[4] S. Beale, D. Sanderson and J. Kruger, Evaluation of the telecare development programme: Final report, 2010, [online] available at: http://www.scie-socialcareonline.org.uk/profile.asp?guid=84c830fd-7a8f-4f12-9ab7-84fc1aab5097 [accessed on 01.11.10].

[5] J. Brett, S. Staniszewska, C. Mockford, K. Seers, S. Herron-Marx and H. Bayliss, The PIRICOM study: A systematic review of the conceptualisation, measurement, impact and outcomes of patient and public involvement in health and social care research, 2010, available from: http://www.ukcrc.org/systematic-review-on-ppi-in-clinical-research/ [accessed 06.10.10].

[6] M. Campbell, R. Fitzpatrick, A. Haines, A.L. Kinmonth, P.D. Sandercock and T.P. Spiegelhalter, Framework for design and evaluation of complex interventions to improve health, *BMJ* **321** (2000), 694 (Published 16 September 2000).

[7] P. Coyte and D. Holmes, Health care adoption and diffusion in a social context, *Policy, Politics and Nursing Practice* **8** (2007), 47–54.

[8] J. Cunnett, Putting people at the heart of public services: Can we make it a reality this time? *The International Journal of Leadership in Public Services* **2**(4) (2008), 15–21

[9] Department of Health, 2007, available from: http://www.dh.gov.uk/en/index.htm [accessed on: 05.08.10].

[10] Department of Health, Building the information core: Implementing the NHS plan, 2001, [online] available from: http://www.dh.gov.uk/en/Publicationsandstatistics/Publications/PublicationsPolicyAndGuidance/DH_4005249 [accessed on 06.08.10].

[11] Department of Health, Information for health: An information strategy for the modern NHS 1998–2005. Executive summary, 1998, [online] available from: http://www.dh.gov.uk/en/Publicationsandstatistics/Publications/PublicationsPolicyAndGuidance/DH_4002944 [accessed on 06.08.10].

[12] Department of Health, Information for social care framework for improving quality in social care through better use of information and information technology executive, 2000, [online] available from: http://www.dh.gov.uk/en/Publicationsandstatistics/Publications/PublicationsPolicyAndGuidance/DH_4008909 [accessed on 06.08.10].

[13] Department of Health, Making healthier choices, 2004, available from: http://webarchive.nationalarchives.gov.uk/+/www.dh.gov.uk/prod_consum_dh/groups/dh_digitalassets/@dh/@en/documents/digitalasset/dh_4120792.pdf [accessed on 06.08.10].

[14] Department of Health, National Standards, Local Action: Health and social care standards and planning framework 2005/06-2007/08, Department Of Health, England, 2004, [online] available from http://www.dh.gov.uk/en/Publicationsandstatistics/Publications/PublicationsPolicyAndGuidance/DH_4086057 [accessed on 06.08.10].

[15] Department of Health, Our health, our care, our say: A new direction for community services, Department Of Health, England, 2006, [online] available from: http://www.dh.gov.uk/en/Publicationsandstatistics/Publications/PublicationsPolicyAndGuidance/DH_4127453 [accessed on 06.08.10].

[16] Department of Health and Social Services and Public Safety, Information and Communications Technology Strategy, Department of Health, Social Services and Public Safety, Northern Ireland, 2005, [online] available at: http://www.dhsspsni.gov.uk/ict-strategy.pdf [accessed on 06.08.10].

[17] Department of Health, Social services and public safety, a healthier future; a twenty year vision for health and wellbeing in Northern Ireland. Department of Health, Social Services and Public Safety: Northern Ireland, 2005, [online] available from: http://www.dhsspsni.gov.uk/healthyfuture-main.pdf [accessed on 06.08.10].

[18] Department of Health, The NHS improvement plan: Putting people at the heart of public services, Department Of Health, England, 2004, [online] available from: http://www.dh.gov.uk/en/publicationsandstatistics/publications/publicationspolicyandguidance/dh_4084476 [accessed on 06.08.10].

[19] Department of Health, Working together with health information: A partnership strategy for education, training and development, 1999, [online] available from: http://www.dh.gov.uk/en/Publicationsandstatistics/Publications/PublicationsPolicyAndGuidance/DH_4008598 [accessed on 06.08.10].

[20] Engineering and Physical Science Research Council, [online] available at: http://www.epsrc.ac.uk/about/progs/healthcare/Pages/default.aspx [accessed on 03.02.11].
[21] Europa: Activities of the European Union, The Amsterdam Treaty, 2008, [online] available at: http://europa.eu/scadplus/leg/en/s50000.htm [accessed on 25.09.10].
[22] Europa glossary: Lisbon Strategy, [online] available at: http://europa.eu/scadplus/glossary/lisbon_strategy_en.htm [accessed on 25.09.10].
[23] European Commission, Competitiveness and Innovation Programme, 2010, [online] available at: http://ec.europa.eu/cip/ [accessed on 01.11.10].
[24] European Commission, eEurope 2005: An information society for all, European Commission, Brussels, 2005, [online] available at: http://ec.europa.eu/information_society/eeurope/2002/news_library/documents/eeurope2005/eeurope2005_en.pdf [accessed on 05.08.10].
[25] European Commission, eHealth priorities and strategies in European countries, European Commission, Brussels, 2007, [online] available at: http://ec.europa.eu/information_society/activities/health/docs/policy/ehealth-era-full-report.pdf [accessed on 05.08.07].
[26] European Commission, Europe's response to world ageing; Promoting social economic progress in an ageing world, European Commission, Brussels, 2002, [online] available at: http://eurlex.europa.eu/LexUriServ/site/en/com/2002/com2002_0143en01.pdf [accessed on 05.08.10].
[27] European Commission, Joint report on social protection and social inclusion, European Commission, Brussels, 2007, [online] available at: http://ec.europa.eu/employment_social/social_inclusion/jrep_en.html [accessed on 05.08.10].
[28] European Commission, Legal Challenges in eHealth, European Commission, Brussels, 2007, [online] available at: http://ec.europa.eu/information_society/newsroom/cf/itemlongdetail.cfm?item_id=3507 [accessed on 05.08.10].
[29] European Commission, Living labs for user-driven open innovation, 2010, [online] available at: http://ec.europa.eu/information_society/activities/livinglabs/index_en.htm [accessed on 01.11.10].
[30] European Commission, What is eHealth? European Commission, Brussels, 2007, [online] available at: http://ec.europa.eu/information_society/activities/health/whatis_ehealth/index_en.htm [accessed on 03.02.2011].
[31] European Commission, What is eHealth? European Commission, Brussels, 2007, [online] available at: http://ec.europa.eu/information_society/activities/health/whatis_ehealth/index_en.htm [accessed on 03.08.10].
[32] Europes Information Society Thematic Portal, [online] available at: http://ec.europa.eu/information_society/activities/livinglabs/index_en.htm [accessed on 03.02.2011].
[33] Europes Information Society Thematic Portal, [online] available at: http://ec.europa.eu/information_society/activities/livinglabs/index_en.htm [accessed on 01.11.10].
[34] FarNorth, FarNorth Living Lab, 2010, http://farnorthlivinglab.no/, last accessed September 11, 2010.
[35] K. Feuerstein, A. Hesmer, K.A. Hribernik, K.-D. Thoben and J. Schumacher, Living labs: A new development opportunity, in: *European Living Labs – A New Approach for Human Centric Regional Innovation*, J. Schumacher and V.-P. Niitamo, eds, 2008.
[36] F. Garcia-Lizana and A. Sarria-Santamera, New technologies for chronic disease management and control: a systematic review, *Journal of Telemedicine and Telecare* **13**(2) (2007), 62–68.
[37] Higher Education Funding Council, Research Excellence Framework, 2010, [online] available at: http://www.hefce.ac.uk/research/ref/ [accessed on 01.11.10].
[38] Joint Improvement Team, available from: http://www.jitscotland.org.uk/action-areas/telecare-in-scotland/ [accessed on 06.08.10].
[39] Kent County Council, [online] available from: http://www.kent.gov.uk/adult_social_services/social_services_professionals/partnerships_and_projects/assistive_technologies.aspx [accessed on 02.02.2011].
[40] S. Martin, G. Kernohan, B. McCreight and C. Nugent, Smart home technologies for health and social care support, *Cochrane Database of Systematic Reviews* (4) (2008), Art. No.: CD006412. DOI: 10.1002/14651858.CD006412.pub2.
[41] S. Martin and G. Rankin, Using commercially available technology to assist in the delivery of a person-centred health and social care, *Journal of Telemedicine and Telecare* **8**(2) (2002), 60–62.
[42] A. Martinez, V. Villarroel and P. Puig-Junoy, An economic analysis of the EHAS telemedicine system in Alto Amazonas, *Journal of Telemedicine and Telecare* **13**(1) (2007), 7–14.
[43] E. Marziali, T. Damianakis and P. Donahue, Internet-based clinical services virtual support groups for family caregivers, *Journal of Telemedicine and Telecare* **24**(2–3) (2006), 39–54.
[44] W.J. Mitchell, *Me++: The Cyborg Self and the Networked City*, MIT Press, Cambridge, Mass, 2003.
[45] J.A. Muir Gray, *Evidence-Based Healthcare*, Churchill Livingstone, 2008.
[46] myhealth@age, available at: http://www.myhealth-age.eu/ [accessed on 01.11.10].
[47] NHS Scotland, [online] available from eHealth Scotland: http://www.ehealth.scot.nhs.uk/ [accessed on 06.08.10].

[48] J. Norum, S. Pedersen, J. Stormer, M. Rumpsfeld and A. Stormo, Prioritisation of telemedicine services for large scale implementation in Norway, *Journal of Telemedicine and Telecare* **13**(4) (2007), 185–192.
[49] OFCOM, Next generation services for older and disabled people, 2010, [online] available at: http://www.ofcom.org.uk/about/how-ofcom-is-run/committees/older-and-disabled-people/research/ [accessed 06.10.10].
[50] A. Ohinma and S. Richard, A cost model for videoconferencing in Alberta, *Journal of Telemedicine and Telecare* **12**(7) (2006), 363–369.
[51] V. Patterson, Teleneurology, *Journal of Telemedicine and Telecare* **11**(2) (2005), 55–59.
[52] J. Sanford, H. Hoenig, P. Griffiths and T. Butterfield, A comparison of televideo and traditional in-home rehabilitation in mobility impaired older adults, *Physical and Occupational Therapy in Geriatrics* **25**(3) (2007), 1–18.
[53] P. Seibert, T. Whitmore, P. Parker, F. Grimsley and K. Payne, The emerging role of telemedicine in diagnosing and treating sleep disorders, *Journal of Telemedicine and Telecare* **12**(8) (2007), 379–381.
[54] TRAIL living lab, [online] available at: http://trail.ulster.ac.uk/ [accessed on 01.11.10].
[55] P. Whitten and M. Maureen, Home telecare for COPD/CHF patients: Outcomes and perceptions, *Journal of Telemedicine and Telecare* **13**(2) (2007), 69–73.
[56] Whole System Demonstrators, [online] available from: http://webarchive.nationalarchives.gov.uk/+/www.dh.gov.uk/en/Healthcare/Longtermconditions/wholesystemdemonstrators/index.htm [accessed on 02.02.2011].
[57] World Health Organization, Building foundations for eHealth, World Health Organisation, Geneva, 2006, [online] available at: http://www.who.int/ehealth/resources/en/ [accessed on 03.09.10].
[58] World Health Organization, Building foundations for eHealth, World Health Organisation, Geneva, 2006, [online] available at: http://www.who.int/ehealth/resources/en/ [accessed on 03.08.10].
[59] World Health Organization, Connecting for health. Global vision, local insight: Report for the world summit on the information society, World Health Organisation, Geneva, 2005, [online] available at: http://www.who.int/kms/resources/WSISReport_Connecting_for_Health.pdf [accessed on 03.09.10].
[60] World Health Organization, Declaration of Alma Ata, 1978, available at: http://www.who.int/social_determinants/tools/multimedia/alma_ata/en/index.html [accessed on 01.11.10].
[61] World Health Organization, eHealth, Report by the secretariat, World Health Organisation, Geneva, 2005, [online] available at: http://www.who.int/gb/ebwha/pdf_files/WHA58/A58_21-en.pdf [accessed on 03.09.10].
[62] World Health Organization, Report EB117/15 from the secretariat on eHealth proposed tools and services, World Health Organisation, Geneva, 2006, [online] available at: http://www.who.int/gb/ebwha/pdf_files/EB117/B117_15-en.pdf [accessed on 03.09.10].
[63] World Health Organization, Report EB117/15 from the secretariat on eHealth proposed tools and services, World Health Organisation, Geneva, 2006, [online] available at: http://www.who.int/gb/ebwha/pdf_files/EB117/B117_15-en.pdf [accessed on 03.08.10].
[64] World Health Organization, Resolution WHA58.28 eHealth, World Health Organisation, Geneva, 2005, [online] available at: http://www.who.int/gb/ebwha/pdf_files/WHA58/WHA58_28-en.pdf [accessed on 03.09.10].
[65] World Health Organization, The world health report 2006: Working together for health, World Health Organisation, Geneva, 2006, [online] available at: http://www.who.int/whr/2006/chapter1/en/index.html [accessed on 29.09.10].
[66] World Health Organization, The world health report 2006: Working together for health, World Health Organisation, Geneva, 2006, [online] available at: http://www.who.int/whr/2006/chapter1/en/index.html [accessed on 29.07.10].

Smart Homes as a Vehicle for Ambient Assisted Living

Handbook of Ambient Assisted Living
J.C. Augusto et al. (Eds.)
IOS Press, 2012

doi:10.3233/978-1-60750-837-3-387

Smart Homes as a Vehicle for AAL

Juan Carlos AUGUSTO *
University of Ulster, UK

Abstract. The chapters in this section provide good examples of developments which facilitate Ambient Assisted Living at home and consider the technologies and challenges involved in the development of such systems as well as the way they complement traditional healthcare systems provision.

Keywords. Ambient assisted living, smart homes, innovation, sensing

Introduction

Smart Homes have been at the core of the development of the area of Ambient Assisted Living. This area evolved from the earlier telecare/telehealth services delivered at home which enabled the monitoring of (usually) isolated biometric parameters on a person or a family. The idea of smart homes explores the orchestration of several services related to safety, health, comfort and economy. It blends sensing technology and networking infrastructure with intelligent software which can provide a more holistic analysis of situations which are of specific interest to the occupants of the house and makes decisions in real-time and long-term profiles to enhance the quality of life of those living in the house. Developments with a focus on healthcare, and wellbeing are exemplified through the following chapters:

Designing Ambient and Personalised Displays to Encourage Healthier Lifestyles, by Tatsuo Nakajima and Fahim Kawsar, addresses the important issue of interaction and how a system can be more effective through the use of useful feedback to encourage following a specific lifestyle which has been recognized as beneficial for a specific individual.

Supporting Wellbeing through Improving Interactions and Understanding in Self-Monitoring Systems, by Dana Pavel, Vic Callaghan and Anind Dey, highlights the importance of explanations that help the user understand their routines and how they relate to their wellbeing, these explanations are rich in terms of providing context as well as on the delivery of the message with support of a blend of media which makes the interaction more appealing and understandable.

Sensor Selection to Support Practical Use of Health-Monitoring Smart Environments, by Diane Cook and Lawrence Holder, turns the focus into the core technology of sensing and the effect the deployment of this infrastructure has on machine learning algorithms used to extract user profiles and to understand how they relate to essential lifestyle parameters.

*Corresponding Author: Juan Carlos Augusto. E-mail: jc.augusto@ulster.ac.uk.

Utilization of Cloud Infrastructures for Pervasive Healthcare Applications, by Charalambos Doukas, Thomas Pliakas and Ilias Maglogiannis, highlight the new opportunities arising from cloud computing to implement the concept of Ubiquitous healthcare, the deployment of personal data and the access of that data from various places (home, health centre, traveling, holiday destination, etc.) which can facilitate a more flexible, updated interaction between people and the healthcare system which will be ready to be used in real-time wherever the person is.

Smart Living Environment: Ubiquitous Computing Approach Based on TRON Architecture, by Ken Sakamura, provides an insight on an ambitious Japanase project which supports the use of Ubiquitous Computing across society. It explains developments of smart homes as well as technology which supports people in their interaction with the world outside the home environment. The emphasis is on the engineering of these systems and the lessons collected after years of development and experimentation.

All these developments show the level of maturity of this field where the infrastructure available to the developing teams has evolved into a more reliable stage with a variety of media that can be used to collect and convey information. Intelligent software has been developed which can understand meaningful contexts and take decisions which can potentially help the occupants of a house to improve their health and lifestyles or to be connected with the health system in a more flexible way, whenever and wherever they need it. There are certainly many aspects which are only at experimental stages and many problems which may take considerable effort to solve but progress in the last decade is encouraging and there is hope within the many sectors involved that this technology can improve our quality of life in the future.

Handbook of Ambient Assisted Living
J.C. Augusto et al. (Eds.)
IOS Press, 2012

doi:10.3233/978-1-60750-837-3-389

Designing Ambient and Personalised Displays to Encourage Healthier Lifestyles

Tatsuo NAKAJIMA [a,*] and Fahim KAWSAR [b]
[a] *Computer Science Department, Waseda University, Tokyo, Japan*
[b] *Bell Labs, Belgium and Lancaster University, United Kingdom*

Abstract. In recent years, the deteriorations of living habits like immobilization or unhealthy diet are becoming serious social problems in many developed countries. Even if we know the importance, it is difficult to change our undesirable habits and to maintain a desirable lifestyle. Previous studies have suggested that persuasive technology can play a significant role in persuading individuals for behavioural change. In the article, we discuss the design of persuasive ambient displays aimed at addressing this issue borrowing theories from behavioural psychology. In our design, aesthetic and empathetic expressions are used to represent the visualisation reflecting behavioural feedback of an individual. If an individual's behaviour is leaned towards healthier lifestyle, the display expression is designed to boost his/her positive emotion where as display expression is progressively shifted to increase negative emotion of the individual if he/she does not sustain the desirable behaviour. In this paper, we introduce design principles of our approach and present four case studies to show the applicability of our approach. We also discuss a number of issues uncovered during the design and evaluation of these case studies.

Keywords. Ambient display, persuasive technology, personalisation, better lifestyle

1. Introduction

While the purpose of technology is to bring about positive change in the world, some problems cannot be fixed by simply applying a technological solution. Problems that arise from people's choices and lifestyles are often more effectively addressed by altering human behaviour than by attempting to develop a technological fix. In practice, desirable lifestyle patterns may be challenging for individuals to realize. In these cases, technology can be applied indirectly as a tool to motivate behavioural change. Persuasive media such as books and pamphlets have been used to change people's attitudes and behaviour since ancient times. Recent advances in persuasive technologies such as the Web and mobile phones have had a strong impact on our daily lives [7]. Several previous approaches [14,16] have tried to change an individual's daily behaviour to motivate him/her towards a better lifestyle.

*Corresponding Author: Tatsuo Nakajima, Computer Science Department, Waseda University, Japan. E-mail: tatsuo@dcl.info.waseda.ac.jp.

The objective of our work is to design solutions for an open-ended target group to bring about lifestyle changes in mundane daily activities. We felt that in this area ubiquitous computing technologies could provide new possibilities. Ubiquitous computing is already used in areas such as health, hygiene and food safety to directly address and fix people's problems. We focused on areas where improvement requires a change in voluntary human behaviour. A key promise of ubiquitous computing is that it allows us to design systems that are almost invisible to the user. The systems can obtain input from sensors and computers embedded in everyday objects, and provide calm output through ambient displays integrated into the environment. Considering the ubiquity of such peripheral displays in our environment we see an interesting opportunity to motivate behavioural change for healthier lifestyle by combining persuasive technologies with peripheral displays. To this end, in this article we present an approach grounded to the theory of behavioural psychology to design ambient displays aimed at motivating individual for a healthier lifestyle. We used some basic tenets from operant conditioning [6] as a basic principle for changing a user's habits. The most obvious issue is that the system should include a feedback loop between the user's behaviour and the expression shown on an ambient display.

Expression has a role not only as a representer of information but also as an external motivator for the user's future action. A picture is originally designed to be watched and to have something attractive, but it is also suitable for information visualization [11]. One of the important challenges in ubiquitous computing is how to represent large amounts of information in a calm and unobtrusive manner. Aesthetic expression of the information is also important in order to accept ubiquitous computing technologies in our daily lives. Our approach enhances traditional ambient displays to claim that an ambient display can be used to persuade to change a user's undesirable habits, and keep desirable habits.

In this paper, we discuss how aesthetic and empathetic expressions are effective in persuading a user to change his undesirable habits. In the next section we describe existing behaviour-shaping technologies, and discuss their benefits and limitations. We then present the design principles of our approach discussing the rationales behind our design decisions. Section 4 presents four behavioural-shaping application case studies designed with ambient display systems following our principles: Persuasive Art, Virtual Aquarium, Mona Lisa Bookshelf, and EcoIsland. After that we discuss a range of issues uncovered during our research. Finally Section 6 concludes the paper with avenues of our future work.

2. Related Work

Even though successful specialized computerized solutions for motivating change in behaviour have been demonstrated, their adoption in everyday life remains scarce. The researchers who created Squire's Quest found that it was challenging to find time for the gaming sessions that were intended to alter behaviour [2]. The sessions would also likely have to be repeated in order to maintain the effect. Effecting additional changes, such as improving dental hygiene in addition to teaching better nutritional choices, would require a separate set of sessions. The time requirement placed on the user limits the applicability of this type of serious games for effecting changes in people's lifestyles.

Furthermore, in some areas there may be psychological limits to the ability of education alone to effect behavioural change. Even when a person full-well knows that a particular behaviour is detrimental enough to her long-term well-being to offset any possible short-term benefits, she may still irrationally choose the short-term indulgence. Examples of such behaviour include smoking, over-eating, under-exercising and poor personal care. Future consequences, while widely known, are easily ignored in the present.

To combat these behaviour patterns, commercial software solutions are available that operate on a principle different from education: they turn long-term effects into short-term feedback. For example, so-called "Quit Meters" [24] provide smokers with constant feedback on how much money is wasted and how many minutes of life are lost. "Carb Counters" [23] for Palm handheld devices provide instant feedback on meal choices. Compared to games, quit meters and carb counters do not require setting aside time for game sessions, as their use is intended to happen during normal daily activities. But the feedback they provide lacks the engagement and fun that games strive for, lessening their emotional impact.

Quit meters, carb counters and many lifestyle-shaping games suffer from problems created by self-reporting. Besides being burdensome and time-consuming, reporting one's behaviour to a machine in order to obtain feedback is unreliable: people are known to submit false data, both intentionally and due to cognitive biases. This hampers the system's ability to effect real change. 'Ere Be Dragons' [5] is an example of a serious game that utilizes passive sensors to observe user behaviour. The game's purpose is to encourage the players to partake in a healthy level of physical exercise. Users roam in an outdoor space while the game collects data from heart-rate sensors and GPS devices and renders the game world on a PDA screen. The only self-reported bit of information is player age. As a tool for effecting lifestyle change in mundane daily activities, the concept behind 'Ere Be Dragons' nevertheless suffers from the same problem as Squire's Quest: it requires setting aside significant time and space for gaming sessions. Ubiquitous computing and ambient interaction solutions are intended to relax the time-space requirements of interacting with a computer system. Such systems are integrated into daily environments and seek to utilize peripheral perception capacity to deliver information in an unobtrusive way. An example of this idea is found in the Informative art project, where both the appearance and physical role of information displays is designed to resemble paintings hanging on the wall [13]. However, ambient displays are typically used to deliver outside information to the user, from weather conditions to unread emails. In our work, the goal is to motivate desirable lifestyle changes by making boring tasks fun rather than by just presenting information.

3. Design Principles for Ambient Displays

Traditionally, computational interfaces are confined to conventional displays. However with the emergence of pervasive technologies, displays of different size, shape and form factor are being embedded into our everyday lives. Most of these displays aim to be ambient and peripheral in nature (thus drawing minimal attention) yet delivering the intended information elegantly. These displays, so-called *Ambient Displays* due to their inherent characteristics of being operational in our periphery suit perfectly as the interfaces for persuasive applications aimed at improving our everyday lifestyles. In this section, we discuss different design cardinals to construct ambient displays. However, before moving to the design discussion, let us take a closer look at the process of behavioural change, the primary objective of designing these displays in the context of this work. A better understanding of this process will assist us in addressing the issues that are critical for the successful design of these displays.

Exploring the psychological research, we observe that one of the pioneer model that describes the mechanics of intentional behaviour change is the Transtheoretical Model of Change (TTM). Proposed by Prochaska et al., this model suggests that individuals experience a cycle of stages before achieving the intentional behaviours [28]. In detail, The Transtheoretical Model construes change as a process involving progress through a series of five stages: precontemplation, contemplation, preparation, action and maintenance – until one relinquishes the undesired behaviours.

1. The first stage, pre-contemplation, is where individuals are unaware and uninformed of their problems and have no intention to change the behaviour.
2. In the next stage, contemplation, they are aware of the problem but yet not committed to take action to alter the behaviours.
3. In the preparation stage, individuals form intention and actively plan to take action to address the problematic behaviours.
4. The fourth stage, action is where individuals willingly and actively taking actions to change their behaviours.
5. The last stage is maintenance where individuals try to sustain their actions to keep the new behaviours.

We argue that TTM provides a sound indication of the mechanics of intentional behaviour change. Many people remain in the first two stages of the TTM model regarding problematic lifestyle and possess mental barriers that prevent them from understanding the issue or seeing the benefits of behaviour change. Ambient display as a channel for raising peripheral awareness can address these pre-action stages. In addition, a feedback mechanism that can reflect the impact of later stages can significantly contribute in motivating individuals to sustain healthier lifestyle.

Motivating humans can be classified into two approaches. One is to make users aware of their current situation and the other is to enhance the user's willingness to change his habits. Motivating a change of habits can also be classified into two types. The positive expression style increases a user's positive emotion to motivate a change in the user's undesirable habits. The user feels happy when changing his/her undesirable habits even if the change is challenging and hard. Another type is the negative expression style. This promotes negative emotion to feel a sense of crisis that motivates to change the user's undesirable habits. For instance, if a user looks at himself in a mirror and finds that he is significantly overweight, this may motivate him to do more exercise.

Accordingly, our design principles are primarily driven by ambient display strategies and ambient feedback strategies.

3.1. Ambient Display Strategies

Pousman et al. defined Ambient Information System as the system that [27]

1. Displays information that is important but not critical.
2. Can move from the periphery to the focus of attention and back again.
3. Focuses on the tangible, representations in the environment.

4. Provides subtle changes to reflect updates in information and
5. Is asthetically pleasing.

We agree with their understanding, and consequently have adopted their guidelines in our display strategies which are described in the following:

Representation Fidelity: A major challenge in designing ambient displays is the representation fidelity taking into account how individuals perceive information, manage to sustain attentive to information of interest available in our periphery, and remain aware of changes of information in an unobtrusive way. Too much information potentially degrade conveniences of our daily living, and this inconvenience might lead an individual to ignore the information completely. Henceforth, significant research efforts focused on finding the proper balance between perceptual complexity and information overload, making sure information is provided in an appropriate way. Consulting the theory of semiotics, we can observe three alternatives for representation: Indexical – direct representation, Iconic – representation through related metaphor and Symbolic – abstract representation. Although, a range of previous studies (including ours as we will discuss later in the case study sections) have designed ambient displays with iconic or abstract images [18,9], we consider the ideal design would be a hybrid one, where abstract or iconic representation would be primary visual element that is augmented with minimal indexical representation when needed, reducing the fidelity of information so that it is easier to perceive. This indexical information is particularly important to ensure the intelligibility of the system.

History: It is also important that the representation portrays the temporal gradient of their action so that individuals can apprehend the progress of their behavioural change mechanics. This is a challenging aspect particularly considering the representation fidelity we have discussed earlier. Depending on the visualization technique it might be possible to reflect the progress but for a convincing understanding, abstract and/or iconic representation is not often adequate. However, designing visualization with indexical representation can address this issue. In this case, indexical representation over a time period might not be the primary display content, but could be invoked through user interaction.

Intelligibility: One of the limitations of ambient visualisation is that individuals might not understand why the particular visualisation is displayed and how it reflects his/her actions. Of course with careful design it is possible to formulate a direct connection between users physical actions and corresponding digital representation, but more than often users will feel confused as well as frustrated if the representation is not intelligible enough [22]. Addressing this issue at the representation level is very complicated, and it is often needed that the ambient display system provides visual clue and in some cases clear explanation to users describing the meaning of the representation.

Personalization: Related to the intelligibility of the visualisation, it is also important to place users at the central of the control of the ambient display system. This is particularly important to enable users to personalize their visualisation that reflects their personal likings, taste and values. Personalization is a matured concept that have widely used in different application domains to provide adaptive, custom tailored output. In an ambient display system designed for behaviour-shaping applications, it is important that users can personalize the visual output, this could be as simple as changing the colour, brightness,

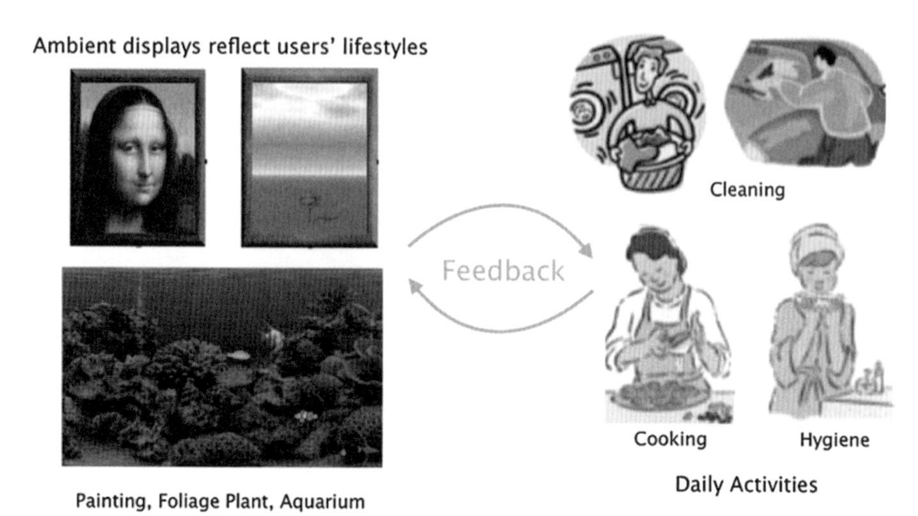

Figure 1. The ambient display system could be described as a kind of mirror, because it reflects something about the user. The display does not show the usual outward appearance, but reflects more personal facts that may otherwise go unnoticed.

transition effect etc., to more complex ones, e.g., modifying the underlying application policy, visualization technique, etc.

Emotional Engagement: The fact that the information is delivered in a non-disruptive way must not mean that it ends up being irrelevant to the user. To effect a change in behaviour in operant conditioning, we must be able to administer some sort of meaningful consequences to the user. We do not have means to effect changes in physical reality (such as threatening the user's family), so would it be possible to make the user care about changes in the internal state of a computer system? Computer games seem to be able to do this. Good games are able to provoke a range of emotional responses, from fun and satisfaction to guilt and discontent. By mimicking the techniques used in computer games, we should be able to build an emotionally engaging visual representation, allowing us to administer punishments and rewards without any physical resources. By "emotional engagement" we do not necessarily mean strong and deep emotional responses, but the simple kicks that make many games interesting and addictive.

3.2. Ambient Feedback Strategy

Ambient feedback as shown in Fig. 1 is intended to be implemented using ubiquitous computing techniques, including sensors and ambient displays, but most implementation details are determined by the needs of a particular application and what behaviour it targets to satisfy the following principles below. To lend a solid framework for feedback design, we referred to elementary behavioural psychology. Behavioural psychology is a discipline dealing with the relationship between behaviour and consequences. It posits that the form and frequency of behaviour can be affected by controlling the consequences. The principle to design the systems consists of the following three components.

Passive observation: One of the key factors limiting the applicability of the earlier solutions to our intended purpose is the various burdens they place on a user, either in the form of time use or effort. To avoid the burdens of self-reporting, the system should be able to passively observe the user's behaviour. To eliminate the need to set aside time or go to a special place, the system should be integrated with normal daily activities. Thus our first design principle is to use observations of the users' behaviour as the system's input, as opposed to using keystrokes or some other proxy behaviour. This also facilitates the delivery immediate feedback, a key factor in the effectiveness of operant conditioning.

Unobtrusive Feedback: To complete the integration of an ambient display into the user's daily living environment, we must also make sure that the notification mechanism of the feedback is appropriate. We refer to Mark Weiser's concept of calm technology: technology that is able to leverage our peripheral perception to deliver information, as opposed to constantly demanding direct attention [33]. Consulting the theory of attention management, we can categorise human attention into three types: inattention, focused attention and divided attention [25,32]. In inattention, objects might not be in our periphery but can still affect our behaviour (e.g., memory recall). In divided attention our attention is distributed over several objects whereas in focused attention, all our attention resources are dedicated on one stimulus. Considering the importance of information visualised in ambient displays we argue that feedback notifcation should operate in the degree of divided attention and should not consume entire attention space.

Focused Domain and Micro Activity: It is important the feedback is provided for a focused domain, and in principle for a micro activity. In some cases the activity might include multiple physical actions. If feedback is provided for multiple activities with an abstract representation it is often difficult to understand which activity is contributing to the visualisation and how. In addition, representing relationship effectively while ensuring the persuasive nature of the feedback is extremely difficult. As previous studies have discussed [34], it is very important to ensure that the feedback is provided for a focused domain so that representation is comprehensive to the users.

Feedback Logic: The feedback logic determines the type of visualization that the system should be giving at any point in time. The decision is reached by comparing the user's pattern of behaviour, as reflected by the context information, with the desired "ideal" pattern. In principle, the closer the pattern is to the ideal, the more positive the feedback. The logic obviously depends on implementation and can be extremely complicated, in particular if it attempts to embrace a detailed psychological model. In operant conditioning, feedback content can be divided into reinforcement and punishment depending on whether behavior is encouraged or discouraged. Reinforcement and punishment are further divided into four types:

1. Positive reinforcement: encouraging a user's behaviour by providing a favourable stimulus in response to it.
2. Negative reinforcement: encouraging a user's behaviour by removing an averse stimulus in response to it.
3. Positive punishment: discouraging a user's behaviour by providing an averse stimulus in response to it.
4. Negative punishment: discouraging a user's behaviour by removing a favourable stimulus in response to it.

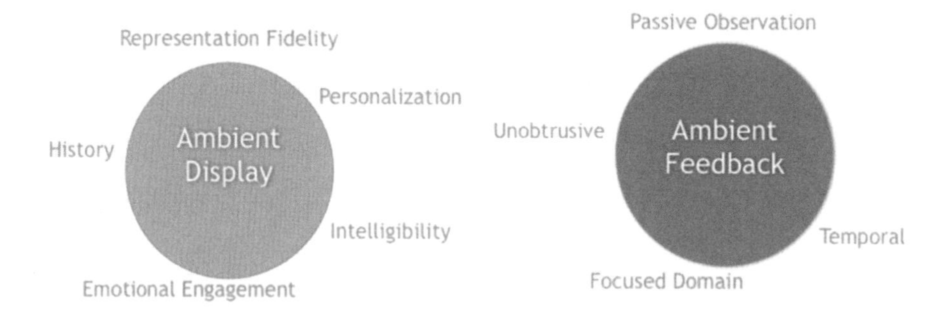

Figure 2. Design principles for Ambient and Personalised Displays.

Another consideration in operant conditioning is scheduling: the temporal arrangement of stimuli in relation to behaviour. The feedback logic has to have a persistent state, so that it facilitates delayed, aggregated and scheduled feedback. In our design we have two types of feedback provision: "Immediate feedback" gives users an immediate clue on the desirability of their actions; "Accumulated feedback" may be used to reflect long-term consequences faster than the real long-term consequences of the behaviour would occur. It can also create an accumulated history for a behaviour that otherwise has little. For example, children (and adults, too) sometimes argue that cleaning one's room is futile, since it will be just as messy again the next week. This could be helped by keeping track of the number of times the room has been cleaned and presenting it in an engaging way. Instead of things seemingly returning to status quo, accumulated feedback shows that actions result in progress.

Figure 2 highlights the different cardinals of our design principles distributed across ambient display and feedback strategies. These design principles provide basic directives for designing ambient displays for behaviour-shaping applications. However, more situated strategy can be adopted in the design depending on the application context and the target activities.

4. Four Case Studies

In this section, we discuss four case studies where combinations of the design principles introduced in the previous section have been applied.

4.1. Persuasive Art

Decorating walls with pictures is common at home. Pictures are a very important way to increase aesthetic feeling in our daily lives. Persuasive Art uses a painting to motivate a user to walk at least 8000 steps every day to keep his/her fit. The number of steps are monitored automatically and stored into a computer. The painting shows the feedback of the current status of the user's exercise to motivate him to maintain desirable habits. Persuasive Art currently offers the following four paintings as shown in Fig. 3. The landscape painting includes a tree that grows and withers, The figure painting is Mona Lisa, the abstract painting has objects that change in size, and the still life picture contains changing number of orbs.

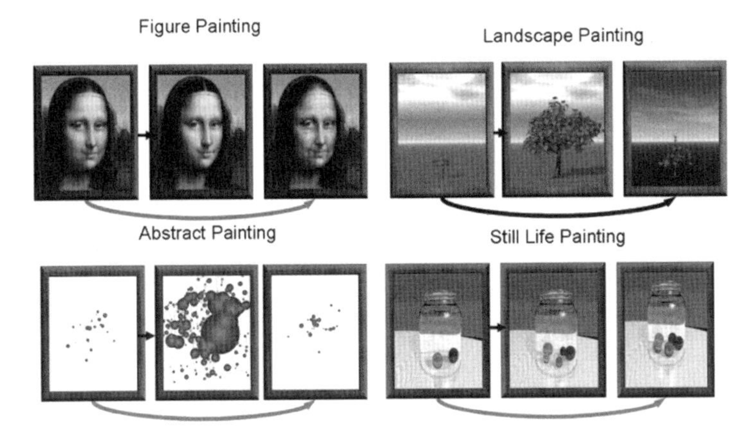

Figure 3. Four alternative Virtual Paintings for Persuasive Art.

When using the landscape painting, the tree's growth is varied according to the user's behaviour. When the user maintains desirable habits by walking daily 8000 step or more, the tree will grow, but if he/she does walk enough, then the tree gradually dies. So, the basic metaphor here is that the increase of healthy activities makes the tree more healthy, but the neglect of the exercise lets the tree die. The other paintings are of similar strategy, i.e., Mona Lisa looks older, object size shrinks, and orb number reduces, all to reflect unhealthy behaviour.

This visualization tries to reduce the information fidelity by adopting a symbolic (abstract) representation, provides history through gradual transition, tends to be emotionally engaging and provides personalization features through multiple paintings. In addition, the metaphors used for the paintings are self explanatory thus exhibiting a minimum level of intelligibility.

The feedback strategy here is temporally accumulative, unobtrusive in the sense that the paintings do not provide too much information consequently draw less attention, and reflect one micro activity, i.e., number of walking steps which is observed passively through an on-body pedometer.

4.2. Virtual Aquarium

Virtual Aquarium shown in Fig. 4 has the objective of improving users' dental hygiene by promoting correct toothbrushing practices. The system is set up in the lavatory where it turns a mirror into a simulated aquarium. Fish living in the aquarium are affected by the users' toothbrushing activity. If users brush their teeth properly, the fish prosper and procreate. If not, they are weakened and may even perish.

In this system, we used a 3-axis accelerometer that is attached to each toothbrush in a household. Since toothbrushes are usually not shared and each accelerometer has a unique identification number, we are able to infer which user is using the system at a given time. Toothbrushing patterns are recognised by analysing the acceleration data. Fig. 4 shows a user brushing his teeth in front of the Virtual Aquarium using a sensor augmented toothbrush. The toothbrush is able to observe how a user brushes his/her teeth passively without requesting extra actions.

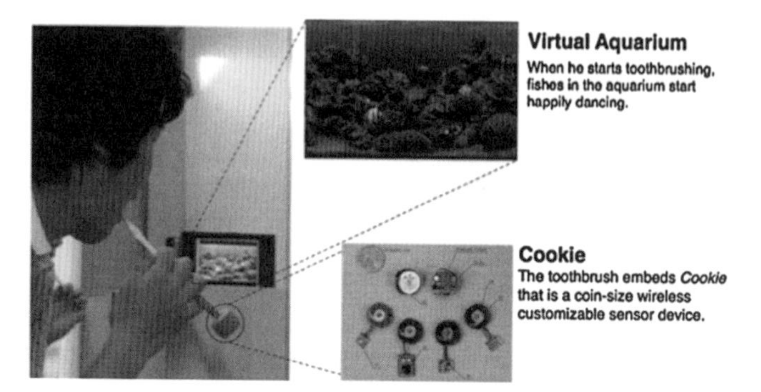

Figure 4. A user toothbrushing in front of a Virtual Aquarium. The toothbrush carries a wireless sensor device that tracks the users' activity.

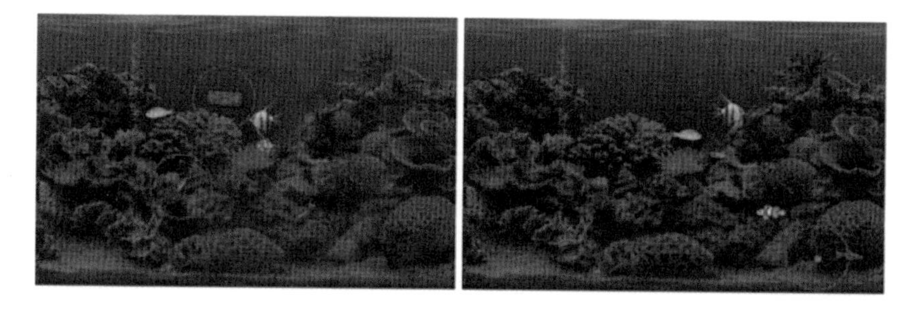

Figure 5. Screen Images of Virtual Aquarium.

The objective of Virtual Aquarium is to promote good toothbrushing practices. In this application, the ideal behaviour was defined as follows: 1) users should brush their teeth at least twice per day; 2) one session should involve at least three minutes of brushing; and 3) brushing should involve patterns that ensure the teeth are properly cleaned. User behaviour is compared to this ideal and translated to feedback as described below.

When a user begins to brush her teeth, a scrub inside the aquarium starts cleaning algae off the aquarium wall. At the same time, a set of fish associated with the user starts moving in the aquarium in a playful manner. When the user has brushed for a sufficient time, the scrub finishes cleaning and the fishes' dance turns to a more elegant pattern. When the user finishes brushing, the fish end their dance and resume their normal activities. Both the activity of the fish and the movement of the scrub are designed in such a way as to give the user hints regarding the correct method of toothbrushing. The left picture in Fig. 5 shows a scene from the aquarium during brushing. However, if a user does not brush his/her teeth sufficiently, the aquarium becomes dirty, and the fishes in the aquarium become sick.

The fish's health is visibly affected by how clean the aquarium is. If a user neglects to brush her teeth, some fish fall ill and may even die. In contrast, faithful brushing may result in the fish laying eggs (the right picture in Fig. 5). At first, the eggs are not very likely to hatch. If the user continues to brush consistently for a number of days in row, the incubation ratio increases. This way, the accumulated feedback gives clues to the correct behaviour and attempts to maintain motivation over a period of time.

This aquarium visualization also tries to reduce the information fidelity by using symbolic (abstract) representation, provides history through gradual transition of the aquarium conditions, tends to be emotionally engaging and playful. In addition, the metaphor used for the aquarium is easy to co-relate with the activity in context, so we consider the application to be intelligible.

The feedback focuses on micro activity, i.e., toothbrushing and is both temporally immediate and accumulative. We also found the feedback to be unobtrusive in the sense that toothbrushing can easily be performed while looking at the aquarium as the feedback is immediate, individuals can actually use the aquarium as a mirror. Finally, the activity is tracked completely passively without any intervention from the user.

4.3. Mona Lisa Bookshelf

Resources shared by a number of people, such as a public toilet or a bookshelf in a research lab, tend to deteriorate quickly in a process called the tragedy of the commons. This happens because each individual derives a personal benefit from using the resource, while any costs are shared between all the users, leading to reckless use. Garret Hardin, the ecologist who popularized the concept, noted that this belongs to the category of problems that cannot be solved by technology alone, requiring instead a change in human behavior [12]. Mona Lisa Bookshelf, is aimed at keeping a bookshelf organized. It tries to encourage users to keep books in order and to return missing books, but also to take books out every now and then for reading. Each book in the shelf is linked with a piece of a digital image of the Mona Lisa. Like a picture puzzle, the image changes according to how the books are positioned. A high-quality flat display placed near the bookshelf shows the image to the users.

The tracking of a user's behavior is based on optically detecting books in the shelf. In the prototype system, visual tags are attached to the spines of the books to facilitate their detection and identification. Visual tags are also attached to the corners of the shelf to determine its dimensions (Fig. 6 (left)). The detection system (Fig. 6 (middle)) comprises the following hardware: a digital video camera (iSight by Apple), a high-resolution digital camera (D50 by Nikon) and two infrared distance detectors (GP2D12 by SHARP). The distance sensors and the digital video camera are used to detect whether a user is manipulating books in the shelf. OpenCV, a real-time computer vision software library, is used to analyze the video signal. As soon as a user is seen leaving the shelf, the high-resolution still camera takes a picture of it and all the books contained within it. Images captured by the still camera are analyzed by the VisualCodes [29] software library, which recognizes the visual tags attached to the books. The system is shown installed in Fig. 6 (right). Each visual code yields data regarding its position, alignment and identity. This is then translated into context information that describes the bookshelf's width and height, which books are currently contained in shelf, and how they are aligned and ordered. This information is then passed to the feedback logic component. The above approach is able to observe how a user uses her bookshelf passively without requesting extra actions to play the game.

In this system, the feedback logic aims to encourage the following ideal behavior: 1) books should be arranged correctly and aligned neatly; and 2) at least one of the books should be read at least once per week. The correct arrangement of the books is pre-programmed, and could be e.g. alphabetical. User behavior is compared to this ideal, and translated to feedback as described below.

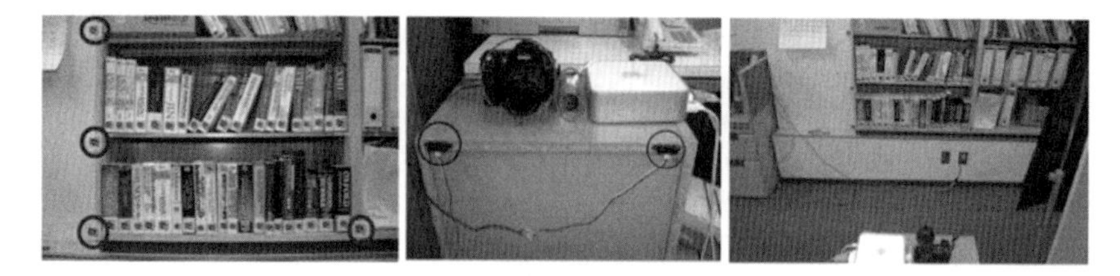

Figure 6. Mona Lisa Bookshelf prototype installation.

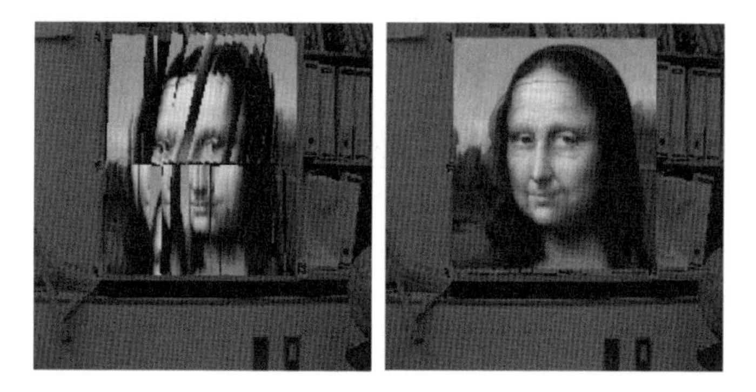

Figure 7. Two example outputs of the Mona Lisa Bookshelf. The image on the left shows that some books are tilted and in the wrong order. Some books are also missing. The image on the right side indicates that none of books have been picked up for a long time.

Mona Lisa Bookshelf also offers two expression styles to return feedback to a user to encourage cleaning his/her bookshelf or reading books in the following ways. When a book is removed from the shelf, the corresponding piece of the Mona Lisa image also disappears. If books are lying on their face or otherwise misaligned, the pieces of the image also become misaligned, distorting the picture. When the books are arranged neatly, Mona Lisa smiles contently. The assumption is that users are aware of how da Vinci's Mona Lisa is supposed to look like, and as when completing a picture puzzle, inherently prefer the correct solution to a distorted image. The feedback thus provides clues and motivation for keeping the bookshelf organized. The left picture in Fig. 7 shows and example of a distorted image. Also, if none of the books are removed from the shelf for over a week, Mona Lisa starts getting visibly older. The right picture shows and example of an aged portrait. As soon as one of the books is removed from the shelf, she regains her youth.

The Mona Lisa painting reduces the information fidelity by using symbolic (abstract) representation, provides history through gradual transition, aesthetically pleasing, emotionally engaging and playful. In addition, the metaphor used for the painting is easy to co-relate with the activity in context, i.e., organising the bookshelf, so we consider the application to be intelligible.

The feedback strategy used in this application is accumulative. The activity is tracked completely passively without any intervention from the user, thus letting users to focus primarily on the activity at hand. This contributes to the unobtrusiveness of the feedback. Finally, the feedback reflects the behaviour of one singular activity, i.e., organising the book shelf.

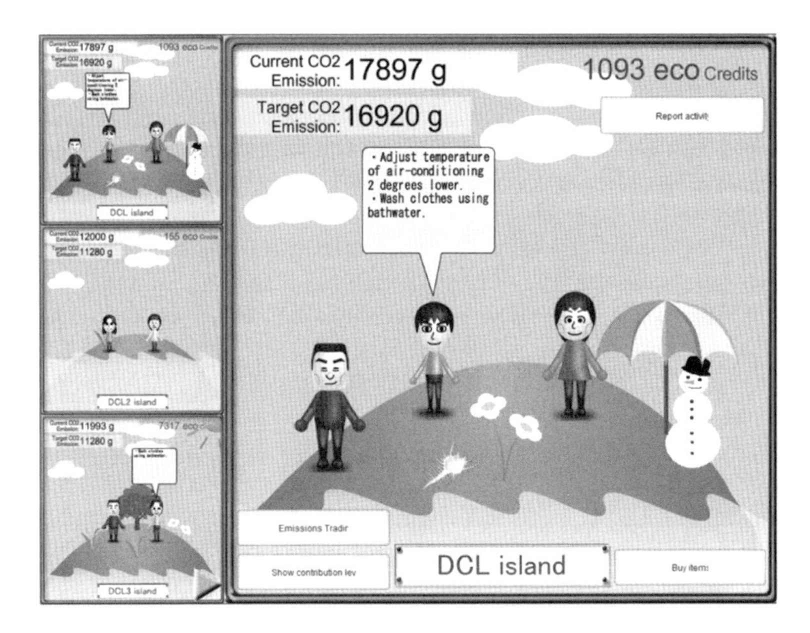

Figure 8. Some Screenshots of EcoIsland.

4.4. EcoIsland

Global warming caused by greenhouse gases released into the atmosphere through the actions of man is believed to be a major threat to the earth's ecology [15]. Efforts to reduce greenhouse gas emissions come in two forms: technological solutions and changes in human behavior. Technological solutions broadly include improving energy efficiency and developing cleaner energy sources. Dramatic changes in human behavior may also be necessary if catastrophic climate change is to be avoided.

Public and private efforts to change individual behavior towards more environmentally friendly practices usually rely on education, but there are psychological limits to the ability of education alone to effect behavioural change. Even when a person full-well knows that a particular behavior is detrimental enough to their long-term well-being to offset any possible short-term benefits, their may still irrationally choose the short-term indulgence. Future consequences, while widely known, are easily ignored in the present.

EcoIsland is a game-like application intended to be used as a background activity by an ecologically minded family in the course of their normal daily activities. A display installed in the kitchen or another prominent place in the household presents a virtual island. Each family member is represented on the island by an avatar (Fig. 8). The family sets a target CO_2 emission level (e.g. national average minus 20%) and the system tracks their approximate current emissions using sensors and self-reported data. If the emissions exceed the target level, the water around the island begins to rise, eventually sweeping away the avatars' possessions and resulting in a game over.

On their mobile phones, the participants have a list of actions that they may take to reduce the emissions: turning down the air conditioning by one degree, taking the train instead of the car, etc. Upon completing an action, a participant reports using the phone, and the water level reacts accordingly. Reported activities are also shown in speech bubbles above the corresponding avatars. A lack of activity causes the avatars to suggest actions. Participants can also see neighbouring islands and their activities in the display, and can list buy and sell offers for emission rights on a marketplace. Trading is conducted using a virtual currency obtained from a regular allowance. The credits are also used to buy improvements and decorations to the island, so successful sellers can afford to decorate their island more, while heavy emitters have to spend their allowance on emission rights.

The general approach from ambient lifestyle feedback systems is to provide a feedback loop for user behavior. The virtual island shown in the display acts as a metaphor and makes the participants conscious of the ecological consequences of their choices and activities. We also tap into social psychology, attempting to exploit *social facilitation* and *conforming behavior* to encourage the desired behavior. Social facilitation is the phenomenon where a person performs better at a task when someone else, e.g. a colleague or a supervisor, is watching [35]. Conforming behavior is the desire not to act against group consensus [1]. EcoIsland's design facilitates these by involving the whole family, and by presenting the participants' activity reports in the speech bubbles and providing contribution charts and activity histories. On the other hand, the fact that the game is played by a family unit instead of an individual means that participants can also agree to assign tasks to certain members.

Lastly, there is the trading system, which is based on the same principle as industry level emissions trading systems: reductions should be carried out in places where it is easiest to do so. A family that finds it easy to make significant reductions can sell emission rights to households that find it difficult due to e.g. location or job. This should make it possible to attain the same amount of total reductions with a lower total cost (measured in disutility), promoting use of the system.

The visualization used in this application is a combination of iconic and indexical, whereas the virtual island metaphorically represents our planet and the labelling within the visualization shows the actual data of the application. The visualization is aesthetically pleasing, emotionally engaging and playful as we have found from our studies. It also reflects the temporal gradient of the activity through progressive transition. In addition, the metaphors used are easy to co-relate with the activity in context, i.e., reducing carbon emission, so we consider the application to be intelligible.

The feedback strategy used in this application is accumulative. In this application the activity is tracked in both passively and through active participation of the users. This participation obviously reduces the degree of unobtrusiveness, however, as we discussed in the design section, tapping into Transtheoretical Model of Change (TTM) [28] we argue that this active participation in fact complements the later stages – preparation and action.

5. Some Experiences with Case Studies

Through the development of these ambient displays, over the years we have gained deeper insights on several issues that are significant for the design of future ambient displays aiming at persuasive applications. Drawing on our experiences in this section we discuss some of these issues which we consider could instigate further work in the field.

5.1. Sensing and Lightweight Interaction

Virtual Aquarium uses a 3D accelerometer to recognise the movement of the user's toothbrush to observe the user's behavior without his explicit interaction. Our experiences show that recognizing the user's behavior with sensors has its limitations in reliability. In Virtual Aquarium and Mona Lisa Bookshelf, we chose to analyze a very simple context that can be implemented in a reliable way. It is very difficult to analyze the user's behavior correctly without heavy-weighted algorithms. Thus, EcoIsland uses a self-reporting method to input what kind of actions the user takes in order to avoid complex behavior analysis.

EcoIsland encourages the user to input his actions to reduce CO_2 emission since he is recognized as an eco-conscious person. However, we believe that lightweight interaction techniques such as using gestures is important in order to compensate implicit interaction for realizing passive observation. The user will be able to input his current action with a minimum cognitive effort. Lightweight interaction can also be used to correct mistakes of behavior analysis. Gesture analysis is easier to compare than general behavior analysis. The combination of explicit interaction with gesture analysis and implicit interaction with sensor data analysis is a very interesting topic and has a critical role in our future researches.

One of the problems in the current case studies is that a user may cheat the analysis of the sensors consciously. For example, in Virtual Aquarium, some users imitated the movement of their toothbrushes in order to make the fishes dancing. There are two approaches to solve this problem. The first approach is to prohibit cheating by increasing the accuracy of the movement analysis. The second approach is to encourage the user not to cheat to use sensors. We are very interested in adopting the second approach in our future case studies. This approach requires the user to think about the merit behind the desirable lifestyle. How technologies can be used to encourage a user to think more deeply is a very challenging issue.

5.2. End User Involvement

As we have shown in all these case studies, one important element of designing ambient display systems is the instrumentation of everyday objects, e.g., toothbrush, bookshelf etc. This puts forth a range of unprecedented opportunities for end-users to manage, co-ordinate, and control these smart artefacts to realize unique, personalized and co-ordinated behaviour within and across devices that were not anticipated by the designers. For instance, an individual might be interested in using Persuasive Art for reflecting toothbrushing behaviour rather than Virtual Aquarium, or composing both. Another end-user might compose a small electrical appliance, e.g., an iron, a kettle, etc. with the Mona Lisa painting (e.g., increase in the energy consumption is reflects by ageing Mona Lisa) to understand and compare its energy consumption to make informed decisions. Such possibilities of software driven personalized behaviour generation with ambient displays signify the transformation of our physical world into a programmable information space and can effectively increase the impact of these displays in changing problematic behaviour. While the technological building blocks for realizing programmable physical space is converging [19], there is a clear need to shift the focus onto end-users. It is essential to empower end-users with an appropriate capacity to program this interactive physical space and enable them to unleash computing enabled creativity capitalizing the possibilities offered by pervasive computing, and ideally this should be done in a Do-It-Yourself (DIY) fashion [20]. For the success of ambient display systems in motivating individual's behavioural change it is very crucial to involve end-users in display and feedback generation process as it is the people who occupy those environments and have the best knowledge about how their physical and computational environments should respond to their activities.

5.3. Persuasive Expression

The user study on Persuasive Art shows that users preferred the tree and the Mona Lisa over the abstract and the still life. The reason given was that more figurative paintings were considered to be more "intuitive". While any visual representation can be used to relay information, shapes that come with pre-attached meanings (e.g. "a tree withering is a negative thing") are more capable of evoking emotional engagement. It is therefore important to remember this third design principle when choosing a presentation metaphor. Tan and Cheok [31] showed that a real creature is found to arouse more empathy than a virtual creature. However, especially in Japan, people feel empathy also to virtual creatures. Fujinami [10] presented that Japanese users feel empathy for even virtual creatures represented as abstract symbols. We sometimes assign different meanings to a real creature and a virtual creature because we know the differences between them. We need to investigate the effect of virtual creatures as a persuasive expressions in future case studies.

In the future, it is necessary to consider how the feedback information appeals users without the explanation about the interpretation of the expressions because ambient lifestyle feedback information will appear anywhere to visualize a variety of aspects of our lifestyle. The metaphor visualizing a user's lifestyle helps him to notice the feedback information. The concept of affordance could be a guideline in designing linkages between activities and feedback. Product semantics [21] may be one suitable theory to help how feedback expression affords the meaning of the expression. A user sometimes mistakes to make the meaning of an expression, and this is one of the serious problem to rely on affordance. The user tends to define the non intentional meaning of an expression [3]. For example, an ugly picture may be used to discourage to keep the current undesirable habits, but the picture may encourage to keep the current undesirable habits for some avant-garde people. This is highly depending on the cultures and personalities of the users. It is not easy for a designer to assign a single meaning to a specific expression by all people. We believe that the expression of showing some virtual creatures is more acceptable to most of the people. Of course, each person may love different creatures. Empathetic feeling is a key to design successful ambient lifestyle feedback systems.

There are some very close systems to ambient lifestyle feedback systems. Playful toothbrush [4] shows a virtual teeth representing the current status of the user's toothbrushing. It explicitly shows the goals of the user's behavior. The user continues to use and enjoy the systems until he achieves the goal. However, motivating a user based on a long-term goal is important to maintain desirable lifestyle. The advanced motivation theories [30] help us to develop more effective case studies. It is useful to distinguish a short-term goal and a long-term goal to encourage the change away from undesirable habits and to keep desirable habits. In our case studies, Virtual Aquarium sets a short-term goal to complete sufficient toothbrushing in every night. On the other hand, EcoIsland sets a long-term goal to reduce CO_2 emission. Showing the explicit goal is effective to keep desirable habits until achieving the goal. The goal setting should be carefully designed so as not to stop desirable habits before achieving the goal. The combination of a short-term and a long-term goal is a very effective way to motivate a better lifestyle. Also, it is important to consider how to represent a goal in the expression. In Persuasive Art, the growth of the tree can be reinitialized every week to start a new goal, but it may reduce the sense of achievement in long-term. The relationship between the expression and goal setting should be investigated more in the near future.

5.4. Feedback Control and Emotion

In operant conditioning, feedback content can be divided into reinforcement and punishment depending on whether some behavior is encouraged or discouraged. Reinforcement and punishment are further divided into four types [6]: Positive Reinforcement, Negative Reinforcement, Positive Punishment, and Negative Punishment. Our case studies use the combination of the above four types of feedback. One of our finding is that the balance between positive reinforcement and positive punishment is very important in changing a user's behavior permanently. The user may be bored if the expression offers only positive reinforcement. On the other hand, the user may give up his hope to change undesirable habits when only positive punishment is offered. An appropriate balance is important in order to change the user's behavior permanently.

Jordan classified pleasure into four types: physio-pleasure, psycho-pleasure, socio-pleasure, ideo-pleasure [17]. This classification is a useful tool to design a reinforcement and a punishment. Physical comfort and discomfort are used as reinforcement and punishment to change the user's behavior. For example, a chair may change our comfortability by moving the backrest or arms. In the near future, we are interested in using physio-pleasure to design smart objects that change their shape according to the user's current behavior. In most of our case studies, the user's behavior is changed due to positive and negative emotion caused by the expression representing the user's current behavior. Dancing fishes make the user exited and increase his positive emotion, but when Mona Lisa is getting old, the negative emotion is increased and he feels anxious. Emotion is a very powerful tool to change a user's behavior [8] and we will try to develop a systematic way to use positive and negative emotions. We are going to enhance the use of social aspects into the feedback expression. If all people know the rules, the expression displayed in a public space would put interesting pressure on the user who is the target of the information. In EcoIsland, we have tried to use socio-pleasure as the feedback of the user's activities to reduce CO_2 emission. Social effects are an interesting tool in designing the feedback and need to be investigated more in the near future. Ideo-pleasure is interesting to be used to change the user's attitude in future case studies. The user's long-term good attitude will permanently change his undesirable habits and maintain his desirable habits. Ideo-Pleasure makes it possible motivate the user by himself. He has a belief called self-efficacy that he will be able to achieve his goal. Contemporary arts make us to think deeply about our future like sustainability and peace in the world. We like to consider how to use the expression of contemporary arts to persuade the user to change his attitude in future case studies.

6. Conclusions and Future Directions

In our daily lives, most of our behavior do not return adequate feedbacks. If computer technologies help to return adequate feedbacks to the user, they make him aware of his current lifestyle and he can change undesirable habits and maintain desirable habits easily. In the paper, we introduced a brief overview of ambient lifestyle feedback systems and four case studies. Each case study gave us various insights and we showed several findings with the case studies.

Economic benefit is a strong incentive to motivate the user to change his behavior. We have introduced the “Eco credit” concept in EcoIsland. The user will be encouraged if he has an incentive to get a return for his effort or contribution to reduce CO_2 emission. The user’s activities are monitored by the system and paid to users in order to stimulate their desirable actions. In EcoIsland, a user can use the credit to purchase decorating items or to trade eco-unconscious activities. Thus, the user will be both a consumer and a producer. We believe that we can accelerate the money circulation by adding economical concepts in ambient lifestyle feedback systems.

There are many places to encourage a user to change his/her behavior to motivate a better lifestyle. In our case studies, Persuasive Art and Virtual Aquarium assume that the systems are installed in the user’s house. In the near future, our daily life was become more nomadic and we often stay in hotels for personal or business reasons. In this case, we cannot see the status of the tree or the dancing the fishes. Some participants in the user study in Virtual Aquarium told that they wanted to take care of the fishes even when they were not stay at home. Thus, we believe that the feedback should be reflected in many places such as hotels and public spaces. One of the problem to realize the goal is that the user needs to find which digital expression reflects the feedback of his behavior. However, if we can use a public display to show the feedback of the user’s behavior, it makes it possible to use social factors as positive reinforcement and punishment. Ambient lifestyle feedback systems may be installed everywhere to enhance a variety of our daily activities in future, but we also need to consider whether this is our dream or just a nightmare. Is this really a better lifestyle for the future? Also, using ambient lifestyle feedback systems everywhere may take control of our attitude, which may cause serious ethical problems. The user should have a right to control which behaviors are reflected in expressions. We also need to discuss who chooses expressions to reflect the user’s behavior. Does the system choose expressions automatically? Can the user choose expressions manually? It is important to consider how to reflect the user’s behavior when trying to change multiple behaviours at the same time.

References

[1] S.E. Asch, Opinions and social pressure, *Scientific American*, 1955, pp. 31–35.

[2] T. Baranowski, J. Baranowski, K.W. Cullen, T. Marsh, N. Islam, I. Zakeri, L.H. Morreale and C. de Moor, Squire’s quest! Dietary outcome evaluation of a multimedia game, *American Journal of Preventive Medicine* **24**(1) (2003).

[3] U. Brandes and M. Erlhoff, *Non Intentional Design*, daad, 2006.

[4] Y. Chang, J. Lo, C. Huang, N. Hsu, H. Chu, H. Wang, P. Chi and Y. Hsieh, Playful toothbrush: UbiComp technology for teaching tooth brushing to kindergarten children, in: *Proc. of ACM CHI’08*, 2008.

[5] S.B. Davis, M. Moar, R. Jacobs, M. Watkins, C. Riddoch and K. Cooke, Ere be dragons: Heart and health, in: *Proc. of PerGames 2006*, 2006.

[6] M.P. Domjan, *The Principles of Learning and Behavior*, 5th edn, Wadsworth, 2002.

[7] B.J. Fogg, *Persuasive Technology: Using to Change what We Think and Do*, Morgan Kaufmann, 2002.
[8] B.L. Fredrikson, The value of positive emotions: The emerging science of positive psychology is coming to understand why it's good to feel good, *American Scientist* **91** (July–August, 2003).
[9] J. Froehlich et al., UbiGreen: Investigating a mobile tool for tracking and supporting green transportation habits, in: *Proc. of CHI 2009*, 2009, pp. 1043–1052.
[10] K. Fujinami and J. Riekki, A case study on an ambient display as a persuasive medium for exercise awareness, in: *Proc. of the 3rd International Conference on Persuasive Technology*, 2008.
[11] L. Hallnas and J. Redstrom, Slow technology – Designing for reflection, *Personal and Ubiqutious Computing* **5**(3) (2001), Springer.
[12] G. Hardin, The tragedy of the commons, *Science* **162** (1968), 1243–1248.
[13] L.E. Holmquist and T. Skog, Informative art: Information visualization in everyday environments, in: *Proc. of GRAPHITE'03*, 2003.
[14] S.S. Intille, J.Nawyn and K.Larson, Embedding behavior modification strategies into a consumer electronics device, in: *Proc. of Ubicomp'06*, 2006.
[15] IPCC. IPCC Fourth Assessment Report: Climate Change 2007, http://www.ipcc.ch/.
[16] N. Jafarinaimi, J. Forlizzi, A. Hurst and J. Zimmerman, Breakway: An ambient display designed to change human behavior, in: *Proc. of ACM CHI'05*, 2005.
[17] P.W. Jordan, *Designing Pleasurable Products: An Introduction to the New Human Factors*, Routledge, 2002.
[18] K. Kappel and T. Grechenig, Show-me: Water consumption at a glance to promote water conservation in the shower, in: *Proc. Persuasive Technology 2009*, 2009, pp. 1–6.
[19] F. Kawsar, K. Fujinami and T. Nakajima, A document centric approach for supporting incremental deployment of pervasive applications, in: *Proc. of the 5th Annual International Conference on Mobile and Ubiquitous Systems: Computing, Networking and Services (MobiQuitous 2008).*
[20] F. Kawsar, K. Fujinami and T. Nakajima, Deploy spontaneously: Supporting end-users in building and enhancing a smart home, in: *Proc. of the 10th International Conference on Ubiquitous Computing (Ubicomp 2008)*, pp. 282–291
[21] K.Krippendorff, *The Semantic Turn: An New Foundation for Design*, CRC Press, 2005.
[22] B.Y. Lim, A.K. Dey, D. Avrahami, Why and why not explanations improve the intelligibility of context-aware intelligent systems, *Proc. of 27th International Conference on Human Factors in Computing Systems (CHI)*, 2009.
[23] List of diet and nutrition software for Palm [online, February 27, 2007], http://www.handango.com/SoftwareCatalog.jsp?siteId=1&platformId=1&N=96804+95712.
[24] List of quit smoking meters [online, February 27, 2007], http://www.ciggyfree.com/ODAT/index.php?option=com_content&task=view&id=205&Itemid=25.
[25] A. Mack, Perceptual organization and attention, *Cognitive Psychology* **24** (1992), 475–501.
[26] T. Nakajima, V. Lehdonvirta, E. Tokunaga and H. Kimura, Reflecting human behavior to motivate desirable lifestyle, in: *Proc. of ACM Designing Interactive Systems '08*, 2008.
[27] Z. Pousman and J. Stasko, A taxonomy of ambient information systems: Four patterns of design, in: *Proc. of AVI 2006*, 2006.
[28] J. Prochaska and W. Velicer, The transtheoretical model of health behavior change, *Am. J. of Health Promotion* **12**(1) (1997), 38–48.
[29] M. Rohs, Visual code widgets for marker-based interaction, in: *Proc. of ICDCS Workshops: IWSAWC'05*, 2005.
[30] J. Reeve, *Understanding Motivation and Emotion*, 4th edn, Wiley, 2005.
[31] R.K.C. Tan and A.D. Cheok, Empathetic living media, in: *Proc. of ACM Designing Interactive Systems '08*, 2008.
[32] A. Treisman, Distributed attention, in: *Attention: Selection Awareness and Control*, 1993, pp. 5–35.
[33] M. Weiser and J.S. Brown, Designing calm technology, December 21, 1995 [online, February 27, 2007], http://www.ubiq.com/hypertext/weiser/calmtech/calmtech.htm.
[34] A. Woodruff, J. Hasbrouck and S. Augustin, A bright green perspective on sustainable choices, in: *Proc. of CHI 2008*, 2008, pp. 313–322.
[35] R.B. Zajonc, Social facilitation, *Science* **149** (1965), 269–274.

Handbook of Ambient Assisted Living
J.C. Augusto et al. (Eds.)
IOS Press, 2012

doi:10.3233/978-1-60750-837-3-408

Supporting Wellbeing Through Improving Interactions and Understanding in Self-Monitoring Systems[1]

Dana PAVEL[a,*], Vic CALLAGHAN[a] and Anind K. DEY[b]
[a] *School of Computer Science and Electronic Engineering, University of Essex, UK*
[b] *Human-Computer Interaction Institute, Carnegie Mellon University, USA*

Abstract. We use computing devices at work, at home and on the go. We generate huge amount of data that is stored (either temporarily or permanent) on our machines or on remote servers. There is a lot of value in this information and some of it is already further exploited by many external parties. So, if others consider our information important why don't we take proper advantage of it? How can we use the information we generate to our own advantage? How can we use this information to improve our lives and support our wellbeing? And how can we create better environments that will be able to offer more personalized and engaging interfaces supporting such diversity of information? We offer here our answer to such questions by presenting the MyRoR system with its main goals of better supporting self-understanding and offer more natural interfaces for information visualizations, based on personalized and interactive stories.

1. Introduction

Wellness and *wellbeing* are terms used more and more these days in various contexts but what do they actually mean? A quick Internet search will bring up various definitions, more or less vague. In most instances, wellness and wellbeing are associated with being healthy and happy, even though, as discussed in [28], in reality these states include subjective perceptions meaning that an ill person can have a sense of wellbeing while a seemingly healthy person might not have it. The limitations of these terms come mainly from the fact that most of the time *health* refers to physical aspects, even though definitions that are more complex have existed for a long time. Most prominently, the WHO (World Health Organization) Constitution, defines health as "*a state of complete physical, mental and social well-being and not merely the absence of disease or infirmity*". However, with chronic diseases becoming a huge problem in our societies, more understanding is necessary for determining not only how to treat them but also how to prevent them. The necessity to understand what influences such chronic diseases broadens the concepts of wellbeing and wellness and they become more holistic. We give here just a few examples of the multiple aspects of wellness[2]: in [12], Corbin et al. define wellness as a "multidimensional state of being, describing the

[*] Corresponding Author: Dana Pavel, Wivenhoe Park, Wivenhoe, Essex, U.K. E-mail: dmpave@essex.ac.uk.
[1] This work is part of the PAL research project (http://www.palproject.org.uk), funded by UK's TSB and EPSRC under the project number TP/AN072C.
[2] For further readings on wellness-related literature we recommend [27] and [33].

existence of positive health in an individual as exemplified by quality of life and a sense of well-being". In [2], wellness is described as having 7 components: physical, social, emotional, intellectual, spiritual, occupational and environmental. Other dimensions mentioned in [13] are financial, mental and medical. As mentioned before, the increased focus on wellness and its multiple facets was necessary in order to create a more preventive focus of healthcare systems and individuals. While wellbeing is more of a *state* of feeling well (overall), wellness can be seen as a *life goal*, which includes self-responsibility and a daily process of making lifestyle decisions and dealing with various aspects covered by the components described above [28]. There is now much more understanding of the impact our daily lifestyle choices have on our wellbeing and healthcare systems do consider the aspect of making people more aware and informed as very important in the strategy of dealing with the problem of chronic diseases [6,14,61]. The advances in wearable technologies as well as the realization that self-monitoring systems help people become more aware and even change their behaviors [15,19] have helped create many solutions that deal with various health aspects. However, most of the existing systems focus on physical health recording and monitoring and pay little attention to other dimensions, much as the views on health discussed above. We will present some of these existing solutions in Section 2.

In this article we argue that it is time to take advantage of the varied data available through our smart environments and move from focusing only on *what* happened towards *why* it happened. We believe that by using self-monitoring technologies that are able to create a more detailed and complex picture of our lives, we will be able to address the wellbeing at a holistic level and not only by looking at various separate aspects. Our aim is to create systems that support users in self understanding and self reflection. We discuss the challenges presented by dealing with different types of information, especially in terms of modelling and visualization and we introduce our approach for creating interactive, personalize and informative systems. As a case study, we introduce our system approach and we discuss its design and implementation together with a user experiment. We conclude with a discussion of our results so far, our ongoing work and future plans.

2. Background and Motivation

Lifestyle choices affect our lives in multiple ways but most evident is their role in chronic diseases. Chronic diseases is a generic name for various health conditions that, once acquired cannot be cured but just managed. According to the World Health Organization (WHO), chronic diseases are the leading cause of illness and death in the world [61], posing a considerable financial and emotional burden on patients and their support networks. Some of the most common chronic diseases are coronary heart disease (CHD), cancer, renal disease, diabetes and mental health. In 2005 in UK there were more than 17.5 million people living with at least one chronic condition and it is estimated that by 2030 the incidence of chronic disease in the over 65s will more than double [14]. Many people are diagnosed with more than one chronic disease and sometimes one condition becomes a risk factor for another one. One important aspect is that chronic diseases are not only a problem of elderly, as people from various age groups are now affected, a situation mainly caused by changes in our lifestyles. Certain lifestyle-related factors, such as smoking, alcohol, physical inactivity, diet (irregular meals, salty or fatty foods) and psychosocial stress, have a proven impact on chronic diseases, which also means that they have become the main targets for preventive healthcare programs [6,61]. Prevention plays an important role both in avoiding acquiring a disease, as well as for avoiding worsening of an existing condition. Lifestyle management support can have a significant impact as most of the patients living with chronic diseases fall into the low risk category, which means that, with the right support, they can learn how to manage their disease [14].

Various programs for inducing and supporting preventive behaviours have been implemented using various channels, such as printed material, TV and radio campains or through healthcare providers offering advice to patients, e.g., on what to eat in order to reduce cholesterol or how to avoid living a sedentary life. The advances in wearable monitoring systems allow for an increased offering in solutions that can record, store (either locally or remotely), and analyze patient data. Using such systems for outpatient monitoring benefits both healthcare systems and patients, as patients can live normal lives and avoid hospitalization. The importance of empowering both patients and medical staff with more objective information obtained through outpatient self monitoring systems is emphasized in recent reports such as [19]. The same report also documents a continuous shift in attitudes both of patients and medical staff towards using such technologies, especially as they become more unobtrusive and as their benefits (both social and economical) are better understood. A large number of the 1000 people interviewed in [19] (in UK, ages from 16+) were already using various means for self diagnosis (60%) and a significant number of people (over 60%) were interested in monitoring their own health, particularly for various parameters such as cholesterol and blood pressure.

Using wearable systems for outpatient monitoring accrues multiple benefits, for all parties involved. We include here some of the existing self-monitoring systems[3].

2.1. Lifestyle Management and Self-Monitoring Technologies

The increased availability of wearable and unobtrusive sensing devices, either based on specialized systems or on widely available mobile devices such as smart phones, has made it possible to create more sophisticated self-monitoring systems both for clinical and lifestyle scenarios. In this section we intend to take a look at some commercially available self-monitoring systems, the types of users they aim to support and how they usually work. We separate the existing systems on two major health categories: physical and mental health.

2.1.1. Physical Health

2.1.1.1. Movement (Physical Activity, Fall Detection, Energy Expenditure)

Systems that measure movement can have both medical and lifestyle applications. GPS and 3-axis accelerometers integrated into wristwatches, pedometers, pendants and smartphones are used both for measuring how much and how fast a person moves and for detecting falls. Some of the most popular fitness-related devices are produced by Garmin and Polar and they usually include a heart monitor that allows for keeping track of the effort level. Products such as WristCare (from Vivago) [62] and SenseWear BMS [43] allow for creating movement activity profiles for a certain user and then detecting and signalling abnormal patterns. The WristCare also integrates skin tempera-

[3] More information on studies using such systems (including benefits) can be found in [15], a report published by the Department of Health in UK in 2005–2006.

ture and skin conductivity sensors and it uses a few initial days to learn what is "normal" for the user and send alarms when the values change.

For more assistive scenarios, fall detection systems such as Philips' LifeLine [38] and Wellcore Emergency Response System [59] allow for monitoring as well as alerting in emergency situations. Usually, such solutions include various options to determine who and how to alert in emergencies. These systems mainly work in home scenarios, as they connect through the main phone lines.

As phone applications become more and more popular and smartphones now include sensors such as GPS and accelerometer, various applications for fitness as well as assistance have started to appear (e.g., iFall for Android [25], Sports Tracker for Symbian [48], or Nike+iPod [36]).

2.1.1.2. Heart Rate/Blood Pressure Monitoring

Given that heart-related conditions top the list of chronic diseases a large selection of systems exist for recording and monitoring of such data. Data usually recorded is blood pressure, heart rate, pulse, heart rate variability and ECG. The data recording can be done at certain times or continuously, by using heart monitoring devices, most of them provided through hospitals or primary healthcare providers.

Examples of heart monitoring systems are: t+ blood pressure (OBS Medical) [37], Medixine's Chronic Disease Clinic [30], HealthBuddy (from Bosch Healthcare) [24], and CardioNet solutions. For most of the existing solutions, data is stored on a remote server and analysed by nurses, doctors, clinicians, etc. Patients might be able to add certain notes, symptoms, and so on, and receive certain feedback from medical staff.

Certain sensing devices such as the Alive Heart and Activity Monitor [1] also provide finer granularity data through ECG recording and they can connect to other recording devices (e.g., mobile phones) through Bluetooth.

2.1.1.3. Food/Calories Intake/Weight Management

Solutions for recording food and calories intake can range from manual to fully automated. In the manual mode, the user has to record what she ate during the day and how many calories it contained.

There are now multiple applications for iPod/iPhones and Android phones that can help people keep track of what they eat (e.g., CalorieCounter for iPhones).

The HealthBuddy system [24] provides a middle solution where the user is prompted to use a compatible scale that can send information to the hub through Bluetooth. The device also includes an interactive and supportive questionnaire that helps users record more information about their eating patterns.

More automated solutions can be built based on reading RFID tags attached to food items or based on scanning barcodes and determining their caloric value using web services.

2.1.1.4. Diabetes Support

In such systems patients usually record blood glucose measurements, timestamps as well as information related to administering insulin. In most of the systems, the patient manually performs the measurement, recording and insulin delivery. Some of these solutions are Medixine's Chronic Disease Clinic [30], t+ diabetes from OBS Medical [37] and HealthBuddy [24] that provide support in various ways and combine recording with visualizing and medical support.

However, new systems have recently appeared where certain or all steps of the process have been automated. For example, the MiniMed from Medtronic [32] can use under skin sensors for automated and continuous glucose monitoring and an automated insulin pump. Less invasively, the Calisto GlucoBand [8] wristwatch can use bio-electromagnetic resonance to measure and monitor blood glucose levels.

2.1.1.5. Asthma and COPD (Chronic Obstructive Pulmonary Disease)
While some symptoms might be similar, asthma is more common in patients under 35 years old while COPD is mainly induced by smoking and environmental pollutants and is more common in patients over 35. As both asthma and COPD involve problems with the air flow, the main parameter monitored by systems addressing them is the peak flow information. Other parameters monitored for COPD patients are the forced expiatory volume in one second (FEV) and the blood oxygenation levels (SpO2). Usually, these parameters can be manually recorded by the patients in an electronic diary, together with certain observed symptoms. Data is stored on a server where medical staff can examine it and give feedback to the patient (e.g., t+ asthma and t+ COPD solutions from OBS Medical [37]). An interesting system is Medixine's Health Forecasting [31] focused mainly on preventing weather related crisis, by sending alerts based on weather forecast, as there are observed correlations between certain weather conditions and an increase of asthma and COPD-related hospital admissions.

2.2. Mental Health

Even though mental health is extremely important and a large number of people will suffer from a diagnosable mental condition at some point in life [53], the area remains poorly addressed by self-monitoring technological systems. Systems such as HealthBuddy [24] provide a certain support for depression patients, by using an interactive questionnaire and prompting for a periodic recording of blood pressure. Most of the self-monitoring methods for depression focus on keeping manual mood diaries.

2.2.1. Memory Support

Various systems exist for helping patients with memory problems keep track of their medication. Most of the systems allow patients or their carers to pre-program alarms for times when certain pills should be taken. Some of them also store pills and include sensors that record when the pillbox was opened, such as the Daily Alarmed PillBox from PivoTell [34]. Some systems can even communicate with a mobile phone if the pillbox has not been opened at the scheduled time, such as the SIMpill [45].

Various research projects have also used camera-based systems, such as SenseCam, for supporting patients with more advanced memory problems [29].

2.2.2. Relaxation Systems

Stress is part of our lives and various methods exist to address it, most of them based on relaxation techniques. Biofeedback systems offer technological support for such processes. The systems we looked at employ various sensors and methods. The main sensors used are for measuring GSR (skin conductivity), heart rate, heart rate variability, and EEG (electrical brain activity).

Various visualizations and interaction methods are employed to allow for controlling the measured parameters. For example, certain systems use game-based interfaces allowing users to control functionalities in the games through controlling their physiological parameters (e.g., Journey to Wild Divine [26] and products from SmartBrain Technologies [47]). Other systems use sounds, lights or charts for allowing users to become aware of their stress levels as well as enable their control (e.g., GSR2 Biofeedback Relaxation System [23], StressEraser [50], Resperate [41], emWave PSR [17]).

2.3. Trends in Lifestyle Management

Many of the existing health monitoring system providers chose to create integrated health hub devices that allow for recording more than one parameter and even include small screens that can be used for various types of communicating with a patient. Most of the health hubs available combine two or more of the physiological parameters mentioned above. For example, the HealthBuddy [24] can integrate data received from various compatibles devices such as digital scales, blood pressure monitors, digital blood glucose level readers, etc., and it has a display used for asking questions, prompting for values or tasks, giving encouragements and advices.

Similar systems are provided by Viterion Telehealthcare (Viterion 100, Viterion 200) [57] and TeleMedCare, whose TMC Home [54] collects information from various devices as well as using questionnaires to gather more information from users. Its health hub also has video capabilities to facilitate communication between the patient and the monitoring medical staff. Tunstall Lifeline provides various solutions for telecare/telehealth addressing conditions such as COPD, CHF (Chronic Heart Failure), CDM (Chronic Disease Management), diabetes and coagulation issues, by allowing it to integrate multiple sensors with their hub [56].

Sensor vests are another type of integrated systems. Vivometrics and Xenetec were producing such systems but they seem to have disappeared, so it is not clear how popular such systems proved to be.

As seen, most of the available solutions focus on recording and monitoring physiological parameters. The market is extremely segmented and based on proprietary devices and formats. There is however a certain drive to create interoperable solutions, such as the Continua Health Alliance [11]. In most cases user data is sent to remote servers to be stored and analyzed by nurses or clinicians. These self-monitoring systems are mainly targeted at patients with existing health conditions and focus mainly on prevention of worsening conditions or detecting emergency situations. Systems are mainly provided by hospitals.

Mobile phones are some of the most pervasive computing devices and they can now be used for collecting, interpreting, visualizing as well as remotely sending and accessing information. More and more mobile-based applications appear everyday allowing people to keep track of various lifestyle-related aspects: heart rate, exercising, blood glucose levels, etc. It is now possible to also integrate various sensors with mobile phones, such as the Alive Heart and Activity Monitor [1] or the Nike+iPod. Companies such as MobiHealth [35] even provide whole solutions around mobile phones that can measure multi-lead ECG and EMG, plethysmogram, pulse rate, oxygen saturation, respiration and core/skin temperature through an Android phone.

Within the research community there have been multiple projects focused on developing wearable and integrated self-monitoring systems or platforms for distributed wellness data collection, some of them being described in [51,55,63].

However, looking at available lifestyle management systems, there seem to be very few systems that support users in understanding why something happened. Correlations between physiological data recorded and events that might have triggered certain changes are mostly based on recollections, subjective and prone to various memory errors. In most cases, patients can monitor certain physiological data but have no idea what context the data was collected in and what might have affected their wellbeing.

We believe that the number of self-monitoring systems used and owned by individuals will continue to grow, driven by an increased availability of sensors and sensor-based applications as well as by the higher degree of acceptance towards digitally recording life experiences that can be observed in younger generations [52].

3. Towards an Integrated Lifestyle Management System

3.1. Our Approach

We believe that a lifestyle management system should be able to create a holistic, if not comprehensive picture, of a user's daily experiences. As we showed in the previous section, there are currently multiple systems that address various aspects of users' health. However, what we believe is missing, is a system that helps users better understand what the relation is between the monitored parameters and what is going on in their lives.

Through our work we seek to go beyond just recording certain physiological parameters and create lifestyle management systems that better support people in understanding of *what* happened and *why* it happened. For creating such a system we build on existing sensing solutions and focus on collecting data that we generate through our everyday use of computing devices. Data we produce while using computers at home, at work or on the go is important because it creates a picture about what we like, what we do, who we interact with and where we go. In our work we focus on all aspects of creating such system, from information gathering to information visualization. One of the most important aspects of our work is to design fun and interactive interfaces that allow users to become part of the process of collecting, creating, and interpreting information so that reflective processes can be properly supported, much aligned with Shneiderman's view [44]. We also build on existing studies that show relations between what we do during the day and our wellbeing, such as [6], studies showing that people *do* like to think back and reflect on what happened and why they feel a certain way, such as [39,49] and studies showing that future generations of adults will probably be more open to monitor and record their lives [52]. We aim for creating a piece of *calm technology* [58], where *periphery*-based recordings of user context can be brought together into a supportive and engaging *center*-based interface.

Though the current trend seems to be that more and more "cloud" services collect user-related information either for adapting functionalities or delivering customized information, our aim is to design and build systems that can make use of our information but also allow us to control what, where and why such information is stored, as well be aware of what it is used for.

Even though we consider collecting more user information, we are not making the case for a Big Brother type of society. Our approach is more about empowering end users rather than giving the power to collect and correlate our data to "cloud" entities. Our goal is to support individuals in understanding the influence daily activities have over their health. For this, we set out to collect, interpret, correlate and visualize information that can make people aware of their health, where health is seen as a complex picture that includes physical, mental, emotional and social aspects.

3.2. Main Scenario

To better exemplify what types of systems and interactions we envision we present here a user scenario.

Mary is 53 and she has developed a heart problem. She can still live her life normally but her doctor advised her to take it slow and pay more attention to her lifestyle. To make it easier, Mary is using the MyRoR system, which can record various activity data from her personal devices and correlate all information into a daily story view, so that she can see how certain activities performed during the day impact her physiological state, especially her heart condition. The system helps her remember what happened during the day and allows her to record her own thoughts regarding the events as well as her reactions. For example, the other evening Mary tried to figure out why she felt unusually tired. By using the MyRoR system, she could see that she had lots of meetings and skipped lunch. One meeting was especially demanding, as her colleague George kept interrupting her presentation, as usual, which annoyed her. The system not only helps her to better understand her own behavior, but also allows her to access some of the information when she talks to her doctor so together they could identify potential risk factors.

3.3. System Requirements

Though we include discussions on choices regarding our system design and implementation throughout the article, we summarize here the main requirements guiding our overall system work:

1. Minimize the amount of sensors a user has to wear;
2. Tap into available information that can be used to describe multiple relevant aspects of user's daily activities;
3. Build upon existing monitoring systems by integrating and correlating their data: There are now multiple systems available addressing various aspects. It is unrealistic to think that they will go away so a better approach is to make it possible to incorporate their data. This might not always be possible, as one way to differentiate is to create proprietary formats, but it seems to be that most of these systems can export data in certain widely used formats, such as XML. Certain ongoing efforts towards interoperability between medical devices such as Continua Health Alliance [11], give us some hope that in the future integrating various monitoring devices might get easier;
4. Work based on realistic scenarios, where monitoring systems cannot provide a comprehensive picture of users' lives. It would be impossible and probably also very intrusive to try to record all our daily activities, so it is better to assume that self-monitoring systems will have to function based on incomplete information;
5. Reasoning engines should not replace users and medical professionals. Even though self-diagnosis through Internet search seems to become more and more popular [19], it is not something that we aim for at least not to the extent that it replaces human interactions. We should allow people to become part of the in-

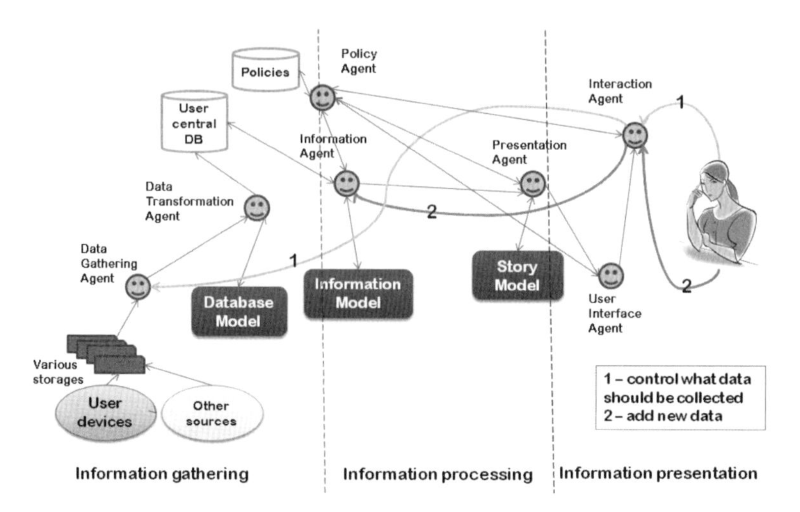

Figure 1. Multi agent system view.

formation gathering and interpretation. Such system should support users in understanding not present them with ready-made conclusions;

6. Create better interfaces and interaction paradigms. This is one of the biggest challenges, as the more and diverse information we add to the system the harder it becomes to visualize it in a comprehensive way. Current systems do not possess appropriate visualization means, as they mainly focus on time-based charts or map-based representations. So, how do we make these systems more comprehensive, interactive and engaging?

3.4. MyRoR System Design

We will further discuss certain aspects of such system along three main information lifecycle: gathering, processing and visualization. Figure 1 presents a multi-agent view of our system along such components.

The *Data Gathering Agent* is responsible for collecting data from various input sources. Such sources can include various devices used by the user during the day (e.g., work machine, home machine, mobile phone, etc.) as well as external content servers providing user-related data, such as emails and calendar events. The data collection can be done both asynchronously and in real time, according to the intended scenario. We have so far mainly focused on the asynchronous mode, as we are more interested in providing support for user reflective behaviors. Throughout this chapter we will consider this type of information gathering.

The *Data Transformation Agent* performs various operations on input data available in differing formats and in multiple local storages, such as: data conversion (e.g., from bytes to values), data clustering, filtering, storing into a user database, including its optimization (for time and space), and Database Model management. The *Database Model* contains information about the database structure and governs the storage operations. Unlike many existing lifestyle management systems described above that collect and send data to remote servers, we focus on creating a user-controlled information storage that better addresses privacy concerns as well as fit the single user centric view of the current system. Ongoing work in the PAL project looks into implementing various levels of access to such storage, depending on the situation and scope.

Data collected into the central database is processed by the *Information Agent* through various specialized modules. Various types of information processing take place, such as *filtering* in order to discard useless or faulty information, *interpretation* of existing information, *aggregation* of two or more types of data in order to create higher-level concepts, as well as *correlation* of two or more types of data according to certain interesting features derived through data analysis. The initial data, the newly created information and the rules for information processing are contained in the *Information Model*.

As discussed before, capturing such a diverse and large amount of information allows for creating a better picture of what has happened and why but also brings in big challenges in terms of presenting such information to the user. For various reasons discussed later, we have decided to use a combination of story-based and advanced chart-based visualizations for conveying recorded information to the user. The *Presentation Agent* has the role of assembling information into a story format, according to the *Story Model*.

The *User Interface Agent* is responsible for creating various information visualizations. Since the system is envisioned as being highly interactive, the *User Interface Agent* and *Interaction Agent* need to work together in order to: (1) allow the user to see and manage what is being collected; (2) allow the user to query for specific information; (3) allow the user to add new information as either annotations to existing data or new data altogether; (4) allow the user to customize the user interface to better reflect their personality; (5) take into account certain device capabilities, especially for scenarios that involve remote access to the system.

It is important to note that Fig. 1 includes a larger scope than currently addressed in our implementation, as it also reflects work on policy based information transactions currently done in the PAL project [46]. The *Policy Agent* is responsible for managing policies related to information usage, as well as various user preferences, and will become increasingly important once other information usages involving external parties are added to the system.

3.5. System Implementation

In this section, we describe the current implementation of our MyRoR system along the main information areas mentioned before.

3.5.1. Information Gathering

The decisions made regarding the information collected and sources used were governed by the requirements described in Section 3.3. Some of the most important criteria are that: (1) collected information can provide useful support for self-understanding and reflective behaviours; (2) system can deal with both static and mobile scenarios spanning various spaces and situations; (3) system should include commonly used user devices such as PCs, laptops and mobile phones; (4) system should include commercially available sensing devices; (5) number of sensors should be limited both because of the amount of processing they require as well as to prevent creating systems that are too obtrusive or require too much time and effort to attach.

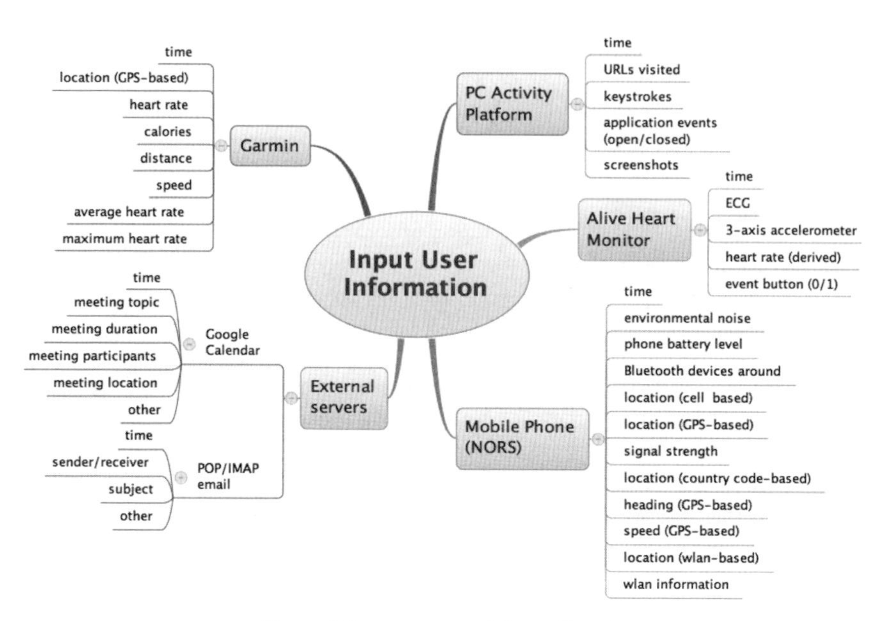

Figure 2. Input sources and data collected.

Figure 2 shows what input sources we have now and what information we are able to collect. The system can collect information from both physical (raw data) and logical sensors (interpreted data).

Here are more details about the main sources we are using:

- Garmin ForeRunner 305 is a popular wristwatch-like device used for fitness-related monitoring. The device is capable of providing heart rate and GPS-related information, raw as well as interpreted (e.g., distance, speed, etc.). A chest belt monitor provides heart rate information. Data is collected and stored on the device in Garmin's own file format, TCX, an XML-based format using a specific Garmin XML Schema. The files are currently stored onto the user's machine over a USB interface. More recent versions of such devices are able to synchronize data with a computer automatically;
- Mobile phone (Symbian-based mainly such as Nokia N97 or Samsung Omnia HD) running NORS platform [55], a mobile Java-based sensing platform that implements various sensor handlers allowing data collection of phone data as well as from attached Bluetooth(BT)-enabled sensors. The NORS platform collects data in its own file format. The file can be stored on a PC either through Bluetooth or over GPRS;
- The Alive Heart and Activity Monitor is a small wearable sensing device developed by Alive Technologies [1]. The device can measure ECG through 2 skin electrodes, and 3 axis accelerometer data. It also provides an event button that can be used by a user for various purposes, such as annotating certain interesting moments, making it easier for the system to find meaningful events. The data is recorded on an internal SD card. It can also be collected via Bluetooth through the NORS platform on the mobile phone and also directly recorded on a desktop through BT (e.g., for stationary scenarios when the user is at the computer);

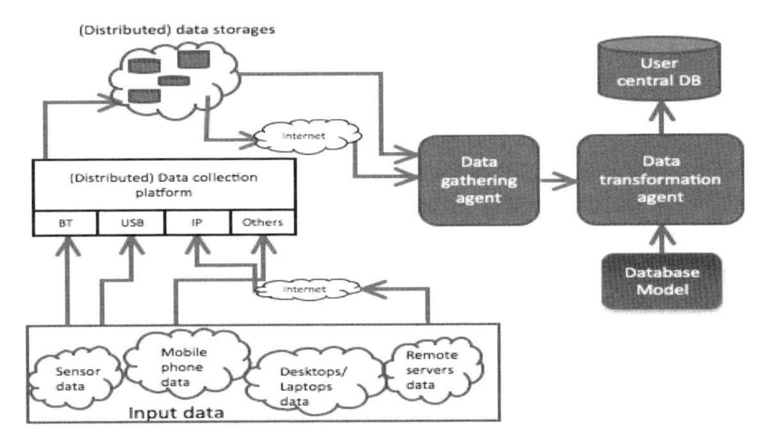

Figure 3. Data collection platform.

- A PC activity platform that provides various types of information related to user's activity context. Currently, the platform is Windows-based mainly for the sake of experimenting, but this is not to be considered a limitation of the system. We tested multiple existing activity platforms and decided to use the ActualSpy (http://www.actualspy.com/) platform, because it can record data on the local machine in open formats, and it allows for user awareness. The platform provides URLs visited (useful to determine web as well as search activity), applications used and associated events (i.e., application started, run, and closed), user name (helpful to differentiate between multiple users), keystrokes (can be used to search for certain keywords in order to determine interest as well as counted for activity intensity), as well as screenshots (timer-based images that can be used to create a comprehensive picture of currently used applications);
- External servers are used to provide more social activity information, such as emails sent and received and calendar information. We currently have modules that collect emails from POP3 and IMAP servers as well as obtain information from a user's Google Calendar (assuming the person uses such calendar, of course). These modules can obtain information on-demand and such information is not necessarily stored in the database but used in understanding a user's social context as well as activities and interest. Information obtained from such servers can be filtered based on time ranges and keywords. Currently, by using an Android phone, we are also able to add call and sms activity information to the Google calendar.

Figure 3 shows a platform view of the information collection process. *The Data Collection Platform* component comprises of various modules gathering data from multiple distributed sources, over various technologies (e.g., Bluetooth-BT, USB, IP) and storing it into distributed data storages.

The input data can be stored onto sensing devices, sensing gateways (such as phones), personal computers or remote servers. The Data Gathering Agent needs to know where the input data resides, collect it and pass it to the Data Transformation Agent for processing and storing into the central user database. We discuss some of the issues we have encountered in building this platform in Section 4.

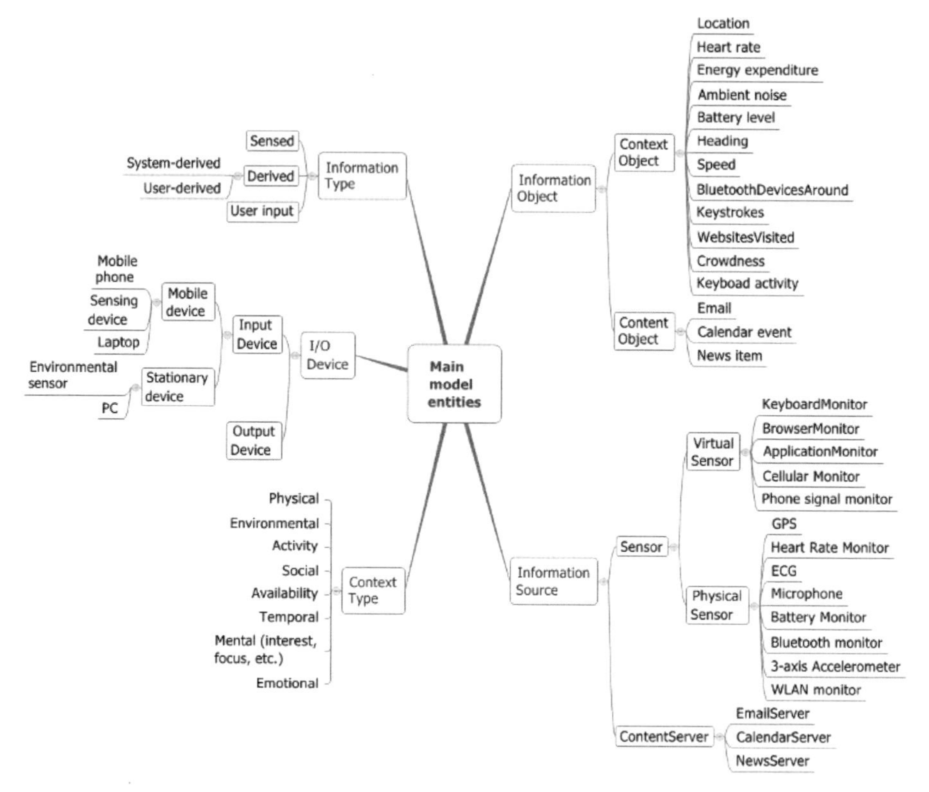

Figure 4. Main entities in the information model.

3.5.2. Information Processing

The Information Model captures both raw and processed information as well as relationships between them (i.e., how processed information has been obtained). A representation of the main objects included in the model is shown in Fig. 4.

The mind map model presented in Fig. 4 is used to create the semantic model and the relationships between the entities.

An important phase in the modeling process is to identify which features should be extracted from the available information. Figure 5 shows what information can be derived based on available initial data and how initial and derived information are combined to create the various types of user context [16].

The contexts we consider are:

- *Physical context*: location information (absolute, relative and at various granularity levels) obtained from various types of sensors – e.g., GPS, cell information, country code, wifi, meeting location, BT vicinity, as well as derived information such as distance, speed or heading.
- *Social context:* information about a user's social activities, obtained from sensors (e.g., BT devices) or social communication tools such as emails, calendar, and chat programs.
- *Emotional context*: information about a user's emotional state obtained from physiological sensors, such as ECG and heart rate, and through virtual sensors, such as keyword-based filtering of registered keystrokes, email content, etc.

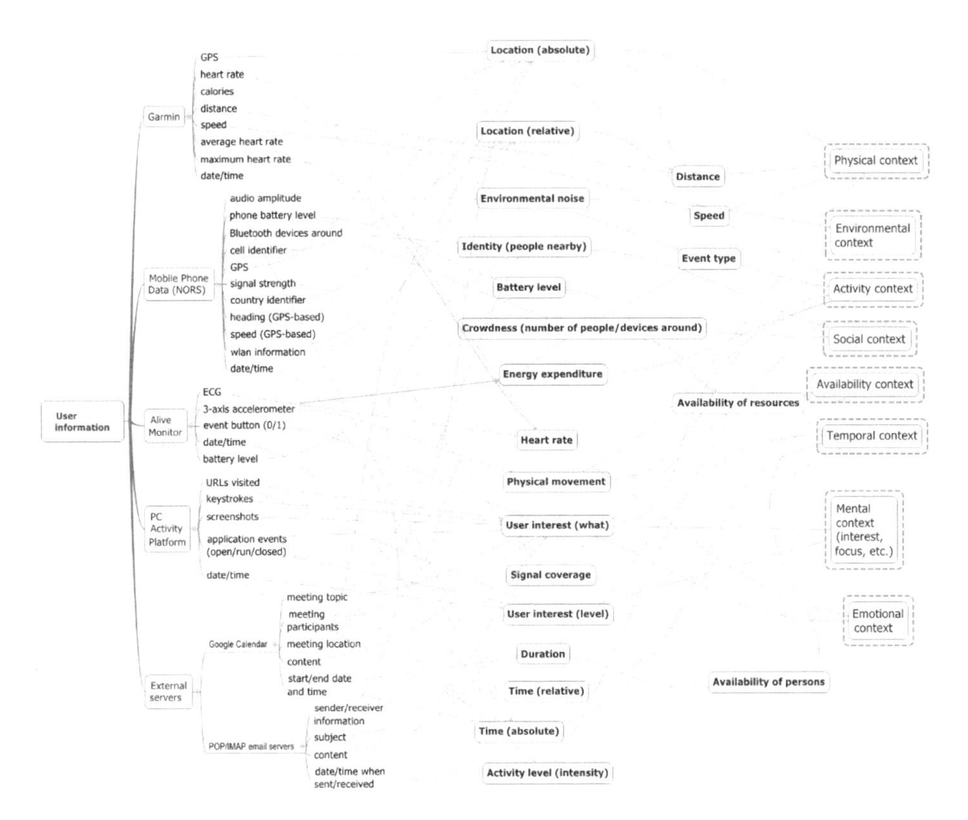

Figure 5. Information processing.

- *Mental context*: information about a user's interest both as topic and as intensity level, derived through web activity, applications used, keyword-based filtering of keystrokes, emails and screenshots.
- *Activity context:* information about what was the user doing derived from physical sensors, such as accelerometer data and GPS, as well as from applications used, web activity, screenshots and calendar information.
- *Availability context:* information regarding availability of people or devices
  - the availability of devices is determined through Bluetooth vicinity, battery level, signal coverage (if device is a mobile phone);
  - the availability of people can be determined through identifying people around, through checking calendar information. Furthermore, other types of context information (e.g., mental, activity) can be used for determining if a person should be interrupted or not.
- *Environmental context*: information about environment parameters that can affect users, such as noise, temperature or lighting.

An appropriate balance has to be found between having too much abstraction and allowing transparency. Allowing end user access to certain unprocessed or lightly processed data can also generate abstractions that a system designer might not have considered or could not even consider due to incomplete information. For example, in our initial scenario, the system can realize that Mary's heart rate increased, her voice pitch raised and deduct that she was getting angry. However, Mary's status could also be a reaction to an increase in room temperature or to being in a crowded environment rather than anger. Her emotional state might also have been influenced by other hidden parameters, current or historical, such as previous experiences related to people present, etc. In such situations it is better to show the user through the interface that something unusual happened at a certain moment during the day (e.g., based on her heart rate and voice pitch changes) and let her deduct what exactly happened and why, by allowing access to other collected information (e.g., who else was there, what else happened around the same time, etc.). With all the advances in emotion recognition, it is still hard to determine with certitude what the user feels, especially when considering real world settings (as opposed to controlled research laboratory experiments), as described by Picard et al. in [40].

3.5.3. Information Presentation and Usage

Our exploration of interactive information systems and natural ways of presenting life experiences led us to *stories* as a means of relating information to humans. Stories offer a way of organizing information as collections of meaningful events brought together either by following a timeline or a certain topic or character, as described by Brooks in [4]. Related work in this space has mainly focused on computer assisted storytelling [7] or on creating stories based on image annotations [3]. An inspiration for our work on creating fun and interactive environments based on collected context data is the Affective Diary project [49], where the focus was on creating better visualizations for self-monitoring systems.

In our system, we explore this type of story-based information presentation from simple to more complex structures enabled by a modeling process that takes information from the *Information Model* and arranges it into a story-based representation, according to the *Story Model* (see Fig. 6).

The main elements of a story, as described in Fig. 6 are:

- Characters or actors: the entities that take part in the story, being them humans or other living beings. The characters have various roles and are connected by certain relationships.
- Storyline: this is the plot of the story and it is formed by a sequence of meaningful events. An event can be described in terms of the context types defined above and the "*meaningfulness*" of an event can be determined through observing certain changes in contexts.
- Setting of the story: includes important elements that create the setting of a story or of an event, such as time, place, weather, etc.
- Theme of the story: places a certain emphasis on one or more types of contexts. For example, it focuses the story more on physical movements or on emotional changes, etc.
- Point of view: it determines how the story should be told. For example, we are currently mainly considering the case when the system creates a story as a diary, where the main user (the one the data refers to) is also the main consumer. However, in the future, we would also like to look at cases where the story can be customized by its main user to be shown to other people.

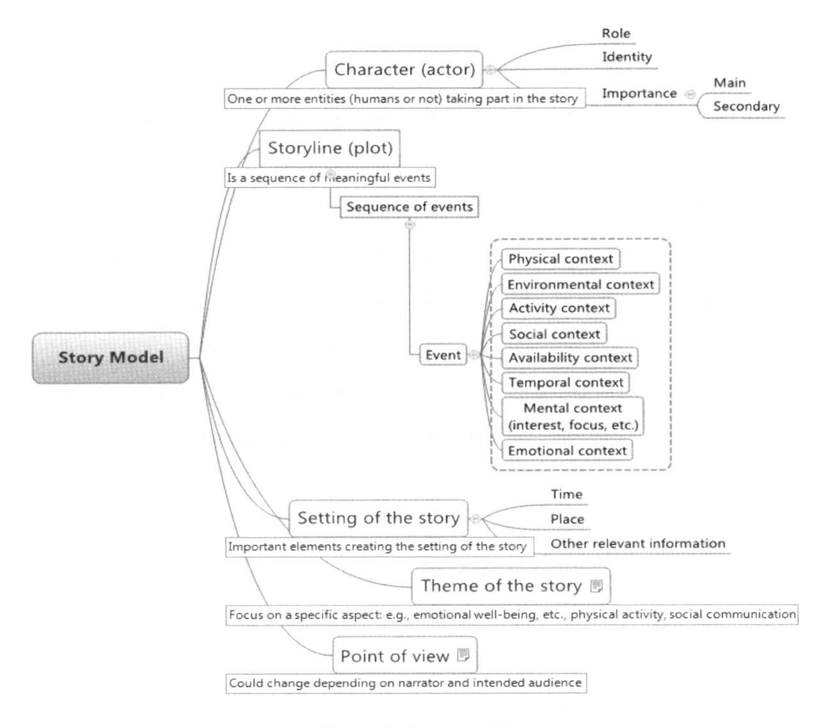

Figure 6. Story model.

The story creation is done by the *Presentation Agent,* working together with the *Information Agent* in order to determine what events are *meaningful* as well as use recorded context information to fill in the other elements of the story. An example of a meaningful event is given in our scenario: Mary's meeting, her presentation and her increased heart rate. In this event, Mary is the main character with the other meeting participants being secondary characters. Through zoom-in functionalities, Mary has access to all information recorded during the meeting. She can also add her own annotations to the story (e.g., explain why she thinks she felt so stressed during the meeting). The annotations become part of the story and will be available to her when she reflects on the information in the future. This makes the story evolve in a subjective, human way, as feelings and explanations can change based on remembering things in a different way.

After considering multiple environments and libraries such as Alice, Scratch, Greenfoot [22], Prefuse, Piccolo and PHPGraphLib, we have decided to use Scratch [42] as well as Google Visualizations [21] to develop various ways of creating and representing stories.

Scratch is a Squeak-based environment (Fig. 7) created as a way of making programming fun for kids. It has been developed by the Lifelong Kindergarten group at MIT Media Lab.

The reason we have eventually decided to use Scratch is that it provides an easy way to create rich media stories, where images, colours, texts, sounds and animations can easily convey the multidimensional sense of change within a sequence of events.

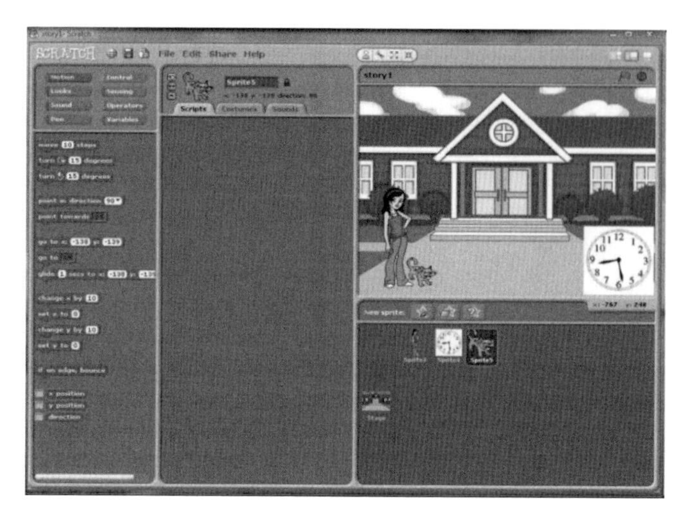

Figure 7. Scratch environment.

The various types of context represented within an event (see Fig. 6) can be visualized by using multiple types of media provided by such an environment (see Fig. 8). Scratch allows users to add and customize images, record voice annotations, add audio, create movements, change appearance of characters (which can be used to convey a sense of mood and activity changing), and change backgrounds (can be used to show environmental and physical changes).

Time can also be conveyed in Scratch in various ways, such as using a sequence of clock images (see Fig. 7) or by using an animated time line. Each character or object (called sprite) used in creating a Scratch story can be individually customized and controlled through parallel running scripts.

Our vision is to create a system that can offer both high-level, summarized view of information as well as allow access to more lower-level recorded data in order to increase user understanding. For this reason we have decided to use both stories and graphs. For creating more detailed visualizations we use Google Visualizations and correlate two or more types of data. The visualizations are embedded into a diary-like interface (see Fig. 9) built within a WordPress environment, one of the most commonly used blogging platforms [60]. The next section presents in more detail how collected data is interpreted and visualized as part of a user experiment.

4. Case Study

4.1. Experiment

To better exemplify the type of system we envision and the challenges we have encountered, we present here a user experiment that collected various types of user information over a few hours. In this scenario, the user is a PhD student having a board meeting and the experiment follows the user through the hours before the meeting, during the meeting and after the meeting. The table below shows what kind of data the system recorded during the experiment. During the experiment the user moved from home to university, around the campus, in the meeting room and then back home.

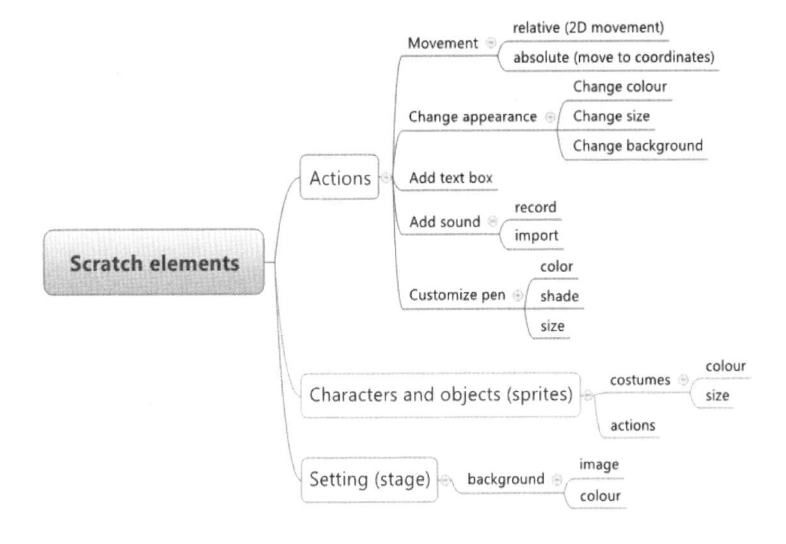

Figure 8. Main elements in Scratch.

Input source	Input data
Alive monitor	ECG, 3 axis accelerometer, event button
Phone (with NORS)	Audio amplitude, Bluetooth devices around, GPS, cell ID, battery information
PC activity platform	Web activity, applications used, keystrokes

4.2. Visualizations

All the visualizations created based on the collected data are accessible via a Wordpress-based system, in order to create an environment that is familiar, portable and based on available and commonly used technologies. The Wordpress interface integrates with our MySQL user backend database and we have created various PHP and Javascript programs that access, interpret and visualize collected data.

A widget PHP script runs to check if new data is available in the database. If data is available for a certain day then the script creates posts that allow the user to access the data by using various visualizations of the data (raw and interpreted), including the story created based on the data.

4.2.1. Detailed Visualizations

In the current version of the system interface, individual posts are created for each source (see Fig. 9), as we are currently using this version to organize and have access to collected data as well as test various visualizations and interpretations. Future versions might have a different interface.

In Fig. 10 we have included various visualizations for data such as heart rate, ambient noise levels, number and name of BT devices around, GPS coordinates, event button, keystrokes, applications used and web activity. In some of the visualizations, we were

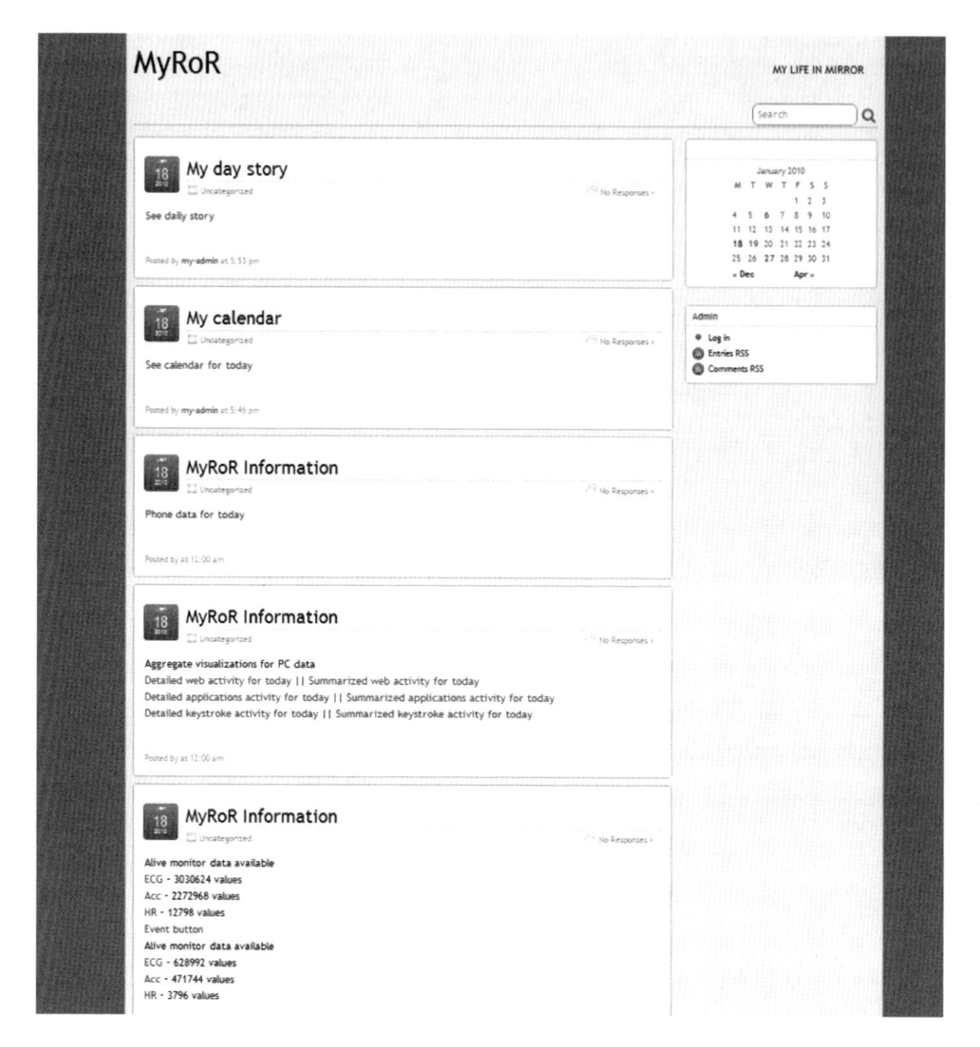

Figure 9. User interface to MyRoR system.

able to correlate certain data, such as GPS and time, number of BT devices, time and BT names, and heart rate and annotations based on certain conditions by using the AnnotatedTimeLine API and the MAP API offered by the Google Visualizations. More detailed information can be obtained by using the table representations (Fig. 10f), where full detail of captured data is available (i.e., time of collection, URL and window caption). Summarized visualizations, focused on giving an overall picture of words, are created by using word cloud API (h and g). Such summarized visualizations give a clear indication of what the user's focus was during the recording period.

While such visualizations can give a very good picture of various aspects of user's context at the time of the recording, it is very hard to combine them all into a summarized format based on graphs or maps. That is the main reason why we believe that stories are the appropriate format to create compressed and user-friendly interfaces.

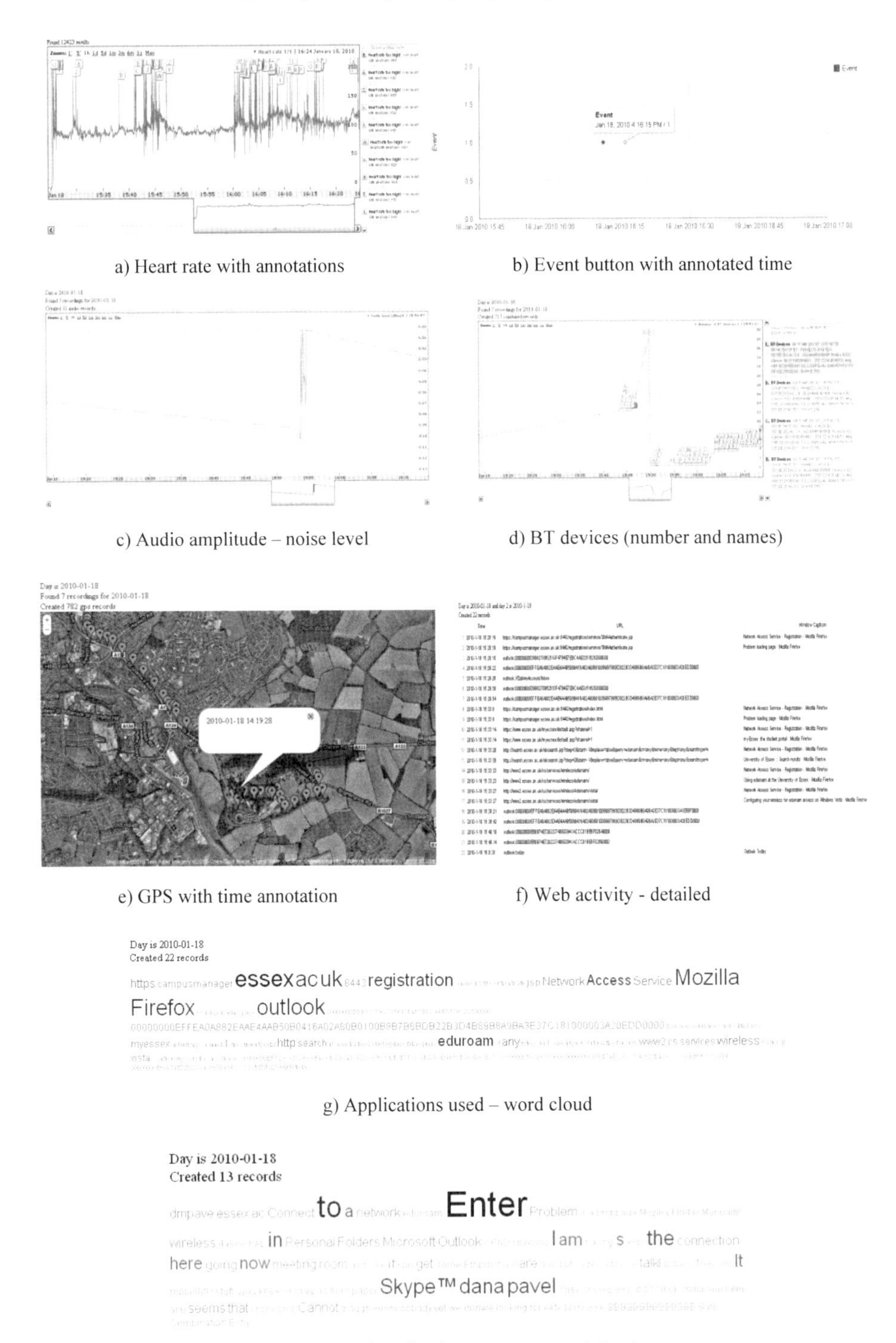

a) Heart rate with annotations

b) Event button with annotated time

c) Audio amplitude – noise level

d) BT devices (number and names)

e) GPS with time annotation

f) Web activity - detailed

g) Applications used – word cloud

h) Keys and application context – word cloud

Figure 10. Various visualizations.

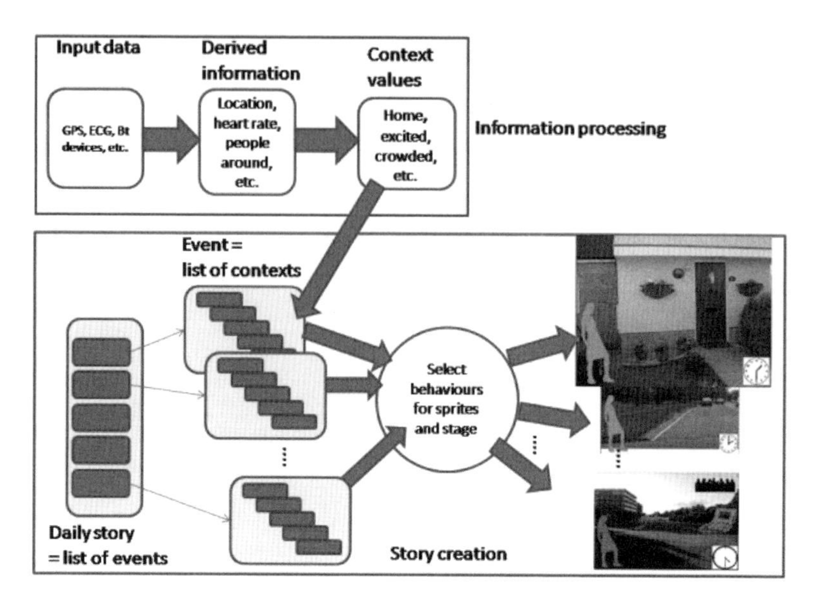

Figure 11. Story creation process.

4.2.2. Building the Story

For creating the story, we have used BYOB (http://byob.berkeley.edu/), which implements certain extensions to Scratch while keeping the same main interface and concepts. The main reason we use this environment is that it allows lists of lists. Lists are collections of elements, much like arrays. You can see in Fig. 11 how this feature is used.

The collected information is used to create derived information and create values for the contexts described above. The context values are then written in files that correspond to the list of lists structure described in Fig. 11. The daily story we create is a list of events, where each event is defined by the various aspects of context and each context has one or more values. The values given to contexts are used to create the graphical representation of each event by using features offered by the Scratch environment.

The story is created through running various parallel scripts that test for keywords (i.e., context values) and then determine the behaviours of the various sprites selected to make up the story and the selection of the background.

The user has a lot of freedom to decide what colours, sprites, and backgrounds to choose. For example, in our story the Home location is shown as a background of user's house (Fig. 11) and the university location with a picture of the campus (Fig. 12). Driving is shown by changing the background (Fig. 12) though it can also be shown by using a car as a sprite. Current time is shown through various clocks. The meeting is shown through a sprite (Fig. 12). The user has the option to select an own sprite as her avatar and she can customize its colour to reflect the emotional context: in this case the user decided to choose green for energetic (during driving and at home) and red for excited (during the PhD board). The appropriate sprite is then chosen based on the heart rate. Having such freedom to map emotional states to colours removes the ambiguity issues around personal interpretations of certain colours [49].

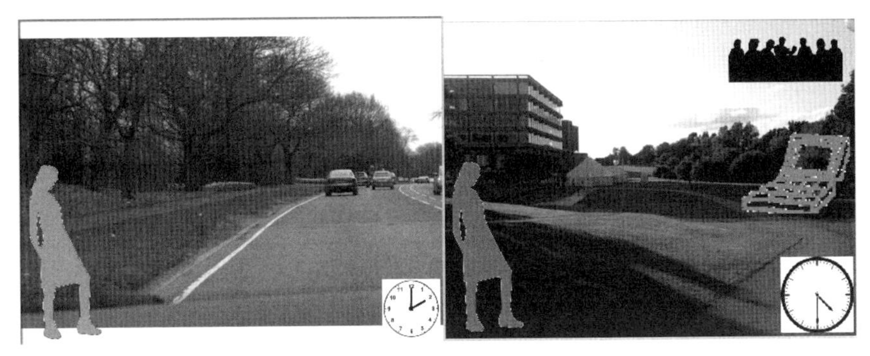

Figure 12. Two screenshots for two events: Driving and having a meeting at the university.

The blog interface allows us to group various types of visualizations and media together, so that the user has access both to higher-level representations, such as stories, and to more detailed one, such as graphs, tables, maps and word clouds. Another major advantage is that users can add their own notes and thoughts, which could be reflections based on visualizations as well as usual blog entries. Using the calendar as an entry point follows our thinking of creating daily stories and makes it easy to show which days have available data, as based on our experience, the data collection happens quite sparsely and it is usually motivated by the expectation that something a bit more unusual will happen during that day.

The blog can also be accessed from mobile devices (e.g., by using Wordpress apps on Android and iPod/iPhone), which makes it easy to access notes and visualizations as well as add new ones while on the go. More importantly, the whole environment can run within user's own environment. We are currently using XAMPP which provides an Apache server and a MySQL database running on user's machine and also allows external exposure for remote access to the whole environment.

4.3. Lessons Learned

In building our data collection platform we came across various issues, some of them quite expected and often encountered when building life loggers. We present here some of our preliminary results. Further experiments will be performed in the near future.

One of the main ones is related to *data size*. Some of the data collected, especially from ECG and accelerometer, generate a large amount of information, as they are sampled very often (300 samples/second for ECG and 75 samples/second for accelerometer). In order to avoid huge database sizes, we decided to create binary file repositories for ECG and accelerometer data and only store pointers to these files into the database. Hence, raw data is still preserved for further processing (e.g., heart rate determination based on ECG or activity context based on accelerometer data) but database size is substantially reduced. Writing to the database is a very time-consuming operation, especially for data sampled quite frequently. Hence, we use buffered writing operations in order to improve the data storing performance. Data size is also an issue for creating visualizations as the Google Visualization we used (Annotated Time Line) and other libraries seem to have problems representing such an amount of values so we had to vary the sampling steps depending on how many values were to be displayed.

Another important issue is the existence of various formats and synching methods used by our data sources, which requires a considerable effort when building the data gathering modules. Certain standardization efforts [11] should improve the situation but it still remains a major issue when building such a system.

In terms of battery life, the Alive monitor can record for a few days of intermittent operation but phones do not last more than a day, especially when GPS recording is involved.

Because of using multiple devices we found time correlation very challenging, as their clocks can differ from seconds or minutes (mainly due to imprecise clock operation) to hours (when time zone changes). Some devices can use time zones and others cannot. For example, the Alive Monitor cannot have any time zone set. Because of such issues, special care needs to be taken in correlating gathered data and certain assumptions need to be made (e.g., the Alive monitor timezone is always GMT+0).

We have discussed before the challenges to visualize such diverse information by using currently available means. This is due to sampling differences (as data is not usually sampled at the same intervals) but also format issues, as number data fits in various ranges and string data is hard to represent.

In our data collection experiments, we have been focusing on a single user recording data in various situations such as at home, at work, or on the go. Our preliminary findings show that: (1) it is unrealistic to assume that people would wear or even remember to switch on devices all the time (e.g., Garmin requires an explicit Start/Stop action); (2) the incentive of using such system depends on how eventful the day is expected to be; (3) attaching wearable electronics such as a heart monitor belt is still not comfortable enough to allow for permanent data collection; (4) the accuracy of data highly depends on where and how the sensors are placed, a person's posture or movement.

5. Conclusions and Future Work

In this chapter we have focused on what we see as necessary improvements to existing lifestyle management self-monitoring systems in order to make them more informative and interactive. In the process, we have looked at various existing systems and we believe that what is missing in most such systems is a focus on supporting users reflect and understand *why* something has happened. For that, we need to not only focus on physiological and location data but also on other types of context data that can offer a better picture into what our activities and interests were at a certain point in time. In our system we have collected and correlated physiological and location data with various data we generate through our daily use of computing devices, data that creates a more complex picture of what our social, emotional, and mental activities were. The motivation behind this type of data collection comes from multiple studies showing links between what we do during the day, our lifestyles and our wellbeing and wellness.

We have also found that recording such varied data involves multiple challenges in terms of data collection, processing and visualization. Our exploration in more engaging and natural types of interfaces capable to correlate and summarize recorded user context brought us to story-based representations of data collected. For creating our vision of such stories we have made use of existing environments and technologies, allowing us to address important design criteria such as making use of various media, allowing the user to personalize stories the way they want, using familiar interfaces appropriate for a digital diary and allowing for both local and remote access of information stored within user's trusted environment.

When building our system we have considered various existing user studies and results with similar solutions and also tried to create something that *we* would use. Therefore, our initial user experiments were mainly designed to deal with the inherent issues introduced by building up the whole system, from data collection to data visualization. Future work includes further user experiments focused on various aspects, such as: (1) selection of further information that can better support self reflection and self understanding; (2) personalization of stories through various means: colours, audio, images, text; (3) using such system in specific health areas, such as bipolar disease; (4) introducing a persuasive dimension [18] into the stories.

References

[1] Alive heart and activity monitor, http://www.alivetec.com/products.htm (accessed 13 September 2010).

[2] D. Anspaugh, M. Hamrick and F. Rosato, *Wellness: Concepts and Applications*, 7th edn, McGraw-Hill, 2008.

[3] A. Aris, J. Gemmell and R. Lueder, Exploiting location and time for photo search and storytelling in MyLifeBits, Microsoft Research Technical Report, MSR-TR-2004-102, October 2004.

[4] K. Brooks, Do story agents use rocking chairs? The theory and implementation of one model for computational narrative, in: *Proc. of the 4th ACM Conference on Multimedia,* November 1996.

[5] J. Bruner, *Acts of Meaning*, Harvard University Press, Cambridge, MA, 1990.

[6] J. Burton, WHO healthy workplace framework and model: Background and supporting literature and practices, February 2010.

[7] D. Byrne and G.J. Jones, Towards computational autobiographical narratives through human digital memories, in: *Proc. of the 2nd ACM International Workshop on Story Representation, Mechanism and Context*, October, 2008.

[8] Calisto Glucoband, http://www.calistomedical.com/?cat=14 (accessed 13 September 2010).

[9] CardioNet patient solutions, http://www.cardionet.com/patients_01.htm (accessed 13 September 2010).

[10] B. Clarkson, K. Mase and A. Pentland, The familiar: A living diary and companion, in: *Proc. of Computer-Human Interaction*, ACM, New York, NY, USA, 2001, pp. 271–272.

[11] Continua Health Alliance, http://www.continuaalliance.org (accessed 13 September 2010).

[12] C.B. Corbin, R. Lindsey, G. Welk, *Concepts of fitness and wellness: A comprehensive lifestyle approach*, McGraw-Hill, Boston, 2000.

[13] Definition of Wellness website, http://www.definitionofwellness.com/index.html (accessed on 10 September 2010).

[14] Department of Health, Improving chronic disease management, electronic publication, 3 March 2004 (accessed online 13 September 2010).

[15] Department of Health, Supporting self-care – A practical option: Diagnostic, monitoring and assistive tools, devices, technologies and equipment to support self care, published 21 April 2006, http://www.dh.gov.uk/en/Publicationsandstatistics/Publications/PublicationsPolicyAndGuidance/DH_4134006 (accessed 13 September 2010).

[16] A.K. Dey and G.D. Abowd, Towards a better understanding of context and context awareness, in: *Proc. of HUC '99*, 1999.

[17] emWave, http://www.heartmathstore.com/item/6300/emwave-personal-stress-reliever (accessed 13 September 2010).

[18] B.J. Fogg, *Persuasive Technology: Using Computers to Change what We Think and Do*, Morgan Kaufmann, San Francisco, CA, 2003.

[19] Friends Provident and Future Foundation, Visions of Britain 2020: Health and wellbeing, published July 2010.

[20] J. Gemmell, G. Bell, L. Gordon, D. Roger, S. Drucker and C. Wong, MyLifeBits: Fulfilling the memex vision, in: *ACM Multimedia '02*, December 1–6, 2002, Juan-les-Pins, France, pp. 235–238.

[21] Google visualizations, http://code.google.com/apis/visualization/documentation/gallery.html (link accessed 5 May 2010).

[22] Greenfoot, http://www.greenfoot.org/ (link accessed 5 May 2010).

[23] GSR2 Relaxation Monitor, http://www.bio-medical.com/product_info.cfm?inventory__imodel=T2001&gclid=CNe9qo-kiaQCFUkrDgodhXOkHQ (accessed 13 September 2010).
[24] HealthBuddy, http://www.bosch-telehealth.com/content/language1/html/5578_ENU_XHTML.aspx (accessed 13 September 2010).
[25] iFall article, http://www.imedicalapps.com/2010/04/ifall-android-medical-app/ (accessed 13 September 2010).
[26] Journey to wild divine – The passage, http://www.wilddivine.com/servlet/-strse-72/The-Passage-OEM/Detail (accessed 13 September 2010).
[27] T.G. Kirsten, H.J. van der Walt and C.T. Viljoen, Health, well-being and wellness: An anthropological eco-system approach, *Journal of Interdisciplinary Health Sciences* **14**(1) (2009), Article #407.
[28] B. Kozier and G. Erb, *Fundamentals of Nursing: Concepts, Process and Practice*, 8th edn, Pearson Education, published January 2008.
[29] M.L. Lee and A.K. Dey, Lifelogging memory appliance for people with episodic memory impairment, in: *Proc. of the 10th International Conference on Ubiquitous Computing*, 2008.
[30] Medixine Chronic Disease Clinic, http://www.medixine.com/do.xsp?viewType=viewinfoview&objectType=complextype&directoryType=simple&complextypeOID=1219667445_463_13315 (accessed 13 September 2010).
[31] Medixine Health Forecasting, http://www.medixine.com/do.xsp?viewType=viewinfoview&objectType=complextype&directoryType=simple&complextypeOID=1219666324_854_8ce9 (accessed 13 September 2010).
[32] Medtronic MiniMed, http://www.minimed.com/products/index.html (accessed 13 September 2010).
[33] G. Miller and L. Foster, Critical synthesis of wellness literature, under the British Columbia atlas of wellness, http://www.geog.uvic.ca/wellness/ (accessed 5 October 2010).
[34] MiniTell daily alarmed box from PivoTell, http://www.pivotell.co.uk/Order_MiniTell_Daily_Alarmed_Pill_Box.htm (accessed 13 September 2010).
[35] MobiHealth, http://www.mobihealth.com/services/en/mh_mobile.php (accessed 13 September 2010).
[36] Nike+iPod, http://www.apple.com/ipod/nike/ (accessed 13 September 2010).
[37] OBS Medical, http://www.obsmedical.com/products (accessed 13 September 2010).
[38] Philips lifeline solutions, http://www.lifelinesys.com/content/home (accessed 13 September 2010).
[39] R.W. Picard, *Affective Computing*, MIT Press, Cambridge, MA, 1997.
[40] R. Picard, E. Vyzas and J. Healey, Toward machine emotional intelligence: Analysis of affective physiological state, *IEEE Transactions on Pattern Analysis and Machine Intelligence* **23**(10) (October 2001), 175–1191.
[41] Resperate, http://www.resperate.com/us/welcome/index.aspx (accessed 13 September 2010).
[42] Scratch environment, http://scratch.mit.edu (link accessed 5 May 2010).
[43] SenseWear BMS, http://www.sensewear.com/BMS/solutions_bms.php (accessed 13 September 2010).
[44] B. Shneiderman, *Leonardo's Laptop: Human Needs and the New Computing Technologies*, MIT Press, Cambridge, MA, USA, 2002.
[45] SIMPill, http://www.simpill.com/ (accessed 13 September 2010).
[46] J. Singh and J. Bacon, Event-based data dissemination control in healthcare, in: *Proc. of eHealth 2008*.
[47] SmartBrain Technologies, http://www.smartbraintech.com/ (accessed 13 September 2010).
[48] Sports tracker for symbian, http://www.sports-tracker.com/ (accessed 13 September 2010).
[49] A. Ståhl, K. Höök, M. Svensson, A. Taylor and M. Combetto, Experiencing the affective diary, *Journal of Personal and Ubiquitous Computing* **13**(5) (June 2009), 365–378.
[50] StressEraser biofeedback, http://stresseraser.com/ (accessed 13 September 2010).
[51] M. Sung and A. Pentland, LiveNet: Health and lifestyle networking through distributed mobile devices, Technology 2–4.
[52] D. Tapscott, *Grown Up Digital: How the Net Generation is Changing Your World*, McGraw-Hill, New York, 2008.
[53] The Future Vision Coalition, A future vision for mental health, Report published July 2009.
[54] TMC Home from TeleMedCare, http://www.telemedcare.com.au/index.php?option=com_content&view=article&id=3&Itemid=8 (accessed 13 September 2010).
[55] D. Trossen and D. Pavel, NORS: An open source platform to facilitate participatory sensing with mobile phones, in: *Proc. of MobiQuitous*, 2007.
[56] Tunstall Lifeline Connect Telecare, http://www.tunstall.co.uk/assets/Literature/Portfolio/portfolio__issue_20.pdf (accessed 13 September 2010).
[57] Viterion Telehealthcare, http://www.viterion.com/products.cfm (accessed 13 September 2010).
[58] M. Weiser and J. Seely Brown, The coming age of calm technology, Xerox PARC paper, October 1996.
[59] Wellcore emergency response system solutions, http://www.wellcore.com/buy/ (accessed 13 September 2010).

[60] WordPress, http://wordpress.org/ (link accessed 6 October 2010).
[61] World Health Organization (WHO), Preventing chronic diseases: A vital investment: WHO global report, published 2005, accessed online 13 September 2010.
[62] WristCare, http://www.istsec.fi/eng/Emikakoti.htm (accessed 13 September 2010).
[63] L. Zeng, P. Hsueh and H. Chang, Greenolive: An open platform for wellness management ecosystem.

Handbook of Ambient Assisted Living
J.C. Augusto et al. (Eds.)
IOS Press, 2012

doi:10.3233/978-1-60750-837-3-434

Sensor Selection to Support Practical Use of Health-Monitoring Smart Environments

Diane J. COOK* and Lawrence B. HOLDER
School of Electrical Engineering and Computer Science,
Washington State University, Pullman WA, USA
{cook,holder}@eecs.wsu.edu

Abstract. The data mining and pervasive sensing technologies found in smart homes offer unprecedented opportunities for providing health monitoring and assistance to individuals experiencing difficulties living independently at home. In order to monitor the functional health of smart home residents, we need to design technologies that recognize and track activities that people normally perform as part of their daily routines. One question that frequently arises, however, is how many smart home sensors are needed and where should they be placed in order to accurately recognize activities? We employ data mining techniques to look at the problem of sensor selection for activity recognition in smart homes. We analyze the results based on six data sets collected in five distinct smart home environments.

Keywords. Activity recognition, feature selection, feature construction, machine learning

Introduction

A convergence of technologies in data mining and pervasive computing as well as the increased accessibility of robust sensors and actuators has caused interest in the development of *smart environments* to emerge. Furthermore, researchers are recognizing that smart environments can assist with valuable functions such as remote health monitoring and intervention. The need for the development of such technologies is underscored by the aging of the population, the cost of formal health care, and the importance that individuals place on remaining independent in their own homes.

To function independently at home, individuals need to be able to complete Activities of Daily Living (ADLs) [15] such as eating, dressing, cooking, drinking, and taking medicine. Automating the recognition of activities is an important step toward monitoring the functional health of a smart home resident. When surveyed about assistive technologies, family caregivers of Alzheimer's patients ranked activity identification and tracking at the top of their list of needs [17].

In response to this recognized need, researchers have designed a variety of approaches to model and recognize activities. The generally accepted approach is to model and recognize those activities that are frequently used to measure the functional health of an individual [19]. The challenge that researchers and practitioners face is

*Corresponding Author: Diane J. Cook. E-mail: cook@eecs.wsu.edu.

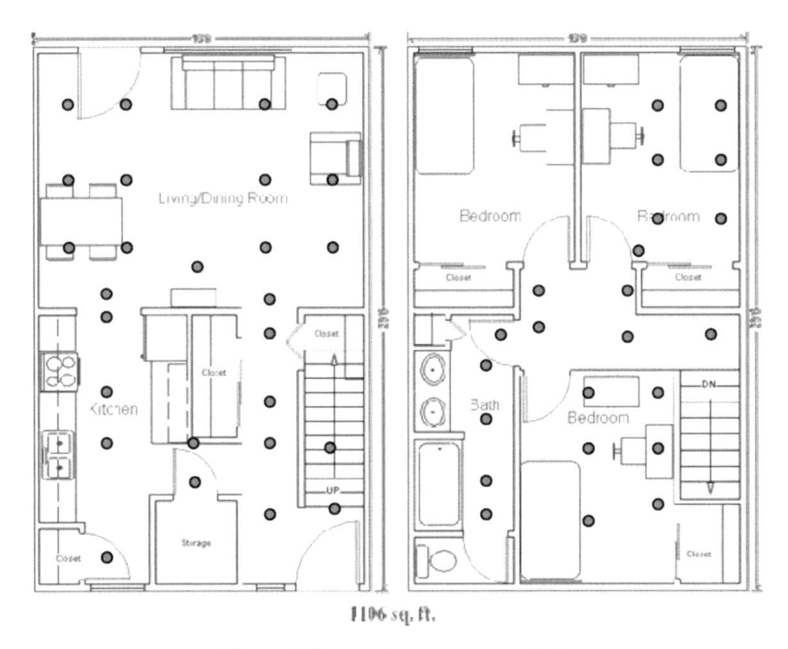

Figure 1. Kyoto smart apartment testbed.

deciding how many smart home sensors are needed and where they should be placed to perform this activity recognition task. This is not a straightforward decision. A greater density of sensors provides more pinpointed information on exactly where and when interactions with the environment occur. On the other hand, the addition of sensors imposes more energy consumption and cost constraints. In addition, when more sensors are used then the representation is more complex, thus a greater amount of training data is needed to accurately learn activity models. In this paper, we explore methods of selecting and positioning sensors in a smart environment and implement our approach in the context of the CASAS Smart Home project [15].

1. Datasets

To test our ideas, we collected sensor events from five physical testbeds. The first testbed, referred to as Kyoto and shown in Fig. 1, is a two-bedroom CASAS apartment located on the Washington State University campus. The apartment is equipped with motion sensors positioned on the ceiling approximately 1 meter apart throughout the space. In addition, we have installed sensors to provide ambient temperature readings, and custom-built analog sensors to provide readings for hot water, cold water, and stove burner use. Voice over IP captures phone usage, contact switch sensors monitor the open/closed status of doors and cabinets, and pressure sensors monitor usage of key items such as the medicine container, cooking tools, and telephone. The first dataset in this environment represents 138,039 events collected by 71 sensors monitoring 16 activities. The second represents 5,312 events collected by 24 sensors monitoring 5 activities.

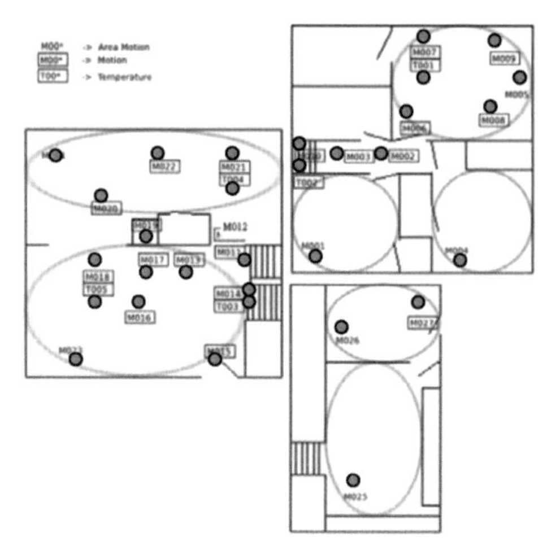

Figure 2. Cairo smart home which housed an older adult couple with a cat.

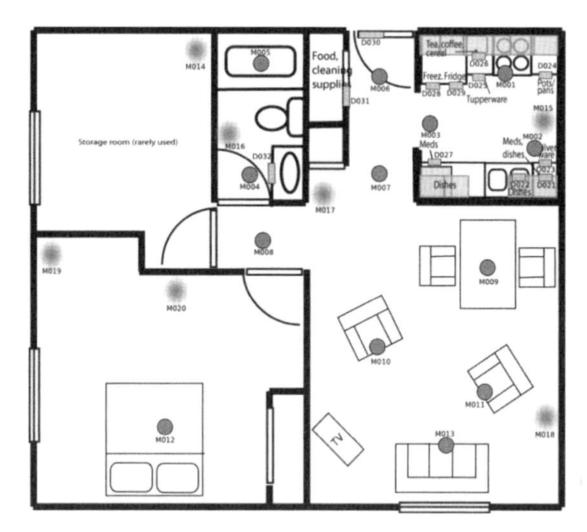

Figure 3. Bosch-1 smart apartment which housed a single older adult resident.

The second testbed, referred to as Cairo (see Fig. 2), is a two-bedroom, two-story home. Here we collected 726,534 events from 27 sensors monitoring 13 activities for two residents. Environments three through five (shown in Figs 3–5) are single-resident apartments that are part of an assisted care facility. Each of these sites contains motion sensors throughout the space as well as door contact sensors in key areas. We monitor 11 activities in each of these three apartments and the number of sensor events is 371,925 for the first apartment, 254,920 for the second, and 164,561 for the third. Sensor data for each of the environments is captured using a sensor network that was designed in-house and is stored in a SQL database. Our middleware uses a jabber-based publish/subscribe protocol as a lightweight platform and language-independent middleware to push data to client tools with minimal overhead and maximal flexibility.

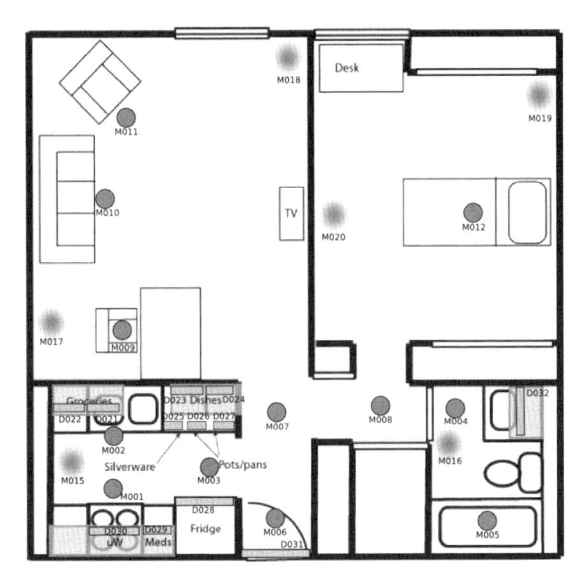

Figure 4. Bosch-2 smart apartment which housed a single older adult resident.

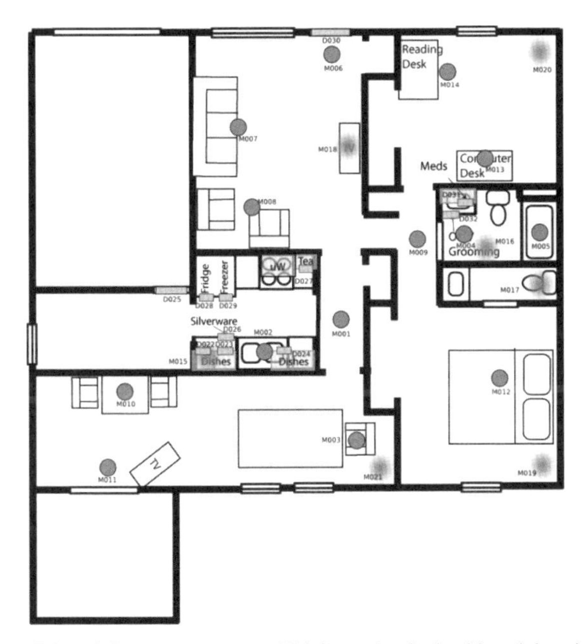

Figure 5. Bosch-3 smart apartment which housed a single older adult resident.

2. ADL Recognition

We treat a smart environment as an intelligent agent that perceives the state of the resident and the physical surroundings using sensors and acts on the environment using controllers in such a way that the specified performance measured is optimized [3]. Researchers have generated ideas for designing smart environment software algorithms that track the location and activities of residents, that generate reminders, and that react to hazardous situations. A few smart environment projects with physical testbeds now exist [1,3,5,7,20]. Resulting from these advances, researchers are now beginning to recognize the importance of applying smart environment technology to health assistance and companies are recognizing the potential of this technology for a quickly-growing consumer base.

Activity recognition is not an untapped area of research. Because the need for activity recognition technology is great, researchers have explored a number of approaches to this problem. The approaches differ according to the type of sensor data that is used for classification, the model that is designed to learn activity definitions, and the method that is used to annotate sample data.

Sensor data. Researchers have found that different types of sensor information are effective for classifying different types of activities. When trying to recognize actions that involve repetitive body motions (e.g., walking, running), data collected from accelerometers positioned on the body has been used [11]. Other activities are not as easily distinguishable by body position and in these cases, researchers [12,14] observe the smart home resident's interaction with objects of interest such as doors, windows, refrigerators, keys, and medicine containers. Other researchers, including Cook and Schmitter-Edgecombe [4], rely upon motion sensors as well as item sensors to recognize ADL activities that are being performed. In addition, some researchers such as Brdiczka et al. [2] video tape smart home residents and process the video to recognize activities, though this can introduce challenges for technology acceptance and the computational expense of processing the data.

Activity models. The number of machine learning models that have been used for activity recognition varies almost as greatly as the types of sensor data that have been tested. Naïve Bayes classifiers have been used with promising results for activity recognition [2] by identifying the activity that corresponds with the greatest probability to the set of sensor values that were observed. Other researchers, including Maurer et al. [11], have employed decision trees to learn logical descriptions of the activities. Gu et al. [6] use the notion of emerging patterns to look for frequent sensor sequences that can be associated with each activity as an aid for recognition. Alternative approaches have been explored by other researchers to encode the probabilistic sequence of sensor events using Markov models, dynamic Bayes networks, and conditional random fields [10,14].

In our approach we employ a hidden Markov model (HMM) to recognize possibly-interleaved activities from a stream of sensor events. A HMM is a statistical model in which the underlying data source is not itself observable but can be linked to another set of stochastic processes that produce the sequence of observed features. Because the model is Markovian, the conditional probability distribution of any hidden state depends only on the value of a finite number of preceding hidden states. The value of an observable state depends only on the value of the current hidden state.

In our HMM we let the hidden states represent activities. The observable states represent the sensors whose values are observed via the recorded sensor events. The probabilistic relationships between hidden nodes and observable nodes, and the probabilistic transition between hidden nodes, are estimated by the relative frequency with which these relationships occur in the sample data corresponding to the activity cluster. An example hidden Markov model for the activities Prepare Meal, Medicine Dispenser, Watch DVD, and Write Birthday Card is shown in Fig. 6. Given an input sequence of sensor events, our goal is to find the most likely sequence of hidden states, or activities,

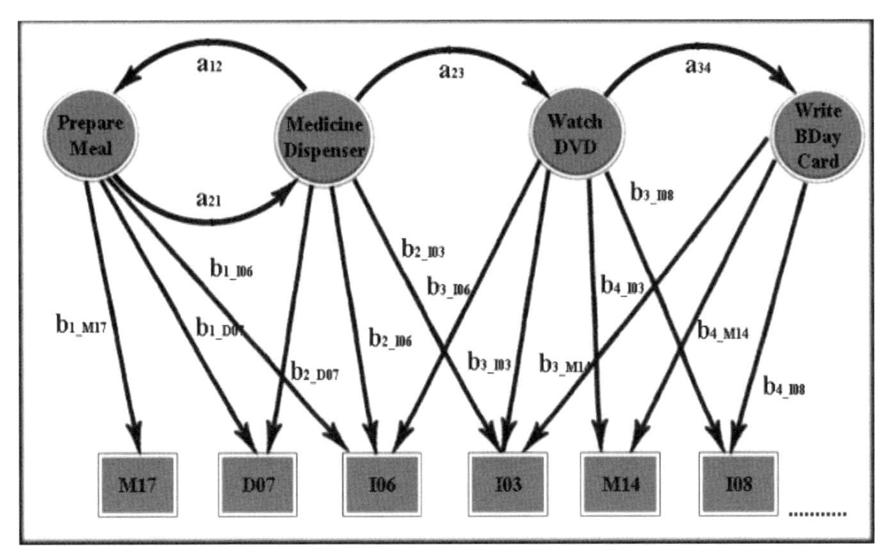

Figure 6. HMM for an activity recognition task with four hidden states (activities) and a set of observable nodes that correspond to possible sensor events.

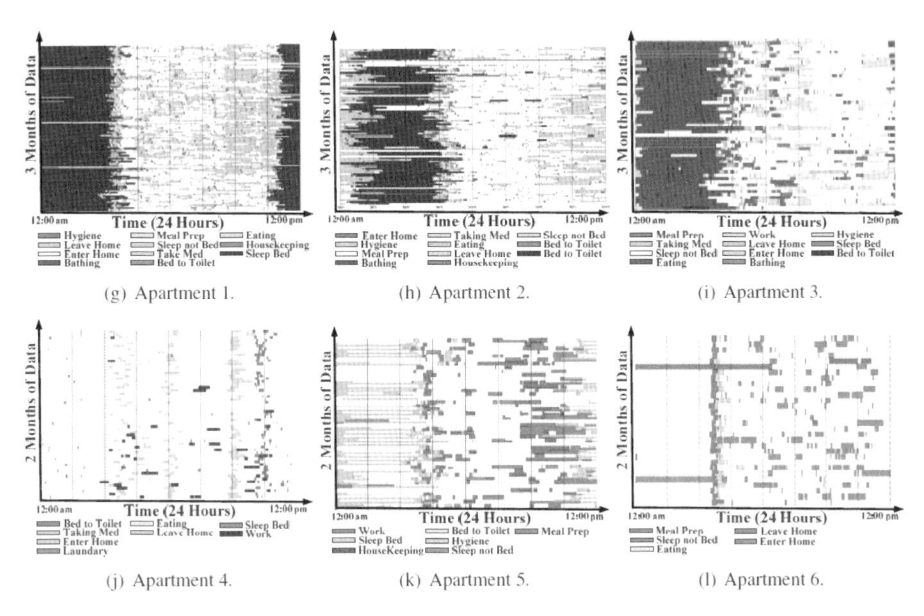

Figure 7. Bosch-3 smart apartment which housed a single older adult resident.

which could have generated the observed event sequence. We use the Viterbi algorithm [18] to identify this sequence of hidden states. The graphs in Fig. 7 plot activities that are observed in the various smart homes over a period of time. The x axis indicates the hour of day and the y axis indicates the day within the observation period.

3. Sensor Selection

In this book chapter we address three questions pertaining to the selection, placement, and focus of sensors in a smart environment that is used for activity recognition:

1. Which sensors from among an available set are needed to produce optimal activity recognition results?
2. Can sensors be clustered together to form a new, smaller set of sensors that do not sacrifice recognition accuracy?
3. Can general rules be gleaned about sensor selection and placement in smart environments?

To address the first question we draw from the wealth of literature on feature selection in the field of machine learning and data mining. A variety of approaches have been explored by researchers including wrapper approaches [9] which select features based on which combinations perform best on sample data and filter approaches [8] which apply external criteria to select sensors.

In this study, we employ the filter-based criteria of mutual information (MI) [13] to rank sensors and we systematically evaluate the effect of removing sensors with low MI values on activity recognition performance. In this case we are choosing sensors which best discriminate the activities. The MI calculation of sensor s for a set of activities A is shown in Eq. (1).

$$MI(s,A) = \sum_{es \in values(s)} \sum_{a \in A} P(es,a) \log(P(es,a) / P(es)P(a)) \tag{1}$$

The second question is analogous to the idea of feature construction in machine learning. In particular, when motion sensors are placed in an environment their range of observation is manually restricted in order to provide focused movement information in the space. If we merge neighboring sensors together we can replace the pair of sensors with a single sensor associated with a larger range of view. Thus the approach we take for feature construction is to perform hierarchical clustering on the sensors, selecting the set of clusters that perform the best and merging sensors within the clusters that share physical proximity in the space.

In the following section we summarize the results of applying these techniques to data collected in our smart environment testbeds. We use the data and the results to make observations that allow us to answer the third question as well.

4. Experimental Results

We hypothesize that feature selection methods can be used to identify the number and placement of sensors to result in the best activity recognition accuracy. We also postulate that a larger number of sensors does not always result in higher performance. Not only does an increase in sensors add to the cost of smart environment creation and the ongoing energy usage, but it can sometimes actually degrade performance because more labeled training data is needed in order to adequately learn the more complex concept that is a function of the increased number of sensor variables.

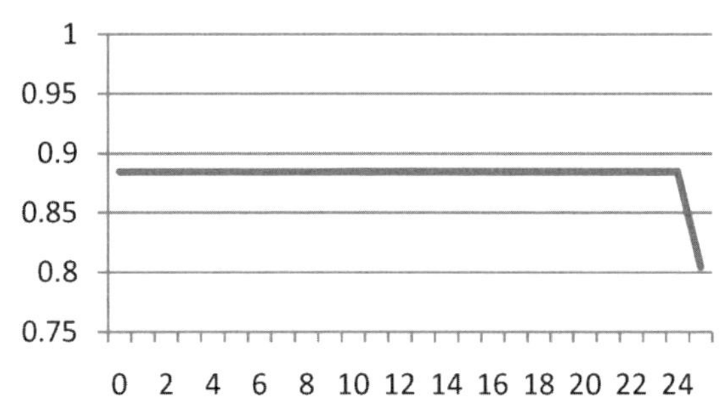

Figure 8. Activity recognition accuracy (vertical axis) as a function of the number of sensors that are removed from the environment (horizontal axis) for the Kyoto 1 smart apartment testbed.

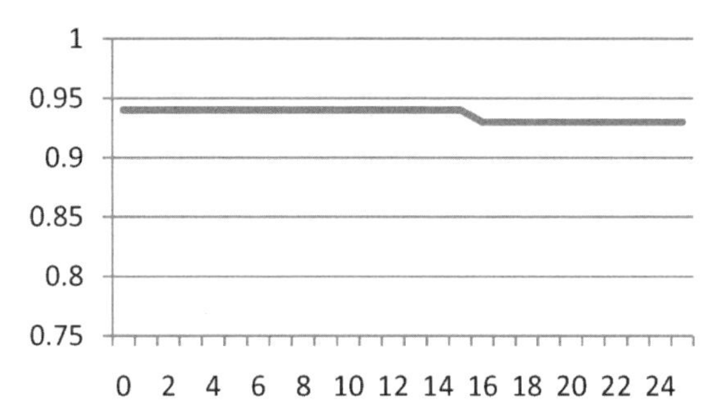

Figure 9. Activity recognition accuracy as a function of the number of sensors that are removed from the environment for the Kyoto 2 smart apartment testbed.

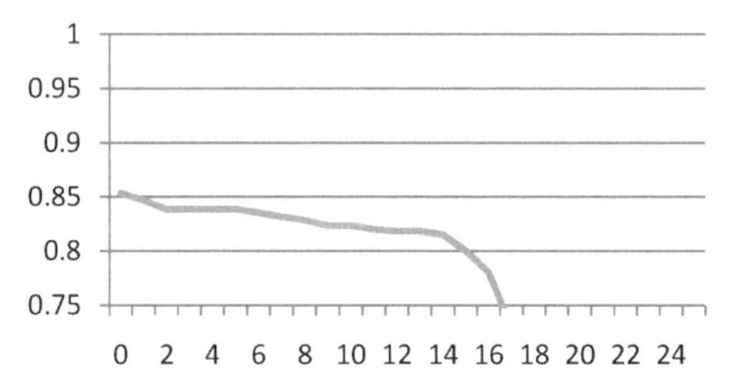

Figure 10. Activity recognition accuracy as a function of the number of sensors that are removed from the environment for the Cairo smart apartment testbed.

Figures 8–13 graphs activity recognition performance for each test when all of the sensors are used and when sensors are removed in nondecreasing order of MI value. As the graphs show, there is an overall decrease in accuracy as sensors are removed. However, the decrease does not always happen right away. In fact for both Kyoto datasets the accuracy stays constant even when up to 15 sensors are removed from consideration. In addition, in some cases accuracy increases as sensors are removed. For example, the accuracy increases from 0.857911 to 0.859831 when sensors are removed from the Bosch-2 dataset.

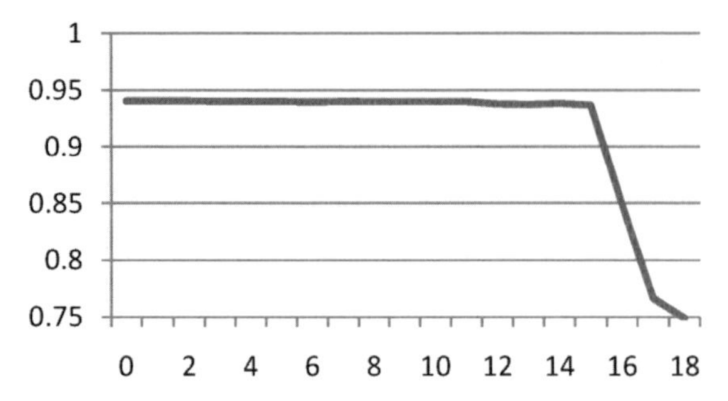

Figure 11. Activity recognition accuracy as a function of the number of sensors that are removed from the environment for the Bosch-1 smart apartment testbed.

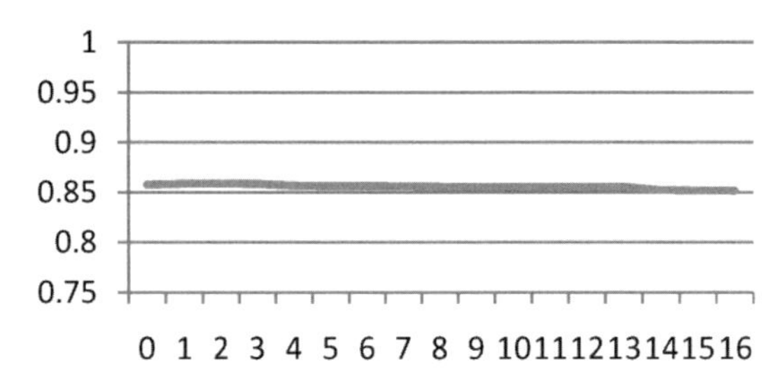

Figure 12. Activity recognition accuracy as a function of the number of sensors that are removed from the environment for the Bosch-2 smart apartment testbed.

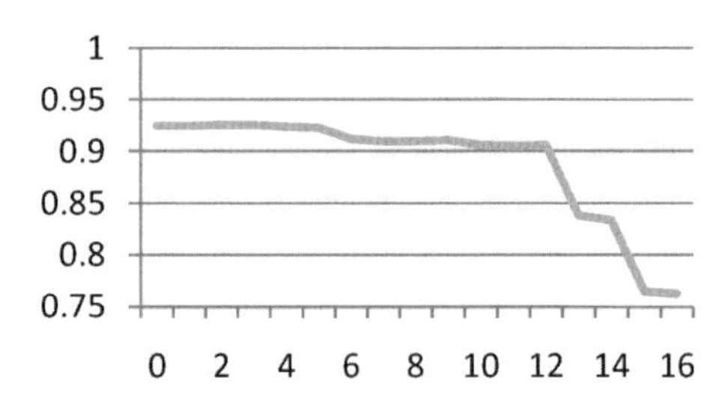

Figure 13. Activity recognition accuracy as a function of the number of sensors that are removed from the environment for the Bosch-3 smart apartment testbed.

Next, we evaluate our clustering algorithm on the same six datasets. The results are graphed in Figs 14–19. This approach is different than sensor selection because the merged sensors act as one new sensor. The individual sensor information is not lost but no distinction is made between each of the sensors that are members of the same cluster.

Our criterion for terminating the clustering algorithm is a subsequent degradation in activity recognition accuracy. Figures 14–19 show a large reduction in the needed number of sensors for some of the environments. This occurs particularly in the Kyoto testbeds, which is not surprising because this environment contains the greatest density of sensors. The environment also contains a number of special-purpose sensors for light, temperature, and water usage. Almost all of the special-purpose sensors were not removed in the feature selection step but were merged with other sensors in the clustering

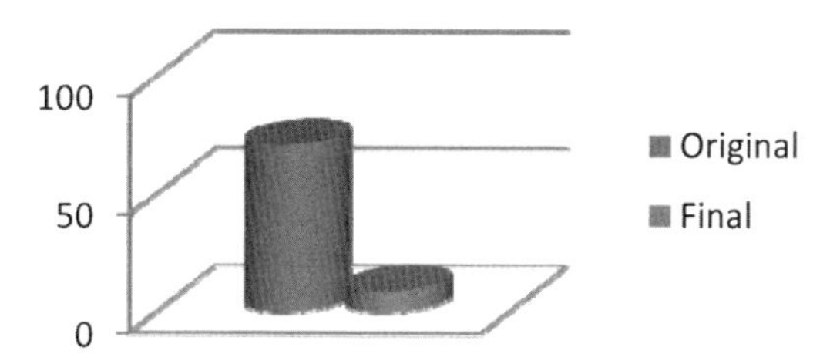

Figure 14. The original number of clusters found in the Kyoto 1 environment and the final number of distinct clusters that result from the clustering algorithm without any decrease in recognition accuracy.

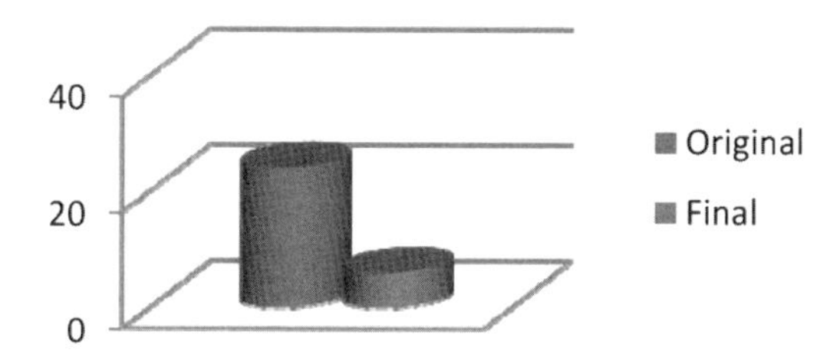

Figure 15. The original number of clusters found in the Kyoto 2 environment and the final number of distinct clusters that result from the clustering algorithm without any decrease in recognition accuracy.

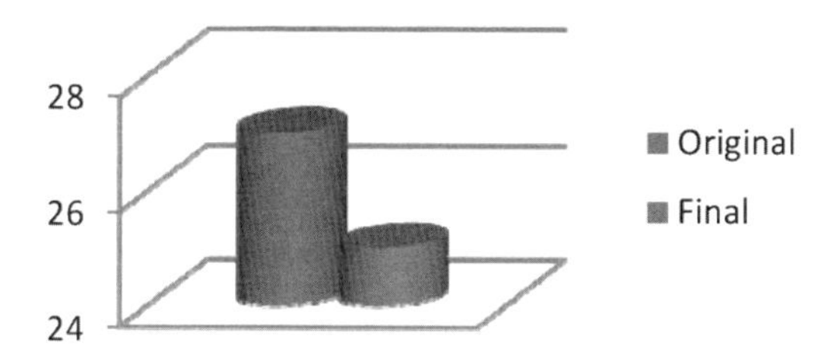

Figure 16. The original number of clusters found in the Cairo environment and the final number of distinct clusters that result from the clustering algorithm without any decrease in recognition accuracy.

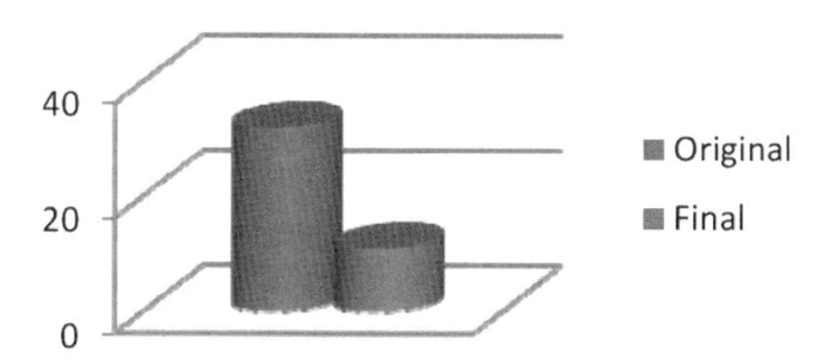

Figure 17. The original number of clusters found in the Bosch-1 environment and the final number of distinct clusters that result from the clustering algorithm without any decrease in recognition accuracy.

algorithm. As with the feature selection step, every one of the testbeds realizes an initial *increase* in recognition accuracy with the clustering algorithm. In each case, however, as more sensors are clustered the accuracy eventually declines.

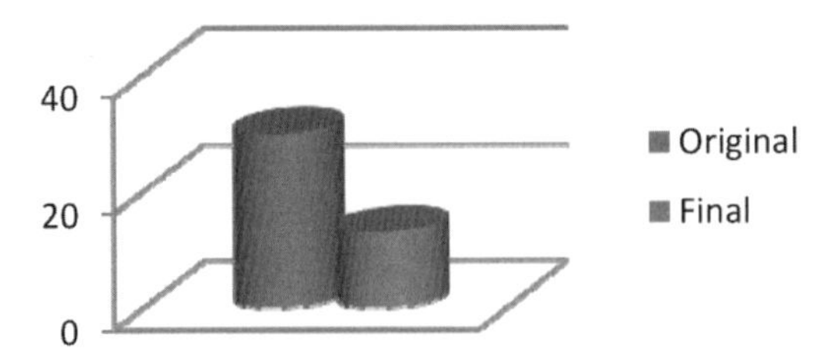

Figure 18. The original number of clusters found in the Bosch-2 environment and the final number of distinct clusters that result from the clustering algorithm without any decrease in recognition accuracy.

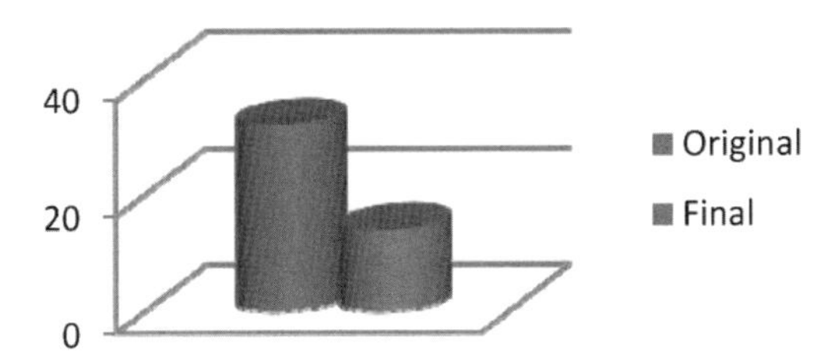

Figure 19. The original number of clusters found in the Bosch-3 environment and the final number of distinct clusters that result from the clustering algorithm without any decrease in recognition accuracy.

5. Sensitivity to Recognition Algorithm

The results from the first set of experiments clearly indicate that the adage "the more the better" does not apply to sensor selection for activity recognition. In fact, in these experiments not only were a large number of sensors not needed, but in many cases the algorithms performed better with a smaller number of sensors covering larger spaces.

We next consider the question of whether the results of these experiments are specific for a particular type of modeling and recognition algorithm. In order to determine whether the results are generalizable to multiple learning algorithms, we run the activity recognition algorithm on these smart environment databases for three learning algorithms: the original hidden Markov model, a naïve Bayes classifier, and a linear-chain conditional random field classifier. In each case we test the performance of the algorithm using 3-fold cross validation and apply it to the database using the original set of sensors and using the final set of sensors as indicate by the sensor selection and clustering algorithms. If the results of these algorithms are generalizable then the accuracy of each of the algorithms will not degrade when they are applied to the smaller set of sensors.

As the results in Figs 20–30 show, the reduction in sensors does not dramatically change the predictive accuracy for any of the classifiers or any of the datasets. The results sometimes degrade and sometimes improve. The largest decrease in accuracy results for the database in which the greatest reduction was made in the number of sensors. This indicates that sensor reduction should be applied more conservatively if the feature selection process is intended to be used for more than one model and not customized to a specific learning model.

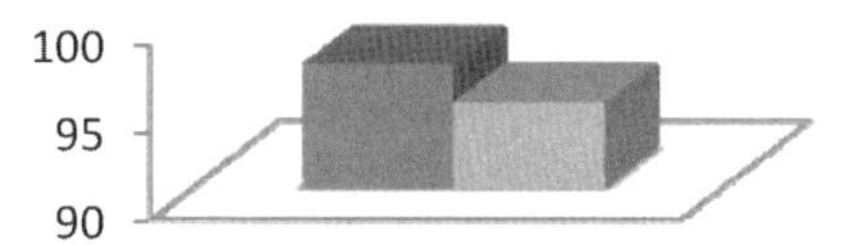

Figure 20. Activity recognition accuracy for the Kyoto 1 dataset with a naïve Bayes classifier applied before and after applying clustering-based feature selection and construction.

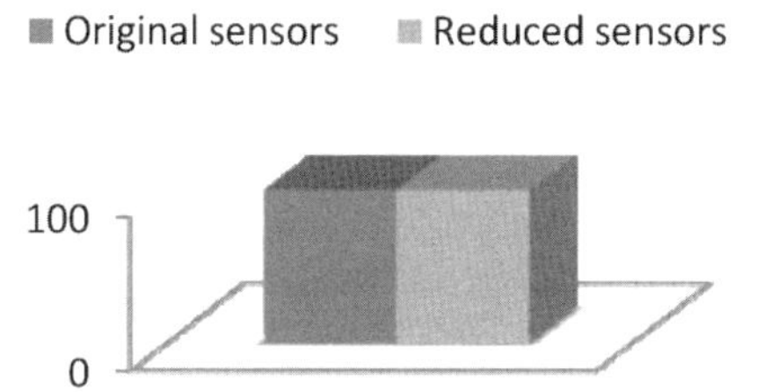

Figure 21. Activity recognition accuracy for the Kyoto 2 dataset with a naïve Bayes classifier applied before and after applying clustering-based feature selection and construction.

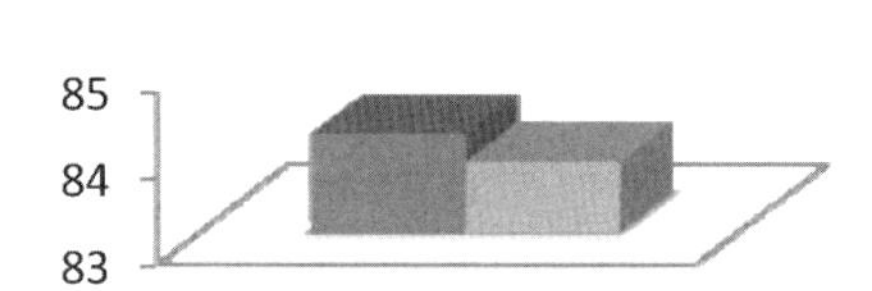

Figure 22. Activity recognition accuracy for the Cairo dataset with a naïve Bayes classifier applied before and after applying clustering-based feature selection and construction.

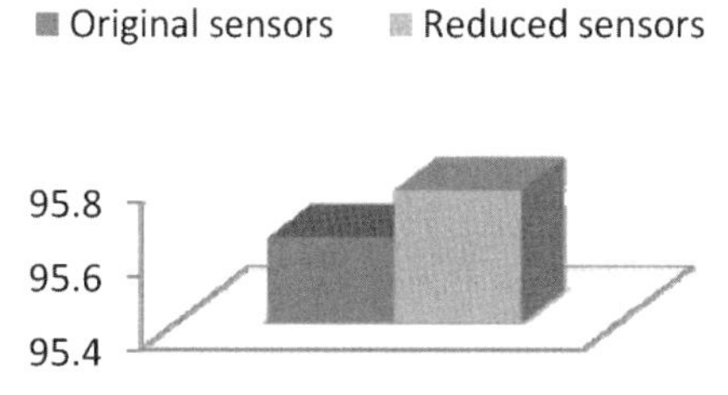

Figure 23. Activity recognition accuracy for the Bosch-1 dataset with a naïve Bayes classifier applied before and after applying clustering-based feature selection and construction.

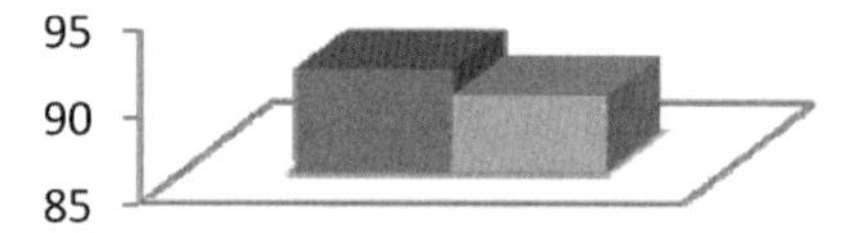

Figure 24. Activity recognition accuracy for the Bosch-2 dataset with a naïve Bayes classifier applied before and after applying clustering-based feature selection and construction.

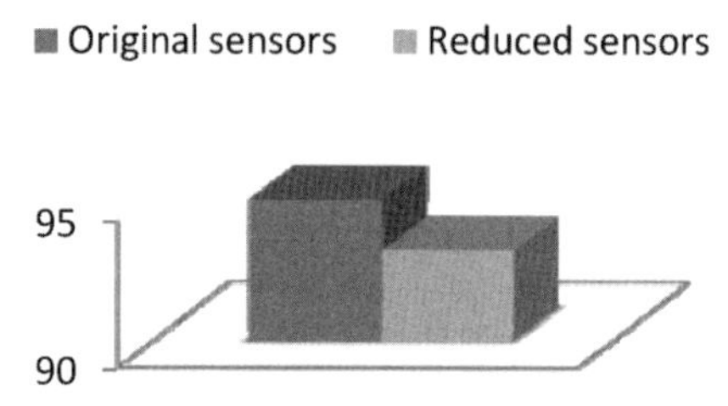

Figure 25. Activity recognition accuracy for the Bosch-3 dataset with a naïve Bayes classifier applied before and after applying clustering-based feature selection and construction.

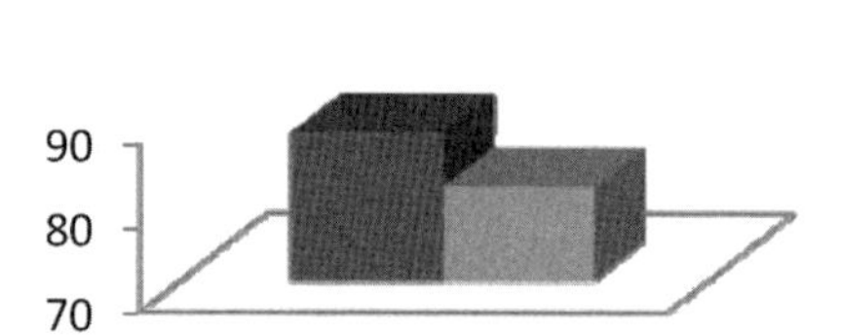

Figure 26. Activity recognition accuracy for the Kyoto 1 dataset with conditional random fields applied before and after applying clustering-based feature selection and construction.

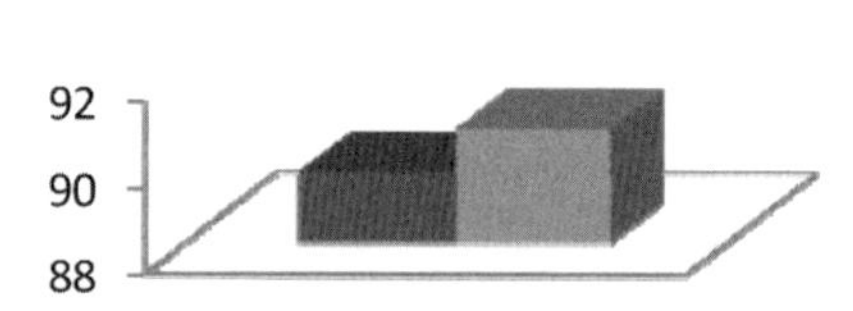

Figure 27. Activity recognition accuracy for the Kyoto 2 dataset with conditional random fields applied before and after applying clustering-based feature selection and construction.

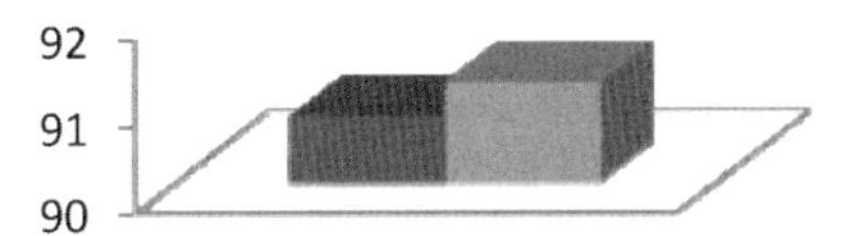

Figure 28. Activity recognition accuracy for the Cairo dataset with conditional random fields applied before and after applying clustering-based feature selection and construction.

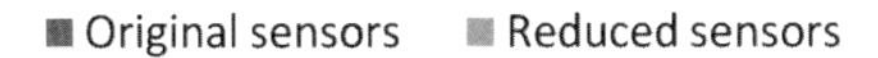

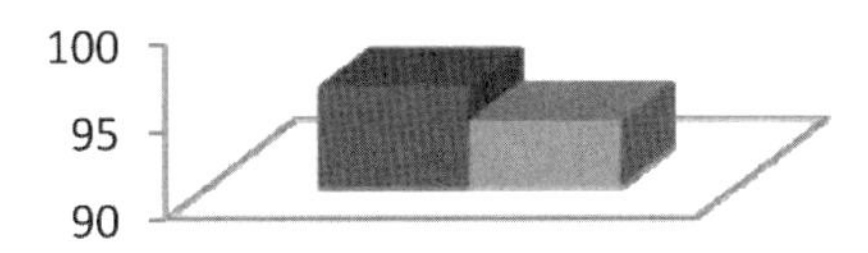

Figure 29. Activity recognition accuracy for the Bosch-1 dataset with conditional random fields applied before and after applying clustering-based feature selection and construction.

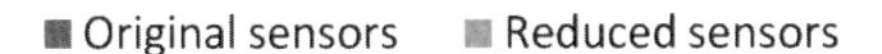

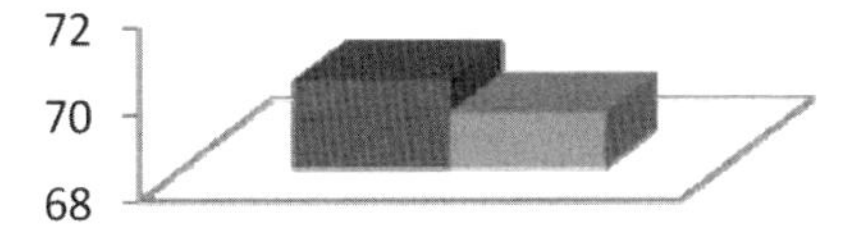

Figure 30. Activity recognition accuracy for the Bosch-2 dataset with conditional random fields applied before and after applying clustering-based feature selection and construction.

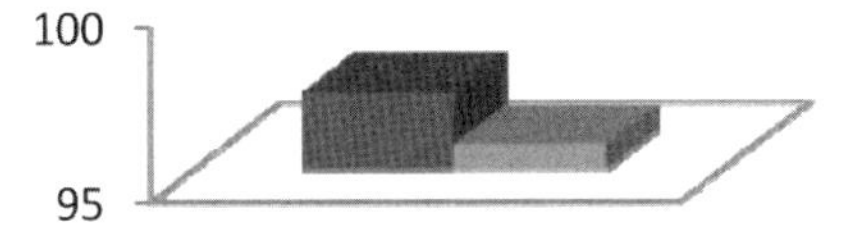

Figure 31. Activity recognition accuracy for the Bosch-3 dataset with conditional random fields applied before and after applying clustering-based feature selection and construction.

6. Heuristics for Sensor Placement

Based on our observations in processing data from the smart environment testbeds, the following features have a noticeable influence on the learned activity model for a particular space:

- The size of the area that is covered by the sensor.
- The number of other sensors (of any type) that overlap coverage areas with this sensor.
- The amount of resident movement that occurs in this area (labeled as low, medium, or high).
- The type of sensor that is being considered.

Using these features to describe the sensors, we created a database of all of the sensors found in the five testbeds. We then labeled them as high value, medium value, or low value based on how quickly they were removed in our MI step or merged in our clustering step. We fed the database as input to a decision tree algorithm to see if it could learn the value of the sensors and also to see the rules that would be generated by the algorithm.

The decision tree algorithm learned these three classes with 67% accuracy. The rules that were generated by the decision tree algorithm were fairly intuitive and actually make use of all of the features we listed above. The rules are summarized here as:

- If there is little movement in the area, the value of the sensor is low; particularly if it is not a motion sensor (the value is medium for motion sensors when other sensors are nearby).
- If there is a medium amount of movement in the area then the value of the sensor (of any type) is medium.
- If there is a large amount of movement in the area then the value of a motion sensor is high, while the value of any other type of sensor is medium.

From these results we see that motion sensors in general provide the greatest value for activity recognition. In practice we have found that special-purposes sensors for water, light, door usage, burner usage, and phone usage assist in our tracking the steps of an activity but rarely provide discriminative power in differentiating between activities. These rules also indicate that rooms with a greater amount of movement need more sensors. The results of the feature selection and feature construction experiments are consistent with this rule: Sensors found in guest bedrooms and closets tended to be the first to be pruned, whereas sensors in the kitchen and living room / TV area were generally kept and not quickly merged with others.

The next experiment we would like to try in the future is to use these heuristics to not only select and to merge existing sensors but to actually change the exact position and coverage of sensors in a smart environment. It would also be useful to consider additional features in the selection process, such as the number and type of activities that need to be recognized and tracked.

7. Conclusions

In order to provide robust activity recognition and tracking capabilities for smart home residents, researchers need to consider techniques for identifying the activities to recognize and track. In this work we examine the issue of selecting and placing sensors in a smart home in order to maximize activity recognition accuracy but minimize the number of sensors that are purchased, installed and maintained. Our study results indicate that a larger number of sensors is not always desirable, not only for the sake of cost but even for recognition accuracy. Feature selection and construction techniques can be used to determine an optimal number of sensors for a particular environment and to generalize rules for initial section and placement of sensors.

Ultimately, we want to use our algorithm design as a component of a complete system that performs functional assessment of adults in their everyday environments. This type of automated assessment also provides a mechanism for evaluating the effectiveness of alternative health interventions. We believe these activity profiling techniques are valuable for providing automated health monitoring and assistance in an individual's everyday environments.

References

[1] G. Abowd and E. Mynatt, Designing for the human experience in smart environments, in: *Smart Environments: Technology, Protocols, and Applications*, D. Cook and S. Das, eds, Wiley, 2004, pp. 153–174.

[2] O. Brdiczka, P. Reignier and J. Crowley, Detecting individual activities from video in a smart home, in: *Proceedings of the International Conference on Knowledge-Based and Intelligent Information and Engineering Systems*, 2007, pp. 363–370.

[3] D. Cook and S. Das, *Smart Environments: Technology, Protocols, and Applications*, 2004, Wiley.

[4] D. Cook and M. Schmitter-Edgecombe, Assessing the quality of activities in a smart environment, *Methods of Information in Medicine* **48**(5) (2009), 480–485.

[5] F. Doctor, H. Hagras and V. Callaghan, A fuzzy embedded agent-based approach for realizing ambient intelligence in intelligent inhabited environments, *IEEE Transactions on Systems, Man, and Cybernetics, Part A* **35**(1) (2005), 55–56.

[6] T. Gu, Z. Wu, X. Tao, H. Pung and J. Lu, epSICAR: An emerging patterns based approach to sequential, interleaved and concurrent activity recognition, in: *Proceedings of the IEEE International Conference on Pervasive Computing and Communication*, 2009.

[7] A. Helal, W. Mann, H. El-Zabadani, J. King, Y. Kaddoura and E. Jansen, The gator tech smart house: A programmable pervasive space, *IEEE Computer* **38**(3) (2005), 50–60.

[8] K. Kira and L. Rendell, The feature selection problem: Traditional methods and a new algorithm, in: *Proceedings of the National Conference on Artificial Intelligence*, 1992.

[9] R. Kohavi and G. John, Wrappers for feature subset selection, *Artificial Intelligence* **97**(1–2) (1997), 273–324.

[10] L. Liao, D. Fox and H. Kautz, Location-based activity recognition using relational Markov networks, in: *Proceedings of the International Joint Conference on Artificial Intelligence*, 2005, pp. 773–778.

[11] U. Maurer, A. Smailagic, D. Siewiorek and M. Deisher, Activity recognition and monitoring using multiple sensors on different body positions, in: *Proceedings of the International Workshop on Wearable and Implantable Body Sensor Networks*, 2006, pp. 99–102.

[12] E. Munguia-Tapia, S.S. Intille and K. Larson, Activity recognition in the home using simple and ubiquitous sensors, in: *Proceedings of Pervasive*, 2004, pp. 158–175.

[13] H.C. Peng, F. Long and C. Ding, Feature selection based on mutual information: Criteria of max-dependency, max-relevance, and min-redundancy, *IEEE Transactions on Patterns Analysis and Machine Intelligence* **27**(8) (2005), 1226–1238.

[14] M. Philipose, K. Fishkin, M. Perkowitz, D. Patterson, D. Fox, H. Kautz and D. Hahnel, Inferring activities from interactions with objects, *IEEE Pervasive Computing* **3**(4) (2004), 50–57.

[15] P. Rashidi and D. Cook, Keeping the resident in the loop: Adapting the smart home to the user, *IEEE Transactions on Systems, Man, and Cybernetics, Part A: Systems and Humans* **39**(5) (2009), 949–959.

[16] B. Reisberg et al., The Alzheimer's disease activities of daily living international scale (ASL-IS), *International Psychogeriatrics* **13** (2001), 163–181.

[17] V. Rialle, C. Ollivet, C. Guigui and C. Herve, What do family caregivers of Alzheimer's disease patients desire in smart home technologies? *Methods of Information in Medicine* **47** (2008), 63–69.

[18] A. Viterbi, Error bounds for convolutional codes and an asymptotically-optimum decoding algorithm, *IEEE Transactions on Information Theory* **13**(2) (1967), 260–269.
[19] V. Wadley, O. Okonkwo, M. Crowe and L.A. Ross-Meadows, Mild cognitive impairment and everyday function: Evidence of reduced speed in performing instrumental activities of daily living, *American Journal of Geriatric Psychiatry* **16** (2007), 416–424.
[20] G.M. Youngblood and D. Cook, Data mining for hierarchical model creation, *IEEE Transactions on Systems, Man, and Cybernetics, Part C* **37**(4) (2007), 1–12.

Handbook of Ambient Assisted Living
J.C. Augusto et al. (Eds.)
IOS Press, 2012

doi:10.3233/978-1-60750-837-3-451

Utilization of Cloud Infrastructures for Pervasive Healthcare Applications

Charalampos DOUKAS[a], Thomas PLIAKAS[b] and Ilias MAGLOGIANNIS[a,*]
[a] *University of Central Greece*
[b] *Nokia Siemens Networks*

Abstract. Cloud computing has been receiving much attention as an alternative to both specialized grids and to owning and managing data centers. It represents a new way, in some cases a more cost effective way, of delivering enterprise IT. Ambient Assistive Living Applications (AAL) and pervasive health application require also the collection and processing of heterogeneous data from various data sources. In this context cloud computing provides an attractive IT platform to reduce the cost of building e-health or AAL systems and in terms of both ownership and IT maintenance burdens for many medical practices and to enable techniques for advance process of their data without the need of hosting the processing power. The concept of cloud computing complies with the emerging trend to move from the economy of ownership to the economy of use. The field of pervasive and ubiquitous healthcare services requires that resources and information can be available anywhere and anytime, since the rapid and safe exchange and disposal of large amounts of information at the point of care is needed. Enabling the access to healthcare ubiquitously not only will help to improve healthcare as the data will always be accessible from anywhere at any time, but also it helps reducing the costs drastically. In this chapter we provide an overview of the cloud computing architectures that enable pervasive health applications and discuss the medical data management issues that arise in the cloud. Finally a prototype application called @HealthCloud is presented. The specific application enables pervasive healthcare information management system for mobile devices utilizing Cloud Computing and Android Operating System (OS).

Keywords. Pervasive health information management, cloud computing, Android platform

Introduction

Pervasive healthcare systems focus towards achieving two specific goals: the availability of e-health applications and medical information anywhere and anytime and the invisibility of computing [39]. Applications and interfaces that are able to automatically process data provided by medical devices and sensors, exchange knowledge and make intelligent decisions in a given context are strongly desirable. Natural user interactions with such applications are based on autonomy, avoiding the need for the user to control every action, and adaptivity, so that they are contextualized and personalized, delivering the right information and decision at the right moment [9]. Mobile pervasive

*Corresponding Author: Dr. Ilias Maglogiannis, University of Central Greece Department of Computer Science and Biomedical Informatics Papasiopoulou 2–4, PC 35100 Lamia, Greece, Tel. +30 22310 66931, Fax. +30 22310 66939. E-mail: imaglo@ucg.gr.

healthcare technologies can support a wide range of applications and services including mobile telemedicine, patient monitoring, location-based medical services, emergency response and management, personalized monitoring and pervasive access to healthcare information. The latter can provide great benefits to both patients and medical personnel. During a check-up, for example, patients can use a handheld device to upload their personal medical history and insurance data into their healthcare provider's database, reducing the effort required to enter such detailed information manually. Alternatively, such information can be downloaded from a Web-based health information system with proper authentication. Patients are able likewise to use mobile devices to update their personal and family medical history and physician contacts, receive alerts to take prescribed medications, check for drug interactions, or dynamically change restrictions on who can access their health data.

However, the realization of pervasive health information management through mobile devices introduces several challenges:

- Data storage and management: Storing such sensitive data raises issues about physical storage (e.g., the location of data) and availability; data must always be available and accessible from different platforms (devices and operating systems) and locations (supporting mobility). Proper management of healthcare data also requires maintenance procedures (e.g., backups, etc.). Thus, data storage and management requires proper design and utilization of several storage and computational resources.
- Interoperability and availability of heterogeneous resources: Healthcare data consists of heterogeneous data (e.g., clinical data, medical images, health records, etc.) acquired from and stored into different resources (e.g., electronic health record systems, radiology information systems, laboratory information systems, etc.). An aggregate access to aforementioned data from mobile devices involves the establishment of mechanisms that provide global access to the latter resources seamlessly.
- Security and privacy: Securing healthcare data involves security and encryption mechanisms both at the data storage elements and the transmission links. Protocols and mechanisms used must be compliant with the majority of operating systems and device types. Permission control must be carefully designed and deployed for prohibiting unauthorized access to sensitive data assuring privacy.
- Unified and ubiquitous access: Provide users with proper interfaces for accessing data from different platforms (e.g., mobile devices, web, etc.) and infrastructures (e.g., public or private networks, etc.) using a single entry point.

One potential solution for addressing all aforementioned issues is the introduction of Cloud Computing concept in electronic healthcare systems. Cloud computing has been receiving much attention as an alternative to both specialized grids and to owning and managing data centers. It represents a new way, in some cases a more cost effective way, of delivering enterprise IT. The increasing adoption rate of cloud computing is currently driving a significant increase in both the supply and the demand side of this new market for IT. Many healthcare providers and insurance companies today have adopted some form of electronic medical record systems, though most of them store medical records in centralized databases in the form of electronic records. Typically, a patient may have many healthcare providers, including primary care physicians, specialists, therapists, and other medical practitioners. In addition, a patient may use multiple healthcare insurance companies for different types of insurances, such as medical, dental, vision, and so forth. Currently, each healthcare provider typically uses its private datacenter for Electronic Health Records (EHRs). Sharing and process information between healthcare practitioners across administrative boundaries is translated to sharing information between EHR systems. The interoperation and sharing among different EHRs has been extremely slow due to cost and poor usability, which have been cited as the biggest obstacles to adoption of electronic health care.

This book chapter aims to present the key issues for enabling the management of pervasive healthcare applications and data utilizing cloud infrastructures. The chapter begins with an overview of the health cloud notion, followed by an introduction into cloud management issues. Section 3 discusses solutions for protecting patient data and privacy in cloud environments and Section 4 describes distributed processing of data. Sections 5 and 6 present @HealthCloud, a prototype application that enables pervasive healthcare information management system for mobile devices utilizing Cloud Computing and Android Operating System (OS). Finally, Section 7 concludes the chapter.

1. Health Cloud Overview

Cloud computing provides an attractive IT platform to reduce the cost of EHR systems in terms of both ownership and IT maintenance burdens for many medical practices and to enable techniques for advance process of their data without the need of hosting the processing power. It is widely recognized that cloud computing and open standards are important to streamline healthcare whether it is for maintaining health records, monitoring of patients, managing diseases and cares more efficiently and effectively, or collaboration with peers and analysis of data. The concept of cloud computing complies with the emerging trend to move from the economy of ownership to the economy of use. The field of pervasive and ubiquitous healthcare services requires that resources and information can be available anywhere and anytime, since the rapid and safe exchange and disposal of large amounts of information at the point of care is needed.

Enabling the access to healthcare ubiquitously not only will help to improve healthcare as the data will always be accessible from anywhere at any time, but also it helps reducing the costs drastically. Several studies have demonstrated that the limited access to patient-related information during decision-making and the ineffective communication among patient care team members are proximal causes of medical errors in healthcare [23,27]. Thus, the pervasive and ubiquitous access to healthcare data is considered essential for the proper diagnosis and treatment procedure. Cloud Computing is also a model for enabling convenient, on-demand network access to a shared group of configurable computing resources (e.g., networks, servers, storage, applications, and services) that can be rapidly provisioned and released with minimal management effort or service provider interaction.

Based on cloud service models, we can divide healthcare cloud systems into three layers:

- Applications in the cloud (Software as a Service – SaaS). This layer provides capability for consumers to use the provider's applications running on a cloud infrastructure. For instance, the applications are accessible from various client devices through a thin client interface such as Web browser. The consumer does not manage or control the underlying cloud infrastructure including network, servers, operating systems, storage, or even individual application capabilities. In this type of cloud service model, the security and privacy protection is provided as an integral part of the SaaS to the healthcare consumers.

- Platforms in the cloud (Platform as a service – PaaS). This layer offers capability for consumers to deploy consumer-created or acquired applications written using programming languages and tools supported by the cloud provider. The consumer does not manage or control the underlying cloud infrastructure including network, servers, operating systems, or storage, but has control over the deployed applications and possibly application hosting environment configurations. In this type of cloud service model, two levels of protection for security and privacy are required. At the lower system level, the cloud provider may provide basic security mechanisms such as end-to-end encryption, authentication, and authorization. At the higher application level, the consumers need to define application dependent access control policies, authenticity requirements, and so forth.
- Infrastructure in the cloud (Infrastructure as a Service – IaaS). This type of cloud service model provides the capability for consumers to provision processing, storage, networks, and other fundamental computing resources, in which consumer is able to deploy and run arbitrary software, including operating systems and applications. The consumer does not manage or control the underlying cloud infrastructure but has control over operating systems, storage, deployed applications, and possibly limited control of select networking components (e.g., host firewalls). In the Infrastructure cloud model, the healthcare application developers hold full responsibility for protecting patients' security and privacy.

We can also use the cloud deployment models below to give the taxonomy of healthcare clouds.

- Private cloud. The cloud infrastructure is operated solely for a healthcare delivery organization. It may be managed by the organization or a third party and may exist on or off premise. In this type of cloud deployment model, the cloud provider provides the same capability in terms of security and privacy protection as those in the EMR system running by such an organization.
- Hybrid cloud. The cloud infrastructure is shared by several organizations and supports a specific community that has shared concerns (e.g., mission, security requirements, policy, and compliance considerations). It is most likely managed by the third party or the content organizations and may exist on or off premise.
- Public cloud. The cloud infrastructure is made available to the general public or a large industry group and is owned by a cloud service provider. In this deployment model, the healthcare application developers and consumers hold full responsibility for protecting patients' security and privacy.

Much of pervasive healthcare is transactional, for instance registering an individual, monitoring a patient at home, getting access to electronic patient record data etc. Yet transactions are only the operational expression of an understanding of the patient, and a set of goals and plans for his treatment.

2. Cloud and Data Management Issues

The expansion of this IaaS market is leading to a rapid increase in the complexity, and users have to face when they strive to acquire resources in a cost-effective manner in such a market, while still respecting their application-level quality of service (QoS) constraints. Continuing standardization efforts in virtualization technology and IaaS offerings will further increase the options available to a consumer when acquiring resources "in the cloud". This issue is exacerbated by the fact that consumers often also own private IT infrastructure, especially for healthcare organizations where security of data is important. Through the creation of hybrid clouds [33], one can use this internal infrastructure in tandem with public cloud resources, thereby capitalizing on investments made, and catering for specific application requirements in terms of data confidentiality, security, performance and latency.

Due to the current lack of support tools to deal with the inherent complexity of cost-optimal resource allocation within such a hybrid setting, this process is error-prone and time-consuming. In addition, a structured approach is required that caters for optimizing such resource allocations in a multi-consumer context. Indeed, the addition of volume or reservation-based price reductions in the pricing options of public cloud providers allows for the further reduction of costs if an organization collectively engages in delivery, contracts for its entire user base. This differs from the practice of allowing users to individually acquire resources from cloud providers.

2.1. Data and Resources Management and Scaling

Presuming the existence of large integrated medical of data, another major challenge is in managing those data, in an efficient, secure and cost effective way. Some of the important dimensions of medical information management include the data semantics and annotation.

Raw data almost never speak for themselves, and their interpretation inevitably relies on metadata – annotations to the primary data that provide the necessary context. For example, the primary data for the human genome consist of a sequence of some 3 billion nucleotides. Metadata associated with the primary data help scientists to identify significant patterns within those data – a given sequence might be annotated as a gene or a regulatory element. Metadata could also be used to trace the provenance or lineage of data. For example, the value of certain data in an electronic health record could be enhanced if the data included information about the conditions under which certain data were obtained (e.g., physician observations of a patient's description of symptoms might be accompanied by video and audio recordings of the session with the patient in a pervasive health environment). With metadata, a primary problem is the design and development of tools to facilitate machine-readable annotations in large databases. The same problem exists in patient monitoring and home care applications, where sensors and vital signal monitoring devices produce huge amounts of streaming data.

2.2. Information Extraction from Large Amount of Heterogeneous Medical Data

New techniques are needed for mining information from such streaming data concerning patient status, emergency situations or even medicine names, and disease names from visual or textual notes, and for generating automatic linkages between different relevant entities. Such extraction would make it possible to piece together a larger picture automatically while pulling information from multiple heterogeneous data and information sources. Extraction of data from tables and figures in reports is another example of a useful information extraction capability.

3. Security and Privacy Issues

Research on the various security issues concerning healthcare information systems has been heated over the last few years. ISO/TS 18308 standard gives the definitions of security and privacy issue for EHR [4]. The Working Group 4 of International Medical Informatics Association (IMIA) was set up to investigate the issues of data protection and security within the healthcare environment. Its work to date has mainly concentrated on security in EHR networked systems and common security solutions for communicating patient data [7]. The European AIM/SEISMED (Advanced Informatics in Medicine/Secure Environment for Information Systems in MEDicine) project is initiated to address a wide spectrum of security issues within healthcare and provides practical guidelines for secure healthcare establishment [8,16,26]. US HHS (Health and Human Services) recently published a report about personal health records (PHRs), aiming at developing PHRs and PHR systems to put forward a vision that "would create a personal health record that patients, doctors and other health care providers could securely access through the Internet no matter where a patient is seeking medical care."

In healthcare clouds the term "patient-centric" is commonly used, which is a term used mostly in community/hybrid healthcare systems. Hybrid healthcare system offers an open platform for patient to collect, store, use, and share health information in a controlled manner with ubiquitous accessibility. It also offers secure storage and management of patients' EHRs for multiple applications (e.g. disease treatment, lab research, insurance, and other social-networking applications). Most of the community healthcare cloud service models, such as Microsoft HealthVault and Google Health, adopt a centralized architecture with patient-centric views. By patient-centric, it means that the information stored in the community EHR system is imported by patients and only can be made available to a variety of applications under the control of patients.

The common security issues shared by healthcare cloud applications are ownership of information, authenticity, authentication, non-repudiation, patient consent and authorization, integrity and confidentiality of data.

- Ownership of information: In general, the owner is defined as the creator of the information. Establishing the ownership of the information is necessary for protection against unauthorized access or misuse of patient's medical information. The "owner" can refer to the person responsible for the information or the organization creating and storing the information. The term of "owner" may refer to "creator", "author" and "manager" of the information.
- The "Creator" indicates the person generating the data. In healthcare system, practitioner or laboratory staff is the creator of medical data about a patient. "Author" means the person or entity responsible for the content of the information. In healthcare system, author is the creator of the information, be it the clinician or the organizations, which the creator belongs to. "Manager" is for the person or entity responsible for management, provision and protection of

information. In patient-controlled healthcare system, manager is the patient self. While in decentralized healthcare system, manager may refer to a trusted third party, who is authorized by the patient or healthcare providers. The ownership of information can be protected through a combination of encryption and watermarking techniques.

- Authenticity and Authentication: Authenticity in general refers to the truthfulness of origins, attributions, commitments, and intentions. Authentication is the act of establishing or confirming claims made by or about the subject are true and authentic. The authentication of information can pose special problems, especially man-in-the-middle (MITM) attacks, and is often implemented with authenticating identity. Most cryptographic protocols include some form of endpoint authentication specifically to prevent MITM attacks. For instance, Transport Layer Security (TLS) and its predecessor, Secure Sockets Layer (SSL), are cryptographic protocols that provide security for communications over networks such as the Internet. TLS and SSL encrypt the segments of network connections at the Transport Layer end-to-end. Several versions of the protocols are in widespread use in applications like web browsing, electronic mail, Internet faxing, instant messaging and voice-over-IP (VoIP). One can use SSL or TLS to authenticate the server using a mutually trusted certification authority. In a healthcare system, both for healthcare information offered by providers and identities of consumers should be verified at the entry of every access.
- Non-repudiation: Non-repudiation implies one's intention to fulfill its obligations to a contract. It also implies that one party of a transaction cannot deny having received a transaction nor can the other party deny having sent a transaction. Electronic commerce uses technology such as digital signatures and encryption to establish authenticity and non-repudiation.
- Patient consent and authorization: Patient can allow or deny sharing their information with other healthcare practitioners or CDOs. To implement patient consent in a healthcare system, patient may grant rights to users on the basis of a role or attributes held by the respective user.
- Integrity and confidentiality of data: Integrity means preserving the accuracy and consistency of data. In the health care system, it refers to the fact that data has not been tampered by unauthorized use. The International Organization defines confidentiality for Standardization (ISO) in ISO-17799 as "ensuring that information is accessible only to those authorized to have access". Confidentiality is one of the design goals for many crypto systems and made possible in practice by the techniques of modern cryptography. Confidentiality can be achieved by access control and encryption techniques in EHR systems.
- Availability and utility: For any EHR system to serve its purpose, the information must be available when it is needed. This means that the computing systems used to store and process the EHR data, the security controls used to protect it, and the communication channels used to access it must be functioning correctly. High availability systems aim to remain available at all times, preventing service disruptions due to power outages, hardware failures, and system upgrades. Ensuring availability also involves preventing denial-of-service attacks, and preserving utility of EHR data. Utility here refers to the ability to

preserve the usability of EHR data after exercising and enforcing security and privacy protection and HIPPA compliance.
- Audit and archiving are two optional security metrics to measure and ensure the safety of a healthcare system. Audit means recording user activities of the healthcare system in chronological order, such as maintaining a log of every access to and modification of data. Auditing capability enables prior states of the information to be faithfully reconstructed. Archiving means moving healthcare information to off-line storage in a way that ensures the possibility of restoring them to on-line storage whenever it is needed without the loss of information [17].

Regarding patient data safety, the Health Insurance Portability and Accountability Action (HIPAA) [22] provides national minimum standards to protect an individual's health information. HIPAA covers Protected Health Information (PHI) which is any information regarding an individual's physical or mental health, the provision of healthcare to them, or payment of related services. PHI also includes any personally identifiable information, including for example Employer Identification Number, social security number, name, address, phone number, medical condition when linked to a patient, and some types of billing information.

HIPAA's privacy rule regulations include standards regarding the encryption of all PHI in transmission and in storage. The same data encryption mechanisms used in a traditional computing environment, such as a local server or a managed hosting server, can also be used in virtual computing environments. HIPAA's security safeguards also require in-depth auditing capabilities, data back-up procedures and disaster recovery mechanisms. Health cloud infrastructures should support established security standards in order to be exploitable at an operational level. Commercial clouds such as the Amazon cloud discussed later on this chapter already comply with this requirement.

4. Distributed Processing of Pervasive Healthcare Data in Cloud Infrastructures

The development of pervasive health-care systems is a very promising area for commercial organizations active in the health-monitoring domain. The considered pervasive infrastructure creates numerous business opportunities for players like emergency medical assistance companies, the telecommunication operators, insurance companies, etc. Numerous portable devices are available that can detect certain medical conditions – pulse rate, blood pressure, breath alcohol level, and so on – from a user's touch. Many such capabilities could be integrated into a handheld wireless device that also contains the user's medical history. All the latter produce a vast amount of data that need to be distributary managed and processed within a cloud infrastructure.

The distribution of tasks in a cluster for parallel processing is not a new concept, and there are several techniques that use this idea to optimize the processing of information. The Map-Reduce paradigm [14], for example, is a framework for processing huge datasets of certain kinds of distributable problems using a large number of computers (nodes), collectively referred to as a cluster. It consists of an initial Map stage, where a master node takes the input, chops it into smaller or sub-problems, and distributes the parts to worker nodes, which process the information; following there is the Reduce stage, where the master node collects the answers to all the sub-problems and combines them to produce the job output. The process is illustrated in Fig. 1.

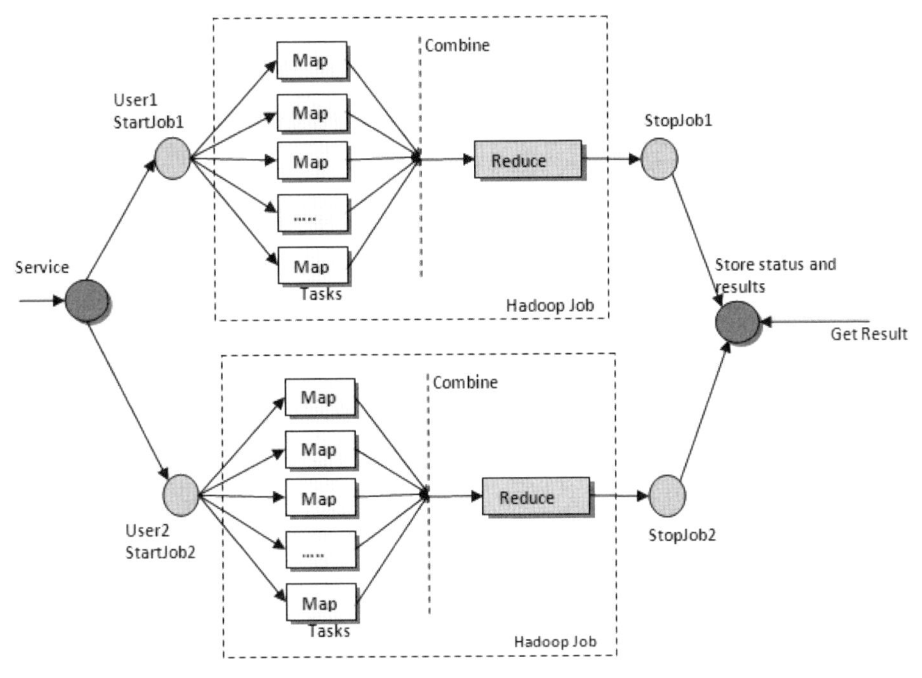

Figure 1. Map Reduce Architecture.

A popular Map-Reduce implementation is Apache's Hadoop [5], which consists of one Job Tracker, to which client applications submit Map-Reduce jobs. The Job Tracker pushes work out to available Task Tracker nodes in the cluster, which execute the map and reduce tasks.

However, despite being a very appealing and efficient technique for processing large volumes of data, there are a number of challenges associated with the deployment of Map-Reduce architectures. One of them is the required infrastructure. To make the process truly effective, one needs several machines acting as nodes, which often requires a large upfront investment in infrastructure.

This point is extremely critical in situations where the processing demand is seasonal. In addition, fault tolerance issues and the need of a shared file system to support mappers and reducers make the deployment of a Map-Reduce architecture complex and costly.

In cases where there is a seasonal computation demand, the use of public Clouds, for information processing and storage, is emerging as an interesting alternative. The Hardware as a Service (HaaS) [10] paradigm relieves the burden of making huge investments in infrastructure, and at the same time supports on-the-fly resizing of resources, and adaptation to current needs.

With a public Cloud, one can quickly make provision for the resources required to perform a particular task, and pay only for the computational resources effectively used. This is good solution, not only because it deploys faster, as opposed to having to order and install physical hardware, but it also optimizes overall costs, as resources can be released immediately after the task is completed.

One of the largest providers in the public Cloud is Amazon AWS, with its Elastic Cloud Computing (EC2) [1] and Simple Storage Service (S3) [31] services. Amazon EC2 is a web service interface that provides resizable computing capacity in the cloud, allowing a complete control of computing resources and reducing the time required to obtain and boot new server instances. This feature is of particular interest because it allows applications to quickly scale up and down their processing and storage resources as computing requirements change. Amazon S3 provides a simple web services interface that can be used to store and retrieve data on the web, and provides a scalable data storage infrastructure.

In the specific case of applications requiring parallel processing using Map-Reduce architecture, one may also use the Elastic Map Reduce, which implements a hosted Hadoop framework running on the infrastructure of Amazon EC2 and Amazon S3.

The Map-Reduce architecture is an interesting approach, once it is versatile enough to be deployed in both environments. However, the Map Reduce architecture isn't generic enough to be used in all classes of problems that deal with large amounts of data to be processed, once there are some issues that are not addressed efficiently, such as the use of different Reduce algorithms for some specific pieces of information, or the chunk ordering before the Reduce step.

A good example where Map-Reduce could be generalized is the compression of high definition video files and especially for medical video, which requires intensive information processing. In this compression process, streams of audio and video are processed with different algorithms, and there is a great correlation between subsequent video frames, especially when there is temporal compression. The order in which pieces of audio and video are recombined after having been processed must also be taken into account so as to avoid that significant distortions are incorporated in the output. Moreover, issues such as fault tolerance, security and scalability need to be thoroughly considered, so that the proposed architecture becomes robust enough to meet the requirements of different video compression applications.

4.1. Distributed Video Processing

Video compression refers to reducing the quantity of data used to represent digital video images, and is a combination of spatial image compression and temporal motion compensation. Video applications require some form of data compression to facilitate storage and transmission. Digital video compression is one of the main issues in digital video encoding, enabling efficient distribution and interchange of visual information.

The process of high quality video encoding and analysis is usually very costly to the encoder, which, and require a lot of production time. When we consider situations where there are large content volumes, this is even more critical, since a single video may require the server's processing power for long time periods. Moreover, there are cases where the speed of publication is a critical point. Video and biosignals acquisition are typical pervasive applications in which time is crucial, so that every second spent in data encoding may represent information loss and delays.

We note that the higher the quality, i.e., the bitrate of the video output, the lower the speed of encoding. In order to speed up encoding times, there are basically two solutions. The first one is to augment the investment in encoding hardware infrastructure, to be used in full capacity only at peak times. The downside is that the infrastructure will be idled the remaining of the time.

The second solution is to try and optimize the use of available resources. The ideal scenario is to optimize resources by distributing the tasks among them evenly. In the specific case of video encoding, the intuitive solution is to break a video into several pieces and distribute the encoding of each piece among several servers in a cluster. The challenge of this approach is to split, as well as merge video fragments without loss in synchronization.

4.2. Dynamic Resource Allocation in Hybrid Clouds

In a data center, the primary goal of a dynamic autonomous resource management process is to avoid wasting resources as a result of under-utilization. Such a process should also aim to avoid high response times as a result of over-utilization, which may result in violation of the service level agreements (SLA) between the clients and the provider. Furthermore, it needs to be carried out continuously due to the time variant nature of the workloads of application environments.

At a high level, this process can be decomposed into two separate, and inter-dependent phases:

1. The *first phase* consists of defining a mapping between the application's service level and resource level requirements. Resource level requirements are generally derived from SLAs based on certain parameters such as response time, throughput, etc.; whereas, resource level requirements are often outlined as CPU usage, memory, bandwidth, etc. As the workload of an application changes in time, this mapping is used to determine the amount of resources that should be assigned to each component – encapsulated in VMs – in order to satisfy the terms outlined in the SLA. This phase also requires performance modeling and demand forecasting for applications. The accuracy of the output from this first phase has direct effects on the accuracy of the configuration produced in the second phase.
2. The *second phase* involves the computation and application of a new configuration by distributing the resources in a data center among the VMs that represent application environments. The configuration is computed based on the output of the mappings produced in the first phase. Maintaining this configuration is a resource allocation problem and is generally defined as a Knapsack Problem [37] or as a specific variant of it, namely Vector Bin Packing Problem [2], both of which are known to be NP-Hard. This phase consists of selecting a suitable configuration from a solution space with respect to a set of criteria. The criteria are used to define the quality of the solution in terms of certain requirements such as satisfying SLAs, overall data center utilization, and the overhead of applying an alternative configuration. The methods to be adopted in this phase need to be flexible so that the providers can easily redefine the configuration goals by adding new criteria or tuning the importance assigned to them.

In the second phase, certain constraints and limitations need to be taken into consideration.

Two of these are the time-spent during the selection of a new configuration, and the feasibility of it. Due to the time variance in workloads, a new configuration must be computed in a reasonable amount of time so that it is not stale under the current conditions. The selected configuration must also be feasible in terms of the number migrations necessary. The number of migrations that can be performed in a data center still has limits with the current technologies.

5. A Case Study of a Pervasive Health Cloud Application: The @HealthCloud

This section discusses the main features of the @HealthCloud application and presents implementation details. The prevalent functionality of the application is to provide medical experts and patients with a mobile user interface for managing healthcare information. The latter interprets into storing, querying and retrieving medical images (e.g., CT scans, MRIs, US etc.), patient health records and patient-related medical data (e.g., biosignals). The data may reside at a distributed Cloud Storage facility, initially uploaded/stored by medical personnel through an HER (Electronic Health Record) or a PHR (Personal Health Record) system. In order to be interoperable with a variety of Cloud Computing infrastructures, the communication and data exchange has to be performed through non-proprietary, open and interoperable communication standards.

@HealthCloud utilizing Web Services connectivity and Android OS supports the following functionality:

- Seamless connection to Cloud Computing storage utilizing Web Services and the REST API [30]: The main application allows users to retrieve, modify and upload medical content (medical images, patient health records and biosignals). The content resides remotely into the distributed storage elements but access is presented to the user as the resources are located locally in the device (see Fig. 2(e)).
- Patient Health Record Management: Information regarding patient's status, related biosignals and image content can be displayed and managed through the application's interface (see Fig. 2(a)).
- DICOM image viewing support: The DICOM [36] medical image protocol is supported. Medical images are decoded and displayed on the device among with the information stored into the file's header (see Fig. 2(b)).
- JPEG2000 viewing support: JPEG2000 [3] standard has already been widely used for the coding of medical images. It supports lossy and lossless compression, progressing coding and Region of Interest (ROI) coding [15]. The progressive coding allows the user to decode large image files at different resolution levels according to available network bandwidth optimizing this way network resources and allowing image acquisition even in cases network availability is limited (see examples in Fig. 2(c) and Fig. 2(d)). The code for performing wavelet decoding on mobile devices in [25] has been modified to support the JPEG2000 standard on the Android platform.
- Image annotation support: User can annotate medical images using the multi-touch functions of the Android OS. The annotation information is stored separately and retrieved automatically every time the image is retrieved.
- Proper user authentication and data encryption: User is authenticated at the Cloud Computing Service with SHA1 [38] hashing for message authentication and SSL [29] for encrypted data communication.

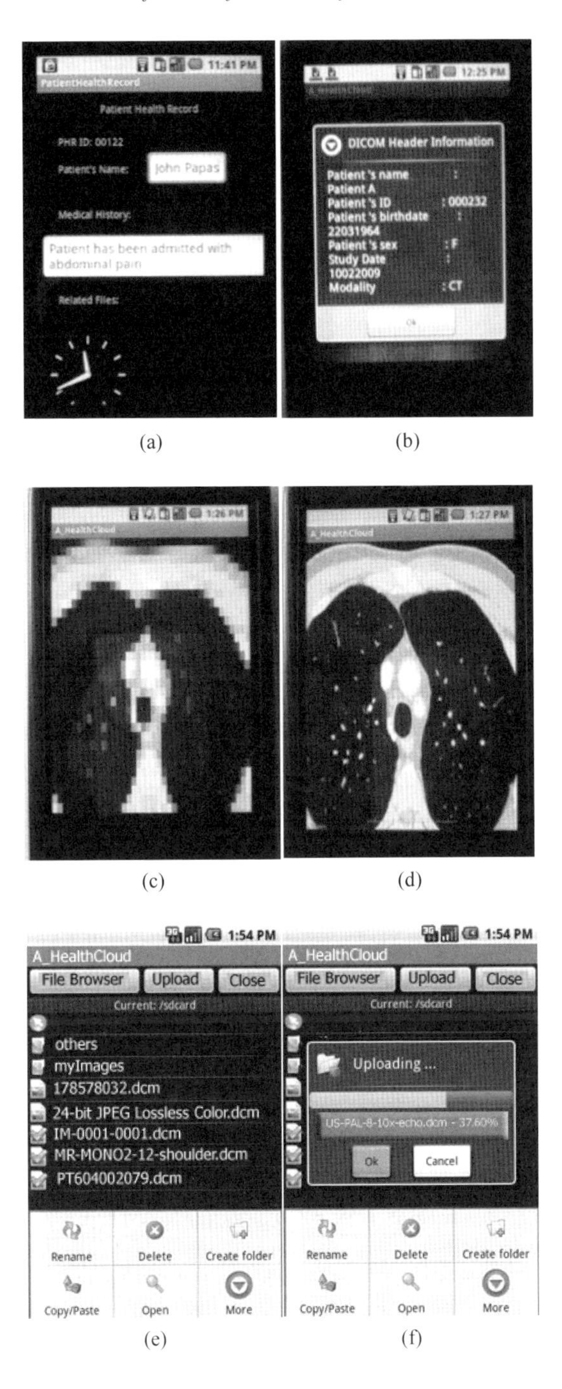

Figure 2. Screenshots of the @HealthCloud mobile application: a) Displaying a patient health record, b) illustration of DICOM header extraction, c) JPEG2000 progressive decoding of a CT scan at frist resolution level (out of five), d) final output of JPEG2000 progressive decoding of a CT scan, e) The main application interface displaying available files on the Cloud and available operations, f) illustration of the uploading procedure of a file into the Cloud.

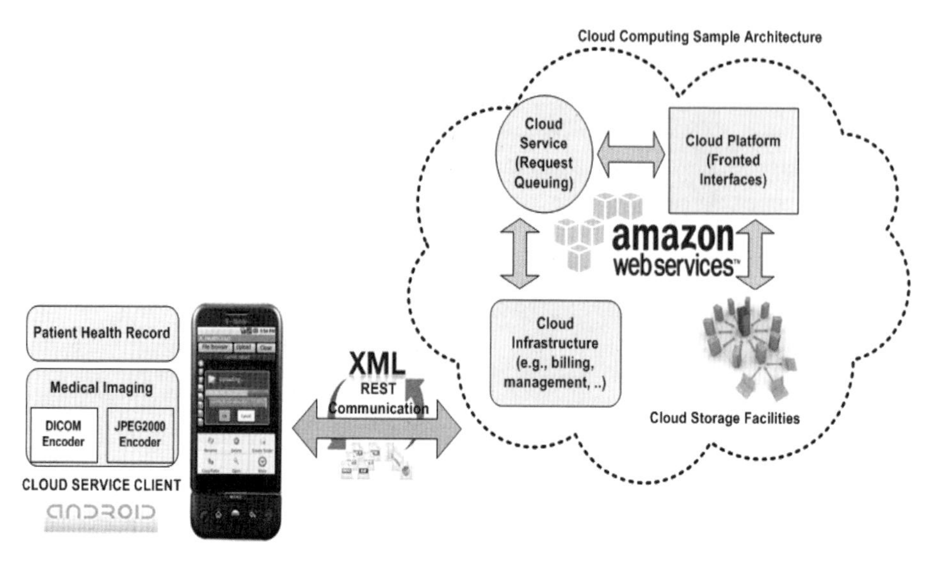

Figure 3. Illustration of the proposed system architecture.

The main components of a Cloud Computing Service usually are [28] the platform front-end interface that communicates directly with users and allows the management of the storage content. The interface can be a web client or a standalone application. The Cloud Storage Facilities manages the physical infrastructure (e.g., storage elements) utilized for managing data and is also responsible for performing maintaining operations (e.g., backing up data, etc.) The Cloud Platform interface is also connected to the Cloud Service module, which is responsible for accepting and queuing user requests. Finally, the Cloud Infrastructure module manages user account, accessibility and billing issues.

Previous work by authors [25] has demonstrated the applicability of mobile devices into retrieving medical image data from remote repositories wirelessly utilizing proper content coding (i.e., wavelet compression with region of interest support). The mobile application used has been initially developed using Java for mobile devices (J2ME [20]) and communication for data exchange was performed using Remote Method Invocation (RMI [21]). This work has been now extended to include the functionality of communicating with Cloud Computing platforms and support communication through Web Services. In this context, @HealthCloud has been developed based on Google's Android mobile Operating System (OS) [35] using the appropriate software development kit (sdk). Android is a mobile operating system running on the Linux kernel. Several mobile device vendors already support it. The platform is adaptable to larger and traditional smartphone layouts and supports a variety of connectivity technologies (GSM/EDGE, CDMA, EV-DO, UMTS, Bluetooth, and Wi-Fi). It supports a great variety of audio, video and still image format, making it suitable for displaying medical content. Finally, it supports native multi-touch technology, which allows better manipulation of medical images and generally increases the application's usability.

The Cloud Service client running on Android OS consists of several modules. The Patient Health Record application acquires and displays patient records stored into the cloud. The Medical Imaging module is responsible for displaying medical images on the device. It decodes images in DICOM format displaying both image and heard information data. When JEPG2000 compression is used, the appropriate sub-module decodes the image.

The communication with the Cloud is performed through an implementation of Web Services REST API that is supported natively by Android. Web Services are emerging as a promising technology to build distributed applications and is suitable for creating Cloud Computing client applications. It is an implementation of Service Oriented Architecture that supports the concept of loosely-coupled, open-standard, language – and platform-independent systems. Web services provide several technological and business benefits, a few of which include application and data integration, versatility, code re-use and cost savings. The inherent interoperability that comes with using vendor, platform, and language independent XML technologies and the ubiquitous HTTP as a transport mean that any application can communicate with any other application using Web services. Web services are also versatile by design. They can be accessed through Web-based client interfaces, other applications including mobile ones and other Web services.

Data in Cloud are seamlessly stored and presented to the user as if they reside locally. This means that the Cloud repository is presented as a virtual folder and does not provide the features of a database scheme. In order to provide the user with data querying functionality, medical records and related data (images and biosignals) are stored into a SQLite [37] file. SQLite is the database platform supported by Android. The file resides into a specific location at the Cloud and is retrieved on the device every time user needs to query data. The query is performed locally and the actual location of the data in the cloud is revealed to the applications. The database file is updated and uploaded into the Cloud every time user modifies data, respectively.

5.1. Utilizing Amazon S3 Cloud Computing Service

For the realization of the mobile pervasive healthcare information management system the Amazon Simple Storage Service (S3) has been utilized. The main reason for selecting the specific Cloud Computing platform is that it is a commercial service well established and used successfully in several applications [2]. It provides users with several interoperable web interfaces for managing data (SaaS model) and developers with the ability to create their own applications for accessing the latter (PaaS model) and is suitable for managing healthcare information.

5.1.1. Security Issues and HIPAA Compliance

The Amazon S3 Service as a part of AWS provides a reliable, scalable, and inexpensive computing platform "in the cloud" that can be used to facilitate healthcare customers' HIPAA compliant applications [13]. HIPAA's privacy rule regulations include standards regarding the encryption of all PHI in transmission and in storage. The same data encryption mechanisms used in a traditional computing environment, such as a local server or a managed hosting server, can also be used in a virtual computing environment, such as Amazon S3. Using Amazon Web Services (AWS), customer's system administrators can utilize token or key-based authentication to access their virtual servers. Amazon EC2 creates a 2048 bit RSA key pair, with private and public keys and a unique identifier for each key pair to help facilitate secure access.

Table 1. Transmission time of medical images using Amazon S3 Cloud Service and different network types

Image Type (encoding)	File Size (MB)	Time (secs)	
		3G Network	*WLAN Network*
OT (24-bit JPEG2000 Lossless Color)	6.8	42.532	7.894
CT (Uncompressed)	0.528	4.023	2.382
CT (JPEG2000)	0.102	1.223	0.892
MR (JPEG Lossless)	0.721	9.738	3.894
PET (JPEG2000 Lossy)	0.037	0.923	0.793
Ultrasound (sequence of 10 images, JPEG2000 Lossless)	0.487	3.892	3.251

Using Amazon S3, access can be easily controlled down to the object level. The system administrator maintains full control over who has access to the data at all times and the default setting only permits authenticated access to the creator. Read, write and delete permissions are controlled by an Access Control List (ACL) associated with each object.

HIPAA's security safeguards also require in-depth auditing capabilities, data back-up procedures and disaster recovery mechanisms. AWS services contain many features that help customers address these requirements. Amazon S3 provides a highly available solution for data storage and automated back-ups. By simply loading a file or image into Amazon S3, multiple redundant copies are automatically created and stored in separate data centers. These files can be accessed at any time, from anywhere (based on permissions) and are stored until intentionally deleted by the customer's system administrator. Using Amazon S3, customer's data is replicated and automatically stored in separate data centers to ensure reliable data storage with a service level of 99.9% availability and no single points of failure [13].

6. @HealthCloud in Practice: Initial Evaluation

In order to prove the system's usability, some initial experiments evaluating the system's performance have been conducted. Experiments concern the time needed to transmit data to the Amazon S3 Cloud storage service. Due to the fact that textual data like a patient's health record or a biosignal sequence do not consist of large data files and do not require high bandwidth, the presented results involve the transmission of medical images. The @HealthCloud application as presented in previous sections has been used on a HTC G1 [19] mobile phone running Android OS version 1.6. A number of medical images of different modalities (MR, CT, PET, OT and Ultrasound) and different file sizes have been used. The transmission times are displayed in Table 1. As indicated, two different wireless network infrastructure types have been utilized; a WLAN and a commercial 3G Network.

The performance of both WLAN and 3G networks can be easily biased by traffic and other network conditions, since commercial networks have been utilized in both cases. Also, the response time of the Amazon S3 Cloud service can play an important role on the total transmission time. However, the acquired results can be considered as indicative since the experiments reflect a real case scenario where the specific service and commercial wireless networks are utilized in order to transmit medical data. In addition, the time needed to decode and present the specific images used in the experiments has been measured. For the HTC G1 mobile phone used, the time needed by @HealthCloud to display uncompressed CT images at a resolution of 512 × 512 pixels was 0.52 sec, compressed CT images with JPEG2000 coding at a resolution of 512 × 512 pixels was 4.53 sec. The time needed to decode OT images compressed with JPEG2000 at resolution of 3072 × 2048 was 21 sec. and 7.5 sec. for a sequence of 10 ultrasound images of 600 × 430 pixels.

7. Conclusions

The technological advances of the last few years in mobile communications, location- and context-aware computing has facilitated the introduction of pervasive healthcare applications. The sharing of medical information resources (electronic health data and corresponding processing applications) is a key factor playing an important role towards the successful adoption of pervasive healthcare systems. Moreover, due to the mobility of the patients and the medical personnel, healthcare networks are increasingly equipped with capabilities to share healthcare-related information among the various actors of electronic health. In this context the concept of Cloud Computing will attract the interest of scientists, developers and industrial partners working in the field of biomedical informatics. Cloud computing has been receiving much attention as an alternative to both specialized grids and to owning and managing data centers. It represents a new way, in some cases a more cost effective way, of delivering enterprise IT. The increasing adoption rate of cloud computing is currently driving a significant increase in both the supply and the demand side of this new market for IT.

References

[1] Amazon Web Services Developer Community, http://developer.amazonwebservices.com/connect/servlet/KbServlet/downloadImage/1632-102-188/figure5.png.
[2] Amazon's AWS Success Case Studies, http://aws.amazon.com/solutions/case-studies/.
[3] G. Anastassopoulos and A. Skodras, JPEG2000 ROI coding in medical imaging applications, in: *2nd IASTED Int. Conf. Visualization, Imaging and Image Processing (VIIP2002)*, Malaga, Spain, Sept. 2002.
[4] ANSI, ISO/TS 18308 Health Informatics-Requirements for an Electronic Health Record Architecture, ISO 2003.
[5] Apache Hadoop, http://hadoop.apache.org/mapreduce/.
[6] M. Armbrust, M. Fox, R. Griffith et al., Above the clouds: A Berkeley view of cloud computing, in: University of California at Berkeley Technical Report no. UCB/EECS-2009-28, February 10, 2009, pp. 6–7.
[7] R. Bakker, B. Barber, R. Tervo-Pellikka and A. Treacher, Communicating health information in an insecure World, *Proceedings of the Helsinki Working Conference* **43**(1) (1995), 2.
[8] B. Barber, D. Garwood and P. Skerman, in: *Security in Hospital Information Systems, Security and data protection programme presented at the IMIA WH10 Working conference*, Durham, 1994.
[9] J. Birnbaum, Pervasive information systems, *Communications of the ACM* **40**(2) (1997) 40–41.
[10] N. Carr, Here comes HaaS, 2006, http://www.roughtype.com/archives/2006/03/here_comes_haas.php.
[11] D. Cearley, Hype Cycle for Cloud Computing, Gartner report number G00 168780, 2009.
[12] Cloud Computing – Web-Based Applications That Change The Way You Work And Collaborate Online, 2009.
[13] Creating HIPAA-Compliant Medical Data Applications with Amazon Web Services, White Paper, available online at: http://awsmedia.s3.amazonaws.com/AWS_HIPAA_Whitepaper_Final.pdf.
[14] J. Dean and S. Ghemawat, MapReduce: Simplified data processing on large clusters, in: *OSDI*, 2004.
[15] C. Doukas and I. Maglogiannis, Region of interest coding techniques for medical image compression, *Engineering in Medicine and Biology Magazine, IEEE* **26**(5) (Sept.-Oct. 2007), pp. 29–35.
[16] S.M. Furnell and P.W. Sanders, Security management in the health-care environment, in: *MEDINFO'95, Proceedings of the eighth World Congress on Medical Informatics*, R.A. Greenes, H.E. Peterson and D.J. Protti, eds, Canada, pp. 675–678.

[17] D. Garets and M. Davis, A HIMSS Analytics White Paper. Electronic Medical Records vs. Electronic Health Records: Yes, There Is a Difference, January 26, 2006, http://www.himssanalytics.org/docs/wp_emr_ehr.pdf.
[18] F. Hermenier, X. Lorca, J.M. Menaud, G. Muller and J. Lawall, Entropy: A Consolidation Manager for Clusters, in: *VEE'09: Proceedings of the 2009 ACM SIGPLAN/SIGOPS International Conference on Virtual Execution Environments*, 2009, pp. 41–50.
[19] HTC G1 mobile phone, http://www.htc.com/www/product/g1/overview.html.
[20] Java for Mobile Devices, http://java.sun.com/javame/index.jsp.
[21] Java Remote Method Invocation, http://java.sun.com/javase/technologies/core/basic/rmi/index.jsp.
[22] C. Krager and D. Krager, *HIPAA for Health Care Professionals (Paperback)*, Delmar Cengage Learning, 1st edn, February 11, 2008, ISBN: 1418080535.
[23] L.L. Leape, Error in medicine, *J. Am. Med. Assoc.* **272** (1994) 1851–1857.
[24] H. Linden, D. Kalra, A. Hasman and J. Talmon. Inter-organization future proof HER systems – A review of the security and privacy related issues, *International Journal of Medical Informatics* **78** (2009), 141–160.
[25] I. Maglogiannis, C. Doukas, G. Kormentzas and T. Pliakas, Wavelet-based compression with ROI coding support for mobile access to DICOM images over heterogeneous radio networks, *IEEE Transactions on Information Technology in Biomedicine* **13**(4) (July 2009), pp. 458–466.
[26] A. Patel and I. Kantzavelou, Implementing network security guidelines in health-care information systems, in: *MEDINFO'95. Proceedings of the eighth World Congress on Medical Informatics,* Vancouver Trade and Convention Centre, Canada, pp. 671–674.
[27] J.T. Reason, *Human Error*, Cambridge University Press, Cambridge, 1990.
[28] G. Reese, *Cloud Application Architectures: Building Applications and Infrastructure in the Cloud,* O'Reilly Media, Paperback, April 17, 2009, ISBN: 0596156367.
[29] E. Rescorla, *SSL and TLS: Designing and Building Secure Systems (Paperback)*, Addison-Wesley Professional, October 27, 2000, ISBN: 0201615983.
[30] L. Richardson, S. Ruby and D.H. Hansson, *Restful Web Services (Paperback)*, O'Reilly Media, May 2007, ISBN: 0596529260.
[31] S3 Amazon Simple Storage Service (S3), http://aws.amazon.com/s3/.
[32] O. Shimrat, *Cloud Computing and Healthcare*, San Diego Physician, April 2009, pp. 26–29.
[33] B. Sotomayor, R.S. Montero, I.M. Llorente and I. Foster, Virtual infrastructure management in private and hybrid clouds, *IEEE Internet Computing* **13**(5) (2009), 14– 22.
[34] The AmazonTM Simple Storage Service, http://aws.amazon.com/s3/.
[35] The Android mobile OS by GoogleTM, http://www.android.com/.
[36] The Digital Imaging and Communications in Medicine (DICOM) standard, http://medical.nema.org/.
[37] The SQLite Database Engine, http://www.sqlite.org/.
[38] US Secure Hash Algorithm 1 (SHA1), http://www.faqs.org/rfcs/rfc3174.html.
[39] U. Varshney, Pervasive healthcare, *IEEE Computer Magazine* **36**(12) (2003) 138–140.
[40] W. Vogels, A head in the clouds – The power of infrastructure as a service, in: *First workshop on Cloud Computing in Applications (CCA'08)*, October, 2008.
[41] M.A. Vouk, Cloud computing – Issues, research and implementations, in: *30th International Conference on Information Technology Interfaces*, June, 2008, pp. 31–40.
[42] W.E. Walsh, G. Tesauro, J.O. Kephart and R. Das, Utility functions in autonomic systems, in: *ICAC'04: Proceedings of the First International Conference on Autonomic Computing*, IEEE Computer Society, 2004, pp. 70–77.

Handbook of Ambient Assisted Living
J.C. Augusto et al. (Eds.)
IOS Press, 2012

doi:10.3233/978-1-60750-837-3-469

Smart Living Environment: Ubiquitous Computing Approach Based on TRON Architecture

Ken SAKAMURA*
Professor, Graduate School of Interdisciplinary Information Studies, The University of Tokyo
Director, Ubiquitous Networking Laboratory, Division of Yokosuka Telecom Research Park, Inc.

Abstract. Smart houses that use the results of the ubiquitous computing have been built to assist the residents including the physically-challenged. Similar technological infrastructure is now being applied at the urban landscape level to create a smart town or city to help the citizens including the challenged. Such future infrastructure will become more important as the underlying technology becomes affordable. Assisted living environment will be richer thanks to the services offered by ubiquitous computing, or the IoT.

Keywords. Intelligent house, smart house, smart city, embedded computers, ubiquitous computing, the Internet of Things (IoT)

Introduction

A concept of a system in which computers, sensors, and actuators are embedded into every object, and objects exchange information with each other via networks to achieve a particular goal, is drawing global attention.

In a project called TRON Project which started from 1984, we probably became the first in the world to propose this concept, by the name of "Computing Everywhere" [6,8]. To realize this concept, we have actively conducted researches on fundamental topics and application issues. Since then, many similar concepts have been proposed, and today this concept is called "Ubiquitous Computing" [2,16].

Concepts called "Pervasive Computing," "Calm Computing," or "Invisible Computting" in the United States also refer to the similar idea [9]. What these terms mean is that by embedding computers into various objects, people no longer recognize computers as such. In Europe, names such as "Smart Environment" and "Ambient Intelligence" are also used. These terms invoke an image of the environment becoming more sophisticated.

Today, this concept is increasingly called "the IoT: the Internet of Things" around the world. This is because many research groups and projects including the CASAGRAS project conducted by the EU FP7 [3] adopted this term to describe the concept of their vision of the future in which every object has an embedded computer inside

*Corresponding Author: Ken Sakamura. E-mail: ken@sakamura-lab.org.

and is connected to a network. In China, the term "物聯網," a literal Chinese translation of the IoT, is becoming familiar [10].

Based on the background as noted above, we shall explain how we have created ubiquitous environments with TRON, our original computer system architecture for embedding into physical objects, along with the resulting effects and advantages. It has a strong impact on assisted living environment as the readers shall see.

1. TRON and Computing Everywhere

TRON is an acronym of "The Real-time Operating system Nucleus" [12]. It is a specification for computers to be embedded into objects. To realize the "Ubiquitous Computing" concept, TRON Project first aimed to establish an environment for developing advanced computer-embedded devices, which was not popular yet back in 1984, at a lower cost and with higher quality. The set of TRON specifications have been developed to achieve this goal, and operating systems based on this specification are all capable of real-time processing. Today, operating systems based on the TRON specification is widely used in Japan, including engine controls for Toyota automobiles, RF controls for mobile phones, digital camera controls, printers, video cameras, VCRs, etc., all in all holding 60 percents of market share in the country. In addition to its performance, technical information is fully disclosed and the license is free of charge. These advantages have made TRON specification OS the de facto standard of embedded systems [4].

TRON Project is now a generic term for various activities which aim for realization of computing everywhere. The term TRON is used as the general indication of everything that the project is working on.

2. TRON Intelligent House

2.1. Thousand Computers in a Single House

To test ahead the future living environment where ubiquitous computing is commonly applied, we created "TRON Intelligent House" [7,18].

TRON Intelligent House was built at the end of 1989 as an experimental house in Roppongi, Tokyo (Photos 1 and 2). Using technology available at the time, this experimental house tried as much as possible to realize a living environment of the future, created by the ubiquitous computing technology, in which every element and facility, such as doors, ceilings, and walls, is embedded with computers and connected to the network. The entire house had about 400 main subsystems with computers, and about 1,000 computers were used in total including the ones used for smaller units.

Networks were spread all over the house, categorized into sensor systems, telephony systems, video information systems, audio control systems, and subsystems for each facility. Data was managed by the house server installed at the basement (Fig. 1).

Some people lived in this house for three years, collected various data, and conducted experiments assuming unusual events such as computer failure, fire, or housebreaking. Unfortunately, the actual facility cannot be seen now, because it was disassembled to reuse the site.

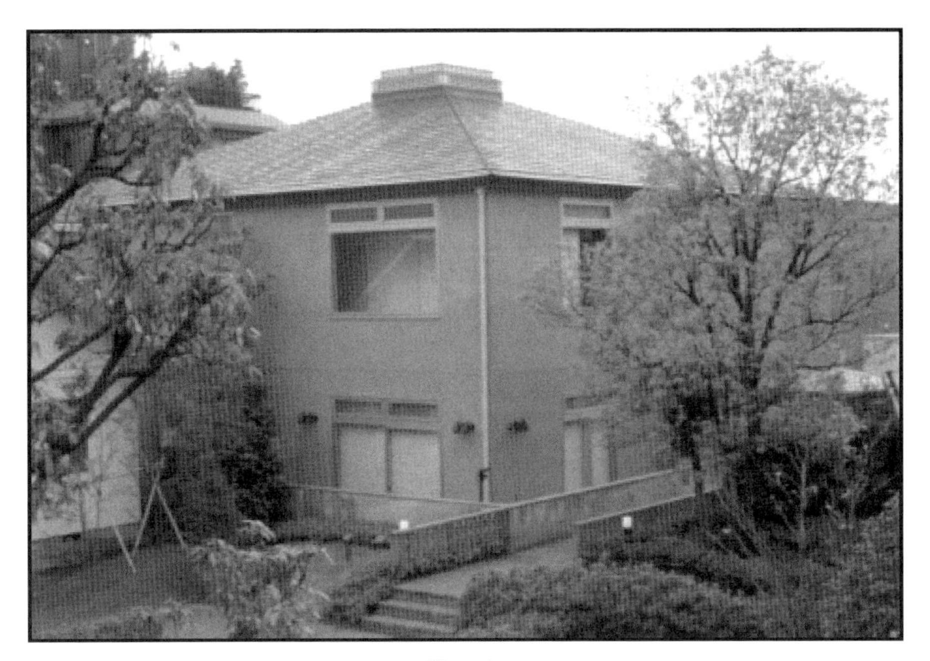

Photo 1.

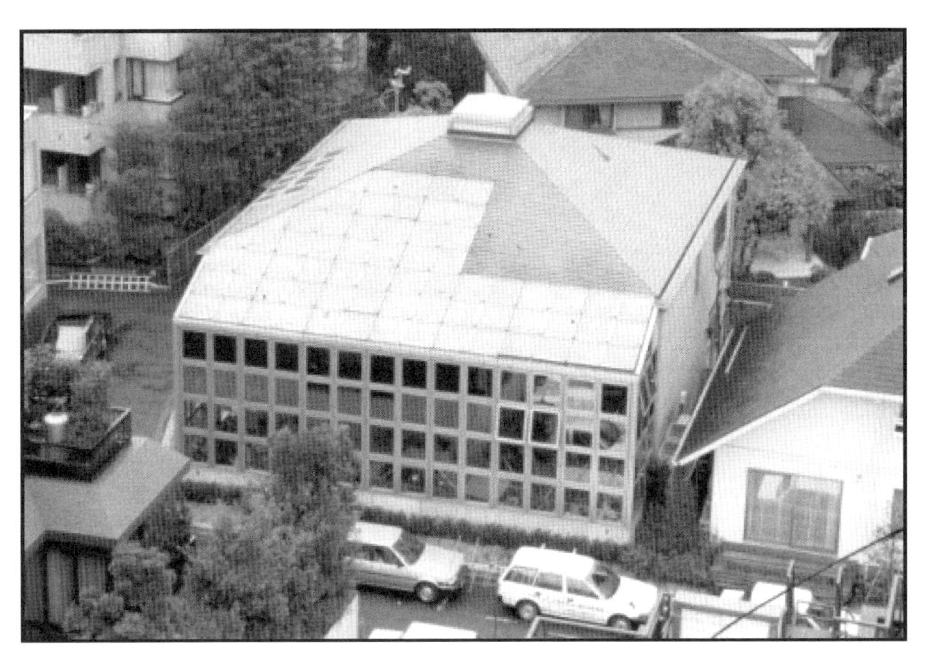

Photo 2.

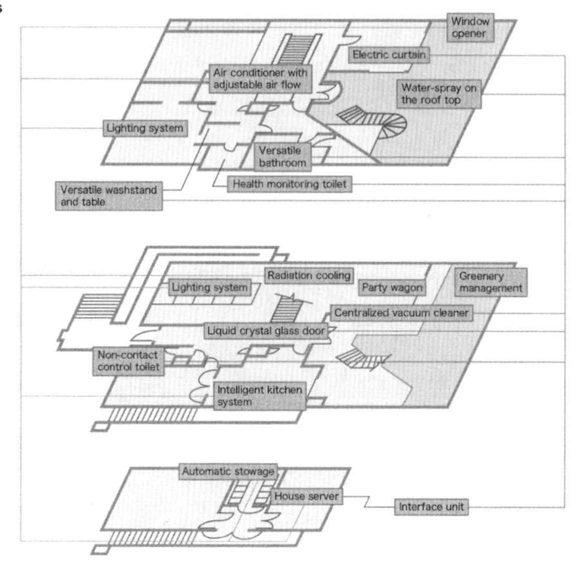

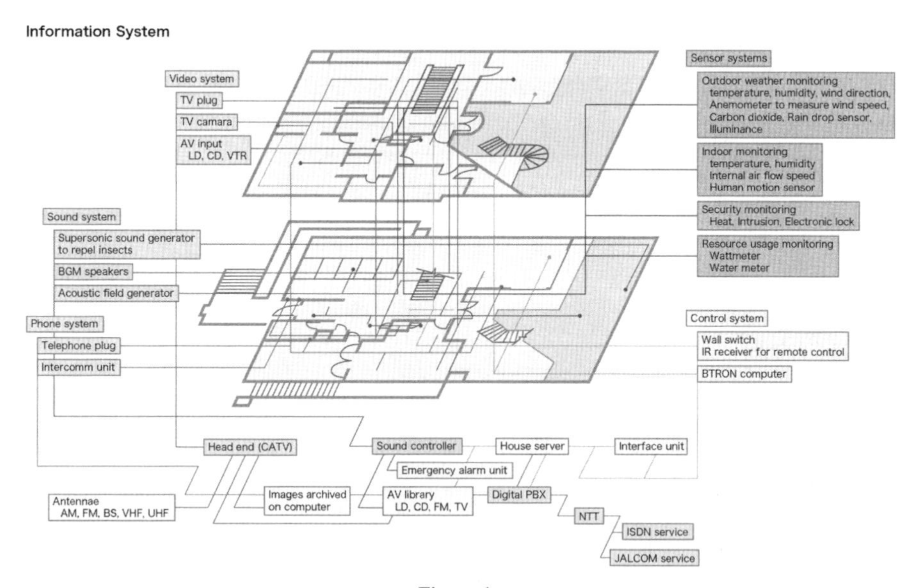

Figure 1.

2.2. Networked House

This house could be distinguished from other “electric houses of the future” by the fact that it was a networked house based on networks. By being connected to each other via networks, the subsystems were capable of operating in a coordinated manner.

For example, by passing information from an alarm system to a lighting system, actions such as turning the light on automatically when a person enters the house, and turning it off when no one is in the house, were easily configured on the software. By

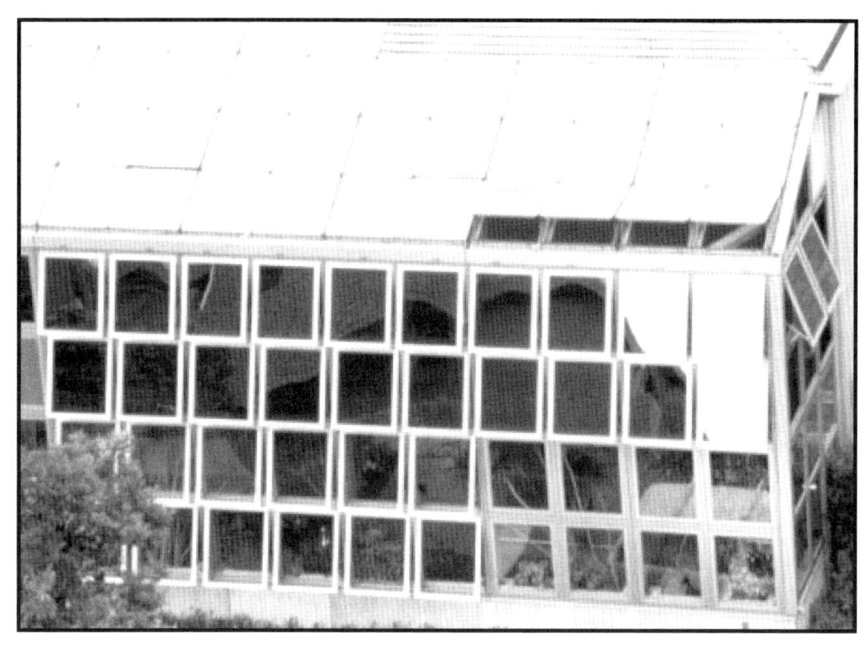

Photo 3.

sending sunlight data to the lighting system but also to an air conditioning system, the management of the temperature became more efficiently done. By letting the air conditioning system know that the sound level of the music being played by AV (Audio and Video) system is just entering into a pianissimo, the air conditioning system could temporarily switch itself to a quiet operation. This allows the music to be heard undisturbed by other noises.

The house might open up its windows when the wind is blowing comfortably outside. But once the ambient environment condition becomes harsh, it might close the windows and automatically run the air conditioning system (Photos 3 and 4). When a lighting scene is selected, this information might be passed to the audio control system, which would select a background music matching the mood and change the sound field processor settings. The volume of audio equipment around a telephone might be turned down when someone is using the telephone. As such, cooperative behavior beyond the borders of the subsystems has many possibilities.

As seen above, networked houses utilize each computer-controlled facility to bring comfort to people, not separately but in a cooperative manner.

2.3. Time-Space Design

In the conventional framework of "architecture" with the main focus on the "static form," there may be a school of thought that regards facilities, etc., are often necessary evil from the viewpoint of establishing an "architectural beauty."

However, in houses of the future featuring many embedded computers, we think "architecture" should be considered from the "time-space" (spatiotemporal) point of view, which combines space on one axis and time (implemented as features) on another axis.

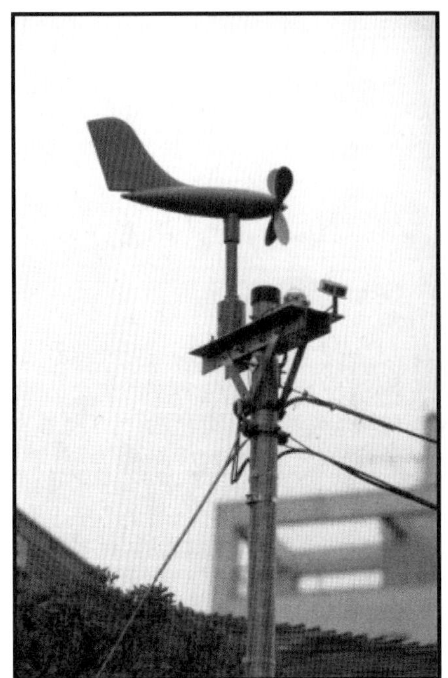

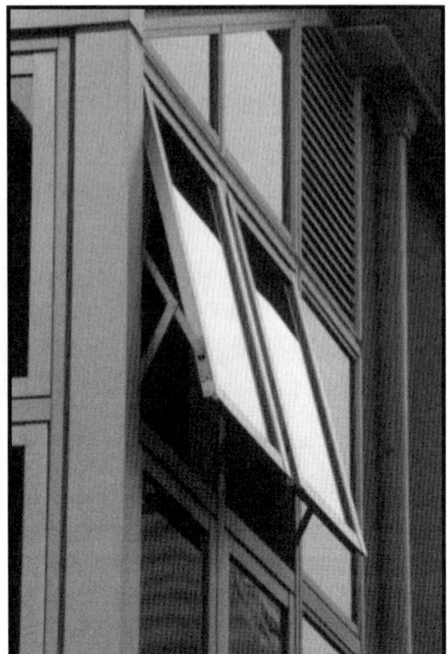

Photo 4.

For example, the Intelligent House mentioned before had a semi-open space, large enough to be called a garden and even featured a second-floor veranda and trees (trees and flowers were grown by a computer-managed hydroponics system) (Photo 5). This space was created by covering the garden part of a common house with a glass wall and ceiling, computer-controlled to open up and close depending on the ambient condition at the moment. In other words, when the glasses were open, the space looked like a garden, and when closed, it looked like a giant sunroom.

This house was built at the heart of Tokyo. Large estate was not available, and surrounding landscape and air were not good for the most of the time. This semi-open space works as a capsule to protect people and plants in such unfriendly environment of the city. Here, the important point is that the semi-open environment is not complete closed; it is ready to open whenever the unfriendly conditions of the neighborhood is disapper.

Since the garden was not completely outside, strong separation between interior and the semi-open space was not required. The borders were dynamic, and mutually possible to penetrate from both sides. For example, in the TRON Intelligent House, part of the kitchen was created in the garden, and the garden penetrated to the stairs that led to the bathroom at the second floor (Fig. 2).

Here, a "static form" does not exist. This space presents a "dynamic form" as an essence of housing, or in another words, "time-space."

Our greatest finding from designing this experimental house was that, designing networked houses in the future means designing "time-space." Automatic computer operations were designed to change environment settings gradually, so that they don't stand out conspicuously and are not noticed as much as possible to hide them.

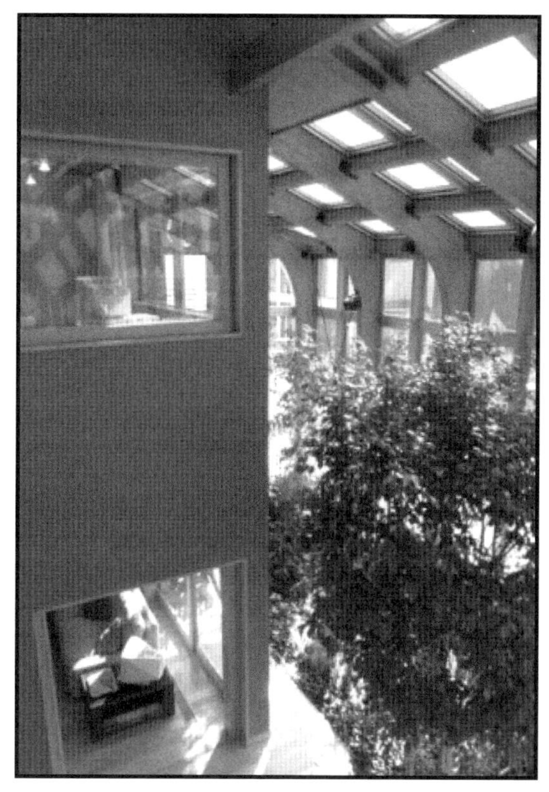

Photo 5.

3. New Technology Available for Intelligent Houses

More than 20 years have passed since this Intelligent House experiment. Now, a networked house based on such a concept is available at an affordable cost. In other words, the technology in the world finally caught up with our concept after 20 years.

The most important point is that computers had become increasingly smaller and higher in performance. For example, the TRON Intelligent House had a workstation server installed at the machine room in the basement (Photo 6), but now a several hundred dollar PC can serve the purpose. Various subsystems required a PC for implementation with the technology at that time. But now it is possible to configure the required function on a single chip including network connection. Building an intelligent house is now possible at an affordable cost, less than one tenth of the experimental house.

Another notable technology for realizing an intelligent house is the progress in networking technology. The TRON Intelligent House already had a problem with tremendous wiring, and we learned the hard way that this problem must be solved in order to spread the use of networked houses. Partly due to the thickness of the LAN (local area network) cable available at that time, an enormous space was consumed by vast wires running through the framework of the building. We even had to make some of the beams thicker (Photo 7) because its strength decreased at the holes for passing the cables through.

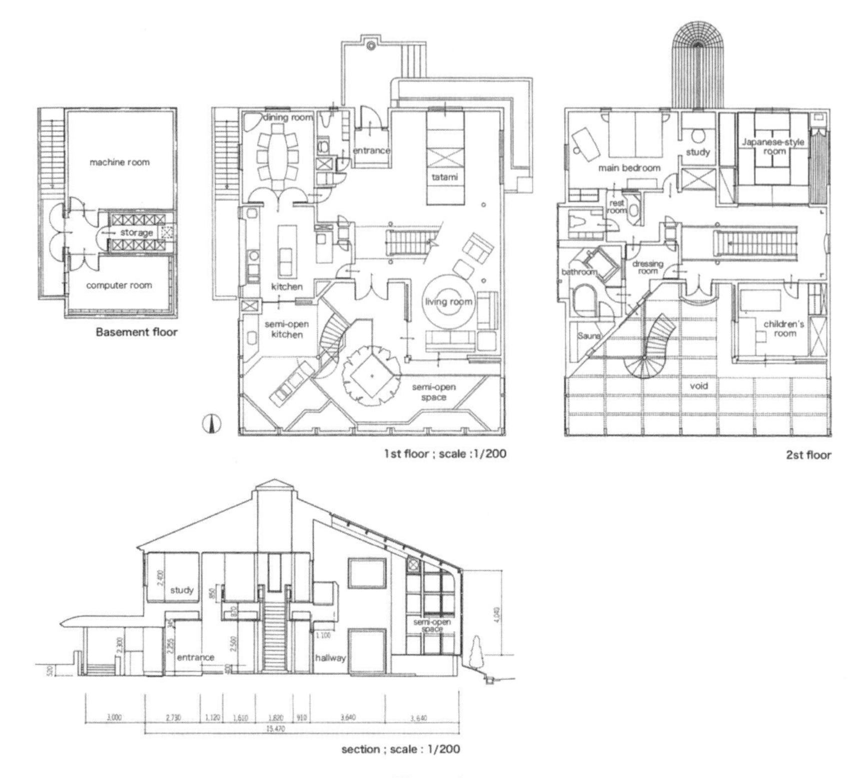

Figure 2.

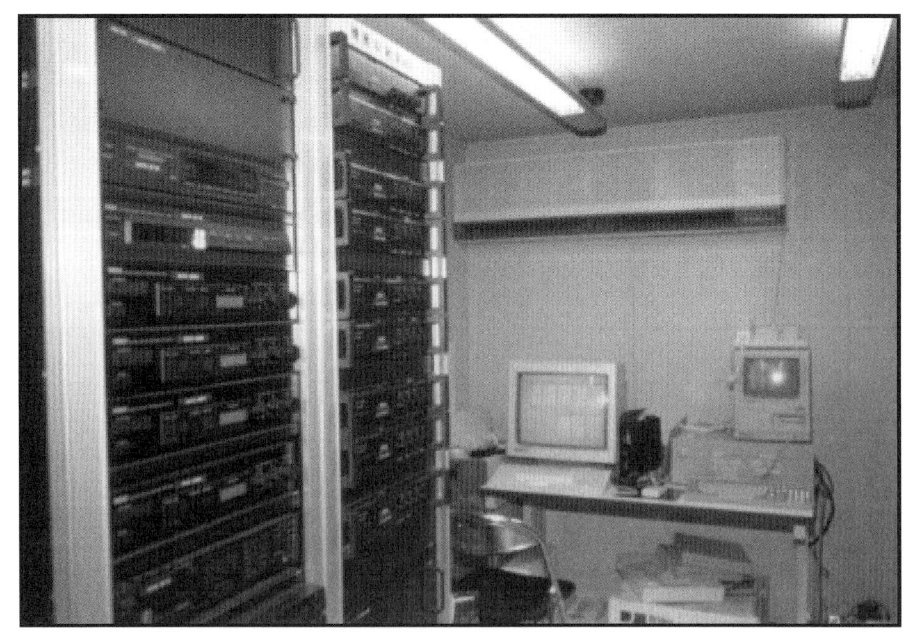

Photo 6.

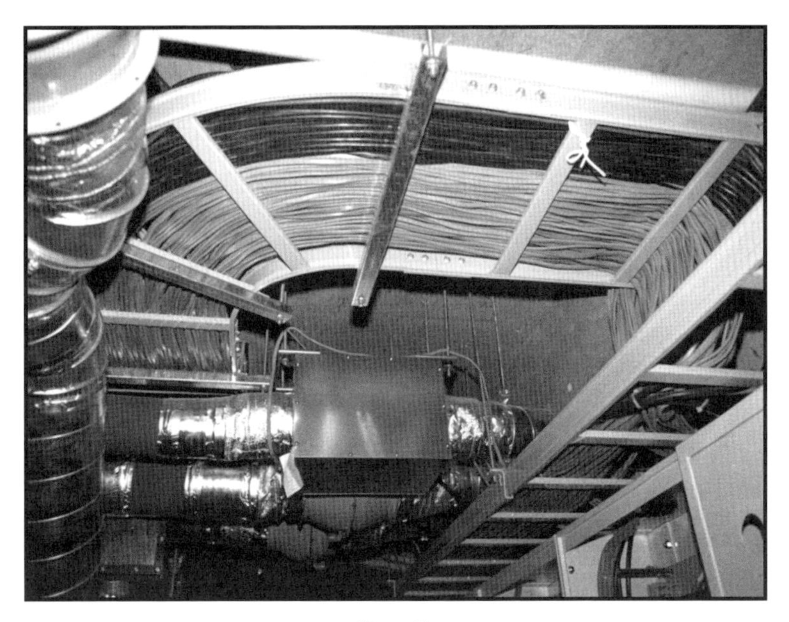

Photo 7.

Since Japanese houses tend to be generally higher in space cost, if electrical pipe shafts similar to a full-spec intelligent building should be prepared, the already small floor area will soon be too small and oppressive. With neighboring houses so near and setback regulation so strict, installing a floating floor would result in people's heads stuck at the ceiling.

In such housing environment, a rapid growth of wireless networking technology is drawing attention. The spread spectrum communication technology enables noise-resistant and high-speed digital communication by combining multiple frequencies. Thanks to this technology, a fast wireless network that rivals the traditional wired network has become possible. Taking easiness of installation and movement into concern, such wireless networking technology is important for domestic use.

When using such wireless network widely, information security technology will be particularly important. For this reason, cryptography will be essential. The technical standard for cryptography should be defined so a nonprofessional person who buys a new facility can set up a strong encrypted environment easily and surely.

Basic technology is about to be established, but issues remain. There is no standard for facilities separately installed in subsystems to perform a cooperative distributed action. Several standards have been proposed about in-house networking and audio-visual specifications, but nothing is established that is capable of advanced cooperation beyond the bounds of manufacturers. Ideally, many possibilities should be tested to converge into a de facto standard, but if standards are not unified for a long time, such as in the past example of VHS and Beta-max video standards, the demerits will be felt by many for a long. In order to avoid such situations where possible technological convenience cannot be enjoyed, the standardization of information exchange, e.g. protocols and data formats, between facilities is very important [5].

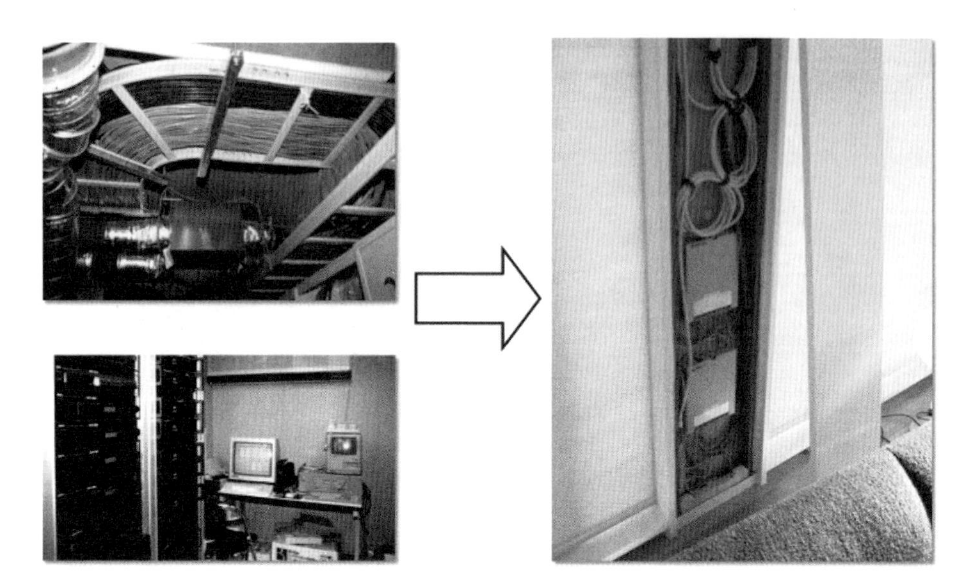

Photo 8. From 1989 to 2004.

4. History of Intelligent House Implementation

In order to contribute to the solution, after the first TRON Intelligent House, we built further experimental houses, namely PAPI in Nagoya in 2004 [1,17] and u-home in Taiwan in 2009 [19].

From the perspective of implementation, for PAPI we distributed processors in various locations and adopted LAN wiring and succeeded to get rid of vast wires (Photo 8). And, based on further device improvement, we created u-home in Taiwan to study the feasibility of implementation at an affordable cost and introduce intelligent housing to the market.

While technology change is a large factor, in the 21st century, down-to-earth features such as eco-friendliness and energy saving have begun to draw attention. These are very different from the features focused at the time of designing the first TRON Intelligent House more than 20 years ago. Environmental changes are also enormous. In Japan, because industry-wide energy saving took place since the Oil Crisis of 1973, there is not much room left for saving more energy in the industry sector. Therefore, for Japan to demonstrate energy saving performance to the world, household energy consumption must be reduced. The enormous earthquake that affected the Tohoku region of Japan on Mar. 11, 2011 resulted in power supply shortage, further leading to this direction.

To encourage energy saving, it is not enough to implement a system to switch off the light when no one is around. First of all, residents must be educated to be aware of energy saving. This is why "visualization" of energy consumption is beginning to draw attention. Experiments show that a person on a diet is likely to lose weight if he/she gets on the scale every day and record the weight. This is because people tend to make

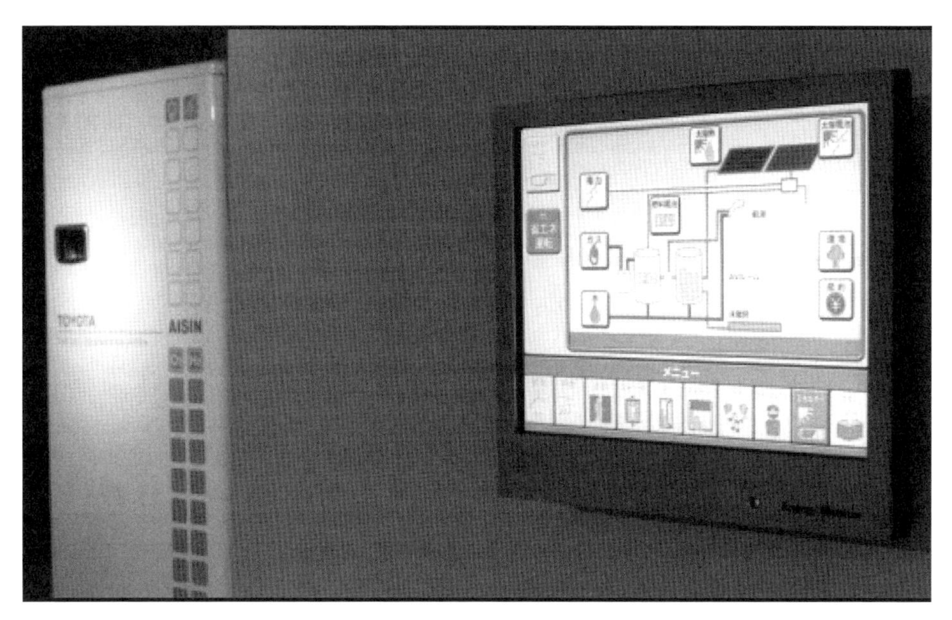

Photo 9.

an effort only when they are able to see the result. Therefore, we began an experiment to mount sensors to newly built houses to measure detailed energy consumption and feedback the results to the residents to see how much energy can be saved by being aware of the consumed amount (Photo 9).

Performing such an experiment requires detailed measurements to learn which living activity is causing energy consumption and how much, and household power meters are insufficient for this purpose. At least, the detailed power consumption data for each room is required, and preferably the data for which device is consuming how much energy should be measured.

Furthermore, even if the concept is good, energy saving cannot be achieved unless the facilities for implementing such features are supplied at a low cost. Therefore, we used TRON specification real-time OS, which has small memory footprint with network capabilities, to create devices such as a power outlet with energy consumption monitoring at a cost of only 1.5 times the conventional device.

According to the results of several experiments, performed by mounting a monitor to every electrical appliance in 10 households where people live, and by providing energy saving advices, comparing with the average energy consumption rate of their neighboring households, the households were able to save around 20 percents of energy usage.

5. Ubiquitous ID Architecture

5.1. Bridging Virtual and Real Worlds

What is the ideal society that we want to realize through ubiquitous computing?

Imagine a social infrastructure which has a vast number of computers embedded in real-world environment such as objects and places. Status of our surrounding is au-

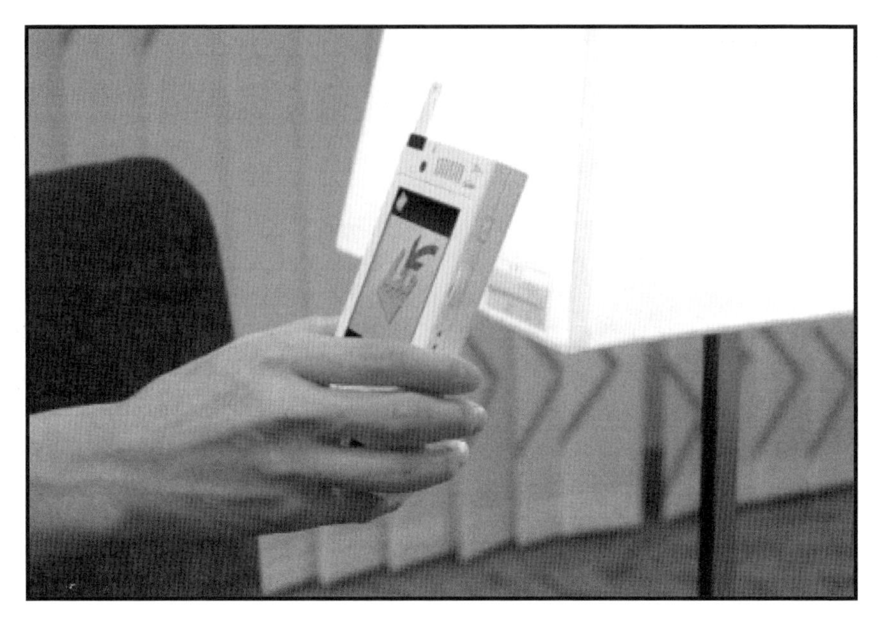

Photo 10.

tomatically recognized as much as possible, and users can enjoy, in particular time and place, the information or service ideally tailored for them without the user's being aware of it not to mention the needs for intentional operation. Such computing paradigm is called ubiquitous computing (and other names such as calm computing, etc.).

Philosophically, this can be described as "infrastructure for bridging virtual and real worlds."

The Internet has now become so popular that if you know any keyword that is associated with a topic, you can use search engines to get a vast amount of information about the topic.

However, what if there are no keywords whatsoever?

In the reception room of our laboratory, there is a tree. I often ask the visitor what kind of tree it is, and most of the time the answer is "I don't know." In this case, even if I pass an Internet terminal to the visitor, finding out the name of the tree without a keyword will be difficult.

However, if objects are tagged and thus can be identified in the world of computer network, the fact about the object can be easily found.

I am currently leading concerted efforts to tag everything. For example, each product can be given a computer-readable tag during the manufacturing phase. Even natural objects will be tagged when someone discovers them and finds out what they are.

Now back to the example of the tree, in our approach, it is tagged when brought into the office. Information regarding the type of the tree will be stored on the server accessible via the computer network. When "Ubiquitous Communicator (UC)," a terminal to read electronic tags, is held up to this tag – in the future, this function of reading electronically tagged data will be implemented on mobile phones – the information associated with the tree can be fetched from the server (Photo 10). Thus the real and virtual worlds are bridged.

Photo 11.

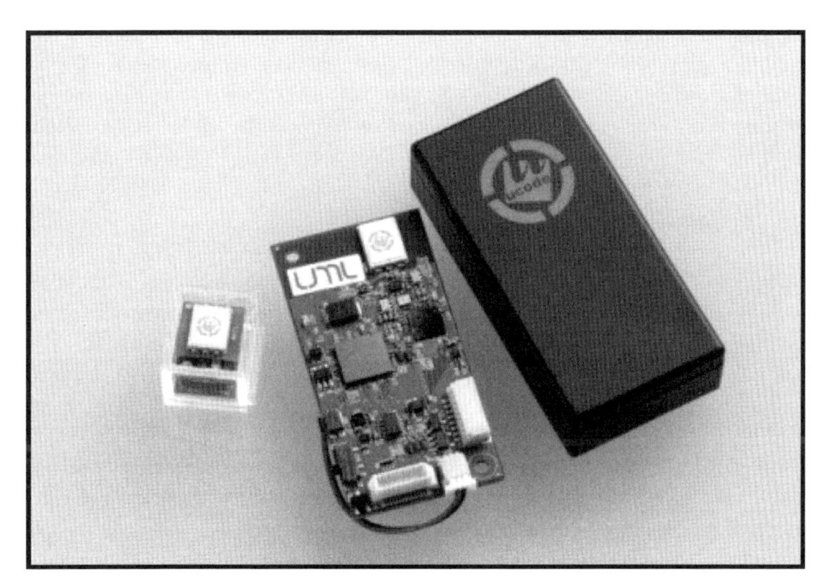

Photo 12.

Application of tags to real world objects, and fetching information based on tags is the major concept of bridging the virtual and real worlds.

5.2. Establishment of Tagging Technology

During the past several years, passive RFID tag technology has been drawing attention. A passive RFID tag is a kind of electronic tag without power source. Aside from electronic tags, barcodes are also an important technology for tagging (Photo 11).

Battery-powered active tags are also one of the hot topics today. Our laboratory has developed an active tag technology named Dice (Photo 12), which features a communication method named UWB that permits low power operation and allows transmission over a long distance. Sized roughly 1 cm dice, the current version can last up to a little less than 10 years with a lithium button cell. Furthermore, this system features anti-collision of up to 1,000 objects at a time, which means it can recognize 1,000 objects simultaneously. By using a battery, the tag can be equipped with sensors; for example, measuring ambient conditions such as temperature.

When we explain about attaching small electronic tags to objects and locations, one of the most frequently asked question is: "Is all information contained in that small electronic tag?" The answer is no. Actually, tags for distinguishing objects only store a number. But please note that this number, called ucode, is a unique number in the whole world. Ubiquitous Communicator reads this unique number and sends it to servers on the computer networks, and we will eventually learn the content information of the objects.

This is called Ubiquitous ID Architecture [14,15].

The virtual world contains plenty of information. To know how information in the virtual world corresponds to the real world, we attach a tag that is associated with the information to real-world objects and locations. If we succeed in standardizing this technology, objects and locations in the real world, across the borders of companies, organizations, and industries, will become an infrastructure that works as a bridge to the virtual world. When such infrastructure is established, various kinds of innovation that utilizes the infrastructure will emerge, and we will be able to realize many activities that we have never achieved before, such as helping the physically-challenged, at low cost.

5.3. A Simple Number without Any Loaded Meaning

To recognize a condition or status of our surrounding, we must know "what" the object is, or "where" the location is. This is all based on "identification." In order to recognize real-world objects, we must be able to identify that A and B are different.

Every objects, locations, concepts, and ideas to be identified will be assigned a ucode, an individual identification number. Everything we want to identify must be numbered.

However, please note that our concept do not number people. This is because tagging people and having the environment read the information from their tags bears a very complicated problem in terms of privacy and security.

In this case, requests should be provided to the environment from the people.

Elevators these days often have audio guidance announcing: "Third floor," "Fourth floor," "Door will open," and "Door will close." Some people might feel this guidance annoying. If nobody needs the audio guidance, it does not need to be output. However, the audio guidance allows the visually-challenged to ride on the elevator by themselves, and thus this is very commendable from the universal design point of view.

In this case, I think it's not good to attach a tag to a person and let the elevator read the information on the chip to recognize that a visually-challenged person is inside. Our design approach is that if a person wants audio guidance, he/she should be able to send a request to the elevator to receive information irrespective of whether the person is visually-challenged or not.

The terminal owned by a person reads information from the surrounding environment and understands the status or condition, and then sends requests for available services on behalf of the user. Allowing this is an issue of design philosophy and/or ap-

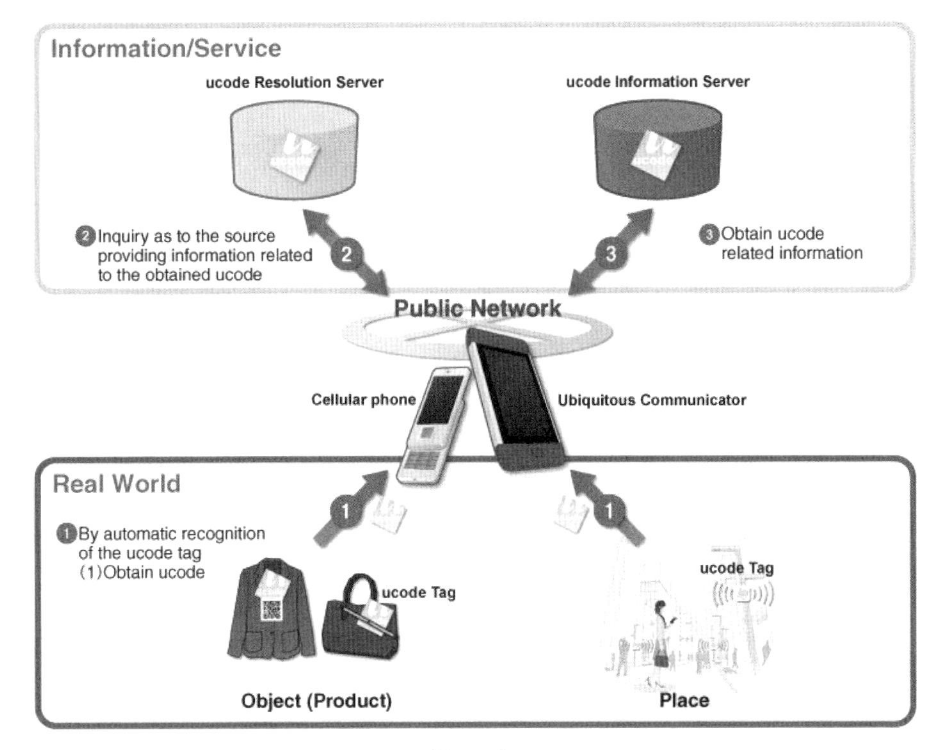

Figure 3.

proach. It is important to define why and how the assistive technology is designed from the standpoint of design philosophy. Just because computers are used in our environment does not necessarily mean that there is a problem of violation of privacy or weakness of security. It is important to look at the design philosophy and the basic design behind the computer systems in our environments.

The terminals use the individual identification number called ucode to read the information of the environment and learn the status or conditions. While ucode is a unique identification number that can be identified within an open and universal network, it is not a semantic code. An example of semantic code is a product barcode on every commercial product. The manufacturer and the nationality of the product will be indicated just by reading the barcode.

However, meaning of a ucode cannot be identified by just reading the code. When a ucode is sent to Ubiquitous ID Center via a network, the Center returns the reference to the corresponding information, thus enabling the user to obtain the relevant information. This mechanism is similar to cloud computing (Fig. 3).

The design philosophy of the ucode that is not a semantic code, says "semantics is to be defined in a cloud." This means that a ucode is an "identifier independent from the administration structure of the society." This is very important, since semantics, when embedded on tags, might lead to various problems.

Conventional notations of objects and locations employ a "hierarchical structure." The problem is that it reflects the administration structure of the user organizations: the rules established by cities, states, and national governments to make administration of objects and locations easier for the users in the public sector are reflected in the hierar-

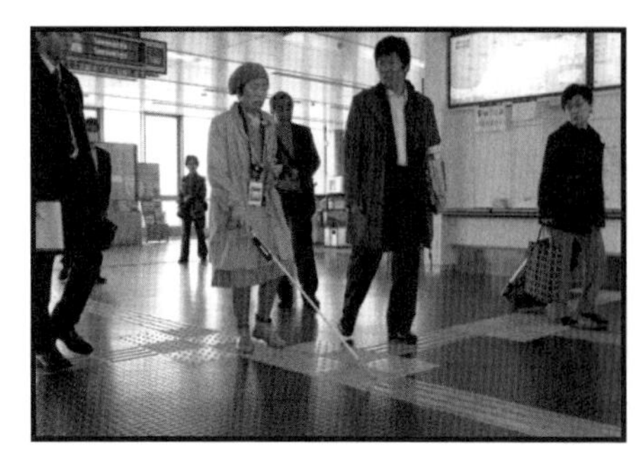
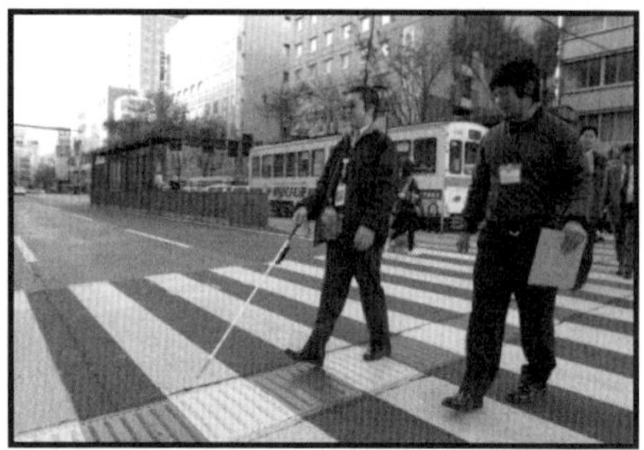

Photo 13.

chical structure of notations used there, for example. Because administration methods and rules are reflected "as is" in the hierarchical information structure, the relevant notation, the data format used for identification, might be unusable in different organizations, countries, or different applications for the same users.

Let us state this again since it is important. Meaningful numbers defined by a particular organization for a particular set of objects cannot be used easily by other organizations, countries, or private corporations.

The system we are trying to create features identification numbers that can be shared across organizations on the other hand. For this, it is not appropriate to include semantics, or meaning, in the numbers stored in tags. This is why a simple number without any other loaded meaning is used for identification in our approach [13,21].

5.4. Feasibility Study Experiments

To spread the applications of ubiquitous computing around the world, we are running many projects to embed chips to various objects and locations. (See [14,15,20] for more detailed explanations of the systems mentioned in this and the following sections.)

First of all, let me introduce "Free Mobility Assistance Project," conducted with the Ministry of Land, Infrastructure, Transport, and Tourism (MLIT). The project attempted to organize information for the challenged to walk by himself/herself. This is considered to be important in Japan, which is facing aging society with declining birth rate.

The feasibility study experiment for the Free Mobility Assistance Project has been run in Aomori, Sakai (Osaka), Kobe (Hyogo – Photo 13), Kumamoto, Wakayama, Nara, Shizuoka, and Tokyo. In this experiment, pedestrians are guided using the electronic tags embedded in the sidewalk and active tags mounted on building walls and on the street lampposts. The system serves as a pedestrian navigation using audio guide and maps on the screen for able-bodied people, and a sightseeing guide is added for tourists. On the other hand, the same infrastructure is used to guide wheelchair users along a route without steps or with elevator to help them, and to escort visually-challenged users using audio guidance to the desired location even if this is his/her first visit. To guide the visually-challenged, positional precision must be especially high on corners and pedestrian crossings. For this purpose, we are conducting an experiment to give the visually-challenged a real-time and precise guidance, by embedding RFID tags to the

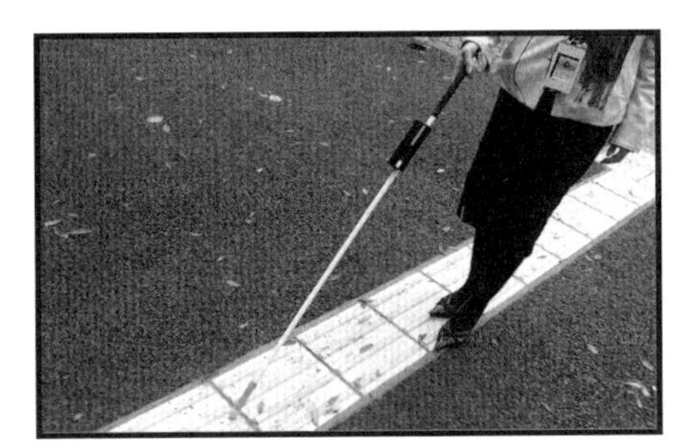

Photo 14.

key guidance blocks on the roads. The white cane carried by the visually-challenged will read the ucodes. The canes are equipped with an antenna and capable of sending the ucode to their mobile terminals (Photo 14).

We are also running experiments to detect whether or not the tags embedded in the road have failed or not, and to figure out how to reduce costs for maintenance.

Other experiments include automatic transmission of tourist information in Chinese, English, Japanese, and Korean when tourists arrive at the site, automatic streaming of a video in which the owner of the store explains his/her product whenever someone stands in front of that product, and displaying of a 3-D map to show what is ahead.

One experiment that gained much good reputation is the Ueno Zoo (Photo 15) experiment. This has been put into practical use to meet many requests of the visitors daily. With this system, users can see a video in which the zoo director himself guides visitors in the zoo, and when a user stands in front of an animal, he/she will be explained about the animal and the date when it came to the zoo. This system turned out to be very popular among the visiting children.

The Tokyo Ubiquitous Technology Project in Ginza experiment started in Dec. 2006 (Photo 16). In Ginza, for example, users can view from underground a panorama photo of view above ground. When they arrive at the subway station, the time table is displayed. This is part of a long-term study lasting for five years conducted jointly with the Tokyo Metropolitan Government, for bringing ubiquitous computing environment to a practical use in a real-world city. By creating a general-purpose ubiquitous computing environment in Ginza, we are capable of running various application experiments. This infrastructure can be used as a general-purpose research environment for any registered users. Various private experiments using the infrastructure have been conducted so far [11].

A very important aspect regarding such experiments is a decision on who should be given what, and not just the embedding of tags. Adults and children, foreign visitors and local residents, are not satisfied with the same content.

Lately, electronic tags based on the NFC standard are embedded on street lights, which can be used from mobile phones capable of reading NFC tags. This has many applications. For example, in case of emergency, people will be able to know information about evacuation routes and shelter areas. On normal occasions, the data about the store in front of the user might be given. This system is also created based on the philosophy of universal design.

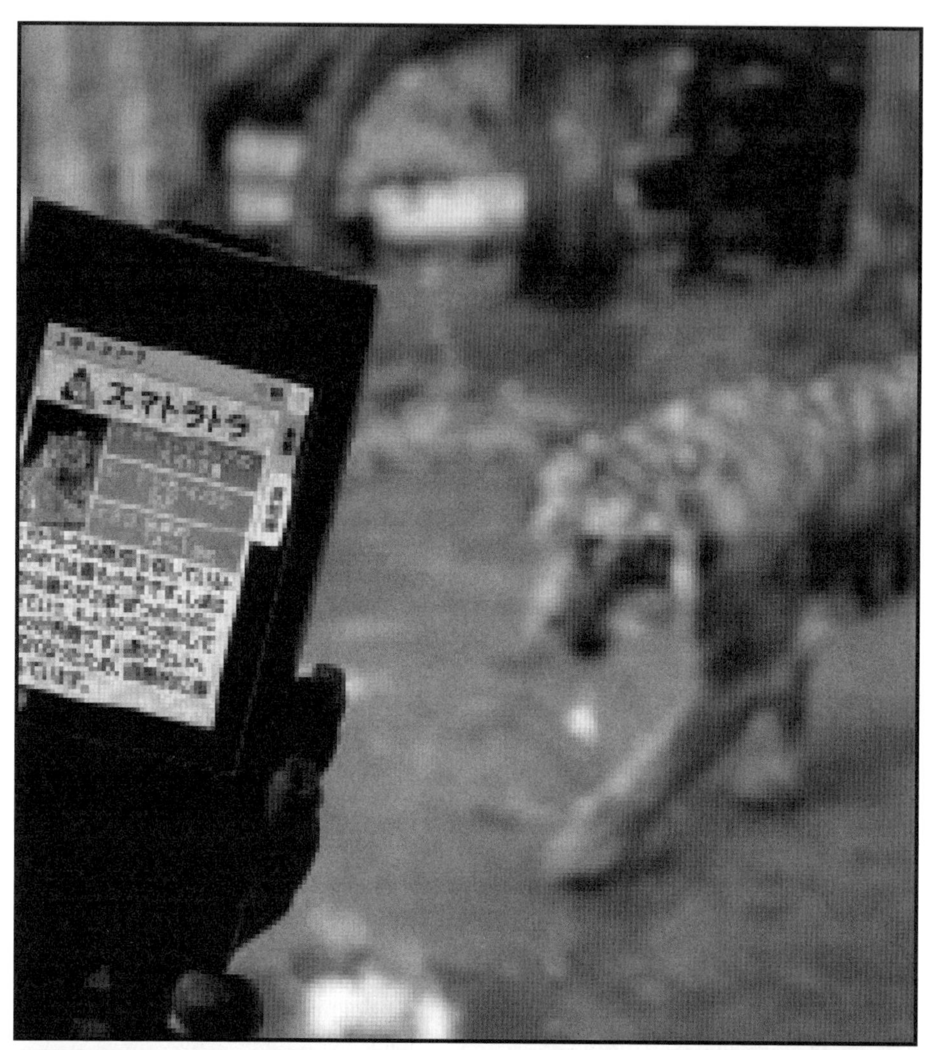

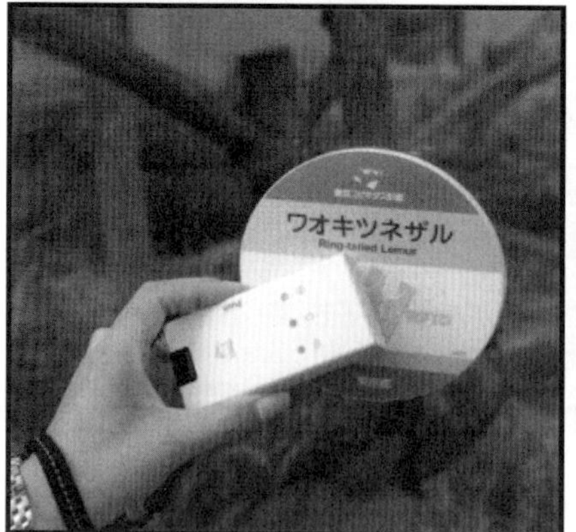

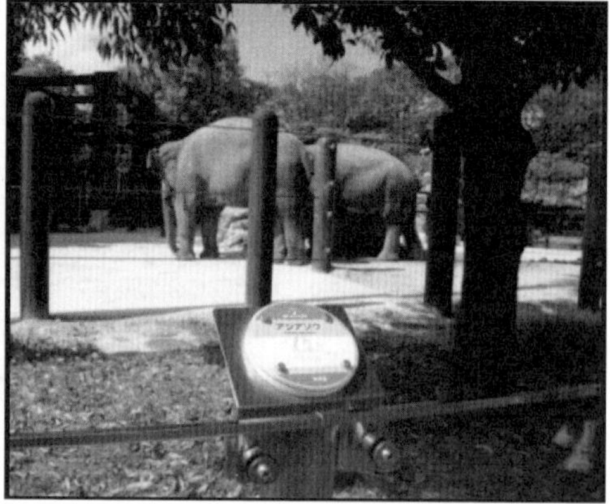

Photo 15.

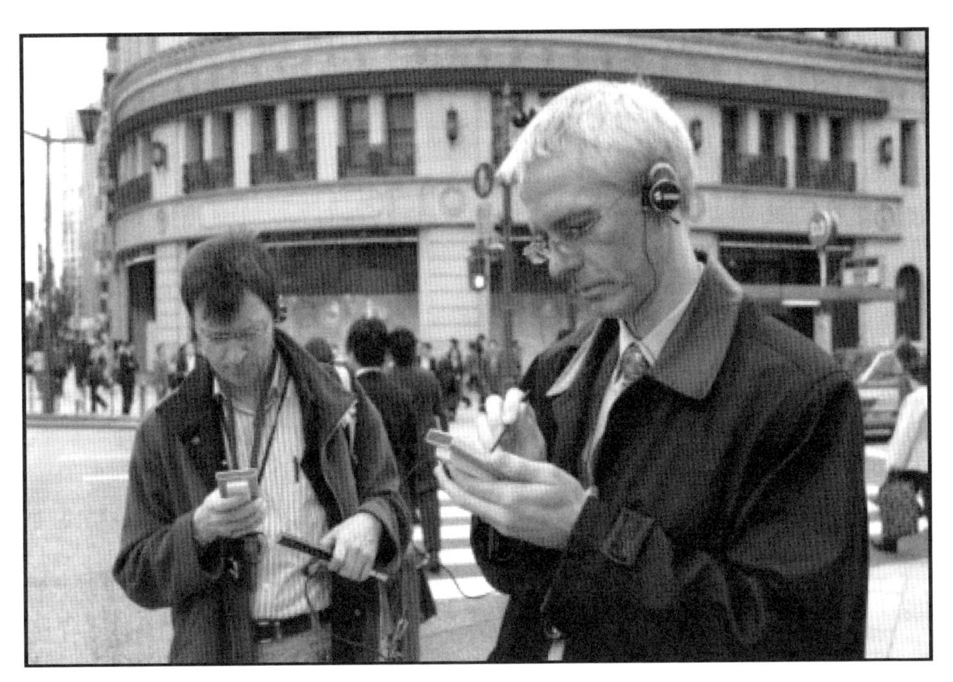

Photo 16.

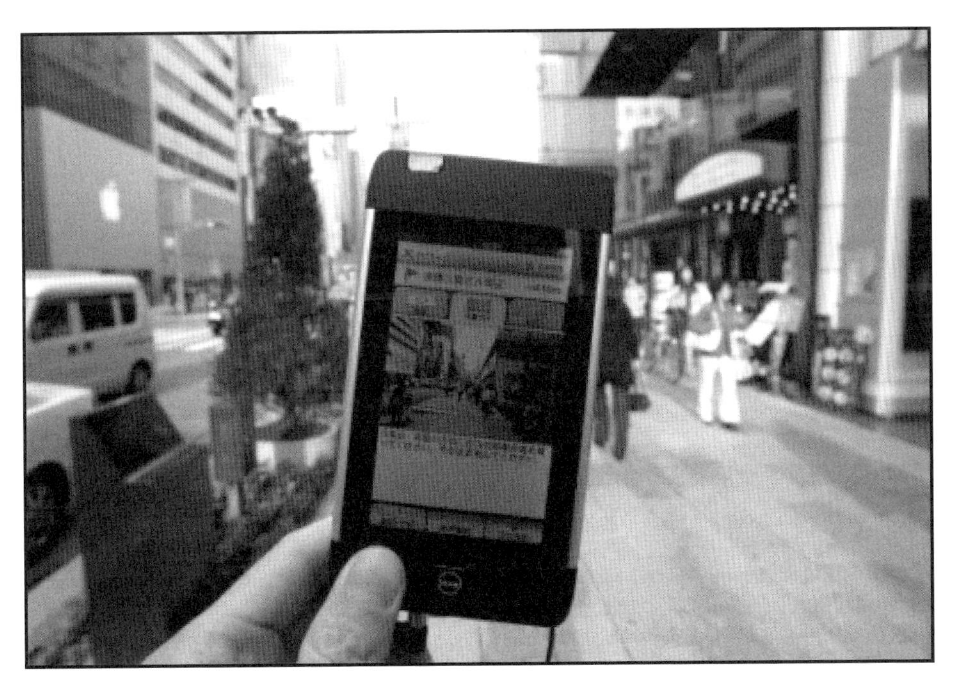

Photo 17.

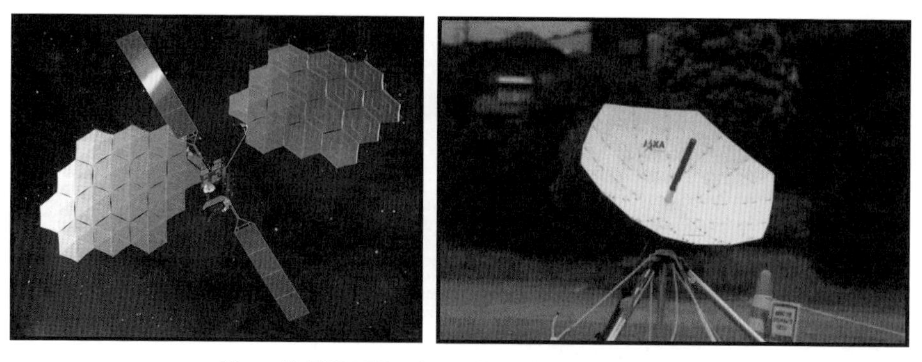

Photo 18. ETS-VIII and a small portable ground station.

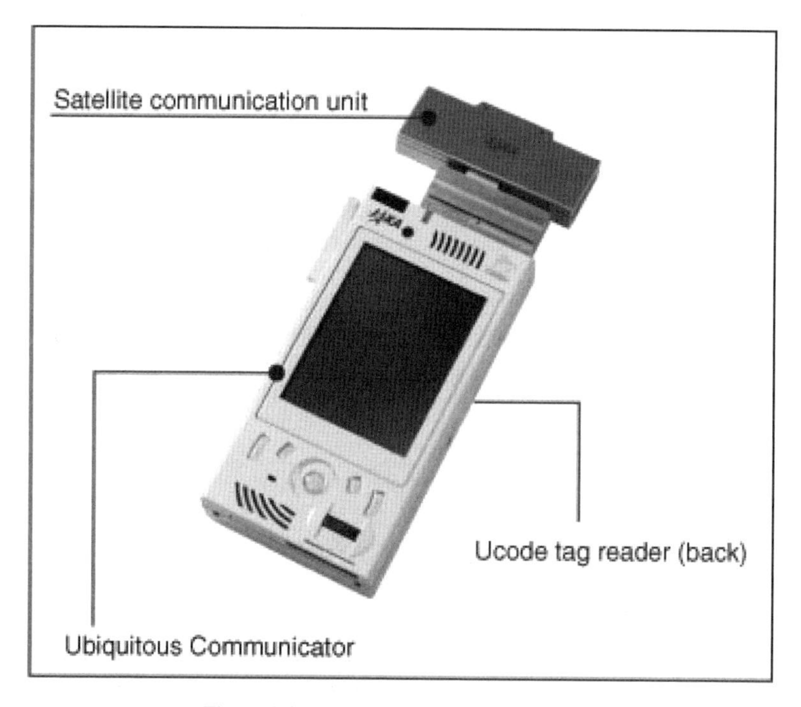

Figure 4. Satellite communication unit for UC.

5.5. From Feasibility Study Experiment to Practical Use

In a joint experiment with Japan Aerospace Exploration Agency (JAXA), we have succeeded to develop a small device to communicate directly via Ubiquitous Communicator to the digital information communication satellite ETS-VIII. ETS-VIII has a pair of antennas, about the size of two tennis courts, and thus a small unit on the ground can communicate with it directly. In this experiment, we assign ucodes to houses. In case of disaster, the residents would be able to send information such as which houses are destroyed via the satellite, so the government could get the idea of damages to the houses (Photo 18, Fig. 4).

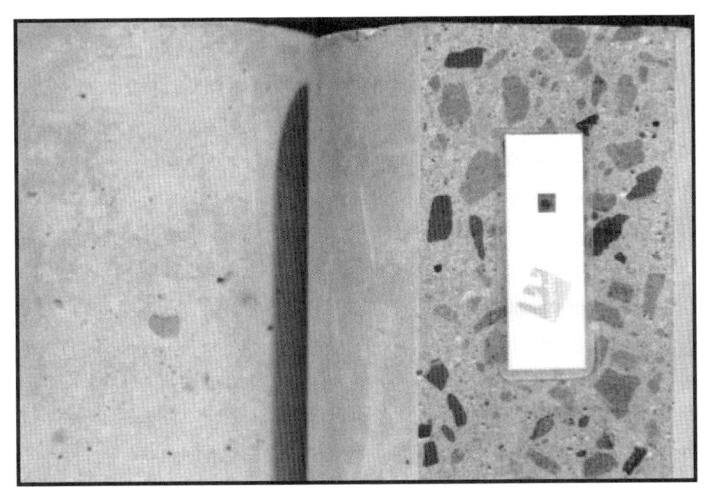

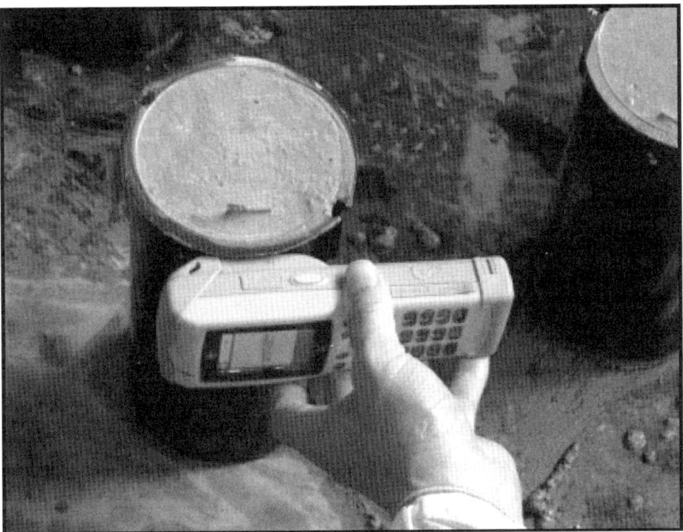

Photo 19.

If many ucodes are embedded in a building, in case the building is unfortunately destroyed, a robot can go into the building and read ucode information to send the information about which part of the building has collapsed. Particularly in case of disaster, ucodes will be of great use even when GPS is not accurate enough.

We have also succeeded in an experiment to embed RFID tags into cement and use them (Photo 19), as announced by Sumitomo Osaka Cement Co., Ltd. and YRP Ubiquitous Networking Laboratory. ucode tags are embedded at the production phase of the cement. By accessing the ucodes, information such as the manufacturer and strength of the cement or the design drawing of the building can be obtained even after years. This system has been created for long-term maintenance of cities.

6. Summary

TRON Project is a completely open project. Its application is not limited to assistive technology, but we feel it is important to organize a universal informational structure to create a social environment where assistive technology can be used widely at a lower cost. The Internet is also not limited to assistive technology, but because of its high versatility, it has spread widely in the society, and relevant devices and systems became available at a lower cost, and as a result, became useful as the basis of assistive technology. To bring this methodology beyond the world of information technology to the real world, we are trying to establish the "infrastructure for bridging virtual and real worlds." This is our ubiquitous ID architecture.

Although the project still needs time to spread its application all over the world, it is making a steady progress. We hope our experimental cases can serve as a reference for the future assistive living environment construction.

References

General Web sites
Ubiquitous ID Center: http://www.uidcenter.org/
T-Engine Forum: http://www.t-engine.org/

[1] A House of Sustainability: PAPI, Special Issue of A+U (Architecture and Urbanism), December 2005, Japan Architect Co., Ltd., ISBN4-900211-60-5 C3052.
[2] J. Begole and R. Masuoka, Search for Eden: Historic perspective and current trends toward the ubiquitous computing vision of effortless living, *Information Processing Society of Japan Magazine* **49**(6) (2008), 635–640, Original English version [online] available: http://www.parc.com/research/publications/details.php?id=6469.
[3] CASAGRAS Project web, http://www.rfidglobal.eu/.
[4] Interview: A Conversation with Jim Ready, ACM Queue, April 1, 2003, [Online] Available: http://queue.acm.org/detail.cfm?id=644261.
[5] N. Koshizuka and K. Sakamura, Ubiquitous ID: Standards for ubiquitous computing and the internet of things, *Pervasive Computing* **9**(4) (October–December 2010), 98–101.
[6] J. Krikke, T-Engine: Japan's ubiquitous computing architecture is ready for prime time, *Pervasive Computing, IEEE Computing Society* **4**(2) (April-June 2005), 4-9.
[7] D. Normile, From Japan: Intelligence with classic style, *Popular Science* (September 1990), 58–61.
[8] K. Sakamura, TRON – Total Architecture, in: *Proceedings of Architecture Workshop in Japan '84*, Information Processing Society of Japan, August 1984, pp. 41–50.
[9] See for example, Pervasive Computing magazine, Published by IEEE Computer Society.
[10] H. Sundmaeker, P. Guillemin, P. Friess and S. Woelffle, Vision and Challenges for Realizsing the Internet of Things, March 2010, CERPP-IOT.
[11] Tokyo Ubiquitous Technology Project, online available: http://www.tokyoubinavi.jp/index_en.html.
[12] TRON Project 1987 Open Architecture Computer Systems, Springer Verlag, ISBN 97803877002.
[13] Ubiquitous ID Center, Ubiquitous ID architecture, 910-S002-0.00.24, [online] available: http://www.uidcenter.org/.
[14] Ubiquitous ID Center, Ubiquitous ID Technologies 2009, [online] available: http://www.uidcenter.org/.
[15] Ubiquitous ID Center, Ubiquitous ID Technologies 2011, [online] available: http://www.uidcenter.org/.
[16] M. Weiser, *The Computer for the 21st Century*, Scientific American, 1991.
[17] YouTube Ubiquitous ID Center Channel, PAPI: The 2nd TRON Smart House In Japan, [online] available: http://www.youtube.com/watch?v=vyhO6y2nUOU.
[18] YouTube Ubiquitous ID Center Channel, TRON Smart House, [online] available: http://www.youtube.com/watch?v=7jPKEyM44GU.
[19] YouTube Ubiquitous ID Center Channel, u-Home, [online] available: http://www.youtube.com/watch?v=nfd1ecaVenY.

[20] YouTube Ubiquitous ID Center Channel, uID Application, [online] available: http://www.youtube.com/watch?v=Y193LQUZqW4.
[21] YouTube Ubiquitous ID Center Channel, uID_Architecture, [online] available: http://www.youtube.com/watch?v=mo8s2S78EOc.

Applications of Ambient Assisted Living in Rehabilitation

Handbook of Ambient Assisted Living
J.C. Augusto et al. (Eds.)
IOS Press, 2012

doi:10.3233/978-1-60750-837-3-495

Introduction to Section on AAL for Rehabilitation

Reiner WICHERT*
Fraunhofer-Allianz Ambient Assisted Living, Darmstadt, Germany

Abstract. Rehabilitation techniques in Ambient Assisted Living, which concentrates on supporting persons with special needs, is viewed as one of the most promising areas of AAL (Ambient Assisted Living). Thus these technologies for rehabilitation constitute a major research area within AAL research. A large number of new technologies have been developed in R&D projects for rehabilitation in recent years. Lots of project results in form of applications and prototypes have been developed. This section contains important work on technologies to support people with chronic obstructive pulmonary disease, on robotics for remote motor rehabilitation, smart home technologies to help people with cognitive impairments, Tele-Rehabilitation approaches, Cardiac Rehabilitation solutions and Computer Vision Access Technologies, but all focused on Ambient Assisted Rehabilitation. Authors from Northern America, Australia and Europe highlighted their work in Ambient Assisted Rehabilitation in the following six chapters.

Keywords. AAL, cardiovascular disease, rehabilitation, case study, stroke, robotics, virtual environments

Content

The following chapters describe the main challenges in AAL rehabilitation. One of the most emerging fields in this area is Tele-Rehabilitation. Therefore the first chapter "ICT Infrastructures for Tele-Rehabilitation" aims to optimize the process of rehabilitation by using efficient information exchange methods between different stakeholders. It describes the relevance of this field with regard to medical and business aspects. Here the focus lays on cost-effective medical treatment processes and financial savings in the health care system. For this reason an architectural approach with its building block components will be suggested which are able to serve together as a toolbox for efficiently implementing Tele-Rehabilitation applications, which have been implemented in several projects.

The second chapter "AAL in Cardiac Rehabilitation" illustrates individually adapted physical exercise training under medical supervision as an important building block in the rehabilitation and secondary prevention for patients with cardiovascular diseases with help of AAL technology. Lifelong exercises are a necessity to avoid further cardiac events. Here training within the home environment seems to be an appropriate approach. The chapter shows how the risk of an adverse cardiovascular event could be reduced by an individually adjusted exercise training application. It describes the components controlling a training session, which needs to recognize critical patient

* Corresponding Author: Reiner Wichert. E-mail. reiner.wichert@igd.fraunhofer.de.

states through a continuous monitoring of vital signs and the according reaction. The system allows detecting heart issues further in advance and makes it possible for the system to react before further medical issues actually arise.

The next chapter "Smart Home Technologies for People with Cognitive Impairment: An Affordable, Rehabilitative Approach" examines functional assessment for living at home and provides a model for retrofitting existing homes for inexpensive smart home solutions. It additionally describes available tools for improving home-based everyday support. Psychosocial implications of smart home utilization e.g. why therapists are strongly urged to learn about smart home technologies and to appropriately facilitate their use in helping people live safely and independently at home will be illustrated.

The chapter "AAL Technologies in Rehabilitation – Lessons learned from a COPD Case Study" shows that existing R&D lacks treatment of organizational issues related to AAL technologies e.g. re-engineering of existing work practices, training and on-the-job learning of care personnel and support for collaborative workflows. It outlines the research methodology used in order to identify the key technology goals of the AAL research programmes. To achieve this it analyzes the results from European R&D projects within the area of rehabilitation, in terms of technologies, services, requirements and scenarios, which is then used to identify potential gaps between European AAL roadmaps and funding goals and additionally discusses the findings from the COPD@Home project.

Sensors, Virtual Reality, and robotic systems have been increasingly useful for augmenting traditional motor rehabilitation techniques and thus for the remote monitoring of individuals in a number of environments. Therefore the fifth chapter "Assisted Ambient Living Applied to Remote Motor Rehabilitation" present exciting results from current literature, as well as their own work, that indicate promising directions for ambient assisted living techniques in the field of stroke rehabilitation. Such monitoring can lead to increased quality of life. It discusses how AAL techniques can be used to provide motor rehabilitation in ambient environments to individuals who have suffered from stroke and focus on various rehabilitation techniques for stroke that make use of robotics, sensors, virtual reality, and other technologies to transfer clinical practices and techniques to individuals in ambient environments.

This section ends with the chapter "Home-based computer vision access technologies for individuals with severe motor impairments" which introduces contactless home-based access technologies that exploit computer vision via cameras, operating in the visible or infrared light spectrum. For individuals with severe disabilities, home-based access to communication, computer and environmental controls can prove to be a non-trivial challenge. Here the user interacts with the environment using gross movements of the limbs, trunk or head and via gestures. After introducing the fundamentals of each technology, clinical illustrations of how these technologies have been applied in the home or community setting will be described. The chapter concludes with a discussion of the pros and cons and the limitations of computer vision-based access technologies.

Reflection

Even a lot of very good approaches have yet been realized in the area of rehabilitation in AAL, the market breakthrough has still not been achieved. A few gaps can be deducted from recent projects and concluded from the following chapters of this section e.g. the missing support for learning and training of users, the up to now low support for collaboration among different organizational units in the rehabilitation process, and the worse integrality of solutions with legacy systems. A related issue is also the lack of research on the services that will be enabled based on the technological solutions. A stronger service orientation of the approach will help to move the whole technology solutions into a cloud-based approach, driven by the metaphor of "Reha-Apps from an AAL-eHealth-Store". As a result, patients will be able in the future to access rehabilitation services on demand.

On the other side at the current point in time such systems are still in a prototype state and more research will be needed to raise them to product level. Furthermore, legal limitations such as medical device certification and emergency guidelines have to be taken into account. Nevertheless systems using context based vital sign estimation are apparently safer even today than using no alarm management at all and leaving the patient out alone.

The further chapters will provide more insights on these conclusions and will explain why these implications have been deducted.

Handbook of Ambient Assisted Living
J.C. Augusto et al. (Eds.)
IOS Press, 2012

doi:10.3233/978-1-60750-837-3-498

ICT Infrastructures for Telerehabilitation

Wolfgang DEITERS*, Oliver KOCH, Thomas KÖNIGSMANN and Sven MEISTER
Fraunhofer Institute for Software and Systems Engineering, Dortmund, Germany

Abstract. Telerehabilitation is an emerging field that aims at optimizing the process of rehabilitation by using efficient information exchange methods between different stakeholders. A wide range of technologies have been developed to facilitate this exchange using monolithic application architectures. These architectures are often the reason why projects fail due to disproportionate investment of money and time as well as lack of knowledge. In this paper, we present an overview of projects in the field of telerehabilitation and telemedicine based on the so called CHOPIN architecture, a toolbox for composition of telemedical services into high quality applications. It facilitates reuse and leverage of existing services and components, thus reducing costs and work efforts with each new application that is implemented on the basis of CHOPIN. Our future prospects will focus on even stronger service orientation of the approach developing the whole technology towards a cloud-based approach driven by the metaphor of "Reha-Apps from an AAL-eHealth-Store".

Keywords. Telerehabilitation, infrastructure, platform, telemedicine, SOA

1. Introduction

Ambient Assisted Living (AAL) technology is mainly being discussed in the context of demographic change, aiming to support elderly people to live independently in their homes for as long as possible. One major field of application is providing medical services or observing vital body parameters (such as blood pressure, heart beat rates etc.) in order to monitor physical conditions or diseases.

However, many of these services were not specifically developed for elderly people, but they are as important for them as for any other person suffering from diverse illnesses. Taking this into account, the importance of considering AAL technology and telemedicine as an overall concept becomes evident.

Within the following paper, we therefore want to extend the scope of AAL applications towards telemedicine, especially telerehabilitation, due to the relevance of this field with regard to medical and business aspects. An AAL based approach towards telemedicine could not only considerably improve quality of medical treatment of a patient. It could also contribute to cost-effective medical treatment processes and financial savings in the health care system.

The paper is organized as follows: In the next section we discuss the range of telerehabilitation services, followed by a look at related work, i.e. applications that have already been developed. In Section 3 we present an architecture for telerehabilitation applications. This architecture and building block components are able to serve together as a toolbox for efficiently implementing telerehabilitation applications supporting

*Corresponding Author: Wolfgang Deiters. E-mail: wolfgang.deiters@isst.fraunhofer.de.

specific diseases. Section 4 illustrates different applications. These applications have partly been employed as use cases defining requirements for developing the architecture. The implementation is partly based on the architecture. In this way our architecture has been developed and evaluated in an incremental way, driven by concrete applications. Finally, we conclude by summing up and indicating future steps.

2. Range of Telerehabilitation Services/Applications

The relevance of telemedicine applications in the healthcare sector has grown over the last 10 years [2,18]. Telemedicine is understood as the delivery of medical services (diagnosis, therapy, control etc.) to patients or clinicians/therapists/care providers by bridging geographical and/or temporal distances via telecommunication networks and/or the internet. By analogy with the wide range of medical services a great variety of telemedicine application areas has evolved, e.g. telecardiology, teleradiology, teledermatology, telepathology, teleneurology or telepsychiatry.

A further application area is telerehabilitation. In a simple form of definition, telerehabilitation can be described as the delivery of rehabilitation services over telecommunication networks and/or the internet. The different aspects and specific characteristics of telerehabilitation become particularly clear by looking at the approaches of the American Occupational Therapy Association (AOTA) and the Telerehabilitation Research Unit of the University of Queensland:

"*Telerehabilitation is the clinical application of consultative, preventative, diagnostic, and therapeutic services via two-way interactive telecommunication technology.*" [17]

"[...] *the provision of conventional rehabilitation services at a distance using telecommunication technology as the service delivery medium. It is an alternate means of providing all aspects of care including the interview, physical assessment and diagnosis, intervention, maintenance activities, consultation, education and training to clients at remote locations.*" [13]

Basically the "tele" aspect of telerehabilitation is not thus limited to specific diseases or indications. In practice there are certainly limitations of transforming conventional rehabilitation services into telerehabilitation services. The key aspect of these services is the virtualization of the communication relation between clinicians/therapists/care providers and patients. So, the following fields of application have indicated a significantly high benefit of supporting this relation and enabling these innovative services:

- Cardiac Rehabilitation (e.g. myocardial infarction, by-pass operation).
- Neurological Rehabilitation (e.g. traumatic brain injury, stroke, Parkinson's disease, spinal column injuries).
- Sports Medical Rehabilitation (e.g. sports injuries or war wounded).
- Oncological Rehabilitation.
- Psychiatric Disorder (e.g. depression, anorexia).
- Rehabilitation for Hearing-impaired People.
- Language Disorders, Speech Impediments and Dysphasia.
- Psychosomatic Rehabilitation (especially addicts).

Telerehabilitation has many advantages for patients and also for clinicians/ therapists/care providers. Modern telecommunication technologies and internet services facilitate innovative rehab services [3]. Transport costs and time can be saved for both, patients and the health care system. This also has a potential environmental impact by reducing travel expenses (according to "green healthcare"). Telerehabilitation services which are available in a 24/7-mode, can ensure continuity of patient care. They also improve the ability to monitor timing, intensity and sequencing of rehabilitation intervention. The positive effects of reducing healthcare costs and enabling patients to *convalesce* in their home environment should also not be underestimated [15].

From a technical point of view different technologies are used to facilitate a wide range of telerehabilitation services. These technologies can be differentiated into image-based technologies, sensor-based technologies, virtual environments and virtual reality [13]. Image-based technologies, especially videoconferencing, which were one of the first developed telerehabilitation services, are widespread and used especially in sparsely populated regions and countries. Sensor-based technologies enable the remote monitoring of rehabilitation-relevant physical parameters (e.g. cardiological parameters or motion parameters). Initiatives like the Continua Health Alliance [5] are deeply engaged in defining generally accepted standards for the communication and integration of these "biosignals" into healthcare scenarios. Virtual reality-based telerehabilitation systems use three-dimensional virtual environments. These environments can be displayed to patients via computer monitors or fully-immersive environments (head-mounted displays or haptic feedback devices). Patients have to perform specific movements in the context of their rehabilitation program.

One key barrier for the further diffusion and extension of the range of telerehabilitation services is their reimbursement. Private and public authorities are still reluctant to finance corresponding services. Some of the research (Chapter 2) set the focus on demonstrating the equivalence of telerehabilitation assessment and therapy to in-person assessment and therapy.

3. Related Work

As a sub discipline of telemedicine the history of telerehabilitation is closely connected to the history of telemedicine. Although the first beginnings of telemedicine research date back to the 1950s, the breakthrough came with the introduction of low-cost high-speed internet connections, high-performance computer hardware and innovative sensor technologies at the beginning of the 21st century. In 1998 the first Rehabilitation Engineering Research Center (RERC) on telerehabilitation was founded by the U.S. American National Institute on Disability and Rehabilitation Research (NIDRR).[1]

Ever since different medical facilities, rehabilitation centers and research institutes in North America, Australia and Europe have started research on the different aspects of telerehabilitation. Examples for such organizations are in the United States the Rutgers Telerehabilitation Institute RERC on Telerehabilitation, the Rehabilitation Institute of Chicago or the National Rehabilitation Hospital in Washington DC, in Australia the University of Queensland or in Germany (as example for Europe) the Institut für angewandte Telemedizin (IFAT).

[1] http://mcn.ed.psu.edu/dbm/newsletter3/DeRuyter_AAC_RERC.pdf.

The focus of telerehabilitation research projects varies depending on the main objective of the research activities:

1. As already mentioned the reimbursement of telerehablitation services depends on the equivalence of conventional rehabilitation and telerehabilitation. So, some of the research projects try to demonstrate for example the comparability of therapeutic success based on web-based training or face-to-face therapy sessions.
2. Development of new telerehabilitation services or service aspects by integrating innovative technologies (e.g. virtual reality, telehaptics). These services do have an extended range of functions in comparison with conventional rehabilitation services. They can contribute to improving the quality of rehabilitation.
3. Building new data collection systems to digitize information that a therapist can use in practice. Especially medical sensor technologies increase the amount of data and information. Because of the huge amount of available data, it might be necessary to implement appropriate information logistic functions to avoid information overload.

One or more of these objectives can be found in every research project concerning telerehabilitation. The variety of telerehabilitation projects of the United States, Australia and Germany should give an exemplary insight into the range of telerehabilitation projects:

- PlayStation 3-based telerehabilitation for children with hemiplegia (Rutgers University):
  Researchers from the University of Indiana and the Rutgers University modified a PlayStation 3 game console to help children with hemiplegia to improve their hand functions. Because of the resulting telerehabilitation station children can play customized therapy-orientated games. Researchers can oversee the participants' session data.
- Telerehabilitation enhanced wellness program in spina bifida (RERC on Telerahabilitation, University of Pittsburgh):
  One project at the University of Pittsburgh aims to develop specially designed applications for smartphones supporting persons with spina bifida and other disabilities with cognitive deficits in their daily life. The study wants to show that wireless telerahabilitation tools will improve the self-management of health routines and conditions.
- Internet multidisciplinary assessment following traumatic brain injury (University of Queensland):
  The University of Queensland has various projects in the field of telerehabilitation. The projects are mostly designed to help people with diseases in rural Australia or other remote locations. The goal of one project for example is to determine the feasibility and accuracy of performing multidisciplinary assessments of patients with traumatic brain injury via the internet using videoconferencing.
- Internet assessment of upper limb range of motion following stroke (University of Queensland):
  Another project at the University of Queensland wants to demonstrate the ability to measure the upper limb range of motion in people who have had a stroke via the internet with a recently developed internet-based goniometer.

- Saphire:
  The software developed at the clinic of Herzogenaurach in cooperation with the company Evosoft Tele Care in the Saphire project offers the possibility to compile existing and proved training software in the fields of neurolinguistics and neuropsychology to an individual training package for patients. After an appropriate briefing the patients can train at home and the therapist gets the automatically generated data of training time, duration and achievements.

4. Architecture

Driven by different projects in the area of telemedicine and AAL we recognized that there exists a large number of software-architectural realizations. Nevertheless, only a small proportion of projects are realized in practice. Frequent reasons for the failure of other projects are the lack of working business models, knowledge deficits regarding the characteristics of the healthcare domain, and monolithic application architectures that make continuous software maintenance, adaptations to changing demands, and interoperability with other systems necessary. These modifications are highly expensive and difficult to realize.

We conclude that single telemedicine projects, which want to meet all requirements mentioned before tend to fail [10]. It is hardly feasible to concentrate on the application-specific functionality while also investigating aspects of interoperability and stakeholder autonomy; this especially applies to small and medium-sized companies. Consequently, the demand for a common framework arises that provides the basis for various telemedical applications by implementing application-independent, basic functionalities.

To facilitate the implementation of telemedicine and AAL projects, new methodologies and technologies in software-development have to be researched. Based upon two projects named E-Health@Home and Telemedizin-Repository the FraunhoferInstitute for Software and Systems Engineering began to define and develop a service-oriented framework for telemedicine- and AAL-services. The framework is called CHOPIN [11] (Composition of Healthcare services through Open Platform Integration) and has to fulfill the following characteristics:

- The framework should not be a universal world model but highly specialized to the domain of telemedicine and AAL.
- The framework is based on the idea of encapsulating business logic into services to facilitate the reuse of software. A service defined and developed for a scenario should be reusable.
- The framework makes no claim to be complete. It defines a scaffold to develop telemedicine and AAL services in a time- and cost-efficient way.
- The framework has to offer a set of methodologies to foster its continuous evolution.

Furthermore, the framework has to take into account requirements like data security and privacy, interoperability, modularity, overcoming technical barriers, ensuring autonomy of stakeholders and the adaption to business models.

Referring to Fig. 1, the resulting concept for the framework consists of three layers called horizontals which are interconnected using two layers called verticals. It conse-

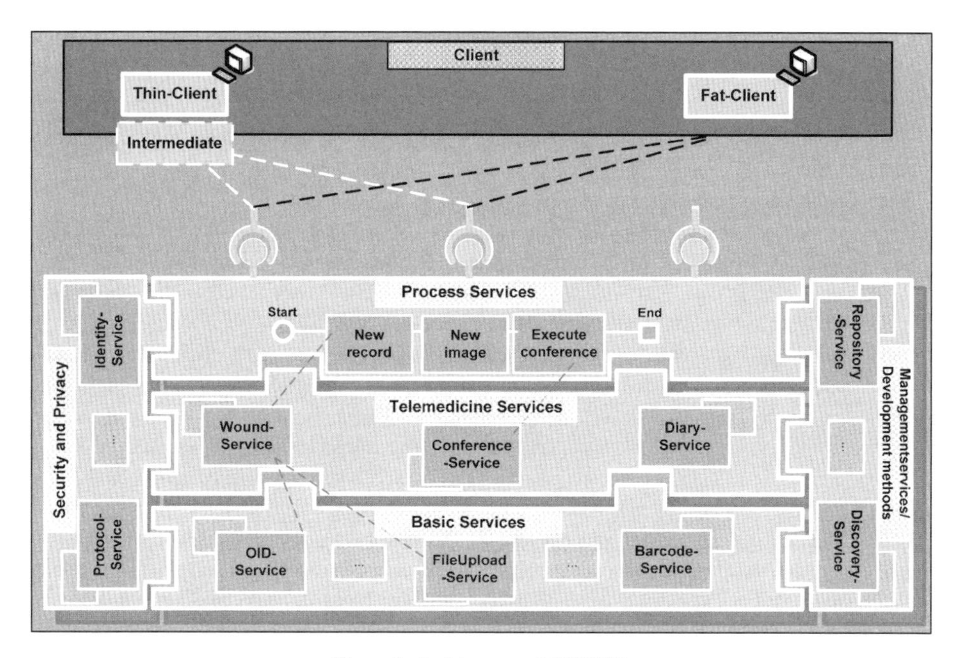

Figure 1. Architecture of CHOPIN.

quently relies on modular, distributed development of services [6], reuse, and decentrally organized collaboration networks. Some of the above-mentioned requirements have already been fulfilled on an architectural level.

The horizontal layers represent three levels of granularity which should be used to develop telemedicine and AAL services. In *principle*, the basic service layer wants to integrate services with a high potential for being reused. Basic services provide functionality, which does not require a domain-specific dimension. They represent the smallest unit of the framework that is the maximum level of decomposition of an application. In contrast to basic services, telemedicine services on the next higher layer are closely related to the healthcare domain and are often developed with regard to specific telemedical applications. They act as an orchestrator of basic services and require a minor percentage of implementation. By employing process-oriented telemedicine services, the framework provides methods for orchestrating services according to the requirements of the respective setting. Process-oriented telemedicine services envelop process fragments that are not supposed to represent complete processes but manageable components that can be used by various telemedical applications. These services do not normally have implementation parts but orchestrate telemedicine services based on expert knowledge.

Besides the horizontals, the verticals are the second pillar of the framework. They are rather a set of methodologies and concepts than implementations. For now the framework consists of two verticals, one representing security concepts and one containing management and development methodologies which are initially composed of:

- Requirements-Engineering: Only a project with a well defined catalogue of requirements can lead to a successful product [9,10]. Especially projects in the healthcare sector need the expertise of heterogeneous project teams. There are technical experts who have to work together with physicians and other skilled experts. CHOPIN defines a methodology to gather requirements in a structured and comprehensive way. Once gathered, they are classified, structured and saved in a requirements-repository so that they are reusable. Over the years the repository becomes a knowledge base with invaluable expert know-how.

- Software development process: There is a need for a well-defined software development process using service-based technologies. The typical models like the waterfall model or the spiral model do not reflect the development process. In the last few years enhanced research activities in this area produced new software development processes, adapted to the needs of service-oriented architectures. CHOPIN functions as a repository that collects those new processes and makes them comparable. By now two processes named Service-Oriented Modeling Framework (SOMF) and Service-Oriented Design and Development (SOAD) are the preferred ones [16].
- Security and privacy concepts: In Germany a large amount of regulations protects the privacy and security of personal data [4]. Particularly health data have to be protected against abuse. To ensure a secure transport of data, IT-infrastructures have to take advantage of confidentiality, integrity, authenticity, availability, validity, reliability, traceability, legal liability and non-deniability concepts. The chances given by the modularity of the framework also create security issues for example: How can a secure transport be guaranteed in a loose coupled world of services? The security-concepts indicated in the vertical pillar of the framework describe how the requirements mentioned above could be fulfilled. They are based upon existing standards like the WS-* family and proofed technologies like Public-Key-Infrastructures [1].

5. Applications

The CHOPIN framework presented in Section 4 is based on experience gained while developing telemedicine applications. The framework summarizes expertise and best practices for IT solutions in the health care market. In the following sections we will present some of these applications that were realized using the CHOPIN approach. With the help of these applications we want to show, how such a framework can improve the development process to reduce costs and other expenses.

In a first step we will introduce the "wound consultation", which was the first application that was realized with the framework. This application was used to gather requirements and collect practical experiences in the usage of such frameworks. In a second step, an application for "back pain" is introduced to show how existing components taken from the "wound consultation" can be used to speed up the development of applications that addresses other indications and participants. As third application the "digital companion" is presented. We will demonstrate how the framework can be used for a redevelopment of (older) existing telemedicine applications to bring them to the state-of-the-art of science and technology. Finally, we show an application in the area of the "alternative health care market". We believe that this is a very promising field for new telemedicine services that will greatly profit from the proposed framework.

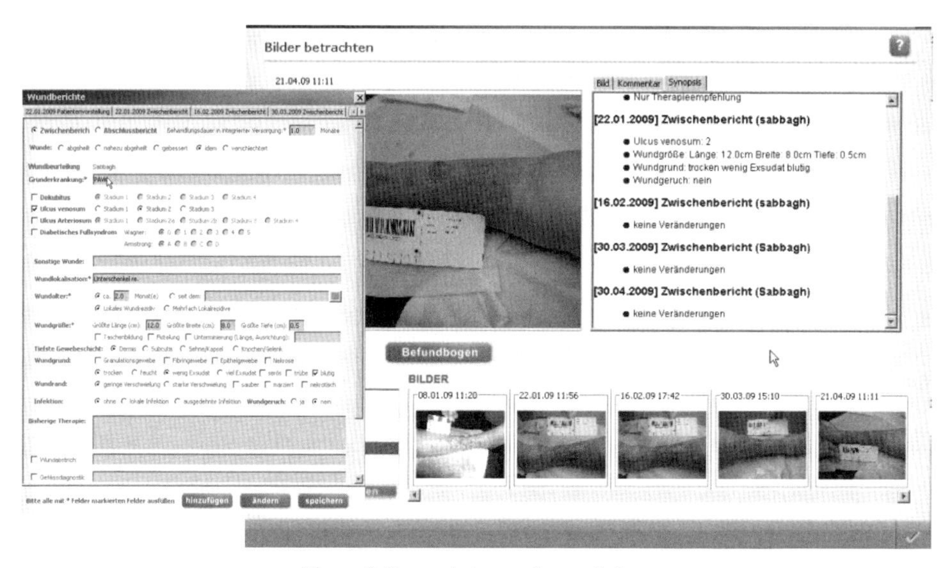

Figure 2. Screenshot wound consultation.

6. Wound Consultation

Due to aging population and significant growth in incidence of diabetes mellitus, the number of patients with wound healing problems is continually increasing. Frequently, wound management requires multidisciplinary expert knowledge over a long period of time. The first application that was developed based on the CHOPIN framework was a telemedical wound consultation. In December 2008, the hospital "Evangelisches Krankenhaus Witten" and a local network of doctors "Ärztliche Qualitätsgemeinschaft Witten" started to use this tool. Patients with chronic wounds had the opportunity to participate in a telemedical wound consultation, where different physicians from the hospital and the local network of doctors could access wound pictures and medical findings. Aim of the wound consultation was to collect the expertise of different disciplines like dermatologist, experts on diabetes and surgeons to enhance therapy plans and give fast response of different experts. In connection with the cooperation of the hospital the objective was to improve the information flow between the hospital and the attending physician.

This kind of telemedicine application is well known and good documented in the community. As a first application, it was a proof of concept for the CHOPIN framework and a source for requirements analysis. The software is based on a Java Web Start Client that is connected to a telemedical application platform, based on a Glassfish Application Server. A Java based client was chosen because the patient master file, medical findings and wound pictures need an encryption that was realized by software certificates.

The telemedical application platform delivers the following services:

- a health record (based on eFA [12]) where all data (patient master file, medical findings, wound pictures, diagnostic findings for the wound picture) are stored. This component is one of the core elements of this application and realizes the security specification that is given by the eFA,

- a bar code generator and reader, which allows an automatic allocation from pictures to wound records,
- an automatic white balance and adjustment of picture size,
- a task list for each physician,
- a printable wound history,
- standardized wound documentation sheets,
- PDF generator.

Since 2008 more than 300 patients have been registered in the wound consultation. The quality of the treatment has improved and the costs have decreased due to the fact that fewer specialists have been contacted. In addition, the number of patients transported to hospital by ambulance services has been reduced.

7. Back Pain

Back pain is a very common complaint. About three in four adults will experience back pain during their lifetime. The number will probably increase in the future because of the aging population and the problem of obesity. Depending on the severity level of a spinal disease, the medical treatment can be a long-running process, in which a number of different healthcare specialists participate.

In order to facilitate the cooperation between stakeholders and to contribute to patient empowerment, a telemedical application was developed that based on the following functional requirements:

- Appropriate visualization of treatment plans for physicians and patients.
- Change of states of treatment processes by physicians.
- Possibility to customize treatment plans to individual needs of patients.
- Integration of value-added services for physicians and patients (e.g. process-oriented and quality-ensured information supply, appointment reminders, secure conversation and message delivery etc.).

Health professionals get access to the application via web browser. Patients get access by using a mobile device, e.g. an iPhone. Furthermore, an access via home television was realized using remote control for interaction (set-top-box). Elderly people have the possibility to employ the telemedical application at home.

Following the component-based approach basic services (health record, security, authorization) from the wound consultation application are used. So the focus was set on the realization of the treatment plans.

In order to provide a common view for physicians and patients on the treatment of spinal diseases, we specified an electronic treatment plan consisting of three types of elements. Milestones divide the plan into treatment sections, such as diagnostics, minimal-invasive therapy, surgery, rehabilitation, after-care and prevention. Each section consists of a sequence of treatment steps that describe medical tasks and are connected via sequential control flow constructs. After each milestone, it is possible to flexibly choose the next treatment section. Both, electronic treatment plans as well as treatment steps correspond to XML documents. In this way, it is possible to refer to HL7 basic data types and to establish a basis for interoperability. For each treatment step, it is possible to define telemedical services. In our current implementation, we realized an

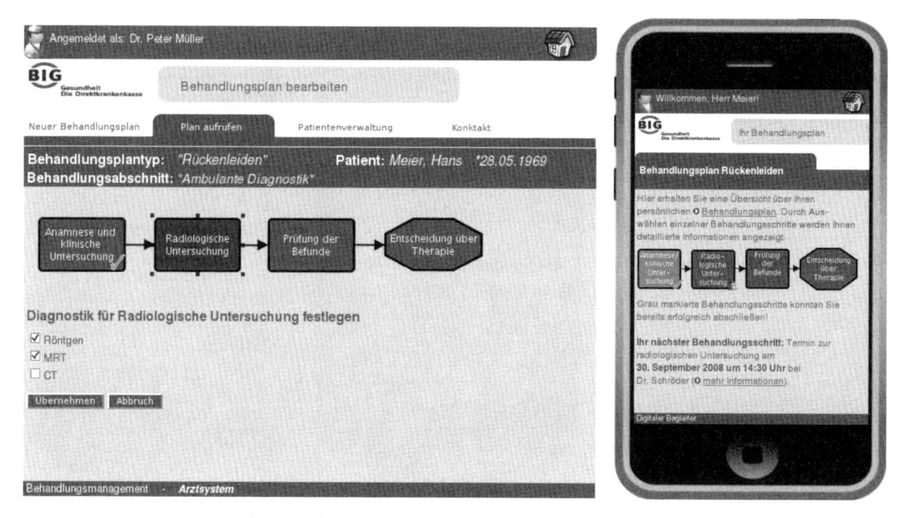

Figure 3. Screenshot Web-Client and mobile device.

information service providing qualified information for patients according to treatment steps, an appointment reminder service for patients and a message service that facilitates communication between physicians and patients.

This application was implemented/developed on behalf of a German health insurance company using CHOPIN. The concept is not limited to the management of spinal diseases, but can be transferred to other diagnoses.

8. Adiposity/Obesity

Digital health companions describe information logistics systems, which assist patients with chronic diseases in their daily life and try to support them to live healthier. The adiposity companion which supports adipose patients after hospital treatment in the follow-up period is one example for such an information system.

The Gelderland clinic comes with over 15 years experience in the hospital treatment of patients with adiposity caused by psychosomatic reasons. The clinic observed that the positive results (weight loss, attitude change) achieved in their special treatment programs could not be kept up over a longer period. In spite of highly motivated patients they are often overstrained in their daily life and risk to fall back into old behavior patterns.

In 2003 the Gelderland clinic and Fraunhofer Institute for Software and Systems Engineering started working on a personalized adiposity companion (in the form of a PDA), which should be used by patients in the follow-up period after hospital adiposity treatment. Newly learned behavior patterns in the hospital treatment are also trained "at home" by dialog transmitted self control techniques and psychological help.

In 2003 the first digital health companion was developed. Because of lacking important telemedicine communication and security standards a redevelopment using the CHOPIN approach was necessary. The idea behind the redevelopment was to extract existing source code and encapsulate it into reusable telemedicine services. The digital companion is based on plenty of smaller telemedicine applications like a protocol of

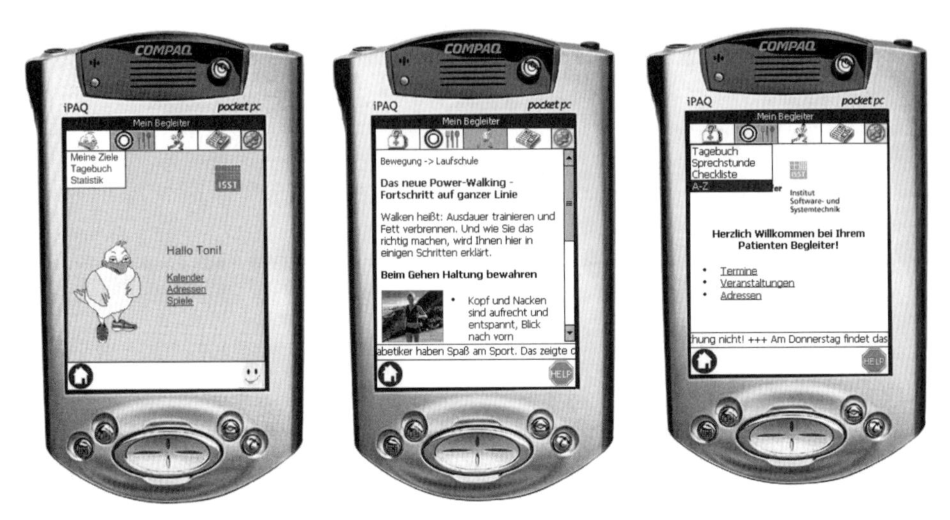

Figure 4. Screenshots digital companion.

ADL (Activity of Daily Living), food and sport plans, communication services, behavior checklists, cookbook and many more. Over 20 services were identified that are necessary for this kind of telemedicine support.

The primal implementation based on a typical three-tier architecture using a special client implementation for the mobile device. The main task was to transfer this architecture to the service-oriented CHOPIN approach. The redevelopment of the digital companion required the following steps:

- Replacement of the "middleware" that was responsible for the communication between server and mobile device. This includes basic components like authentication and authorisation of patients and therapists, communication protocol and security features.
- Identification of the services and restructuring of the server components of the application. Definition of Web Service interfaces for the identified components.
- The transformation of the user interfaces that were implemented in C++ for the windows mobile platform and are now transformed to the XML GUI description Language XAML.

The reimplementation is still in development and will be finished mid 2011. The application will be used for a clinical trial to evaluate long term effects of this application supporting adipose patients.

9. Alternative Health Care Market

As a result of the demographic change the German healthcare system is longing for a reorganization of medical care. Healthcare insurances mainly financing healthcare services will probably not be able to ensure quality and fair distribution of medical care within the next years. High-quality treatment to reduced prices/costs is needed. The healthcare system reacts – a so called second healthcare market takes root. In contrast

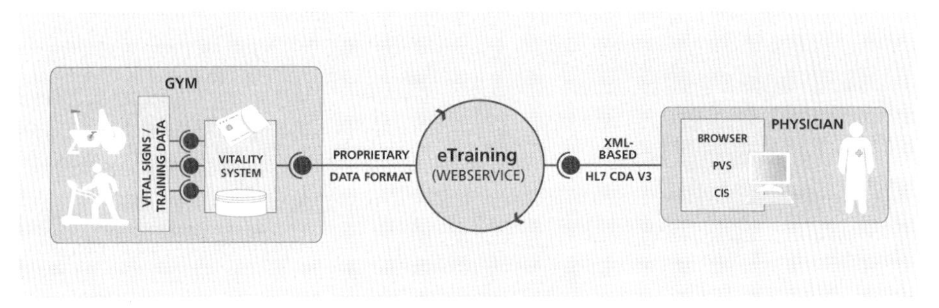

Figure 5. eTraining.

to the first healthcare market where healthcare insurances finance healthcare services, the second healthcare market is driven by the idea of financing healthcare services by private individuals themselves. Especially within the scope of prevention and rehabilitation the elderly (generation 50+) are willing and able to finance the maintenance of their health on their own. In the long term, the second healthcare market promises to reduce the follow-up costs for the healthcare system. So that new healthcare services from the second healthcare market could be integrated into existing medical healthcare processes. Russel [14] shows the high potential of telerehabilitation as a clinical tool for physiotherapists. Also Engbers [7] explains how networking using ICT could improve care. But in order to achieve this, the information chain between both healthcare markets has to be standardized and quality-assured. Therefore the Fraunhofer Institute for Software and Systems Engineering is working on intelligent software services and standards, based on the architecture described in Section 4 to enable cross-sectoral communication.

In cooperation with ERGO-FIT, a German manufacturer of fitness equipment, the Fraunhofer Institute for Software and Systems Engineering shows how training in fitness studios can be integrated into the process of rehabilitation. Today's fitness equipment has a lot of sensors to monitor the execution of training and vital signs. Examples are the range of motion, the pulse or the used amount of weight. First a bridge is necessary to communicate the above mentioned data needed by physicians to specialized staff of the first healthcare market. Second there has to be some kind of document which defines exercises for a given rehabilitation goal i.e. endurance training. Based on the CHOPIN approach we developed a secure data interface, whose main component is a data model of a training plan (named eTraining) based on HL7 CDA (Fig. 5). Especially the security modules from CHOPIN are reused.

HL7 [8] is a widespread international standard for data exchange in the healthcare sector, which implies that this kind of data can easily be integrated into existing healthcare systems of a surgery or a hospital. With the aid of eTraining you can document the training which consists of training sessions, exercise groups, exercises and series on two different layers. There is one layer for planning training activities and one for recording the execution of the planned activities. The software developed for ERGO-FIT to communicate with the underlying data interface is shown in Fig. 6. There are two different views, one for a physician and one for the performer.

Within rehabilitation a physician uses eTraining to plan training activities related to the rehabilitation goal. Supported by the program, even elderly patients are able to perform the training units independently. During execution eTraining records relevant training values. A physician, sports scientist or trainer can compare the planned activi-

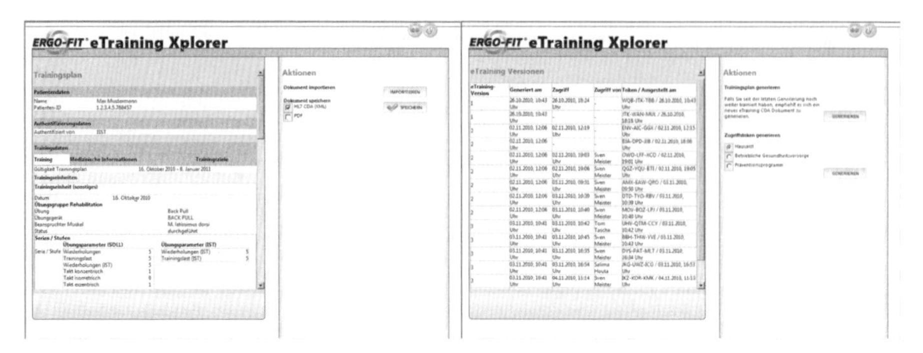

Figure 6. Left: HTML-formated eTraining CDA for a physician; Right: View of generated eTraining versions for the performer of exercise.

ties with the training results. Deviation from the expected values signals that the rehabilitation process has to be revised. This implies that the therapeutic process of rehabilitation is being optimized and personalized faster, which saves time and money. Furthermore, eTraining can be employed as monitoring instrument for insurers, in order to verify if and how training units were performed.

10. Summary and Conclusion

Within this paper we have taken an extended view onto AAL technology, discussing its relevance for supporting rehabilitation processes people have to undergo after medical illnesses. We have proposed an architecture that, together with building blocks, can serve as a toolbox for efficiently implementing telerehabilitation applications. The architecture is strongly influenced by practical applications. We have started to derive requirements from already developed applications for the architecture of telerehabilitation services. In later projects we have used the architecture in concrete implementations. Thereby it has been evaluated and improved.

Our future work will concentrate on an even stronger service orientation of the approach moving the whole technology into a cloud-based approach, driven by the metaphor of “Reha-Apps from an AAL-eHealth-Store”. As a result, patients will be able to access telerehabilitation services on demand. On the other hand, a scalable technology will be available to providers of healthcare services, as well as a distribution mechanism towards patients and users. Of course, due to the high sensitivity of personal health data, special focus has to be kept on data security and safety issues.

References

[1] O. Boehm and R. Kuhlisch, eCR Security Architecture 1.2 – Services and Interfaces, Fraunhofer ISST, 2008.

[2] J.A. Brebner, E.M. Brebner and H. Ruddick-Bracken, Experience-based guidelines for the implementation of telemedicine services, *Journal of Telemedicine and Telecare* **11**(Suppl. 1) (2005), 3–5.

[3] D.M. Brennan, S. Mawson and S. Brownsell, Telerehabilitation: Enabling the remote delivery of healthcare, rehabilitation and self management, *Stud. Health Technol. Inform.* **145** (2009), 231–248.

[4] M. Bultmann, R. Wellbrock, H. Biermann, J. Engels, W. Ernestus, U. Höhn, R. Wehrmann and A. Schurig, *Datenschutz und Telemedizin – Anforderungen an Medizinnetze*, 2002.

[5] Continua Health Alliance, http://www.continuaalliance.org/index.html, last access: 05. November 2010.
[6] W. Dostal, M. Jeckle, I. Melzer and B. Zengler, *Service-Orientierte Architekturen mit Web Services*, Elsevier, 2005.
[7] L. Engbers, H. Bloo, R. Kleissen, J. Spoelstra and M. Vollenbroek-Hutten, Development of a teleconsultation system for communication between physiotherapists concerning children with complex movement and postural disorders, *Journal of Telemedicine and Telecare* **9** (2003), 339–343.
[8] HL7: HL7 Version 3 Standard, http://www.hl7.org/v3ballot/html/welcome/environment/index.htm, last access: 05. November 2010.
[9] K. Pohl, *Requirements Engineering – Grundlagen, Prinzipien, Techniken*, dpunkt.verlag GmbH, Heidelberg, 2008.
[10] H.F. Rashvandt, E.L. Hines, D. Illiescu and R.J. Green, Integrated Telehealth – Requirement and implementation, in: *Advances in Medical, Signal and Information Processing*, 2006.
[11] C. Reuter, T. Köngismann, S. Meister, S. Houta and J. Neuhaus, CHOPIN: Toolbox for composition of telemedical services, in: *Telehealth and Assistive Technology*, 2009.
[12] C. Reuter, J. Neuhaus, J. Caumanns and O. Boehm, Die elektronische FallAkte. Ein Standard für die einrichtungs-übergreifende Kommunikation, in: *Telemedizinführer Deutschland 2009*, A. Jäckel, ed., 2009, pp. 157–162.
[13] T. Russel, Telerehabilitation: A coming of age, *Australian Journal of Physiotherapy* **55**(1) (2009), 5.
[14] T.G. Russell, Establishing the efficacy of telemedicine as a clinical tool for physiotherapists: From systems design to a randomised controlled trial, PhD Thesis, School of Health and Rehabilitation Sciences, The University of Queensland.
[15] L.H. Schopp, J.W. Hales, G.D. Brown and J.L. Quetsch, A rationale and training agenda for rehabilitation informatics: Roadmap for an emerging discipline, *NeuroRehabilitation* **18**(2) (2003), 159–170.
[16] O. Thomas, K. Leyking and M. Scheid, Serviceorientierte Vorgehensmodelle: Überblick, Klassifikation und Vergleich, in: *Informatik Spektrum*, Springer, Berlin (Heidelberg), 2009.
[17] L. Wakeford, P. Wittman, M. White, M. Wesley and M. Schmeler, Telerehabilitation position paper, November/December 2005, *American Journal of Occupational Therapy (AJOT)* **59**(6) (2005), 656.
[18] P.M. Yellowlees, Successfully developing a telemedicine system, *Journal of Telemedicine and Telecare* **11**(7) (2005), 331–335.

Handbook of Ambient Assisted Living
J.C. Augusto et al. (Eds.)
IOS Press, 2012

doi:10.3233/978-1-60750-837-3-512

AAL in Cardiac Rehabilitation

Frerk MÜLLER[a,*], Myriam LIPPRANDT[a], Marco EICHELBERG[a], Axel HELMER[a], Clemens BUSCH[b], Detlev WILLEMSEN[b] and Andreas HEIN[a]
[a] *OFFIS – Institute for Information Technology, Oldenburg, Germany*
[b] *Schüchtermann-Schiller'sche Kliniken, Bad Rothenfelde, Germany*

Abstract. Individually adapted physical exercise training under medical supervision is an important building block in the rehabilitation and secondary prevention for patients with cardiovascular diseases. Ambient assisted living technology permits such training to be carried out in the familiar home environment while at the same time reducing the risk of an adverse cardiovascular event. Against this background this article describes the requirements of a system for cardiac tele-rehabilitation at home and in particular discusses the components controlling a training session, which needs to recognize critical patient states through a continuous monitoring of vital signs and react accordingly. Furthermore, the health related data collected during such exercise training sessions provides useful information for patient care. Results need to be made available to the cardiologist responsible for follow-up e.g. in the form of structured training reports. The challenges involved in integrating data acquired at home with the professional healthcare IT infrastructure based on vendor-independent medical IT standards are also discussed.

Keywords. Ambient assisted living, cardiovascular disease, cardiac rehabilitation

Introduction

Cardiovascular diseases (CVD) are the leading cause of death in the world [47], and cause nearly half of all deaths in Europe (48%) and in the EU (42%) [2]. Due to demographic change ("ageing society"), the prevalence of CVD is expected to increase in the future, which means that they will be one of the major burdens of diseases that need to be addressed with sustainable prevention programs. The treatment of people with chronic diseases over their lifetime costs 3.5 times as much compared to the treatment of others, and accounts for 80% of all hospital bed days and 96% of home care visits [36]. One important factor for the health outcome of CVD patients after an acute event or cardiac surgery is cardiac rehabilitation. According to the European Association for Cardiovascular Prevention and Rehabilitation (EACPR), ambulatory (outpatient) rehabilitation programs are needed in order to achieve the comprehensive goals of cardiac rehabilitation and maintain them over time [10]. One key aspect of such ambulatory rehabilitation is exercise training, which can reduce further deterioration of the disease and prevent expensive readmission. For high-risk CVD patients, however, supervision and monitoring by health professionals are required.

Currently patients in Germany with severe CVD after acute treatment receive an in-patient rehabilitation program of 3 to 5 weeks. During this time the health status

[*] Corresponding Author: Frerk Müller, OFFIS – Institute for Information Technology, Escherweg 2, 26121 Oldenburg, Germany. E-mail: frerk.mueller@offis.de.

required for a reintegration of the patient should be achieved. Therefore, the restoration of the patient's physical capabilities through an exercise adapted to the patient's individual condition is in focus of the rehabilitation treatment. Furthermore, patients receive training and consultancy with regard to reducing the avoidable risk factors.

However, after a cardiac event, lifelong secondary prevention is absolutely crucial to avert further deterioration of the disease, maintain at least the current health status and improve the cardiac prognosis. Currently only 50% of all patients participate in phase II rehabilitation in Europe, according to the Euroaspire study [27]. The American Heart Association (AHA) as well as the European Association of Cardiovascular Prevention and Rehabilitation (EACPR) define core components for a lifelong secondary prevention of cardiac heart disease. The prevention aims to enhance the modifiable cardiac risk factors which are weight management, nutritional counseling, blood pressure management, lipid management, smoking cessation and physical activity counseling [4,38,43].

After a cardiac event and the following phase II rehabilitation, cardiac risk factors are well adjusted. But several studies have shown that one year after discharge the risk factors are comparable to the time before the cardiac event and in some cases even deteriorate (PIN [45], PROTECT [46], Euroaspire [27]). These data are elevated from patients participating phase II rehabilitation. It can be assumed that for the 50% of all patients not taking part in any rehabilitation the risk factors will deteriorate in the same manner or even worse. Recently the Euroaspire III – study published the data from 22 European countries, 13935 patient records were reviewed and 8966 patients were interviewed. The aim was to determine how the ESC guidelines on cardiovascular prevention are being followed in clinical practice [26,27]. The results showed a prevalence of 38% obesity[1], 60,9% of raised blood pressure $\geq$ 140/90 mmHG ($\geq$ 130/80 in people with diabetes), 46,2% had raised cholesterol concentration and 28% reported diabetes mellitus. Physical activity has only been evaluated by questionnaire. Even so only 33.8% of patients reported some regular exercise to improve their personal health.

Regular physical activity and exercise training have a positive influence on risk factors like hypertension, diabetes, obesity and dyslipidemia, which are not sufficiently treated already six month after a cardiac event as shown before. The American College of Sports Medicine, the American Heart Association, the European Society of Cardiology and the German Society of Rehabilitation and Prevention recommend a minimal amount of physical exercise for at least five times a week for 30 minutes in moderate intensity [4,38,43]. However those guidelines only suggest physical endurance exercise in general. Several studies have shown that an individualized exercise regime will even increase the effect of physical activity. A controlled, on personal needs adjusted training can optimize the secondary prevention. An ideal way for controlled training is a bicycle ergometer. Here the exact power and time can be adjusted and different physical parameters like heart frequency, ECG, oxygen saturation, blood pressure can be easily monitored. For high risk patients monitored exercise is strongly recommended and is standard in phase II rehabilitation.

Typically an exercise session on a bicycle ergometer is divided in three or five phases. It starts with a warm-up phase, which is normally preset on an individual low intensity (approximately 30–40% of the individual maximal performance). The amount of time depends on the total time of the exercise session (e.g. three minutes within a total time of 30 minutes). The second part brings the intensity to its training load in a

[1]Defined as BMI $\geq$ 30 m^2/kg.

linear way (within a 30 minutes exercise unit it would take two minutes to raise the exercise load). The next part is the actual training. It lasts at least 20 min. and it is adjusted to the individual need. The forth and fifth section are congruent to the warm-up and the developing phase in time and load but vice versa. Very weak patients would exercise with so-called interval training. It is divided in three phases (warm-up, training and cool-down). The training is characterized with alternation of low intensity and high intensity loads, typically divided in two to one interval meaning, e.g. 40 seconds on low intensity and 20 seconds on high intensity load, plus three to five minutes of continuous low load as warm-up and cool-down phase.

Many heart centers today offer so-called "cardiac sports groups" where patients can train regularly under professional supervision as a means of secondary prevention. While urban areas provide a sufficient offer of cardiac sports groups, only a small number of such groups are offered in rural regions, requiring participants to accept significant journeys. In this context the introduction of telemedical supervision systems for exercise training at home seems reasonable [34]. The long-term benefits of telemedically supervised rehabilitation have been demonstrated [29].

This article is structured as follows. First, an overview of the state of the art for telemedical supervision systems (Section 1.1), the relevant medical IT standards (Section 1.2), and existing projects in this field (Section 1.3) are presented. The following Section 2 presents the core components of a system for an individually adjusted exercise training at home for patients with cardiovascular diseases. The core components are the home gateway (Section 2.2), the clinical supervision system (Section 2.2), an actuator based training control system (Section 2.3) or an actuator-less training control system (Section 2.4). The article ends with a conclusion and outlook (Section 3).

1. State of the Art

In this section the state of the art in telemedical supervision systems for use at home as well as relevant IT standards for interoperability in home environment and in between actors of the health system are described.

1.1. Telemedical Supervision Systems

Systems for training in home environment encompass medical devices for rehabilitation as well as devices for fitness and personal exercises as these groups of devices are dominating the marked for health dependent training devices in the home environment.

For individual fitness exercises many commercial products are available. These are in most cases integrated in small devices such as watches and can be used for data logging as well as for computer aided coaching during the training session.

Polar Electro Oy [40] is one of the most established companies for such devices. Polar offers devices for several types of sports activities, including cycling, running, and horseback riding (including measurement of vital signs of the horse) as well as different exercise goals such as muscle strengthening or endurance. The Polar "RS800CX Pro Training Edition PREMIUM", which is one of the leading products of this vendor offers heart rate measurement, heart rate variability measurement, a stride sensor, a cadence sensor for cycling, atmospheric air pressure sensor for altitude measurement and a GPS sensor for measurement of track position and speed. This information is aggregated to higher level information such as fitness level, individual heart rate

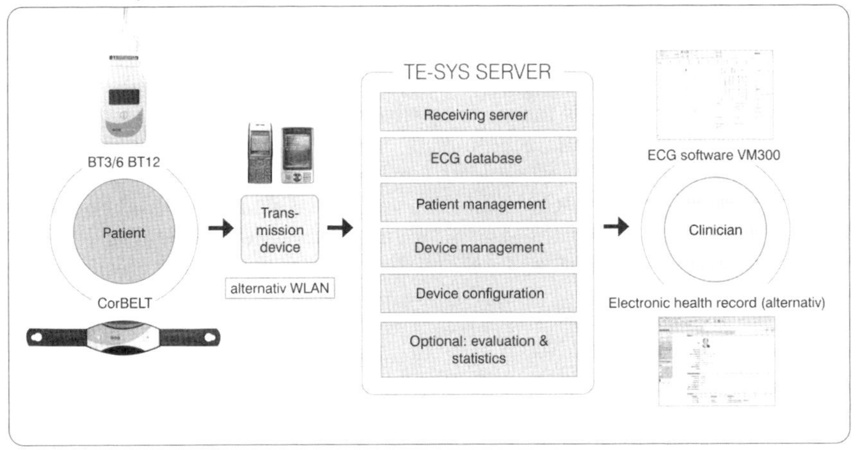

Figure 1. Overview of the Corscience TE-SYS system for ECG telemonitoring.

training zones and fitness progress. In combination with the "Polar Pro Trainer 5" training software, analyzing, planning and diary keeping of training sessions is possible. Polar also provides devices for group trainings like the Polar "Cardio GX" [39]. This system contains a base station that can connect up to 28 cardio transmitters for transmitting heart rate measurements using Bluetooth technology. In combination with a notebook or a personal digital assistant (PDA), Polar software can be used to monitor vital signs in real time, e.g. during soccer training or during ergobike exercises. This enables a professional to optimize the training of a group. Also non-stationary training can be performed with the system. The transmitter is able to store vital sign measurements, so data can be evaluated by the coach "offline" after the training session. All systems described in this section so far are "fitness devices", developed to support healthy people during training sessions, but do not support medical services for cardiac patients.

The Corscience TE-SYS system is an application for ECG telemonitoring. It consists of several small devices to transfer measured ECG data to a remote monitor system, for example in a hospital. In Fig. 1 an overview of the TE-SYS system is shown. Three different ECG sensor systems based on Bluetooth technology are available. The BT 3/6 and BT12 (upper left corner) are standard ECGs using adhesive leads placed on the patient's body whereas the Corscience CorBELT (lower left corner) is a single-channel ECG event recorder implemented as a thorax belt that can be easily handled also by non-professionals. These Bluetooth sensors transfer there measured data to a mobile phone that operates as a transmission device and forwards the ECG data via GPRS or wireless LAN to the TE-SYS server. Within the server the data is stored and accessible through a graphical front-end. The Bluetooth ECG can also be configured by the TE-SYS server, for example thresholds for ECG events can be set. Currently tachycardias and VF/VT, bradycardias, absolute arrhythmias and pauses are detected as events. With the graphical ECG viewer "VM300" the data should be checked by a medical professional. This system can be used in rehabilitation to monitor cardiac patients, but is not capable of supervising patients autonomously.

In addition to monitoring devices also services for cardiac monitoring are available on the market. SHL Telemedicine is such a company [42]. A central part of the company is a telemedical call-center for cardiac monitoring. Customers of the company receive a personal health record stored at the company, plus telemedical devices such as a 12 lead ECG, a blood pressure sensor, a weight and a blood analysis station. All devices are able to transmit their measurements directly to the "Medical Monitoring Center". Costumers may call in and ask for medical help. All employees of the monitoring center are trained professionals and able to read an ECG correctly. In case of emergency situations, an emergency call will be placed by the monitoring center. All information stored in the personal health record including ECG measurements, blood pressure, and weight can be made available to the medical emergency team and may save important time in case of an emergency. Beside this all data and data history are always available to the costumer and can be used for further analysis.

1.2. Interface Standards for Telemedical Supervision

The application of AAL concepts in cardiac rehabilitation requires that vital parameters be recorded, processed and evaluated in the home environment and, if necessary, forwarded to health professionals for further follow-up. Typical vital parameters that need to be recorded during cardiac rehabilitation training are electrocardiogram (ECG), oxygen saturation, and blood pressure. In the case of training on an ergometer additionally the device parameters (speed, load) need to be monitored and controlled. In a typical set-up, two networks with different purpose and capabilities are needed: A "personal area network" (PAN, also referred to as "body area network") in the immediate environment of the patient, and a wide area network connecting the patient with the IT infrastructure of the health professionals supporting the cardiac rehabilitation. The use of vendor independent interface standards for the various components that need to be connected is desirable since it adds flexibility to a system by making it much easier to add or exchange components. In the following we discuss the most important interface standards in this domain. It should be noted, however, that although related standardization activities have significantly advanced in the last few years (most notably through the work of the Continua Health Alliance [9]), market adoption is still fairly limited. This means that system developers need to be prepared to also support proprietary interfaces at least for some time, and in fact all vital parameter monitoring devices used during the research projects on which this article is based required implementation of proprietary protocols.

1.2.1. Personal Area Network

The recording of vital parameters requires sensors with direct contact to the human body. It is obviously not efficient (in terms of energy consumption, RF exposure and also in economic terms) to provide distinct wide area network interfaces such as WLAN or GSM separately in each sensor. Therefore, the sensors are instead equipped with means for short distance communications to a "hub" or "base station". The base station receives sensor input, provides means for local data processing and, where needed, the capability to forward raw sensor data or summarized recordings over a wide area network to the health professionals supervising the rehabilitation.

Sensors are connected to the base station either through cables (RS-232 serial line or universal serial bus, USB) or in a wireless manner. The transport layer protocols (covering the four lower layers of the OSI network reference model [22]) used for wireless connections are either Bluetooth (IEEE 802.15.1) [5,18] or, to a lesser degree,

ZigBee [48]. More specifically, the Bluetooth specification defines a number of so-called "profiles", three of which are relevant for vital parameter monitoring: the "serial port profile" [6], which emulates a serial connection and is supported by many existing devices, and the "health device profile" [7], which supports the multiplexing of data coming from multiple sensors over a single connection. Furthermore there is "Bluetooth low energy technology", published as part of the latest Bluetooth specification profile [5], which promises significantly lower energy consumption and, thus, longer battery life. In general wireless sensors are more comfortable to put on and wear, especially if the user moves a lot, as during exercise training. However, they also have disadvantages: they are necessarily battery powered (whereas cabled sensors may provide power over the connection cable), requiring more or less frequent change of batteries, which can become an inconvenience if there are many sensors and, thus, many batteries. Furthermore, the pairing process between sensor and base station required by the Bluetooth protocol and the utilization of the intensively used 2.4 GHz band may both contribute to communication failures between sensor and base station – a problem that does not exist with cable bound sensors.

The most important standardized application layer protocol (covering layers 5 to 7 of the OSI reference model) for vital parameter monitoring in personal area networks is the ISO/IEEE 11073 family of standards [23]. Originally developed to provide plug-and-play interoperability between vital parameter monitors and other devices used in intensive care units within a hospital, these standards have been adapted to the needs of personal health applications. In brief, ISO/IEEE 11073 allows a network consisting of multiple „agent systems" (sensors and actuators) and one "manager system" (the base station) to be established. The manager can query the status of each agent and, where possible, adjust settings through "Get" and "Set" messages, and agents can provide sensor data and status update through "Event-report" messages. This enables a "real-time" streaming (in soft real time) of vital parameters from multiple sensors to the manager system. The standard provides definitions for mandatory and optional data structures (properties, attributes) to be supported by specific device categories such as scale, pulse oximetry or ECG so both that vendor independence and plug-and-play interoperability can be achieved. So-called profiles govern the binding of the application layer protocol to a specific transport protocol and transmission technique, such as a binding to USB or to Bluetooth using the medical profile. As noted above, the adoption of ISO/IEEE 11073 in the market is still fairly limited, although the increasing number of devices available indicates that this situation may improve over the next few years.

1.2.2. Wide Area Network

A wide area network connects the base station of the personal area network to the IT infrastructure of the health professionals supervising the patient's health status and progress. Depending on the application scenario, again either cable-bound or wireless connections can be used – GSM (global system for mobile communications) or UMTS (universal mobile telecommunications system) for wireless connections over cellular networks and "classical" communication technologies such as telephony landlines (modem), ISDN (integrated services digital network), TV broadband cable or DSL (digital subscriber line) for cable-bound communication. Obviously mobile and outdoor applications will require the use of wireless connections, whereas applications in the home environment (such as ergometer training) can also be connected more inexpensively over cable (possibly using a wireless local area network – WLAN – within the home to simplify cabling), which is typically less expensive (especially if the infrastructure is already available in the home environment) and provides higher bandwidth.

In all cases the transport layer communication protocol is TCP/IP, which can be routed either over dedicated point-to-point connections (e.g. ISDN) or through the public Internet, if appropriate measures for safeguarding the communication are taken. This includes the use of an encryption protocol such as secure socket layer (SSL) [14] or transport layer security (TLS) [11] with an appropriate choice of ciphersuite (i.e., algorithms for key exchange, encryption and message digests) to guarantee the confidentiality and integrity of the communication, as well as the use of certificates or other reliable techniques to provide an authentication of communicating systems and thus prevent so-called "man in the middle" attacks. Systems that can detect emergency situations (such as a cardiac infarction) furthermore need to be able to reliably raise alarms, which typically requires the use of redundant communication channels (e.g. both cable based Internet access and communication over GSM or UMTS).

On application layer, it would theoretically be possible to also use ISO/IEEE 11073 and thus forward raw vital parameters in real time. While this may be a useful feature in some cases (e.g. when a doctor wants to remotely supervise a "live" training session in order to adjust the training program according to the vital parameter readouts), this use case is certainly the exception and not the norm. Patients who are discharged from "traditional" in-patient or ambulatory rehabilitation and become eligible for an "extended" rehabilitation through AAL techniques should be sufficiently stable in order to perform rehabilitation exercises at home without real-time supervision (which would generally not be available at all without the development of remote monitoring techniques). Furthermore, the provision of medical staff for a "live" supervision of all patients doing rehabilitation exercise at home would not be feasible for rehabilitation clinics. Therefore, the base station needs to provide sufficient "intelligence" (i.e. signal processing capabilities) to supervise the vital parameters locally during a training session and adjust the training load or stop the training when vital parameters exceed predefined maximum or minimum values. As long as the training is proceeding normally and no adverse events are discovered, the health professionals will most likely not be interested in individual vital parameters, but rather in a summary of the training sessions since the last review and possibly in the visualization of trends in the development of relevant parameters over time. In the case of adverse events, checking the vital parameters will be necessary, but rather in a retrospective manner and not "live" in real time. This means that the data exchanged over the WAN interface needs to be organized in a rather document-centered manner where recordings over a certain period (typically a single training session) are transmitted and can be reviewed en bloc, and not individually. However, the system's capability to compute trends in parameters over several training sessions requires individual vital parameters to be identifiable and "extractable" from these documents in an automated way, which precludes the use of simple documents formats such as PDF documents or web pages. Instead, a document format permitting a semantic annotation of data is needed.

One standard format well suited for this purpose is the Clinical Document Architecture (CDA) [17] developed by the HL7 organization. CDA is an XML based document format consisting of a structured document header describing metadata about the document such as the author, subject, and document type, and a document body consisting of one or more sections. Each section must have a title and contain human readable content (the so-called "narrative block"), and may additionally contain semantic markup information providing machine-readable equivalents to the section header and content. So-called CDA templates define additional constraints on this generic document format for specific use cases, i.e. the sections needed for a certain document type, the content and format for each section, and the semantic mark-up where required. CDA documents can easily be visualized – there is an official style sheet developed by HL7 converting each syntactically valid CDA document into a simple web page – but can contain sufficient machine-readable semantic annotation to make vital parameters identifiable and extractable within the larger document.

One notable CDA template that is important for the applications discussed in this article is the Continuity of Care Document (CCD) [16], which defines a collection of section templates intended as a core dataset of the most relevant administrative, demographic, and clinical data about a person's healthcare in the context of one or more episodes of care. An extension of the CCD format co-developed by HL7 and the Continua Health Alliance is called Personal Health Monitoring Report (PHMR) [19]. The PHMR is specifically intended for the storage and transmission of data from homecare monitoring, i.e. the supervision of vital parameters in the home environment. It permits the transmission of either a summary of results or of a complete set of vital parameters. Additionally textual information and graphs (e.g. trend curves) can be embedded. A similar CDA template that is also based on CCD and intended for the exchange between health information managed by the patient himself or herself and health professionals is the Exchange of Personal Health Records (XPHR) integration profile defined by IHE [20].

Since the Clinical Document Architecture does not define any transmission protocol for network transmissions, several application level protocols are possible. The Continua Health Alliance recommends the use of the IHE Cross-enterprise Document Reliable Interchange (XDR) integration profile [21], a communication protocol based on Web Services, and ebXML [37] for the encoding of metadata, encrypted with TLS. In our projects we have also successfully used the Devices Profile for Web Services (DPWS) [37], a set of implementation constraints for the Web Service specifications ("WS-*") that enable secure Web Service based messaging and is optimized for use with resource constrained devices.

Finally, the vital parameter sensor producing the by far largest amount of data in the context of cardiac rehabilitation is the ECG. While it is possible to include ECG data into CCD documents, the data volume and the fact that the textual representation of ECG in XML format is rather inefficient may justify the use of a dedicated format for ECG. For this sensor type, a number of standard formats with efficient binary encoding exist, including Digital Imaging and Communications in Medicine (DICOM) Waveforms [35], the Standard Communication Protocol for ECG (SCP-ECG) [12], and the European Data Format (EDF) [25].

1.3. Projects on Cardiac Rehabilitation in the Home Environment

Several research projects have been performed in the field of cardiac phase II rehabilitation in a telemedical setting. For high risk patients as well as for patients with a low compliance, a telemedical setting is expected to improve the patient's adherence (compliance) to the therapy. In the SenSAVE (sensor assistance for vital events) project [32] medical sensor data is collected in everyday life situations. With a central processing unit the vital data gathered are transmitted to a server. This unit is also the user interface for the patient to show the measured vital data. The server processing the information is accessible to physicians through a web application and displays the medical information gathered. TEMONICS (telemonitoring with cardiorespiratory systems) focuses on an interdisciplinary integrated system to monitor patients with cardiovascular diseases using smart textiles [1]. The PRECARE project developed a system consisting of a patient centered monitoring and a processing and storing system. The PRECARE process focuses on health prevention more than health care. Patients should be enabled to play an active role in their convalescence [28]. In MyHeart [15] the development of smart textiles for preventive care application for a specific user group is the main objective to collect vital data from a patient. Furthermore, five application areas are addressed where main risks could arise, that is: "CardioActive", "CardioBalance", "CardioSleep", "CardioRelax", and "CardioSafe". HeartCycle [41] provides a disease management application that comprises a direct patient loop to support the daily treatment and a professional loop that assists medical professionals in decision making (e.g. care plan). SAPHIRE [8] and OSAmI [31] concentrate on a telemonitoring exercise regime based on a bicycle ergometer. In OSAmI, in addition to the indoor training patients are equipped with a mobile device that enables them to perform outdoor activities such as nordic walking or jogging.

2. Medical Applications in the Home Environment for Cardiac Rehabilitation

2.1. Scenario

As described above, after an acute cardiac disease a patient passes through a stationary rehabilitation program that aims at improving an individually defined degree of fitness to avoid a new relapse. After the in-patient phase the achieved health status can only be sustained and further developed through a medical supervised rehabilitation phase III that a patient should continue lifelong.

The tele-rehabilitation of patients with cardiovascular disease takes place in the home environment. The patient is equipped with an ergometer bicycle and a set of medical sensors like an ECG, blood pressure, oxygen saturation and pulse sensor to monitor the heart frequency. Through a computer system the sensor data can be analyzed during a training session to control the ergometer load and to avoid any overload of the patient. Also an alarm system must give feedback about the current health state while exercising. The needs of an individualized training plan that is adapted over time makes a connection to a clinic necessary. Also training reports including all vital parameters and medical events like alarms must be transmitted to the clinic after every training session. The training reports represent the patient's health status, history and fitness level. Based on this information, a medical supervisor could review every training report to generate a new appropriately adapted training plan that can be transmitted back to the home-based rehabilitation system. For interoperability reasons, the gathered vital parameters should be transmitted in a standard format as discussed in Section 1.2. In addition to the bicycle ergometer training, a tele-rehabilitation application should support different sport activities that can be performed to increase the physical fitness level, such as nordic walking. The challenge in the development of such a system is to adapt from the laboratory conditions into the tele-rehabilitation system at home. The characteristics of a clinical setting give complete control and information about the patient's health status during the training phase. This allows progress monitoring, emergency detection and adaption of exercise levels for a medical professional without being face-to-face with the patient all the time.

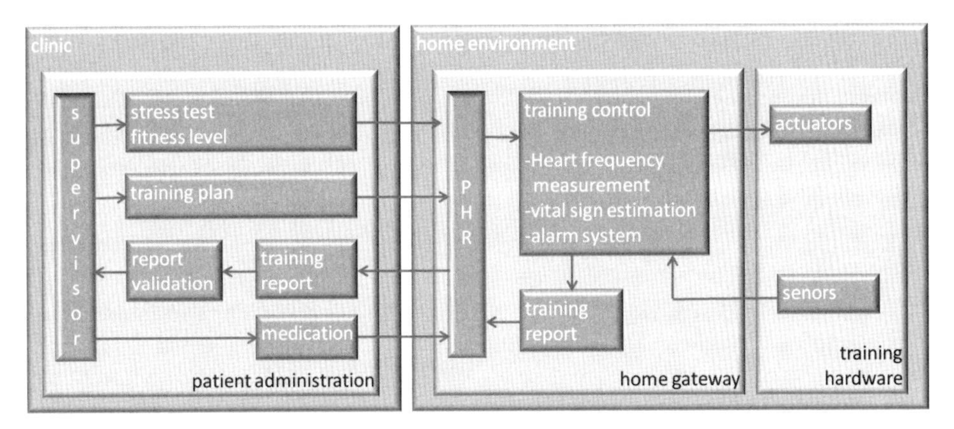

Figure 2. General structure of a cardiac rehabilitation device for the home environment.

2.2. General Structure of a Cardiac Telemedical Device

In the following we introduce the general structure of a telemedical exercise system for cardiac patients in phase III rehabilitation at home, including the related processes within the hospital as well as in the home environment and give a brief overview of processes needed to fulfill the requirements of such a system. The basic system structure is shown in Fig. 2.

For training within the home environment data exchange between the training device in the home environment and the medical professional in the clinic is necessary. On the left side of the figure, the clinical parts of the process are shown whereas the right side shows the basic structure of the system within the home environment. During the rehabilitation a repeating circle of information exchange has to be followed. The supervisor sets up a training plan for an individual patient based on the results of a stress test (left side of the figure). Next to the training plan and the results of stress test, medication and diagnosis is stored into the personal health record (PHR) of the patient in the home environment (center of the figure). Using this information the training device can be configured and supports the patient in performing his exercises. During the training the device monitors the vital signs of the patient and guides him or her through the training session. Additionally the system is performing a vital sign estimation basing on the stress test results and medication as this is mainly affecting the vital signs on a given load. The vital sign estimation is necessary to support the alarm system to figure out whether a vital parameter is out of range or not. If a certain threshold is exceeded the training device has to stop the exercise and calm the patient down before serious heart problems occur. Once a training session has ended the training report is generated and stored in the system's personal health record (PHR). This report consists of vital data measurement like rest measurement and measurements of heart frequency, ECG, blood pressure and oxygen saturation during the training synchronized with the load of the patient over time. The report can be accessed and validated by the doctor (lower left corner of the figure). Validation of the training results then leads to an adaptation of the training plan, which is updated on the PHR and leads to a new configuration of the training device. At this point the circle is closed.

This scenario is based on an "offline" training session performed without real-time presence of a medical professional. Besides this scenario it is also possible that all vital data recorded during the training session is streamed in real time into the hospital where a medical professional can monitor one ore even more patients at a time performing a training session. This allows the doctor to step into the running session and adapt parameter of the training. This can be useful if a patient does not feel well during the exercises or if the doctor wants to have direct feedback from the patient on changes of the training plan such as an increased target heart frequency. If the training plan adaptation leads to the results the medical professional expected, the changes can be stored into a new training plan acting as the new plan for further offline training sessions.

Two major interfaces are essential for such training systems. The first interface can be found between the home gateway and the training hardware (centre and right part of the figure). As this should be easy to handle for the patient, wireless communication is useful. In particular, sensors placed on the patient body should not be wired. Such interfaces are described in Section 1.2.1. Standards like the Bluetooth health device profile can be used to decouple the training control component of the home gateway from vital sensors and actuators e.g. an ergometer bicycle. The second even more important interface can be found between the home environment and the hospital. Several clinical IT-Systems have to provide the training control system with the necessary information. To standardize this communication, a well-defined interface has to be set up. This also enables different companies to develop training devices that can be connected to one clinical system.

2.2.1. Personal Health Records for Medical Applications in the Home Environment

Patients who are performing cardiologic rehabilitation training often also suffer from additional diseases such as diabetes mellitus or high blood pressure (hypertension). The treatment of such diseases demands the intake of diverse medications that could cause effects on the patient's vital parameters during a training session (e.g. beta blockers). In addition, data such the patient's sex, age, and weight or body fat percentage are important for the training plan. Further relevant information can only be obtained through supervised medical assessments, e.g. in a rehabilitation clinic. Such controlled settings and the presence of medical staff permit the execution of medical tests that could otherwise potentially lead the patient into a critical health state.

Systems for automatic training control depend on this information for the definition and update of boundary values (e.g. for the triggering of alarms) to provide a safe rehabilitation training. This shows that training systems at home have to process more information than obtainable during the training itself. Commonly the information is scattered over the IT systems of different actors in the health care system or could only be delivered by the patient himself. Besides the aggregation of the required data, the provisioning and their communication is an unsolved problem in general (see Section 1.2).

One way to tackle this issue is the usage of a Personal Health Record (PHR). According to the Markle Foundation, the PHR "... is an Internet-based set of tools that allows people to access and coordinate their lifelong health information and make appropriate parts available to those who need it" [24]. PHR systems supporting controlled rehabilitation training have to combine the data that could influence the patient's rehabilitation training and provide it as a model of the patient's medical state. A PHR could also manage results from the rehabilitation training itself and provide them to the medical supervisor as well as to the patient. In addition to other positive aspects such as the empowerment of the patient (see [33] and [3]), the aggregated data could be used for other medical systems to improve the quality of their services. Furthermore, the PHR could provide mechanisms for a standardized communication of the patient's health data or training reports, it could assist physicians for the creation of exercise plans, manage the training schedules and presentation of the exercise plan to the patient in an appropriate manner. For cardiac rehabilitation the results of the stress test, the medication as well as the training plan are the most important information.

2.2.2. Phase II Stress Test as Basis for the Device Parameter Estimation

At the end of phase II rehabilitation, an exercise stress test is mandatory. It is performed typically either on a treadmill or bicycle ergometer. During this test vital data like ECG, heart frequency, blood pressure and oxygen saturation are monitored. Based on the results of the test exercise physiologists can adjust a training for individual patients. A load test follows clinical guidelines defining the test including step size, step length and other parameters. Besides the fact that the test is used as diagnostic tool for measuring patient fitness, the results of such a test can be used to measure heart frequency reaction on load changes as parameter estimation for a heart frequency based controller. In Fig. 3, the result of a so-called "modified Naughton" treadmill test is shown. The data was recorded by clinical software during the performance of a load step test with 2 minute steps each with increasing step size. The test ended at 220 Watts, which is depending on the individual patient.

This step test can be used to estimate the parameters of a heart frequency based controller. The reaction of the heart frequency on load changes is interpreted as an impulse response whereas the impulse response is the output signal of a system as reaction on a Dirac impulse [44]. In system theory this reaction is used to characterize linear time invariant systems. This approach was studied in the project Ambient Intelligence [30]. Within this project a scenario for heart frequency based training for cyclists was developed. The parameter set of the controller, estimated by evaluation, was not individual, but identical for all cyclists. As an outcome of this evaluation it was figured out that the parameter set could not be used for untrained persons and that the standard step test is not an appropriate method to estimate a parameter set for untrained persons. Especially the step length of 3 minutes (a different step test protocol than the one presented in Fig. 3) was too short, because the heart frequency of untrained persons reacts more slowly and often heavier on load changes than heart frequency of a well trained person. In conclusion, the parameter estimation for a heart frequency based controller for untrained persons is generally feasible, but requires an adaptation of the standard load step tests.

2.2.3. Structure of a Training Plan for Cardiac Rehabilitation

In addition to information about the medication and the results of the stress test, a training plan is needed to perform a training session. This plan is developed by the doctor and individually fitted to the patient. It contains a course of actions depending on training method, vital sign ranges / thresholds and information about heart rate issues.

In Fig. 4, a general overview of the three major training methods is shown. All training methods contain a warm-up phase and a cool-down phase that are load driven. The warm-up is always starting with a constant load until a defined point in time. In the second part of the warm-up the load increases until the target load defined by the medical professional is reached. The cool-down phase is analogue. The load decreases for a

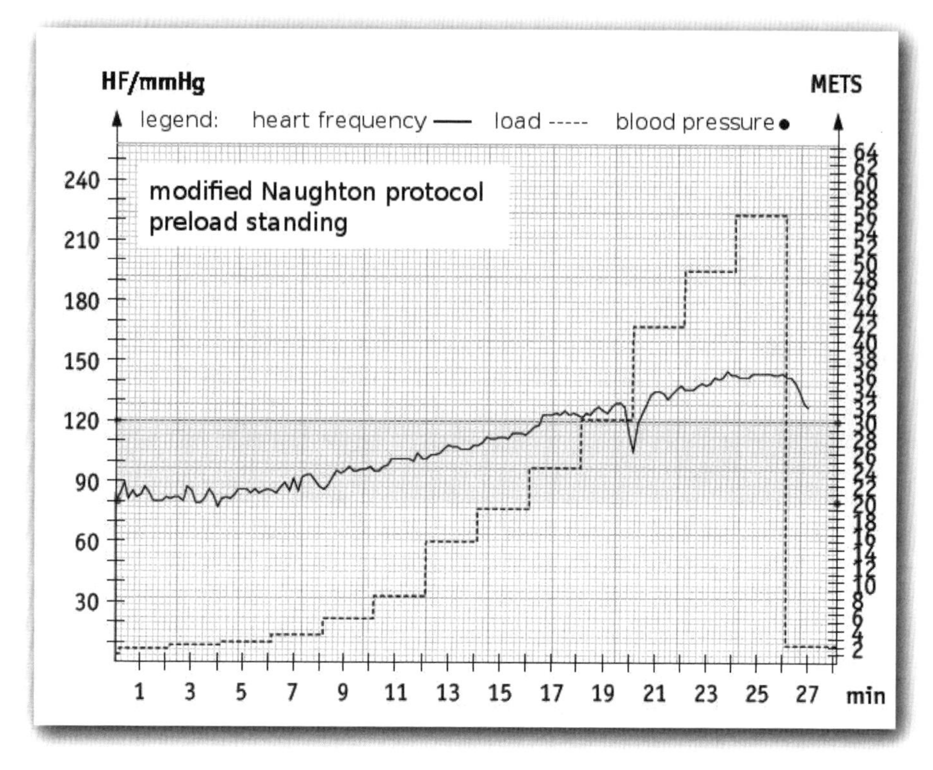

Figure 3. Results of a load step test including load, heart frequency and blood pressure.

defined time to a defined target load and is left constant until the end of the training. The load stages of the training methods vary. Figure 4b shows a load based training method with constant load. Within the load stage the load is left to a constant value not depending on any vital parameter unless a threshold is exceeded. This would lead to an abort of the training session. The training method shown Fig. 4c is interval based load training. The load is changing during the load stage from high to low for several times defined by the medical professional. This leads to heart frequency changes, but does not depend on them. The third training method is a heart frequency based training method shown in Fig. 4a. Like in the first and second training method, the warm-up and cool-down stages are load driven, but the third training method is depending on a target heart frequency within the load stage. A control system adapts the load on the patient in the background to control the heart rate. The heart frequency controller can be configured by the results of the stress test.

In order to set up a system to perform these kinds of training methods in the home environment, a complex structure of controlling systems has to be implemented. These structures are described in the following.

2.3. Actuator Based Devices for Cardiac Rehabilitation Exercises

In the last section the general structure of a rehabilitation device for the home environment was pointed out. The data flow between clinic, home gateway and exercise hardware was described as well as the structure of the training plan and the fitness level

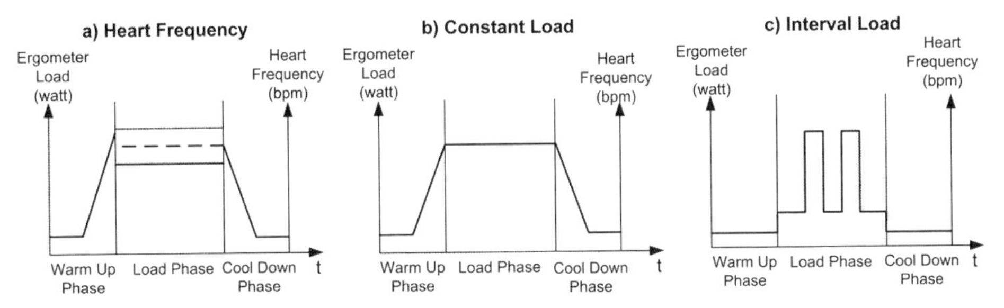

Figure 4. General layout of the three major training methods: a) describes a heart frequency based training whereas during load phase the dashed line represents the target heart rate and the solid lines upper and lower load limits, b) and c) are load based training methods.

parameter estimation. This section focuses on the training control system performing the exercise and the way the provided data is used during the training session to keep the patient in a stable health state.

In general two types of training control systems have to be taken into account. The first one is actuator based and the second one operates in an actuator-less manner. Actuator-less devices are devices that cannot directly influence the patient by load changes whereas an actuator based training control system is able to control the load on the patient body. For example during a walk a device can only recommend to change load by increasing / decreasing walking speed whereas during an ergometer bicycle training the force needed to rotate the primary shaft is controllable by an eddy current brake. This section focuses on actuator based devices. Ergometer bicycle training is used as an example.

The basic structure of the training control system is a control loop as know from automatic control engineering [44]. In such a control loop a desired target parameter is permanently compared to the current target parameter value and the delta is fed to a control system to process changes on control parameter which will affect the physical system and therefore the target parameter in a predictable manner. Such a target parameter could be e.g. the heart frequency which is affected by changing the load on the patient as the described control parameter.

In Fig. 5, the training control system is described. The information needed to configure the device is provided by the vector $\vec{\sigma}$, which is fed from the PHR (upper centre of Fig. 5). This information includes a patient model with personal information such as age, weight, sex and size as well as information about the individual fitness level already explained in Section 2.2.2. Also medication is important information as it can have influence on vital signs such as heart frequency changes affected by beta blockers, which may cause the target heart rate not to be reached even if load is increased more and more. This could lead to dangerous behavior of the training control, because the patient would be lead to overstrain. The whole information of $\vec{\sigma}$ will be fed to the vital sign estimation (lower left part of the control system) to process a prediction of the vital signs of the patient regarding the current load on the patient. During the stress test described in Section 2.2.2 the body reaction of the patient is measured and stored in a mathematical model to calculate an estimation of the vital signs based on the input $\vec{\sigma}$ and the load currently affecting the patient. Next to $\vec{\sigma}$ the training plan $\vec{Tp}(k)$ is fed from the PHR to the training control system (left side of Fig. 5). Within this vector the target values for vital signs depending on discrete time *(k)* are defined for the duration of the training session as well as vital sign thresholds. The vital sign measurements

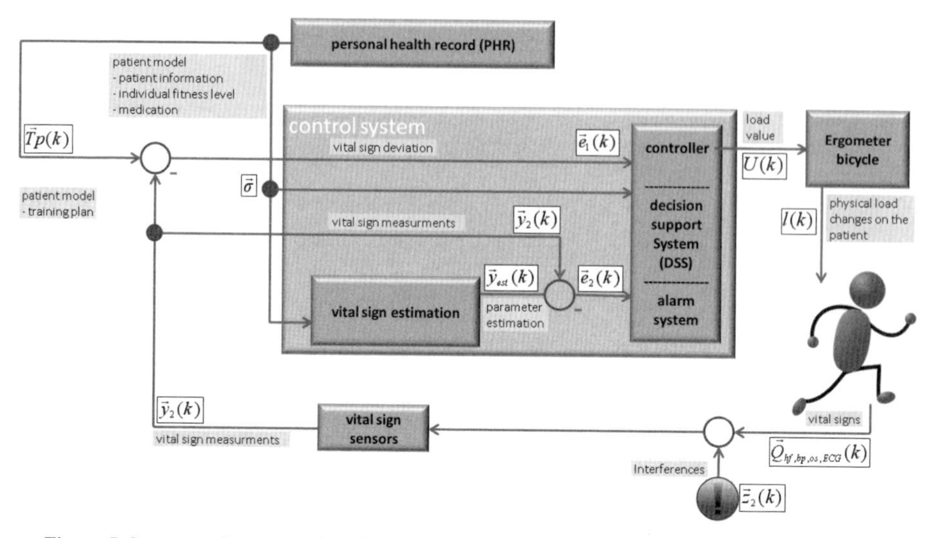

Figure 5. Structure of a actuator based training control system based on ergometer bicycle exercises.

$\vec{y}_2(k)$ gathered by the system (lower left corner) during the session are subtracted from the training plan $\vec{Tp}(k)$ to the control deviation $\vec{e}_1(k) = \vec{Tp}(k) - \vec{y}_2(k)$. As an example the heart rate can be used. If during a training session at a defined point in time the heart frequency target is 120 BPM (as part of $\vec{Tp}(k)$) and was measured at 100 BPM (as part of $\vec{y}_2(k)$) the control deviation of the heart frequency would be 20 BPM (as part of $\vec{e}_1(k)$). This is analog to all measured vital signs e.g. blood pressure or oxygen saturation.

$\vec{e}_1(k)$ is than fed to the decision support system that consists of two major blocks: The controller for handling the vital signs themselves and an alarm system for detecting emergency situations. By interpreting the control deviation $\vec{e}_1(k)$ the decision support system (DSS) is able to calculate the correcting variable $U(k)$ and adapts the eddy current brake on the ergometer bicycle to change load $l(k)$ on the patient (upper right corner). This will lead to new vital signs $\vec{Q}_{hf,os,bp,ECG}(k)$ of the patient, measured by the vital sign sensors influenced by the disturbance variable $\vec{z}_2(k)$ to $\vec{y}_2(k) = \vec{Q}_{hf,os,bp,ECG}(k) + \vec{z}_2(k)$. Following the heart rate example from above, the current heart rate was 20 BPM slower than the target heart rate. Therefore, the load on the patient has to be increased, for example $U(k) = U(k-1) + 30[Watt]$. In this example, the load is increased by 30 Watt. Depending individually on the patient, the vital signs will change. The heart rate is expected to rise. The result $\vec{y}_2(k)$ is used afterwards to calculate the control deviation $\vec{e}_1(k)$ for the controller as already described above and secondly to calculate the estimation deviation $\vec{e}_2(k) = \vec{y}_{est}(k) - \vec{y}_2(k)$ whereas $\vec{y}_{est}(k)$ is the result of the vital sign estimation and $\vec{y}_2(k)$ represents the actual measurement. If the vital sign estimation meets the results of the measurement, $\vec{e}_2(k) = 0$ is given. The greater the absolute value of $\vec{e}_2(k)$, the greater an indication of an alarm. $\vec{e}_2(k)$ is then fed to the alarm block of the decision support system (DSS). If the deviation of a vital sign and the estimation exceeds a certain threshold, an alarm will be raised and influence the controller part of the DSS. This could be an abort of the training session, but also a notification to adapt the load in a certain way. For example because of the load increment by 30 Watts, it is expected that the heart frequency will also increase. If this assumption fails because of medication (e.g. beta blocker), then the estimation deviation will increase also because the current heart rate remains fairly constant whereas the estimation increases and the alarm system will notify the controller system when reaching the limit.

This control loop controls the whole training session among all stages of training (warm-up, load stage, cool-down), but the target parameter could change during the exercise. If for example heart frequency based training should be performed, the target parameter during the load phase is the heart rate whereas the warm-up and cool-down phase are load driven and do not depend on the heart rate. During load driven training the vital sensor is mostly used for vital sign deviation measurements to detect emergency situations.

2.4. Actuator Less Devices for Cardiac Rehabilitation

For cardiac rehabilitation in the home environment, outdoor activities should be also taken into account, especially since cardiac patients need to perform regular training sessions for the rest of their life. In addition to indoor ergometer bicycle training outdoor training such as walking can be a motivating alternative, but outdoor activities lead to new challenges as these require an actuator-less training control system. There are many devices for outdoor exercises available on the market to coach people during their training session, but for cardiac rehabilitation not all requirements are met. In particular the alarm system needed to avoid further heart problems is not available in such devices. Most devices measure heart frequency and throw an alert when exceeding defined heart rate thresholds, but these thresholds are not linked to the environment. For example, if a person is running at the beach, a heart rate of 140 BPM may be a valid value, but if the person is walking on the street the same value may be an indication for an emergency. Therefore, environmental information like outdoor temperature, patient speed, step frequency, slopes or subsurface consistence (e.g. sand or grass) are necessary information to figure out whether vital parameters are inline or not. Therefore, for outdoor training the vital sign estimation for ergometer exercises as described in see Section 2.3 has to be extended by further input values including information about the environment and the patient himself or herself.

2.4.1. Basic Structure of a Load Estimation Map for Route Planning

As already described the environment during the walking exercise is not as predictable as in ergometer training. Therefore, it is necessary to pre-process a-priori as many parameters as possible before the training. This increases the quality of the vital signs estimation and comfort level during the training. To enhance the quality of a training session it is very useful to plan the route in a way that environment changes do not disturb the training or – even better – do support it. Therefore, a load estimation map has to be generated.

In Fig. 6 an example of a load estimation map is shown. Such a map is pre-training knowledge used to plan the route for the exercise. For planning a track, a map has to be annotated with environment information about every road section that could be part of the training. Figure 6 gives an example of an annotated map. The track sections marked in closely dotted lines are tracks with a hard subsurface whereas widely dotted track sections represent soft subsurface. Grey bars on a track define slopes with a specified angle and direction. Every track section can be used to define a target route. This is analog to a modern navigation system where speed limits are annotated to the streets to

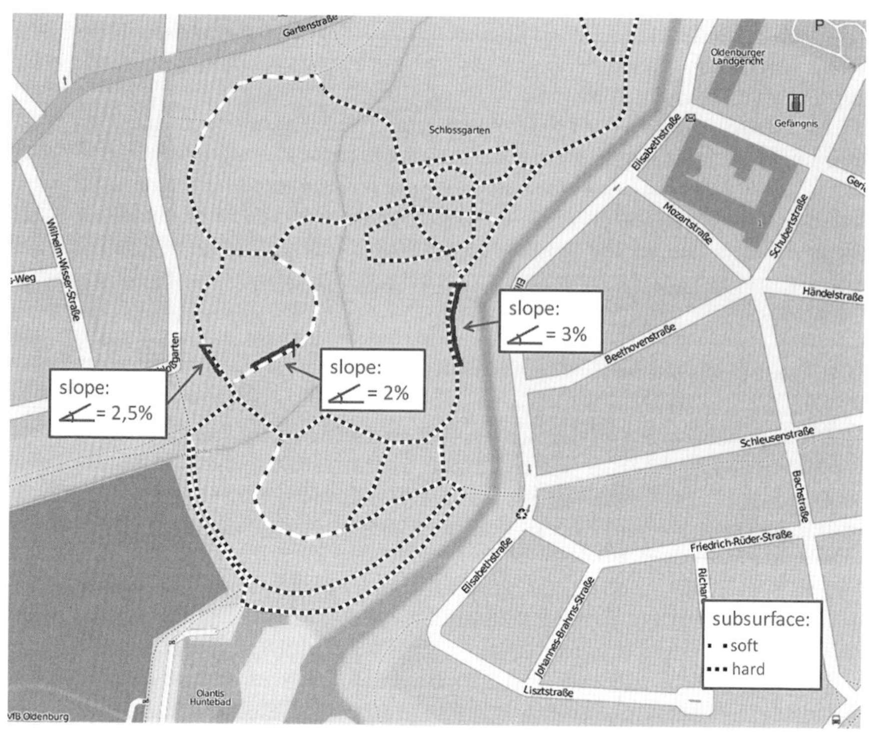

Figure 6. Example of a load estimation map. Widely dotted tracks are marked as soft subsurface whereas closely dottedba tracks show hard subsurface. Grey bars mark slopes in direction and angle. The map is based on Open Street Map data [13].

plan driving time. In this case the annotations should provide information about the subsurface (hard or loose), because this will affect the body reaction. For example running on sand with a given speed will be more exhausting than running with the same speed on grass. Furthermore, the slope of a track section is important. Running up a hill is more exhausting than running with the same speed on the same altitude level. This information has to be taken into account during training time as otherwise in the worst case the training would have to be aborted. For example, running up a steep slope during warm-up will cause the heart frequency to increase quickly because of the high load on the patient. In this case the vital sign limits set for a warm-up will most likely cause the training to be aborted. A similar reasoning applies to the subsurface. In the best case the route is planned such that the environment is used to support the training, for example by placing a slope on the track at a point in time where heart frequency should actually increase. Therefore, an intelligent algorithm for training plan generation depending on the load estimation map is necessary.

2.4.2. Individual Behavior Model to Enhance Pre-Training Prediction on Vital Signs

As described above, the load estimation map should be taken into account when planning an outdoor training session in order to increase the quality of the training plan. Furthermore, there are many other variables that should also be included. The vital signs will be mostly determined by the speed of the patient on a given track, but there are inter-individual differences in dealing with environment changes. As an example some patients may try to keep their speed when entering a slope, leading to an increasing heart frequency. Others may be unable or unwilling to keep their speed and thus slow down, which could lead to a fixed (or even decreasing) heart frequency. This behavior has to be measured for each patient individually and adapted into a model for prediction. Normally this model will be adapted with every training session during which the patient uses the system and may also change over time. By using the load estimation map in combination with a model to predict user behavior on environment changes, the quality of vital sign estimation in pre-training state for route planning will increase.

An abstract description of the behavior model is presented in Fig. 7. $U_R(k)$ is an audio/visual command of a PDA-based device informing the patient about the expected speed. By an estimated proportional reaction (P element in upper centre) on the speed command the patient should accelerate or decelerate to $v_{des}(k)$ which represents the desired speed. Because of the environment, this speed can be affected, for example when running on sand. Therefore, an attenuation element was placed in the path (element in the centre of the figure). $v_{act}(k)$, which is the actual speed as the result on the attenuation, can be integrated by an integration element (left centre in the figure) to the actual position on track $\vec{P}_{x,y,z}(k)$. This actual position is then fed back to the attenuation element, because the attenuation depends on the position on track. It is also assumed that in addition to the attenuation the human behavior does include some kind of self-control that causes an attempt to adapt the speed. In the abstract description of the behavior the self-control is added as speed deviation $e_v(k) = v_{des}(k) - v_{act}(k)$ and fed back to the proportional element P on the upper center of the figure. It is also assumed that $v_{act}(k)$ is affecting the body reaction in combination with temperature $T_{area}(k)$ to vital signs like heart frequency $hf(k)$, oxygen saturation $os(k)$ and blood pressure $\vec{bp}(k)$ which can be measured by vital sign sensors under addition of disturbance of $z_{2..4}(k)$. The position $\vec{P}_{x,y,z}(k)$ of the patient is also measured by a GPS sensor under addition of disturbance variable $z_1(k)$. After extraction of the parameter set to configure the P-element and the attenuation element, the model can be applied to the load estimation map. As a result of the load estimation map, a non-individual load index for a track section is generated and individualized by combination with the predictive behavior model as described here. This information will afterwards not only be used for planning, but also during the training session for vital sign estimation to detect emergency situations.

2.4.3. General Structure of a Training Control System for Actuator-Less Devices

From a classical automatic control engineering point of view it is not possible to implement a control loop without an actuator, because this control element is responsible for propagating the calculated changes to the physical control path – without it no controlling is possible. To avoid this problem the classical control loop has to be extended within the training control system for actuator-less devices. The control element is replaced by a "recommendation element" that recommends the patient to change behavior. Since a human being cannot react to the recommendation with the same level of precision as a control element on a value input, the reaction of the recommendation is not reliable. Because of this fact the reaction of the human being on recommendation input has to be measured and fed back to the control system as a second feedback in addition to the vital sign measurements. In Fig. 8 an actuator-less training control system is described for the example of walking. Most functions within this figure are iden-

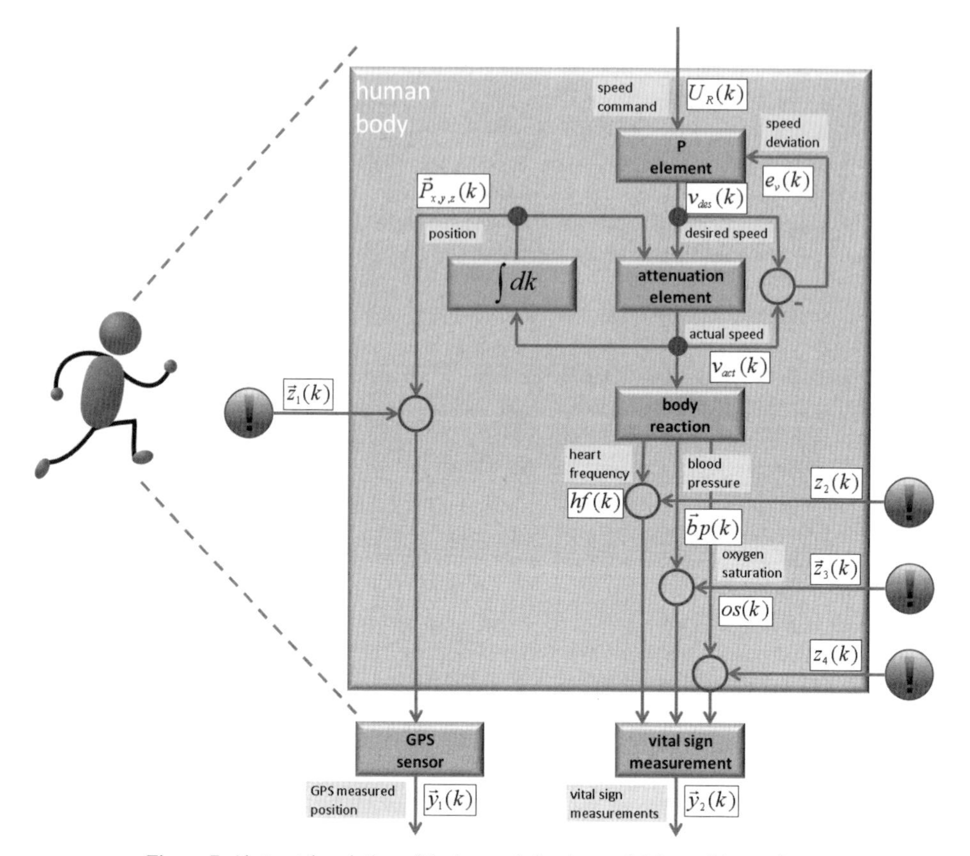

Figure 7. Abstract description of the human behavior model for walking patients.

tical to those of the actuator based training control system (Fig. 5). Therefore, the description focuses on changes and new elements.

As in the actuator based system the information needed to perform the exercise is stored within the PHR and fed to the training control system. The vector $\vec{\sigma}$ still includes all the static data to configure the decision support system (DSS) and the vital sign estimation, but the individual behavioral model already described in Section 2.4.2 extends $\vec{\sigma}$ by additional information. Also $\vec{T}p(k)$ as a function is extended because in addition to the normal training plan information such as vital sign target values and limits, the pre-arranged GPS track is also part of this training plan. As in the actuator based system the control deviation $\vec{e}_1(k) = \vec{T}p(k) - \vec{y}_2(k)$ is the difference between the training plan $\vec{T}p(k)$ and the vital sign measurements $\vec{y}_2(k)$. The controller block of the DSS then calculates the control variable $U(k)$, which is a speed and not a load value as in the actuator based system. This value is transferred to the PDA (upper right corner), which uses the data to issue a audio-visual recommendation to the patient, thus coaching him or her to run faster, slower or even to stop the training session because of an emergency situation. The reaction of the patient on the recommendation is tracked by the position of the patient as well as by vital sign changes. The GPS position is measured as $\vec{y}_1(k) = \vec{P}_{x,y,z}(k) + \vec{z}_1(k)$ whereas $\vec{P}_{x,y,z}(k)$ is the real position in a 3D environment and $\vec{z}_1(k)$ is the disturbance influence. $\vec{y}_1(k)$ is fed to a derivative ele-

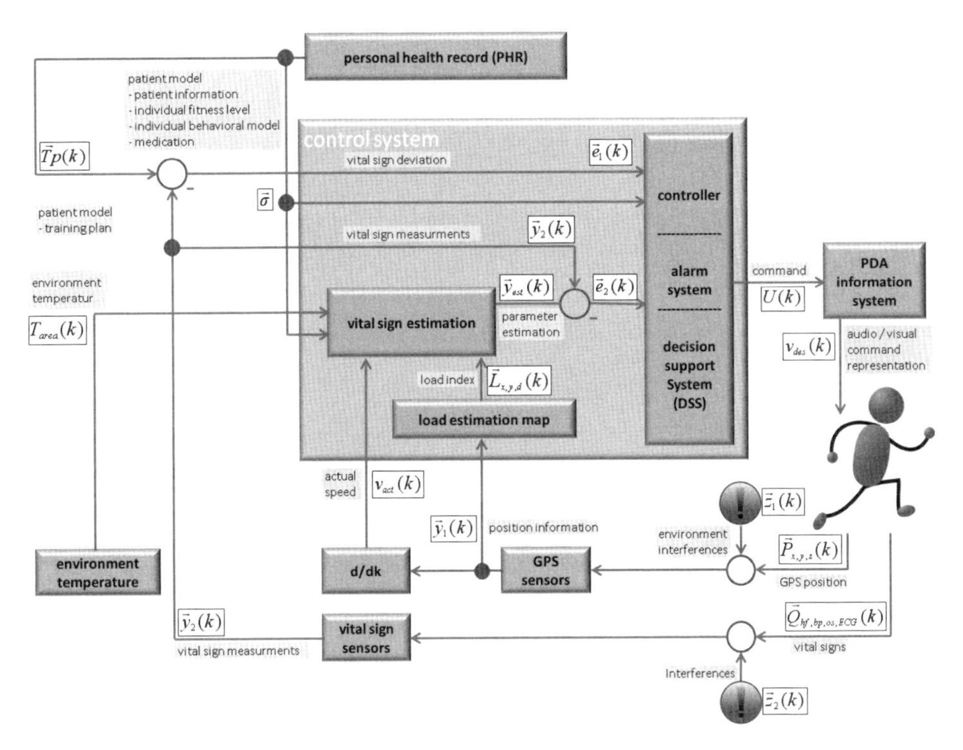

Figure 8. Description of an actuator-less training control system for walking.

ment that calculates $v_{act}(k) = y_1'(k)$, e.g. the actual speed of the patient. The position is also fed to the load estimation map (centre of the figure), which was already explained in Section 2.4.1 for route planning. In this case it is used for run-time vital sign estimation. The load index $\vec{L}_{x,y,d}(k)$ depends on the vertical and horizontal position on the map and the direction of the patient because of slopes. The load index $\vec{L}_{x,y,d}(k)$ as a result of the load estimation map at a given position and direction in combination with the results of the fitness test and temperature $T_{area}(k)$ leads to $\vec{y}_{est}(k)$ by using the vital sign estimation. The estimation deviation $\vec{e}_2(k) = \vec{y}_{est}(k) - \vec{y}_2(k)$ is used afterwards to detect alarm situations, like in the actuator based training system. As this is a description of a control loop the circle is closed at this point and repeated until the end of the training session.

In summary, a system that includes measurements of the environment and the vital signs for performing a vital sign estimation based on individual patient information, as outlined above, is a necessary prerequisite for an implementation of a telemedical exercise system for the home environment when taking into account the medical background on cardiac patients.

3. Conclusion and Outlook

In the field of cardiac rehabilitation, lifelong exercises are a necessity to avoid further cardiac events. Therefore, training within the home environment seems to be an appropriate approach. To set-up an appropriate system for phase III rehabilitation, many technical and medical requirements have to be met. To enable a communication between health system participants using the clinic IT infrastructure and systems of the home environment, a personal health record following vendor-independent standards like CDA should be used. This will also allow vendors to implement devices independently from each other.

Furthermore, devices for cardiac rehabilitation within the home environment have to respect health issues that would normally be handled by the medical professional during the exercise within the hospital. Therefore, complex training control systems have to be implemented. To fulfill the requirement that such a system has to monitor and control vital signs (e.g. heart frequency as a target parameter) of a patient, it is necessary to estimate the parameters based on information such as the results of a stress test, the medication and other "pre-existing" knowledge. This allows heart issues to be detected further in advance and, therefore, makes it possible for the system to react before further medical issues actually arise. In addition to the well-controlled circumstances of an ergometer bicycle training where the load on the patient can be directly defined, actuator-less systems can be implemented to coach a cardiac patient during outdoor exercises. For the estimation of vital signs in such an environment additional measurements have to be made, for example the temperature within the training area, the speed of the patient as well as the subsurface of the track. Environment variables like the subsurface can be measured in advance and stored as a load estimation map for route planning algorithms. To increase the precision of such a system a human behavior model has to be fitted to the patient individually, which will permit more concrete planning of the route as well as a higher precision for the vital sign estimation and, therefore, a stable alarm system with low failure rate.

Although the systems described in this article are intended for cardiac rehabilitation, they could rather easily be adapted to patients with other health issues where context based vital sign estimation is applicable. At the current point in time such systems are still in prototype state and a more research will be needed to raise them to product level. Furthermore, legal limitations such as medical device certification and emergency guidelines have to be taken into account. Nevertheless systems using context based vital sign estimation are apparently safer even today than using no alarm management at all and leaving the patient out alone.

Acknowledgement

This work was funded in part by the German Ministry of Education and Research within the research project "OSAMI-D" (grant 01 IS 08003) and in part by the Ministry for Science and Culture of Lower Saxony within the Research Network "Design of Environments for Ageing" (grant VWZN 2420/2524).

References

[1] I. Alich, B. Kotterba, B. Dömer et al., TEMONICS – Telemonitoring with cardiorespiratory systems – Teleüberwachung von Lungen – und Herz-Kreislauf-Patienten, in: *Tagungsband Ambient Assisted Living, 1. Deutscher AAL-Kongress*, Berlin, Germany, 2008.

[2] S. Allender, P. Scarborough, V. Peto et al., European heart network: European cardiovascular disease statistics, 2008 edition.

[3] M. Ball, C. Smith and R. Bakalar, Personal health records: Empowering consumers, *J. Healthc. Inf. Manag.* (2007), 76–86.
[4] B. Bjarnason-Wehrens, K. Held, E. Hoberg et al., Deutsche Leitlinie zu Rehabilitation von Patienten mit Herz-Kreislauferkrankungen (DLL-KardReha), *Clinical Research in Cardiology Supplements* **2**(3) (2007).
[5] Bluetooth Special Interest Group, Specification of the Bluetooth system 4.0, 2009.
[6] Bluetooth Special Interest Group, Specification of the Bluetooth system 1.1, part K.5 serial port profile, 2001.
[7] Bluetooth Special Interest Group, Specification of the Bluetooth system, health device profile, 2008.
[8] C. Busch, C. Baumbach, D. Willemsen et al., Supervised training with wireless monitoring of ECG, blood pressure and oxygen-saturation in cardiac patients, *J. Telemedicine Telecare* **15** (2009), 112–114.
[9] Continua Health Alliance, Continua design guidelines, version 1.0, October 2008.
[10] U. Corrà, P. Giannuzzia, S. Adamopoulos et al., Executive summary of the position paper of the working group on cardiac rehabilitation and exercise physiology of the European Society of cardiology (ESC): Core components of cardiac rehabilitation in chronic heart failure, *European Journal of Cardiovascular Prevention and Rehabilitation* **12** (2005), 321–325.
[11] T. Dierks and E. Rescorla, The transport layer security (TLS) protocol, version 1.2, IETF proposed standard RFC 5246, 2008.
[12] EN 1064:2005 Health informatics – Standard communication protocol – Computer-assisted electrocardiography.
[13] FOSSGIS e.V., OpenStreetMap Homepage, http://www.openstreetmap.de/ (accessed 2010-06-23).
[14] A.O. Freier, P. Karlton and P.C. Kocher, The SSL protocol, version 3.0, 1996.
[15] J. Habetha, The MyHeart project – Fighting cardiovascular diseases by prevention and early diagnosis, *Conf. Proc. IEEE Eng. Med. Biol. Soc.* (2006), Suppl:6746-9.
[16] Health Level Seven, HL7 implementation guide: CDA release 2 – Continuity of care document (CCD), 2007.
[17] Health Level Seven, The HL7 clinical document architecture (CDA) release 2, 2005.
[18] IEEE 802.15.1:2005 IEEE Standard for Information technology – Telecommunications and information exchange between systems – Local and metropolitan area networks – Specific requirements, Part 15.1: Wireless medium access control (MAC) and physical layer (PHY) specifications for wireless personal area networks (WPANs).
[19] Implementation guide for CDA release 2.0: Personal healthcare monitoring report (PHMR), Draft standard for trial use, release 1, 2008.
[20] Integrating the Healthcare Enterprise, IHE patient care coordination (PCC) technical framework, revision 5.0, 2009.
[21] Integrating the Healthcare Enterprise, IT infrastructure technical framework, revision 6.0, 2009.
[22] ISO/IEC 7498-1:1996 Information technology – Open systems interconnection – Basic reference model: The basic model.
[23] ISO/IEEE 11073-00000:2006 Health informatics – Point-of-care medical device communication – Framework and overview.
[24] D. Kaelber, S. Shah, A. Vincent et al., The value of personal health records, *Journal: CITL (Center for Information Technology Leaderchip)* **144** (2008).
[25] B. Kemp, A. Värri, A.C. Rosa et al., A simple format for exchange of digitized polygraphic recordings, *Electroencephalography and Clinical Neurophysiology* **82** (1992), 391–393.
[26] K. Kotseva, D. Wood, G. De Backer et al., Cardiovascular prevention guidelines in daily practice: A comparison of EUROASPIRE I, II, and III surveys in eight European countries, *Lancet* **373** (2009), 929–40.
[27] K. Kotseva, D. Wood, G. De Backer et al., EUROASPIRE III: A survey on the lifestyle, risk factors and use of cardioprotective drug therapies in coronary patients from 22 European countries, *European Journal of Cardiovascular Prevention and Rehabilitation* **16** (2009), 121–137.
[28] B. Kotterba, M. Ashauer, B. Schöller et al., Überwachung von Patienten mit Herz-Kreislauf-Erkrankungen, in: *Tagungsband Ambient Assisted Living, 1. Deutscher AAL-Kongress*, Berlin, Germany, 2008.
[29] H. Körtke, R.G. Heinze, K. Bockhorst et al., Telemedizinisch basierte Rehabilitation: Nachhaltig von Nutzen, *Dtsch. Arztebl.* **103**(44) (2006).
[30] A. Le and O. Gabel, Bericht des Forschungsschwerpunktes Ambient Intelligence: Entwurf eines Reglers für das AmI-Szenario Assisted Training, project report, 2008.
[31] M. Lipprandt and M Eichelberg, W. Thronicke et al., OSAMI-D: An open service platform for healthcare monitoring applications, in: *Proc. 2nd International Conference on Human System Interaction*, 2009, 139–145.

[32] A. Lorenz and R. Oppermann, Mobile health monitoring for the elderly: Designing for diversity, *Pervasive and Mobile Computing* **5** (2009), 1–22.
[33] Markle Foundation, Connecting americans to their health care: Final report working group on policies for electronic information sharing between doctors and patients, Markle Foundation, 2004
[34] O. Nee, A. Hein, T. Gorath et al., SAPHIRE: Intelligent healthcare monitoring based on semantic interoperability platform: Pilot applications, *IET Communications* **2** (2008), 192–201.
[35] NEMA Standards Publication PS3, Digital imaging and communications in medicine (DICOM), national electrical manufacturers association, Rosslyn, VA, 2009.
[36] J. Nobel and G. Norman, Emerging information management technologies and the future of disease management, *Disease Management* **6**(4) (2003), 219–231.
[37] Organization for the Advancement of Structured Information Standards, OASIS/ebXML registry information model specification v3.0, 2005.
[38] M.F. Piepoli, U. Corra, W. Benzer et al., Secondary prevention through cardiac rehabilitation: From knowledge to implementation, A position paper from the cardiac rehabilitation section of the European association of cardiovascular prevention and rehabilitation, *European Journal of Cardiovascular Prevention and Rehabilitation* **17** (2010), 1–17.
[39] Polar Electro Oy, Polar cardio Gx product description, http://www.polar.fi/us-en/b2b_products/club_solutions/polar_cardio_gx/polar_cardio_gx (accessed 2010-06-23).
[40] Polar Electro Oy, Polar homepage, http://www.polar.fi/en (accessed 2010-06-23).
[41] H. Reiter and N. Maglaveras, HeartCycle: Compliance and effectiveness in HF and CAD closed-loop management, *Conf. Proc. IEEE Eng. Med. Biol. Soc.* (2009), 2009:299-302.
[42] SHL Telemedicine, SHL homepage, http://www.shl-telemedicine.com/ (accessed 2010-06-23).
[43] S.C. Smith, J. Allen, S.N. Blair et al., AHA/ACC guidelines for secondary prevention for patients with coronary and other atherosclerotic vascular disease: 2006 update, *Circulation* **113** (2006), 2363–2372.
[44] H. Unbehauen, *Regelungstechnik I. Wiesbaden,* Friedr. Vieweg & Sohn Verlag, 2005.
[45] H. Völler, H. Hahmann, H. Gohlke et al., Effects of inpatient rehabilitation on cardiovascular risk factors in patients with coronary heart disease, PIN-Study Group, *Dtsch. Med. Wochenschr.* Jul. 9 **124**(27) (1999), 817–823.
[46] B.D. Weatherley, G. Cotter, H.C. Dittrich et al., Design and rationale of the PROTECT study: A placebo-controlled randomized study of the selective A1 adenosine receptor antagonist rolofylline for patients hospitalized with acute decompensated heart failure and volume overload to assess treatment effect on congestion and renal function, *J. Card. Fail.* **16**(1) (2010), 25–35.
[47] World Health Organization, fact sheet N°317, cardiovascular diseases (CVDs), updated 2009, http://www.who.int/mediacentre/factsheets/fs317/en/print.html (accessed 2010-06-23).
[48] ZigBee Standards Organization, ZigBee specification, Document 053474r17, 2007.

Handbook of Ambient Assisted Living
J.C. Augusto et al. (Eds.)
IOS Press, 2012

doi:10.3233/978-1-60750-837-3-535

Smart Home Technologies for People with Cognitive Impairment: An Affordable, Rehabilitative Approach

Tony GENTRY, PhD OTR/L*
Department of Occupational Therapy, Virginia Commonwealth University
Richmond, VA, USA

Abstract. People with disabilities related to cognitive impairment may be excellent candidates for smart home and ambient technologies that support safety and functional independence. Fortunately, many of the tools that may be leveraged to provide these supports are available and affordable in the consumer marketplace and can be readily implemented within the context of a rehabilitation therapy program. This chapter examines: (1) functional assessment for living at home, (2) a model for retrofitting existing homes for inexpensive smart home solutions that are focused on safety and functional independence, (3) a range of consumer tools available for improving home-based everyday support, (4) psychosocial implications of smart home utilization, and (5) issues surrounding funding for these technologies.

Keywords. Assistive technology, smart home, cognition, disability, rehabilitation

Introduction

Research into advanced smart home and ambient assistance technologies to support people with disabilities in home settings is progressing rapidly. A recent comprehensive review [5] lists 38 ongoing university-based projects that are investigating technologies ranging from sophisticated models of home automation to computer-based user monitoring and guidance (in some cases provided by a robotic caregiver). Focus areas include physiological response capture, behavior prediction, context-specific cueing, and a range of statistical analysis packages intended to provide just-in-time home-based support for people with mobility, sensory or cognitive challenges.

While this burgeoning research holds great promise for providing individualized home supports for people with disabilities, few advanced products have yet found their way to the consumer marketplace. Fortunately, however, it is possible to provide effective smart home supports utilizing readily available and affordable devices. Smart homes of this nature include – among many others – the smart apartments in the Hereward College student dormitories in Coventry, England [8], Imagine! Corporation's Bob and Judy Charles Smarthome in Boulder, Colorado, USA [4] and the Woodrow Wilson Rehabilitation Center's smart cottage for people with brain injury in Fishersville, VA, USA [10]. Each of these dwellings incorporates suites of consumer-based technologies that include, among other devices: (1) remote controlled or automated

*Corresponding Author: Tony Gentry. E-mail: logentry@vcu.edu.

lighting and appliances utilizing Electronic Aids to Daily Living (EADL), (2) safety alert systems, (3) task reminder messaging, and (4) smartphone applications that extend home-based support to community activities (such as wayfinding, shopping and job support).

Though the use of smart home technologies among people with disabilities is spreading worldwide, there has been very little outcomes-based research examining the effectiveness of this rehabilitation strategy. A Swedish team reported that eleven people with brain injury who each lived alone for one week in a cottage equipped with voice-controlled appliances, caregiver alert bracelets, and a computer-based task reminder system learned how to operate the technologies and felt the smart home improved their sense of self-efficacy [9]. Seven people with brain injury followed a similar research strategy at the Woodrow Wilson Rehabilitation Center Smart Cottage, which is equipped with *low-tech* environmental organizers, caregiver alert devices, automated lighting and appliances, fire and water safety products, and smartphone-based reminder systems. Each of the seven lived successfully in the cottage for one week, having learned to incorporate the smart home technologies into their daily routines [10]. Rigby, Ryan et al. [19] reported that a group of adults with cervical spinal cord injury were able to utilize EADL at home and functioned more independently than a matched group without remote controlled appliances. A recent Cochrane review [14], however, determined that these preliminary studies do not provide enough evidence to support smart home use for people with disabilities. We do not yet have results from a rigorously controlled research study examining consumer-based smart home use with any disability population.

As the studies just reported suggest, people with cognitive impairment may be excellent candidates for assistive technologies that incorporate smart home and ambient applications. These tools may be leveraged to make homes more readily accessible and safer, while reducing the need for caregiver support. They may encourage functional independence in task behaviors such as taking medications and managing hygiene, diet, exercise, home chores and community engagement. Proper utilization of home-based assistive technologies may also reduce the need for nursing home placement, allowing people with disabilities to rehabilitate at home and age in place. Fortunately, many of the tools that may be used to provide these layers of support are available and affordable in the consumer marketplace. They can be readily implemented within the context of a rehabilitation therapy program.

In this chapter, we will examine: (1) functional assessment for living at home, (2) a model for retrofitting existing homes for inexpensive smart home solutions that are focused on safety and functional independence, (3) a range of consumer tools available for improving home-based everyday support, (4) psychosocial implications of smart home utilization, and (5) issues surrounding funding for these technologies.

1. Cognitive Challenges

Though each person with a cognitive disability has a quite individual set of strengths and weaknesses, memory impairment is a relatively common feature of brain injury, neurodegenerative diseases – such as multiple sclerosis and Alzheimer's disease – and many mental illnesses. People with memory impairment may forget to turn off stoves or water faucets, may follow medication routines inconsistently, may have difficulty following home management, diet and exercise plans, and may face diverse challenges in community engagement, school and work settings. Cognitive skills related to memory impairment include difficulty initiating, sequencing or completing tasks, multitasking, prioritizing activities and being aware of safety risks in the home. Any of these difficulties may make independent living problematic. Fortunately, technologies exist to assist with these difficulties.

2. Assessing the Home Needs of a Person with a Cognitive Impairment

A number of well-researched tools are available to help the rehabilitation therapist determine a need for therapeutic intervention in the home. Cognitive assessments that examine the cognitive skills used in everyday life include: (a) The Rivermead Behavioral Memory Test – Extended [25], (2) the Behavioral Assessment of Dysexecutive Syndrome [24], (3) The Test of Everyday Attention [20], and (4) the Executive Function Performance Test [3], among others. Each of these tools exhibits ecological validity, in that it simulates activities a person would be expected to perform in everyday life, and assesses levels of support needed for success at these activities. While they do not offer prescriptive recommendations for home adaptations, they provide useful information for the therapist in determining which functional areas may require support. Therapists are advised to supplement these tests with in-home observations, that may include cooking, cleaning, shopping, medication routines, money management and other everyday tasks, since functional performance on tests and in clinics often differs from that observed in a familiar home setting. Home visits may also include interviews with clients and caregivers focused on delineating areas of functional dependence and human supports available in the home.

A therapist may choose to conduct a generic home safety evaluation at this time, examining the environment for accessibility and safety. Home safety assessments are traditionally offered for people with mobility challenges or sensory impairment, with a primary focus on improving access. Typical recommendations include improved lighting, wheelchair ramps, widened doorways, tub benches and rails, lowered shelving and stair-lifts. EADL, such as motion-controlled lighting or remote-controlled appliances, are sometimes recommended as energy saving features. As we will discuss, many of these familiar adaptations may also play a role in smart home design for people with cognitive impairment.

It is important to remember that a participatory evaluation process, in which a home occupant self-identifies functional needs, tries out recommended adaptations in the home environment, and suggests changes, as needed, while a therapist provides support, follow-along and training, can lead to the right fit for each person. The English research consultancy Smart Thinking offers a free, downloadable program [6] that provides a step-by-step decision tree for working collaboratively in matching smart home technologies with clients. Their CUSTODIAN system is based on the admirable philosophy that smart homes should be "appropriate, enabling, empowering, rehabilitative and stimulate independence".

3. Model of Affordable Smart Home Design

Therapists have at their disposal a rich repertoire of tools to assist their clients with cognitive impairment at home, ranging from *low-tech* adaptations such as organization strategies and paper-and-pen reminders, through *mid-tech* devices such as alarm clocks and automatic coffee pots, to *high-tech* tools that can automate home lighting, heating and task cueing and "think" for the home occupant. Homes that incorporate low-tech safety and cognitive assistance features (examples are stair railings and an organized, de-cluttered living space) may be termed "proto-smart homes".

Electronic solutions may be usefully stratified using the Aldrich classification of smart home design [1], which ranks five levels of technological utilization.

Level one smart homes incorporate intelligent objects, such as doors or window shades that open via a remote control switch or appliances that operate by timer or electronic eye. Suites of these intelligent appliances can make homes more accessible for mobility-impaired occupants and safer for those with cognitive impairment.

Level two homes utilize wired or wireless in-home networks for information exchange, such as computer-controlled thermostats or lighting. They are often used to automatically optimize energy use in the home, but can relieve cognitively-impaired occupants of the responsibility for managing home appliances, while also offering task cues via computer-mediated reminder systems.

Level three homes include electronic networks that reach beyond the home for information exchange (these are often called "connected homes"). People with cognitive impairment may utilize a connected home strategy to provide for automatic bank deposits and bill-paying, automated grocery shopping and/or access to off-site caregivers via telephone, videophone or email.

Level four homes (known as "learning homes") are linked to computers that analyze patterns of activity and manage appliances accordingly. A learning home network, for example, may monitor community energy use, cueing the home occupant of the most energy efficient time to operate appliances such as dishwashers and laundry machines. This strategy may also be used to remotely analyze information from passive monitors in the home, utilizing this information to control lights and appliances, provide context-appropriate task cues for occupants or warn off-site caregivers of irregularities in an occupant's daily routine that may signal a fall or other problem. A few of the learning home suites now in use will be discussed later in this chapter.

As previously described, research centers around the globe have begun exploring the frontiers of cognitive support that may be provided by learning homes; they are developing *level five* "aware homes" that incorporate monitors, computer links and learning algorithms to anticipate human needs and intervene accordingly. Aware homes, at this writing, are still in the research phase, though marketable versions may be just years away.

Therapists clearly have many proto-smart home and smart home options to consider for clients with cognitive impairment who wish to live more safely and independently at home. Each client will require an individualized suite of technologies to address her/his functional challenges, based on preserved functional ability, personal goals, human supports available and financial resources. The remainder of this chapter will provide a model for making these recommendations.

4. Outfitting a Safe, Smart Home

Working with a client and caregiver to select and implement the right suite of home adaptations can be daunting, but it can be helpful to consider the primary categories of functional challenges faced in the home, matching tools and strategies to those needs. In addressing home-based cognitive challenges, therapists are advised to consider the following categories of need: (1) safety, (2) falls risk, (3) forgetfulness and inattention, (4) medication management, (4) general health, (5) sleep hygiene, (6) diet, (7) exercise, (8) home maintenance, (9) money management and (10) community engagement. Let us explore each of these categories, examining technologies that can assist a person in functioning more independently in each area.

4.1. Safety

Safety risks are the most often-cited reason for people having to leave their homes for supported living environments, but a judicious and individualized blend of adaptations may help keep a person with cognitive disability safe at home. Typical concerns and recommended strategies follow.

4.2. Falls Risk

Therapists have many tools at their disposal in addressing falls risk. Proto-smart home recommendations often include ambulation aids and home exercise routines intended to address balance and functional endurance. Home adaptations may include, among other things: (1) improved lighting, (2) removal of pathway obstacles, (3) changes in furniture heights, (4) stair-lifts or stair railings, and (5) tub benches and rails in the bath. Some sort of regular caregiver check-in system – such as a daily phone call – is recommended for people at falls risk. Electronic adaptations may incorporate *level one* consumer technologies, such as motion-activated lighting or a medical alert paging bracelet. In some cases, a *level four* monitoring system that can respond to deviations in a person's home routine may provide an extra measure of assurance. Examples include the monitor-response systems offered by a trio of private companies in the U.S., each of which charges a monthly fee to the user. *Rest Assured* [18] installs video observation cameras and motion sensors in the home. Observers stationed at off-site video monitors counsel occupants via home-based videophones, contact caregivers or alert emergency medical teams when a fall or other problem is noted. As one might expect, this model has been sharply criticized for its intrusion on personal privacy. *Sound Response* [2] addresses this criticism by eliminating video cameras, relying entirely on motion detectors, smoke alarms and door security sensors. Off-site observers compare signals sent by these detectors to an occupant's typical daily routine and send help if deviations are noted that may signal a fall or other problem. *Quietcare* [17] does away entirely with human observation, relying on a computer server to analyze home-based sensor readings and trigger alerts if unusual deviations in a person's daily routine are noted (see Fig. 1 below).

Connected and learning home systems such as these offer some assurance for people who are at falls risk and as supports for those with cognitive impairment, but weaknesses include gaps in observed data and historically slow arrival times by community-based emergency response teams. A person who has fallen may lie on the floor for hours awaiting the system's decision to act and the arrival of a helper. In considering the use of these systems, each client will need to make informed decisions about personal privacy, comfort with off-site supervision and the risk of response-time delays.

4.3. Forgetfulness and Inattention

Memory and attention deficits can lead to a number of safety risks in the home. Perhaps the most dangerous risk is in the kitchen, where leaving a pan on the cook stove

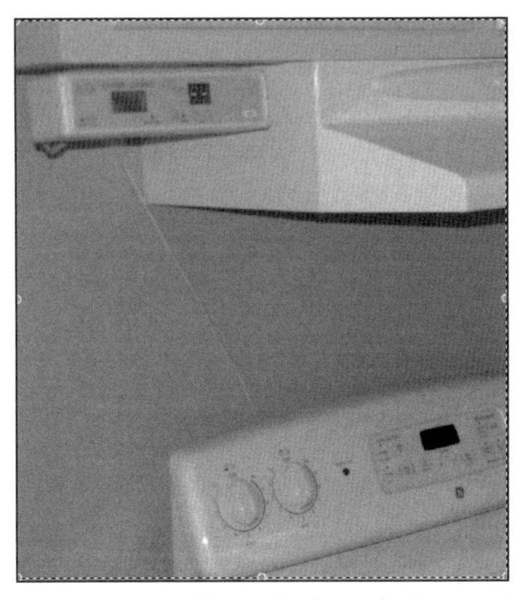

Figure 1. General Electric *Quietcare* system diagram showing passive home monitors, computer server for activity analysis and links to offsite caregivers.

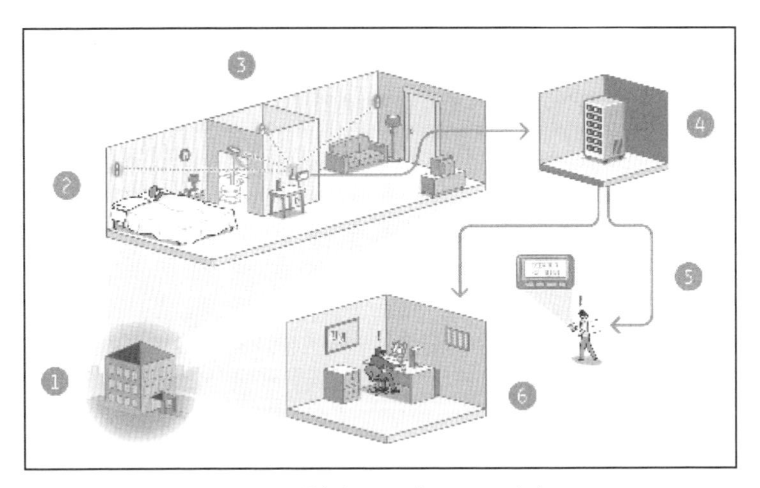

Figure 2. *Stoveguard* kitchen monitor mounted above stove.

can start a house fire, where leaving a faucet running can flood the house, and where inattention to food spoilage dates can lead to illness. Some occupants may wander away from home and get lost. A comprehensive home safety assessment should examine these risks for a particular client, with steps taken to avoid them. In many cases, proto-smart home solutions can be useful. For instance, choosing to use a microwave oven rather than a cook stove can address the risk of fire. In other cases, *level one* kitchen monitors can help. One such device, the *StoveGuard* [22] (see Fig. 2), serves as an electronic eye in the kitchen. The wall-mounted device – connected directly to an electric stove's power supply – turns off the stove if movement in the kitchen is not detected in a pre-selected amount of time.

An inexpensive solution to water spillage risk is a water leak alarm [13]. These battery-powered, palm-sized devices can be placed under a sink, next to a bathtub or washing machine, or behind a toilet, for instance. Any spillage of water sounds a piercing alarm, alerting a resident to turn off the faucet. Awareness of food spoilage dates can be improved by the utilization of timer bands [7], which can be affixed to bottles, jars or other packaging. These devices beep or blink when a preprogrammed food spoilage date is reached.

As an element of home safety evaluation, occupational therapists should examine other safety risks, identifying escape routes, setting up emergency one-touch numbers on client telephones, rehearsing with clients the use of fire extinguishers, and making sure that smoke and carbon monoxide alarms are in proper working order. In some cases, the use of a voice recorder smoke alarm [23] can be effective. This device replays a pre-recorded message when smoke is detected, telling the occupant what to do, rather than simply sounding an alarm.

Many people with cognitive impairment are at risk for wandering away from home or getting lost in the community. Fortunately, most cell-phones now have homing beacons or add-on applications that are readily accessed via Internet by off-site caregivers, showing device location on a map. Free-standing, matchbook-sized homing beacons [28] can be secured in garments for the use of people who do not have phones. Some allow caregivers to pre-set electronic fence parameters in the neighborhood, launching a cell-phone text message alert if the user wanders outside of those parameters. An inexpensive, door-activated digital recorder [16] can cue the person to collect her/his coat, cell-phone, personal digital assistant (PDA) and keys before leaving the house. Similarly, a door-activated paging device can signal an offsite caregiver that an occupant has left the house.

4.4. Medication Management

Patients with neurological conditions are often prescribed powerful medications that influence brain chemistry. Failing to take the proper dosage can lead to illness and hospitalization, so it is essential that these individuals follow a strict medication routine. For people with memory impairment, reminder alarm pillboxes can help. Hundreds of varieties are on the market, ranging from one-dose beepers that fit in a pocket to multi-dose desktop units (such as the *MD2* shown in Fig. 3 [15]) that send text messages to off-site caregivers if a medication dose is ignored. Typically, an off-site caregiver programs these devices, filling day-and-time tagged compartments with an appropriate dose. In this way, the cognitively-impaired consumer only needs to respond to the alarm and take the medication when it sounds. Clinicians are urged to keep a demonstration kit of various reminder alarm pillboxes on hand to try out with clients, as each person's needs are different. The web-based store www.ipill.com sells hundreds of medication reminders at all levels of complexity. People who use cell-phones or PDAs may prefer timed text message reminders or calendar alarm prompts rather than electronic pillboxes.

4.5. General Health

Consumer technologies may be leveraged to help people with cognitive challenges manage sleep hygiene, diet and exercise. Many of these technologies utilize connected home tools such as Internet-linked computer programs, thus requiring basic familiarity with computers and Internet navigation.

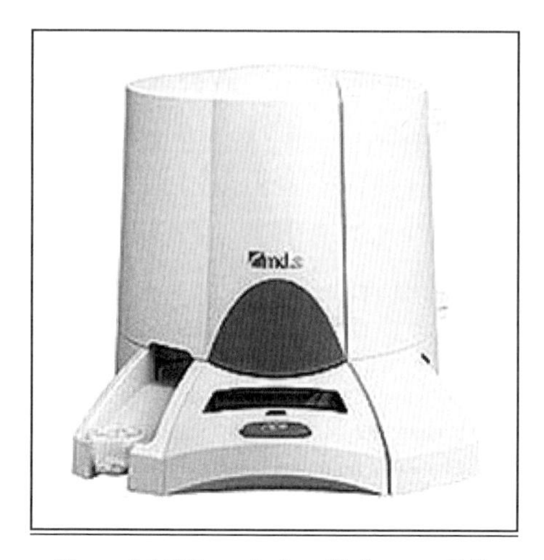

Figure 3. MD2 monitoring pill dispenser [15].

4.6. Sleep Hygiene

Sleep disorders are great thieves of cognitive function; many cognitive rehabilitation therapists start their interventions with sleep management, in order to help maximize a client's cognitive ability. Discussion of comprehensive sleep therapy is outside the scope of this chapter, but there are home-based tools available that can help a person monitor and self-manage sleep challenges. The *Zeo Personal Sleep Coach* [27] is a consumer product that includes a bedside sleep monitor and a headband worn while in bed. The device tracks brainwaves and movement during sleep, providing information on sleep quality and providing Internet-based coaching tips for improving it. For just $4.99 (US), the Sleep Cycle [21] application for accelerometer-equipped smart-phones tracks and graphs movement, providing users with a rough picture of their sleep quality to help in exploring therapeutic options.

4.7. Diet

Many people with cognitive disability have difficulty managing diet, because they forget to eat or forget that they have already eaten. The challenges of menu planning, shopping and preparing a meal can prove overwhelming for these people. Fortunately, reminder alarms on cell-phones or PDAs can be programmed to provide a mealtime cue. Therapists are advised to work closely with clients in the kitchen, simplifying and organizing cooking tools, teaching sequencing strategies for food preparation, and making the kitchen as safe as possible. Smart-phone applications can readily assist in the creation of menus from food on hand in the pantry, assist with shopping lists, and offer step-by-step photographic or videophonic cooking instructions. Calorie tracking applications can serve as diet coaches.

4.8. Exercise

After sleep and diet, exercise is probably the most important factor in maintaining both general and cognitive health, yet people with cognitive impairment may forget to exercise, may not know what to do, or may fear over-exercising. Therapists are advised to assess a client's physical health and prescribe a healthy daily exercise routine. PDA-

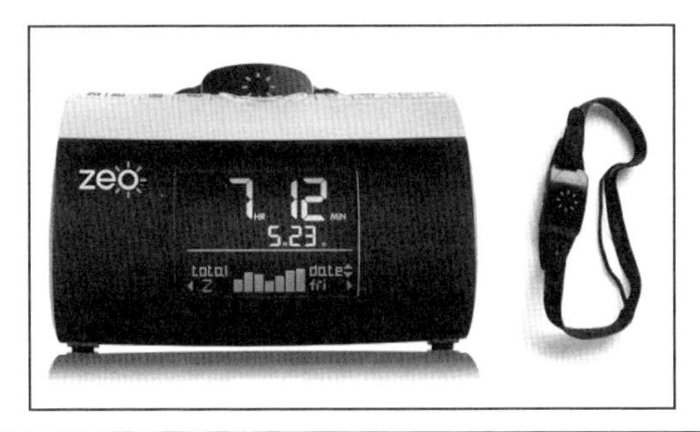

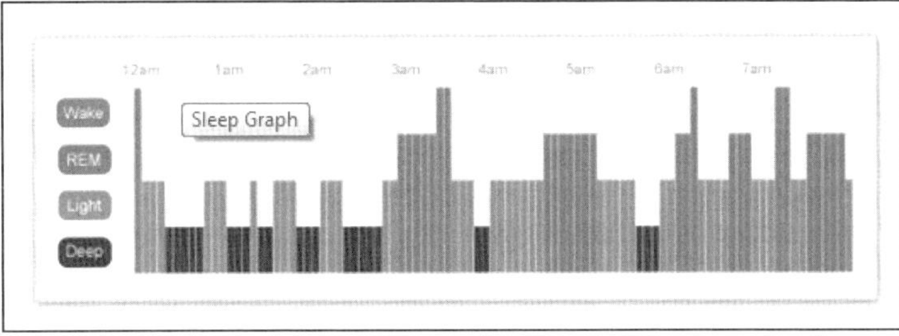

Figure 4. Zeo Sleep System desktop monitor and headband, with example of a weekly sleep quality graph [27].

based reminder alarms may cue a person to exercise, exercise DVDs or athletic activities played on motion-monitoring gaming systems (such as the *Nintendo Wii*, *Microsoft Xbox Kinect* or *Sony Playstation Move*) may be used at home to guide exercise, and a wide range of software applications may be utilized to record exercise progress. Participation in exercise groups at local health clubs may promote both physical and social well-being, though dance classes and other group-based workouts can provide overwhelming sensory stimulation for some people. Quieter group-based activities, such as running, swimming or yoga may work better in these cases.

4.9. Home Maintenance

Managing the home typically incorporates an individualized suite of proto-smart home and smart home adaptations. Low-tech organization strategies following the motto "a place for everything and everything in its place" may include drawer subdividers, a table near the front door where the occupant empties her/his pockets of keys, phone and other items on entering the house (refilling them on the way out), a wall calendar and shopping list. Weekly routines for cleaning, laundry, yard-work and home maintenance should be set up with reminder cues on cell-phone or PDA. Videos of the home occupant performing complex tasks can be loaded onto these portable devices, and referenced as needed if elements of a task are difficult to recall. Occupants may benefit from portable device-based home organization applications (such as *Home Routines* [11]) that allow for structured cueing, task timers and task completion checklists. Some appliances – refrigerators, furnaces, and washing machines, for instance – may be purchased with in-dwelling reminder alarms that signal the occupant when filter replacement or other maintenance is needed. These *level two* smart home features can be especially useful for people with cognitive impairment.

EADL products can be connected to personal computer software to automate appliances and lighting patterns in the home. When linked to readily deployed EADL

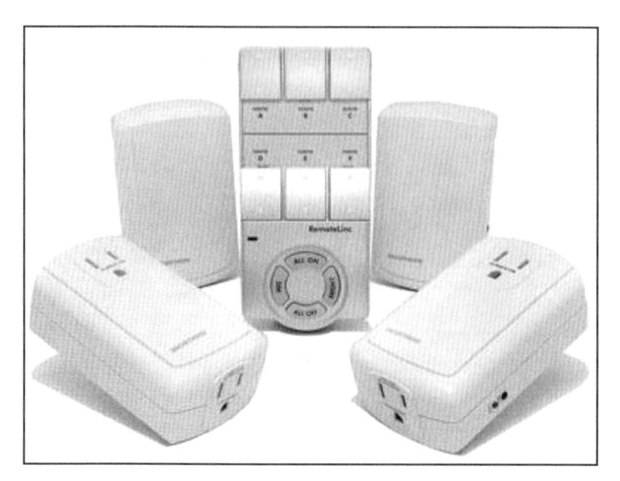

Figure 5. *Insteon* Electronic Aids to Daily Living modules and controller.

modules in the home, *Level three* computer-based software such as the $x - 10$ *Active-Home* [26] or *Insteon Houselinc Two* [12] packages can be programmed to automatically optimize the use of thermostats, lighting and other appliances to reduce energy costs. Creative users of these programs can build morning wake up and bedtime routines that incorporate lighting and voice recorded cues for the cognitively impaired. Timed lamp blinks can be used as unobtrusive medication or task reminders. Connecting EADL control software to Internet-linked computers can allow appliance management by offsite caregivers.

4.10. Money Management

Automated bill-paying and direct deposit bank accounts are ubiquitous *level three* smart home technologies that can prevent people with cognitive impairment from forgetting to pay rent or other important utility bills. Many people utilize personal computer or PDA-based money management software, to help keep track of income and expenditures. By linking this software to credit card, earnings and other accounts, money management can become a nearly hand's free operation.

4.11. Community Engagement

Smart home technologies can help people with cognitive impairment function more safely and independently at home, but occupants may feel trapped or homebound if similar tools are not available for cognitive support in the community. Fortunately, cell-phones and PDAs can be outfitted to address safety and functional independence concerns outside the home. As noted, these devices can be loaded with applications that include person-locators, task and medication reminders, shopping lists, task-sequencing videos, wayfinding solutions (via GPS map or video) and other cognitive supports intended for community access. Therapists are advised to recommend speed dial numbers for caregivers and medical staff, and to introduce and train clients in the use of community access applications in a stepwise manner, so as not to overwhelm them with too many features at once. Clients should be given the opportunity to try out these tools on semi-supervised community outings, in order to test their efficacy and accessibility, before attempting outings on their own.

Table 1. Examples of Affordable Consumer-Level Smart Home Technologies

Product	Vendor	Price (USD)
Basic set of *Insteon* EADL modules for overhead lights, lamps and thermostat	www.insteon.net	300
Insteon Houselinc2 EADL computer controller	www.insteon.net	150
Motion-controlled outdoor lights (front and back doors)	www.lowes.com	100
Stoveguard stove monitor	www.stoveguard.ca	250
Leak Frog water leak alarm (4)	www.gadgeteer.com	20
Vocal Smoke Alarm	www.smarthome.com	60
Food Spoilage Bands (6)	www.smarthome.com	30
Apple Ipod Touch	www.apple.com	219
Miscellaneous cognitive support applications for *Ipod Touch*	www.apple.com	100
One-week medication alarm pillbox	www.ipill.com	25
Nintendo Wii Game Console and Sports Games	www.nintendo.com	250
Total		1504

Table 2. Example of Fee-based Smart Home Services

Product	Vendor	Initial Setup (USD)	Monthly Fee (USD)
Rest Assured passive monitoring system	www.restassuredsystem.com	800	1000
Medical Alert Pendant	www.medicalert.com	0	30
Total		800	1030

4.12. Group-Based Application Testing

As computer-based and handheld lifestyle applications proliferate, therapists may find that offering a series of group-based instructional sessions for clients with cognitive disability may allow them to try out a variety of potentially useful phone or PDA-based applications, explore their use at home, and compare results with other group members. This stepwise method allows for gradual introduction of instructional applications, training in their use, and home trials that may help clients more successfully integrate these tools into their everyday routines.

5. Funding Smart Home Technologies

The proto-smart home and smart home applications discussed in this chapter are relatively inexpensive and easily retrofitted into existing homes. Motion-activated lighting, EADL, and safety devices such as the *Stoveguard* can be installed by an electrician in an afternoon. Therapists with expertise in assistive technology and cognitive disability are essential, of course, to facilitate assessment, device selection, implementation and follow-along. Though the needs of every person will differ, the equipment used in a generic smart home for a person with cognitive impairment – incorporating *level three* technologies – may cost no more than $2500 (USD) (see Table 1).

Including *level four* monitor-response technologies adds a monthly fee ranging from $800–1400 (USD) (see Table 2). In many cases, therapeutic intervention and purchase of home-based technologies are supported by third party payers, especially when those payers recognize that living at home costs them much less than funding a client in a group living environment.

6. The Quest for the Perfect Smart Home

As we have discussed, there are diverse technological means available to support people with cognitive disability in their homes. People with mild cognitive impairments may find that an individualized suite of these tools provides the support needed for safe and independent function without caregiver intervention; people with more severe impairments, however, must still rely on off-site or – in some cases – in-home caregivers to supplement proto-smart home and smart home technologies. When a caregiver is available for weekly visits, it can be helpful to develop a checklist of tasks to be conducted during that visit. The checklist may include: (1) filling a reminder pillbox and setting reminder alarms; (2) discussing the past week's activities, with a focus on adherence to sleep, diet, exercise and home maintenance routines (perhaps reviewing PDA-based applications that have been used to record daily activity); (3) collaborating with the home occupant on planning activities and home maintenance chores for the following week, and setting reminder messages on cell-phone or PDA for those activities; and (4) checking batteries and electrical connections for EADL and safety tools (such as a *Stoveguard*, water overflow monitor and food expiration tags).

Caregivers who cannot make weekly visits can sometimes utilize phone calls or videophone calls to accomplish these tasks, directing the home occupant to perform them while on the phone. Written instructions or PDA-based videos demonstrating these smart home maintenance activities can supplement telephonic instruction. If difficulties related to the smart home technologies are noted, the prescribing therapist should be called in to collaborate on making adaptations, as needed.

In cases where severe cognitive impairment precludes independent living, smart home technologies can still provide a level of support for safety and functional independence greater than that offered by a human caregiver alone. Reminder messages can free the caregiver of constant nagging over medication routines and everyday chores, person locator tools can reduce the risk of a wandering person getting lost, and safety products can protect the house and its occupants from fire and water damage. Smart home tools in these cases reduce caregiver burden and reduce overall anxiety in the family.

We do not yet have any suite of smart home technologies that guarantees safety and functional independence for people at every level of cognitive impairment. Instead, we have tools that allow a person with cognitive impairment to live independently when things go well and to fail safely, with a safety net, when they do not. Even here, it must be noted, that no system is perfect. Electronic devices fail, Internet servers go down, caregivers may be out of touch when needed, and emergency response times vary. Each family must take on the responsibility of determining what level of electronic surveillance and support is comfortable for them, while identifying caregivers who will participate in the smart home intervention and take part in maintenance and troubleshooting tasks.

Some cognitive conditions are degenerative; others can be remediated. In either case, a client's needs will change over time. Therapists should expect to provide follow-along assistance periodically to reassess functional needs and recommend adaptations. Caregivers should be coached to be alert for any degeneration in functional safety or performance. At the same time, technologies that support safe and independent home dwelling constantly evolve. All team members must stay alert to the arrival of new products that may serve the needs of clients at home.

7. Psychosocial Implications of Smart Homes

When considering the recommendation of smart home technologies for a person with cognitive impairment, one must keep in mind that the client: (1) may not be fully aware of her/his functional challenges, (2) may prefer human supports over technological supports, (3) may not want to have any changes made to the home, and (4) may be frightened by or indisposed to technological solutions to everyday problems. Because people often perceive their homes as sanctuaries, as extensions of their own personalities, and as private domains, any recommendation may be perceived as an unwelcome intrusion. Therapists must respect this position. Issues of insight and awareness of cognitive deficit can be addressed by collaborating with a family member or caregiver who has a realistic appraisal of the client's functional skills. Working as a team, the therapist, client and caregiver can map out everyday challenges and try out solutions that may incorporate elements of human support, proto-smart home and smart home interventions. Each technology should be introduced on a trial basis, with training and follow-along provided, in order to see whether it works as hoped and is accepted in the home. (As noted, the *CUSTODIAN* decision tree can be useful in negotiating client acceptance of home adaptations.) In this way, each person may be guaranteed an individualized suite of cognitive supports that can adapt over time, as technologies evolve and as cognitive support needs change.

8. Conclusion

Research into advanced home-based monitoring and cueing technologies for people with disabilities is advancing rapidly, though outcomes-based research on the efficacy of smart home technologies for this population lags. It is apparent, however, that smart home technologies may be leveraged to promote safety and functional independence for people with cognitive impairment. An ever-growing catalogue of home-based tools is available to address safety, medication management, health, home maintenance and community engagement, and a suite of these technologies can be both inexpensive and readily retrofitted into existing homes. Rehabilitation therapists are strongly urged to learn about smart home technologies and to appropriately facilitate their use in helping people live safely and independently at home, despite cognitive disability. As noted, in working with people in the intimacy of their home environments, knowledge of assistive technology theory and application must be supplemented by an assessment, provision and follow-along process that recognizes the functional goals, unique habits and psychosocial needs of the end user. This process appears more likely to assure long-term adoption of any smart home technology solution. In light of the current paucity of outcomes-based research in this area, investigators are urged to pursue rigorous studies that will explore the efficacy, adoption characteristics and cost-effectiveness of smart homes with populations that have cognitive impairment and/or other disabling conditions.

References

[1] F. Aldrich, Smart homes past, present and future, in: *Inside the Smart Home*, R. Harper, ed., Springer, London, 2003.

[2] L.R. Barrett, Electronic watchdog keeps developmentally disabled safe, *Wisconsin State Journal* **1** (December 2003), http//www.waisman.wisc.edu/news/soundresponse.html, last access: 28 February 2011.

[3] C.M. Baum, T. Morrison, M. Hahn and D.D. Edwards, *Executive Function Performance Test*, Washington University, St. Louis, 2007.
[4] Bob and Judy Charles Smarthome, http://www.imaginesmarthomes.org/BOULDER.htm, last access: 28 February 2011.
[5] M. Chan, D. Esteve, C. Escriba and E. Campo, A review of smart homes – Present state and future challenges, *Computer Methods and Programs in Biomedicine* **91** (2008), 55–81.
[6] Custodian, http://www.smartthinking.ukideas.com/CUST%20Index.html, last access: 28 February 2011.
[7] DaysAgo Timer, http://www.smarthome.com/915dam.html, last access: 28 February 2011.
[8] G. Dewsbury and J. Linskell, Smart home technology for safety and functional independence: The UK experience, http://www.smartthinking.ukideas.com/Articles.html, last access: 28 February 2011.
[9] A. Erikson, G. Karlsson, M. Soderstrom and K. Tham, A training apartment with electronic aids to daily living: Lived experiences of persons with brain damage, *American Journal of Occupational Therapy* **58** (2004), 261–271.
[10] T. Gentry and M. Breister, Outcomes from a trial of smart home technologies for adults with brain injury, *Brain Injury* (in press).
[11] Home Routines, http://www.homeroutines.com, last access: 28 February 2011.
[12] Insteon Houselinc, http://www.insteon.net/2412UH-houselinc2-usb-interface.html, last access: 28 February 2011.
[13] Leakfrog Water Alarm, http://the-gadgeteer.com/2005/09/28/ideative_leakfrog_water_alarm/, last access: 28 February 2011.
[14] S. Martin, W.G. Kernohan, B. McCreight and C. Nugent, Smart home technologies for health and social care support (review), The Cochrane Collaboration, 2009, http://www.thecochranelibrary.com, last access: 28 February 2011.
[15] MD2 Monitoring Pill Dispenser, http://www.ipill.com, last access: 28 February 2011.
[16] Motion-activated Digital Recorder, http://www.lhb.org, last access: 28 February 2011.
[17] Quietcare: Living Independently, http://www.gehealthcare.com/usen/telehealth/quietcare/proactive_eldercare_technology.html, last access: 28 February 2011.
[18] Rest Assured System, http://www.restasuredsystem.com, last access: 28 February 2011.
[19] P. Rigby, S. Ryan, S. Joos, B. Cooper, J. Jutai and E. Steggles, Impact of electronic aids to daily living on the lives of persons with cervical spinal cord injuries, *Assistive Technology* **17** (2005), 89–97.
[20] I.H. Robertson, T. Ward, V. Ridgeway and I. Nimmo-Smith, *The Test of Everyday Attention*, Pearson, New York, 1994.
[21] Sleep Cycle, http://www.mdlabs.se/sleepcycle, last access: 28 February 2011.
[22] Stoveguard, http://www.stoveguard.ca, last access: 28 February 2011.
[23] Vocal Smoke Alarm, http://www.smarthome.com/7563/Vocal-Smoke-Alarm/p.aspx, last access: 28 February 2011.
[24] B. Wilson, N. Alderman, P.W. Burgess, H. Emslie and J.J. Evans, *Behavioural Assessment of the Dysexecutive Syndrome*, Pearson, New York, 1993.
[25] B. Wilson, J. Cockburn and A. Baddelay, The *Rivermead Behavioral Memory Test-Extended*, 2nd edn, Thames Valley Test Company, Bury St. Edmunds, England, 1991.
[26] $x - 10$ Activehome, http://www.x10.com/automation/x10_ck11a.htm, last access: 28 February 2011.
[27] Zeo Personal Sleep Coach, http://www.myzeo.com, last access: 28 February 2011.
[28] Zoombak Personal GPS Locator, http://www.zoombak.com/products/universal, last access: 28 February 2011.

Handbook of Ambient Assisted Living
J.C. Augusto et al. (Eds.)
IOS Press, 2012

doi:10.3233/978-1-60750-837-3-549

AAL Technologies in Rehabilitation – Lessons Learned from a COPD Case Study

Babak A. FARSHCHIAN[a,*], Kristine HOLBØ[b], Marius MIKALSEN[a] and Jarl REITAN[b]
[a]*SINTEF ICT, Norway*
[b]*SINTEF T&S, Norway*

Abstract. AAL technologies for rehabilitation constitute a major research area within AAL research. A large number of novel technologies and applications has been developed in R&D projects. Our focus in this paper is to see how these technologies support innovation in the field. We document how these technologies and innovations meet the requirements driven by our sample project, called COPD@Home, carried out in the Norwegian settings. We outline the participatory design methodology used in COPD@Home. We document the resulting requirements. We then analyze the definition of AAL provided by some European strategy documents, and briefly survey a number of EU-funded projects in the field. We provide a gap analysis between the requirements from COPD@Home and the results from the surveyed EU-funded R&D projects. Our findings show that existing R&D lacks proper treatment of organizational issues related to AAL technologies such as re-engineering of existing work practices, training and on-the-job learning of care personnel, and support for collaborative workflows. In general we also see a lack of focus on service innovation as an inherent part of the current technological developments in AAL.

Keywords. AAL, COPD, rehabilitation, needs driven innovation, case study, ICT, lessons learned

Introduction

Chronic obstructive pulmonary disease (COPD) is a collective term for conditions in which the chronic constriction or collapse of minor airways causes increased resistance in the airways. Sufferers from this condition have difficulty in breathing even when they are at rest. The limitation of airflow is poorly reversible and usually gets progressively worse over time. Its final stages lead to pulmonary failure with chronic lack of oxygen than can lead to problems in concentrating, dizziness, chest pain, and finally, heart failure [11]. The primary cause of COPD is tobacco smoke (through tobacco use or second-hand smoke). The disease now affects men and women almost equally, due in part to increased tobacco use among women in high-income countries. COPD is not curable, but treatment can slow the progress of the disease. According to World Health Organization [22] an estimated 210 million people have COPD worldwide. More than 3 million people died of COPD in 2005, which is equal to 5% of all deaths globally that year. Almost 90% of COPD deaths occur in low- and middle-income countries. Total

*Corresponding Author: Babak A. Farshchian, SINTEF, S.P. Andersensvei 15B, NO-7465, Trondheim, Norway. E-mail: babak.farshchian@sintef.no.

deaths from COPD are projected to increase by more than 30% in the next 10 years without interventions to cut risks, particularly exposure to tobacco smoke.

A patient with COPD at an advanced stage may suffer from three to four acute exacerbations per year [23]. During these attacks, the patients become seriously ill and must be hospitalized immediately for advanced medical treatment. These acute relapses are often caused by viral or bacterial infections of the airways, but they can also be triggered by reactions to allergens, non-specific irritants, changes in the weather, atmospheric pollution, etc. The frequent deteriorations, with repeated long stays in hospital affect their life situations.

The case of COPD is highly relevant for AAL (Ambient Assisted Living). This was made clear as the initial AAL call for proposals [6] identified COPD as one of the conditions where early detection and efficient management through AAL technology can contribute radically to individual well-being and economic sustainability.

We will describe the results from the COPD@Home project that set out to use state-of-the-art methodologies within system and product design in order to create concepts, technologies and services that could be used by all the involved stakeholders. Our overall approach was to combine these methodologies with input from existing innovation projects within the field of AAL in order to identify the potential for truly useful technologies.

Our overall research goals are summarized as follow:

- Identify the key technology goals of the AAL research programmes by analyzing the technology characteristics as described in strategic documents.
- Collect and analyze a body of empirical knowledge about the needs of the stakeholders in the area of rehabilitation, with a focus on COPD.
- Analyze the results from European R&D projects within the area of rehabilitation, in terms of technologies, services, requirements and scenarios. This is then used to identify potential gaps between European AAL roadmaps and funding goals, the requirements found in COPD@Home, and what is done in reality in existing R&D the projects in Europe (within the area of rehabilitation).

The focus of our research is on AAL technologies and services for supporting physiological rehabilitation outside formal care institutions. Rehabilitation in medical terms denotes the process of assisting someone to improve and recover lost function after an event, illness or injury that has caused functional limitations. Rehabilitation is a major field within health, promoting recovery for people after events such as stroke, spinal cord injury, orthopedic surgery, and traumatic brain injury. Rehabilitation engineering, of particular interest for AAL and our research, is "*the systematic application of engineering sciences to design, develop, adapt, test, evaluate, apply, and distribute technological solutions to problems confronted by individuals with disabilities*" [21].

This paper is organized as follows. First, in Section 2, we outline the research methodology used in order to answer the above research goals. Second, in Section 3, we will report our findings from the analysis of key AAL technology characteristics, the findings from the COPD@Home project, and the review of some selected EU research projects. In Section 4 we discuss our findings. Finally, in Section 5, we show the limitations of our study and describe our plans for future research.

1. Methodology

Due to the pioneering nature of AAL technologies used for rehabilitation of COPD patients in Norway, the methodology employed by the project was that of new product development, combined with a review of existing solutions in the European R&D scene. This means that the project followed two parallel but interconnected activities:

- One group of researchers led a user-centered and needs-driven innovation process where new product concepts were developed in close cooperation with the intended users.
- Another group of researchers did an analysis of the nature of AAL and a review of ongoing initiatives funded in parts by the European Commission. The findings from this group were exchanged with the first group in order to provide a pool of ideas for new concepts.

This approach was selected because of two reasons. First, the project wanted to bring in ideas from European R&D initiatives working on AAL solutions for rehabilitation. These ideas were used in the exploration phases of the project as described later. Second, we intended to do a gap analysis of what our project found to be real, empirically validated user needs, compared to what other European initiatives focused on as central needs. This gap analysis can be useful decision-making information for future funding in this area, both nationally in Norway and at a European level. Although our project is limited in size and scope, the user-driven focus involving real COPD patients and professionals can bring insight into this complicated area of AAL research.

The following two sections will describe the specific methodologies followed by these two activities.

1.1. User Involvement in the Fuzzy Front-End of Innovation

Product design has traditionally been focusing on explicit and observable user needs and technical information related to a rather defined product. Due to new demands, there is a shift from simply designing products to designing solutions for tacit and latent needs and experiences and for societal needs. Co-Design and participatory design are promising tools for coping with this new design challenge.

As pointed out by e.g. Sanders et al. [16], Steen et al. [17] and Koen et al. [9], most approaches to innovation focus on user involvement only after there is a clear value proposition established for a product or a service. Evidence shows however that there is a need for user involvement already before a value proposition is defined, i.e. in the fuzzy front end of innovation. The fuzzy front end of innovation is referring to the early stages of a project where context, ideas and concepts are explored. This is therefore a critical stage for the evolving new design processes. The front end describes activities to be worked out before an idea or a concept is selected for further development. The goal is thus to arrive at the decision about what to design. The starting point of this phase is typically open-ended questions like: how can persons with dementia improve their quality of life? Or how can children's experiences during hospitalization be improved? In our case the initial question was: How can we improve the situation for COPD patients?

The open-ended questions imply that in this phase the scope of the succeeding development process is not decided. The final solutions may be e.g. new products, procedures, services, new organization forms, or a combination of all these. New technology

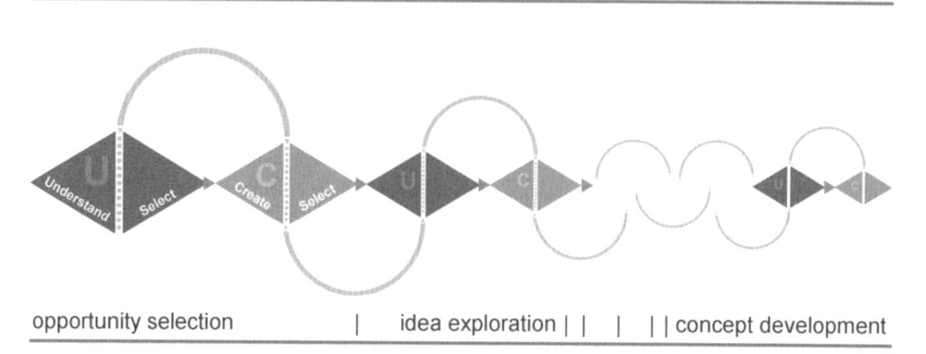

Figure 1. Structuring of the fuzzy front end in COPD@Home.

can be an important part of a new concept, but a concept can also be created by making useful solutions based on well-known technologies or non-technological knowledge. Because of the high level of uncertainty and complexity, the front end is often referred to as being fuzzy.

According to Sanders et al., the fuzzy front end is an isolated iterative process with a gradual transition to the following product development stages. When a concept is chosen during the fuzzy front end, the following processes may adhere to any traditional development process, as described by Darrel Rhea in Design research: methods and perspectives [15].

The question is then: How can we organize the fuzzy front end in such a way that it will result in good product concepts addressing real needs? A lot of novel solutions get developed but never used. How can we avoid creating the wrong product or service in the first place? Using proper methods to reduce the fuzziness in the front end might be the most efficient way to reduce costs and the risk for failure in a project. Most of these methods inevitably involve users.

The project group has based their process on a traditional product development methodology [18], and divided the fuzzy front end into three iterative phases: *Opportunity selection*, *idea exploration* and *concept development*, inspired by Koen et al. [9] and as shown in Fig. 1. Each phase has one or more cycles of "understand and create", with an associated "select" phase in order to gradually focus the process. The process differs somewhat form traditional methodologies, because of a broad, fuzzy starting point, involvement of users in defining the scope, and a focus on exploring needs thoroughly before concepts are developed.

While early phases focus on ideas and concepts, the more we move to the right of the figure the more tangible the results become. The method employs early prototypes in order to explore the main needs: Early prototypes developed and tried out in focus groups are used to collect feedback on the product/service ideas. The prototypes are often low-tech and are used mainly to trigger feedback.

Continuous cycles of understanding and creation within each phase open for input from outside. This is where the project group connected to other European projects through a review of their ideas and results.

1.2. Survey of European Research Results

The project group also did a survey of the results from a number of European projects. The goal was two-folded. First, we wanted to get some ideas about the opportunities provided by modern AAL technologies. This is a valuable input to all the three phases in the development process (Fig. 1). Second, we were interested in finding out whether a structured method for the fuzzy front end would result in different types of solutions than using other methods, such as scenario-based development, commonly used in e.g. European R&D projects.

In order to narrow the scope and make the review task manageable, we concentrated on projects that were partly funded by the EC. The projects were identified using online databases of the European Commission. We did a review of the material available on the public web sites of these projects. We did not contact the projects directly in order to obtain supplementary information, but will do this as a future research activity.

In order to spot overlaps and differences we did a point-by-point analysis of each project. We evaluated the projects based on the characteristics of AAL technologies being developed by the projects (see Section 1 for these characteristics) and based on the emerging needs of the COPD@Home project. Our findings are shown in the following sections.

2. Findings

The findings are organized into four sections. First we describe the findings from an early product development process, divided into opportunity selection, idea exploration and concept development [9,18]. Then we will present the findings from our review of selected European projects.

2.1. Identification of AAL Technology in Rehabilitation Characteristics

In order to investigate the status of the research done in AAL (Ambient Assisted Living) technologies for rehabilitation, we needed to have a clear understanding of the term in general, and also what characterizes AAL rehabilitation technology in particular. The generic term AAL was coined by the European Commission as part of the AAL Joint Programme. In this Programme, AAL is defined as an agenda for "*cultivating the development of innovative ICT – based products, services and systems for the process of ageing well at home, in the community and at work, therefore improving the quality of life, autonomy, the participation in social life, skills and the employability of elder people and reducing the costs of health and social care*" [20].

While being very generic, the above definition suggests that AAL is about *ICT* (Information and Communication Technology) as an enabler of wellbeing. More information on the particular technology characteristics for use in e.g. rehabilitation are given in the first AAL call that had as its main topic "*innovative ICT based solutions for elderly persons with identified risk factors and/or chronic conditions*" [6]. Furthermore, the same call text sheds more light on what characteristics AAL technology should have: "*Specific attention should be made to the adaptation of generic tools to the specific conditions of a given elderly person and his/her immediate environment including informal and formal carers. Co-morbidity situations also require the developing of integrated technological solutions addressing the multi-faceted nature of the elderly*

Table 1. AAL technology characteristics

AAL Technologies should	be ICT-based products, services or systems
	support ageing well at home, in the community and at work
	be interoperable
	be evolvable according to their always changing settings
	be unobtrusive with respect to daily life activities
	be highly reliable and provide safeguard against failure
	not be too power demanding
	be based on wearable/ubiquitous sensors for monitoring physiological and other parameters
	provide information to remote users, e.g. families and clinicians
	assist to make an exact diagnosis and to identify correct therapies and to intervene at the right time

and the evolution of the solution with his/her evolving condition in a flexible and appropriate way. Developed systems should be unobtrusive, highly reliable and low power demanding."

The AAL roadmap developed by AALIANCE [20] acknowledges that management of chronic diseases plays an important role in the context of assistive living. The roadmap also highlights that "*tele-monitoring patient status and self-management of chronic pathological conditions (e.g. COPD), represents the most evident, short-term outcome of Research and Technology Development (RTD) in the domains of Ambient Assisted Healthcare, rehabilitation and long-term care.*"

By analyzing the above sources, we found that they assign a set of AAL technology characteristics. These are shown in Table 1.

Some of these characteristics are generic and can apply to any modern technology, while some are more specific and demonstrate a very specific vision of AAL drawn by the authors of the mentioned documents. The AALIANCE roadmap defines rehabilitation services as one possible scenario for AAL: "*Technological rehabilitation services can help patients effectively and frequently carry out rehabilitation tasks in clinical rehabilitation centers and also at home*" [20]. Examples of AAL rehabilitation technologies from the AALIANCE are:

- Memory supporting proper medication (e.g. smart dispensers).
- ICT support for rehabilitation training (e.g. monitoring, education, robot assistance).
- Monitoring and sharing of physiological parameters (sensors).

2.2. Analysis of Empirical Knowledge of the Needs of the Stakeholders in the Area pf COPD Rehabilitation

In Norway, which is the country of our case study, there are about 1.2 million smokers, of who around 250.000 suffer from COPD. It is one of the most frequently occurring and rapidly increasing diseases. Every year, some 9000 people in Norway acquire COPD. In 2005, more than 15.000 patients were hospitalized for COPD. Most of these were 65 years old or more, an age group that is increasing in number.

Patients with serious COPD and incipient lung failure require advanced treatment and follow-up. In 2005, the average length of stay for such patients at St. Olavs' Hospital in Trondheim, Norway (the site for our case study) was 7.9 days, while the aver-

Table 2. Stakeholders in COPD@Home

Primary users	COPD patients, personnel at the healthcare services and family doctors by the municipality and personnel at rehabilitation centers and Department of Pulmonary Diseases at the hospital.
Secondary users	Next of kin, managers at municipality and hospital like departments of economics, interaction, IT etc.

age for other pulmonary patients was 5.3 days. After hospitalization, patients need from eight to 12 weeks of reconvalescence. Patients with COPD are one of the largest groups of “revolving door” patients, and are major consumers of health services. The Department of Pulmonary Diseases at St. Olav’s Hospital has 700 inpatients with COPD relapses every year, half of which are “repeaters”.

On the basis of the disease statistics, and the constant pattern of relapses and hospitalizations of COPD patients, the Department of Pulmonary Diseases at St. Olav’s Hospital has long since noted the need for innovation, and initiated a number of research and innovation projects. The principle objective of these projects is to reduce the number of hospitalizations of patients with COPD. It is desirable to improve the home-based treatment of such patients, as it would raise the efficacy of the health services while improving the quality of life for the patients themselves. The aim for these projects is to bring about earlier mobilization, better treatment in familiar surroundings with greater security, and finally, a higher level of competence in the local health care services.

2.2.1. Opportunity Selection

In the opportunity selection phase, the project group focused on activities related to the open-ended question “How can we improve the situation for COPD patients?”

The question was gradually broken down into more specific ones such as “What are the major needs within the area of COPD, due to prevention, early symptom registration, making diagnoses, identify correct therapies, emergency, rehabilitation and home situation?”

This large scope was selected because the needs related to COPD patients were assumed to be both complex and connected. Their needs are forming a whole (a person’s everyday life) that should be approached as is and not as isolated needs which would probably lead to incompatible solutions. Since the topic is extensive, there was at the same time a need to prioritize one or several main challenges for further development.

2.2.1.1. Understand

In this phase we intended to identify an open-ended list of opportunities for users to use technology. The project had several groups of users, as shown in Table 2. (Note that primary and secondary denotes here a different grouping than the one used by the European AAL program e.g. in [20].)

In order to answer the initial question, the different users were asked to tell about their lives (COPD patients) and their work with COPD patients (professionals). Their stories were told through semi-structured interviews. In addition, literature reviews were conducted. The information from the data collection was sorted in groups belonging to different phases of COPD disease management, ranging from prevention to home situation. The interviews were organized as show in Table 3.

Table 3. Overview of informants

Prevention	Interview with 2 doctors at the Department of Pulmonary Diseases at the hospital
Early symptom registration	Interview with 2 doctors at the Department of Pulmonary Diseases at the hospital
Making diagnoses	Interview with 2 doctors at the Department of Pulmonary Diseases at the hospital
Medical treatment	Interview with 2 doctors, 1 oxygen nurse, 1 physiotherapist at the Department of Pulmonary Diseases at the hospital and 2 engineers responsible for oxygen concentrator and equipment at the Department of Medical technology at the hospital
Rehabilitation	Interview with leader at rehabilitation institute and COPD patient at institution
Home situation	Interview with 4 COPD patients at home, observations at home and interview with next of kin

Table 4. The four most promising topics for improving situation for COPD patients

Need for new solutions in preventive health measures
Need for new solutions for early COPD diagnose
Need for new solutions for oxygen treatment at home
Need for new solutions for home-based treatments

2.2.1.2. Create

Based on the results from the first "understand" phase, the project group focused on high-level brainstorming activities related to the initial open-ended question "How can we improve the situation for COPD patients?"

The information from the open-ended interviews and literature review resulted in several possible topics. The four most promising topics identified are listed in Table 4.

The underlying criteria for selecting a topic as a follow-up project were the following: 1) A potential for improving the lives of COPD patients, 2) A potential for making the health care sector more efficient, and 3) A potential for growth in the Norwegian AAL industry. Based on these criteria for selection, two of the above topics, i.e. the need for new solutions for home-based treatment and for better oxygen treatment, have been followed up in separate projects.

2.2.2. Idea Exploration

The target for this activity was to identify the needs related to watching over COPD patients at home, and to create ideas related to these needs.

2.2.2.1. Understand

Similar to the opportunity selection activity, data collection was conducted through literature review, interviews and observation, but this time more in- depth on a narrower topic identified in the first iteration, i.e. the situation at home. The interviews were semi-structured and included a wide selection including COPD patients, home care nurses, and specialists at the hospital (i.e. primary users). Interviews with next of kind and friends (secondary users) were also performed.

An extraction of needs and questions based on the data collection was then carried out in workshops with the secondary specialists. This exercise resulted in a list of major needs, and several important questions that could not be answered through interviews, observations or workshops. For both the stakeholders and the project group, it was dif-

Table 5. Main needs needing solving and main questions raised

Main needs	Main questions discovered
Symptoms of disease worsening should be discovered early.	Which symptoms should be registered? How should these symptoms be registered? How often should the registrations be done? Which roles should the different stakeholders have?
Effective treatment system when a worsening is discovered.	Will COPD patients be able to watch over themselves? Is it important that the professionals and the patients know each other? Will there be an information overload? Will a better monitoring system reduce the number of hospitalizations?

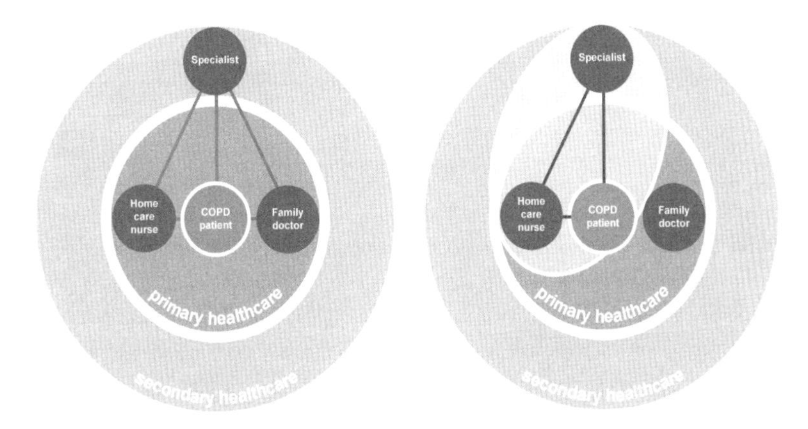

Figure 2. Stakeholder map (to the left) and selected stakeholders for the pilot study (to the right).

ficult to envision needs related to future solutions. In addition, the COPD patients are severely ill, and in-depth interviews and observations were difficult to accomplish. This is a general methodological problem for AAL solutions, especially in cases where main users have physical or cognitive impairments.

The in-depth investigation of the topics revealed some main needs to be solved, and some questions to be answered.

2.2.2.2. Create

Since the early research activities discovered more questions than answers and specific requirements, different scenarios with different stakeholders were worked out in order to create a low-tech pilot prototype. Within this activity, a map was drawn, showing the stakeholders, and their possible interactions, as shown in Fig. 2.

Based on these maps, COPD patients, secondary specialists and home care nurses were selected as primary stakeholders. COPD patients were not assigned any responsibility in the first low-tech pilot. The secondary specialists were assigned responsibility as experts and COPD advisory service. The home care nurses were responsible for monitoring the patients and activating treatment. At this phase it was clear that the home care nurse was to be a major user for the first low-tech pilot. This identification of main stakeholders resulted in more specific list of requirements and ideas for possible solutions to be created, as shown in Table 6. Based on these needs, an intervention with a low-tech pilot solution was created. The pilot was designed to study the main questions discovered in the "understand" phase. The intervention design, the paper

Table 6. Main needs and solutions

Main needs	Needs of home care nurse	Low-tech pilot solution
Symptoms of disease worsening should be discovered early	Knowledge about COPD	*COPD School*: held by the secondary specialists, developed to give the home care nursing staff training in diagnosing the progress of COPD
	Frequent registration of symptoms and progress	*COPD Diary*: in paper form for registration of the progress of the disease, The diary is kept at home, and used by the nurses
Effective treatment system when a worsening is discovered	Easy access to a patient's treatment description	*Guidance*: A detailed instruction in the COPD Diary – about the disease, the patient and the treatment
	Easy access to expertise	*COPD Central*: this is a reception apparatus that has been set up at the Department of Pulmonary Disease at St. Olav's Hospital

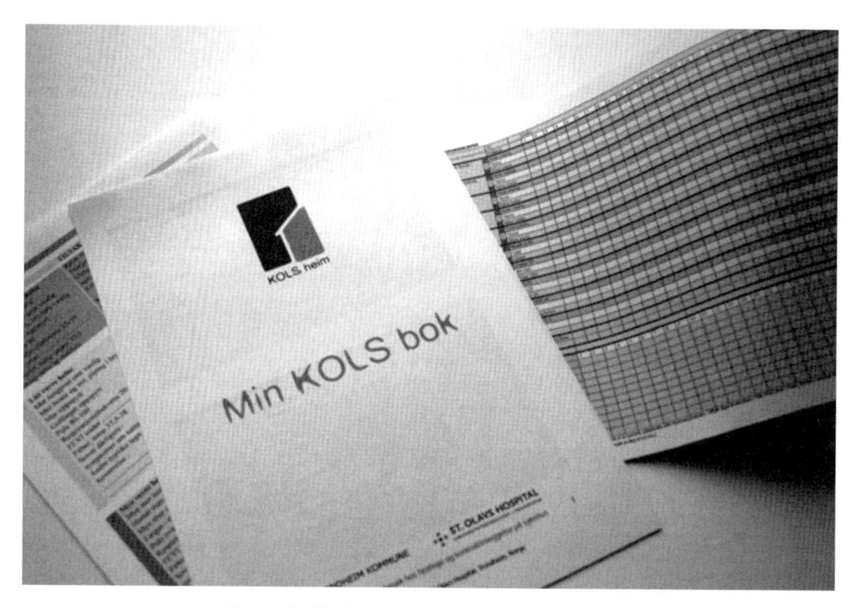

Figure 3. The low-tech prototype COPD Diary.

forms and the instructions about treatment were developed in a co-design process with the designers and the secondary specialists. The physicians had the final word concerning which symptoms to be registered, and how the instructions should be formed. The nurses were responsible for completing measurements of high professional quality and understandable for their colleagues in the home care services. Since the process was iterative, most decisions regarding the intervention and the related products and processes were taken during workshops with the project team.

Hospital at home schemes can be safely used to care for patients with acute exacerbations of COPD who would otherwise be admitted to hospital. Clinicians should consider this form of management, especially as there is increasing pressure for inpatient beds in the United Kingdom [13]. In the intervention, home care nurses visit the COPD patients regularly to follow up the progress of the disease, which is recorded in a COPD Diary. In the event of relapse, the central is contacted by mobile telephone,

Table 7. Research methods used to answer last round of questions

User group 1	COPD patients and next of kin, offered COPD Home as a new services	Semi-structured interviews with 5 patient and 2 next of kin Direct observations of the new services at homes Cultural probes, that allow COPD patient themselves to document their needs Drama workshop, role-playing with the patient and nurse- assisted monitoring at home
User group 2	Home care nurse at the municipality	Semi-structured interviews with 4 home care nurses who had used the new services Direct observations of 2 nurse-assisted monitoring at home Drama workshop, role-playing with 4 nurse-assisted monitoring at home.
User group 3	Nurses at the Department of Pulmonary Diseases at the hospital, responsible for the COPD central	Semi-structured interviews, one by one and groups with 3 nurses at the COPD central

and the center decides which extra measures need to be set in motion. At this stage, the pilot, as described in Table 6, consisted of a paper-based COPD Diary and a normal phone-based COPD Central. In addition, training and education of home care nurses was done in a COPD School.

2.2.3. Concept Development

In the second iteration we focused on getting feedback from the first phase's low-tech pilot, and expanding to include the last stakeholder in the loop, i.e. the COPD patient. Further development of the low-tech pilots and collection of feedback on how these pilots were used gave us further insight into the major needs related to the home situation. An obvious result was the challenge of creating technology that could be used by the patients themselves.

The results from this phase were intended to be specifications of ICT-based AAL technologies and concepts. The COPD@Home project did not intend to develop any of these technologies, but to share the ideas and concepts with the Norwegian AAL industry.

2.2.3.1. Understand

The basis for the Concept Development phase was a study of the early pilot solution, with the intention to investigate stakeholders' satisfaction and needs for further improvements, for follow-up and treatment of COPD at home. The involved stakeholders were asked to answer the questions:

- What are the major satisfactions with the new pilot solution?
- What are the major areas for improvement?

The research methods that were used to answer the last round of questions and to clarify more specific requirements for AAL technologies are shown in Table 7.

All user statements and items of information were analyzed with the aim of identifying user needs and requirements to develop an improved solution. All of the information gathered from the user groups was partly transcribed. The first step was done by

Table 8. Main questions and main findings

Main questions	Main findings
What are the major satisfactions with the new pilot solution	Home care nurses are satisfied with the easy access to decision making support at the COPD Central
	Home care nurses are satisfied with the easy access to patient's treatment description in the COPD Diary
	Home care nurses are satisfied with increased responsibility and development of knowledge throguh COPD School
	Patients are satisfied with supervision in registration of medical condition
What are the major needs for improvement	Easier daily registration of medical condition Reduction in the number of parameters for registration More discrete procedure for monitoring – possibility to hide results Easier format for registration – the COPD Diary is bothersome A new solution which can reduce the number of home visits for home care nurses
	Better assistance in registration of medical parameters
	A new registration system which gives easy access to a patient's treatment description for home care nurses, family doctor and hospital.

sorting the statements and activities into topics, by using language processing, and classifying user statements through color-coding. These topics were then evaluated in terms of their importance and relevance to the solution, and the result was a series of activities with their associated requirements. Table 8 shows some of the major findings.

2.2.3.2. Create

Based on the Understand activity, the most important areas of improvement were highlighted. From here, several holistic future scenarios involving AAL technologies were developed. Potential industrial partners were screened. A co-design and development working group consisting of representatives from the municipality of Trondheim, Department of Pulmonary Diseases at the hospital, Department of Interaction at the hospital and Department of ICT at The Regional Health enterprise was conducted to further detail the technological solutions. Product designers at SINTEF facilitate the creative process of designing the technology. Some of the preliminary results denoting new technological solutions are shown in Table 9.

Results from this activity have been presented for the steering group of COPD@Home for evaluation and selection of a preferred solution. Important criteria for selection have been: Quality of life improvements for COPD patients, improving the efficiency in the health care, coincidence with existing strategy for development in municipality and hospital, cost benefit, industries accomplishment etc.

2.3. Review of Related European Research

In this section we will provide our preliminary results from an ongoing systematic review of EC-funded projects in the area of rehabilitation and management of chronic diseases. At this initial stage our intention was not to do a thorough analysis of each project's results. What was important for us was 1) whether the overall objectives of each project, and the reported use cases, were in line with a set of overall requirements (from EC's AAL definition and from our own COPD@Home project) and 2) whether there were any innovative technologies either developed/used or planned to be developed by the projects that could be useful for COPD@Home.

Table 9. Suggestions for rehabilitation technology

Main questions	Main findings	New solution
What are the major satisfactions with the new pilot solution	Home care nurses are satisfied with a easy access to decision making support	Support for communication with experts ad the COPD center through various channels (e.g. PDA, TV, PC, phone)
	Home care nurses are satisfied with the easy access to a patient's treatment description in the COPD – book	Treatment description should be easily available and easily updatable and new knowledge becomes available (e.g. on an online portal with easy editing possibilities)
	Home care nurses are satisfied with increased responsibility and development of knowledge	Allow for continuous education of existing and new home care nurses (e.g. e-learning solutions)
	Patients are satisfied with supervision in registration of medical condition	Education programs for patients, easy-to-use ubiquitous measurement technologies (e.g. e-learning solutions, automatic measurements through integrated sensors)
What are the major needs for improvement	Easier daily registration of medical condition	Personnel or support with use of technology
	Reduction in the number of parameters for registration	Possibly integration of ubiquitous sensor technologies
	More discrete procedure for monitoring – possibility to hide results	Sensor technologies, privacy enhancing technologies
	Easier format for registration – the COPD Diary is bothersome	Multi-modal interfaces for easy interaction
	A new solution which can reduce the number of home visits for home care nurses	A combination of new technologies, but also organizational level re-engineering
	A new registration system which gives easy access to a patient's treatment description for home care nurses, family doctor and hospital.	Centralized patient record systems, integrated with multi-modal interfaces

Our review includes mainly projects supported by the EC AAL joint programme because these projects have a shorter time-to-market than e.g. IST projects. We also looked into a number of ICT PSP projects that are actually in the phase of commercializing their services and products. The AAL Joint Program funded projects we reviewed are a2e2 [1], Agnes [2], Amica [3], Health@Home [7], IS-ACTIVE [8], PAMAP.ORG [12], and RGS [14]. From the eTen/ICT PSP program we have currently reviewed DREAMING [5] and NEXES [10]. From the ICT FP7 programme we reviewed only CHRONIOUS [4], which showed to be of relevance for rehabilitation and chronic diseases.

Our review is based on a set of generic questions we ask regarding each project. The questions are listed in the Appendix A. These questions are mainly aimed at identifying the vision and overall research and innovation areas of each project, and the nature of expected results from each project. A set of these questions is based on the definition of AAL provided by EC's AAL-related documents (Table 10 in Appendix A). A second set of questions is based on our findings from the COPD@Home project. Some of the questions in the two sets were overlapping (e.g. the need to do ambient-based measurements), but there are also a number of distinct questions. E.g. COPD@Home found that learning and knowledge management was an important factor for the project, a factor which does not seem to be emphasized in EC's definitions of AAL. Or, EC's

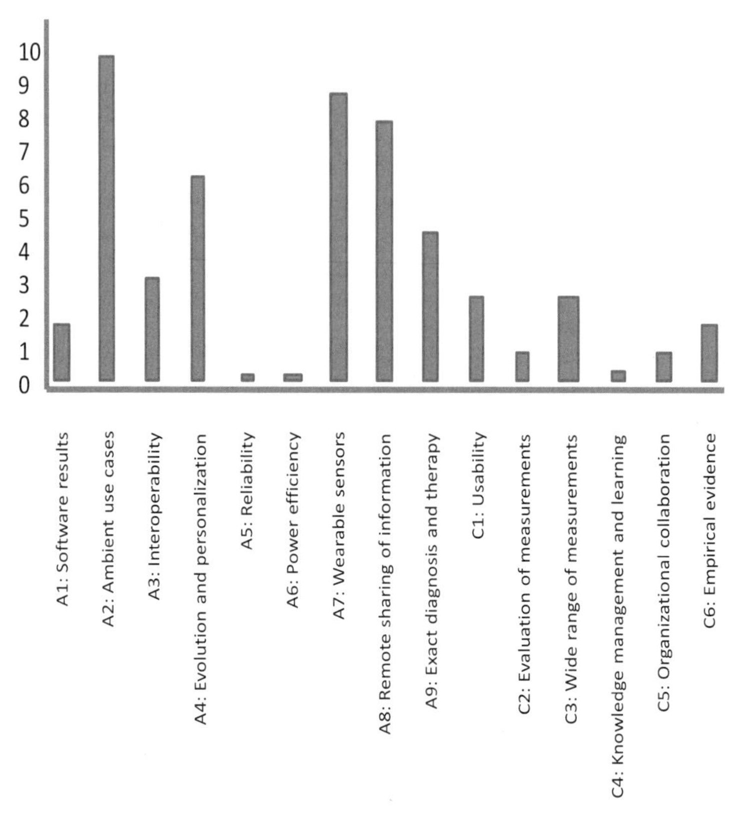

Figure 4. The number of projects claiming to address each of the questions.

definition of AAL includes technical aspects such as reliability and power consumption that were not directly posed by COPD@Home.

The questions, due to their generic nature, were answered using yes or no. We based our answers on the information we found on the projects' web pages and publications. At this stage we were not interested in the details of the solutions, only overall focus and expected results. The graph in Fig. 4 shows the answers to the questions. We have anonymized the answers' connection to the individual projects.

As we can see, for some aspects of AAL and rehabilitation there is a uniform coverage, or lack of such, in the reviewed projects. For instance, all projects satisfy the "Ambient" requirement and focus on scenarios that include home and natural habitat of the users (Question A1). On the other hand, aspects such as reliability and power efficiency are apparently not handled at all by the reviewed projects (A5 and A6). This is a concern since most of the projects promise results that can be commercialized within 1–2 years or less. We also noticed that only a few of the projects make available software results, or even designs of their concepts and architectures (A1). This might be due to the immaturity of the results. But it comes natural to us to expect that publicly funded projects should make parts of their results publicly available. Interoperability is also an aspect that is only partially addressed (A3). This is also a major concern regarding commercialization. Health care service providers are definitely not interested in new and isolated tools and platforms, and wish to integrate with their existing tools.

Almost all of the reviewed projects provide some solution for collecting data through ambient sensors (A2, A7). In addition, local or remote access to collected data is provided by many of the projects (A8). We also see a quite high level of reported adaptation of raw data to the necessary decision making parameters (A9). However, most projects are focusing on a limited set of sensors, which in realistic settings will not provide a holistic and correct view of the condition being monitored. Most conditions are not measurable or candidate for monitoring based on a few isolated biological or physical parameters. We consider this as a general research challenge for AAL research and infrastructure.

Additionally, although some pre-processing and adaptation/integration of data is reported, there is very little reported empirical evidence regarding the usefulness of such adaptations with respect to decision making (C2). In general, only a few of the projects report any empirical validation of the concepts and services that are developed (C6). This might be a major concern for practitioners who want to adopt the solutions. Empirical validation is often a must for any research that borders medical conditions, and the lack of such will be a major hamper for innovation in the field.

An interesting mismatch we see between our requirements and the work done by the R&D projects is a seemingly total lack of attention to organizational aspects. For instance, none of the projects report results related to learning and knowledge management (C4). And only one project reports results on organizational coordination and process level innovation (C5). These are major concerns regarding the probability that the solutions will be adopted by the organizations they are intended for. For instance, most of the product and service concepts that are being developed can be considered high-tech. This means that home care personnel or elderly without technical background will need to be continuously trained in using these technologies. Additionally, most of these concepts are potentially disruptive and will require major modifications to existing organizational structures. This might include changes in power structures, budget distributions, incentives etc. that each can be an obstacle to innovation.

3. Discussion

AAL technologies operate in complex settings involving multitude of stakeholders and organizations. The target end users, i.e. the elderly and their relatives, constitute a varied group of people with a wide range of needs. Our research has focused on cases where the elderly are clearly defined as patients with chronic diseases under rehabilitation. Although this scoping arguably simplifies the settings, our findings show that European R&D has a rather narrow focus, addressing only portions of the overall picture.

The model employed by many of the reviewed projects is that of a closed technological system for monitoring of biological and contextual parameters. Ranges of novel sensors are used to collect information from home, and to deliver that information to caregivers. The projects demonstrate the potential of such technologies in a wide range of scenarios. However, it appears to us that the available results are still in the early stage of research in form of proof-of-concept demonstrators. From a technological point of view, aspects such as reliability, ease of use, and power efficiency are apparently not in focus.

For our COPD@Home project, sensors and remote access to health parameters were of high importance. But they were at the same time not the only aspects pointed out by our users as being important. In order for these technologies to innovate in the marketplace, a wider set of requirements will have to be fulfilled. What seems to be missing is a focus on the organizational aspects of AAL. Examples of such organizational aspects include: Re-engineering of existing processes and services as a result of novel solutions (such as home-based monitoring), support for learning and training of users (such as home care personnel, the elderly and their next of kin), support for collaboration among different organizational units involved in the rehabilitation process, and the existence of solutions that can be integrated with legacy systems (such as electronic health records). A related issue is the lack of research on the services (clinical and non-clinical) that will be enabled based on the technological solutions. In this sense, the results from the European projects will solve only a small part of the problems that COPD@Home is facing. Ranges of aspects related to innovation in the marketplace are still missing.

There is an underlying assumption in the reviewed projects (and seemingly in EC's definition of AAL) that the patients can play an active role in the management of their own disease. In COPD@Home this assumption does not hold. The studies patients were in a physical condition that made it necessary to involve relatives or other formal or informal caregivers. The activities involved in measuring COPD-related parameters in COPD@Home were not complicated, but the physical condition of the patients made it necessary to have third parties helping them with these simple operations. An acute need then arose related to the training of caregivers with no pre-existing expertise in the field. Our users point out distribution of knowledge about chronic diseases as a major requirement. We believe technologies such as e-learning and knowledge management solutions can play a crucial role here.

4. Limitations of the Study and Plans for Future Research

The reported study of COPD patients represents only a first step in a series of such studies necessary in order to generalize the results and to compile a list of definite requirements. We also need to evaluate more advanced services and prototypes in real settings in order to validate our own results. In particular, we have only started to explore the organizational and collaboration aspects of rehabilitation at home. A number of studies are planned and requests for funding are prepared. We hope to be able to report on our further studies in the future.

The review of the European R&D projects was done with a number of simplifications. Although we focused our review mainly on projects funded under the AAL Joint Programme, we are aware of a number of other relevant R&D projects, e.g. under the Framework Programme 7. In particular a number of highly ambitious projects are looking into developing common platforms for AAL, which hopefully will address a number of raised technological issues including interoperability. Our review also limits itself to the publicly available information from project web sites and publications. This limitation was necessary at this stage in order to get an overview of the overall focus of the individual projects. We acknowledge that a more thorough study will be needed in the future. Due to commercialization aims of almost all of the reviewed projects, we expect that some of our findings might not be accurate due to the confidentiality of the results from the projects. For instance, stable and interoperable solutions developed in some projects might be strong candidates for commercialization. We plan to extend our review into a more systematic review, involving participants from the reviewed projects.

Acknowledgement

COPD@Home was initially launched by InnoMed in cooperation with St. Olav's Hospital and the Trondheim County. The Norwegian Health Directorate and Innovation Norway financed the project. The review of European projects was partly funded by the European integrated project universAAL. We thank all the involved people in COPD@Home for their cooperation.

Appendix A. Evaluation Criteria and Their Sources

Regarding ID: A denotes AAL Roadmap, while C denotes COPD@Home. For overlapping requirements we have chosen to denote the source with more elaborate definition of the criteria.

Table 10. Requirements from EC's AAL Joint Programme and related documents

ID	Requirement	Metric
A1	Does the project produce ICT based solutions?	Is there any software being made available by the project?
A2	Does the project emphasize support at home, in the community, and at work?	Are there use cases or services supporting activities at home, in the community, or at work?
A3	Does the project produce interoperable solutions?	Are technological and user-interaction aspects of interoperability covered in any use cases?
A4	Does the project emphasize development of evolvable technology?	Are there any use cases for evolution and personalization?
A5	Does the project emphasize reliability of produced technology?	Are there any use cases, plans or test cases related to evaluating the reliability of developed solutions?
A6	Does the project emphasize low power solutions?	Are low power consumption use cases available?
A7	Does the project produce wearable sensors for measuring parameters?	Are wearable sensor use cases defined by the project?
A8	Does the project support remote sharing of information among users of different groups?	Are there any use cases developed for allowing remote access to information?
A9	The information should assist to make an exact diagnosis and to identify correct therapies and to intervene at the right time.	Are there any use cases related to diagnosis, identify therapy, and or intervention at the right time?

Table 11. Requirements from the COPD@Home project

ID	Requirement	Metric
C1	Does the project emphasize multimodal and extremely easy-to-use interfaces?	Are there novel user interaction concepts being developed? Are there any use cases emphasizing ease of use?
C2	Does the project emphasize high level of measurement quality?	Are there any empirical results available related to the quality of measurements?
C3	Does the project emphasize measurement of a wide range of parameters?	Are there use cases demonstrating variety of sensors and measurable parameters?
C4	Does the project emphasize knowledge management and learning?	Are there use cases and services for facilitating knowledge management and learning?

Table 11. (Continued)

ID	Requirement	Metric
C5	Does the project emphasize cross-organizational collaboration and coordination?	Are there use cases and services for facilitating cross-organizational collaboration and coordination?
C6	Does the project support any scientific methodology for collecting empirical evidence?	Are empirically inclined methods described/mentioned/used?

References

[1] a2e2 Consortium: a2e2 – AAL call 1 project, http://www.a2e2.eu/.

[2] Agnes Consortium: Agnes – AAL call 1 project, http://agnes-aal.eu/site/.

[3] Amica Consortium: Amica – Autonomy, Motivation & Individual Self-Management for COPD patients – AAL call 1 project, http://www.amica-aal.com/.

[4] Chromius Consortium: Chronius – FP7 project, http://www.chronious.eu/.

[5] Dreaming Consortium: Dreaming – Home, http://www.dreaming-project.org/.

[6] European Commission: Call AAL-2008-1 – Ambient Assisted Living, 2008.

[7] Health@Home Consortium: Health@Home Project – Home – AAL call 1 project, http://www.health-at-home.eu/.

[8] IS-ACTIVE Consortium: IS-ACTIVE – AAL call 1 project, http://www.is-active.eu/.

[9] P.A. Koen, G.M. Ajamian, S. Boyce, A. Clamen, E. Fisher, S. Fountoulakis, A. Johnson, P. Puri and R. Seibert, The Fuzzy Front End for Incremental, Platform, and Breakthrough Products, in: *The PDMA Toolbook for New Product Development*, John Wiley & Sons, Inc., 2002.

[10] Nexes Consortium: NEXES: Supporting Healthier and Independent Living for Chronic Patients and Elderly, http://nexeshealth.eu, 2009.

[11] NHLBI/WHO workshop report: Global Initiative for Chronic Obstructive Lung Disease: What You Can Do About a Lung Disease Called COPD, 2002, http://www.efanet.org/copd/documents/9c_GOLD_PATIENT_GUIDE.pdf (accessed 2/5/2011).

[12] PAMAP.ORG Consortium: PAMAP.ORG – AAL call 1 project, http://www.pamap.org/.

[13] F.S.F. Ram, J.A. Wedzicha, J. Wright and M. Greenstone, Hospital at home for patients with acute exacerbations of chronic obstructive pulmonary disease: Systematic review of evidence, *BMJ* **329** (2004), 315.

[14] RGS Consortium: Rehabilitation Gaming System – AAL call 1 project, http://specs.upf.edu/rgs/.

[15] D. Rhea, *Bringing Clarity to the "Fuzzy Front End", Design Research: Methods and Perspectives*, MIT Press, 2003, p. 350.

[16] E. Sanders and P.J. Stapper, Co-creation and the new landscapes of design, *CoDesign* **4** (Mar. 2008), 5–18.

[17] M. Steen, L. Kuijt-Evers and J. Klok, Early user involvement in research and design projects – A review of methods and practices, in: *23rd EGOS Colloquium (European Group for Organizational Studies)*, 2007, pp. 5–7.

[18] K. Ulrich and S. Eppinger, *Product Design and Development*, McGraw-Hill/Irwin, 2003.

[19] G. Van Den Broek, F. Cavallo and C. Wehrmann, *AALIANCE Ambient Assisted Living Roadmap*, IOS Press.

[20] G. Van Den Broek, F. Cavallo and C. Wehrmann, *Ambient Assisted Living Roadmap*, IOS Press (2010).

[21] Wikipedia: Rehabilitation engineering – Wikipedia, the free encyclopedia.

[22] World Health Organization factsheet: Chronic obstructive pulmonary disease (COPD), http://www.who.int/mediacentre/factsheets/fs315/en/ (accessed 2/5/2011).

[23] A.M. Yohannes, Palliative care provision for patients with chronic obstructive pulmonary disease, *Health and Quality of Life Outcomes* **5**, 17.

Handbook of Ambient Assisted Living
J.C. Augusto et al. (Eds.)
IOS Press, 2012

doi:10.3233/978-1-60750-837-3-567

Assisted Ambient Living Applied to Remote Motor Rehabilitation [1]

Eric R. WADE [a,*] and Avinash PARNANDI [b]

[a] *University of Southern California, Division of Biokinesiology and Physical Therapy, USA*

[b] *Texas A&M University, Department of Computer Science, USA*

Abstract. Of late, sensors, virtual reality, and robotic systems have proven increasingly useful for augmenting traditional motor rehabilitation techniques. We present exciting results from current literature, as well as our own work, that indicate promising directions for ambient assisted living techniques in the field of stroke rehabilitation.

Keywords. Ambient assisted living, stroke, rehabilitation, robotics, virtual environments

Introduction

AAL techniques that make use of robotics, sensors, and information technology have been shown to be useful for the remote monitoring of individuals in a number of environments. For individuals living with motor or cognitive deficits, such monitoring can lead to increased quality of life. Here, we extend the discussion to talk about how AAL techniques can be used to provide motor rehabilitation in ambient environments to individuals who have suffered from stroke. We will focus on various rehabilitation techniques for stroke that make use of robotics, sensors, virtual reality, and other technologies to transfer clinical practices and techniques to individuals in ambient environments. We will describe foundational work in this area before suggesting tools and techniques to advance the field.

To discuss the utility of AAL techniques in stroke rehabilitation, it is necessary to first understand stroke and the resulting deficits it causes. Stroke affects a large percentage of the population worldwide, with over 9 million people affected annually, many of whom go on to live with motor and cognitive deficits [25]. Recovery after a stroke can be divided into three stages. The first stage is the *acute* stage, which lasts on the order of hours (~72 hours) (see Fig. 1). This phase is primarily focused on: ascertaining the type, location, and cause of the stroke; the prevention of other health complications; and

[1]This work was supported by Award Number U01NS056256 from the National Institute of Neurological Disorders and Stroke. The content is solely the responsibility of the authors and does not necessarily represent the official views of the NINDS or the NIH. This work is also supported by NSF CNS-0709296 grant for "CRI: IAD – Computing Research Infrastructure for Human-Robot Interaction and Socially Assistive Robotics" and NSF IIS-0713697 grant "HRI: Personalized Assistive Human-Robot Interaction: Validation in Socially Assistive Robotics for Post-Stroke Rehabilitation" and NIH grant U01NS056256-02.

*Corresponding Author: Eric R. Wade, Center for Health Professionals (CHP), 1540 Alcazar St., Room G30, Los Angeles, CA, USA. Email: erwade@alum.mit.edu.

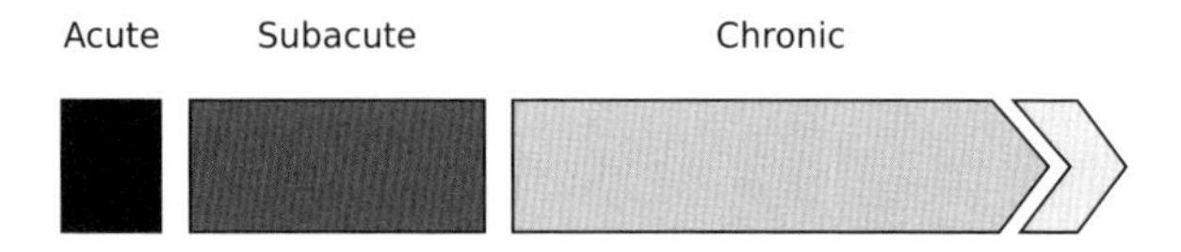

Figure 1. The three stages of recovery for individuals post-stroke.

the stabilization of vital signs. The next phase is the *subacute* phase; during this phase, individuals are inpatients and/or outpatients in the hospital or clinical facility, nursing home, or their own home. They receive physical therapy from trained physical and occupational therapists (PTs and OTs). This phase usually lasts on the order of months (~6 months). Finally, there is the chronic phase. In this phase, individuals no longer receive any guided physical therapy, and by and large, are on their own in terms of recovery activities. Often, they will have a recovery plan prepared by their PT or OT, but receive no more supervision.

1. VR and Robotics for Motor Assessments

Information gained from AAL techniques will be critical to interventions for the subacute phase of stroke recovery. In the short-term, these techniques can be used to obtain sensitive, quantitative measures of performance that may give insight into the resulting deficit. These quantitative data supplement existing outcome measures, and give us a better understanding of recovery in the clinical setting. In the long term, the automation of assessments can be used to obtain longitudinal measures of ability well into the chronic phase. This will lead to better determination of optimal clinical practices and techniques for the subacute phase of recovery. These points are further explored in the following.

1.1. Obtaining Performance Measures Currently Left Uncollected

Subjective measures of performance are commonly used to assess motor capability after stroke. However, objective measures are necessary to evaluate the relative efficacy of therapeutic interventions. The development and use of objective measures is a necessary component of evidence based medicine (EBM). Evidence based medicine can be defined as the use of scientific evidence to reach medical decisions [23]. These measures can be both quantitative (e.g. movement time) and qualitative (e.g. motion smoothness). The reliability and validity of these measures must be established before they can be used to describe clinical outcomes. Once these are established, extensive training is required to ensure that these assessments are administered consistently and accurately. This is often time consuming (in terms of the time to train individuals, and the time required to administer them). As a result, many researchers have focused on technological approaches to validate and/or supplement data obtained from existing assessments.

An example of the use of AAL techniques to supplement existing measures is demonstrated by Leibowitz et al. [12]. Leibowitz developed a VR system to measure proprioceptive sensing ability. The system, shown in Fig. 2, was designed so that individuals could move their hands in a 2D plane; their eyes were covered to remove any visual feedback. Participants were asked to align the palms of their hands over one another. During the interaction, the experimenters moved the participant's left hand to a

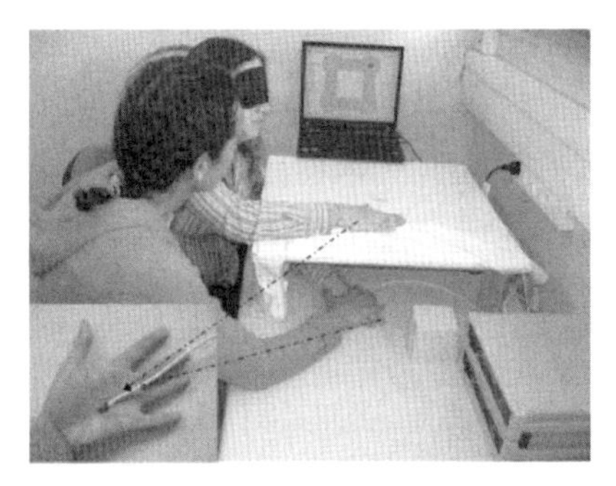

Figure 2. Virtual reality setup used by Leibowitz to measure proprioception. Adapted from [12].

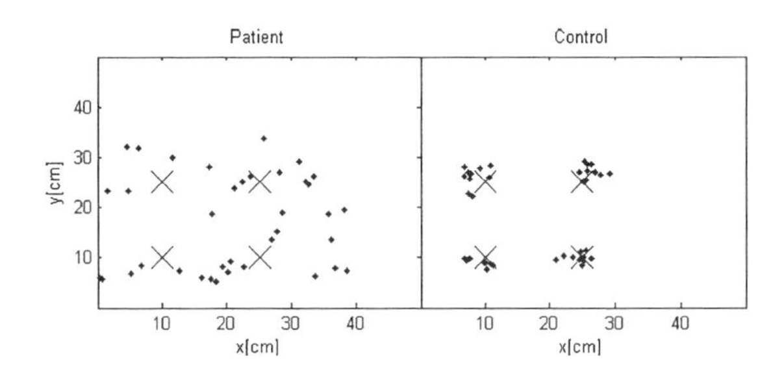

Figure 3. Relative difference outcomes for controls and individuals post-stroke in the Leibowitz study. Adapted from [12].

predetermined location, and the participant would then attempt to move the right hand to the corresponding location, but on a parallel 2D plane. Using an electromagnetic sensing system, the researchers tracked the error (Euclidean distance) between the two palms. The researchers collected error data from 9 non-disabled controls and 22 individuals post-stroke; the comparison between groups is shown in Fig. 3. The plots indicate that the "patient" group had more error between palms (and thus, less proprioceptive sensing ability).

In the study, the experimenters also administered a standard proprioception measure, the timed up-and-down test. Remarkably, the up-and-down test indicated that only 10 of the 22 "patients" had deficits. However, the VR system error data demonstrated significant differences between all individuals post-stroke and the non-disabled controls. While the clinical importance of these subtler measures has not been established, they can be used to provide feedback to individuals regarding progress during rehabilitation.

Another example of the potential of AAL techniques is demonstrated by Kim et al. [11]. The goal of Kim's study was to compare outcomes of different conditions of locomotor training. They had two aims; the first was a comparison of visual imagery and kinesthetic training. Visual imagery training consists of picturing (but not performing) actions as a mechanism of task practice, whereas kinesthetic training involves actual performance of the activity. The second aim was to determine the effect of auditory feedback (provided during practice) on performance. The authors employed a randomized crossover design with 2 variables (training type and auditory feedback), each with 2 levels. In this experiment, the task training consisted of four sessions, each with a different type of locomotor training (separated by at least 24 hours to allow for washout). The researchers used a standard outcome measure knows as the timed up and go (TUG) test, developed by Shumway-Cook [19]. This test consists of an individual standing, walking 3 steps, turning around, and sitting down again. As the name implies, the entire test is timed. In addition, the authors measured EMG signals on the quadriceps, hamstring, tibialis anterior, and gastrocnemius muscles, and used marker-based motion capture techniques to capture kinematic features of motion.

Interestingly, the TUG test showed no significant pre/post differences for any participants. However, the EMG signal at the hamstring during swing phase and for the gastrocnemius muscle during stance phase indicated significant improvement for all participants ($p < 0.05$). Similarly, the kinematic data indicated significant pre/post differences in sagittal plane knee range of motion ($p < 0.05$). Once again, AAL techniques captured performance changes to which the standard instrument was not sensitive. The interesting question alluded to earlier is how *clinically* significant these changes are. To answer this question, many researchers evaluate the minimal clinically important difference (MCID), which is a measure of how much change is needed to have a measure of clinical importance (either functionally, or to the individual with the deficit). There has been much discussion of this idea; while not fully explored here, the argument can be made that, even if such detectable differences lack clinical significance, in the rehabilitation domain, it is well known that individuals are motivated by trends indicating positive (sometimes incremental) improvement. In other words, though these differences may not be clinically significant, they can be used as feedback for participants, to indicate that they are making progress with their recovery. This feedback can contribute to intrinsically motivating patients to practice and perform rehabilitative activities. For example, in a rehabilitation setting, though an individual cannot get up more quickly, the fact that their peak EMG signal is consistently changing may provide them with motivation to continue practicing and improve performance over time.

1.2. The Need for Quantitative Standardized Objective Measures of Function

In the stroke domain, two widely used assessments are the Wolf Motor Function Test (WMFT) assessment, and the Fugl-Meyer (FM) assessment [18,24]. Both measure the timing and quality of motion as individuals perform a battery of gestures and actions. The clinician times gestures using a stopwatch, and also scores performance according to a *functional ability* (FA) score. For each gesture, the FA score is measured on a 0–2 point scale (WMFT) or a 0–5 point scale (FM), and depends on motion smoothness, ease, and other observed characteristics. Both assessments are valid and reliable, but require thorough training of the clinician to be properly administered. Naturally, many researchers have attempted to determine quantitative ways of obtaining these scores to reduce the associated time burden.

An interesting example is the work of Colombo et al. [1]. Colombo's group was interested in observing performance on a robot-assisted virtual reality (VR) task, and determining a relationship to functional assessment scores. In their experiment, individuals post-stroke played a game in which they guided a cursor on a computer screen. Seven participants interacted with a robot providing assistance at the wrist; 7 others interacted with a robot providing assistance at the shoulder and elbow. The outcome measures were the robot score (a measure the amount of assistance provided by the robot), movement accuracy, and mean movement velocity. The apparatus is shown in Fig. 4. Results in-

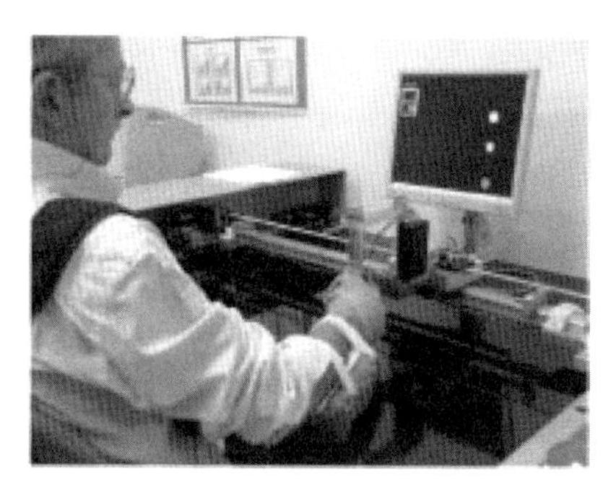

Figure 4. Robot and virtual reality setup used by Colombo et al. to obtain kinematic measures of performance. Adapted from [1].

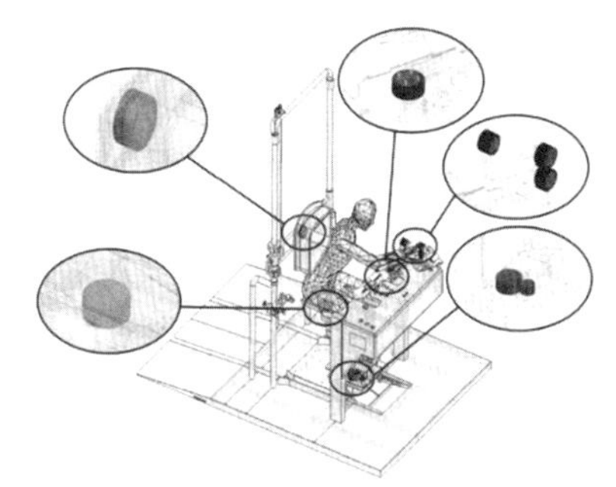

Figure 5. Sensor apparatus used by Van Dijck et al. to obtain kinematic and dynamic measures during real-world task performance. Adapted from [2].

dicated that individuals working with both robots improved on the task, but not significantly. However, the investigators were also interested in determining if any correlations existed between outcome measures. Their work indicated moderately significant correlation between robot measures (robot score, velocity) and upper extremity FM scores.

Though individuals were performing a non-functional task, this provides evidence that certain kinematic and dynamic measures correlate with the outcomes of the FM assessment. One logical improvement on this method is to evaluate how well *functional tasks* might be correlated with such outcomes. This approach was followed by Van Dijck et al. [2]. Van Dijck and colleagues were interested in obtaining performance measures during real-world functional tasks. To do so, they created a robotic apparatus that allowed people to sit and perform a number of tasks. The apparatus was instrumented with a number of force and torque sensors below the seat, at the upper back, at the ankle, the wrist, and the fingers (see Fig. 5). For a task such as "reach and pick up the cup," the apparatus obtained quantitative kinematic and dynamic measures (angular velocity, angular deviation) for each participant. The researchers recruited 57 non-disabled individuals and 57 individuals post-stroke, though only 16 individuals post-stroke were used for the FM assessment correlations. All participants performed a battery of tasks modeled on activities of daily living (ADLs) such as drinking from a glass and turning a key.

This study had a number of interesting outcomes. First, the authors validated the sensitivity of their apparatus to non-disabled and disabled individuals. They were able to compare performance curves between the groups using a mutual information technique

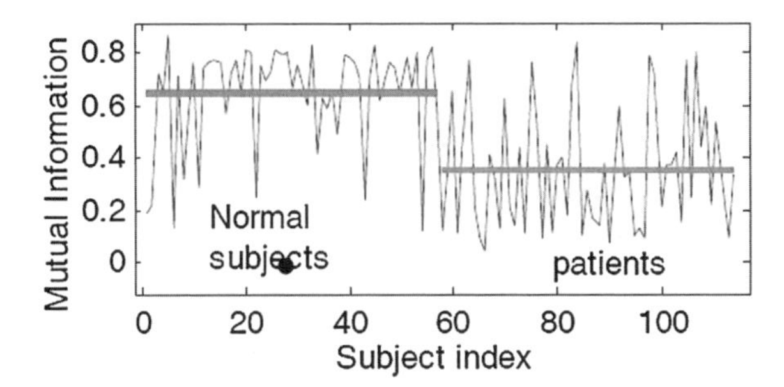

Figure 6. Relative measures of mutual information between limbs for non-disabled individuals and individuals post-stroke. Adapted from [2].

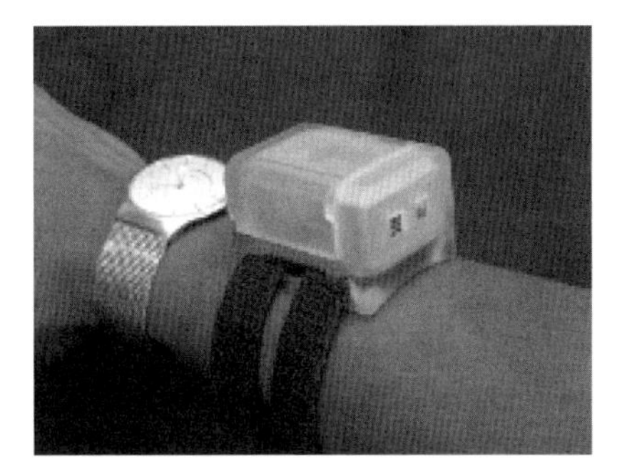

Figure 7. Inertial measurement unit used by Parnandi et al. to capture wrist motion.

(a measure of entropy between two signals). As shown in Fig. 6, there was a distinction between the mutual information between the thumb and index finger for the two groups. Further, they showed correlation between angular deviation and both the upper extremity and global FM scores (Pearson coefficient of 80.29% and 76.6%, respectively). The authors were able to not only use the system to distinguish between non-disabled and disabled individuals, but also use functional tasks to predict FM assessment scores.

A number of researchers have attempted a much more direct approach – specifically, instrumenting individuals while performing the various functional assessments. The quantitative sensor readings obtained from such wearable sensors can be used as predictors for the functional assessment score determined by the trained clinician. In our work, we used a custom inertial measurement unit (IMU) to measure performance during the WMFT [16]. An IMU contains inertial sensors such as accelerometers, rate gyroscopes, and magnetometers (see Fig. 7). These devices have been increasingly used for activity recognition due to their non-invasive nature and ease of use. In our study, we placed an IMU on the user's wrist during the administration of the WMFT (Fig. 8). We used the accelerometer and rate gyro signals to obtain a number of features, including signal kurtosis, skewness, mean, variance, approximate entropy, RMS of jerk, and power. These characteristics were used to train a Naïve Bayes classifier that was used as a predictor for the clinicians' ratings. Such a classifier makes use of a feature vector (e.g. kurtosis) to develop a classifier that uses the maximum a posteriori (MAP) decision rule to distinguish between classes of outcomes. The 'outcomes' were the clinicians' scores. Using this technique, we obtained significant correlation for one participant and

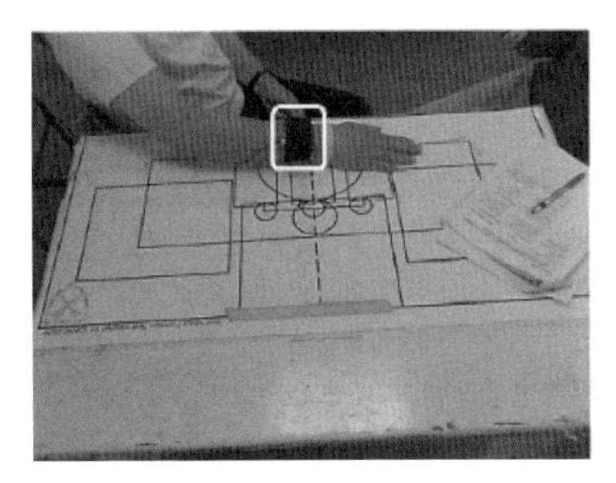

Figure 8. Experimental setup used by Parnandi et al. to correlate inertial measurement unit signal features and WMFT scores.

moderately significant correlation for another. The trial is ongoing, and with a larger population, we expect to strengthen our model.

1.3. Summary

To summarize, AAL techniques can prove quite useful in the subacute phase of stroke when used in conjunction with standard assessments. It is important to note that, much of this discussion generalizes beyond stroke. Particularly, this discussion is relevant to periods when individuals suffering from motor deficits are in clinics or assisted living facilities as inpatients or outpatients. In all cases, standard outcome measures are administered to assess ability or changes in ability. The used of quantitative AAL techniques will allow us to obtain correlates to measures that have been otherwise shown to be valid and reliable. Further, these techniques can extract previously unobservable differences in progress or treatment outcomes. Ultimately, both of these contributions will lead to better rehabilitation practices, for the clinic and the home.

2. Functional Recovery in the Home

For most individuals, the chronic phase is the longest phase of stroke recovery. Many go on to live for a decade or longer after the onset of stroke [7]. The considerations for AAL in this period are drastically different from those of the subacute phase simply because individuals typically receive no supervised care. This is where AAL can make a significant impact; neuroplasticitiy remains long after the onset of stroke. In fact, it is believed that individuals are capable of learning for the duration of their lives. However, it is also known that individuals are susceptible to the phenomenon known as 'learned non-use' [22]. This term refers to the portion of a motor deficit due not to nervous system damage, but to a learned suppression of movement of the affected limb. For example, when an individual tries to use the stroke-affected limb to perform a task, their motor deficit may render task performance difficult. The individual still wants to accomplish the task, and may do so using the non-affected limb. Without constant reminders to try to incorporate the affected limb, this phenomenon can be extremely detrimental.

In order to counter the effects of not having supervised rehabilitation, AAL should be used to encourage functional recovery in the home. This area has not been explored

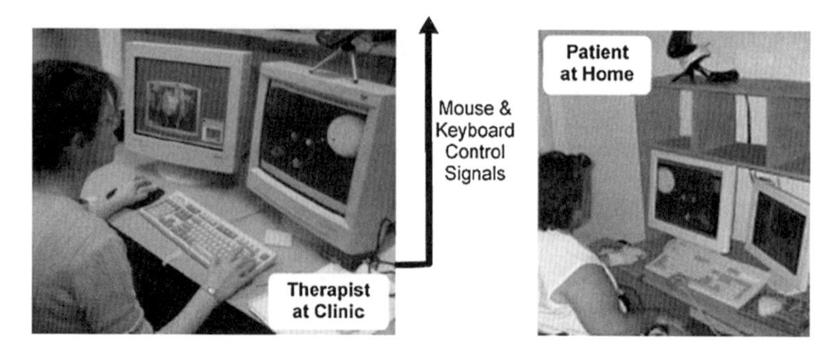

Figure 9. Experimental setup used by Holden et al. to determine the efficacy of a remotely supervised home-based rehabilitation tool. Adapted from [8].

greatly simply because home-based interventions must be validated in a controlled, clinical setting before they can be deployed. Nonetheless, there has been research into the technical feasibility of such systems.

2.1. Increasing the Duration, Intensity, and Quality of Training in the Home

AAL techniques can be used to increase the quality, duration, and intensity of in-home task practice. As an example, Holden et al. developed a system to evaluate a computer based virtual game [8]. Therapists in a clinical setting created and supervised a functional task game practiced by the participants in their own homes. The goal of the study was to determine the technical feasibility of the system, and to determine if the effects of this remote practice would last. Individuals practiced various 'real-world' tasks such as placing an envelope into a mailbox, pulling up a sleeve, and more. Eleven individuals post stroke in the chronic phase of recover (all over 6 months post-stroke) were recruited for the study. The experimental setup can be seen in Fig. 9.

To determine the efficacy of the system, pre/post WMFT, FM, measures of grip strength, and shoulder flexion were obtained. Participants showed statistically significant improvements, even at four months follow up, on all outcome measures excluding grip strength. In this case, the lack of a control group makes it difficult to argue conclusively that outcomes were due to the virtual environment (VE) interaction. Regardless, this project demonstrated the technical feasibility of having a home-based rehabilitation framework supervised remotely by clinicians, using a relatively simple task and interface. One can imagine an adaptation of this technique wherein individuals perform their practice tasks, and a clinician evaluates performance at fixed intervals to provide occasional updates as to how the individual should change or augment their practice schedule.

2.2. Provide a View of Short- and Long-Term Effects of Interventions

With home-based tools, individual progress can more easily be tracked over longer time scales. This idea was explored in another feasibility study wherein the authors introduced various methods to monitor and motivate individuals in the home setting. Like Holden, Reinkensmeyer et al. developed a PC based rehabilitation framework for hand and arm recovery using a hand-held joystick (see Fig. 10) [17]. The authors used a web-based battery of tests, games, and data to provide motivation and performance information. The participant performed a number of tasks designed to train speed, coordination, and

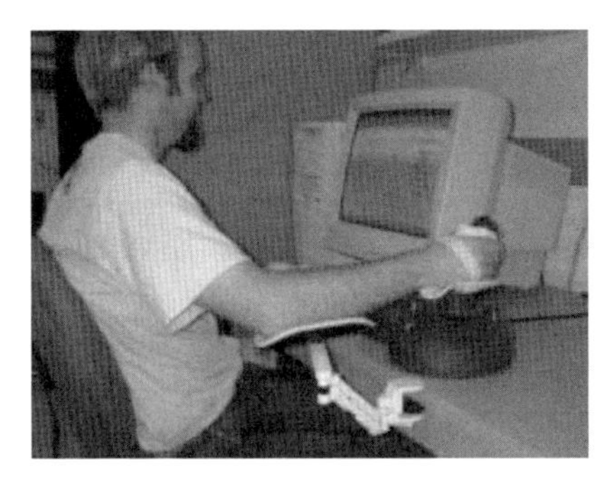

Figure 10. Experimental setup used by Reinkensmeyer et al. to determine the efficacy of a remotely supervised home-based rehabilitation tool. Adapted from [17].

strength. The system provided status tests to evaluate user functional ability (speed and strength). It also provided therapeutic games that challenged different motor abilities. To provide motivation, charts were available so individuals could track their progress over time. In addition, a separate page allowed the therapist to view user progress and augment the exercise regimen remotely. The authors piloted the system with a single participant, who showed no clinically (or statistically) significant improvements, though he did increase scores on the Chedokee-McMaster Upper Extremity Scale.

Again, this study was primarily a technological feasibility study, but it was also important that the experimenters devoted significant effort to determining how to motivate and encourage individuals. For AAL applications to be successful rehabilitation tools, it is important to remember that individuals will be using and interacting with computer interfaces and other technologies for very long periods of time. It is necessary to determine what types of interfaces are most appropriate and user-friendly, but will also be capable of maintaining user interest.

3. Monitoring and Motivation in the Home

The question of monitoring and motivation in rehabilitation deserves some discussion. As with any in-home intervention, individuals are not always compliant with the prescribed regimen. This has been demonstrated with pharmacological interventions [3]. Though, with rehabilitation, there is often intrinsic motivation to comply in order to improve motor capability, any long-term home-based care must have a mechanism for monitoring and motivating individuals.

In addition to the low cost PC and sensor based AAL techniques we've mentioned, a new research domain known as socially assistive robotics (SAR) may be valuable for monitoring and encouraging long-term compliance. Socially assistive robotics is a research field wherein robots are used in a hands-off manner to influence individuals through social means [4]. SAR has been applied to research with a number of populations including those affected by Autism Spectrum Disorders (ASD), obesity, Alzheimer's and dementia, and stroke [4,10,14,16,20,21].

One advantage of SAR is the use of physically embodied agents. Many individuals, when seeing a robot, are curious about how the robot functions, and how they might interact with it. In past studies, individuals have demonstrated an attraction to a variety of

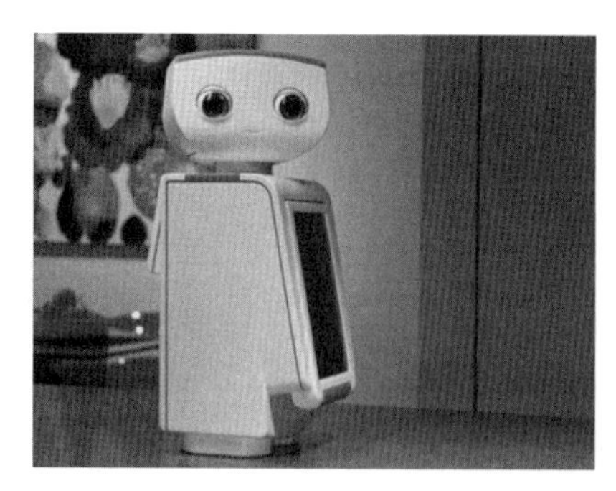

Figure 11. The Intuitive Automata autom™ robot.

robots and assigned them human-like characteristics [5,9,10,13]. Of course, to be useful, a robot needs to be more than visually interesting. When developing the early version of the *autom* robot (see Fig. 11) for his PhD thesis, Kidd sought to determine if, all things being equal, physical embodiment contributed to a higher quality interaction and better outcomes [10].

Kidd et al. designed a study to evaluate the role of embodiment in a weight loss study. The researchers divided individuals into three groups of 15; the groups were tasked with tracking their weight loss progress using either a paper log, a computer-based log, or a robot-based log. As outcomes, Kidd evaluated how long individuals maintained the exercise program, and responses to a custom questionnaire. The results were telling; individuals in the robot group worked with the system significantly longer than the computer group ($p < 0.05$) and significantly longer than the paper log group ($p < 0.01$). Participants also rated the robot highly according to the Working Alliance Index (WAI), a measure of shared goals between therapist and patient. This is one of many studies that have alluded to the fact that robots with human-like characteristics can take advantage of their physical presence and embodiment to elicit desired outcomes. When considering long-term compliance with in-home interventions, taking advantage of this embodiment may be critical.

In our own work, we have investigated this question in the domain of stroke rehabilitation. In a study published in 2007, Matarić et al. initiated a pilot study of an autonomous robot designed to monitor and encourage participants during the performance of functional task practice [14]. Two individuals post-stroke interacted with a mobile robot while performing a book shelving task and a range-of-motion exercise task (see Fig. 12). The robot had three modes of interaction; one provided feedback through sound effects (beeping), one through synthetic voice, and one through pre-recorded human voice. During task performance, the robot verbalized whenever and individual shelved a book or moved their limb. While this study did not focus on motor outcomes, an encouraging outcome was the acceptance of the robots by the individuals. A follow-up study investigated the role of embodiment by comparing interactions with a physical robot, a physical robot viewed remotely, and a computer simulation of a robot. Results indicated that individuals preferred the physically embodied robot.

These pilot results were used to formulate a study focused on a more direct application of clinical techniques in the stroke domain by an SAR agent. The study was designed to evaluate the ability of a humanoid robot to provide knowledge of results (KR) and encouragement during the performance of an upper-extremity functional task game [15].

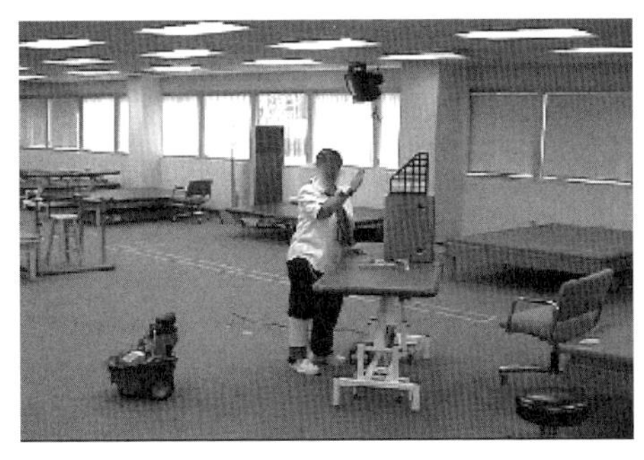

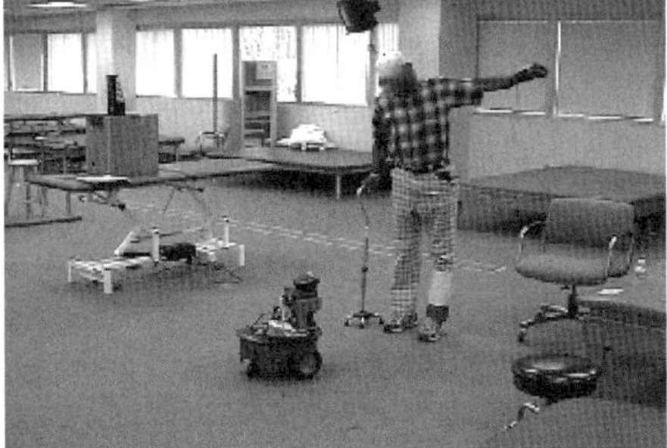

(a) Participant shelving magazines (b) Participant performing a motor rehabilitation task

Figure 12. Experimental setup used by Matarić et al. to evaluate user responses to a socially assistive robotic coach. Individuals performed a variety of tasks while being monitored by a mobile robot.

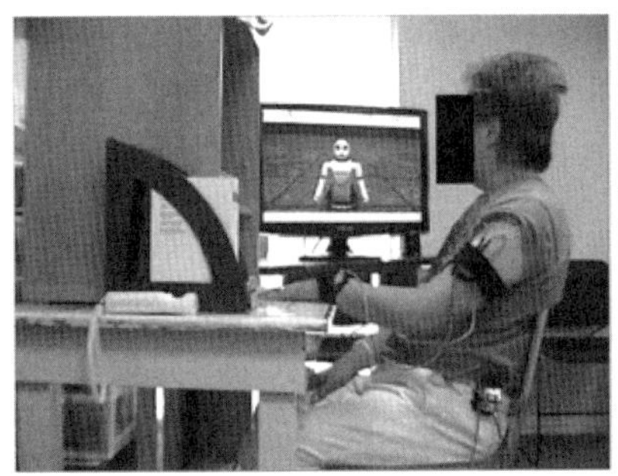

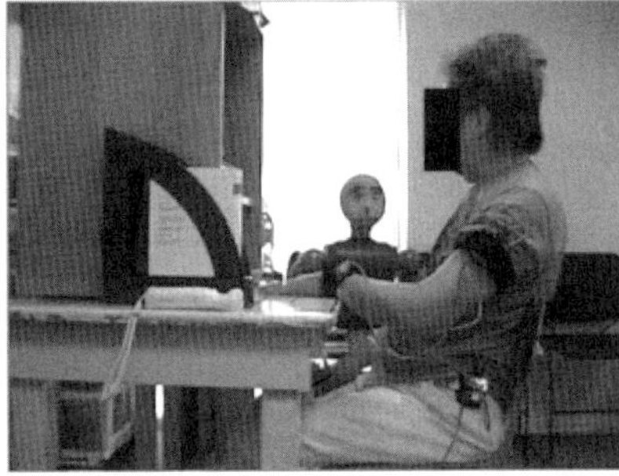

(a) SAR robot simulation (b) SAR robot

Figure 13. Experimental setup used by Mead et al. to evaluate the role of embodiment during the performance of functional task practice.

In a pilot study of the human-robot interaction framework, three participants performed a shelving task with both a humanoid robot and a computer simulation of the same robot (see Fig. 13). Individuals indicated a preference for the physical robot.

The robot was used in a follow up study to provide KR and guide participants as they performed a wire puzzle game (see Fig. 14 (a)). Individuals interacted with the robot during three 45-minute practice sessions. From session to session, the puzzle difficulty increased (where 'increased difficulty' is directly related to the puzzle length and the number of 90° turns). Within a session, task difficulty was incremented by changing the wand with which the participant performed the task (the wand with the largest ring diameter was easiest, while the wand with the smallest ring diameter was the most difficult) (see Fig. 14 (b)). The purpose of using the wire puzzle game was to have a functional, upper extremity practice task with variable difficulty levels. Variable difficulty levels were used to tune the task challenge level to participant ability. According to the challenge point framework, adapting the challenge level to a participants' ability may increase the amount of learning resulting from task performance [6]. While individuals performed the task, the robot monitored the number of errors (contacts between the wand ring and the puzzle) and total movement time; these were provided verbally to the user as KR at the completion of each bout. The study indicated that the SAR robot was capable

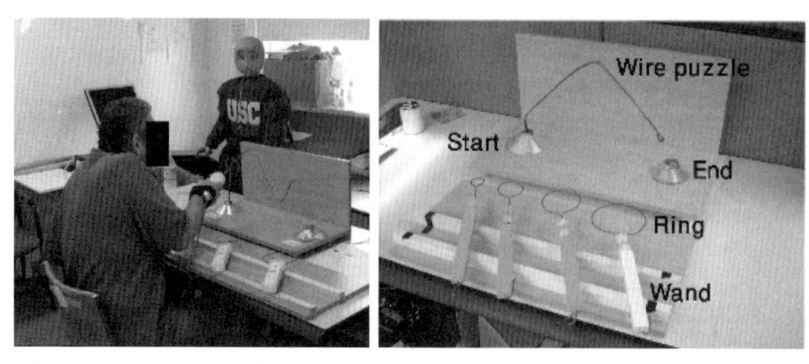

(a) Study participant performing the wire puzzle (b) Wire puzzle and wands of varying difficulty

Figure 14. Participant and puzzle used in an ongoing stroke recovery study.

of guiding the motor task practice session. While preliminary data did not indicate any pre/post functional outcomes, it is encouraging that we can use this framework to validate and determine best practices for techniques known to work in human-human interactions. For instance, the quantitative nature of these systems allows for methodological manipulation of parameters (e.g. schedule and frequency of KR) to determine optimal conditions for bringing about positive functional outcomes in populations suffering from motor deficits. We look forward to adapting this framework to a number of other tasks and interactions to determine the generalizability of this approach.

4. Conclusions: Looking Ahead

We feel very strongly about the potential for AAL techniques in motor rehabilitation. Broadly speaking, progress in this field requires (1) validated rehabilitation techniques and (2) technologies and systems that function in the real world. With respect to the first point, evidence based medicine techniques lead to better understanding of the conditions of practice that are best for obtaining functional outcomes. After determining which conditions of practice lead to the best outcomes in a population, the next logical step is to determine how these therapies can be moved into the AAL domain. This is where the second point, above, becomes relevant. The convergence of the medical and engineering domains is leading to products that have the kinds of functionality required for AAL (power, battery life, wireless transmission, and others) and can make use of clinical best practices.

Future progress in motor rehabilitation requires continued interaction between these domains. The most logical first step is a focus on the time when individuals are available to interact with the clinician on a regular basis; as inpatients and outpatients. Due to the novelty of AAL research, it is necessary to have a period wherein systems can be deployed while mechanisms for continued evaluation and debugging remain in place. This means the clinicians, engineers, and therapists designing the AAL systems need to be in constant contact with the end-users, which includes the participants and patients.

Logically, the area where there is the most potential for these systems is the ambient setting, or the patients' homes. Because individuals are often receiving little to no monitoring, supervision, or rehabilitation in this setting, there is a large gap between what we know to be beneficial and what is actually being provided. Unfortunately, this area is the great unknown – there are many variables for which we cannot control that exist in the home. So intelligent approaches to monitoring not just the participant, but also the functionality of the system and the user's environment are necessary. Successfully doing so will lead to a dramatic impact on the quality of life and functional recovery of individuals in their homes and in other ambient environments.

We must recognize that the positive effects of AAL for rehabilitation are clinical, financial, economic, and social. Moving to a more holistic model for rehabilitation that accounts for the big picture, rather than 'snapshots' of individual ability, will give us a better understanding of how our best practices translate to real-world outcomes.

Acknowledgements

Thanks to all the members of the USC Interaction Laboratory (Maja J. Matarić) and the USC Motor Behavior and Neurorehabilitation Laboratory (Carolee J. Winstein) [24,18].

References

[1] R. Colombo, I. Sterpi, A. Mazzone, C. Delconte, G. Minuco and F. Pisano, Measuring changes of movement dynamics during robot-aided neurorehabilitation of stroke patients, *IEEE Trans. Neural Syst. Rehabil. Eng.* **18**(1) (2010), 75–85.

[2] G.V. Dijck, J.V. Vaerenbergh and M.V. Hulle, Posterior probability profiles for the automated assessment of the recovery of stroke patients, in: *Proc. of AAAI*, 2007, pp. 347–353.

[3] S. Ellis, S. Shumaker, W. Sieber, C. Rand and the Pharmacological Intervention Working Group, Adherence to pharmacological interventions: Current trends and future directions, *Controlled Clinical Trials* **21**(5) (2000), S218–S225.

[4] D.J. Feil-Seifer and M.J. Matarić, Defining socially assistive robotics, in: *Proc. of International Conference on Rehabilitation Robotics*, Chicago, IL, 2005, pp. 465–468.

[5] T. Fong, I. Nourbakhsh and K. Dautenhahn, A survey of socially interactive robots, *Robotics and Autonomous Systems, Special Issue on Socially Interactive Robots* **42** (2003), 143–166.

[6] M.A. Guadagnoli and T.D. Lee, Challenge point: A framework for conceptualizing the effects of various practice conditions in motor learning, *J. Mot. Behav.* **36**(2) (2004), 212–224.

[7] H. Hannerz and M.L. Nielsen, Life expectancies among survivors of acute cerebrovascular disease, *Stroke* **32**(8) (2001), 1739–1744.

[8] M.K. Holden, T.A. Dyar and L. Dayan-Cimadoro, Telerehabilitation using a virtual environment improves upper extremity function in patients with stroke, *IEEE Trans. Neural Syst. Rehabil. Eng.* **15**(1) (2007), 36–42.

[9] M.J. Johnson, X. Feng, L.M. Johnson and J.M. Winters, Potential of a suite of robot/computer-assisted motivating systems for personalized, home-based, stroke rehabilitation, *J. NeuroEngineering and Rehabilitation* **4**(6) (2007), 1–17.

[10] C.D. Kidd, Designing for long-term human-robot interaction and application to weight loss, MIT Thesis, 2008.

[11] J.S. Kim, D.W. Oh, S.Y. Kim and J.D. Choi, Visual and kinesthetic locomotor imagery training integrated with auditory step rhythm for walking performance of patients with chronic stroke, *Clin. Rehabil.* (2010).

[12] N. Leibowitz, N. Levy, S. Weingarten, Y. Grinberg, A. Karniel, Y. Sacher, C. Serfaty and N. Soroker, Automated measurement of proprioception following stroke, *Disabil. Rehabil.* **30**(24) (2008), 1829–1836.

[13] R. Looije, M. Neerincx and F. Cnossen, Persuasive robotic assistant for health self-management of older adults: Design and evaluation of social behaviors, *Int. J. Human-Computer Studies* **68** (2010), 386–397.

[14] M.J. Matarić, J. Eriksson, D.J. Feil-Seifer and C.J. Winstein, Socially assistive robotics for post-stroke rehabilitation, *J. NeuroEngineering and Rehabilitation* **4**(5) (Feb 2007).

[15] R. Mead, E. Wade, P. Johnson, A.B. St. Clair, S. Chen and M.J. Matarić, An architecture for rehabilitation task practice in socially assistive human-robot interaction, in: *Proc. of 19th IEEE International Symposium in Robot and Human Interactive Communication*, 2010.
[16] A. Parnandi, E. Wade and M.J. Matarić, Motor function assessment using wearable inertial sensor, in: *Proc. of IEEE EMBS*, 2010.
[17] D.J. Reinkensmeyer, C.T. Pang, J.A. Nessler and C.C. Painter, Web-based telerehabilitation for the upper extremity after stroke, *IEEE Trans. Neural Syst. Rehabil. Eng.* **10**(2) (2002), 102–108.
[18] J. Sanford, J. Moreland, L. Swanson, P. Stratford and C. Gowland, Reliability of the fugl-meyer assessment for testing motor performance in patients following stroke, *Phys. Ther.* **73**(7) (1993), 447–454.
[19] A. Shumway-Cook, S. Brauer and M. Woollacott, Predicting the probability for falls in community-dwelling older adults using the timed up & go test, *Phys. Ther.* **80**(9) (2000), 896–903.
[20] A. Tapus, M.J. Matarić and B. Scassellati, The grand challenges in socially assistive robotics, *IEEE Robotics and Automation Magazine* **14**(1) (2007), 35–42.
[21] A. Tapus, C. Tapus and M.J. Matarić, The use of socially assistive robots in the design of intelligent cognitive therapies for people with dementia, in: *Proc. of International Conference on Rehabilitation Robotics*, 2009.
[22] E. Taub, G. Uswatte, V.W. Mark and D.M. Morris, The learned nonuse phenomenon: Implications for rehabilitation, *Eura Medicophys.* **42**(3) (2006), 241–256.
[23] S. Timmermans and A. Angell, Evidence-based medicine, clinical uncertainty, and learning to doctor, *Journal of Health and Social Behavior* **42**(4) (2001), 342–359.
[24] S. Wolf, P. Catlin, M. Ellis, A. Archer, B. Morgan and A. Piacentino, Assessing wolf motor function test as outcome measure for research in patients after stroke, *Stroke* **32** (2001), 1635–1639.
[25] World Health Organization, Burden of disease statistics, 2010. http://www.who.org.

Handbook of Ambient Assisted Living
J.C. Augusto et al. (Eds.)
IOS Press, 2012

doi:10.3233/978-1-60750-837-3-581

Home-Based Computer Vision Access Technologies for Individuals with Severe Motor Impairments

Tom CHAU [a,b,*], Negar MEMARIAN [c], Brian LEUNG [a], Deborah TREHERNE [e], David HOBBS [d], Breanna WORTHINGTON-EYRE [f], Andrea LAMONT [a] and Michele PLA-MOBARAK [g]

[a] *Holland Bloorview Kids Rehabilitation Hospital, Toronto, Canada*
[b] *Institute of Biomaterials and Biomedical Engineering, University of Toronto, Canada*
[c] *The Hospital for Sick Children, Toronto, Canada*
[d] *School of Computer Science, Engineering and Mathematics, Flinders University, Adelaide, Australia*
[e] *Alzheimer's Australia South Australia*
[f] *Disability SA, Department for Families and Communities, Government of South Australia, Australia*
[g] *Universidad Iberoamericana, Mexico City, Mexico*

Abstract. For individuals with severe disabilities, home-based access to communication, computer and environmental controls can prove to be a non-trivial challenge. In this chapter, we introduce a family of home-based access technologies that exploit computer vision via one or more cameras, operating in the visible or infrared light spectrum. These technologies are non-contact, requiring no devices to be attached to the user. We present two major categories of access: corporeal access whereby the user interacts with his or her environment using gross movements of the limbs, trunk or head; and orofacial access where the user connects to the environment via gestures of the mouth. After introducing the fundamentals of each type of access technology, we provide clinical illustrations of how these technologies have been applied in the home or community setting. The chapter concludes with a discussion of the merits and limitations of computer vision-based access technologies.

Keywords. Access technology, computer vision, thermal imaging, rehabilitation

Introduction

Individuals with severe motor impairments often have difficulty interacting with the people and objects in their environment [11]. Access to communication and environmental interaction is important for social engagement, recreation, and academic progress, among other developmental domains [3]. While there exists a plethora of mechanical and

*Corresponding Author: Tom Chau, Holland Bloorview Kids Rehabilitation Hospital, Toronto, Ontario, M4G 1R8, Canada. E-mail: tom.chau@utoronto.ca.

electrophysiological switches designed to facilitate interactions, some of the common challenges of physical switch-based access include:

1. difficulty targeting a switch even when positioned well within reach, possibly due to involuntary or poorly coordinated movements;
2. inability to release a switch once activated, for example, due to spasticity;
3. difficulty mustering the force required to activate a switch due for example, to hypotonia;
4. tendency to activate a switch multiple times as a consequence of hyperkinetic movement;
5. positioning the switch safely and consistently, especially when harnessing head and facial movements;
6. limited range of motion due for example to spasticity or joint contractures [25], and
7. lack of universal and comprehensive access assessment [3].

Etiologies leading to such disability may include spastic quadriplegic cerebral palsy [13], neurodegenerative diseases [5], neuro-genetic disorders [6] and spinal cord injury [8], among other conditions. To address this issue, access technologies have been designed to translate the intentions of a user with profound physical impairments into functional activities such as communication, environmental interaction [23] and play [14]. As such, access technologies can enhance the usability of external devices such as electronic communication aids and environmental control systems. Access technologies are ideally unobtrusive to the user, context-aware and adaptive to changing user needs and abilities [20]. As many individuals use access technologies in the home setting, the potential integration of these technologies into personal living environments bears natural appeal. Home-based access technologies can thus be considered an emerging subset of ambient-assisted living technologies. In this chapter, we introduce a genre of home-based access technologies that exploit cameras and image processing to provide users with access to computers, music-making and communication aids. It is important to mention that many other genres of access technologies exist, including for example, mechanical switches, infrared sensing, electromyographic switches, and brain-machine systems. The interested reader is referred to [23] for a review.

1. Technology Paradigm

The general technology paradigm for home-based computer vision access technologies is summarized in Fig. 1. One or more cameras are situated in the personal living environment to capture specific activities of the user. For the purposes of this chapter, we will focus on motoric activities although certain autonomic responses can also be non-invasively monitored via specialized cameras (e.g., thermal imaging). When the user is in the field of view of a camera, image processing algorithms are invoked to detect targeted movements, which when present, are translated into appropriate outputs (e.g., visual and/or auditory feedback). In Fig. 1, the user is interacting with an embedded display in the wall of his home. The display is offering possible messages for transmission to a communication partner. To select the desired message, the user produces a targeted motion (e.g., finger movement or an intentional eye blink), which is captured by

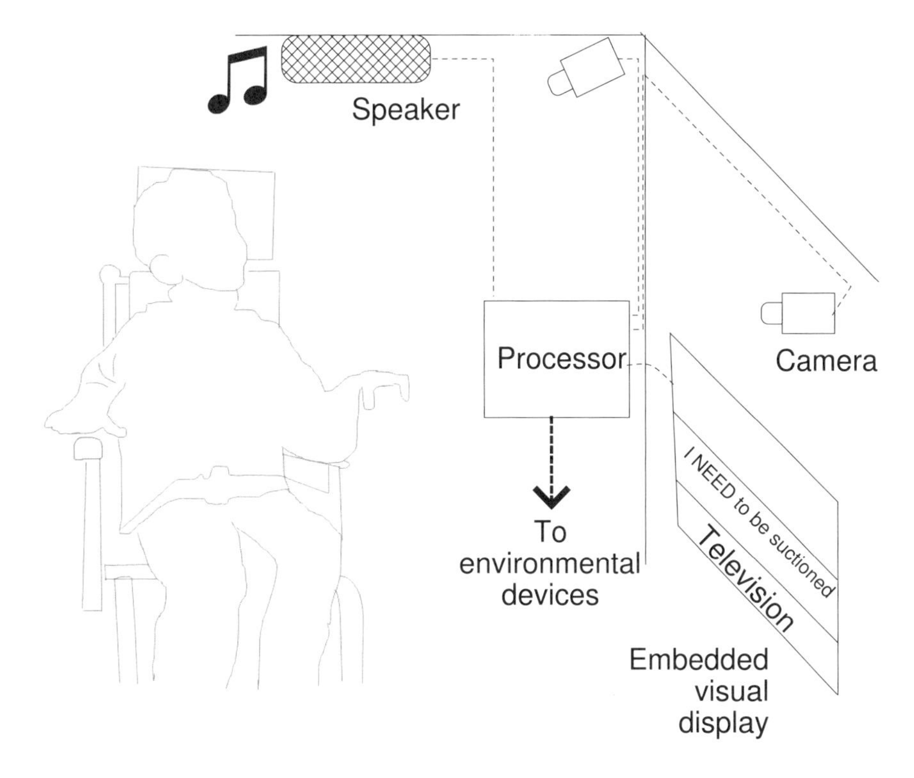

Figure 1. Overall system concept for home-based computer vision access technologies.

one or more cameras and interpreted by algorithms in the processing unit. Once the gesture has been interpreted, the appropriate output (e.g., voice output via environmentally-embedded speakers) is generated. The same set-up can clearly be used for various environmental interactions (e.g., operating lights or entertainment system in the house, or activating a tele-homecare system). In the ensuing sections, we will exemplify systems which harness gross or fine *bodily* movements (i.e., corporeal access), and systems which exploit more subtle *orofacial gestures* (i.e., orofacial access).

2. Corporeal Access

When an individual has extant physical movement, visible light cameras can be used to capture those movements. In the simplest scheme, motion within a targeted area of space can be used to activate an external device (e.g., voice output communication aid, motorized blinds, video door answering system, television or room lighting system).

2.1. Simple Motion Detection

Suppose an enclosed region of space around an individual is demarcated as a potential zone of activation. As shown in Fig. 2, these zones serve as virtual objects because they exist only in the computer-generated environment. The accumulated pixel by pixel difference between the corresponding virtual objects in successive RGB images can be used

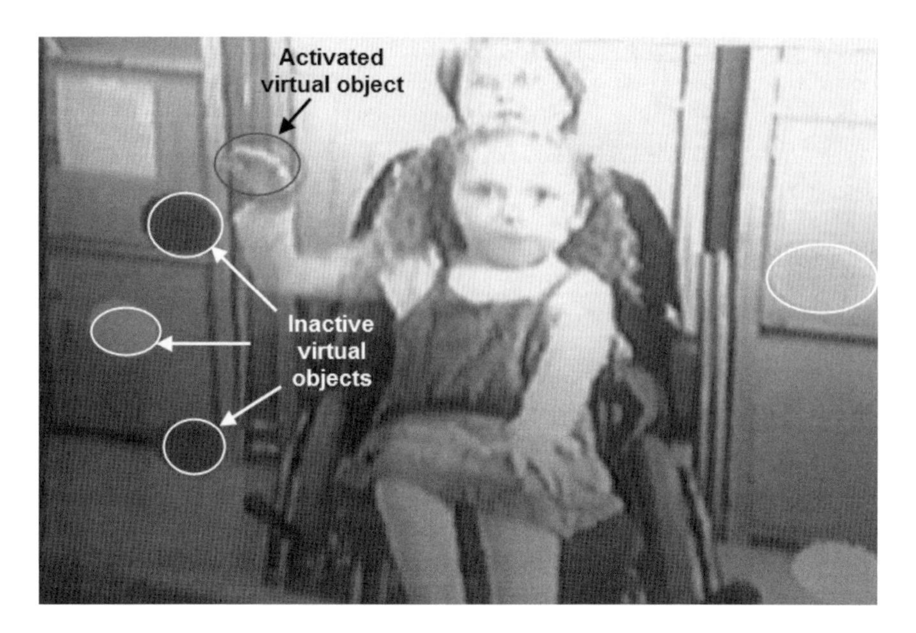

Figure 2. Example of gross motor interaction with a single-camera access system. The on-screen shapes are augmentations of the real environment, which respond aurally and visually when the child interacts with the demarcated space. In this application, the child is engaged in active music-making.

to define the amount of localized activity at the current instant in time. This activity can be normalized by the maximum possible activity for a region of the same size (i.e., the maximum pixel intensity multiplied by the number of pixels in the region). A threshold of activity beyond which motion is considered to be present is required. In [24] and [1], the following threshold is used

$$\text{Threshold} = \frac{1}{2}\left[1 - \tanh\left(\frac{\text{Sensitivity}}{100} \times 6 - 3\right)\right] \tag{1}$$

where $Sensitivity$ is an adjustable parameter between 0 (least sensitive) and 100 (most sensitive) for the virtual object in question. In addition to a threshold of activation, it is frequently useful to also set dwell times to accommodate for unsteady or involuntary movements. A dwell time is the minimum amount of time that an object needs to exhibit suprathreshold activity before the object is deemed activated. Dwell times thus preclude accidental activation on the assumption that unintentional movements will generate momentary suprathreshold motion. To provide a deeper sense of control over the nature of the activation, so-called velocity control can also be implemented. In other words, the quality of the movement can be used to control the volume (i.e., MIDI velocity) of the auditory feedback produced upon activation of a virtual object. In our studies, one possible dynamic determination of the volume of activation, $V_{Activation}$, can be realized as follows

$$V_{Activation} = \frac{1}{2}V_o(1 - e^{-2\delta}) \tag{2}$$

where V_o is the user-configured maximum volume for the object, and δ is the relative activation, namely,

$$\delta = k\left(\frac{\text{Activity} - \text{Threshold}}{\text{Threshold}}\right) \tag{3}$$

where k is an empirically derived scaling constant.

While access systems based on visible light cameras are inexpensive, small and highly portable, they are plagued with illumination challenges. From one environmental setting to the next, lighting differences can be quite dramatic, requiring calibration of any colour-based detection scheme. In the systems depicted in Figs 2 and 4, an illumination compensation scheme was implemented to mitigate the need for manual adjustment of virtual object sensitivities from one lighting environment to the next. The basic idea was to use stored values of room luminance and manually tuned virtual object sensitivities from one environment, to predict new sensitivity values in environments with different illumination levels. Let Y_{new} denote the pixel-averaged luminance of the new environment, derived by averaging the luminance component of each pixel in the YCbCr color space. Further, $a = 0.0125$ and $b = 3$ are constants determined from the limits of sensitivity (ranges between 0 and 1) and luminance (ranges between 0 and 240 arbitrary units). If Y_o and S_o represent the luminance of the original environment and sensitivity level set in that environment, then the new sensitivity can be estimated by

$$S_{new} = e^{-Y_{new}\gamma a+b} \tag{4}$$

where

$$\gamma = \frac{3 - \log(S_o)}{aY_o} \tag{5}$$

In other words, as luminance increases, sensitivity decreases accordingly in an exponentially decaying fashion.

Lighting challenges can also occur even within a single environment that is illuminated by a combination of natural and artificial light. Given variable cloud cover, the level of natural light may vary even within a short period of time. Some practical guidelines for dealing with illumination challenges have arisen from one author's (D. Hobbs) extensive experience with setting up a single-camera motion detection-data projector combination in a classroom environment. Typically, classrooms are illuminated by both natural and artificial lighting, and the level of the former cannot be modulated due to an absence of shades or curtains. The key principle is that the camera should face a well-illuminated user while the projection display is best viewed with minimal lighting. These principles are exemplified in [14], where the projection screen is placed against the natural light source such that the projection surface is minimally affected by natural light. The user is located in front of the screen, facing the natural light and hence is adequately illuminated. Finally, the camera is positioned with its back to the natural light source.

2.2. *The Bloorview Virtual Music Instrument*

The Bloorview Virtual Music Instrument is an example of a corporeal access solution exploiting simple motion detection. With the Bloorview Virtual Music Instrument, simple motion detection is combined with sensory feedback to provide augmented environments for various applications in the hospital, home and community setting. An augmented environment is one in which the properties of the real environment are enhanced via the superposition of interactive virtual objects [7]. To create an augmented environment that supports functional interaction, the Bloorview Virtual Music Instrument defines several virtual objects in the space reachable by the user, as exemplified in Fig. 2. Each virtual object possesses its own response properties, including the sensitivity and dwell times introduced above. In addition, each object can be assigned graphical and acoustic behaviors. Graphical behaviors provide visual feedback to the user, confirming positive activation. For example, the virtual object may become transparent or translucent, rotate, vibrate or translate upon activation. Likewise, acoustic behaviors provide the user auditory feedback corresponding to activation. These may include a single tone, a set of tones (i.e., a chord) or a snippet of a digitized sound file. In Fig. 2, the child is interacting with an augmented musical environment (the Bloorview Virtual Music Instrument), where each virtual object represents a musical note. The child's raised arm is activating one virtual object resulting in the production of a single tone in the timbre of a grand piano, while the other inactive objects remain silent. In the version shown here, the system offered a 3 octave musical range, 128 MIDI instruments, configurable dwell-on and dwell-off times and velocity control. In the following paragraphs, we summarize clinical applications of the Bloorview Virtual Music Instrument with children and older persons.

One of the first studies with the Bloorview Virtual Music Instrument aimed to quantify the usability of simple motion detection-based corporeal access in the context of music education. Using the augmented musical environment, 6 children (3 with cerebral palsy and 3 with spinal muscular atrophy) aged 4.4 ± 1.3 years participated in 6 weeks of music education sessions at a pediatric rehabilitation hospital. Each session was 0.5 hour in length. Children were also given specific augmented environment templates each week and a copy of the computer vision software so that they could practice for 0.5 hours per day at home. By the end of the 6 weeks, all children were able to achieve matched colour activation (i.e., reaching to a virtual object on the basis of a verbal colour cue) and a minimum sequence of at least 10 virtual notes [7].

With its roots in music therapy, the Bloorview Virtual Music Instrument has been deployed in a complex continuing care unit in a pediatric rehabilitation hospital in Canada as a bedside access technology. As seen in Fig. 3, the entire system has been implemented on a mobile, self-powered computer cart, akin to the COWs (Computers-on-Wheels) commonly found in hospitals. In this particular embodiment of the Bloorview Virtual Music Instrument, there are two displays, one for the patient lying in the hospital bed and one for the attending therapist standing at bedside. With the articulating arm, the user display can be inclined, raised, lowered or otherwise positioned to suit the viewing preference of the patient. Likewise, the camera is mounted on a flexible Loc-Line hose to maximize positioning options. Being self-powered, the entire unit can be conveniently wheeled from room-to-room.

A recent study in a school setting aimed to determine an access solution for a child with severe spastic cerebral palsy and cortical vision impairment. With the Bloorview Virtual Music Instrument, the activation of a virtual object can be configured to trigger a switch or a specific behavior of an external device (e.g., mouse click for computer access). This type of interfacing was pursued in this study, as depicted in Fig. 4. Here, the child is scanning through a list of "blank" options to arrive at a specific song on a music player. He scrolls through the list using the virtual "go" button, which is located lateral to his wheelchair tray. Note that this is a virtual button, floating in space. Once the child arrives at the desired song, he uses his virtual "select" button, positioned on

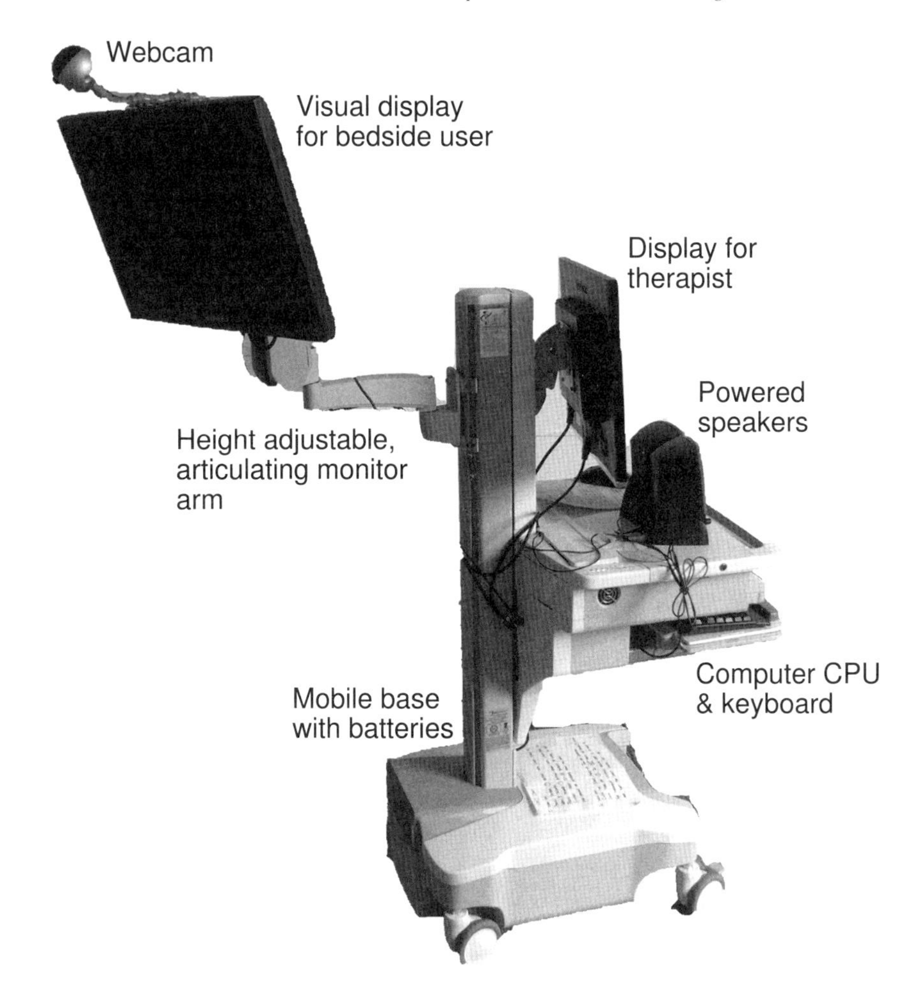

Figure 3. Bloorview virtual music instrument "on-a-pole". This compact, self-powered, self-contained deployment of a motion-detection based corporeal access solution allows children to participate in music making using whatever movements they can generate, while lying in a hospital bed.

his wheelchair tray, to play the selected song. This dual-switch scheme was developed in collaboration with teachers and therapists. The goal was to emulate the mechanical dual-switch set-up with which the child was already familiar, while reducing the physical effort of precise targeting and potentially offering greater postural and switch positioning flexibility.

A trial was conducted in Adelaide, South Australia, at a specialized school for children and young adults ranging in age from 5–21 years of age with intellectual and multiple disabilities [14]. Eight students with multiple disabilities were trialled with the Bloorview Virtual Music Instrument to stimulate physical movement and alertness over an 8-week period. Sessions were 20 minutes in length and were conducted individually, at the same time, and in the same location each week. Session goals were established and monitored over the trial period. The number of shapes, colours and sounds presented during each 20-minute session was gradually increased during the trial and students were scored on a scale of 1 (low response observed) to 10 (high response observed) for each

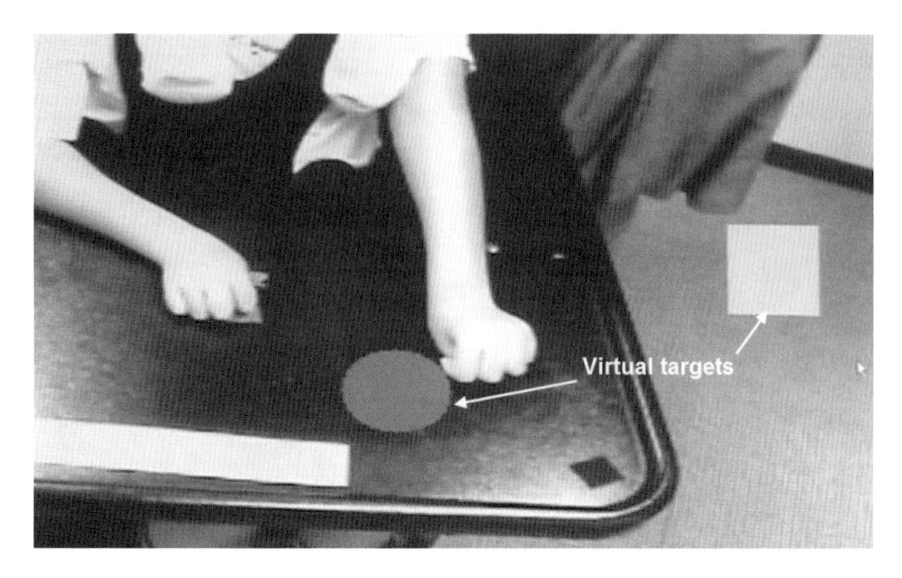

Figure 4. An example of camera-based switch access using the full arm. The circular virtual shape superimposed on the client's tray represents "select" while the square virtual shape floating in space represents "go".

of the session goals. The response was scored by observing the students' overall reaction to the images and sounds presented to them, as well as their ability to follow simple instructions (for example, "show me the red one").

Consistent exposure to the Bloorview Virtual Music Instrument appeared to show improvements in the students' general alertness, behaviour, communication and concentration. Teachers and assistants reported improvements in the students' general behaviour following the sessions – improvements that remained for several days. Since sessions were conducted on a fixed day and time, teachers who were not involved with the trial described the students' anticipating sessions and becoming more alert and excited around the session time. Staff at the school commented that, in conjunction with traditional teaching methods, the system was also a dynamic way to promote, accelerate and consolidate the learning of colours and shapes.

Students at the school were exposed to the Bloorview Virtual Music Instrument in an "integrated" manner, to compliment traditional teaching. Given the customizable nature of the system, typically static lessons and therapy activities could become dynamic and engaging, as the auditory and acoustic aspects of the Bloorview Virtual Music Instrument was used to teach concepts such as big and small, shapes, and colours. Students were also encouraged to create their own music template (i.e.: choosing the shapes, colours and sounds they want), providing practice in making requests and gaining communicative competence through a non-threatening and fun activity.

The Bloorview Virtual Music Instrument system was also trialled as a behavioural outlet for students with ADHD (attention deficit hyperactivity disorder), obsessive disorders, Autism and difficult/harmful behaviours. Students were able to release anger and energy in a safe and effective way through gross movement (such as 'star jumps' or running and jumping in the augmented area), sound and physical activity. Several students at the school had regular sessions with the system specifically for this purpose, with noticeable improvements in their general behaviour. Teachers reported that certain students were calmer yet more alert following the Bloorview Virtual Music Instrument sessions and that they were achieving associated learning goals (i.e.: colour and shape recognition) more efficiently.

In Adelaide, South Australia, the Bloorview Virtual Music Instrument system has also been applied in an aged care facility with residents with dementia. Residents fulfilling one or more of the following criteria were targeted:

- resistive to physiotherapist when investigating range-of-motion
- resistive to participation in activities
- demonstrated general lack of interest/motivation
- of the mindset that they could not do anything more
- willing to assume leadership role in group activities
- willing to explore new activities.

Twelve residents were recruited. Initially, residents participated in one-on-one sessions. They were introduced to the technology via repeated hand-over-hand demonstration of virtual object activation with single-tone auditory feedback. This guided activation would continue until they were able to activate a virtual object independently, as depicted in Fig. 5. The initial one-on-one sessions allowed therapists to assess individual abilities. Subsequent to a few individual sessions, residents graduated to group sessions. The group activities involved physical exercises, including sitting exercises that targeted the upper body and balance exercises that entailed standing with the aid of a frame or chair.

The key observations from these sessions are summarized below.

1. The technology encouraged movement. Residents explored different movements with either minimal or no prompting from staff.
2. The technology facilitated the exploration of range-of-motion with residents who otherwise were resistive to making voluntary movements.
3. Interest and curiosity among residents and staff alike were piqued by the technology. Residents would gather around those using the system and staff were overwhelmed by the residents' responses and the ease with which normally withdrawn residents could be engaged.
4. Residents exhibited a sense of achievement through their smiles when they voluntarily activated sounds and demonstrated encouragement of others by spontaneously applauding each participant during group sessions.
5. Residents were encouraged to think about what was going on and how to coordinate their movements to activate the sounds. Some residents expressed their creativity and imagination by experimenting with different body and facial gestures.
6. The simplicity of the interface made the system particularly appealing for patients with dementia.
7. Residents enjoyed seeing themselves on the large display.

The last observation reverberates with "renarcissization" efforts [2] aimed at improving the self-image of patients with dementia. In fact, the observed empowerment, interest and engagement of the residents closely echo the patient response reported by Benveniste et al. [2] who deployed a virtual keyboard for music-making in small groups of 3 to 4 older adult patients along with a caregiver. In [9], personalized stimuli based on a person's self-identity were identified as among the most engaging for a large cohort of nursing residents with dementia. While the stimuli used in that study related to the participant's past

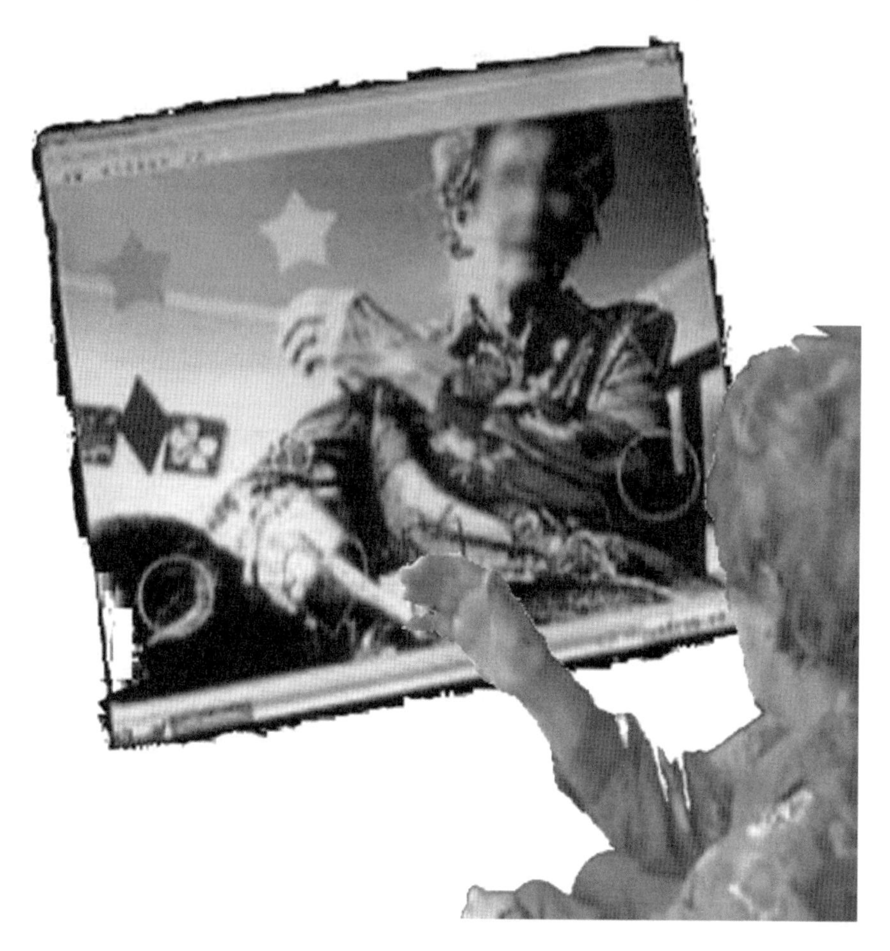

Figure 5. A resident with dementia using the "Bloorview Virtual Music Instrument" motion detection system via arm movements while in a seated posture.

identity with respect to family, occupation, hobbies or interests, the visual feedback (i.e., dynamic mirror image of one's self) of the Bloorview Virtual Music Instrument may have provided residents a similarly familiar stimulus and thus was inherently engaging [10].

The key technical challenges of using the motion detection system in a nursing home setting were related to the learning curve for the associated peripheral hardware, namely, the data projector in this case, and setting up the appropriate augmented environment templates (i.e., placement and configuration of virtual objects). Further, when residents were gathered prior to equipment set-up, they became restless, suggesting that the equipment should be ready to run prior to collecting the residents.

2.3. Motion Primitive Detection

While the previous section has described environmental interactions using simple motion detection (i.e., detecting the presence or absence of motion), one can also decode specific patterns of movement using a single camera. In other words, in addition to detecting the presence of motion, we can also decipher the specific trajectory of movement. Here we describe the dynamic binary frame of reference method introduced in [12]. The method is founded on the rationale that complex movements can be decomposed into a sequence of simple motion descriptors, such as left, right, up and down. Hence, only a coarse image of movement is required to capture the general direction of movement at any instant in time. The method begins with a highly down-sampled image of 16×12 pixels of the scene. The first difference of successive image frames yields an apparent motion matrix at each sampling instant. The apparent motion image sequence is highly susceptible to noise variations from frame to frame. Dilation with a 3×3 cross structuring element expands candidate motion regions while a subsequent logical AND between successive expanded motion frames effectively eliminates apparent motion due to noise.

The difference between successive expanded motion frames yields matrices with partial trajectories, the sum of which provides an estimate of the actual motion trajectory. This final "trajectory" matrix has entries with only 3 possible values, i.e., $\{-1, 0, 1\}$, denoting respectively, the initiation of movement, no movement and the termination of movement. From these entries, directional motion primitives can be derived. For example, if the movement starts on the left and terminates on the right of the image, then the motion descriptor is "Right", suggesting motion towards the right. Likewise, if the movement starts on the top and terminates at the bottom of the image, the motion descriptor is "Down", signifying downward motion. In the left panel of Fig. 6, we exemplify a trajectory matrix where the motion is diagonal from top left to bottom right of the image. The associated motion descriptors in this case would be "Right" and "Down". In this way, a complex gesture can be defined as a sequence of motion descriptors. The right panel of Fig. 6 shows a 12-year old patient with muscular dystrophy who had difficulty communicating as a result of a tracheosotomy. She was equipped with a custom-developed voice output device with a small vocabulary of basic medical (e.g., I need to be suctioned, I am in pain) and emotional (e.g., I am scared) needs. In this image, she is creating a counter-clockwise circular gesture, G, described by a sequence of motion descriptors

$$G = \begin{Bmatrix} L & L & R & R \\ U & D & D & U \end{Bmatrix} \tag{6}$$

In the above, the first column denotes a "Left" and "Up" diagonal gesture while the second column describes a "Left" and "Down" diagonal gesture, and so on. Piecing together the four primitive motions, we have a rough description of a counter-clockwise circular gesture. In this application, the patient used the clockwise and counter-clockwise gestures to navigate (scroll forward/backward) a pictorial grid of messages on a custom-developed electronic voice output device.

With the dynamic binary frame of reference method of motion detection, a gesture database can be assembled by concatenating motion primitives, without training data. When the above processing is applied to a live video stream, a continuous sequence of trajectory matrices are generated, from which a chain of motion descriptors can be derived. A gesture is identified when there is a match between any finite length subset of motion descriptors and a database sequence of motion descriptors. The agreement between candidate gestures and those stored in the database can be ascertained using some distance metric such as the Hamming distance, for discrete-valued strings.

The chief advantage of motion primitive detection is that a custom set of gestures can be defined for each individual without the need to provide training data to the computer. While the above case exemplified finger gestures, gross motor gestures (such as full

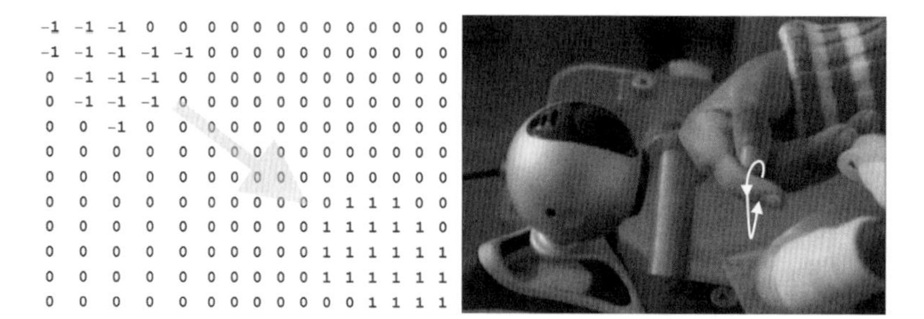

Figure 6. Example of single-camera motion primitive application. The left panel portrays a 16×12 trajectory matrix of diagonal motion towards the bottom-right of the image. In the right panel, the user is creating a counterclockwise finger gesture to scroll backward on an electronic communication aid.

arm movement) are equally viable. The most limiting constraint perhaps however, is the demand for repeatable movements on the part of the user. The system does offer a degree of robustness in that the candidate gesture does not necessarily need to match a database entry exactly, primitive by primitive. Nonetheless, given that each gesture is only made up of a small number of primitives, there is clearly a limit to the variation in the motion primitive sequence. In this light, individuals with a small repertoire of repeatable movements, such as in muscular dystrophy, are more appropriate candidates for motion primitive detection than individuals, for example, with hyperkinetic cerebral palsy, who may have less reliable movements.

3. Orofacial Access

3.1. Multiple Camera Tongue Switch

When a user only has control over muscles involved in mastication, facial expression or tongue movement, cameras can be used to detect specific orofacial gestures. One example of such a system is reported in [15], where three, low cost web cameras were positioned around a child's environment to non-invasively detect tongue protrusion. Specifically, a center camera faced the child while two peripheral cameras were pointed at the user at 45° angles, as shown in Fig. 7. The system was designed for a child with spastic quadriplegic cerebral palsy with intact cognition but without any independent mobility or functional communication. Previous attempts to deploy access technologies that tapped into limb or head movements had been unsuccessful due to spasticity triggered by the effort to exert control, positioning challenges and involuntary head movements. A non-contact camera-based solution was conceived as a means of harnessing tongue protrusions, his most reliable, controlled movement. To address the child's variable head position, multiple cameras were deployed.

The basic system design consisted of three independent replications of a single-camera algorithm. Briefly, in each camera instance, the user's face was localized via skin colour segmentation and automatically followed from frame to frame via the CAMSHIFT colour tracking algorithm. Exploiting the typical red colour saturation of the lips and tongue, the child's mouth was localized from the face sub-image. Based on the rationale that the protruded tongue generates a larger number of saturated red pixels than would occur due to typical baseline fluctuations, the change in the count of saturated

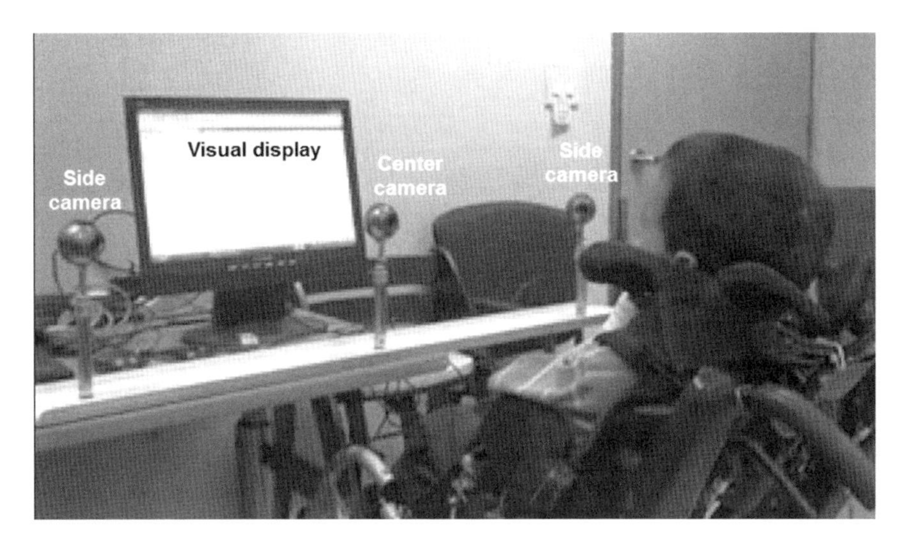

Figure 7. Depiction of multiple camera system designed to detect tongue protrusions regardless of head pose of child. In this application, the child's tongue protrusions serve as a computer mouse click.

red pixels served as an indicator of tongue protrusion. Finally, a measure of the quality of the frontal view was estimated on the assumption that a frontal view would result in the mouth being close to the bisecting line of the bounding rectangle of the face.

The multiple camera tongue protrusion system was evaluated over a period of several weeks in the classroom at the child's school. The child completed 5 sessions of single-switch picture-matching activity. The average sessional sensitivity and specificity both exceeded 80%. Of particular interest is the fact that in 3 of 5 sessions, the peripheral cameras identified the majority of tongue protrusions, affirming their added-value to the overall detection system. Following the research study, a portable home-use version of the system was created for this child. For this purpose, three webcams were mounted on his wheelchair tray.

3.2. Infrared Thermographic Detection

While we presented an illumination compensation scheme, variable lighting between environments remains a challenge for visible light systems. To circumvent this issue, infrared thermal imaging, which is immune to fluctuations in ambient lighting levels, was introduced as an alternative vision-based access technology [17] for the unobtrusive detection of orofacial gestures. In the following, we summarize an algorithm for thermographic detection of mouth opening gestures [16] when the user's head is within the camera's field of view, but not necessarily facing the camera dead on.

Given that the face is generally warmer than the surrounding environment, face localization can be achieved by the simple process of segmenting "warm" pixels followed by the selection of the largest round blob. Likewise, the interior of the mouth is typically warmer than the surrounding regions of the face. Hence, a second thresholding of the warmest pixels in the face yields candidate mouth objects. Lastly, because mouth opening involves motion, two-dimensional motion tracking can be used to isolate warm regions that are in motion. The above procedure will yield candidate objects that are not open

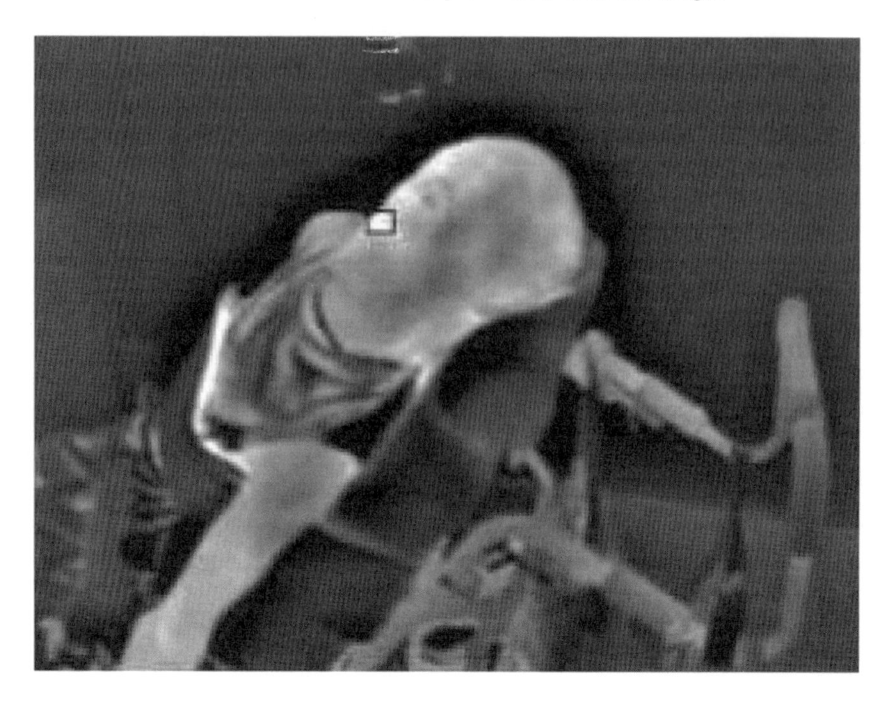

Figure 8. Example of thermal image of client performing a mouth opening gesture. The superimposed rectangular outline over the mouth indicates a positive detection.

mouths. To eliminate non-mouth objects, a series of size, morphological and anthropometric filters can be applied. The concurrent validity of this thermal access technology was established in able-bodied adults using a conventional chin switch as the gold standard in a single-switch number identification activity [16]. In a recent study [19], with a 26 year old male with spastic quadriplegic cerebral palsy, an average correct rate of activation of 90% an average response time of 2.4 s was achieved on a stimulus-response test where the participant was repeatedly cued visually and aurally by the computer to activate the switch (i.e., open his mouth). Likewise, with a single-switch scanning word-matching activity, the individual achieved up to an 80% correct activation rate and response time of 11.7 s over a 6-month period. Figure 8 is a thermal image exemplifying the client's use of the thermal access technology. Because this access technology was well-tolerated by the client, a subsequent home version of the technology was created using a portable, handheld thermal camera (RAZ-IR SX/PRO). The client now uses this technology in his home for navigating electronic books and for computer access.

In a recent clinical evaluation of facial thermography as an access pathway among seven individuals with severe disabilities, the following contraindications were identified [18]. In the physiological domain, frequent body temperature fluctuations, seizures and pain were problematic. The former issue compromised detection consistency while the latter two issues made it difficult for the clients to maintain stable postures. In the motor realm, involuntary movements, muscle spasms or hyper- or hypotonia encumbered the creation of orofacial gestures, while atypical mouth posture and uncontrolled drooling obfuscated mouth detection. Thus, while facial thermography is appealing given its insensitivity to ambient lighting and environmental clutter, physiological and motor contraindications ought to be considered prior to home deployment.

In addition to detecting explicit orofacial gestures, infrared thermal imaging has demonstrated potential for uncovering passive communication cues, such as facial skin temperature changes. In a recent study with 12 able-bodied asymptomatic adults [22], temporal, spectral and time-frequency features derived from frontal infrared thermal images of the face were used to discriminate between self-reported affective states in response to a standardized emotionally-rated picture system. In particular, using genetic feature selection and Fisher linear discriminant classifier, mean adjusted accuracies between 70–80% were reported for the differentiation between baseline infrared images and those associated with either high arousal, low arousal, high valence or low valence stimuli. According to information theoretic measures, the periorbital and nasal regions tend to encode the most information about facial skin temperature changes [21]. These findings suggest that in a home monitoring system, the general affective state of the resident may be periodically and inconspicuously ascertained via thermal imaging. States of elevated stress, fear or confusion may be of particular interest from a care perspective.

4. Discussion

4.1. Merits and Limitations of Computer Vision Access Technologies

Among the most attractive features of a computer vision-based access solution is its non-contact nature. With conventional mechanical switches, positioning is often a formidable challenge, particularly for switches targeting head or facial movements. For those with involuntary movement, safety is also a concern. For example, involuntary hyperextension of the neck may lead to forceful contact with a switch that is mounted to the wheelchair headsupport. In addition to skin abrasions, there is a risk of injury to the eyes. If the switch is disturbed from its original position due to involuntary movement or if the user's posture changes, then repositioning is necessary, again requiring trial and error. With a computer vision-based access solution, positioning of devices on or near the user becomes a moot point. However, there is still the challenge of positioning a camera such that it consistently captures the motion of the access site. This positioning task can also be a non-trivial challenge when the user's posture or head position is frequently changing, and may necessitate the use of multiple, strategically located cameras, as in [15].

In addition to positioning and safety, another notable challenge posed by conventional mechanical switches is the need to apply adequate force for activation. For children with hypotonia and spasticity, this can be an insurmountable challenge. While there exists mechanical switches with variable force thresholds for activation, there is then the tradeoff between ease of activation and preponderance of accidental activations. For others, generating an adequate force is possible, but extremely effortful. As a consequence, the individual fatigues very quickly and is not able to use the switch throughout the day. A related issue is that of switch release. Some individuals can activate the switch but have difficulty releasing the switch. For example, for a conventional button switch mounted on a wheelchair tray, deactivation requires an anti-gravity movement, which can be much more challenging than the gravity-assisted motion of activation.

Computer vision-based access does offer a hygenic advantage. There is no need for routine cleaning. Risk of infection is mitigated as no devices are placed on the user or inside the user's mouth. Nonetheless, a chief disadvantage is the lack of haptic feedback.

With mechanical switches, the natural sensorimotor loop is closed with the tactility of switch depression and the accompanying audible "click". While the auditory feedback can be easily emulated through software, the mechanosensation of mechanical switch interaction is not readily reproducible. Arguably, it may be more difficult for novice switch users, especially those without consistent contingency awareness, to grasp the concept of switch activation by voluntary movement, when there is no haptic feedback. Indeed, recent literature has suggested that haptic feedback can enhance the learning of certain motor tasks, such as the visuo-manual tracking of unfamiliar letter trajectories [4].

Although we have proposed a luminance filter above to automatically compensate for lighting changes between environments, lighting remains a significant challenge for vision-based access systems. With the multiple camera tongue switch for example, the ability to discern "tongue protrusions" on the basis of heightened regional redness is very much a function of ambient brightness. While thermal cameras overcome this fundamental limitation of visible light cameras, they are nonetheless several orders of magnitude more costly. As a consequence, it is not economically practical at present to have a multiple thermal camera system as suggested in [18] to account for varying user poses.

Acknowledgements

The authors would like to acknowledge various funding agencies, including, KidsAction Research, Bloorview Children's Hospital Foundation, the Natural Sciences and Engineering Research Council of Canada, The Lions Club of Charles Sturt in Adelaide, South Australia, Australia and Novita Children's Services, Adelaide, South Australia, Australia.

References

[1] H. Ahonen-Eerikainen, A. Lamont and R. Knox, Rehabilitation for children with cerebral palsy: Seeing through the looking glass – Enhancing participation and restoring self-image through the virtual music instrument, *International Journal of Psychosocial Rehabilitation* **12**(2) (2008), 41–66.

[2] S. Benveniste, P. Jouvelot and R. Pequignot, The MINWii project: Renarcissization of patients suffering from Alzheimer's disease through video game-based music therapy, in: *9th International Conference on Entertainment Computing*, Vol. 6243, Seoul, South Korea, 2010, pp. 79–90.

[3] S. Blain, P. McKeever and T. Chau, Bedside computer access for an individual with severe and multiple disabilities: A case study, *Disability and Rehabilitation: Assistive Technology* **5**(5) (2010), 359–369.

[4] J. Bluteau, S. Coquillart, Y. Payan and E. Gentaz, Haptic guidance improves the visuo-manual tracking of trajectories, *PLoS One* **3**(3) (2008), e1775.

[5] A. Brownlee and M. Palovcak, The role of augmentative communication devices in the medical management of ALS, *Augmentative and Alternative Communication* **22**(6) (2007), 445–450.

[6] S.N. Calculator and T. Black, Parent's priorities for AAC and related instruction for their children with angelman syndrome, *Augmentative and Alternative Communication* **26**(1) (2010), 30–40.

[7] T. Chau, H. Schwellnus, C. Tam, A. Lamont and C. Eaton, Augmented environments for paediatric rehabilitation, *Technology & Disability* **18**(4) (2006), 167–171.

[8] W.L. Chen, A.A. Liou, S.C. Chen, C.M. Chung and Y.L. Chen, A novel home appliance control system for people with disabilities, *Disability and Rehabilitation: Assistive Technology* **2**(4) (2007), 201–206.

[9] J. Cohen-Mansfield, M.S. Marx, M. Dakheel-Ali, N.G. Regier and K. Thein, Can persons with dementia be engaged with stimuli, *American Journal of Geriatric Psychiatry* **18**(4) (2010), 351–362.

[10] J. Cohen-Mansfield, K. Thein, M. Dakheel-Ali and M.S. Marx, The underlying meaning of stimuli: Impact on engagement of persons with dementia, *Psychiatry Research* **177**(1–2) (2010), 216–222.

[11] A. Craig, Y. Tran, P. McIsaac and P. Boord, The efficacy and benefits of environmental control systems for the severely disabled, *Medical Science Monitor* **11**(1) (2005), RA32–39.
[12] J.M. De La Rosa Estanol, Robust recognition of communicative intent in unconstrained environments, Master's Thesis, University of Toronto, 2005.
[13] B. Hemsley, S. Balandin and L Togher, I've got something to say: Interaction in a focus group of adults with cerebral palsy and complex communication needs, *Augmentative and Alternative Communication* **24**(2) (2008), 110–122.
[14] D.A. Hobbs and B.L. Worthington-Eyre, The efficacy of combining augmented reality and music therapy with traditional teaching: Preliminary results, in: *Proc. of the 2nd International Convention on Rehabilitation Engineering and Assistive Technology (i-CREATe)*, Bangkok, Thailand, 2008, p. 4.
[15] B. Leung and T. Chau, A multiple camera tongue switch for a child with severe spastic quadriplegic cerebral palsy, *Disability & Rehabilitation: Assistive Technology* **5**(1) (2010), 58–68.
[16] N. Memarian, A. Venetsanopoulos and T. Chau, Validating an infrared thermal switch as a novel access technology, *Biomedical Engineering OnLine* **9**(38) (2010), 11.
[17] N. Memarian, T. Venetsanopoulos and T. Chau, Infrared thermography as an access pathway for individuals with severe motor impairments, *Journal of Neuorengineering and Rehabilitation* **6**(11) (2009), 8.
[18] N. Memarian, T. Venetsanopoulos and T. Chau, Body functions and structures pertinent to infrared thermography-based access for clients with severe motor disabilities, *Assistive Technology* **x**(x) (2011), in Press.
[19] N. Memarian, T. Venetsanopoulos and T. Chau, Client-centred development of an infrared thermal access switch for a young adult with severe spastic quadriplegic cerebral palsy, *Disability and Rehabilitation: Assistive Technology* **6**(2) (2011), 179–187.
[20] A. Mihailidis and G. Fernie, Context-aware assistive devices for older adults with dementia, *Gerontechnology* **2**(2) (2002), 173–189.
[21] B.R. Nhan and T. Chau, Infrared thermal imaging as a physiological access pathway: A study of baseline characteristics of facial skin temperatures, *Physiological Measurement* **30**(4) (2009), N25–N35.
[22] B.R. Nhan and T. Chau, Classifying affective states using thermal infrared imaging of the human face, *IEEE Transactions on Biomedical Engineering* **57**(4) (2010), 979–987.
[23] K. Tai, S. Blain and T. Chau, A review of emerging access technologies for individuals with severe motor impairments, *Assistive Technology* **20**(4) (2008), 204–219.
[24] C. Tam, H. Schwellnus, C. Eaton, Y. Hamdani, A. Lamont and T. Chau, Movement-to-music computer technology: A development play experience for children with severe physical disabilities, *Occupational Therapy International* **14**(2) (2007), 99–112.
[25] H.Y. Wang, Y.H. Ju, S.M. Chen, S.K. Lo and Y.J. Jong, Joint range of motion limitations in children and young adults with spinal muscular atrophy, *Archives of Physcial Medicine and Rehabilitation* **85**(10) (2004), 1689–1693.

Ambient Assisted Living Initiatives

Handbook of Ambient Assisted Living
J.C. Augusto et al. (Eds.)
IOS Press, 2012

doi:10.3233/978-1-60750-837-3-601

Preparation and Start-Up Phase of the European AAL Joint Programme

Michael HUCH*
Interim Director of the AAL Joint Programme 09/2007 – 11/2009
Coordinator of the AAL169 support action project 09/2004 – 12/2006

Abstract. Research and development in the context of home-based ICT applications – in combination with services – that aim to increase the self-determined and independent life of older persons is today known under the name of Ambient Assisted Living. This text gives a brief historical background how the AAL Joint Programme (AAL JP) was established and thus helped to spread the term over Europe and to the rest of the world.

Keywords. Ambient Assisted Living research and development, Joint Programme, Article 169 (185), coordination of national R&D

1. Introduction

This text describes the administrative process of setting-up the Ambient Assisted Living Joint Programme during the period 2003 to 2007 and sketches some managerial problems during the initial implementation phase.

The perspective focuses on a governance angle and does not cover the content orientation of the AAL Joint Programme. The identification and selection processes for the call for proposals under the AAL JP was driven by highly devoted representatives of the AAL partner states – and resulted in meanwhile four calls for proposals under the AAL Joint Programme.

Needless to say that the complex and highly political process of establishing the AAL Joint Programme on the European level heavily contributed to the establishment national funding schemes in parallel, e.g. the “benefit” programme in Austria or several national AAL calls in Germany.

The following five contributions in this section describe AAL research initiatives that span from a more concept-oriented project to development projects to large scale deployment pilots. Various schemes on European or the respective national levels provided the funding. The text arrangement follows the route from research to market in the following order:

The “universAAL” project is funded under the EU’s 7th Framework programme (FP7). It aims to develop a quasi-platform aiming to establish a common understanding and starting point for technical AAL solutions.

The IS-ACTIVE project is funded under the 1st call of the AAL Joint Programme. This project develops a technical system enabling the management of chronic conditions.

*Corresponding Author: Michael Huch. E-mail: michaelhuch@web.de.

LiKeIT is a research project funded under the Austrian benefit programme and describes a technical system capable of monitoring the activities (Lifestyle) of older persons.

SmartSenior is currently the "biggest" AAL project funded in Germany that works on a broad scope of technical and non-technical issues. It brings together renowned research organisations with leading industry and telecoms.

The Spanish contribution from Tecnalia presents a whole range of research projects implemented at this outstaying research organisation. Funding stems from FP7, the AAL JP as well as national Spanish resources.

It is a very pleasant obligation for me to express my gratitude to all authors and researchers having contributed to this section on AAL projects of the AAL Handbook.

2. Inventing the Term Ambient Assisted Living – AAL

Trends to pervasive or ubiquitous computing, ambient intelligence enabled by smart microsystems, smart home applications, or telematics addressed to improving the quality of life (as under the EU's 4th Framework Programme) – the ingredients that led to the establishment to new research, development and innovation funding programme Ambient Assisted Living were indeed manifold.

It was back in December 2002, when Strese firstly used the term "Ambient Assisted Living" in a non-paper [16]. For some time already, VDI/VDE Innovation + Technik GmbH managed the Microsystems Technologies R&D funding programme on behalf of the German Ministry of Education and Research, and Strese drafted his concept paper in order to sketch the field of a very promising new application area for microsystems technologies: the phenomenon of demographic ageing. In this very short paper of four pages only, the essential philosophy of Ambient Assisted Living, i.e. the "extension of the independent life of older persons in their own preferred environment assisted by technical means" was noted for the first time. Interesting enough, the concept also envisaged the cooperation between the EU and national German level, arguing correctly the wide international occurrence of demographic ageing.

Already in 2000, the EU Research Commissioner, Philippe Busquin, demanded the creation of the European Research Area (ERA). In essence, ERA is about to overcome the fragmentation of the European R&D landscape and one of the foreseen instruments for its achievement is a more intense R&D cooperation – and thus coordination – of the Member States of the European Union. The legal basis for this cooperation was article 169 of the EU treaty (after an amendment of the treaty now known as article 185) which "enables the EU to participate in research programmes undertaken jointly by several Member States, including participation in the structures created for the execution of national programmes" [5].

3. Preparatory Action for the AAL Joint Programme

During 2003, a project proposal was prepared under coordination of VDI/VDE-IT, which aimed at creating a European level R&D cooperation of Member States in the "ICT and Ageing" area. Early October 2003, the proposal was submitted to the 2nd call for proposals under the ICT cooperation programme of the 6th European Framework Programme for research and technological development (FP6). This proposal was supported by nine project partners: Three research ministries, three national programme managing agencies and three research organisations. The proposal received very high evaluation scores and after its successful negotiation the project started its operation on 01.09.2004, coordinated by the author of this text. The following quote for the FP6 database introduces the objective of the project: "The objective of the specific support action "Ambient assisted living" is to prepare an Article 169 initiative in the field of "Small and smart technologies for ambient assisted living" …

Ambient Assisted Living as a concept aims at prolonging the time, people can live in a decent way in their own flat by increasing their autonomy and self-confidence, the discharge of monotonously everyday activities, to monitor and care for the elderly or ill person, to enhance the security and to save resources. The Article 169-initiative in the field of "Small and smart technologies for ambient assisted living" undertaken jointly by several Member states will tackle the major challenges Europe has to face. It will stimulate the development of products and services for societies being characterised by demographic changes. It will improve policy co-ordination in a field where the innovation process has to be accompanied and stimulated by public authorities because of its social dimension" [3].

The so called "AAL169" support action project produced two main documents: In 2005 (revised in March 2006), the report "Europe Is Facing a Demographic Challenge – Ambient Assisted Living Offers Solutions" [15] consistently developed the political justification for a new major policy intervention in the area of demographic ageing. In September 2006, the orientation for a future R&D funding programme on Ambient Assisted Living was finalised [12]. This paper provided the ordo-liberal justification for investing public money into the area of ICT for elderly, presented the thematic scope and developed advanced ideas for the procedural division of labour within the new funding programme. The last part was of special importance as the AAL Joint Programme – as it was called at the point of its start – is heavily based on administrative work performed by the national representatives of the participating states, while the central level administration was meant to be as "light" as possible, leaving mainly the central call announcement and evaluation as the tasks to be performed there.

The programme theme remained stable in scope from the beginning of the preparatory action. However, the European cooperation and most importantly the Finnish experience with similar programmes, led to an increased consideration of the importance of services and business models rather than a deep technological substance. It is until today that the AAL Joint Programme is less a technology development programme, but rather a programme that develops new applications incl. the business models, and uses technologies as important input.

Until today, the following graphic – again introduced by Strese – tend to define the areas of activity of the AAL JP. The indicated areas represented in the graphic stand for needs and demands of the older population. It was soon decided that any call for proposals under the AAL JP would address one or a clever combination of any of the "bubbles" of the graphic.

The selection of call topics combined for the

- 1st call the topics "Health & Wellness" and "Home Care"
- 2nd call the topic "Social Interaction"
- 4th call the topic "Mobility".

It was only the 3rd call that deviated from this approach by addressing the psychological foundation of becoming a well being person. It is probably due to the vagueness

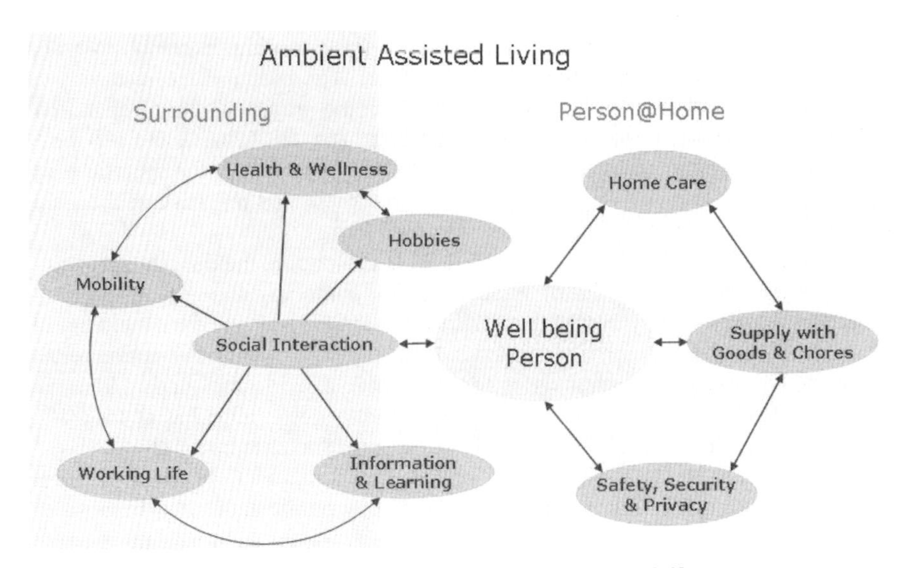

Figure 1. Needs and demands of an elderly person [13].

of imagining appropriate research activities under this call, entitled "ICT-based Solutions for Advancement of Older Persons' Independence and Participation in the "Self-serve Society" that a considerable delay for the approval by the AAL General Assembly occurred.

4. Political Decision Making Processes Towards Establishing the AAL JP

4.1. The Member States Level

While the EU funded project "AAL169" ended at the end of 2006, the process of establishing the AAL JP – with more and more Members States joining the group – continued. Already in the course of 2005 it became clear during intense reflections between the representatives of four article 169 candidate initiatives with EU Commission staff, that an "Article 185 TFEU (ex-Article 169 TEC) initiative will require the establishment or existence of a Dedicated Implementation Structure (DIS). In practice, the Commission will conclude a Delegation Agreement with the corresponding DIS" [4].

Hence, in order to benefit from the expected substantial European co-funding to the AAL Joint Programme, the Member States were forced to establish such a DIS, i.e. a structure that could close legally binding contractual obligations between the participating Member States and the European Commission.

The representatives of the AAL initiative finally decided in favour of founding an international association in Belgium. This model promised an easy set-up process but also proofed to best allow the participation of non-EU states as Israel, Norway and Switzerland, all three having expressed their willingness to join the initiative. Belgium as the country of residence was chosen for mainly two reasons: The closeness to the European Commission and the fact that it was neither one of the three most supportive countries in the process, Austria, Finland and Germany.

With the support of a Belgian lawyer, statutes/draft-by-laws were drafted that fulfilled the legal minimum criteria for an international association. In parallel, Rules of Internal Order provided more details on rules, roles and responsibilities of the various AAL bodies and actors, i.e. the AAL General Assembly as the ultimate decision making body, the Executive Board and the Programme Management, consisting of the Central Management Unit and National Contact Persons, were finalised.

Throughout the year 2007, the Member States were concerned in seeking approval from their organisational hierarchies and drafting the mandate for the respective national delegates who finally signed the official documents during the foundation act of the AAL Association on 19 September 2007.

One of the duties at this day was the election of the first AAL Executive Board. Intentionally organised as a bottom-up process, each country participating in the AAL JP could nominate a member for the Executive Board. However, none of the elected members had to proof his/her professional capability for the job, so rather former engagement in the constitutional process combined with European geographical balance were more important than anything else. It spoke for both, the positive cooperation climate among the AAL states but at the same time already a lack of professional experience that a last minute candidature nomination was accepted and finally six instead of the earlier announced five members were elected into the Executive Board.

4.2. The European Union Level

Compared to the process of founding the association with finally 14 founding members, the constitutional process to formally adopt an article 169 initiative on the European level was even more demanding: Each Article 169 initiative had to be set up via the co-decision procedure of the European Parliament and of the Council following a proposal from the Commission itself.

But before this proposal was actually published, the European Commission took two preparatory and at the same time reassuring steps on the maturity of the initiative: In order to get a substantiated feedback on the dimension of the AAL research field and the research community, a specific AAL call was launched under the 6th call for proposals of the IST theme of FP6 with a deadline in April 2006 and a budget provision of 40 Mio. € [1]. The Commission never discussed the usage of the term "Ambient Assisted Living" for this call with the representatives of the AAL Joint Programme initiative nor sought their approval for doing so. While this call certainly made a big step to establish the understanding of AAL as a research topic, at the same time it also strongly associated AAL research to the EC level. Even today, researchers speak of the EU's AAL Joint Programme, although this is wrong and misleading: The AAL JP is a programme of 23 European Union member states and associated states. Only organisations from these states are eligible for funding. The "eligibility" message was not successfully transported to the proposers of the 1st call under the AAL JP and consequently led to a high number of ineligible (for funding – they could have participated without funding) organisations.

The response rate to the EU's call under FP6 was overwhelming: More than 200 proposals were submitted to this call, resulting in a tremendously high oversubscription: Only a fraction of submitted projects could be selected for funding under this call. Last doubts at the EU level on the substance of the AAL research potential resolved.

The second step of reassurance concerned the collection of the Member States' political and financial commitments. In April 2007, the then EU Commissioner for the

Information Society, Viviane Reding, sent letters to all European Member States, asking them to return their political commitment (if at all and which public body would participate) including the provision of the financial annual contribution (meant as a long-term commitment) regarding their participation in the AAL Joint Programme. With answers received from about 15 states, the EC started the political decision process with the following milestones achieved on its way:

14.06.2007: The Commission adopted the European Action Plan for "Ageing Well in the Information Society" that included the proposal to support the AAL Joint Programme [6].

23.11.2007: The Competitiveness Council of the European Union agreed on a general approach towards the AAL Joint Programme [8].

24.01.2008: The Ambient Assisted Living Joint Programme initiative was unanimously approved by the European Parliament's Industry Committee (ITRE) [9].

13.03.2008: The European Parliament approved the Commission's proposal with great majority [10].

23.06.2008: The Council adopted the participation of the European Commission in the Ambient Assisted Living Joint Programme [7].

It is probably not false to consider this political process to be overly complex and exaggerated in relation to its financial impact: The AAL JP is a RTD programme with an annual expenditure of about 50 to 60 Mio. €. This sum is about the magnitude of a topical line under the ICT cooperation topic of the Framework Programme. The individual sum for the 23 participating countries started from only 100.000 € per annum (!) and reached the maximum of 5 Mio. € for Germany. The EC's annual financial contribution is limited to the maximum of 25 Mio. €. Considering the heavy political machinery behind the approval this administrative effort is way out of justification. If any additional Article 185 initiatives are ever about to see the light, European politicians would be well advised to dramatically cut red tape at this occasion. The positive effect of this machinery, though, was the highly visible and repeated usage of the term "Ambient Assisted Living" – however again with the false notation of the EU's leadership in the programme.

It was also odd to learn that none of the representatives of the AAL initiative were ever involved in the whole process, except for an invitation to present the concept at a very brief hearing session in the European Parliament. Some member delegates also had established contacts to their national delegates in the Council, although this process was not formally organised. On the other side, the hierarchy levels represented within the AAL Joint Programme did not surpass the rank of a "head of unit" within one of the participating ministries or the programme agencies. This hierarchy level is not appropriate for political networking in higher European spheres.

Finally, only in December 2008 the contracts between the AAL Association and the European Commission were signed regarding the EC's participation for the period of the AAL Joint Programme from 2008 to 2013. In parallel, a separate contract specified the concrete financial contribution for the 1st call for proposals and the list of obligations (i.e. deliverables) coming along with this. Due to the hectic in the signing process, it was overlooked that the contracts failed to bear the obligatory two signatories from the side of the AAL Association, which is a very well reflected provision stated in the AAL statutes!

5. Managing the Start-Up Phase

The article 169 initiative "Eurostars" [11] that run in parallel to the AAL JP process was taken care of by the already established and well-equipped EUREKA secretariat. In comparison to this, the establishment of the AAL Joint Programme started from scratch. Besides "knowledge" of or "experience" with similar ventures, e.g. the EUREKA programme and several ERA-Net projects [2], there was no whatsoever basis or infrastructure available to start from. The AAL Association was "virtual" in any dimension: There was no personnel, no office room (the formal registration address was provided by the Flemish AAL partner), no IT environment to process or conduct the AAL calls, but solely a small contract with an agency that financed 1.5 persons who provided the elementary services.

Mainly due to highly diverting preferences among its members regarding the future of the AAL Association and the Joint Programme, the Executive Board members failed to create appropriate management capacities: One member preferred the light cooperation as experienced in ERA-NET projects. This would allow an easy dissolution of the association's infrastructure after the end of the funding period. Other members thought of the AAL JP as a long-lasting R&D&I programme whose administration would also take over more and more assignments in a broader context of the AAL area, e.g. by conducting accompanying activities.

This conflict expressed itself also in a delay of important decisions and it was a logic consequence that tensions between the Executive Board and the Central Management Unit (CMU) occured. At that time, the mismatch in capacity between members of the Executive Board and those of the CMU was still with 6 persons to 2.5 persons.

It was considerably underestimated, if not totally neglected by the Executive Board that the CMU, next to its core task of managing the JP was also heavily absorbed in administering the legal and organisational business of the AAL Association itself. Contracts with bookkeepers, auditors, office room, phone companies etc. had to be arranged. Additional contracts from AAL states with the AAL Association drafted and collected. On top, General Assembly meetings (two per year), Advisory Board meetings and, very extensive, meetings of the Executive Board (10 meetings in the first nine months of 2009) had to be prepared and documented.

In March/April 2009, the CMU put pressure on the Executive Board to alleviate the CMU situation. Indeed, the Executive Board took decisions that seemed to reveal a fruitful outcome in many respects: At first, the contract with the external agency was expanded and allowed a strong increase in the CMU's staff capacity. At second, it was decided to endorse the CMU with a decision mandate in order to run core processes more independently. At third, the decision for starting to hire own personnel for the AAL Association was taken. This decision was represented by launching the vacancy note for the AAL CMU Director position in June 2009. This route, however, turned out to be instable, and short-term oriented.

"The biggest concern in relation to the performance of the programme is the operation of the CMU. It is widely seen as being insufficiently responsive, and often ineffective and slow …" [14]. These consequences of the decisions are quoted from the mid-term evaluation report of the AAL Joint Programme, published in December 2010 by an independent panel group.

While the group addressed a number of highly relevant issues, e.g. the request for harmonised participation conditions across the participating states, it had no mandate to investigate the management structures in more detail. The quote above – as justified as it is – gives a very limited picture only as the largest portion of the administrative performance problems must be addressed to the Executive Board. In absence of clear terms and decisive powers – both bodies execute and manage and are thus in constant conflict – a professional management cannot be set up. But for the future of the AAL Joint Programme, the obvious management deficits of the AAL Association must be overcome.

6. Conclusions

The creation of the AAL Joint Programme was a bottom-up driven and very exciting venture that – in the preparation phase – revealed a very cooperative climate among the supporting AAL partner states. The process was based on the belief into drafting the appropriate research topic (addressing demographic ageing) at the right time and the additional motivation by external supporters, e.g. most importantly the EU.

The political co-decision procedure was way out of an appropriate level for an initiative of the limited financial dimensions as the AAL JP: It took too long and caused too high administrative costs – which is especially true for smaller countries.

Instead of starting all infrastructure building from scratch, a contract for the provision of the central services should be preferred. The dissolution of the AAL Association infrastructure and staff will cause much bigger problems and higher expenses than any ending contract.

Governance skills are an upcoming issue for the management structures of the more and more complex European instruments. Not only in case of article 185 initiatives, representatives of the participating states should undergo – before elected in a management body – a selection process that should be based on communicated and transparent criteria. It could be observed that members of the AAL Executive Board were not capable in fulfilling their mandate, either for a lack of skills, interest or time.

As with any other public body: Paid contracts for advisory services for delegates who formerly worked on a honorary basis raise concerns. Such contracts must be managed under clear terms of references and progress openly reported to the existing supervisory body.

References

[1] Forth Update of the IST Work Programme, pp. 7–14, available from http://cordis.europa.eu/fp6/dc/index.cfm?fuseaction=UserSite.FP6DetailsCallPage&call_id=271.

[2] http://cordis.europa.eu/coordination/era-net.htm (cited 31.03.2011).

[3] http://cordis.europa.eu/fetch?CALLER=NEW_PROJ_TM&ACTION=D&DOC=2&CAT=PROJ&QUERY=012ed2883fd3:2a3c:082ed7e6&RCN=71922 (cited 31.03.2011).

[4] http://cordis.europa.eu/fp7/art185/faq_en.html#question12 (cited 31.03.2011).

[5] http://cordis.europa.eu/fp7/art185/home_en.html (cited 31.03.2011).

[6] http://eur-lex.europa.eu/LexUriServ/LexUriServ.do?uri=CELEX:52007PC0329:EN:NOT (cited 31.03.2011).

[7] http://europa.eu/rapid/pressReleasesAction.do?reference=IP/08/994&format=HTML&aged=0&language=EN&guiLanguage=enBest (cited 31.03.2011).

[8] http://www.consilium.europa.eu/ueDocs/cms_Data/docs/pressData/en/intm/97225.pdf (cited 31.03.2011).

[9] http://www.europarl.europa.eu/sides/getDoc.do?language=en&type=IM-PRESS&reference=20080121IPR19252 (cited 31.03.2011).

[10] http://www.europarl.europa.eu/sides/getDoc.do?pubRef=-//EP//TEXT+TA+P6-TA-2008-0098+0+DOC+XML+V0//EN&language=EN (cited 31.03.2011).
[11] http://www.eurostars-eureka.eu/ (cited 31.03.2011).
[12] M. Huch et al., Regulatory frame for the article 169 initiative AAL, final version, 2006, published on http://www.aal169.org/Published/D2_3RegulatoryFrameAAL169.pdf (cited 31.03.2011).
[13] *Ibid.* p. 15.
[14] Independent Panel Group, Interim Evaluation of the Ambient Assisted Living Joint Programme, December 2010, p. 40, published on http://ec.europa.eu/information_society/activities/einclusion/research/aal/interim_review/index_en.htm.
[15] H. Steg et al., Europe Is Facing a Demographic Challenge – Ambient Assisted Living Offers Solutions, 2006, published on http://www.aal169.org/Published/Final%20Version.pdf (cited 31.03.2011).
[16] H. Strese, Ambient Assisted Living, non paper, unpublished, 19.12.2002.

Handbook of Ambient Assisted Living
J.C. Augusto et al. (Eds.)
IOS Press, 2012

doi:10.3233/978-1-60750-837-3-610

The universAAL Reference Model for AAL

Mohammad-Reza TAZARI [a,*], Francesco FURFARI [b], Álvaro FIDES VALERO [c], Sten HANKE [d], Oliver HÖFTBERGER [e], Dionisis KEHAGIAS [f], Miran MOSMONDOR [g], Reiner WICHERT [a] and Peter WOLF [h]

[a] *Fraunhofer IGD, Darmstadt, Germany*
[b] *CNR-ISTI, Pisa, Italy*
[c] *ITACA-TSB, Valencia, Spain*
[d] *Austrian Institute of Technology, Wr. Neustadt, Austria*
[e] *Technische Universität Wien, Vienna, Austria*
[f] *CERTH-ITI, Thessaloniki, Greece*
[g] *Ericsson Nikola Tesla d.d., Zagreb, Croatia*
[h] *Forschungszentrum Informatik, Karlsruhe, Germany*

Abstract. Ambient Assisted Living (AAL) is lacking a reference model that can serve as a basis for understanding the main issues to be addressed without any solution bias. Such a reference model will facilitate consensus-building processes and consolidation efforts towards converging conclusions on AAL infrastructures. The universAAL project, that aims at producing an open platform along with a standardized approach for making it technically feasible and economically viable to develop AAL solutions, has defined a process consisting of four iterations for filling this gap. Here, the results of the first iteration on *a reference model for AAL* are presented.

Keywords. Reference model, AAL service, AAL space, reference architecture, AAL platform, networked artefacts

About universAAL

Production of software infrastructures supporting AAL has been the core topic of a number of EU projects – some already completed, some still running. The legacy of these projects should not be allowed to die after the end of the projects; rather, it is reasonable to promote them and support their evolution and maturation. This idea seems to have played a substantial role in the definition of a specific target in the context of the ICT call no. four of the Seventh Framework Programme of the European Commission in 2009. In its objective 7.1 (ICT & Ageing) target b (Open Systems Reference Architectures, Standards and ICT Platforms for Ageing Well), this call emphasizes that only one project is planned to be funded that is expected to consolidate the state-of-the-art towards an open cross-application *platform* approach. The one project emanated from this context

*Corresponding Author: Mohammad-Reza Tazari, Fraunhofer IGD, Fraunhoferstr. 5, 64283 Darmstadt, Germany. E-mail: saied.tazari@igd.fraunhofer.de.

is called now universAAL, standing for UNIVERsal open platform and reference Specification for Ambient Assisted Living[1]. Since its kick-off in February 2010, community expectations from universAAL are growing very fast, especially when considering that the more recent research funding schemes related to AAL are encouraging converging conclusions and reuse at the level of a core platform.

universAAL employs different processes and tools in order to live up to these expectations:

- A consolidation process of existing platforms in order to converge to a common reference architecture based on a reference model and a set of reference use cases and requirements[2].
- The provision of a reference implementation of a platform that facilitates the realization of AAL systems based on the envisioned reference architecture using an open source license model.
- Enhancing the scope of the platform to a whole infrastructure with appropriate tools for the different stages of developing, advertising, finding, installing, configuring, and adapting AAL solutions, as well as guidelines and tutorials for these stages along with appropriate training materials.

However, all of the above would not help if there is no consensus building process involving a large community composed by representatives of AAL stakeholders. For this reason, universAAL also allocates resources for "community building", which can be understood as an advanced dissemination plan aiming at involving people and organizations external to universAAL that not only are interested to understand the project results but also use, influence, and even maintain them beyond the duration of a four year project, ensuring the sustainability of the project outcomes.

Simultaneously to these ideas, other initiatives were also starting to undertake actions towards organized consensus building processes. For example, the consortium of the PERSONA project[3], that believed to have produced a reusable platform for AAL, was examining the option of incorporating an open association for AAL and donating the software infrastructure developed within the project to it under permissive open source license models. Another example was the initiative by the MonAmI project[4] in [6] suggesting an "Alliance for an AAL Open Service Platform". Also some partners from the SOPRANO project[5] had started to establish openAAL [15]. Most of these parallel initiatives joined together working towards incorporating AALOA – the Ambient Assisted Living Open Association already present in the Web under http://www.aaloa.org – as a federation of projects. Currently, AALOA is being supported by over 70 individuals as well as the projects MonAmI, OASIS, OsAmI-commons, PERSONA, SOPRANO, universAAL, and WASP. The mission statement of AALOA has been defined using a joint dissemination utility, namely the AALOA Manifesto (available under http://aaloa.org/manifesto/),

[1] See http://www.universaal.org.

[2] Insights into the consolidation practice in universAAL have been published in [12].

[3] An EU-IST integrated project of the Sixth Framework Programme from January 2007 to October 2010; see http://www.aal-persona.org.

[4] An EU-IST integrated project of the Sixth Framework Programme from September 2006 to August 2011; see http://www.monami.info.

[5] An EU-IST integrated project of the Sixth Framework Programme from January 2007 to September 2010; see http://www.soprano-ip.org.

that also shares the vision and serves as a call for action. universAAL has committed to promote AALOA using its "community building" resources.

1. What Is a Reference Model and what Is It Good for?

Modeling is about representing things conceptually, possibly in terms of other things that are somehow related to it, e.g., are part of it. In terms of word analysis, a model can be called a reference model if it is factually used as a reference whenever there is need to understand the subject matter of that model. The following two definitions reflect pretty much the same understanding of the term Reference Model:

> **The AGIMO definition:** An abstract framework for understanding significant relationships among the entities of a specific environment, and for the development of consistent standards or specifications supporting that environment. A reference model is based on a small number of unifying concepts and may be used as a basis for education and explaining standards to a nonspecialist. A reference model is not directly tied to any standards, technologies or other concrete implementation details but it does seek to provide a common semantic that can be used unambiguously across and between different implementations [2].

> **The OASIS definition:** A reference model is an abstract framework for understanding significant relationships among the entities of some environment. It enables the development of specific reference or concrete architectures using consistent standards or specifications supporting that environment. A reference model consists of a minimal set of unifying concepts, axioms and relationships within a particular problem domain, and is independent of specific standards, technologies, implementations, or other concrete details. ... The purpose of a reference model is to provide a common conceptual framework that can be used consistently across and between different implementations and is of particular use in modeling specific solutions [9].

The question about "what a Reference Model is" is answered by the above definitions with the phrases "an abstract framework" consisting of "a small number of unifying concepts" or "a minimal set of unifying concepts, axioms and relationships within a particular problem domain" not in the direction of providing any solution – hence avoiding things that are a matter of taste, such as specific standards, technologies, and implementations – but providing "a common conceptual framework" or "semantic" for "understanding significant relationships among the entities of a specific environment". The following uses of a reference model can be highlighted[6]:

- for education and explaining standards to a nonspecialist
- for the development of consistent standards or specifications supporting the modeled environment[7]
- for modeling specific solutions

[6]The first three taken from the above definitions and the remaining ones borrowed in March 2010 from http://en.wikipedia.org/wiki/Reference_model.

[7]The above mentioned Wikipedia entry talks about "standards for both the objects that inhabit the model and their relationships to one another".

- for breaking down a large problem space into smaller problems that can be understood, tackled, and refined so that developers who are new to a particular set of problems can quickly learn what the different problems are, and can focus on the problems that they are being asked to solve, while trusting that other areas are well understood and rigorously constructed
- for improving communication between people
- for creating clear roles and responsibilities
- for allowing the comparison of different things: e.g., how well each of the candidate solutions can be configured to meet the needs of a particular business process

2. Defining the AAL Reference Model in universAAL

In accordance to its mission, universAAL strives for a widely accepted and used reference model for AAL because we believe that the existence of such a model will, according to the above list of uses of reference models, facilitate the process of reaching consensus and finding converging conclusions in such a fragmented R&D area as AAL. To assure a quality level that increases the chances of this reference model to be accepted and used widely, we have defined a process consisting of four iterations:

- In the first iteration, the main focus is on consolidation of existing results from the input projects[8].
- The second iteration mainly concentrates on filling the gaps by adding the universAAL-specific view towards a more stable version of the reference model.
- The third iteration should incorporate any internal and external feedback and close the scope of the reference model.
- And finally, the fourth iteration is supposed to finalize the reference model and deliver it.

An important part of all reference models is a graphical representation. We chose to use concept maps that are frequently used in more recent examples, such as the reference model for service-oriented architectures in [9] and the technical overview of the OWL-S ontology for describing services [13]. Concept maps are simple graphs with nodes representing concepts and arrows between nodes representing their relationships; thus, they directly map to the definition of reference models. The graphical representation of concepts and their interrelationships within concept maps are assumed to help different types of stakeholders to quickly learn about the understanding of the AAL domain.

As of the consolidation method used in the first iteration, we had to accept that none of the input projects was providing any reference model per se. Hence, the representatives of the input projects were asked to provide concept maps that would reflect in a solution- and technology-neutral way the understanding of the AAL domain within their respective projects. After cleaning these concept maps from all hints of any solution or technology, we eventually merged the input maps into one consistent set of concept maps in several iterations of discussion.

In order to bring more structure into the scene, an ordering of the concepts was worked out by first putting the smallest set of concepts that could reflect a basic under-

[8]With "input projects" we refer to the projects Amigo, GENESYS, MPOWER, OASIS, PERSONA, and SOPRANO whose key partners are present in the universAAL consortium.

standing of AAL systems in one concept map serving as the root map, and then organizing the rest of the concepts in a set of subordinate concept maps that provide more details in different directions at a second level[9]. Last but not least, a glossary of some of the main concepts appearing in the concept maps was provided based on the relationships contained in the concept maps while considering also any related definitions already provided by the input projects.

Some remarks should help to better interpret the concept maps before starting to present them in the following section:

- Top-level concepts are drawn as ovals and the second-level concepts as rectangles.
- Reuse of top-level concepts in the related second level maps indicates the connection between the latter maps and the root map.
- Different colours are used to further group the concepts and add some traceability across the concept maps. In particular, each of the following colours should represent an important view on AAL systems: *Grey* represents the business view, *yellow* stands for technology, *green* indicates integration and convergence, and finally *purple* refers to the need for tools and facilities.
- Bold lines and fonts are used to highlight concepts of special importance.
- Exemplary concepts are connected by dashed lines and are not meant to be comprehensive. They are not part of this reference model, but should help to better understand a related main concept.

3. The Consolidated Reference Model from the First Iteration

The first version of the reference model for AAL can be seen as the result of analyzing AAL systems, because we could agree pretty fast on its definition: an AAL System is a socio-technical system for the provision of AAL Services towards wellbeing, mostly by means of networked artefacts embedded in AAL Spaces. In this context, the emphasis of universAAL is on the provision of a reference architecture for AAL Spaces and an implementation of this reference architecture as an AAL platform that facilitates the development and integration of the embedded artefacts.

Therefore, the *Root Concept Map* – see Fig. 1 – concentrates on reflecting this understanding of AAL systems at the highest level of abstraction in a single picture using the fewest possible set of concepts: AAL systems are all about the provision of *AAL Services*. The importance of ambient technologies in the provision of such services is highlighted by putting the concept of *AAL Spaces* and the underlying technologies (*Networked Artefacts*) right in this top level. The *AAL Reference Architecture* and the compliant *AAL Platforms* incorporate the engineering challenges beyond single technologies towards reconstruct-able infrastructures. The *AAL Reference Architecture* identifies the basic building blocks necessary for constructing an *AAL Space*, such as Home, Supermarkets, Cars or Hospitals. Such an AAL Space provides *AAL Services* with the help of embedded Networked Artefacts that implement (or contribute to the implementation of) those AAL Services. The cooperation between Networked Artefacts distributed in an AAL Space is facilitated by an *AAL Platform* that implements the previously mentioned

[9] This way, it is always possible to add further details in a third (and fourth, and ...) level whenever needed as long as the concepts used in the maps do not pose any technology bias.

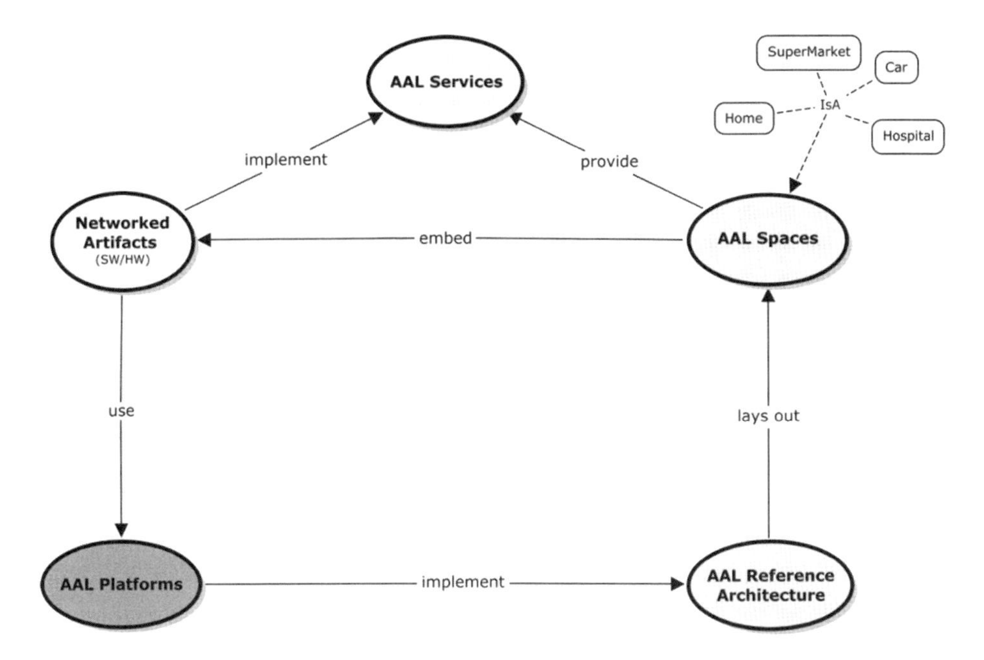

Figure 1. The root concept map.

reference architecture in order to provide for resource sharing and let users experience an integrated world easy to interact with based on natural communication.

Details about the concepts in the root concept map are presented in the next-level concept maps with more contextual information towards the provision of a more precise definition for the related terms. All of the detailed concept maps contain one or more concepts from the root concept map, with the corresponding colour code, as a linking point. In this way it is evident, how the root map and the detailed concept maps relate to each other.

Because of the central role of the AAL Services in the root map, it would be reasonable to first deal with the analysis of this concept. But, in order to be able to provide a definition for AAL services, we must first agree on a common understanding of the term *Service*, which is one of the most ambiguous concepts, especially when it comes to its usage in computer science.

The OASIS reference model for service-oriented architectures (SOA-RM), for example, defines a service as "a mechanism to enable access to one or more capabilities" where capability is understood as "functionality created to address a need." [9]. It, however, also talks about their "invoking", "return values", and "effects" which are normally associated with other terms like function, method, or operation. In the end, it even states that "the service may be talked about in terms of being the capability" [9].

Implementations of SOA actually use the term service as a synonym for each self-contained component that provides an implementation of a shared functional interface; e.g., in OSGi[10] a service is a plain old Java object that implements a shared Java interface and registers itself with the framework, and in the world of Web Services a service is

[10]Originally an abbreviation for Open Services Gateway initiative. An alliance that specifies the OSGi Dynamic Module System for Java. See the pages of the OSGi Alliance at http://www.osgi.org.

a component that implements an interface published in WSDL and is accessible using HTTP/SOAP protocols and exchanges data in XML. Communities dealing with service semantics or its composition and orchestration tend, however, to set this term equal to the operation of a Web service or a single method of an OSGi service; e.g., David Martin, the principle author of OWL-S[11] releases, defines a service as an executable program function [7].

All of the above limit the definition of service to the virtual realm. There are other definitions that provide a more consistent definition of the term service when extending its usage to the real life: In one of his three suggested views, Chris Preist defines service as "the provision of something of value, in the context of some domain of application, by one party to another" [10]. Likewise, Roman et al. define service as the actual value provided to achieve a user's goal, in virtual realm by invoking a computational entity [11]. The two latter definitions would also cover the case of manual and semi-automated services, e.g. many care services that are classified as AAL services. Therefore, the notion of service in universAAL builds on these two latter definitions that are better applicable to different cases when software components provide services to other software components, when humans provide services to each other, and even when software components provide services to humans.

Finally, we agreed that a *Service* can be understood as the embodiment of a specific value addressing a need[12] provided by one party (service provider) to another (service consumer). As a result of consuming a service, the consumer perceives value such as being relieved of a certain task. In the process of providing a service, several (hardware / software / human) resources might be involved; in particular, other subordinate services might be utilized, as well.

The concept map illustrated in Fig. 2 is reflecting this understanding: Both humans and software components can play either of the roles as provider or consumer. We also stress that a service embodies some value which is created by the service provider and perceived by the service consumer. Other concepts that are important in the context of Service, such as service contract and quality, might be added later at a third level of detail. However, we expect to remain compatible with SOA-RM at those levels.

To further underline the provision of services in the virtual realm, the concept of a service utility is introduced. If a service is accessible within the virtual realm, then normally it can be utilized by activating a service utility that triggers a process in which the service provision is eventually performed. Those software components that provide such utilities are called *service components*. Any object that exports a set of methods can be regarded as a service component, where the exported methods (in the virtual realm) would be the *service utilities*. In particular, Web services (or OSGi POJOs) are examples of service components and their operations described in WSDL (or their methods included in a registered Java interface) are the service utilities. Each exported method or operation of a Web Service makes it possible to utilize a service from within the virtual realm. A service utility may directly trigger the process of providing the underlying service or just lead to an arrangement for starting the process at a later point in time[13].

[11] See http://www.ai.sri.com/daml/services/owl-s/.

[12] This is pretty much the same as the definition of a capability in SOA-RM.

[13] The relationship that a Service Component is a Software Component is not shown explicitly in order to keep the concept map tidy.

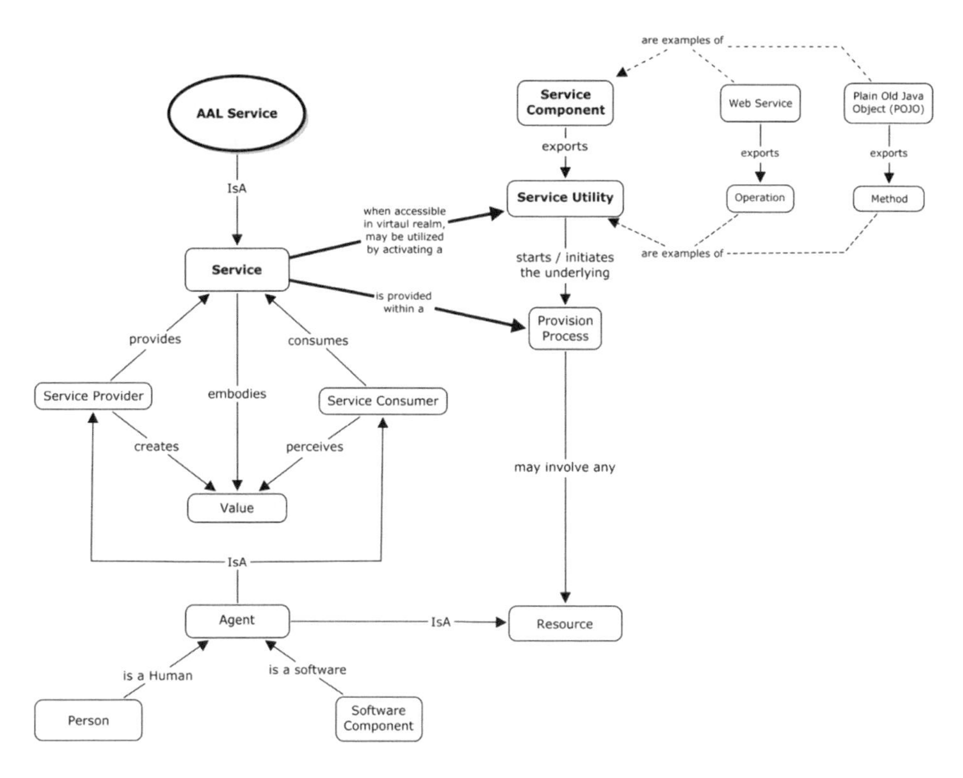

Figure 2. Service concept map.

The domain-specific context of AAL service (illustrated in Fig. 3) helps to better understand the essence of these services as well as the different interests and concerns that various individuals or organizations might have in providing or using such services.

AAL services facilitate social integration and provide assistance which is needed by assisted persons. They are aiming at well-being and comfort of their consumers in their lives, e.g. provision of assistance whenever needed and ensuring social integration in situations of isolation or loneliness. *Assisted persons* are in this way seen as the final beneficiary of the universAAL project. They are the main consumer of AAL Services whose needs are in the centre of designing such services. *Assistance* in the AAL context is defined as provision of relief of a burden either by relying just on resources within an AAL Space (local assistance) or by involving external service providers and their resources (remote assistance). Social integration involves people from each assisted person's personal network, such as relatives, friends, neighbours, and colleagues, who all may also act as *informal caregivers* in the provision of assistance to the assisted person. *Social integration* can be understood as the feeling of belonging to and being useful in the society, in AAL especially with regard to the mentioned stakeholders – generally the circle of people from one's personal network. A *caregiver* is a human resource who has accepted to be involved in the provision of AAL Services, interacts with the assisted person, and might need to access resources provided by AAL Spaces. A *formal caregiver* is defined as a caregiver that is paid for being involved in service provision (e.g., service personnel working for service providers) or are otherwise involved professionally (e.g., skilled volunteers with social commitment).

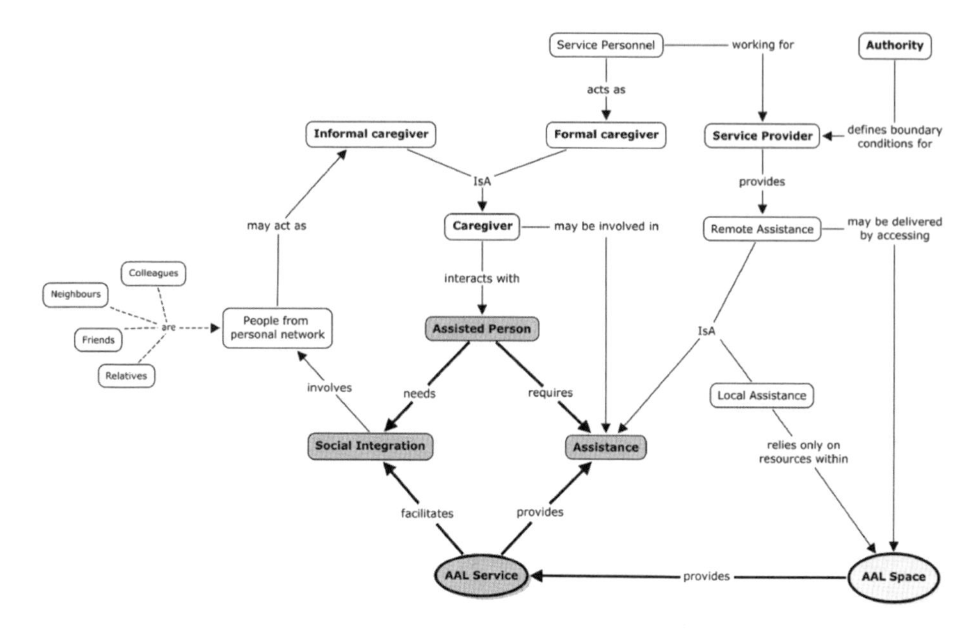

Figure 3. AAL services – The domain-specific context.

Local Assistance that relies only on the resources within an AAL Space would cover mostly fully automated ambient intelligent services provided by service components installed in the AAL Space. Remote Assistance refers to the case of incorporating resources outside the AAL Space possibly in combination with local resources. Remote assistance is usually provided by a *service provider*. Service providers offer their human and technological resources that from the viewpoint of AAL Spaces are considered as "external resources". The boundary conditions for service providers are defined by *authorities*. Boundary conditions are defined for the development, deployment, provision, and usage of AAL Services and involved resources. As such, authorities can be seen as the core part of the quaternary stakeholders identified by the AALIANCE Roadmap (see [14]) who are supposed to work on the economical and legal context of AAL.

Having covered a first analysis of AAL services, it is now time to zoom in on AAL Spaces. AAL Spaces are supposed to be smart environments and since Ambient Intelligence (AmI) is the art / science of creating intelligent environments, we can make use of progresses made in AmI for further understanding the characteristics of AAL Spaces.

According to Aarts and Encarnação in [1], AmI "refers to electronic environments that are sensitive and responsive to the presence of people" and "in an AmI world, devices operate collectively using information and intelligence that is hidden in the network connecting the devices;" they "cooperate seamlessly with one another to improve the total user experience through the support of natural and intuitive user interfaces." In the analysis of the two words comprising the term *Ambient Intelligence*, Aarts and Encarnação state that "the notion of *ambience* in Ambient Intelligence refers to the environment and reflects the need for an embedding of technology in a way that it becomes nonobstrusively integrated into everyday objects. The notion *intelligence* reflects that the digital surroundings exhibit specific forms of social interaction, i.e., the environments

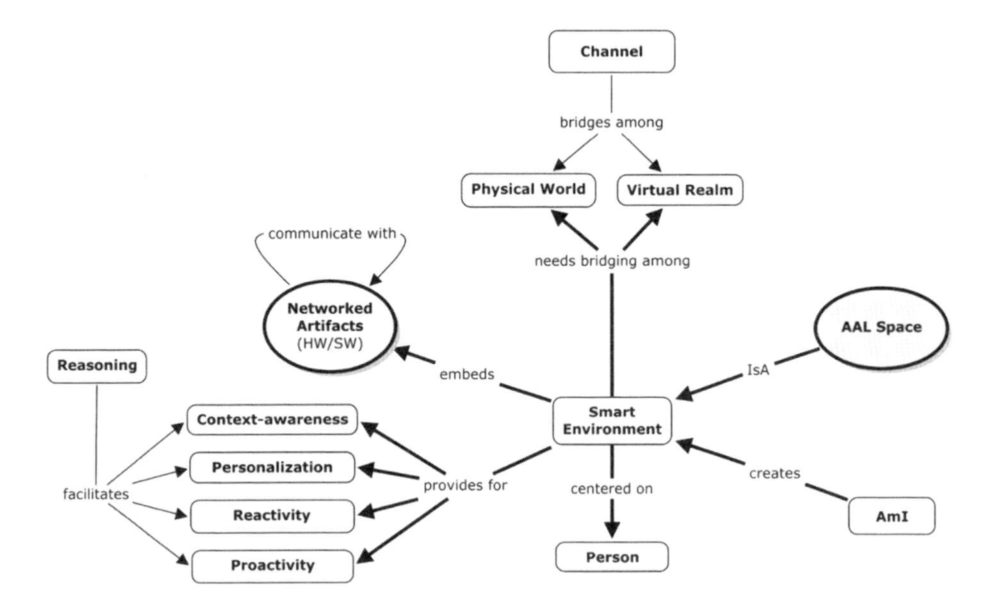

Figure 4. Analysis of AAL spaces.

should be able to recognize the people that live in it, adapt themselves to them, learn from their behaviour, and possibly act upon their behalf." [1]

The development of ambient intelligence systems demands an interdisciplinary approach, borrowing methods and techniques from computing fields, such as Ubiquitous / Pervasive Computing, Context-aware Computing, Human-Computer Interaction (HCI), and Artificial Intelligence (AI). Ubiquitous and pervasive computing refer to the embedding of computational and networking capabilities overall and in all physical things. The embedded artefacts can inter-communicate for providing information and services to each other and specially may provide channels that bridge between the physical world and the virtual realm (cf. [3]). Channel denotes the bridging passage provided by such devices between the physical world and the virtual realm. Depending on the kind of channel opened, a channel might be called a sensing channel (provided by sensors), an acting channel (provided by actuators), an input channel (provided by microphones, keyboards, etc.), or an output channel (provided by displays, loudspeakers, etc.). The virtual realm enlarges the scope of sensitivity and responsiveness so that the notion of *environment* or *space* makes sense in AmI. All this is then employed to serve humans in the environment.

According to AmI, this setup is expected to result in characteristics, such as context-awareness, personalization, reactivity and pro-activity in smart environments (see Fig. 4). That is, smart environments must provide support for acting in a context-aware and personalized way so that responses can be considered to be adaptive. Reaction and pro-action are the two examples of adaptive response that must be emphasized in order for smart environments to live up to what AmI requires. Experience shows that the quality of these four central characteristics can be improved if some sort of reasoning backs them.

To further clarify the notion of channel referred to in Fig. 4, we provide a supplementary concept map (Fig. 5) that also highlights the notion of sensor and actuator always referred to in the context of AmI. However, we would like to emphasize that in

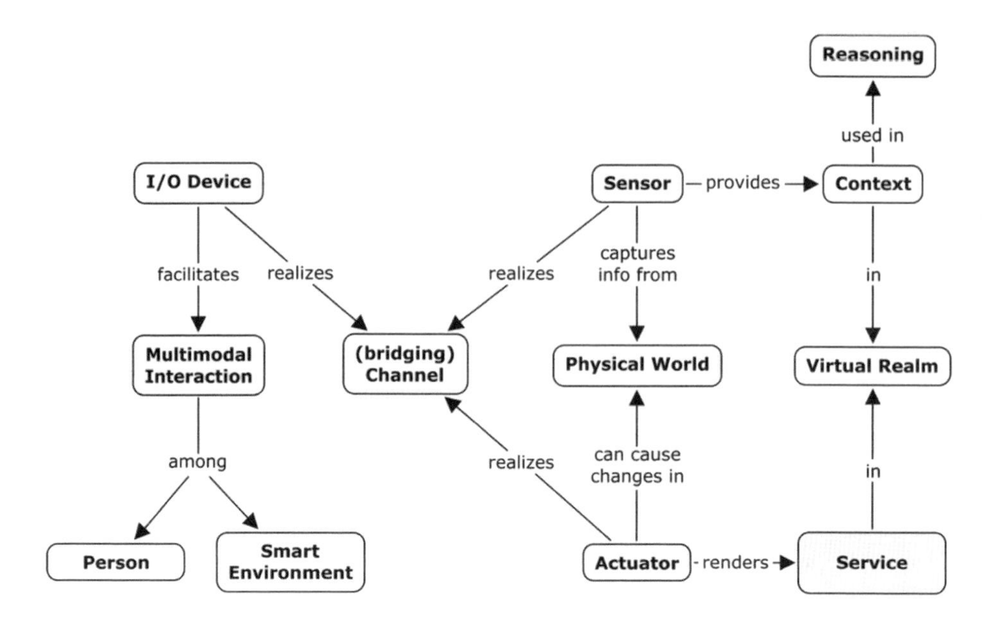

Figure 5. Important categories of devices that realize bridging channels between the physical world and the virtual realm.

addition to sensors and actuators, there are also I/O devices realizing channels between the physical world and the virtual realm that aim at facilitating the interaction between smart environments and humans. This helps to highlight natural interaction as one of the major criteria posed by AmI.

AAL Space is thus defined as a smart environment centred on its human users in which a set of embedded networked artefacts, both hardware and software, collectively realize the paradigm of Ambient Intelligence, mainly by providing for context-awareness and personalization, adaptive reactivity, anticipatory pro-activity, and natural interaction. Smart homes and cars are examples of AAL Spaces. Other important definitions are:

IO Device An abbreviation for input and / or output device. A device that provides an input and / or output channel for facilitating explicit interaction between a smart environment and its human users. Input devices, such as a microphone, a keyboard, or a mouse, can capture an instruction or response that is provided by a human user and represent it in terms of data in the virtual realm. Upon receive of data within the virtual realm that is intended to be presented to human users, output devices, such as displays and loudspeakers, can make it perceivable to the addressed humans.

Context From an AmI *system* point of view, context is data that *can* be shared within a system based on a set of shared models. In reality, the shared models in each system cover only selected areas and therefore context in AmI systems is not comprehensive. There is no guarantee about the availability of all data that is potentially possible to be shared based on the shared models. Even for available data, it might lose its validity after some time is elapsed. Each entity playing a role in the system might have its own partial view on context; such an entity must be fault-tolerant with regard to context use due to the above restrictions regarding the availability and validity of context. This definition focuses on identifying problems to be coped with in AAL systems and makes no statement about an entity's context (cf. Dey's definition of context in [4]). Although the universAAL concept maps highlight the role of info captured by sensors from the physical world and shared as data within the virtual realm, with this definition we make clear that Context may go beyond this.

Context-awareness The quality of incorporating parts of Context when performing actions in the virtual realm. The incorporation of Context is always partial because the shared models are not comprehensive and nevertheless there is usually more data shared as actually used by each single context-aware software component; vice versa, parts of data expected to be available as Context might not be available at runtime or not valid any more.

Peronalization The quality of incorporating knowledge about characteristics, capabilities, and preferences of each individual human user when performing actions in the virtual realm. As a result, the differences between individuals can be accommodated adequately. Personalization can be seen as a special case of Context-awareness since the data representing the knowledge about characteristics, capabilities, and preferences of each individual human user is often classified as a subset of Context.

Reactivity The capability of smart environments to automatically react to certain situations in an adaptive (context-aware and personalized) way.

Pro-activity The capability of smart environments to automatically perform actions that are anticipatory and aim at getting prepared for future situations.

Reasoning Using context for facilitating context-awareness (e.g., inferring and adding new facts to context), personalization (e.g., deducing users' situational preferences), reactivity (e.g., learning from behaviour analysis), and pro-activity (e.g., analysis of correspondence between situations and needs) in smart environments.

Multimodal Interaction The adaptive (context-aware and personalized) utilization of the set of I/O channels available in a smart environment for handling explicit interaction with human users in a natural way. "Multimodal" in this context serves as an abbreviated reference to the potential of performing the interaction using multiple channels in parallel, possibly with a hybrid mix supporting different modalities.

With the concept map illustrated by Fig. 6, we further investigate the question of Stakeholders, this time from a technical point of view. For this purpose, we first emphasize that the networked artefacts referred to so far comprise both networking enabled hardware nodes and software components loadable by certain types of such hardware nodes. This helps to identify manufacturers (as producers of hardware) and developers (as producers of software). In case of networking-enabled nodes, the main issue for manufacturers is the selection of the right communication protocols that help to sell the nodes in several different configurations while keeping the production costs very low. Developers whose main need is the availability of widely adopted platforms that are easy to use (sometimes with the help of appropriate development tools), facilitate the development of the related applications (e.g., rapid development with reduced costs), and help to better market the product.

We also highlight that setting up a complex AAL Space consisting of specialized hardware and software requires certain expertise and knowledge about the available hard-

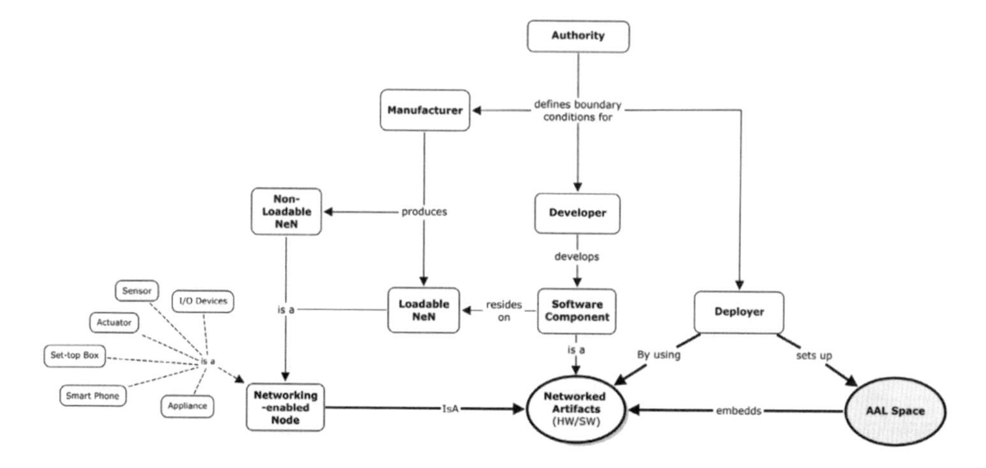

Figure 6. Networked artefacts – Stakeholders concept map.

ware and software. The stakeholders that have this expertise and provide the service of setting up AAL Spaces by using appropriate artefacts are called deployers. Deployers could be seen as special service providers which are experts in the analysis of the needs of the consumers of AAL Services and have a broad knowledge about the available technologies and solutions. They can provide an integrated solution for individuals, set up concrete AAL Spaces on their behalf, and can maintain the resulted AAL system to keep it operational and up-to-date.

Manufacturers, developers and the deployers have to work under the boundary conditions defined by the Authorities.

Networked Artefacts are used to refer to both networking-enabled nodes (in terms of hardware) and software components. Examples of networking-enable nodes are actuators, sensors, I/O devices, appliances, set-top-boxes, smart phones, or more general-purpose computing devices. However, software may freely be loaded only on a subset of the networking-enabled nodes – that we have called Loadable Nodes – as some of the other nodes must be used as packaged by their manufacturers without much further manipulation possibilities. We call this second subset of networking-enabled nodes the Non-loadable Nodes.

The concept map in Fig. 7 describes the concept of middleware which is a central concept for the development of the universAAL platform. It highlights the importance of providing for mechanisms that allow distributed and heterogeneous networked artefacts to interact with each other. The middleware is understood as a software component which ideally has a footprint on all of the networking-enabled nodes. It provides common interfaces that facilitate the integration of other software components and the communication between them. As the middleware hides the distribution and heterogeneity of networking-enabled nodes, developers of software components need not care about the whereabouts of resources they need.

Middleware can thus be defined as (borrowed from [5]) software that ranks among the core of platforms for distributed systems and is responsible for the integration of software components distributed on different nodes and for facilitating the communication among them. For this purpose, middleware hides both the distribution of the system and any possible heterogeneity of its nodes.

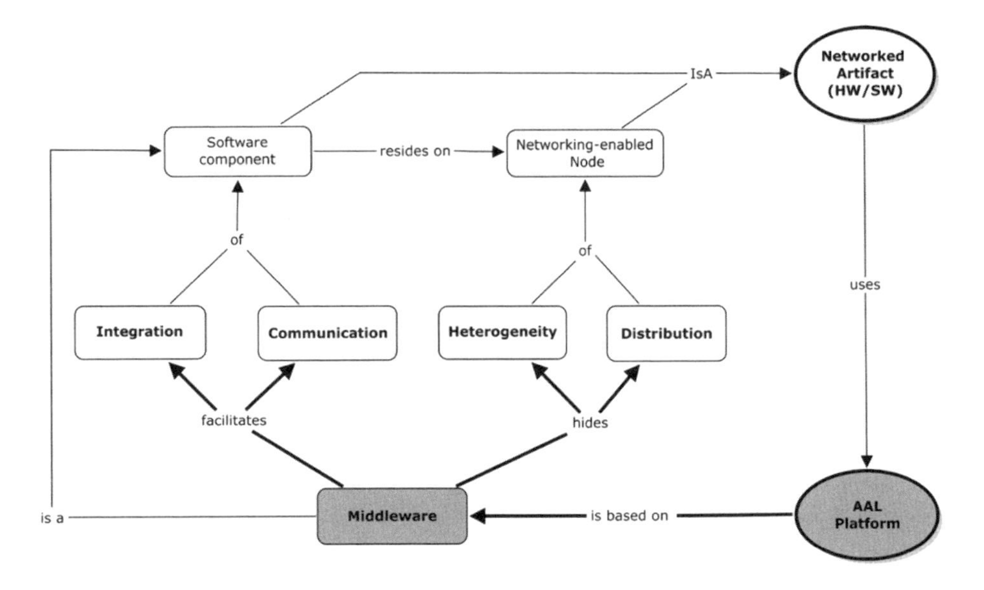

Figure 7. Platform – Middleware concept map.

4. Conclusion

Based on a definition of reference models, we have presented the related universAAL work results in the field of AAL in the previous section. We would like to stress that this is just the outcome of the first iteration in a process consisting of four iterations. Work is going on in three directions for improving this current version (e.g., considering the notion of loadable / non-loadable nodes), extending it (i.e., looking for important concepts that are missing in the root map and / or the second-level maps), and refining (i.e., deciding where we need to add new refinement levels by digging deeper in the second-level concepts).

Classifying the reference model as means for understanding the domain is consistent with the initial assumptions underlying the universAAL description of work. Figure 8 summarizes those assumptions while highlighting the relationships between the expected results of AAL Reference Architecture specification and the reference implementations. This is also consistent with the following definitions adopted from [8]:

Reference Architecture A reference architecture models the abstract architectural elements (building blocks) in the domain independent of the technologies, protocols, and products that are used to implement the domain. It differs from a reference model in that a reference model describes the important concepts and relationships in the domain focusing on what distinguishes the elements of the domain; a reference architecture elaborates further on the model to show a more complete picture that includes showing what is involved in realizing the modelled entities.

Concrete Architecture for Realization By increasing the level of detail in a reference architecture, we can end up with a concrete architecture that specifies all the technologies, components and their relationships in sufficient detail to enable direct implementation.

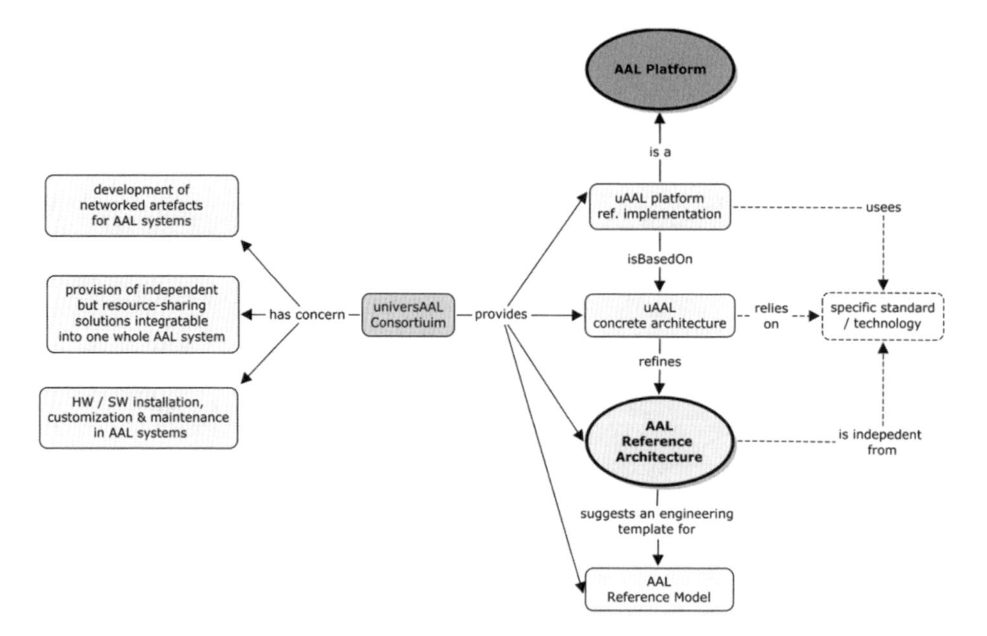

Figure 8. The notion of middleware in universAAL.

universAAL has also finished its first iteration on a reference architecture for AAL that is the result of consolidating the knowledge inherited from the input projects (not discussed here). We are currently finishing the first iteration on the concrete architecture based on which the universAAL platform for AAL is going to be provided.

Acknowledgements

The research leading to these results has received funding from the European Community's Seventh Framework Programme (FP7/2007-2013) under grant agreement n° 247950.

References

[1] E. Aarts and J. Encarnação, Into ambient intelligence, *True Visions: The Emergence of Ambient Intelligence*, Emile Aarts and José Encarnação, eds, Springer, 2006, pp. 1–16, ISBN 3-540-28972-0.

[2] Australian Government Information Management Office (AGIMO), The Australian government business process interoperability framework – Enabling seamless service delivery, July 2007, [online at: http://www.finance.gov.au/publications/agimo/docs/Business_Process_Interoeprabiltiy_Framework.pdf], accessed on: 12.10.2010.

[3] T. Berners-Lee, J. Hendler and O. Lassila, The semantic web, *Scientific American* **284**(5) (2001), 34–43.

[4] A.K. Dey, Understanding and using context, *Personal Ubiquitous Computing* **5**(1) (2001), 4–7, doi:10.1007/s007790170019.

[5] S. Krakowiak, *Middleware Architecture with Patterns and Frameworks*, INRIA Rhône-Alpes, France, 2007, [online at: http://sardes.inrialpes.fr/~krakowia/MW-Book/], accessed on: 12.10.2010.

[6] A. Kung and G. Fagerberg, Alliance for an AAL open service platform, in: *AALIANCE Conference, Malaga, Spain, 11 and 12 March 2010*, [online at: http://www.aaliance.eu/public/aaliance-conference-1/papers-and-posters/4_1_trialog], accessed on: 12.10.2010.

[7] D. Martin, J. Domingue, M.L. Brodie and F. Leymann, Semantic web services, part 1, *IEEE Intelligent Systems* **22**(5) (Sep./Oct. 2007), 12–17, doi:10.1109/MIS.2007.94.
[8] OASIS Open Technical Committee for SOA-RM, Reference architecture foundation for service oriented architecture, Committee Draft 02, Oct. 2009, [online at: http://docs.oasis-open.org/soa-rm/soa-ra/v1.0/soa-ra-cd-02.pdf], accessed on: 09.06.2010.
[9] OASIS Open Technical Committee for SOA-RM, Reference model for service oriented architecture 1.0, August 2006, [online at: http://docs.oasis-open.org/soa-rm/v1.0/soa-rm.pdf], accessed on: 09.06.2010.
[10] Ch. Preist, A conceptual architecture for semantic web services, in: *Proc. of the Third International Semantic Web Conference 2004 (ISWC 2004)*, November 2004.
[11] D. Roman, U. Keller, H. Lausen, J. de Bruijn, R. Lara, M. Stollberg, A. Polleres, C. Feier, Ch. Bussler and D. Fensel, Web service modeling ontology, *Applied Ontology* **1**(1) (2005), 77–106.
[12] M.-R. Tazari, R. Wichert and T. Norgall, Towards a unified ambient assisted living and personal health environment, in: *Fourth German AAL Congress*, Berlin, Germany, 25 and 26 January 2011.
[13] The OWL Services Coalition, OWL-S: Semantic markup for web services, Technical overview, 2006, [online at: http://www.ai.sri.com/daml/services/owl-s/1.2/overview/], accessed on: 11.06.2010.
[14] G. Van Den Broek, F. Cavallo and C. Wehrmann, *AALIANCE Ambient Assisted Living Roadmap*, IOS Press, March 2010, ISBN: 978-1-60750-498-6.
[15] P. Wolf, A. Schmidt, J. Parada Otte, M. Klein, S. Rollwage, B. König-Ries, T. Dettborn and A. Gabdulkhakova, openAAL – The open source middleware for ambient-assisted living, in: *AALIANCE conference*, Malaga, Spain, 11 and 12 March 2010, [online at: http://www.aaliance.eu/public/aaliance-conference-1/papers-and-posters/2_1_uni-karlsruhe], accessed on: 12.10.2010.

Handbook of Ambient Assisted Living
J.C. Augusto et al. (Eds.)
IOS Press, 2012

doi:10.3233/978-1-60750-837-3-626

Managing Chronic Conditions Using Wireless Sensor Networks

Raluca MARIN-PERIANU[a], Juan JIMENEZ GARCIA[a], Stephan BOSCH[a], Mihai MARIN-PERIANU[b] and Paul HAVINGA[a,*]
[a] *University of Twente, The Netherlands*
[b] *Inertia Technology B.V., The Netherlands*

Abstract. Physical activity, therapy and exercising are essential for the management of many chronic conditions. This is why human motion tracking for healthcare applications has received significant attention recently. In this chapter we describe the architecture in which we provide a person-centric healthcare solution for patients with chronic conditions based on the recent advances in wireless inertial sensing systems. We emphasize the role of the home as care environment, by providing real-time support to patients in order to monitor, self-manage and improve their physical condition according to their specific situation.

1. Introduction

In recent years, monitoring the level of daily human activity has gained interest for various medical and wellbeing applications. It has been shown that health condition and quality of life are directly influenced by the amount and intensity of daily physical activity [35]. This is particularly relevant to persons with chronic conditions, such as Chronic Obstructive Pulmonary Disease (COPD), asthma and diabetes [16]. The reason is that persons suffering from chronic conditions enter a vicious circle, in which being active causes discomfort, making them progressively more sedentary, and deteriorating their health. Monitoring the daily activity can stimulate people to perform exercises and to be more active in general by providing feedback and assistance to better manage the physical condition. Apart from medical applications, daily activity monitoring can also be useful for healthy users that want to assess and improve their overall fitness level. Activity monitoring systems can remind, stimulate and motivate people to be more active, especially when used within groups with a competitive nature.

Within the Ambient Assisted Living (AAL) Joint Programme, the IS-ACTIVE project [11] develops a person-centric healthcare solution for persons with chronic conditions – especially elderly people – based on the latest advances in the field of Wireless Sensor Networks (WSNs). WSNs provide distributed sensing and intelligent recognition of activities and situations, as well as simple and ubiquitous feedback modalities, thus taking complex computer interaction out of the loop and breaking the digital divide [17,18]. The home becomes the main care environment, where the users can continuously monitor, self-manage and improve their physical condition according to their specific situation. The IS-ACTIVE consortium designs, builds and tests systems that can be bought and used by the individuals, instead of being the property of health-

[*] Corresponding Author: Paul Havinga. E-mail: paul.havinga@utwente.nl.

care institutions. IS-ACTIVE allows the shift of medical device technology into the mainstream consumer electronics market. This implies that there is a strong focus towards ease of use, integration and pricing.

The IS-ACTIVE system has two key drivers:

- *Paradigm shift in healthcare.* Population of Europe is ageing. The older the population, the higher is the frequency of chronic diseases. This poses an increasing burden on healthcare and social service systems and affects the quality of life by inducing both physical disabilities with frequent hospitalizations and social impairment. There is a need for a paradigm shift from the specialized care centers to the home as self-care environment. Persons with chronic conditions need to be continuously supported in their physical therapy, as the level of physical activity influences directly their status and progress.
- *Technology advances in wireless inertial sensing.* In recent years, miniaturized inertial sensors have become an increasingly popular solution for ambulatory human movement analysis [17]. Furthermore, recent advances in wireless communication and low-power chip design stimulated the development of pervasive technologies, such as wireless sensor and body area networks, foreseen to have a high impact in the wellness and healthcare domains.

Therefore, IS-ACTIVE has a combined solution: intelligent miniaturized inertial sensing systems with wireless communication capabilities. Such systems not only capture the motion parameters of the users, but also self-organize into an ad-hoc, dynamic wireless network, process data locally to extract relevant features, apply distributed inference to assess the physical activity and condition of the users, and eventually provide real-time feedback. The later aspect is of particular importance, as it can increase both the level of awareness and the motivation of following the physical therapy, thus contributing to a better education and self-management of chronic conditions.

IS-ACTIVE results are validated through field trials involving patients suffering from chronic obstructive pulmonary disease (COPD). COPD became the fourth cause of death worldwide due to an increase in smoking rates and demographic changes in many countries. Patients need to manage their chronic condition through extensive physical therapy. However, the physical therapy needs to be adapted to the situation of the patient and according to his/her progress. The field trials that will be carried out at three locations (in Norway, the Netherlands and Romania) will assess the added value of the IS-ACTIVE miniaturized wireless sensing system and reflect back how these objectives are met.

In this chapter we describe the objectives and the associated challenges, the specific innovations beyond state-of-the-art, the general architecture of the system including the various interaction modalities, the current project status and business opportunities.

2. State of the Art – COPD Treatment and Human Motion Tracking

Chronic diseases are the major cause of death and disability worldwide, accounting for 59% of the annual deaths and 46% of the global burden of disease [16,31]. In USA, 45% of the population suffers from at least one chronic condition and 26% from two or more chronic conditions. In 2007, USA spent $1.7 trillion (75% of the total healthcare costs) on chronic conditions. Similar figures hold in Europe, for example in Denmark an estimated 70–80% of healthcare expenses are allocated to chronic conditions. In UK, 8 of the top 11 causes of hospital admissions are chronic conditions. In the central and eastern countries of the European Region, people die from chronic diseases at dramatically younger ages than in western Europe. Due to the overall trend of population ageing, the situation is to become only worse, with the number of co-morbidities increasing progressively with age and achieving higher levels among women.

One of the main factors accounting for almost 60% of the disease burden in Europe is physical inactivity. Our approach is to stimulate patients with chronic conditions to have more and better suited physical activities, through the use of simple to use, yet reliable and entertaining technology. For field trials, the target user group is represented by persons suffering from chronic obstructive pulmonary disease (COPD). COPD became the fourth cause of death worldwide due to an increase in smoking rates and demographic changes in many countries, and is estimated to become the third cause of death in 2020. COPD patients need to manage their chronic condition through extensive physical therapy. However, the physical therapy needs to be adapted to the situation of the patient and according to his/her progress.

Physical activity, therapy and exercising are essential for the management of many chronic conditions. In particular for COPD, a recent study that included approximately 2400 patients showed that regular physical activity reduces hospital admission and mortality [8]. The recommendation that COPD patients should be encouraged to maintain or increase their levels of regular physical activity should be considered in future COPD guidelines, since it is likely to result in a relevant public health benefit.

Therefore, human motion tracking for healthcare applications has received significant attention recently. The most important approaches can be summarized as follows:

- Non-visual tracking
  - Inertial and magnetic sensor based systems, such as MTx [34], G-Link [20], MotionStar [1], Liberty [22].
  - Ultrasonic systems, such as IS-600 Motion Tracker [10].
  - Electromyogram (EMG), such as Biofeedback [19].
  - Glove-based systems, such as CyberGlove [5], PowerGlove [23].
- Visual tracking
  - Marker-based tracking
    - Passive marker-based systems, such as Qualisys [25], VICON [30].
    - Active marker-based systems, such as CODA [4], Polaris [21].
  - Marker-free tracking
    - 2-D systems, such as [3,33].
    - 3-D systems, such as [12,28].
- Robot-aided tracking, such as MIT-MANUS [13], MIME [15], ARM Guide [26], HelpMate [7], Rutgers Ankle [2].

A number of clear limitations and drawbacks of these systems have been recognized in the related literature [35]:

- *High cost and complexity*. Current systems are specialized, utilize expensive, dedicated components and sensors, and require professionals for calibration and often even for operation.

- *Feedback in real-time is missing*, as data is usually processed offline on high-end platforms.
- *Current systems do not provide patient-oriented therapy* and hence cannot yet be directly used in home-based environments.
- *Size and usability*. Current systems are not compact and easy to apply/handle. This aspect is particularly important because patients are expected to have reduced movement abilities.
- *Poor performance in human-computer interface design*. From the practical point of view, an attractive interface will encourage users to carry out the physical therapy.

Starting from these points, we present the following innovations beyond state of the art:

- The ability of capturing motion parameters from a wireless network of relatively cheap and simple sensors.
- The feedback in real-time, by exploiting the distributed processing power available on sensor nodes and the wireless connections that can be established ad-hoc among sensors and the feedback devices.
- The possibility of assisting the patients continuously, in their own environment, instead of periodically, in specialized laboratories.
- The simplification in terms of usability due to the motion-based interfacing, especially with respect to elderly users (low affinity with technology, bad vision, etc.).
- The small scale factor, low-power and low-cost of this distributed solution compared to high-end systems, such as camera-based tracking systems.
- The link to daily objects, which can also be instrumented with wireless sensors, thus providing additional information on the patient condition, as well as leading to more natural or simpler interactions of disabled people with their environment.
- The ability of seamlessly integrating other physiological sensors to the same wireless sensor network system.

3. Architecture

Figure 1 presents the top-level view on the main architectural components taken into account.

We distinguish the following important building blocks:

- *Wireless sensors networks (WSNs)* – the core technology creating a pervasive environment around the user:
    - On-body sensors, such as inertial sensors (used for the analysis of user motions, activity monitoring and exercise coaching) and physiological sensors (used for checking safety limits of user's current condition). The on-body sensors form the Body Sensor Network (BSN).
    - Infrastructure sensors, such as environmental sensors (used for signaling possible adverse environmental conditions with respect to the user specific condition).

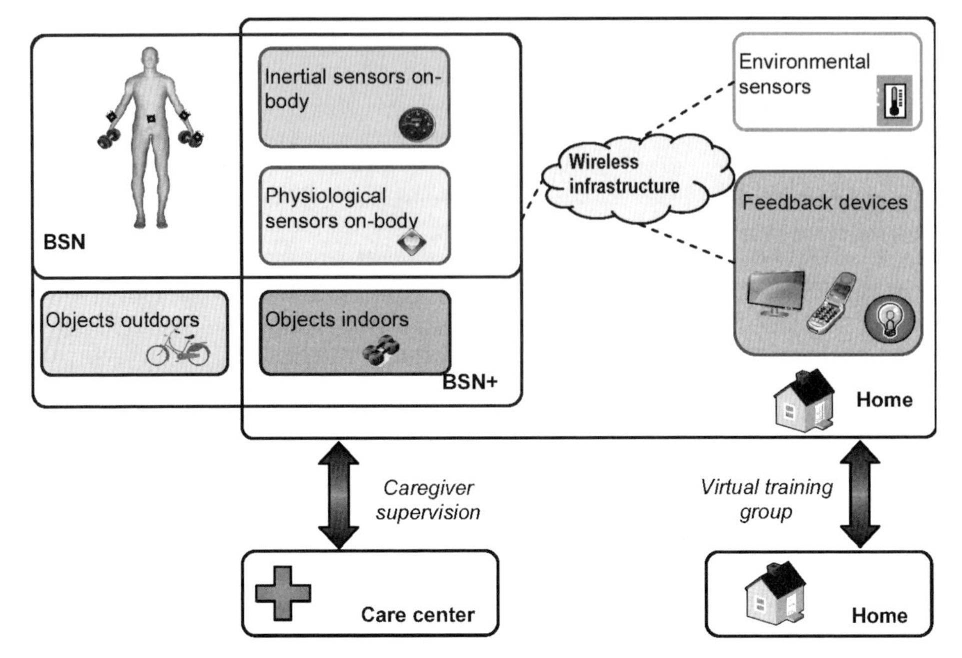

Figure 1. Block diagram of the IS-ACTIVE system architecture.

- *Technology-aided objects (TAOs)* – technology-enhanced daily objects (for indoor or outdoor usage) that contribute to monitoring and assessing the physical training performance of patients. They are mainly graspable objects with which the users carry out training task at home and outdoors. Together, the on-body sensors and TAOs form the Extended Body Sensor Network (BSN+).
- *Feedback devices* – covering all user interaction aspects, providing the information sensed and processed by the WSN in a simple and appealing way to the user. The main objective here is to enhance the user motivation for physical activity.

4. Wireless Sensors Networks (WSNs)

The objective of this section is to describe the hardware and software building blocks of sensor nodes used in the development of the wireless sensor network. Besides, this section includes information about the relevant networking protocols and also considers some of the critical networking issues.

4.1. Sensor Node

A sensor node is the main component of a wireless sensor network and it is capable of performing processing, storage and communication with other nodes in the network [6]. A sensor node has limited hardware resources, including the available power (usually a battery), therefore energy efficiency is an essential requirement for applications running on sensor nodes [9].

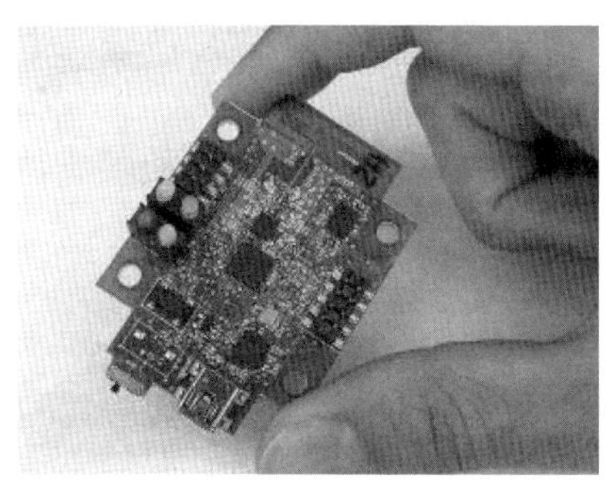

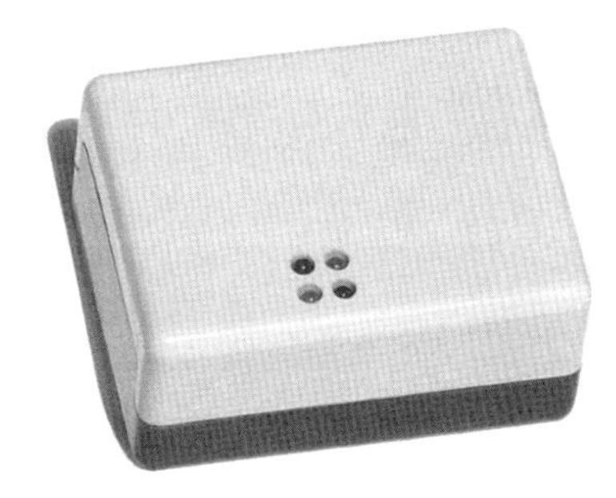

Figure 2. ProMove wireless inertial sensor node [24].

Since one of the main purposes of the system is motion sensing, the wireless sensor node developed in the project is a miniaturized platform – ProMove – that captures and wirelessly communicates full 3-D motion and orientation information and derived motion features through integrated accelerometer, gyroscope and compass sensors (see Fig. 2).

The access to the microcontroller, wireless transceivers and sensors is facilitated by a specific operating system, which is the interface responsible for coordination of activities and management of shared hardware and software resources.

4.2. Sensors Networking

A Wireless Sensor Network (WSN) is composed of sensor nodes that sense several environmental phenomena and form an ad-hoc network for the purpose of collaboratively processing and transmitting the data to the interested parties. A WSN is a self-organizing network that does not need user intervention for configuration or setting up routing paths. Therefore, WSNs can be used in virtually any environment, even in inhospitable terrain or where the physical placement is difficult [27].

Since WSNs differ largely from wireless networks, they require energy-preserving protocols and a suitable model to fit their dynamic topology [29]. Therefore, WSNs do not fully adhere to the ISO-OSI reference model [36].

Sensor nodes are the main building blocks of WSN applications and are mainly battery powered. Changing or recharging batteries at relatively short intervals is impractical and reduces the usability and reliability of these systems. Although the wireless communication standard IEEE 802.15.4 is a popular choice for WSNs due to its low power consumption, the constrained bandwidth utilization is an important problem for the performance of WSNs. Some applications, such as body sensor networks, require synchronized data sampling and communication at high data rates. Taking into account these considerations, the inertial sensor node features:

- Low-power, low-data rate IEEE 802.15.4 compatible wireless communication, for long term sensing and monitoring, e.g. for activity level monitoring applications.
- High-data rate, real-time motion capture networking protocol, for short term, detailed sensor data acquisition, e.g. for algorithm design and evaluation.
- Bluetooth interface for connectivity with off-the-shelf physiological sensors (e.g. heart rate and oxygen saturation) and feedback devices (e.g. smart phone).

Therefore, the ProMove sensor node represents a versatile hardware platform that can be used in all the development phases of the project: algorithm design, algorithm implementation and testing, integration with other sensors and feedback devices and experiments with end-users.

5. Interactive Devices

Interactive devices create a seamless relationship between the end-user's daily life and the sensor-based infrastructure. The latter comprises an invisible technology infrastructure for the patient. In order to incorporate this technology in the user daily life, interactive devices are required to bridge the functionalities of the system with the patient's routines and physical treatment. Interactive devices refer to all those devices with which the end-users interact in different ways to receive suitable and tailored feedback about their physical state and training progress. These devices monitor and evaluate patient's physical state in an unobtrusive way and provide feedback for physical training. They stimulate and encourage physical activity for COPD patients to explore self-monitoring of their physical condition, while improving social and emotional communication with other COPD patients, separated friends and caregivers. Special attention should be taken regarding the people's relationship to new technology and their technology literacy. For instance, it is commonly known that many elderly people are not familiar with technology, demanding a design of simple interfaces with emotional valuable interactions.

A general description about how the user interacts with these devices and what kind of feedback he/she would send and receive from them is depicted in. We categorize the interactive devices in the following way (see also Fig. 3):

- Technology Aided Objects (guidance and training coaching).
- On-Body Sensor devices (monitoring user's vital signs).
- Feedback Devices (communication with caregivers and final feedback).

In the following, we describe the characteristics of these devices and the different nature of the interaction with the user.

5.1. Technology Aided Objects (TAOs)

These objects comprise technology enhancements to monitor and assess the physical training performance of COPD patients. They are mainly graspable objects to coach and guide the patients with their training program (stretching, strengthening muscles, and breathing) at home and outdoors [18], encouraging physical activity and self-monitoring along with virtual training groups. They are meant to persuade COPD patients to follow daily routines and guide them to perform the suggested physical exercises in a correct way. Therefore, these devices provide low-level feedback in the form of immediate and short information while carrying out a physical exercise. It is important to create emotional attachments (trust and value) with playful and pleasurable interactions in order to guarantee daily and long usage. Examples of these devices include: daily objects, fitness equipment or outdoor devices (e.g. bicycle, walking stick) equipped with sensors.

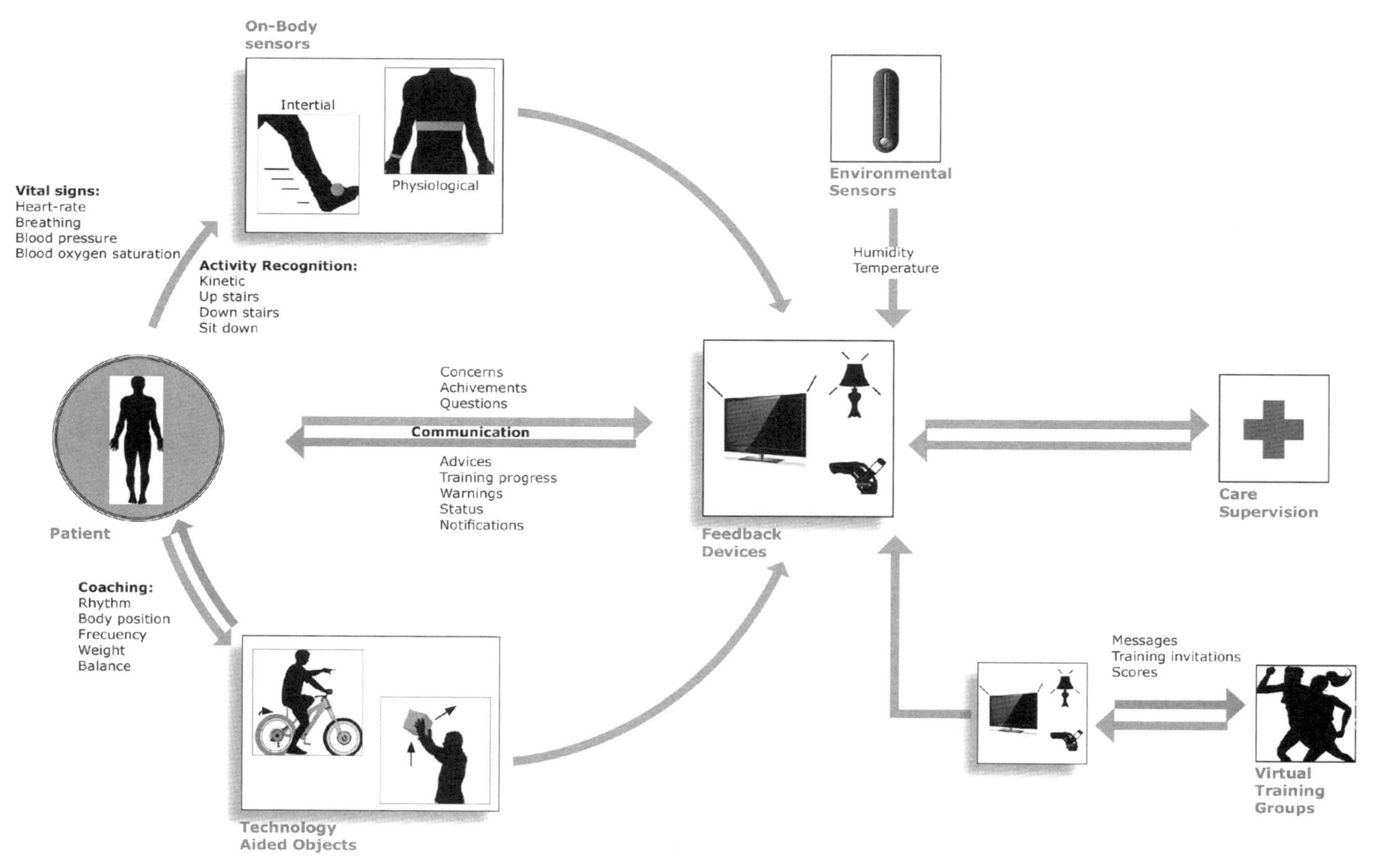

Figure 3. Overview of interactive devices.

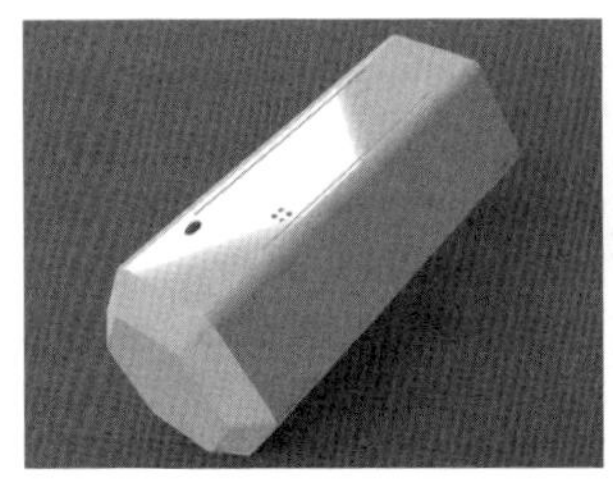
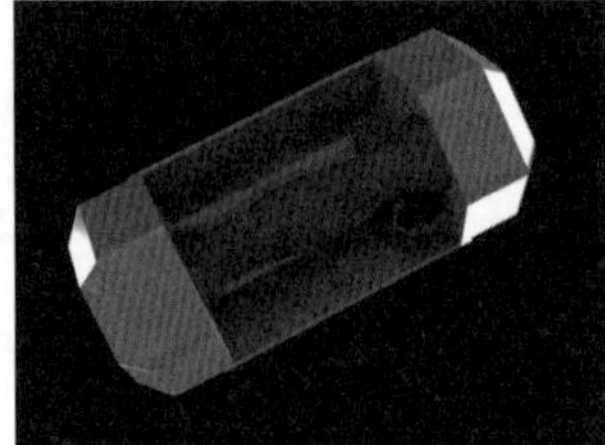
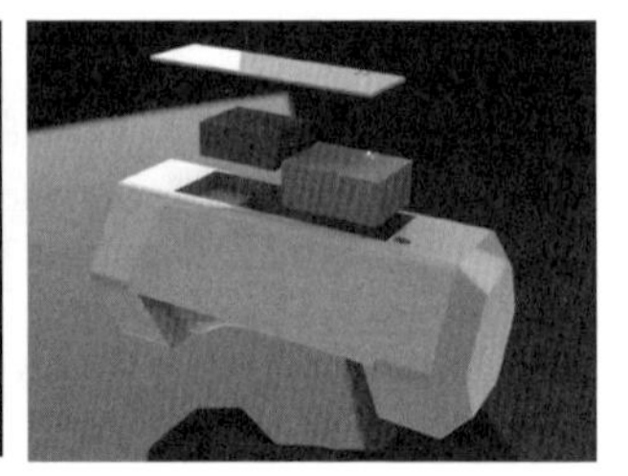

Figure 4. Dumbbell design for COPD patients.

We have designed a dumbbell to be used by COPD patients during their fitness exercises. This TAO incorporates a ProMove node and an oxygen saturation sensor for risk prevention (see Fig. 4).

5.2. On-Body Sensors

These devices are meant to monitor motion and vital signs of people (e.g. heartbeat, breathing, blood oxygen saturation). They are attached to the patient's body in an unobtrusive and comfortable way to wear for long periods. Although they do not have a special shape to interact with the user, and they aim to be invisible for the user and they should encourage patients to use the sensor daily. Therefore, the design should consider a non-invasive measurement of vital signs, simple structure and small size.

We have integrated off-the-shelf heart rate and oxygen sensors with the ProMove sensor node, in order to monitor the patient's status during exercising and thus prevent the risk of exacerbation.

5.3. Feedback Devices

These devices are targeted to manage a high-level feedback for the user in three different ways. Firstly, they are meant to communicate the information sent by the networked system to the user in a form of assessed information about the physical status or training program history. Secondly, they are intended to serve as a communication bridge between caregivers and the patient. Finally, they should enhance motivation for physical activity. In order to translate this feedback to the user, a multi-modal sensory interaction should be applied for these devices by displaying, receiving, accessing and sending information either with visual, auditory or tangible interfaces. For instance, there is a general idea that communicating feedback on already daily-life objects would enable intuitive and natural interactions, increasing the user-acceptance and truthfulness. These objects comprise those already embedded in user's home and life, such as TV, lamps, mobile and computer. It is also important to consider that these devices are meant to serve mainly elderly people, so that simplicity is required to accomplish the interaction with ease.

Feedback can be given when the patient is either inside or outside its home. This poses a question whether the feedback should be integrated into house appliances or it should be a portable device. For the initial experiments, we have chosen two such devices that together meet the requirements for both cases:

1. *Mobile phone.* Mobile phones can be used to access and facilitate the communication between patients, caregivers and friends remotely (outdoors and indoors), while providing feedback about physical status. A mobile phone can

be carried around by the patient and it is thus suitable for giving feedback on activities while the patient is on the move. A disadvantage is that the small screen and touch-based interface might not be suitable to COPD patients as they are unfamiliar with the technology. Elderly patients would find this particularly frustrating due to complex interfaces and usage difficulties, decreasing self-motivation making harder the acceptance of a new device. However, some target users seem to be familiar with integrated technologies (mobile and touch-based interfaces) into their daily life.
2. *Photo frame.* This is an integrated central device into people's daily life and patients are likely to be familiar with it. The photo frame offers an intuitive interface, making it a good opportunity to provide suitable feedback for in-home usage.

We are designing a friendly user interfaces for both mobile phones and photo frames that will be tested for usability and acceptance by COPD patients during the initial experiments. These experiments are expected give insight and motivation about the right feedback devices to be used with the targeted patients group.

6. Functional Overview

In accordance to the requirements analysis, the system architecture supports two main lines of functionality:

- Long-term, *daily physical activity monitoring and stimulation* using wireless sensor networks and intuitive, light-based feedback devices. The system monitors the amount of activity, type of activity, distribution of activity (daily activity pattern), activity intensity and certain types of activities like walking. Patients receive feedback about their activity in order to improve physical condition and quality of life.
- *Physical exercises – training and coaching* – specifically designed for COPD patients, using collaborative intelligence of wireless sensors and a stimulating gaming interface. Interaction and entertaining feedback are essential aspects for convincing patients to perform physical exercises that can be perceived as extremely tiring and tedious in their condition. Patients receive feedback about the right execution of the exercise and safety.

In the following we present the functional architectural overview, with respect to the two lines of functionality mentioned above. The reader is also referred for reference to the top-level architectural view from Fig. 1.

6.1. Activity Monitoring

The main characteristics of this function are the following:

- The primary technical concern is to ensure an optimal trade-off among performance (accuracy of activity monitoring), energy efficiency (for long-term operation of the system) and usability (simple to use, wear etc.).

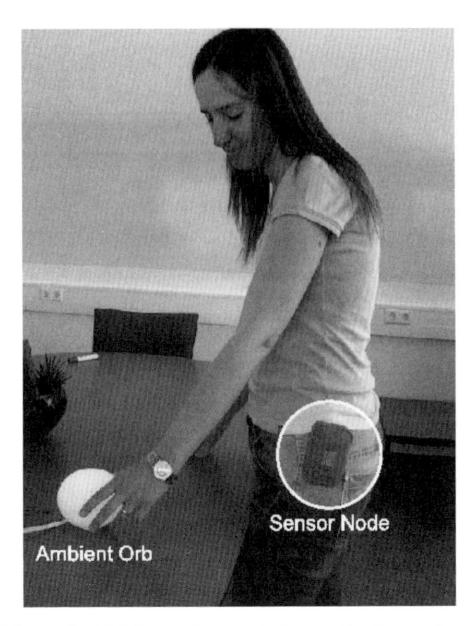

Figure 5. Initial prototype activity monitoring system.

- Because of energy efficiency and usability aspects, only a small subset of sensors from the BSN should be used. For simple activity monitoring, to assess the amount of activity for example, only one sensor node equipped with an accelerometer might be sufficient.
- Feedback should be provided in the form of summaries of long-term assessment of the user activity, but also on a daily basis.
- Summaries of the activity results are primarily targeted for the patient himself, but could be presented to caregivers as well.

Figure 5 shows the prototype activity monitoring system developed in IS-ACTIVE. The subject is wearing a ProMove node at the waist that estimates the energy expenditure by measuring the amount of motion a person performs during daily life. The ProMove node connects wirelessly to a LED-based lamp housed in a diffuse glass orb. The orb glows towards the activity level represented as a color between red and green, where red signifies that the subject was not sufficiently active, while green indicates that the subject has performed enough physical activity during the present day.

6.2. Exercise Coaching

The main characteristics of this function are the following:

- The primary technical concern is to provide accurate interpretation of the user's motions, along with motivating coaching during exercising. Energy efficiency is not a major concern due to the relatively short duration of the exercises.
- The BSN plus TAOs are involved to create a sensor-enhanced exercising experience to the user. Multi-source, multi-type sensor information is needed for accurate tracking of user motion. Additionally, physiological sensors should be in the loop, in order to ensure the safety limits of user's capabilities.

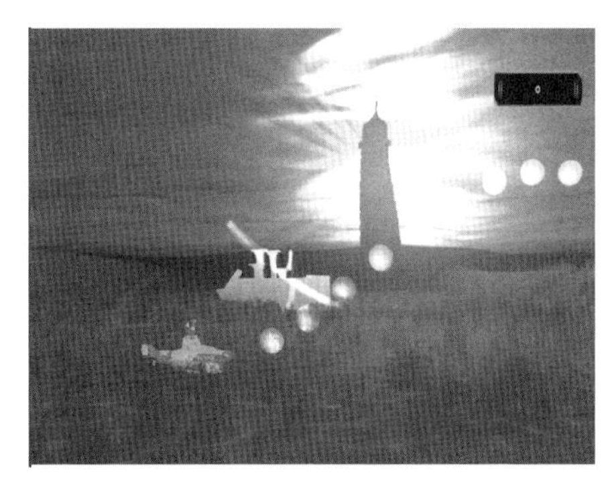

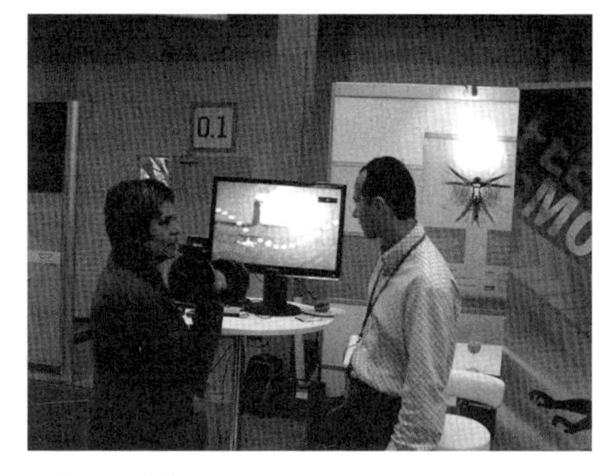

Figure 6. Gaming as exercise coaching.

- Feedback should be provided in a way that stimulates the correct and complete execution of the training exercises.
- The connection with the care center is less relevant. Possibly overall metrics characterizing the performance during training could be reported to the care giver for post-analysis.

Figure 6 shows a prototype game developed. This game is meant to stimulate patients to do exercises with a dumbbell. The up-down movement is detected by the ProMove sensor node attached to a regular dumbbell or embedded in the customized dumbbell presented in Section 5.1. The submarine goes up and down following the movement of the patient's arm and scores points by going through a sinusoidal arrangement of air bubbles. Oxygen saturation readings help prevent the risk of exacerbation: when the oxygen level reaches a certain threshold, the game stops and advises the user to take a break.

7. The Business Perspective

The project consortium aims to valorize the knowledge achieved and the technology developed concerning telemonitoring and coaching of COPD patients and to translate this knowledge into use in daily practice. Pilot programs will be first set up in the three countries involved (The Netherlands, Norway and Romania) to address the adoption of the technology into the COPD treatment program, the impact on the healthcare processes and health status of the patients. Health outcome will be assessed and changes in the health care process compared to the traditional treatment. In addition, privacy [14], patient satisfaction and compliance will be taken into account. If successful, parties with a proven track record in telemedicine service development and COPD care could realize the deployment.

Figure 7 shows the business chain that we foresee for the commercialization of the IS-ACTIVE system. The project partners generate the know-how, technology and validation means. The end users are not only the COPD patients, but they are also represented by family, insurance companies or housing companies. A third-party service provider is necessary for the installation, helpdesk and alarming towards the care center and family.

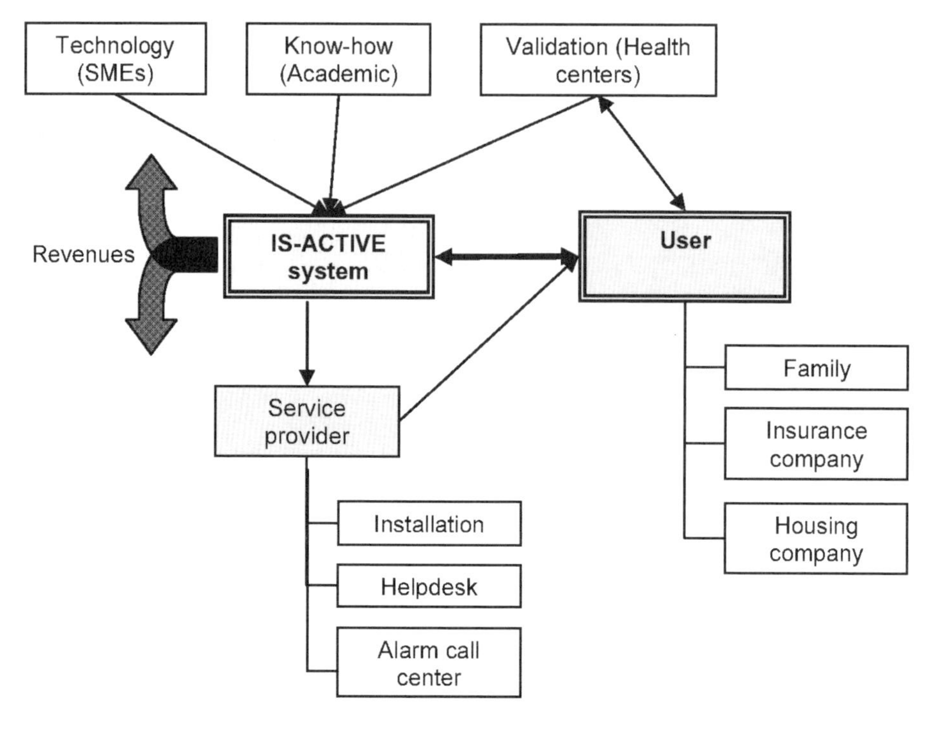

Figure 7. The business chain.

8. Conclusions

This chapter presented an architecture for monitoring, coaching, and stimulating patients with chronicle deceases. We emphasize the role of the home as care environment, by providing real-time support to patients in order to monitor, self-manage and improve their physical condition according to their specific situation.

The use of wireless sensor networking system provide distributed sensing and intelligent recognition of activities and situations, as well as simple and ubiquitous feedback modalities, thus taking complex computer interaction out of the loop and breaking the digital divide. The home becomes the main care environment, where the users can continuously monitor, self-manage and improve their physical condition according to their specific situation.

References

[1] Ascension Technology, http://www.ascensiontech.com/.

[2] R.F. Boian, H. Kourtev, K.M. Erickson, J.E. Deutsch, J.A. Lewis and G.C. Burdea, Dual stewart-platform gait rehabilitation system for individuals post-stroke, in: *Proc. of the International Workshop on Virtual Rehabilitation*, 2003, p. 92.

[3] C. Chang, R. Ansari and A. Khokhar, Cyclic articulated human motion tracking by sequential ancestral simulation, in: *Proc. of IEEE Conference on Computer Vision and Pattern Recognition*, 2003.

[4] Codamotion, http://www.charndyn.com/.

[5] CyberGlove, http://www.vrealities.com/cyber.html.

[6] S. Dulman and P.J.M. Havinga, Operating system fundamentals for the EYES distributed sensor network, *Progress*, the Netherlands, 2002.

[7] G. Engelberger, Helpmate, a service robot with experience, *Ind. Robot. Int. J.* **25**(2) (1998), 101–104.

[8] J. Garcia-Aymerich, P. Lange, M. Benet, P. Schnohr and J.M. Antó, Regular physical activity reduces hospital admission and mortality in chronic obstructive pulmonary disease: A population based cohort study, *Thorax* **61** (2006), 772–778.

[9] P.J.M. Havinga and G.J.M. Smit, Minimizing energy consumption for wireless computers in Moby Dick, in: *IEEE Int. Conf. on Personal Wireless Communication (ICPWC)*, Mumbai, India, IEEE Computer Society, 1997, pp. 306–311, ISBN 0-7803-4298-4.

[10] InterSense, http://www.isense.com/products/prec/is600/.

[11] Is-Active project, http:// http://www.is-active.eu/.

[12] M. Ivana, M. Trivedi, E. Hunter and P. Cosman, Human body model acquisition and tracking using voxel data, *Int. J. Comp. Vis.* **53**(3) (2003), 199–223.

[13] H. Krebs, B. Volpe, M. Aisen and N. Hogan, Increasing productivity and quality of care: Robot-aided nero-rehabilitation, *J. Rehab. Res. Dev.* **37**(6) (2000), 639–652.

[14] Y.W. Law and P.J.M. Havinga, How to secure a wireless sensor network, in: *2nd Int. Conf. on Intelligent Sensors, Sensor Networks and Information Processing (ISSNIP)*, Melbourne, Australia, IEEE Computer Society, 2005, pp. 89–95, ISBN 0-7803-9399-6.

[15] P. Lum, D. Reinkensmeyer, R. Mahoney, W. Rymer and C. Burgar, Robotic devices for movement therapy after stroke: Current status and challenges to clinical acceptance, *Top Stroke Rehab.* **8**(4) (2002), 40–53.

[16] D.M. Mannina and A.S. Buist, Global burden of COPD: Risk factors, prevalence and future trends, *The Lancet* **370** (Sept. 2007).

[17] M. Marin-Perianu, C. Lombriser, O. Amft, P. Havinga and G. Troster, Distributed activity recognition with fuzzy-enabled wireless sensor networks, in: *International Conference on Distributed Computing in Sensor Systems (DCOSS)*, 2008, pp. 296–313.

[18] R.S. Marin-Perianu, M. Marin-Perianu, P.J.M. Havinga and J. Scholten, Movement-based group awareness with wireless sensor networks, in: *5th International Conference on Pervasive Computing (Pervasive)*, 13–16 May 2007, Toronto, Canada, Lecture Notes in Computer Science, Vol. 4480, Springer Verlag, 2007, pp. 298–315, ISBN 978-3-540-72036-2.

[19] C. Mavroidis, J. Nikitczuk, G. Weinberg, B. Danaher, K. Jensen, J. Pelletier, P. Prugnarola, R. Stuart, R. Arango, M. Leahey, R. Pavone, A. Provo and D. Yasevac, Smart portable rehabilitation devices, *J. NeuroEng. Rehab.* **2** (2005).

[20] Microstrain, http://www.microstrain.com/.

[21] Northern Digital Inc., http://www.ndigital.com/polaris.php.

[22] Polhemus, http://www.polhemus.com/.

[23] PowerGlove, http://en.wikipedia.org/wiki/Power_Glove.

[24] ProMove wireless inertial sensor node, http://inertia-technology.com/.

[25] Qualisys, http://www.qualisys.se/.

[26] D. Reinkensmeyer, L. Kahn, M. Averbuch, A. McKenna-Cole, B. Schmit and W. Rymer, Understanding, treating arm movement impairment after chronic brain injury: Progress with the arm guide, *J. Rehab. Res. Dev.* **37**(6) (2000), 653–662.

[27] K. Sohrabi, J. Gao, V. Ailawadhi and G.J. Pottie, Protocols for self-organization of a wireless sensor network, *IEEE Personal Communications* 7(5) (Oct. 2000), 16–27.

[28] J. Sullivan, M. Eriksson, S. Carlsson and D. Liebowitz, Automating multi-view tracking and reconstruction of human motion, in: *European Conference on Computer Vision*, 2002.

[29] L.F.W. van Hoesel and P.J.M. Havinga, A TDMA-based MAC Protocol for WSNs, in: *Proc. of the 2nd International Conference on Embedded Networked Sensor Systems (SENSYS 2004)*, 3–5 Nov. 2004, Baltimore, USA, ACM, 2004, pp. 303–304, ISBN 1-58113-879-2.

[30] VICON, http://www.vicon.com/.

[31] World Health Organization, Chronic Diseases and Health Promotion, Chronic diseases and their common risk factors, Information sheet, 2007, http://www.who.int/chp/chronic_disease_report/media/Factsheet1.pdf.

[32] World Health Organization, Global Strategy on Diet, Physical Activity and Health, Facts related to chronic diseases, 2007, http://www.who.int/dietphysicalactivity/publications/facts/chronic/en/index.html.

[33] C. Wren, A. Azarbayejani, T. Darrell and A. Pentland, Pfinder: Real-time tracking of the human body, *IEEE Trans. Pattern Anal. Mach. Intell.* **19**(7) (1997), 780–785.

[34] Xsens, http://www.xsens.com/.

[35] H. Zhou and H. Hu, Human motion tracking for rehabilitation – A survey, *Biomedical Signal Processing* **3**(1) (January 2008), 1–18.

[36] H. Zimmermann, OSI reference model – The ISO model of architecture for open systems interconnection. 4, s.l., *IEEE Transactions on Communications* **COM-28** (1980).

Handbook of Ambient Assisted Living
J.C. Augusto et al. (Eds.)
IOS Press, 2012

doi:10.3233/978-1-60750-837-3-640

LiKeIT – RFID-Based KeepInTouch Lifestyle Monitoring

Mario DROBICS[a,*], Angelika DOHR[a], Susanne GIESECKE[b] and Günter SCHREIER[a]
[a] *AIT Austrian Institute of Technology GmbH, Safety & Security Department, Vienna, Austria*
[b] *AIT Austrian Institute of Technology GmbH, Foresight & Policy Development Department, Vienna, Austria*

Abstract. Well-being of individuals is influenced by various mental, physical, and social aspects. While some aspects are related to personal predisposition or the environment and thus impossible or hard to change, the personal lifestyle, which can be influenced much easier, has a significant impact on several of these aspects. Frequent physical activity, for example, reduces the risk for heart related diseases and also reduces the risk of severe fractures due to falls. Consequently it is important to maintain a healthy lifestyle, throughout the whole lifespan, especially for elderly people.

When developing solutions for and with elderly people it is important to regard their different experiences, abilities, and needs. Therefore, and as the personal lifestyle may change over time, solutions supporting people in managing their lifestyle have to be flexible and cover different aspects of their lives. Furthermore solutions have to grow with the users, i.e. to be applied for a specific need firstly, but then being extended to satisfy the increased needs of the user e.g. because of changed life circumstances. Doing so, the user can get familiar with the usage of new technologies more easily and learn step-by-step how to use additional functionalities.

In the project *LiKeIT* we aim to develop a flexible solution to support elderly people in managing their lifestyle. In a stakeholder workshop at the beginning of the project physical activity, nutrition/drinking, and health were identified as the key aspects to be supported. We are currently setting up a solution incorporating intuitive data acquisition using Near-Field Communication (NFC), a tablet PC for user interaction, and various sensors, to create a flexible, yet cost efficient solution. To be able to develop an accepted and appropriate application, elderly people are involved in the ongoing development. The final application will not only support people in maintaining their lifestyle by providing them with according information and feedback, but also provide special information for other stakeholders like authorized relatives, caregivers, and physicians.

Keywords. Lifestyle management, telemonitoring, user driven design, acceptance, usability, empowerment

1. Introduction

Due to the expected effects of the global demographic trends, numerous international and national initiatives supporting the research and development of applications for the elderly have been launched [1,3,11]. A main goal of this funding is to preserve and

*Corresponding Author: Mario Drobics. E-mail: mario.drobics@ait.ac.at.

promote the independence of elderly people so that they can stay longer in their familiar environment and become less dependent on the assistance of third parties.

The actual target group for this type of applications – the elderly people – is, however, not clearly defined. Although the process of aging is a gradual one covering many different aspects of life, it is helpful to categorize the target users in some way.

"Previously, the human life-span was divided into three phases: childhood and youth were identified with education and training, adulthood with business and family work, and the third and final phase was the post-professional retirement or 'the age'" [3].

Due to the increased life expectancy in developed countries and the relatively early retirement, the definition of the "elderly" became more differentiated into older people being retired, but still being physically and mentally fit (so-called Go-Goes) and elderly who already suffer from chronic illnesses and are dependent on outside help (so-called Slow-Goes). In nursing science additionally elderly, who are in full care, are defined as so-called No-Goes [3]. When combining Go-Goes and Slow-Goes in one group, a life model with four phases is obtained. The World Health Organization (WHO) defines categories of age in a similar manner on the basis of physical strength as follows:

- **Recently olds**, who are still active and carry out normal activities without support, but can no longer participate in the working life;
- **Olds**, which already coping with difficulties and less able to perform activities;
- **Very olds**, which already have great difficulty at home or no longer cope alone [12].

Common to these classifications is a categorization in terms of health and leisure potential. The WHO further differentiates between the described process of aging according to the above, and the biological aging process. The process of aging has, for example, a significant influence on the likelihood of developing chronic diseases.

1.1. Aspects of the Process of Aging

The process of aging is influenced by the environment, lifestyle, and the presence of chronic diseases which vary with age, but do not represent the age itself. Social and economic factors such as previous occupation, education, residential area, as well as behaviors such as smoking, physical activity, activity in daily life, alcohol consumption, nutrition and social contact are also important aspects in the process of aging [12].

Another important aspect for people of advanced age is not to unnecessarily slip into a situation of dependence – for example due to the treatment of a particular disease. By supporting self-empowerment, elderly people can actively contribute in the design of their treatment and be aware about their own health status and e.g. influence it positively through a more active lifestyle and an appropriate dietary behavior. Thus, the goal of our developments is to improve personal independence by increasing the self-awareness and provide tools which support the users where needed.

1.2. Thematic Coverage

Together with end-users we have identified the following topics as being of high importance in this context:

- **Social Interaction:** Slow-Goes and No-Goes often loose social contact as they are often not mobile enough to participate in social life. Providing tools to communicate and interact with other people is therefore of high interest for these groups.
- **Activity:** Being active is of high importance when getting older as regular activity strengthens the body and thus helps to reduce injuries after accidents and enables people to take care of their own. As for many elderly people household and garden works are a major part of their daily activities, it is important to cover these activities, too, and make people aware in case of decreasing activity.
- **Nutrition:** Eating and drinking behavior have a large influence on the wellbeing of elderly people. In the worst case, this can lead to obesity or malnutrition. It is therefore important to increase the awareness of an adequate and balanced nutrition behavior already at a relatively early age.
- **Health:** Health plays a major role in the life of elderly people suffering from chronic diseases like diabetes, dementia, etc. Simplifying the treatment of those diseases not only eases their everyday life, but can also increase their personal safety by ensuring automatic alarms in case of a deteriorating health status.
- **Safety:** Living alone often causes fear of having an accident and being unable to call for help. This includes falls, accidents in the kitchen, but also general safety e.g. when leaving the home. It is therefore important to provide elderly with tools, which support them regarding these issues and which, in case they cannot call for help on their own, automatically call for assistance.

1.3. Technology for Elderly People

People of advanced age represent a special target group in terms of technology development. Due to their existing experience of life and their past experiences with objects of every daily life (e.g. TV, mobile phones) and the according cognitive-related tasks (e.g. selecting a desired channel, adjusting the volume), fixed assignments of tasks to objects have been done. If an object such as a cell phone (which is associated with the functionality of make a phone call) suddenly is also able to fulfill other tasks, elderly people often react insecure and even skeptical, especially when the target and the additional tasks have not been clearly defined in advance [6].

The problems elderly people encounter when dealing with information and communication technology (ICT) can be summarized as follows:

- Cognitive Complexity: For people of higher age the information processing applied in technical applications is often hard to understand. A simple design of the user interface and the individual modules is necessary.
- Motivation: Motivation covers aspects like attitude, fears, restraint and acceptance. Contrary to the general opinion that elderly people do not want to use new technologies, we have observed in previous projects, that innovative technical applications are accepted and also gained popularity when the benefits of the solution are clearly described and the questions and fears of the users are addressed [6].
- Physical challenges: physical constraints due to the biological aging process, such as decreased mobility of the fingers, impaired vision, impaired hearing

and longer reaction periods affect the applicability of technical aids for the elderly and must be taken into consideration.

Because of these challenges, the following design principles regarding the development of technical applications for elderly people have been identified to be of high importance:

1. Technology shall be designed to support the users, but must not dominate their daily routines
2. Elderly people have individual needs and knowledge in terms of technology, which have to be considered and
3. User interface design must be intuitive and tailored to the needs of the user group, as elderly people are often not used to this type of technological applications.

In applications for people of advanced age, it is also important to consider the tension between support and independence, and between privacy and autonomy. For example, it is not advisable to generate an automatic shopping list with the products lacking in the refrigerator, when the old person still manages the relevant and cognitively demanding task of writing the shopping list. Another example would be a medication reminder for someone, who is still able to take his medication regularly and reliably. Thus, technical applications are primarily intended to compensate for physical deterioration, reduction of cognitive processes, and to support everyday life of elderly people [8].

2. Methods

2.1. User-Centered Design – Stakeholder Workshop

To design a technical application as good as possible for a chosen user group, it is important to involve the users into the planning and development of a product as early and as long as possible. The classical methods of user-centered design as "paper prototyping", which were used by other researchers in this field [9] have considered to be inappropriate in the LiKeIT project, as not only primary and secondary endusers (i.e. endusers and other stakeholders) have been involved, but also lobbyists. To obtain a broad range of possible assistance and prevention strategies for elderly people, a stakeholder workshop with participants from different fields was organized. Participants from the following research fields were involved in the discussion of the different areas of applications and potential solutions:

- Research
- Social science
- Technology
- Nutrition
- Nursing science
- Medicine and
- Retiree lobbyists

The objective of the workshop was to identify the overlap of actual social needs in the health sector and possible IT-based solutions in AAL.

The stakeholder workshop took a non-hierarchical approach and was designed to acknowledge multiple visions, thereby tackling new paths of stakeholder integration, technology development and policy options. The workshop was divided into three question sessions and a group work. In the question sessions moderation cards were handed out to the participants of the workshop. After the questions had been asked, all participants had the opportunity to write their answers to the moderation cards, which were then discussed and fitted on pin boards.
The questions of the three sessions were:

1. What are the crucial events and developments that lead to increased dependency and continuous care?
2. From your experience – what are the shortcomings in the care / support of users in this new phase of life?
3. How could these deficits be prevented?

Grouping the responses from the three question sessions, two topics emerged for the subsequent group work, for which actual ICT solutions would be needed:

- Chronic disease and
- Food and drinking behavior.

2.2. Technologies Used

2.2.1. The Internet of Things

Besides the stakeholder workshop, we explored the technical capabilities to be implemented in a lifestyle management solution for the elderly.

The Internet of Things (IoT), a recent development branch within ICT, facilitates everyday objects with intelligence and thus, offers a suitable infrastructure for a broad range of applications in the field of AAL.
The IoT is a combination of developments and concepts from the fields of:

- Ubiquitous Communication / connectivity,
- Pervasive Computing and
- Ambient Intelligence [5].

The ability of objects to communicate with each other by means of the Internet protocol and to form a network of things, represents the core idea of this development. Prerequisites for the IoT include the availability of broadband solutions for Internet access and wireless local area networks (WLAN) in regular households. Another important technology for the IoT is Radio Frequency Identification (RFID), which is primarily used for the identification of various people and objects of everyday life and for the exchange of data over short distances [7].

2.2.2. KeepInTouch (KIT)

In previous projects we have developed a telemonitoring concept for acquisition and dissemination of health data called "KeepInTouch" (KIT). The intuitive method of data acquisition, by bringing a collector (e.g. mobile phone) close to the appropriate object (e.g. blood pressure meter), provides an intuitive person-machine interface and retains the user's full control on which data is to be transmitted or not. The usability of this approach has already been proven in several case studies for different chronic diseases like diabetes, hypertension, or congestive heart failure as well as in the AAL field [6,10].

KIT is based on various wireless communication technologies such as Bluetooth, ZigBee and near field communication (NFC) and additionally offers the advantages of simple operation and maintainability. Thus, KIT can be used in a wide variety of applications.

3. Results

The stakeholder workshop was attended by a total of 15 participants from research, social science, engineering, food, medicine and nursing science and senior representatives. It was stated, that an essential support for elderly people can be provided by gathering lifestyle and health parameters, process them, eventually visualize them, forward them (to doctors, care givers, etc.), and store them. The direct provision of according user feedback on the collected data is another important aspect for elderly people. As a consequence, self-awareness and self-responsibility of the users should be increased, as they can inquire on their health status by themselves and learn about its relation to their personal lifestyle by receiving according and direct feedback messages. This approach leads to increased safety of the users, as in case of critical situations an alarm can be triggered automatically.

A further objective of the project is to identify opportunities for technical assistance in the area of prevention.

- Primary prevention is concerned with the identification of causes and risk factors for diseases. It addresses social groups (children, men / women, etc.) and includes activities such as vaccinations, awareness campaigns, etc.
- Secondary Prevention: At an individual level, diseases and disabilities are to be identified and treated in time, in order to avoid the risk or deterioration of health. This includes measures for fall prevention, screening for certain forms of disease (breast cancer, prostate cancer), or even screening for malnutrition or regular blood pressure measurements.
- Tertiary prevention: If a disease has already occurred then the tertiary prevention ensures that there is no worsening of the condition or the disease. On the one hand, the negative side-effects of the treatment shall be reduced, while on the other hand the negative consequences of the disease itself shall be mitigated. Tertiary prevention includes rehabilitative activities, social integration, tele-monitoring for chronic diseases, etc.

The use cases covered by the project LiKeIT will focus on aspects related to secondary prevention, but include modules to support tertiary prevention as well.

3.1. Use Cases

3.1.1. Activity and Nutrition

The field of nutrition and drinking also covers aspects like overweight, activity, nutrition related to certain diseases such as e.g. heart failure (these topics are not necessarily age related). Sarcopenia, the degenerative loss of skeletal muscle mass and associated with this, strength, is, however, primarily related to age, but can be influenced by nutrition and activity. Especially women are more vulnerable for sarcopenia and osteoporosis, due to an increases tendency to malnutrition.

During the discussion it was noted, that due to a reduced sense of taste, many elderly people have a preference for sweets they still can taste. This should be considered in the monitoring of nutrition behavior.

The group also discussed which data should be monitored, in order to provide nutritionists and physicians a basis to track the user's health status. A rough indicator might be based on a regular assessment of the user's appetite and body weight. The appetite could, for example, be rated with the categories "high – medium – low" by the users themselves. One possible quantitative measurement would be the usage of plate symbols and associating different plates with low food intake, moderate and large food intake, respectively. Another possibility would be clicking certain icons on a monitor, which refer to different foods (meat, fruits, cereals, etc.). The body weight should be measured regularly (e.g. four times per year).

This approach is, however, restricted by the individual perception which implies the need to consider this information relative to previous reports. Empirical experience has shown that older women eat smaller portions at home. In hospitals or nursing homes, they eat only half portions.

Other possible approaches to monitor the eating behavior in private homes can incorporate sensors mounted on the cutlery drawer, refrigerator, toaster, microwave and oven. This information can then be used to create interaction profiles which provide a good indicator for detecting changes in behavior over time. When "Meals on Wheels" services are used, it can easily be recorded what food is ordered (although this does not necessarily reflect the actual and complete eating behavior). Nevertheless, this data might be combined with some user provided information to obtain a more thorough view on the users eating habits.

Another topic that was discussed in the group was how to design the feedbacks, sent out to the users. Concerning textual feedback messages it was widely agreed, that these messages have to be formulated individually and with great variety. However, they should be easy to grasp. Traffic lights or different symbols (smiley) can provide people a long-term feedback on their lifestyle status. By differentiating the symbols in subcategories, special aspects can be highlighted. A possible grouping could cover nutrition, drinking and activity.

These symbols should be easily and constantly visible and thus provide a discreet reminder to achieve a healthy lifestyle. Such an interface could also be easily extended to remind people on other events, e.g. their regular drug intake.

For the assessment of movement and activity a pedometer or accelerometer, worn throughout the day, seems to be appropriate. While a pedometer only gives very basic information about the steps carried out, an accelerometer can also provide more detailed information about the quality of the activity (walking, running, etc.). With specific accelerometers it is furthermore possible to detect anomalies in the locomotory system.

The group agreed on the fact that such a system has to be modular in order to adapt over time and according to individual needs. Thus, users should be able to start with a simple activity monitoring, and extend the functionality of the system with increasing demand. This also gives users time to get used to the system, as they can focus on one topic at a given time.

The group was also asked, how long a user will most likely be interested in such an application before getting bored and ignoring the provided support. The group was concerned that the effect may wear out after six months to one year and that the focus should then be shifted to another topic (e.g. from activity to nutrition).

3.1.2. Management of Chronic Diseases

For people suffering from chronic diseases like hypertension, chronic heart failure or diabetes, it is of special importance to track not only their health parameters regularly, but also to put this information in context to their current living situation. By combining these two sources of information, a detailed picture of the disease including relevant influences can be obtained. By providing this information in an aggregated way to the user, he/she is enabled to take responsibility about his/her disease and to actively contribute to his treatment.

A major issue is to preserve independence, i.e. to support the users, to actively decide, what data is collected, what purpose the data is used for and who should have access to the data.

It was noted, that for such applications usability – including the way feedbacks are presented, visualization using different bright lights, and acoustic signals, etc. – is of major importance to achieve a high acceptance of the proposed system.

Possible technical applications which might improve comfort for people of advanced age suffering from chronic diseases are for example the integration of the "bio-weather" in daily life to support, e.g. people with high blood pressure. The need to collect health parameters on a regular schedule was also stressed since a uninterrupted collection of health data further allows gaining a detailed picture of the trend of the health state of the user. A change in rhythm of life might be taken as an indication for deterioration of health (of the physical or general condition).

3.2. LiKeIT System Architecture

Lifestyle management for elderly people is to become available to a large group in the near future. Thus, the system architecture was designed using different technologies and components, to support a high degree of flexibility and configurability. Figure 1 shows the proposed system architecture.

To collect measurements from medical devices by the user – i.e. the elderly people – AIT's KeepInTouch technology (KIT) is used. To obtain data from the medical devices and symbol cards, a mobile NFC reader is used. During the trial, an adapted mobile phone will be used for this task. The supported devices are:

- body weight scales,
- blood pressure meters,
- symbol cards with integrated RFID tags,
- pedometers and
- glucose meters.

The lower part of Fig. 1 represents the primary data collection together with the according devices.

Within the project LiKeIT a tablet-PC is used which can be operated via a touch screen as well as by reading in symbol cards using the mobile NFC reader. This Tablet-PC represents the main communication terminal of the system for the user.

In addition to the active data measurement and collection a wireless BlackBox will be placed in the user apartment's reception room, which is often perceived as a location for communication to the outside. This BlackBox will be equipped with a WLAN module and serial ports, which can connect to contact sensors and NFC readers. Contact sensors can for example be used to record, when and how often the house door is

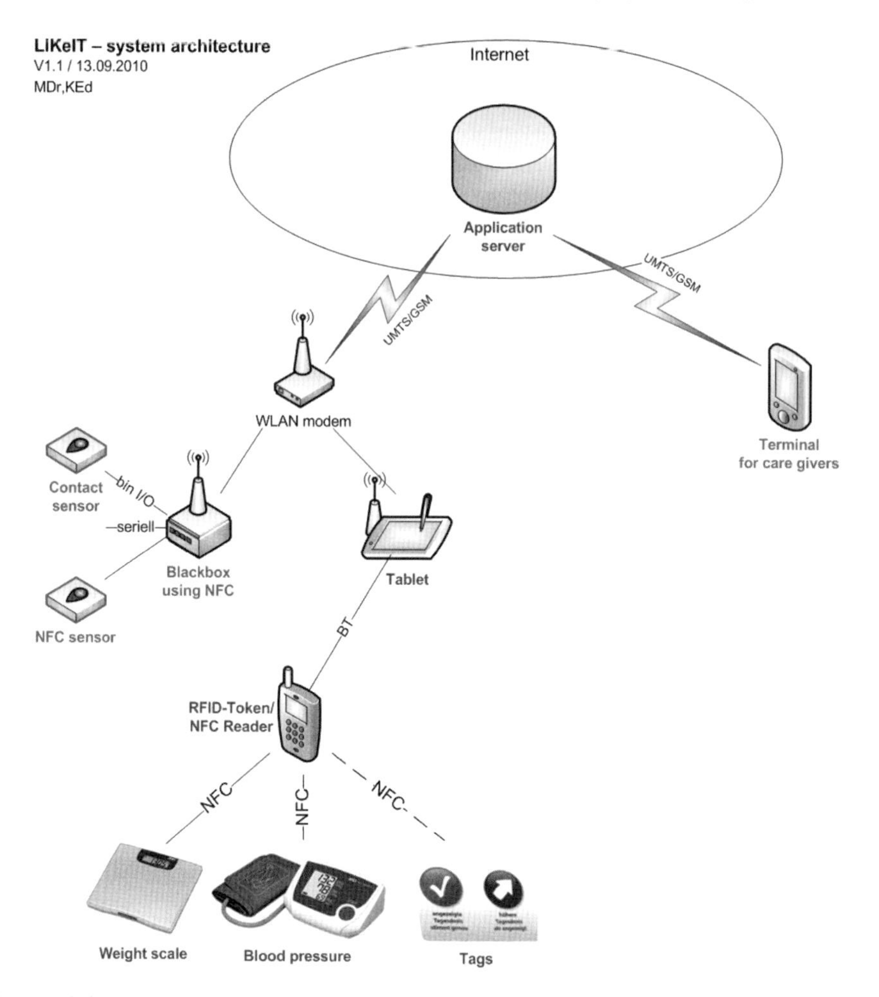

Figure 1. Selected components and system architecture for the collection of lifestyle parameters for elderly people.

opened. The NFC sensor in the apartment's entrance is basically apparent to identify medical and nursing staff.

The data exchange between the BlackBox and the Tablet and the configuration of the BlackBox is done via WLAN. A standard WLAN/UMTS modem is used to communicate with the remote server.

The Tablet-PC also functions as a maintenance terminal, which uses a service interface to communicate with the application server, where the data of the user is stored. Having access to the user's data will enable care givers and physicians to improve their services and to support their clients in a more individual manner.

3.3. Implementation

Currently the platform for the collection of nutrition, drinking behavior and activity data is being implemented. To meet the requirements for an appropriate nutrition and drinking behavior for the elderly, a nutritionist was interviewed to obtain comprehensive information about the lack in nutrients, elderly people are likely suffering from. As quantitative measurements are always very subjective, it was decided to make a qualitative data collection for the nutrient groups "fruit/vegetables", "cereal/potatoes", "milk/milk products" and "meat/fish/egg" and a quantitative collection only for sweets, as well as for the amount of drinking. This data can be captured easily by touching according symbols on the tablet.

For the collection of activity data, three different kinds of activity have been defined: "Garden/household", "Going for a walk" and "Sports", which are differently valuated and multiplied with the time and duration, they were carried out.

Optionally, the health status can be monitored using a blood pressure meter. The health status is then assessed by computing the percentage of measurements in the individual target zone.

This data is then agglomerated by calculating a "vital-index", which reflects the overall status of wellbeing of the elderly person and thus gives feedback on their quality of life. Detailed information on the different categories can be obtained easily, to enhance the people's self-awareness and to increase their motivation towards a healthier lifestyle.

3.4. Next Steps

The system was evaluated by a group of elderly people in the last month. These people were interviewed before and after the test period, to obtain information about their background and expectations, as well as their experiences and ideas for improvement. Based on their feedback, the interface and data capturing is currently being adopted for the second trial period.

4. Discussion

The system architecture shown in Fig. 1 forms the basis for a very dynamic and comprehensive platform for improving the quality of life and safety of elderly people. Using the various interfacing and communication technologies (WLAN, NFC, KIT) the platform can be extended and adopted flexibly to new applications. The usage of such technologies in the context of AAL has been demonstrated by recent Spanish and Chinese developments [2,13].

The user-centered design approach which is being implemented in the project LiKeIT by carrying out stakeholder and focus group workshops, offers the opportunity to collect the requirements of the elderly people and their environment for the software developers themselves. One finding from the stakeholder workshop was that a system for elderly people has to offer a higher degree of customizability. This is reasonable, because elderly people are basically like young ones, just with more experience. This experience allows for giving them more room in their lives to customize an application, which is supposed to support them appropriately.

Furthermore, it is important to clearly define and communicate the purpose of such an application to prevent uncertainty and to ensure broad acceptance. A special focus on physical disabilities is, however, counterproductive and can easily lead to a stigmatization of the users as being old, which does not necessarily mean to be sick. It seems more appropriate to focus on prevention strategies by e.g. monitoring the eating habits and daily activities. Thus, a user can already use such a system during a more active period in life. Later, when different handicaps become present, the system might be expanded with specific assistive components to support the user, allowing a smooth transition into more care oriented applications. This approach also eases the introduction of new technologies, as the user can get familiar with new technologies earlier and not, when he or she is already at a more advanced age and in worse health condition.

The spatial placement in the home of the user for this communication center is advised to be in the kitchen/living room. An Italian study has shown that a spacious kitchen is often used as a welcome point for visitors and as a communication place, while the private rooms or the bedroom rather represent a private retreat [4]. For this reason, it is recommended to store medical instruments like blood pressure, blood sugar meter in the lively kitchen, as the measurement is routinely done in the morning. Additionally the central placement is intended to support a “memory effect” to achieve an active lifestyle and healthy and adequate nutrition. The communication terminal is either in the living room or in the kitchen, depending on the preferences of the user. It should at least provide a relaxed atmosphere so that the terminal can subsequently be used to communicate with the relatives.

The pedometer should either be worn permanently or stored in the entrance of the persons flat. This reminds the person to use the sensor when leaving the home and allows in combination with a NFC sensor to identify the presence/absence of the person. The NFC sensor might furthermore be used to identify not only the users, but also relatives, nurses, and other stakeholders from the surrounding of the elderly.

The other IT components shown in Fig. 1 might be used and placed depending on the preferences of the user and existing infrastructure in the apartment. Generally the placement in this paper is just an advice and should be adapted to the user’s preferences.

It is also planned to make the system accessible for caregivers from the family in the future. Especially daughters, daughters-in-law, and sons often have a bad conscience for not spending enough time with their parents or parents in-law. The mandatory call in the evening with the question of whether the drugs were taken can often be very distressing for relatives. With access to the system through the application server, possibly with a dedicated web interface, relatives authorized by the users can log into the system during the day and see, whether the blood pressure is high or the medication was taken. Thus, the telephone call in the evening is not characterized by medical questions, but can focus on more private and positive topics.

The platform therefore cannot only help to increase the well-being of elderly people, but also those who care about them.

In the project LiKeIT we are currently developing the hardware and software infrastructure with end users intensively involved, so that the specific requirements of the user can be integrated into the final system. As a consequence, ease of use and a simple integration into the daily life of the elderly are main points of development.

Acknowledgements

The project LiKeIT is funded by the “program benefit” from the Federal Ministry for Transport, Innovation and Technology (BMVIT) and is carried out in a collaboration of AIT Austrian Institute of Technology GmbH, TAGnology RFID GmbH, and ilogs, information logistics GmbH.

References

[1] AAL Association, Ambient Assisted Living (AAL) Joint Programme, [Online] [Citation from: September 8th 2009], http://www.aaleurope.eu/.
[2] J. Bravo et al., Enabling NFC technology for supporting chronic diseases: A proposal for Alzheimer caregivers, in: *AmI 2008*, Springer Verlag, Berlin Heidelberg, 2008, pp. 109–125.
[3] Bundesministerium für Verkehr, Innovation und Technologie, Programm benefit, Programmlinie "Demografischer Wandel als Chance", Abteilung III/I 5 Informations und Nanotechnologien, Raumfahrt, Renngasse 5, 1010 Wien, Bundesministerium für Verkehr, Innovation und Technologie, 2008.
[4] Chiara et al., Knocking on elders' door: Investigating the functional and emotional geography of their domestic space, in: *CHI 2009 – Designing for Senior Citizens*, Leonardi, Boston, MA, USA, 2009, pp. 1703–1711.
[5] A. Dohr et al., The Internet of Things for ambient assisted living, in: *Proceedings of Seventh International Conference on Information Technology (ITNG) 2010*, Las Vegas, 2010, pp. 804–809.
[6] M. Drobics, E. Fugger, B. Prazak-Aram and G. Schreier, Evaluation of a personal drug reminder, in: *3rd German AAL Kongress*, Berlin, 2010.
[7] S. Haller, S. Karnouskos and C. Schroth, The Internet of Things in an enterprise context, in: *Future Internet FIS 2008*, Vienna, Lecture Notes in Computer Science (LNCS), Springer, Berlin Heidelberg, 2008, pp. 14–28.
[8] E.D. Mynatt et al., Aware technologies for aging in place: Understanding user needs and attitudes, *Pervasive Computing. Successful Aging* (2004), 36–41.
[9] A. Nischelwitzer et al., Design and development of a mobile medical application for the management of chronic diseases: Methods of improved data input for older people, in: *USAB 2007*, 2007, pp. 119–132.
[10] D. Scherr et al., Effect of homebased telemonitoring using mobile phone technology on the outcome of heart failure patients after an episode of acute decompensation: The MOBIle TELemonitoring in heart failure patients study (MOBITEL), *Journal of Medical Internet Research* **11**(3) (17 August 2009), e34.
[11] H. Steg et al., Europe is facing a demographic change. Ambient assisted living offers solutions, VDI|VDE|IT, Berlin, März 2006.
[12] World Health Organization, Men ageing and health. Achieving health across the life span, World Health Organization, Geneva, 2001. 01WHO/NMH/NPH 01.2.
[13] J.K. Zao et al., Activity orientated design of Health Pal: A smart phone for elders' healthcare support, *EURASIP Journal on Wireless Communication and Networking* (2008), pp. 1–11. Hindawi Publishing Cooperation, Article ID 582194.

Handbook of Ambient Assisted Living
J.C. Augusto et al. (Eds.)
IOS Press, 2012

doi:10.3233/978-1-60750-837-3-652

SmartSenior – Intelligent Services for Senior Citizens

Michael C. BALASCH[a,*], Martin SCHULTZ[b], Christine CARIUS-DUESSEL[b], Dr. Michael JOHN[c], Joachim HÄNSEL[c], Norbert PIETH[c], Thilo ERNST[c], Jörn KISELEV[n], Gerd KOCK[c], Ben HENNIG[d], Klaus F. WAGNER[e], Marten HAESNER[n], Elisabeth STEINHAGEN-THIESSEN[n], Mehmet GÖVERCIN[n] Jan-Peter JANSEN[f], Markus SCHRÖDER[g], Matthias MASUR[h], Tobias LEIPOLD[i], Irina BUSCH[b], Stefan ZEIDLER[a], Dr. Sibylle MEYER[j], Uta BÖHM[j], Christa FRICKE[j], Claudia SPINDLER[k], Harald KLAUS[a], Fabienne WAIDELICH[l], Jens-Uwe BUSSER[l], Wolfgang KLASEN[l] and Katrin MÜLLER[m]

[a]*Deutsche Telekom AG, Innovation Laboratories, Berlin, Germany*
[b]*Telemedicine Center Charité (TMCC), Charité Universitätsmedizin, Berlin, Germany*
[c]*Fraunhofer-Institut für Rechnerarchitektur und Softwaretechnik FIRST, Berlin, Germany*
[d]*Deutsches Forschungsinstitut für Künstliche Intelligenz (DFKI), Saarbrücken, Germany*
[e]*Klinikum Südstadt Rostock, Germany*
[f]*Schmerzzentrum Berlin, Germany*
[g]*Tembit Software GmbH, Berlin, Germany*
[h]*Prisma GmbH, Berlin, Germany*
[i]*Clinpath GmbH, Berlin, Germany*
[j]*SIBIS Institut für Sozialforschung, Berlin, Germany*
[k]*trommsdorff + drüner GmbH, Berlin, Germany*
[l]*Siemens AG, CT T, GTF IT Security, Munich, Germany*
[m]*Siemens AG, Berlin, Germany*
[n]*Forschungsgruppe Geriatrie der Charité Universitätsmedizin, Berlin, Germany*

Abstract. SmartSenior is the largest Ambient Assisted Living research project in Germany, and is scheduled to run from 2009 to 2012. It aims to develop technologically innovative services that will enable older people to continue living in their own homes for longer, and stay independent for longer. SmartSenior is oriented to customers' needs for safety, health, and independence as well as optimum usability. Appliances and services from Ambient Assisted Living (AAL) and (tele-)medicine are integrated into an overall concept to create a comprehensive, modular solution. Research also focuses on the development of role and business models promising effective exploitation and on general issues such as privacy protection and sustainability of AAL services. Selected aspects and current research results of SmartSenior are presented in this article.

* Corresponding author: Michael C. Balasch, Head of Ageing Society/eHealth, Innovation Development, Deutsche Telekom AG, Innovation Laboratories, Ernst-Reuter-Platz 7, 10587 Berlin, Germany. E-mail: michael.balasch@telekom.de.

Keywords. Ambient assisted living, audiovisual services, chronic pain, cooperative business models, data privacy, data privacy laws, emergency assistance, falls, health management, independent living, interactive physical therapy environment, interoperability, multimodal user interface, multimorbidity, older people, pain diary, physical activity, quality of service, safety, sensor, smartphone application, security at home, serious games, social communication, standards, stroke, sustainability, testbed, transparency, telemedicine, telemonitoring, usability, vital data monitoring

Introduction

Michael C. BALASCH
Deutsche Telekom AG, Innovation Laboratories, Berlin, Germany

The aim of the SmartSenior research project is to develop technologically innovative services that will enable older people to continue living in their own homes for longer, and stay independent for longer. The project provides intelligent living environments that help older people to maintain their quality of life in terms of health, social interaction and financial position.

The project brings together a total of 28 partners, including large corporations, research institutes and small and medium-sized enterprises (SMEs). It is the largest Ambient Assisted Living project co-funded by the German Federal Ministry of Education and Research (BMBF) currently running in Germany.

SmartSenior is based on an integrated overall concept comprising health, security, services and communication solutions with standardized and intuitive user interfaces. By linking new technologies with social networks, the project aims to enhance and optimize care and comfort for older people.

Research in the project focuses on three main questions:

- How can senior citizens maintain their mobility and stay safe when on the go?
- How can senior citizens stay healthy – and get well quicker when they do get sick?
- What do senior citizens need to remain independent and to be able to stay in their own home environments for longer?

Differing qualities of life can be attributed to the scenarios “Be safe on the go”, “Get well and stay healthy” and “Live independently at home for longer”. In essence, this means that in the event of an emergency, life-preserving medical procedures are carried out as soon as possible. However, the organization of long-term medical prevention, alongside treatment and therapy, also needs to be optimized. In addition, SmartSenior also strives to maintain extensive autonomy for senior citizens. The aim here is to make life in a familiar environment easier, both in the home and while interacting socially with other people and service providers. Not least, the aim is to significantly enhance the level of comfort and quality of life of senior citizens through new communications solutions, innovative aids to mobility and assistance systems.

Chapter Overview

In the first chapter, we will introduce the project SmartSenior – Intelligent Services for Senior Citizens, outline its mission, scenarios and applications, the key aspects of development and the strengths of the project.

The broad, overarching approach of the project means that we are unable to cover all aspects in detail in this article. Consequently, in the following chapters focus on some selected applications and on overarching topics with fundamental relevance.

Telemedical services will be provided to SmartSenior users in a wide range of scenarios, especially in the case of emergencies. In the second chapter, we outline the potentials and benefits of such services. In order to verify functionality and reliability, a testbed has been created for telemedical applications, as described in Chapter 3. This is followed by two chapters introducing applications from the health application area, covering stroke and fall patients as well as patients with chronic pain. In all SmartSenior scenarios, audiovisual communication plays an important role in enhancing interactions with doctors, care personnel, service providers, family members, and the neighbourhood. These applications and user requirements are described in Chapter 6. Integrated Ambient Assisted Living technologies allowing users to stay in their own home for as long as possible are the main focus of Chapter 7 – including the design of appropriate role and business models, which are crucial for transfering to the market at the end of the research project.

The last two chapters deal with two vital issues in the telemedicine and AAL sector: data privacy protection and the sustainability of AAL services.

1. The AAL Project SmartSenior – Intelligent Services for Senior Citizens

Michael C. BALASCH
Deutsche Telekom AG, Innovation Laboratories, Berlin, Germany

SmartSenior is the largest Ambient Assisted Living research project currently running in Germany. The kick-off was in July 2009; the project is scheduled to run for three years. It aims to develop technologically innovative services that will enable older people to continue living in their own homes for longer, and stay independent for as long as possible. The outcomes of the project will provide intelligent technologies and services to help older people maintain their quality of life, in terms of health, social interaction and financial position.

1.1. Motivation

The proportion of older people among the total population in Germany is rising. It is more important than ever before to maintain senior citizens' standard of living. Independence, mobility, safety and health are significant factors for quality of life of older people.

The demand for services to aid independent living is growing at a rapid rate. In 2008, some 32.2 million people (39% of the German population) were aged 50 or older. During the course of demographic change, the number of 50+ households will grow by 50% over the next ten years [25]. The 50+ generation is financially well-off (net income approx. € 740 billion in 2008 [36]) and willing to spend on the areas of life that are important to them.

Very often, the products and services available on the market for the 50+ generation are characterized by limited availability, poor integration and high costs. There is no integrative solution available which accommodates the varying individual needs of the target group. Furthermore, existing concepts for the use of medical equipment and services for private use, for example, lack consistency and ease of use. This represents a major hurdle to widespread user acceptance.

1.2. Mission and Scenarios

The SmartSenior project is involved in the development of new technologies to create integrated and intelligent environments, aimed at maintaining a high standard of living in old age and enabling older people to lead an independent life, carefree in their own homes for as long as possible. Drawing on the basic needs of safety, health and independence, SmartSenior activities focus on three areas:

1.2.1. Be Safe on the Go

The project aims to develop safety-enhancing, intelligent emergency detection/assistance systems, and integrate such systems into automobiles, with a view to safeguarding individual mobility. Currently, such efforts are concentrating primarily on an emergency management system with vehicle-based functionality for precise localization, automatic transmission of key medical data and an emergency stop assistant.

1.2.2. Get Well and Stay Healthy

New services are being developed in the areas of prevention, treatment and rehabilitation, and existing services are being integrated into the emerging comprehensive system. This work will culminate in an overarching system, covering various different areas of life that monitors and manages vital parameters and helps to detect, manage and prevent emergencies. Specific areas of application include fall prevention, stroke rehabilitation, pain management and telemedically supported peritoneal dialysis.

1.2.3. Live Independently at Home for Longer

Key areas of research include solutions for enhanced safety and comfort in the home environment. The project is also focusing on devising user-friendly communications tools and options. For example, the user's TV set serves as his or her central channel for communications with various themed portals, such as tenant services. These portals enable communication with service providers and offer telemedical functions. Sensor-based services for controlling and monitoring home-automation functions enhance user comfort and safety.

1.3. Key Aspects of Research and Development

In SmartSenior, the following overarching topics are prioritized:

- Consistent orientation of applications and technologies around the target group's needs.
- Using advanced usability engineering techniques to develop an age-appropriate infrastructure service offering that offers exceptional usability thanks to simple, intuitive user interfaces with a recognizable look & feel.

- Development of inconspicuous microsystem sensors for recording, monitoring and transmitting vital parameters in all the aforementioned applications.
- Provision of a basic platform with targeted and future-safe infrastructure solutions for the joint use of systems by a wide range of AAL applications, thanks to uniform information logistics and cross-organizational data linking.
- Conducting field studies with senior citizens and relevant service providers on acceptance, benefits, costs, longterm feasibility, and sustainability in "living labs", test apartments and externally.

1.4. Strengths of the Project

The approach of SmartSenior is to integrate the various results into an overall concept. Appliances and services from AAL and (tele-)medicine will thus form a comprehensive solution. At the same time, SmartSenior is consistently based around customer needs. The focus is also on the calculation of potentials, with a view to devising business models that promise effective market development.

SmartSenior combines the expertise of 28 partners from industry and academia [46] in a diverse, inter-disciplinary consortium with a regional focus in the Berlin area. Participants include small, highly specialized companies as well as established global players, from information and communications technologies, sensor manufacturers, the entertainment industry, mobility & health services, and care institutions, through to medical equipment suppliers. They are joined by research institutes with a medical and technological focus.

In meeting the complex and divergent requirements of senior living, the special challenge and opportunity for this project lies in the size of the consortium and its diverse composition. Only in this way it is possible to accommodate the broad range of the requirements. The project will cover the entire value-added chain under the motto "Live independently to an old age", thanks to partners in the relevant sectors.

2. Telemedicine for Independent Living

Martin SCHULTZ and Christine CARIUS-DUESSEL
Telemedicine Center Charité (TMCC), Charité Universitätsmedizin, Berlin, Germany

2.1. Introduction

In recent years, the establishment of new stationary and mobile broadband data communications networks, the spread of mobile communications, the growing functionality of home entertainment systems, and the development of new medical sensors has laid the foundation for medical care which is both geographically and temporally independent from the availability of medical expertise.

The linking of the various medical technologies to remote supply systems is known as telemedicine, and has already been implemented throughout almost all areas of medicine. As a result, the lines between telemedicine and "usual" IT-assisted processes in the healthcare system, e.g. in diagnostics, treatment, medical documentation and administration blurred. Therefore telemedical procedures involving the transfer of medical data are found in a wide range of apparatus-based diagnostic and treatment techniques that are well established in the medical world.

Telemedicine is currently taking a step forward in the medical care landscape by the establishment of telemedical centers. It focuses on the patient, who either benefits from the continuous monitoring of medical parameters appropriate to his chronic illness and personalized medical care, or from acute medical assistance, which averts major health threats thanks to prompt intervention.

Additionally, the round-the-clock availability of medical expertise from a telemedical center offers particularly older individuals, or those with specific care requirements, a degree of independence and peace of mind in their everyday lives. These centers can also assist individuals with personal health management, with training and with medical information and education on health issues.

Below, we describe how specific telemedical support services can help seniors and people with specific care needs to lead independent lives in their own homes without relying on conventional, institutional, hospital-centered medicine.

2.2. Telemonitoring

The regular monitoring of medical parameters using telemedical techniques is known as telemonitoring. In medicine, the regular and/or continuous monitoring of parameters is currently indicated for a wide range of medical issues. For example, by analyzing series of measurements, it is possible to gauge the patient's current health status and the efficiency of treatment (e.g. medication), or to avoid potentially threatening situations (decompensation).

2.2.1. Care Requirements for Chronic Illnesses

As a result of demographic development and of continuous improvements in medical diagnosis, the level of resources devoted to the care of patients with chronic illnesses has risen sharply in recent years. According to current calculations, around 80 percent of healthcare expenditure in Germany is allocated to the treatment and care of chronic illnesses [18] with chronic cardio-vascular conditions and chronic metabolic disorders accounting for 49 percent.

In Germany, 27 percent of insured individuals suffer from at least one chronic disease. Many chronic conditions, most of which are irreversible, accumulate as patients get older. Over-64-year-olds account for around 45 percent of total health costs across all illnesses. For chronic conditions such as diabetes, their share is around 60 percent. A similar pattern applies to costs of diseases such as dementia (98 percent), ischemic heart disease (66 percent) and malignant neoplasms (59 percent) [61]. Elderly people's higher frequency of contact with health service-providers in the broadest sense of the word leads to above-average costs for out-patient medical care, as well as for the use of medicines, medical aids and remedies [29].

2.2.2. Effects of Close-Knit Monitoring and Communication

Telemonitoring may take various forms. There are two main types: Wellness and disease management, and independent ambient-assisted monitoring [50]. Whilst the former requires the active involvement of the patient as user, ambient-assisted living solutions make no demands on the patient [66]. Both forms have their advantages. For active disease management, the patient is expected to actively record various data and transmit them to the relevant telemedical center.

In order to make it easier for older patients to use, the equipment must be suitably user-friendly and safe. One typical application area is monitoring within the context of a diabetes management program. Certain infrastructure requirements need to be created for the use of ambient-assisted living solutions. The required sensors are either worn on the body (e.g. in clothing) or positioned in the home. Often data are transmitted and evaluated automatically, which poses various ethical questions and data privacy/data protection issues.

A range of positive effects can be achieved by monitoring specific parameters and via regular communication with the patient. For example, positive effects have been achieved for patients with chronic heart failure by means of one telephone call per week by staff at a telemedical center to enquire about the patient's general state of health and compliance, and to monitor various medical parameters such as blood pressure, electrocardiogram and pulse. Studies to date on the use of telemonitoring indicate enhanced treatment compliance on the part of the patient, a reduction in the rate of hospitalization, and a reduced mortality rate [1].

2.3. Emergency Telemedical Assistance

In addition to the continuous monitoring of medical parameters to control the patient's state of health and treatment efficiency, telemedicine can also assist with the avoidance and treatment of medical emergencies. The main aim of emergency telemedical assistance is to provide a basis for effective first aid by rapidly transmitting emergency medical expertise to the patient or other persons tending to him/her. Additionally, the creation of an organizational and technical/infrastructure framework also gives the patient a sense of security and independence.

2.3.1. Prevention of Emergencies

New sensors, both mobile and worn on the body, for measuring cardiac and circulatory parameters can provide permanent monitoring, based primarily on the development of new, low-energy data communication techniques and innovative compression systems for data transfer. For example, by analyzing a continuous stream of highly accurate sensor data, conclusions may be drawn with regard to the heart's haemodynamics, and could also prospectively facilitate the identification of short-term cardiac decompensation risks. Early therapeutic intervention can help to avoid unnecessary hospitalization [38].

In the future, it will not only be possible to detect, but also to predict, falls by using new motion sensors which are currently being developed and trialed, in conjunction with the relevant data analyses. Measures that address the causes can then be initiated to counteract an increased risk of falling, which in turn can be combined with fall-preventing systems [23,66].

2.3.2. Acute Emergency Management

In the event of a direct deterioration in the patient's state of health, such as acute cardiac arrhythmias or accidents (such as falls), these critical situations can now be detected by sensors worn on the body or located in the environment, which generate alarm messages in the telemedical center via automated control mechanisms. A telemedical center will then initiate the required emergency aid, depending on the specific situation. This could range from instructing the patient directly on what to do, to alerting family members and care assistants or wardens or to calling the doctor or emergency services [23].

2.4. Personal Health Management

Telemedicine can strengthen an individual's awareness of his or her own health and support health self-management. The key requirements for personal health management are:

- Availability of valid information on the risks, causes and consequences of symptoms, disease patterns, correct administration of medicines and activities
- Correct identification of the current state of health
- An understanding of living conditions and their influence on a person's health
- Continuous logging of changes, and the
- Option of feedback and motivation for the patient

Potential application areas include the following:

- Dietary management (diet plans, assessment, nutritional monitoring etc.)
- Physical activity (as a parameter of well-being and state of health, level of fitness)
- Preventive examinations, screening, prevention measures
- Scheduling
- Interactive training, avatars

The early use of such support systems from a young or middle age creates excellent requirements for effective, sustainable use with a high level of acceptance in old age, and in the event of physical impairments due to illness.

2.4.1. Patient Compliance Through Acceptance and Motivation

The majority of older people prefer to remain in their own homes rather than move to a senior residence or a nursing home [71]. At the same time, many patients need support with their daily routine and with rehabilitation measures, and need a contact person for acute questions relating to the administration of medicines [21]. Among older patients, compliance with treatment and medication regimes is often limited, particularly among persons who live alone [22]. The challenge is therefore to motivate older people who live alone to follow their treatment plan and take their medication as prescribed.

Studies on telemonitoring services for chronically sick patients suggest that telemonitoring enhances patients' assessments of their own quality of life and compliance with treatment and medication regimes [67,79]. Merely regular telephone calls from a telemonitoring center can help to boost patient compliance [15]. The compliance rate can be further enhanced by regular audiovisual communication with a doctor or nurse [9]. A telemedical center can remind patients to take their medication, provide audiovisual instruction on rehabilitation measures, and motivate patients to do their exercises; they can also answer any questions on health management, and any deterioration in the patient's state of health can be detected automatically. This provides peace of mind for both the patients and their relatives. Consequently, the center is able to take over some of the duties usually performed by staff in sheltered housing, allowing older people to remain in their own homes.

2.4.2. New Healthcare Concepts – The New Health Market

There have been a number of studies about the economic consequences of telemedicine. Contrary to numerous optimistic predictions of market development, it is difficult, especially for healthcare markets that are financed by health insurance funds, like in Germany, to estimate the extent to which savings or additional benefits for the patient can be generated from telemedical services [4,43]. However, we can assume that the expedient use of telemedicine can help to prevent hospital stays and paramedic visits, while at the same time the patient's health awareness is raising [28,80]. Telemedical monitoring and support of at-risk patients can contribute to an improved quality of life: More examinations and treatments can be carried out on an outpatient basis, patients are released earlier from hospital, and medication can be optimized. Duplicate examinations can be avoided, thanks to inter-sector linking, which in turn saves costs [53].

New healthcare concepts such as disease management programs can benefit from telemedical support [55,72]. At the telemedical center a joint case file with access to relevant data in the event of an emergency ensures optimized patient care. Telemedicine facilitates networking of all parties involved and supports the health professionals [7].

2.5. Conclusion

Telemedicine allows older people to remain in their own homes. However, there are limitations; audiovisual communication is no substitute for the personal proximity of a carer, and telemedicine cannot assist with routine tasks (washing, cooking etc.).

3. Building a Testbed for Telemedical SmartSenior Applications and Services

Dr. Michael JOHN, Joachim HÄNSEL, Norbert PIETH and Thilo ERNST
Fraunhofer-Institut für Rechnerarchitektur und Softwaretechnik FIRST, Berlin, Germany

3.1. The Need for a Testbed to Improve the Quality of Service of SmartSenior Applications

The various applications and systems in the SmartSenior platform are highly complex due to the cross-system interactions. The telemedical applications and emergency services are particularly safety-critical and need thorough quality assurance during the development process in order to meet the required reliability and quality of services in the product phase. For this reason, Fraunhofer FIRST is currently building a testbed for the quality assurance of telemedical alarm and emergency services. The testbed will also be used to integrate new services more easily into the SmartSenior platform.

The approach chosen is to provide a synthetic environment for conformance testing of the developed SmartSenior applications. Within this testbed, the test objects will be validated against the requirements and standards used by the SmartSenior platform. The parameters to be tested differ according to each application's scenario and the technologies used. These parameters can comprise data volume to be transferred, performance, latency, conformity to data exchange protocols, and required quality of service parameters for data exchange. The testbed will cover test processes for home and mobile applications. While testing under real conditions, the accurate functionality and conformance of SmartSenior applications and services will be verified using test protocols.

3.2. Components of the Testbed

The test environment will cover test scenarios and test routines for the validation of accurate transmission of vital data and synchronous streaming of vital data and video communication for mobile and home applications. The conformance and integration tests for vital data applications are currently under development. The quality parameters of the radio technologies in the home environment are tested using stress tests. With regard to localization information in case of emergencies, the focus is on reference tests against technology standards like GPS, optical sensors and ultrasound sensors in order to validate the different accuracy of localization services. These test components cover a wide range of Smartsenior applications and services in the field of Ambient Assisted Living, such as vital data transfer according to the ISO 11073 standard, indoor and outdoor localization for fall prevention and alarm alerts in case of emergency. Test routines for assessing the cognitive skills of older people will also be developed in order to assess their driving abilities. The components of the testbed are shown in Fig. 1.

The components of the testbed are described in more detail in the following sections.

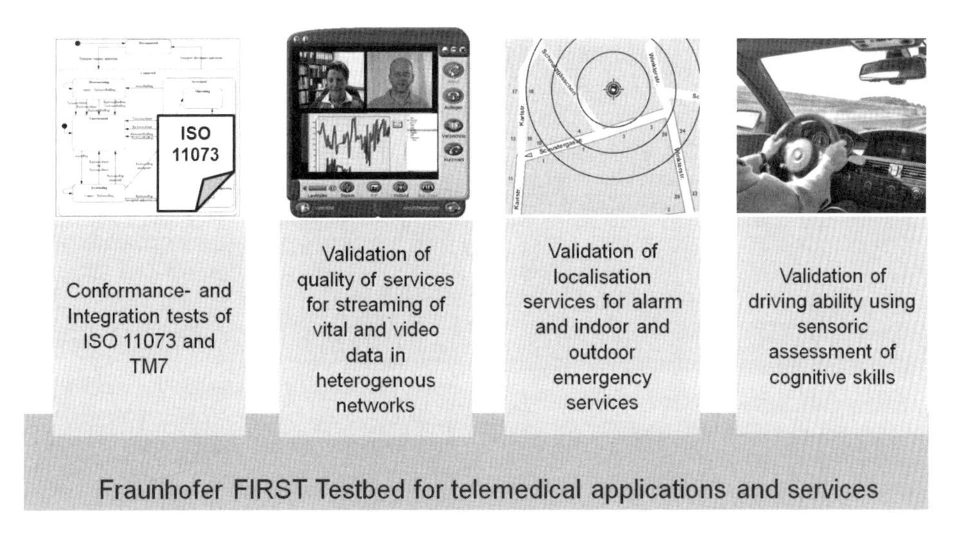

Figure 1. Fraunhofer FIRST Testbed for telemedical applications and services.

3.3. Conformance and Integration Tests for Vital Data Applications

Medical electronic devices are becoming more and more ubiquitous, increasingly dependent on software and, most importantly, more interconnected with one other. Furthermore, connectivity is not restricted to local communication; the advent of telemedical applications has introduced more sophisticated communication protocols. Correct functionality and reliability are clearly the key requirements for medical devices. Since most of the software-based systems cannot be proven to work correctly, both with respect to functionality and required reliability, different approaches need to be taken. In software engineering, quality is ensured by thorough testing on different levels. Although testing is no substitute for proof, tests can raise confidence in the system to a sufficient level where the functionality of the system is highly unlikely to fail and the required level of reliability is met.

3.4. Medical Device Communication and Telemedicine Standards: 11073 and TM7

The interoperability of communicating systems needs open standards. Without these, the benefits of interoperation cannot be felt, since too many adaptations between system specific protocols are required. Furthermore, any adaptation between these different and often proprietary communication protocols introduces potential sources of errors, which in the medical domain is extremely problematic for obvious reasons.

The 11073 family of standards has been created for the transmission of vital data between medical devices. The more recent 11073-20601 standard was introduced to enable easier implementation in conformity with the 11073 standard. The basic standard was found to be too general and complex to be easily implemented. The Continua Health Alliance, a very large consortium of many companies and stakeholders who work with IT systems in the medical domain, has pushed the importance of the 11073-20601 standard to a high degree.

We would also highlight the TM7 standard, which is currently being developed by the SmartSenior consortium in order to cover some identified shortcomings in existing standards. The aim of TM7 is to enable the telemedical operation of medical devices, namely to make them remotely controllable and manageable. It also makes allowance for telemedical factors, such as cost of a connection, time or location. This standard is defined on a level of generality which lies in between standards for vital data communication, audio/video communication and location-based services on the one hand (11073, LOINC, DICOM and GPS) and more complex medical standards like HL7 and IHE which are too general to be implemented in the project context on the other.

Since these two standards play a central role in the project, the project team decided to concentrate the testing activities on the conformance of devices with these standards and on ensuring proper interoperability based on the communication protocols described in the standards. As 11073-20601 is an existing standard, development activities in the project context focused on this area first, and the accompanying testing of 11073-20601 conformance and interoperability was likewise carried out first.

3.5. A Test Concept for Integration and Interoperability Tests for ISO 11073-20601

A tight project schedule made it necessary to have testing available as early as possible. In order to gain a better insight into how the standard would work in practice and to see how well the test approach would perform, the team made use of two existing software implementations which utilize standard-compliant interfaces. One is a demonstration implementation of a virtual thermometer on an Android smartphone device. This demonstrator is publicly available as open source under the name of Morfeo, and conforms to the 11073 thermometer device specialization. The other is a more comprehensive collection of software covering the realization of several so-called Agents for different device specializations and a Manager as the receiver of the vital data. This software collection is known as the Continua Enabling Software Library (CESL).

The CESL was developed by the Continua Health Alliance, which also provides a testing environment. An analysis of this tool's functionality showed that it already comes with a comprehensive collection of tests. In order to create a test suite of test cases of even higher quality, more cutting-edge testing technologies like Model Based Testing (MBT) were applied. MBT only tests the behavioral part of the protocol. For the complex messages that are created for 11073-conformant devices, it is also necessary to test the correct encoding of these messages, i.e. structural testing must accompany the behavioral testing. The NIST (National Institute of Standards and Technology) has realized a tool specifically for this purpose.

The basis of the test concept is therefore defined by the following technologies: the Continua testing tool, MBT tools and the NIST structural tester. The Continua tool has already been applied successfully as it works out of the box. For the MBT tools it was necessary to first choose a tool that would generate tests for the standard, and then create the model itself. The evaluation of several model-based test generators led to the selection of Conformiq Designer, since it is known to come with a well- chosen set of features for generating tests from behavioral models. The connection behavior of the agent as described in 11073-20601 was then modeled. The generation of the full model with all coverage criteria led to the creation of about 400 test cases. The generated tests were executed on the Morfeo software and the CESL agents. Both test executions indicated correct behavior of the tested software.

A second iteration of the test process will focus on better integration of the structural testing software and the tests generated by the model-based testing tool. At the moment, the testing concept is applied to software on devices provided by Prisma GmbH and GHC Global Healthcare GmbH, partners of the SmartSenior project consortium.

The test model covers the 11073-20601 standard. There are plans to widen the model to include more behavioral models arising during the SmartSenior project, and more specifically, to include the models that are created as part of the work being done in the aforementioned TM7 standard development.

3.6. Testing the Quality Parameters of the Radio Technologies

SmartSenior uses different wireless technologies. This is essentially justified due to the fact that the platforms in use must be optimized as "embedded systems" to deal with adapted resources. In the case of universal and relatively high-performance devices, WLAN is usually the preferred short-range technology, while at the sensor level nanoNET and potentially BTLE for BT-medical devices may be considered. Essential selection criteria include availability and ease of integration of the technology itself, required data rates and QoS parameters, software requirements, power requirements for battery devices, and potential locating support. Existing mobile phone networks are used to connect the SmartSenior application to the Service Center TMZ by radio.

In particular, the home environment and the technologies used there may conflict with other application scenarios, since all of them will compete inside one common free ISM radio band. This, for example, is represented by an installed video transmission in the home network with extensive bandwidth usage, and the SmartSenior applications should be able to cope with these important restrictions without failure. As evidence of this in practice, stress tests are required, to validate and document the QoS (Quality of Service) parameters defined in SmartSenior in such expected, typical disturbed environments.

When using the mobile networks in particular, the latency and the transmission standards of the data transmission should be taken into account, i.e. an E2E quality analysis of the communication. It must be noted in principle that due to the locally installed infrastructure, these are only one-off tests and conclusions cannot automatically be drawn regarding the attainable parameters of the technology at each location.

The test environment from the radio-technical viewpoint is realized by test equipment based on PC technology or additionally using "Embedded Devices", which are configured to allow independent test scenarios according to the SmartSenior guidelines, while monitoring and documenting the respective QoS results of the test runs. With respect to the E2E application, data quality and latency are the most important criteria, i.e. the completeness of the data and their time behavior.

As part of the SmartSenior project, some tests had already been carried out that were related to the 2.4 GHz ISM band, which is currently the most widely used ISM radio band. Here, the three technologies WLAN, Bluetooth and nanoNET were tested in all combinations and with different data sets to simulate typical applications. Furthermore, the local placements of parallel active transmitters and receivers were varied to assist with technology selection by comparing the respective results. In addition to the use of configured SmartSenior-device parameters, a validated pseudo video stream with very large data packets was used as a source of interference. WLAN and Bluetooth were used with PC-based IP data transfers. The nanoNET communication was carried out by a completely independent "embedded application" and with recording of the results on one of the PCs. The test runs resulted in a table of QoS parameters in relation to the respective test setups.

As the project work progresses, the current test processes will be refined and further customized to real-world conditions. The goal here is to readily integrate the real devices into test scenarios and verify their performance in relation to the SmartSenior requirements.

3.7. Quality Assurance of Location Services for Emergency Situations

Location technologies such as GPS are already in use to support rescue operations in outdoor areas, where they can be critical for survival in case of emergency. Furthermore, more and more elderly people own devices that are equipped with GPS technology, such as navigation devices and mobile telephones. In a scenario where such an elderly person equipped with a GPS device is not at home and is in need of medical support, the location service provided by the GPS device could make the difference between life and death.

Location technologies for outdoor use are not the only ones that can assist with emergency situations faced by elderly people. Either in everyday life or in situations where they visit a hospital or rehabilitation clinic, they will enter complex buildings. Outdoor location technologies like GPS do not work inside buildings. A requirement analysis of the SmartSenior project revealed that indoor location technologies are needed. It was decided that room precision will ensure the best tradeoff between available precison by the technologies and the accuracy that is needed to locate a person in an emergency. Although these technologies are not available yet, development in this field appears sufficiently rapid to suggest that systems with the required degree of precision will become available during the term of the project.

At the moment, the most promising technology with respect to precision, widespread use and economic aspects is triangulation by wireless networks. This technology will therefore be primarily used for evaluation and validation purposes. Secondary to and alongside triangulation by wireless networks, IEEE 802.15.4.a-based location and ultrasonic location technologies will also be included.

The test concept covers different series of measurements of GPS and WLAN signals in comparison to the IEEE 802.15.4.a localization functionality as well as reference measurements. The reference measurements will be achieved using optical sensors such as time-of-flight cameras and laser scanners or acoustic sensors such as ultrasound. The existing building plans and localization maps will also be taken into account, in order to validate the accuracy of the localization service.

4. Prevention and Rehabilitation of Elderly Stroke and Fall Patients: Concept and Development of an Interactive Trainer

Jörn KISELEV [a], Gerd KOCK [b], Ben HENNIG [c], Michael JOHN [b], Elisabeth STEINHAGEN-THIESSEN [a] and Mehmet GÖVERCIN [a]

[a] *Forschungsgruppe Geriatrie der Charité Universitätsmedizin, Berlin, Germany*

[b] *Fraunhofer-Institut für Rechnerarchitektur und Softwaretechnik FIRST, Berlin, Germany*

[c] *Deutsches Forschungsinstitut für Künstliche Intelligenz (DFKI), Saarbrücken, Germany*

4.1. Introduction

Multimorbidity leads to immobility, declining levels of physical activity and repeated falls in the elderly population [42]. The reductions in muscle mass and cognition associated with aging can be abated or even partially reversed by maintaining and increasing an older person's current level of physical activity. Increases in physical activity lead to a higher quality of life and psychological wellbeing [14,16,73].

Whether or not older people remain active depends on a wide variety of factors, such as subjective self-efficacy, expected effectiveness of physical activity, perceived barriers as well as social support [2,51]. Negative expectations and personal perceptions, frailty, fear of negative experiences, subjective or objective barriers to physical activity and lack of knowledge about the positive effects of physical activity can severely affect one's willingness to be active and greatly increase one's risk of physical inactivity [13,65].

In several focus group studies, Hardy and Grogan (2009) identified six factors that positively influence physical activity [33]. These factors are: "motivation to enhance personal health", "having fun", "social contacts" and, surprisingly, "opportunity for competition". Additionally, focus group members stressed the need for age-adjusted exercise, such as “availability of training facilities” and “coming home before darkness” [33].

Unfortunately, these findings are rarely taken into account by current healthcare systems. In a study by Buttery and Martin [12], only 11% of older people interviewed, who had a Barthel Index (BI) of 9 to 20, were advised by healthcare providers to increase their level of physical activity. Most of the recommendations for increased physical activity observed in the study were of a generic non-individual nature [12]. For this reason, there is an urgent need to develop and implement new concepts for older people. Such concepts should make allowance for the special needs of the elderly population. Moreover, exercises should be monitored to enhance the self-efficacy of the participants and assure that individual goals are being reached. Furthermore, new training concepts should provide participants with an enjoyable training environment that is specifically tailored to the needs of the elderly to ensure their long-term motivation and participation [78].

4.2. Development of a Modular Multi-Sensor System

The SmartSenior project addresses the specifications mentioned above by developing an interactive physical therapy environment to be installed in the homes of elderly people. It comes with a simple-to-use multimodal interface (TV screen, microphone and speaker, wireless control), allows social interaction between the therapist, patient and/or other users (video conference) and can function alone as a kind of virtual therapist.

A variety of devices were investigated for the (real-time) analysis of user motion. Initially, optical devices such as web cams, time-of-flight cameras incorporating PMD (Photonic Mixer Devices) sensors [39], and bio-inspired optical stereo-sensors [30] were tested. However, optical sensors were found to have certain limitations. For instance, we were unable to derive necessary information about the weight distribution of the subject, and motion tracking was only possible within a limited range.

Due to the concept of sensor data fusion, laminar pressure and proximity sensors were also consideredin order to acquire better information about patients’ motion and

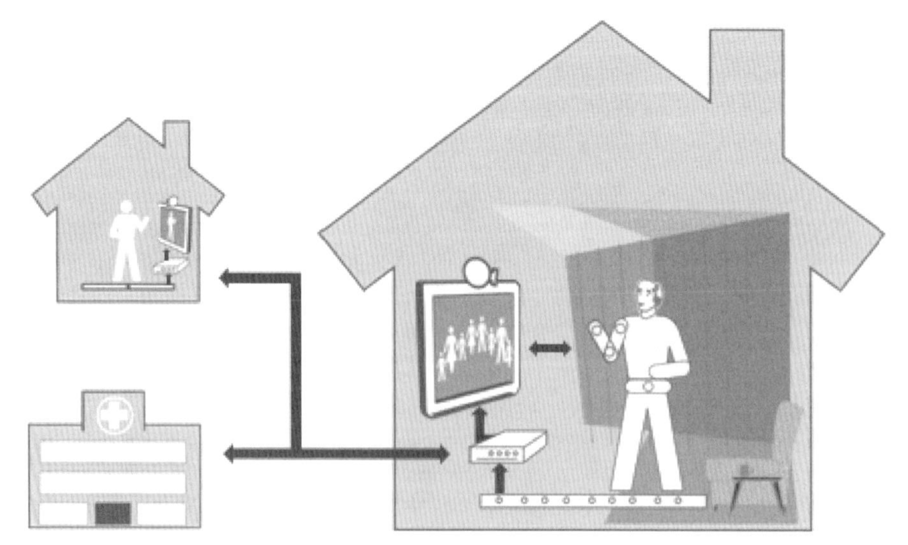

Figure 2. Interactive physical therapy environment.

position. The following devices were used: 1) a high-resolution laminar pressure distribution sensor approximately the size of a mattress (XSensor Body by XSensor Technology Corp.) to measure the dynamic weight of seated, lying or standing subjects, and 2) a specially-designed area rug ("Smart Floor" roughly 10m^2) with a proximity sensor system of lower resolution (SensFloor® by Future-Shape GmbH).

Finally, body-worn sensor units were explored, which use motion-capture technology that is widely used in the fields of film, animation and game productions. The following devices were investigated: the Shimmer wireless sensor platform [41], the MTx multiple motion trackers of Xsens [44] and the pi-node [40] sensor. The combination of accelerometers and gyros in inertial sensor systems has been used successfully in commercial motion-capture body suits. As of late, these technologies have received much attention for use in therapeutic settings. These sensors seem to be especially suited for a vast range of slowly executed physical therapy exercises.

During these exercises, the data from the different sensor systems, model data (skeleton, constraints of human anatomy) and a priori knowledge are fused.

These sensor components provide different types of real-time data. Optical and time-of-flight cameras (ToF) generate two-dimensional images, shape data or three-dimensional depth maps. The depth maps can then be compared with the individual human model data and a priori biomechanical knowledge. Using this knowledge we know which region of the body will be active during the current exercise. The model data incorporates the human anatomy and physical constraints, i.e. information about the bones and joints of a skeleton and about possible degrees of freedom.

The sensor mat data can be used for several purposes. The pressure distribution indicates whether the user is within the given motion volume and also if he or she deviates from the set weight loads for a given joint. For instance, weight distribution and reconstructed 3D skeletons can give hints about possible hip damage. Preventive recognition means that the system can effectively counteract improper use.

The inertial sensors measure acceleration angles with respect to a calibrated reference system. These measurements can be used for redundancy reasons or in cases where the camera(s) cannot "see" the movement. The distribution of force and hence the body load can also be determined using these types of sensor systems (e.g. stress on a joint can be detected via strong negative accelerations). The overall process of sensor fusion and motion analysis is shown in Fig. 3.

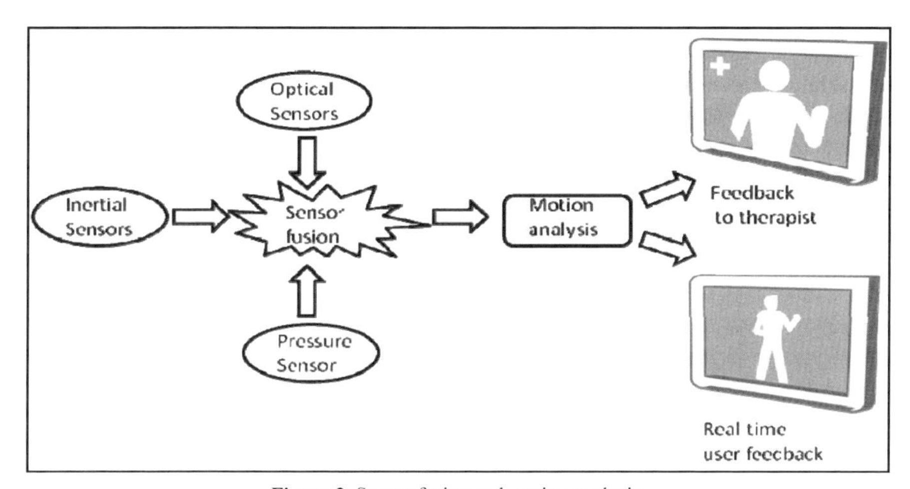

Figure 3. Sensor fusion and motion analysis.

4.3. Development of a Multimodal User Interface

The challenge facing user interface design is that most people in the target group have cognitive limitations or impaired motor skills. Hence, it is important to develop an interaction manager which supports different input and output modalities to customize the system to user limitations, leaving the user free to concentrate on the rehabilitative training.

For this purpose, a multimodal user interface was implemented. The user can use spoken input and output to communicate with the system. The system also supports other interaction options (e.g., it is also possible to control the system with simple operating elements).

The multimodal interface has different input channels, some of which are designed to interact with the user directly. Another channel is used to recognize either correct or incorrect motion (see sensor section). This means that the sensor data can be used to interact with the patient to improve his or her training performance and to motivate the user. Vital signs are also monitored to determine the user's overall fitness levels and gauge the workload of the exercises accordingly. Key information designed to improve and motivate the user is visualized on the game engine, which is also connected with the multimodal interface.

To ensure that the system makes allowance for the limitations of the user, a knowledge base, a so-called ontology, was implemented where different limitations are described and parameterized. It describes the capabilities of an individual user. The system is also customized to user limitations and, additionally, the user has the choice of interacting with the system in his or her preferred manner. The user can concentrate on the exercise for effective and regular training without any distractions by the system itself. Personalized interaction is pivotal to long-term motivation in a systematic training program. Furthermore, to motivate the user for long-term usage, therapeutic assessments are integrated into a game environment for additional motivation especially during game effects.

With the multimodal interface users are free to choose how much information is useful and have the option of selecting their own preferred training method.

4.4. Therapist-User Interface

During the initial contact between a potential user and the supervising physical therapist, a comprehensive assessment of the user's abilities will be performed to give both sides an indication of where to start with the exercise program. Patient-centered goal-setting will be integrated into the process of exercise planning, as well as a more motivating set of exercises. The assessments and the patient-centered goals are re-evaluated at regular intervals.

During a given period of training, all available sensor data can be transferred to the supervising physical therapist, allowing the therapist to monitor the frequency, duration and quality of the exercises performed by each participating user. An automated alert can be automatically generated in case of critical deviations from the instructed motion patterns. Data from each exercise, as well as the user's overall training results, can be interpreted by the therapist to manage and adjust the training program according to the needs and abilities of the user. Furthermore, the available sensor data can be used to complement the initial assessments and to evaluate the user's further progress.

If either the user or the therapist wishes to communicate directly during a given training period, both sides can ask for and initiate AV communication. During any of these video conferences, the physical therapist can directly monitor the quality of the exercises and can discuss changes to the movement patterns as well as changes to the training program with the user. On the part of the user, this communication can be used as needed to ask or discuss any problems with the exercise program, the sensor system or the whole system.

5. The Elderly Patient with Chronic Pain – Improvement in the Quality of Care, Patient Autonomy and Patient Mobility in Rural and Urban Areas Through Integrated New Technologies of the SmartSenior Platform

Klaus F. WAGNER[a], Marten HAESNER[b], Jan-Peter JANSEN[c], Markus SCHRÖDER[d], Matthias MASUR[e], Tobias LEIPOLD[f] and Irina BUSCH[g]

[a] *Klinikum Südstadt Rostock, Germany*

[b] *Forschungsgruppe Geriatrie der Charité Universitätsmedizin, Berlin, Germany*

[c] *Schmerzzentrum Berlin, Germany*

[d] *Tembit Software GmbH, Berlin, Germany*

[e] *Prisma GmbH, Berlin, Germany*

[f] *Clinpath GmbH, Berlin, Germany*

[g] *Telemedicine Center Charité (TMCC), Charité Universitätsmedizin, Berlin, Germany*

5.1. Introduction

Chronic pain – defined as pain of more than six months' duration – affects 17% of the German population [35], especially the elderly [10]. Pain among older adults, which is often undiagnosed and untreated, can lead to depression, fatigue, social isolation, sleep disturbances and impaired mobility [52]. Lower back pain is ranked among the top 3 diagnoses in Germany, with a prevalence of approximately 25% in patients suffering from chronic pain syndromes [24]. Despite improvements in pharmacological and surgical therapy, chronic back pain often remains refractory to therapeutic efforts [56]. Intrathecal drug delivery offers a promising new treatment option for chronic back pain. A small plastic catheter is surgically inserted into the spinal canal (intrathecal space), and connected to a micro infusion pump. Intrathecal drug delivery has been shown to effectively reduce pain in 60–70% of patients suffering from chronic back pain [60].

However, the therapy requires rigorous medical supervision. It is therefore necessary to implement the following measures: (1) user feedback on their well-being; (2) the standardized transmission of vital signs; (3) detection of anomalies; (4) monitoring; and (5) emergency management. These systems are not currently available for pain patients living at home.

Within the SmartSenior project, subproject 3 has the overarching goal of integrating existing and new services in the areas of prevention, treatment and rehabilitation. Currently, its focus is to develop a new approach for treating patients with an intrathecal drug pump by using Ambient Assisted Living-technology. The main components of this phase are a Smartphone pain diary application and a vital signs monitor. Together with complementary services (such as the central collection of data on a web-based server, a 24/7 emergency management system and a telemedicine center), the Smartphone application and vital signs monitor should serve to promote the autonomy of elderly pain patients both in urban and rural areas.

The device interfaces conform to health device communications standards (ISO-IEEE 11073), so that further development of devices, services and applications can easily be integrated into the SmartSenior platform.

5.2. Emergency Care: Integration of a Sensor System and Telemedicine Center

Because the service requires 24/7 readiness, the SmartSenior telemedicine center is of critical importance. It ensures that technical errors are addressed and provides adequate services for the senior.

To avoid overdoses or detoxification, three vital signs are measured: oxygen saturation, heart rate and respiratory rate. The mobile system allows vital data to be acquired and digitalized, while enabling the patient to be fully mobile. The vital sign sensors that the patient wears are miniaturized and have demonstrated high usability among older users. Data packets are transmitted through nodes with local intelligence (BAN, PAN) to the SmartSenior telemedicine center, where they are collected, analysed, and archived in the patient's central record (mdoc®).

In the case of detected vital sign anomalies, the telemedicine center can attempt to contact the senior via audiovisual communication or it can alert a necessary support service. However, in the case of an emergency, the critical vital signs and contact information are transferred to the local pain center, which can trigger a predefined emergency response. In such a case, the "Schnelle Medizinische Hilfe", a patient transport service in Germany that operates as an extension of the local pain center, receives a defined set of patient data and the exact localization (indoor/outdoor) of that patient. The emergency response can also be initiated by the senior himself by pushing the emergency button on his Smartphone or by calling the telemedicine center directly.

5.3. Smartphone Pain Diary Application

A pain diary for the seniors' Smartphone is an important component in the SmartSenior environment for the easy and effective tracking and management of chronic pain conditions. The "Berliner Bogen" is a newly developed pain diary implemented by Prisma GmbH to be easy and convenient for elderly users (e.g. completion time less than five minutes). Characteristic of this new approach is that the pain diary measures the subjective quality of life rather than relying solely on surrogate medical parameters. The senior-friendly GUI of the Smartphone (Windows® Mobile®, more platforms to be added soon) pain diary was developed especially for this age group and allows the easy and secure transfer of information to the central patient record. The pain specialist compares the subjective patient entries with objective vital sign data. He can also carry out modifications by individually updating the data (e.g. by setting different time intervals for filling out the pain diary). The generic diary allows the doctor to add individual questions depending on the patient's current condition.

5.4. The Clinical Pathway Software ClinPath®

Clinical pathways are developed to provide diagnostic and therapeutic medical decision-making support (patient pathways ClinPath®). The pathway software tracks the entire treatment process. After the implantation of an intrathecal drug pump, ClinPath® monitors the process and can offer support to the medical staff treating this patient group. Because there are significant differences between urban and rural health care structures for pain patients, prototypes of these clinical pathways have been implemented in two medical facilities. The "Klinikum Südstadt Rostock" represents an acute clinic in a rural area of Germany, whereas the "Schmerzzentrum Berlin" is an outpatient center for the treatment of pain in an urban setting. The clinical pathway application can be individually configured by pain doctors because it includes all treatment settings (outpatient/day hospital/inpatient). The main goal is to develop a guideline for the treatment of patients with an intrathecal drug pump that is generally applicable but also easily adapted to the specific characteristics of individual medical facilities.

5.5. The Central Electronic Patient Record mdoc®

The data of seniors with chronic pain are saved in a central patient record (mdoc®) consisting of compiled results. The mdoc patient record documents the current status of the senior and can be accessed at any time by the local pain specialist. The medical history data is presented graphically in a clear and comprehensible way so that a physician's attention is immediately called to significant changes in a patients' condition. The mdoc software also includes statistical analysis tools to support the medical staff.

Configurable threshold values (pick-up, alerting) allow alert limits of the vital data to be set individually for each patient in order to reduce the number of false alarms. This system provides the greatest possible benefit for both patients and doctors by the monitoring of vital data of the patients to avoid overdoses or detoxification and ensuring the confidentiality of sensitive data (sensitive information is stored on a central server in the protected environment of the SmartSenior telemedicine center). The data is obtained by a certified and highly efficient data protection system, which allows secure access for local pain specialists in emergency situations at home, at work or during holidays.

5.6. Outlook

First prototypes are currently in development, and usability tests have demonstrated high compliance among the elderly patients with the new technical devices and applications. In 2012, a field test with 40 seniors will be conducted to assess acceptance, benefits, costs and sustainability.

6. Solutions for Social Communications – User Requirements and Market Overview

Stefan ZEIDLER[a], Dr. Sibylle MEYER[b], Uta BÖHM[b], Christa FRICKE[b] and Claudia SPINDLER[c]
[a]*Deutsche Telekom AG, Innovation Laboratories, Berlin, Germany*
[b]*SIBIS Institut für Sozialforschung, Berlin, Germany*
[c]*trommsdorff + drüner GmbH, Berlin, Germany*

6.1. Introduction

The proportion of older people in the population is continuously rising in industrialized countries. In Germany, the proportion of people aged 65 or over is expected to increase from around 32% at present to 50% by the year 2030 (DESTATIS2006). This also means an increase in the number of private households with older people, particularly single-person households.

For example, the DFG research group on "Senior-appropriate technology in the domestic environment (sentha)" [27] found that for older people, the priority is to remain in their own homes for as long as possible. There is little willingness to move to a different location or property, even if they are no longer able to care for themselves independently in their own homes. This opens up a wide range of opportunities for assisted living concepts and the use of smart home technologies and video communications.

A number of studies [57–59] over the past 15 years have revealed that older people are perfectly willing to use innovative technologies to support them in their own homes. Although the acceptance of technology among older people remains lower than that of young people, it is constantly rising. People who have already experienced modern communications technologies at work have a far more positive attitude to such technologies than earlier generations.

Against this background, there are currently a large number of studies aimed at increasing the independence of older people. The current research focus of the Federal Ministry for Education and Research (BMBF), "Ambient Assisted Living (AAL)", plays a particularly prominent role here. One area of research which has not yet been widely explored concerns using innovative technologies to encourage social involvement among older people, particularly with the aid of video communications. Although the changes in communicative behavior prompted by telephone and mobile communications are self-evident and have been researched by social scientists and psychologists for many years, little is known about the potential effects of video communication on the older generation.

In order to be able to successfully develop and market such products and services, however, it is very important to understand the specific requirements of the 55-plus target group. With this in mind, SmartSenior questioned potential users about a variety of service scenarios. We also analyzed of the competition in order to identify the consequences that should be taken into account with any future products based on existing products and services.

6.2. Competition Analysis

The starting point for this survey was to identify criteria for senior-appropriate products and to analyze the competition on a cross-industry basis, with the aim of creating optimum framework conditions and comprehensive suggestions for the development of SmartSenior. The number of new products designed to support older people in their day-to-day lives is constantly growing; the first such products are already on the market. Countless international research projects are dedicated to developing related products.

Our analysis focused on products and projects in the information and communications technology sector, but also made allowance for other sectors (such as robotics) in order to obtain an extensive understanding of products aimed at the elderly. Studies [48] and postings on blogs, forums and social networks were incorporated into our the research. The products and projects thus identified were subsequently analyzed, condensed, evaluated vis-à-vis their relevance for SmartSenior, and selected on this basis.

This research enabled us to identify eight central criteria for senior-appropriate products:

- Appeal,
- Quality,
- Operational controls,
- Intelligibilty,
- Design,
- Level of innovation,
- Reliability,
- Price.

On this basis, more general categories were subsequently defined and used for further analysis:

- Telephone,
- PC,
- TV,
- Platform,
- Medical support,
- Research project,
- Other sectors.

Having identified the criteria for senior-appropriate products and analyzed the competition, we concluded that attention should focus in particular on the following aspects during the development of SmartSenior:

- An attractive design,
- Intuitive operation,
- Robust, stable materials, and
- The option of linking to other equipment.

It is also worth noting that older people do not want the products designed for them to be marketed specifically at senior citizens; however, the use of such products should be adapted to their needs by focusing on clarity, simple operation and intelligibility. In order to attract a broad mass of customers, it is important to pitch it at an affordable entry-level price with a range of optional add-ons.

6.3. User Requirements

The second part of the study analyzed requirements from a user viewpoint. To this end, we presented participants with four different usage scenarios: "Video communication with friends and family", "video communication with the doctor", "watching television together" and "finding new friends/acquaintances".

The results of this study show that senior citizens are not a homogeneous target group, but instead differ widely. Older people's needs for support as a result of age- and health-related restrictions can take just as many different forms as their day-to-day behavior, lifestyles and acceptance of technology. This makes it very difficult to develop intelligent technologies and services for the elderly.

One key finding from our analysis of requirements was that the majority of test subjects tended to be in favor of video communication. The added value of "image" or "video" appeared plausible to those questioned. Almost all respondents had a positive spontaneous impression and could envisage using video communication themselves in some format. For the majority of those questioned, the television as output device was of particular interest. The most convincing arguments were:

- Attractive in a private context.
- Attractive for long distances.
- Convincing for those confined to bed.
- Convincing for those with mobility restrictions.
- Attractive for rural regions/areas with a weak infrastructure.

By contrast, the level of acceptance for the scenarios presented varied widely. The scenarios "Video communication with friends and family" and "Video communication with the doctor" were very positively received, whereas the scenarios "Watching television together" and "Finding new friends/acquaintances" only attracted a low level of acceptance.

The scenario "Video communication with friends and family" was the highest-ranked option, with 78% of those questioned willing to use it. Almost all of the arguments put forward during the discussion were positive; the only fear that was voiced concerned the anticipated additional cost. The following were cited as convincing factors:

- Particularly attractive if the family lives far away.
- Particularly attractive for watching grandchildren and great-grandchildren grow up.
- Attractive as a way of supporting friends and family.
- Attractive as a way of combating isolation and loneliness.
- Encourages shared activities.
- Attractive as a way of showing objects.

The scenario "Video communication with the doctor" was the second highest-ranked option, with 69% of those questioned willing to use it. The invited testers felt that this scenario would become even more attractive as they grew older or more restricted in their mobility. It cannot be concluded unequivocally from this that older or more mobility-impaired groups would be more willing to use the service; an evaluation of the questionnaire suggests that the older the respondent is, the less willing they become to use the service. The most convincing arguments were:

- Video contact is reassuring, especially in case of an emergency.
- Video visits are convenient.
- No waiting involved.
- Data monitoring could make this service more attractive.

The scenario "Watching television together" was ranked in third place, with only 29% willing to use it. The reasons for this are reflected in the everyday habits and lifestyles of the target group. The senior citizens questioned only rarely watch television together with other people from outside the household, and only on special occasions. Conversations while watching television are considered disruptive, and even "Watching television with your partner" was often considered onerous. The main arguments put forward by our testers were:

- Watching television together is rather onerous.

- It is better to watch television separately, then talk afterwards.
- Only suitable for certain groups (sports fans, mobility restrictions, loneliness).
- Only on rare occasions (light entertainment, sports, interest/fan groups).

Least popular was the scenario "Finding new friends/acquaintances", which 23% were willing to use. Respondents evaluated the concept differently depending on whether the service was intended to generate "new friends" or "new acquaintances". Even when aimed at "Finding new acquaintances", respondents still had serious reservations about the concept, and as a way of "Finding new friends", it was largely rejected. The screening of television habits and one-dimensional questions about hobbies are evidently insufficient. We would recommend completely rethinking this concept. It is worth considering whether differentiated personality profiles should be surveyed and depicted in menus. Internet-based dating agency services, or projects such as "Visual communication for senior citizens in Berlin", which tested out a service concept 10 years ago with the aim of promoting and implementing contact between senior citizens via video telephony, could serve as suitable models.

The usage requirements of senior citizens are derived primarily from the television habits of the target group. The following aspects were considered particularly relevant:

- Easy to operate.
- Option of switching off the image.
- Should not detract from the home's aesthetics.
- Video answering machine.
- Mobile camera.
- Privacy setting: e.g. switching from loudspeaker to headset.
- Switching between various terminal equipment (TV, PC, fixed network or mobile telephone).

The test subjects rated the "text line" (61%) as their preferred signaling mode, followed by a photograph of the caller (30%). Only 27% of those surveyed accepted a visual signal that was not linked to the caller. It is important to remember that almost two-thirds of those questioned felt that they needed an additional acoustic signal. This "twin-channel principle" (visual and acoustic signaling) is likewise an important requirement of the universal design, and a component of the usability recommendations of the national and international standardization committees.

The test subjects felt that the following aspects were important:

- Knowing who is calling.
- Twin-channel principle: Visual and acoustic signal.
- Individual signaling settings.
- Receiving a signal even if the television set is switched off.

The "headset" was the preferred speaker variant (46%), followed by "individual device on the table or television" (29%). Mounting a microphone in an item of furniture (e.g. standard lamp) was the least convincing option. It is worth noting that our respondents felt that a headset was not sufficient as the only speaker variant; instead, most would require a headset in addition to one of the other two variants. User requirements:

- Permanently installed near the TV + changeover to headset.
- Alternating between appliances (video TV to fixed-network telephone).

- Proposal: Microphone in the remote control.
- The most convincing arguments for video communication via the TV were.
- Attractive in a private context.
- Attractive for long distances.
- Convincing for those confined to bed.
- Convincing for those with mobility restrictions.
- Attractive for rural regions/areas with a weak infrastructure.

Other phases of the study focused on detailed scenarios such as games, in order to obtain a more in-depth knowledge of the target group.

Acceptance of the other scenarios presented was surprisingly high. The following were the TOP three scenarios in terms of acceptance and willingness to use:

- "Intelligent alarm system",
- "Interactive TV quiz games", and
- "Video-assisted board games".

"Interactive movement games" (ergometer and Wii games) were less well-accepted, although here too, at least half of our subjects were willing to use them. Differences also emerged depending on age- and health-related restrictions and on the variations in day-to-day and leisure behavior, as well as variations in lifestyle and acceptance of technology.

6.4. Conclusion

Overall, we concluded that the test subjects compared the opportunities offered by video communications with fixed network and mobile telephony, and applied the same standards with regard to usage and comfort. They want comparable features as when making a telephone call. PC functions are likewise cited in a comparative way.

Overall, we ascertained that the test subjects want the scenarios presented to complement, rather than replace, their everyday and leisure activities in their current life situation. However, they could envisage the importance of these services for entertainment, social contact and mental and physical fitness increasing as their mobility becomes impaired and/or they have less direct contact with others.

7. Live Independently at Home for Longer: Scenarios and Approaches for Co-Operative Business Models

Harald Klaus

Deutsche Telekom AG, Innovation Laboratories, Berlin, Germany

7.1. Introduction

Most people, particularly as they get older, want to be able to continue living at home despite increasing health restrictions. Technical assistance systems aim to respond to this need by using intelligent technology and innovative services to support senior citizens in their everyday lives and make life safer, more convenient and healthier, as well as helping them to remain in a familiar environment for as long as possible.

At present, the German Government, especially the Federal Ministry for Education and Research (BMBF), is making millions of Euros available to help fund the development of these technologies, in response to the anticipated consequences of demographic change: By 2035, more than half of all people in Germany will be aged 50 or above, and one in three will be over 60. For the majority of these men and women, this period of their lives will open up a wealth of individual opportunities. However, as we grow older, the number of complaints and illnesses also increases, making us reliant on support. Technology alone cannot solve this challenge, but it can make an important contribution.

The goal is to support older people and all those involved in their well-being. As the number of young people available to care for the elderly decreases, the hope is that technical assistance systems will help to ease the pressure on younger family members, enabling them to combine family life, work and caring for elderly relatives. This also includes offering technical support for employees in outpatient and inpatient healthcare facilities and for older employees.

There is already a wide range of impressive applications available that use intelligent, discreet technology to make life easier [3,34,49]. Here are just a few examples:

- Movement sensors detect when a person gets up in the night to use the toilet and automatically light the way to the bathroom.
- When leaving the home, displays on the entrance door warn residents if they have forgotten to switch off the oven or close the window. This helps to avoid house fires and prevent burglaries.
- As well as providing protection and security, the home is often also the place where emergency situations arise. Accidents do not always happen without warning – they often develop from everyday, initially harmless situations where several factors coincide in an unfortunate manner and the individual concerned fails to respond quickly enough. As part of the SmartSenior project, currently the largest of 18 projects being subsidized by the BMBF, an innovative solution is being developed to identify emergencies in the home environment so that potentially dangerous everyday situations can be detected and resolved promptly.
- Assistance systems help to remind people to take their medicines, and automatically adjust the next appointment if they are occasionally forgotten.
- Telemedical assistance systems can automatically monitor vital data and transmit up-to-date readings to a telemedical center in the event of unusual or critical conditions. Continuous logging, evaluation and processing of a senior citizen's vital data provides comprehensive information about their current state of health. Other information (such as the weather or above-average pollen counts in the surrounding area) can also be incorporated to provide additional peace of mind and relief for allergy-sufferers.
- A special access system supports healthcare professionals, and eliminates the need to carry around a large bunch of keys. The monitoring and display of vital data can provide the healthcare team with an insight into a client's vital data records over the past 24 hours, and help them to assess their general state of health.

- Other technical systems are designed to facilitate communications and encourage participation in social life. Image transmission puts people in touch with friends living many miles away, at least on the screen; virtual coffee mornings and family get-togethers are now a technical reality. Bridging distances, cultivating existing friendships and forging new ones helps to improve quality of life while at the same time promoting preventive healthcare: Participating in a social life, be it in private networks, charities, sporting or church contacts, helps people to stay healthy and alert.
- Services for vital data monitoring and the detection and treatment of emergencies can be used both at home and on the move. For users, there are no system interruptions, as these systems work equally well in the home and on the move, thanks to a smartphone; what is more, many people find that it makes them feel more secure, because in case of doubt, they can check that everything at home is OK while they are travelling.
- An electronic diary can be used both at home and on the move to compensate for any cognitive restrictions. Intelligent algorithms provide appointment reminders depending on the location and distance from the next appointment.

A whole new range of products for the home can be derived from the combination of technical assistance systems with innovative services. Local service and communication platforms notify users of events, offers and activities in the surrounding area. In future, the intelligent control of electronic appliances will enable consumers to save money by taking advantage of cheaper night-time electricity rates. Such solutions are no longer confined to the PC. Modern set-top boxes allow this information to be transmitted to the television, so that it can be retrieved from the comfort of the user's armchair, or allow them to participate in activities in the neighborhood.

7.2. Value-Added and Business Roles in AAL Services

The market for assistance systems for the elderly in Germany is currently characterized by many different suppliers of services and products with a complex system of interrelations. The challenges faced by successful business models in the AAL environment can be characterized as follows:

- Technical integration must also be reflected in future business models; in particular, general business models for the privately funded market and the medical and nursing care sectors need to be redefined.
- There is a demand for the development of suitable models for cost and revenue sharing, role distribution and service responsibility throughout the entire value-added chain. The aim must be to cover the entire value-added chain, including all affected sectors, so that sustainable general business models can be defined alongside the technological development.
- The players in non-technical sectors, particularly medical and nursing care insurance companies (who bear the costs) and the housing sector (particularly integration into the existing housing stock) are also equally important.

Simple technical solutions are already widely used as standard. By contrast, providers of more ambitious technologies have thus far failed to dimension their offerings in a way that makes them broadly acceptable to both the cost-bearing organizations and the end customers. This is often because they have tended to focus too strongly on the technical possibilities without giving adequate consideration to the preferences, needs

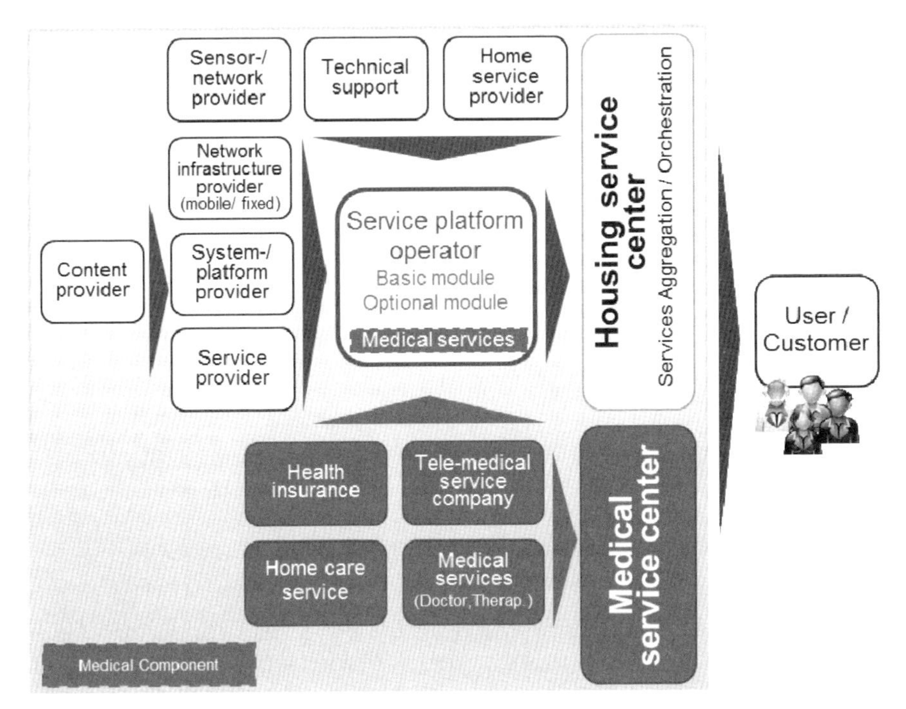

Figure 4. Value-added chain with a housing services company acting as the service aggregator and central point of contact for customers.

and interests of potential users. The technical design must concentrate primarily on the specific customer benefits. Technical solutions will not become successful and well-established unless there is a significant added-value for users. A less pronounced emphasis on technology could offer greater opportunities for implementation here. Additionally, these technical solutions must be coordinated with and linked to the products and services of traditional suppliers.

Generally speaking, business scenarios must not only be viable from a macroeconomic viewpoint, but also for each participating individual. In order to succeed, the framework conditions for successful business models in the AAL environment must be observed. These may be summarized and illustrated by two central aspects:

1. Demographic change and its effects on those market segments that are particularly affected by an ageing society, especially the healthcare market.
2. The need for twofold interconnection, i.e. technical integration and the linking of participating partners.

In future, combinations of multiple services will be offered via integrated service platforms, which should help to increase user acceptance of such services. However, as well as being easy to use, technical components must also be simple to install and maintain. The spectrum of services, from the control of domestic appliances through to the telemedical detection of emergencies, requires coordinated cooperation between numerous partners. The project is currently exploring ways of improving and accelerating the establishment of products and services with certain constellations of the various players involved in the supply process, whereby a central provider of AAL services would be one possible option (cf. Fig. 4).

Developing new business models is particularly challenging where various different participants offer their products and services via shared technical platforms. Additionally, the involvement of telemedical services in the process makes the models more complex, since third parties (e.g. medical and nursing care insurance companies) often finance services but are not themselves the direct beneficiaries of such services.

The results of future business models in the AAL environment to date suggest that a powerful service platform can offer the individual partners a wide range of business and action opportunities, allowing them to respond flexibly to the market and adapt promptly to the various requirements.

8. Data Privacy Protection in AAL Scenarios

Fabienne WAIDELICH, Jens-Uwe BUSSER and Wolfgang KLASEN
Siemens AG, CT T, GTF IT Security, Munich, Germany

8.1. Introduction

In many developed countries, current demographic trends show that the population is growing older. This trend of an ageing society is a worldwide phenomenon: by 2050, one in every five people worldwide will be 60 years or older [64]. One of the biggest challenges for our societies is to adjust to this human paradigm as more and more people live into very old age. This requires technological innovations which help to maintain health and functional capability, overcome social isolation, and extend the time people can live at home by increasing their autonomy, self-confidence and mobility.

"Ambient Assisted Living" (AAL) embraces a range of methods, concepts, products, systems and services which combine new technologies and social environment with the goal of increasing the quality of life of individuals of any age. IT systems play an important role, allowing the supervision of patients under the remote control of physicians and usage of data supplied by sensors and measuring instruments in order to be able to respond fast to emergencies. However, this raises important data privacy and security issues. Indeed, AAL systems must be compliant with national and international laws on data privacy protection. Furthermore, the secure handling of personal data is not only a legal requirement, but is also crucial for the acceptance of AAL solutions by elderly people. The objectives of this paper are to identify general data privacy requirements for AAL systems and to propose appropriate enforcement measures.

8.2. Data Privacy Protection and Its Legal Framework

8.2.1. At the Very Beginning: The German Data Privacy Regulations

In most advanced industrial democracies, data privacy laws only emerged a few decades ago, and were intended to protect information on private individuals from intentional or unintentional disclosure or misuse. In 1970 the German federal state of Hesse enacted the world's first general data protection law in response to concerns about the implications of automated data processing in the public administration [26]. By 1981, all other West German federal states had followed suit with laws regulating data protection in state and local government agencies and in public bodies. In each federal state, observance of the law is controlled by a state data protection commissioner. Additionally, the German Federal Data Protection Act (BDSG), first enacted in 1977 and revised in 2001, 2006, 2009 and most recently in 2010 [31], regulates the handling of personal data which is collected, processed and used in IT systems or collected by public and private bodies and commercial enterprises in a non-automated manner. The office of the Federal Data Protection Commissioner was subsequently created in 1978.

Additionally, further regulations amend both national and state data privacy laws with regard to medical information. Some examples are:

- The German Criminal Code (StGB) [17] which prohibits e.g. unauthorized disclosure of confidential medical and other personal data within §203.
- Federal hospital laws (e.g. LKHG [5]) which handle the protection of patient-related data.
- Federal laws on the public ambulance service (e.g. RDG [6]) which regulate the protection of personal data in case of emergency.

Not only does Germany have one of the longest experiences of data privacy regulation; furthermore, its legal framework was also an important source of inspiration for the European Directive on Protection of Personal Data [20].

8.2.2. The European Directive on Protection of Personal Data

Adopted in 1995, the European Directive on Protection of Personal Data was designed to unify national laws on data protection within the European Community and came into force in 1998. It contains a number of key principles, which Member States were required to transpose into compliant national law.

8.2.3. Data Privacy in the USA

The Privacy Act of 1974 [70] establishes a code of fair information practices that governs the collection, maintenance, use, and dissemination of personal data maintained by federal agencies. However, there are very few mandatory regulations for private bodies and commercial enterprises. European and American concepts of privacy thus differ in important respects. Unlike the European approach to privacy protection, which relies on comprehensive privacy legislation, the U.S. approach relies on industry-specific legislation, regulation and self-regulation.

As a consequence, the so-called US-EU Safe Harbor framework [77] was developed by the US Department of Commerce in order to provide a means for US companies to demonstrate compliance with the European Directive on Protection of Personal Data and thus simplify relations with European businesses. Rather than a law imposed on all organizations in the USA, the Safe Harbor is a voluntary program approved by the EU in 2000 which US organizations can join, having self-assessed their compliance with the principles of the European Directive on Protection of Personal Data.

8.3. Data Privacy Requirements in AAL Scenarios

Personal data is commonly defined as “any information concerning the personal or material circumstances of an identified or identifiable individual (the data subject)” (BDSG §3 [31]). The privacy protection of such data is a crucial issue in AAL scenarios.

Personal data may be of a general nature such as name, date of birth, address, etc. Even indirect data such as car registration number, private phone number, or IP address are classed as personal data. Beside such general data, AAL systems usually handle more specific data such as social insurance data (e.g. social insurance contributions, billing information about received benefits) or medical data which are subject to even stricter privacy requirements. Examples of medical data may include diet plans, measurement values of bodily functions such as pulse or oxygen saturation, diagnostic findings, or any communication between patient and physician. The very fact that a certain patient-physician relationship exists constitutes medical data.

Although national laws may differ from one country to another or even from one federal state to another (e.g. in Germany), it is nevertheless possible to identify various general data privacy requirements for AAL systems, which may be roughly divided into three categories: transparency, legitimate-purpose, and proportionality requirements.

Transparency requirements concern the access rights of the data subject to his data. The data subject must indeed be granted access to his personal data and notified when his data is processed. Data must also be rectified, erased, and blocked if so requested by the data subject. He also has the right to object to the processing of his data. Moreover, the instance which determines the purposes and means of the processing of personal data must provide his name and address, the purpose of processing, the recipients of the data, and all other information required to ensure the processing is fair. Additionally, AAL systems should support audit functionalities.

The second class of data privacy requirements concerns the legitimate purpose of the data processing: personal data may only be collected and processed for specified, explicit and legitimate purposes.

Thirdly, certain proportionality requirements complete the list of general data privacy requirements. Data processing must be adequate, relevant and not excessive in relation to the purposes for which they are collected and/or further processed. Furthermore, any information collected by an individual cannot be disclosed to other organizations unless authorized by law or by consent of the individual. Further general requirements are that data records should be kept accurate and up-to-date, that data must be erased when no longer needed for the stated purpose, and that data collected for different purposes must be processed separately. Finally, data processing must be secure. Personal information must be protected from loss, misuse and unauthorized access, disclosure, alteration and destruction.

These requirements are the minimum set of requirements any AAL system should fulfill. Further specific requirements may be additionally specified by local or national laws on data privacy protection, depending on the place where data is collected, processed or used, the nature of the processed personal data, and the type of institutions involved. For example, vital data such as pulse measured by an AAL device at home and transferred to the telemedicine center of a Berlin public hospital would be subject to both the German Federal Data Protection Act [31] and the Berlin Data Protection Act [32]. Moreover, their confidentiality would also be required under §203 of the German Criminal Code [17].

The legal framework for data privacy protection in AAL scenarios is basically not much different from other domains, but the personal data involved is particularly sensitive. Moreover, security measures must be very carefully chosen to fulfill the requirements without hindering user convenience.

8.4. Data Privacy Protection in AAL Scenarios

Data privacy protection relies on a large variety of organizational as well as technical measures.

Organizationally, a pre-requisite for the collection and processing of personal data in AAL scenarios is the qualified agreement of the subscriber based on comprehensive information. Even a layman must be able to understand which data is collected and for which purpose. The agreement is then documented in a consent form. If the subscriber withdraws his agreement, no further data may be collected or processed; the data already gathered must be erased, or blocked if it must be archived for legal reasons. Even with the subscriber's agreement, data may only be collected and processed if necessary. The use of such data for purposes other than those stated in the agreement is prohibited.

Another organizational measure concerns the confidentiality to be observed by all persons involved in the processing of personal data. Physicians are well aware of their duty to handle medical records confidentially, but assistants (especially non-medical ones such as IT personnel) must be instructed to obey data privacy regulations as well. Any person in contact with personal data must commit to the protection of data privacy and must be trained regularly to raise awareness of data privacy protection requirements and related security measures.

Physical access to buildings and rooms used for data processing, access to data processing systems (e.g. data servers), and digital access to the data itself must likewise be restricted and controlled. Additionally, only physically non-accessible or shielded wires may be used for any communication, which is not cryptographically protected, and the number of persons having access to the systems should be kept to a minimum.

Other organizational measures also help to guarantee the confidentiality of data, such as defining strong password policies, separating responsibilities for installation and data analysis ("blinding"), making sure that data is homogeneous so that its content cannot be guessed through probability checks, or forbidding private data storage media within AAL data centers.

Finally, the availability of data may be provided by the use of backup systems.

Organizational measures are complemented by technical measures. For example, data authenticity and integrity protection may be provided by digital signatures and other cryptographic checksums. A public key infrastructure supports the easy and secure management of security credentials. Also, the authentication of sender and receiver guarantees that transmitted data is received from the correct origin and sent to the legitimate recipient.

Confidentiality requirements may be fulfilled by different security solutions which can be used to complement one other. A strong user authentication process on IT systems and a detailed role and rights management system for authorized users may be combined for access control. Data encryption (based on state-of-the-art cryptographic methods) is explicitly stated in an amendment to BDSG §9 para. 1 [31] as an appropriate measure to prevent unauthorized access to personal data. Pseudonymization is a further mechanism to ensure data confidentiality by removing identifying data in a data record and replacing it with one or more artificial identifiers. This allows the flexible handling of data by reducing the risks of unauthorized access, but also data tracking back to the original person if required by authorized bodies.

To ensure that security mechanisms achieve the expected level of security, security credentials must be properly protected. Confidential security credentials (e.g. passwords, private keys) must therefore be stored in protected memory areas (e.g. chip cards) to prevent unauthorized readout. Even security-related data which is not confidential, such as root certificates, access control lists, etc. must also be protected against unauthorized addition, replacement, and deletion. Password policies defined as organizational measures can also be enforced by automatically checking the compliance of new or changed passwords.

Furthermore, basic security measures such as operating system hardening (deinstallation of unused software, removal of unnecessary user accounts and services, minimal system privileges for essential user accounts and services, closing of unnecessary communication interfaces, installation of virus and malware protection, and continuous software updates) and network separation by installation of firewalls also provide a solid foundation for security measures.

Audit trail is another important technical measure to be adopted. System use must be logged for data protection auditing. Security-relevant events must be automatically recorded in logging files as well. Moreover, these files should be analyzed regularly by an experienced system administrator who should be automatically notified by SMS or email in critical cases.

Nevertheless, there are some cases in AAL scenarios where standard IT security measures may be not sufficient, for example:

- The user has the right to know if recording devices are running and to decide whether they may run. This requires a clear indication of device activity (e.g. an LED displaying camera recording), and a simple, non-cancellable method to switch it off.
- The user's agreement for recording of images or sound in his apartment may be insufficient if there are other persons who are recorded too. Their agreement is required as well, or they must at least be informed in advance about the data collection.
- Storage of personal data in persistent memory (e.g. hard disk) may require encryption even in case of cached data.

8.5. Conclusion

In AAL scenarios, the support of individuals in their daily life as well as in case of emergency by close user interaction and remote supervision requires the collection and processing of large quantities of personal – even medical – data. This raises serious IT security and data privacy issues. To achieve compliance with the legal framework and acceptance by the targeted user community, appropriate data protection measures must be determined and enforced.

We have presented an overview of data privacy requirements and general measures to fulfill these requirements. However, the challenge in a given AAL project is to conduct a careful analysis of the actual system and disclose any unconventional threats and risks. Well-balanced organizational as well as technical measures must then be defined to achieve a uniform level of security and data privacy and thus provide a secure and cost-efficient solution. This is one of our tasks in the SmartSenior research project [47], which focuses on supporting elderly people economically, socially, and medically so that they can remain at home for as long as possible. Together with our project partners, we are currently working out a dedicated data protection concept fulfilling the legal requirements of the German Federal Data Protection Act [31] and the Berlin Data Protection Act [32].

9. Development of Sustainable AAL Services

Katrin MÜLLER
Siemens AG, Berlin, Germany

9.1. Introduction

The development of sustainable AAL services requires a balance between the triple bottom lines of people, planet, and profit. The paper summarizes defined indicators and requirements to be fulfilled in order to identify potential synergies between all three categories and to minimize conflicts between the different goals. AAL services are often customized to specific needs and the utilization depends on the application scenario. At the same time an infrastructure has to be implemented to provide these services efficiently. The paper proposes an assessment model to run scenario based calculations to figure out the influence of the AAL service design. Both developments, the indicators and the assessment model, deliver the backbone of the development of sustainable AAL services.

9.2. Sustainability Indicators

The research on sustainability indicators has been conducted in two parallel streams. The top-down-approach has studied the global, European, national and organizational sustainability agendas and associated measurements and indicators [8,19,63,68], Millenium Development Goals [76], Indicators of Sustainable Development [75], UNECE Sustainable Development Statistics [74], OECD Sustainable Development [11,37,54,62,69]. In a bottom-up approach, AAL application fields considering the three SmartSenior scenarios “safe mobility”, “health services” and “longer independence” as well as stakeholder interests have been analyzed (Fig. 5).

In total 107 indicators have been identified targeting the development of sustainable AAL services. 52 indicators evaluate the regional distribution of the AAL of services. 33 indicators cover the organizational aspects and 22 indicators affect the individual level of the user.

The collected indicators and targets have been evaluated regarding relevance and significance for developing AAL services as well as the possibility to control and influence these aspects. At the same time each indicator has been evaluated if AAL services would support the target of a sustainable development in a positive or negative manner.

44 indicators out of the 107 have to be applied to all AAL applications, 14 indicators are specific to the “safe mobility” area, 28 indicators have to be considered for “health services” and 21 indicators are relevant for “longer independence” services, additionally.

More than half of the indicators are influenced in a positive manner, means providing and using AAL services would contribute to achieve the sustainability target either on a regional, organizational or individual level. Example indicators are: social interac-

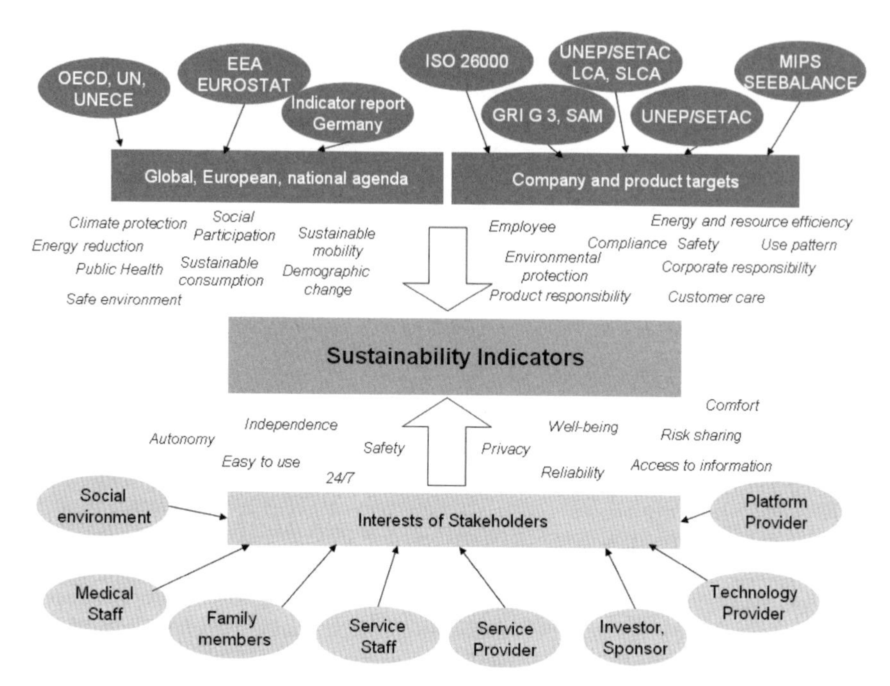

Figure 5. Process of collecting sustainability indicators.

tion and activities, availability and access to services, ratio of population using Internet and computer.

However AAL services might also have ambivalent influence on the sustainable targets and even between the targets conflicts might exist. Especially these indicators have to be monitored carefully during development and implementation of AAL services.

For instance the AAL infrastructure might increase the portion of cost of accommodation on the available household income. The extension of tele-medical services might provide equal opportunities and access to health care solutions, however there is also a risk associated with, by excluding groups of people with disability using the services.

An issue might occur between the requirement of a 24/7 availability and the energy reduction as well as associated green house gas emissions. 24/7 availability requires a certain infrastructure and stand-by demand which result in additional energy demand.

The availability and an increasing number of AAL services might reduce the amount of voluntary engagement, especially if technological and organizational solutions are prioritized and if they are not integrated in existing structures and human relationships.

The following requirements have been defined to improve the sustainability of AAL services:

1. Integrate all stakeholders in service development in order to enable basic services, prevention, treatment and rehabilitation more efficiently and improve acceptance and market penetration.
2. Design reimbursement schemes across the financial structure of the health and care system in order to enable investment in preventive solutions.

3. Tele-medical services shall be combined with appropriated education and training of seniors and patients and their relatives to take over more responsibility on personal health and improve the compliance.
4. Incentives and motivational schemes shall consider the individual habits, life style and daily routines as well as support personal goals.
5. Business models shall integrate and combine public and private financing.
6. Services shall be offered in modular and flexible modules or packages to enable adaptation regarding changing demands depending on the individual context.
7. Services shall be developed in close relation to care takers on-site and shall activate and challenge the seniors to a certain extend supporting their independence in conducting daily activities and to improve the cognitive balance of the person.
8. Non-technical actors shall be integrated very closely and technology shall support their tasks in order to increase acceptance and promotion of the services.
9. Services shall consider the right of privacy, information and data security, informational self-determination.
10. Services shall support the communication and interaction between the actors, service providers, social environment etc. in a transparent and comfortable manner as well as reduce the mental load of caretakers especially in the case if they are family members.
11. Service shall provide the some quality of care with lower cost or better quality at the same cost to be considered in the reimbursement schemes of health and care insurance systems.

9.3. Assessment Model

Often AAL services will require more energy demand and related environmental impacts of the use phase depending on the number of users and the number of services consumed, therefore an environmental assessment has to be provided and the customer and users have to be informed and educated.

Therefore a generic system model has been developed consisting functional building blocks. Depending on the application functional building blocks can be combined and depending on the use pattern the model can be parameterized to evaluate the environmental impact of services.

The model has been applied to tele-medical assisted peritoneal dialysis at home. A first case study has been conducted evaluating one year of service in Germany using a DSL access at home and resulted in a energy demand of ca. 850 kWh and green house gas emission of ca. 467 kg CO2eq.

Figure 6 shows the functional building blocks at home. The measurements are conducted on a daily basis and send to a tele-medical service center for interpretation and storage.

The assessment of AAL services is based on:

- the number and type of components, products and technologies applied and used at home and at the service center.
- the frequency of use (number of measurements, data and measurement cycles) and events occurred requiring an interaction.

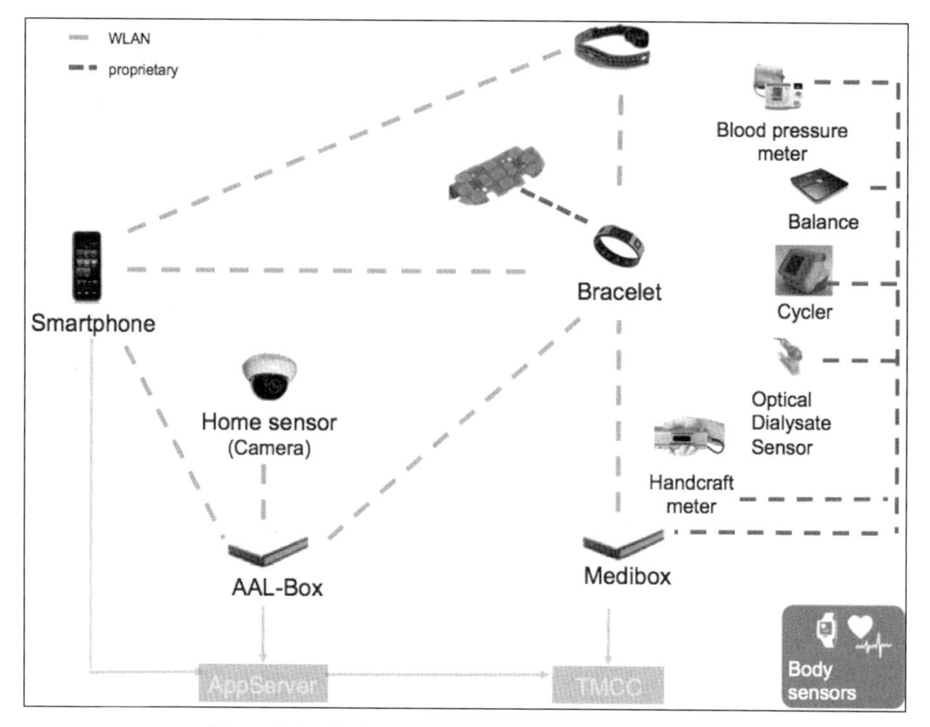

Figure 6. Application scenario – Peritoneal dialysis at home.

The model allows a comparison of different equipment and configurations as well as the influence on measurement cycles, the amount of data transmitted, and the failure tolerance of the system.

Additional to the environmental evaluation of the tele-medical assisted peritoneal dialysis future sustainability indicators have been evaluated in comparison to the traditional dialysis.

Each additional patient who can be treated at home would result in major savings against a treatment at hospital or medical centers. E.g. time saving can be reached up to 60% at the patient site, 20% at hospital, energy demand could be reduced up to 20% and green house gase emissions up to 65%. The tele-medical support could increase the safety of the patient, complications could be identified earlier, which would reduce the hospitalization required and cost associated with.

10. Summary

Michael C. BALASCH
Deutsche Telekom AG, Innovation Laboratories, Berlin, Germany

This article introduced the project SmartSenior – Intelligent Services for Senior Citizens and presented some selected applications, focusing in particular on overarching issues with fundamental relevance.

The project work will continue until autumn 2012. An initial usability evaluation on user interfaces and application modules was completed in winter 2010, the findings from which will be incorporated into future development. Work to integrate all modules started in spring 2011; a comprehensive service environment will be available from autumn 2011. Field tests will be performed in spring 2012 with first results available in early summer 2012. Publications and other selected results will be made public on the project's website www.smart-senior.de [45].

Acknowledgements

The consortium's work in this project is supported and co-funded by the German Ministry of Education and Research (Bundesministerium für Bildung und Forschung, BMBF) as part of its High-Tech Strategy for Germany.

The authors would like to thank all partners within SmartSenior for their cooperation and valuable contribution.

References

[1] R. Antonicelli, P. Testarmata, L. Spazzafumo, C. Gagliardi, G. Bilo, M. Valentini, F. Olivieri and G. Parati, Impact of telemonitoring at home on the management of elderly patients with congestive heart failure, *J. Telemed. Telecare* **14**(6) (2008), 300–305.

[2] B.J. Ayotte, J.A. Margrett and J. Hicks-Patrick, Physical activity in middle-aged and young-old adults: The roles of self-efficacy, barriers, outcome expectancies, self-regulatory behaviors and social support, *J. Health Psychol.* **15**(2) (2010), 173–185.

[3] M. Balasch, Integrierte intelligente Dienste und Dienstleistungen für Senioren, in: *Ambient Assisted Living 2009, 2. Deutscher Kongress mit Ausstellung / Technologien – Anwendungen 27–28 Januar 2009 in Berlin / Tagungsbeiträge*, VDE, Berlin, 2009.

[4] T.S. Bergmo, Economic evaluation in telemedicine – Still room for improvement, *J. Telemed. Telecare* **16**(5) (2010), 229–231.

[5] Berliner Landeskrankenhausgesetz LKHG, 2001, http://www.awb.tu-berlin.de/lv/unterlagen/docs/lv22/Landeskrankenhausgesetz.pdf.

[6] Berliner Rettungsdienstgesetz RDG, 2004, http://www.berlin.de/imperia/md/content/seninn/abteilungiii/vorschriften/rdg.pdf?start&ts=1269427655&file=rdg.pdf.

[7] M. Bethke and J. Overbeck, Chronic care management: Telemedizin in der praxis, *Schweizer Ärztezeitung* **91**(17) (2010), 664.

[8] J. Blazejczak and D. Edler, *DIW Vierteljahrshefte zur Wirtschaftsforschung* **73**(1) (2004), 10–30.

[9] T. Botsis and G. Hartvigsen, Current status and future perspectives in telecare for elderly people suffering from chronic diseases, *J. Telemed. Telecare* **14**(4) (2008), 195–203.

[10] Bundesministerium für Gesundheit, *Gesundheitsberichterstattung des Bundes. Gesundheit in Deutschland 2006*, Berlin, 2006, pp. 34–35.

[11] Bundesministerium für Land- und Forstwirtschaft, Umwelt und Wasserwirtschaft, *Indikatoren Bericht Juni 2009*, Vienna, 2009.

[12] A.K. Buttery and F.C. Martin, Knowledge, attitudes and intentions about participation in physical activity of older post-acute hospital inpatients, *Physiotherapy* **95**(3) (2009), 192–198.

[13] Y. Chen, Perceived barriers to physical activity among older adults residing in long-term care institutions, *J. Clin. Nurs.* **19**(3–4) (2010), 432–439.

[14] W.J. Chodzko-Zajko, D.N. Proctor, M.A. Fiatarone Singh, C.T. Minson, C.R. Nigg, G.J. Salem and J.S. Skinner, American College of Sports Medicine, Position Stand, Exercise and physical activity for older adults, *Med. Sci. Sports. Exerc.* **41**(7) (2009), 1510–1530.

[15] R.A. Clark, J.J. Yallop, L. Piterman, J. Croucher, A. Tonkin, S. Stewart and H. Krum, CHAT study team: Adherence, adaptation and acceptance of elderly chronic heart failure patients to receiving healthcare via telephone-monitoring, *Eur. J. Heart Fail.* **9**(11) (2007), 1104–1111.

[16] V.S. Conn, A.R. Hafdahl and L.M. Brown, Meta-analysis of quality-of-life outcomes from physical activity interventions, *Nurs. Res.* **58**(3) (2009), 175–183.

[17] Criminal Code (Strafgesetzbuch, StGB), as promulgated on 13 November 1998 (Federal Law Gazette I), 945, 3322, http://www.iuscomp.org/gla/statutes/StGB.htm#203.
[18] Deutsche Bank Research, Telemedizin verbessert Patientenversorgung, *Themen International: Aktuelle Themen* **472** (2010), 5 [online available on: http://www.dbresearch.de/PROD/DBR_INTERNET_DE-PROD/PROD0000000000253251.pdf].
[19] Deutscher Bundestag, Enquete-Kommission, *Schutz des Menschen und der Umwelt, Ziele und Rahmenbedingungen einer nachhaltig zukunftsverträglichen Entwicklung: Konzept Nachhaltigkeit – Vom Leitbild zur Umsetzung*, Bundestagsdrucksache 13/11200, Bonn, 1998.
[20] Directive 95/46/EC of the European Parliament and of the Council of 24 October 1995 on the protection of individuals with regard to the processing of personal data and on the free movement of such data, http://ec.europa.eu/justice/policies/privacy/docs/95-46-ce/dir1995-46_part1_en.pdf.
[21] G. Dooghe, Informal caregivers of elderly people: An European review, *Ageing and Society* **12** (1992), 369–380.
[22] M. Dornan and H. Wynne, Drug compliance in elderly patients: Can it be improved?, *Reviews in Clinical Gerontology* **8** (1998), 183–188.
[23] dsn Projekte und Studien für Wirtschaft und Gesellschaft, *Altenwanderung und Seniorengerechte Infrastruktur. Endbericht Teil B. E-Health und E-Care für ein selbst bestimmtes Wohnen älterer Menschen im ländlichen Raum*, Innenministerium des Landes Schleswig-Holstein, Kiel, 2007.
[24] K.M. Dunn, K.P. Jordan and P.R. Croft, Contributions of prognostic factors for poor outcome in primary care low back pain patients, *Eur. J. Pain* **15**(3) (2010), 313–319.
[25] Federal Statistical Office, *Bevölkerung Deutschlands bis 2050. Übersicht der Ergebnisse der 11. koordinierten Bevölkerungsvorausberechnung – Varianten und zusätzliche Modellrechnungen*, Wiesbaden, 2006.
[26] D.H. Flaherty, *Protecting Privacy in Surveillance Societies: The Federal Republic of Germany, Sweden, France, Canada, and the United States*, The University of North Carolina Press, Chapel Hill, Reprint edition, 1992.
[27] W. Friesdorf and A. Heine, eds, *sentha. Seniorengerechte Technik im häuslichen Alltag. Ein Forschungsbericht mit integriertem Roman*, Springer, Berlin/Heidelberg, 2007.
[28] Frost & Sullivan, Strategic analysis of the European telemedicine markets, 2006.
[29] V. Garms-Homolová and D. Schaeffer, Einzelne Bevölkerungsgruppen: Ältere und Alte, in: *Das Public Health Buch. Gesundheit und Gesundheitswesen*, F.W. Schwartz, B. Badura, R. Leidl, H. Raspe, J. Siegrist and U. Walter, eds, Urban und Schwarzenberg, Munich, 2003, pp. 675–686.
[30] H. Garn and M. Krenn, Smart eye – UCOS universal counting sensor, AIT Austrian Institute of Technology, 2009.
[31] German Federal Data Protection Act (Bundesdatenschutzgesetz – BDSG), as of June 2010 http://www.bfdi.bund.de/EN/DataProtectionActs/Artikel/BDSG_idFv01092009.pdf?__blob=publicationFile.
[32] Gesetz zum Schutz personenbezogener Daten in der Berliner Verwaltung (Berliner Datenschutzgesetz – BlnDSG) in der Fassung vom 17 Dezember 1990 (GVBl. 1991 S. 16, 54), zuletzt geändert durch Gesetz vom 30 November 2007 (GVBl. S. 598), http://www.datenschutz-berlin.de/attachments/346/BlnDSG2008.pdf?1200651252.
[33] S. Hardy and S. Grogan, Preventing disability through exercise: Investigating older adults' influences and motivations to engage in physical activity, *J. Health Psychol.* **14**(7) (2009), 1036–1046.
[34] http://www.analytictech.com/ucinet/.
[35] http://www.dgss.org/fileadmin/pdf/ZahlenundFakten_neu.pdf.
[36] http://www.gfk.com/imperia/md/content/presse/pd_kaufkraft_i-2008_dfin.pdf.
[37] http://www.miljo.fi/default.asp?node=15131&lan=en (11/03/2009).
[38] http://www.mstonline.de/foerderung/projektliste/printable_pdf?vb_nr=V3PMM001 (27/09/2010).
[39] http://www.pmdtec.com/fileadmin/pmdtec/downloads/publications/200710_PMD_VDI.pdf.
[40] http://www.research.philips.com/initiatives/orthopedictrainer/en/downloads/pinode.pdf.
[41] http://www.shimmer-research.com/p/products/development-kits/motion-development-kit.
[42] http://www.svr-gesundheit.de/Gutachten/Gutacht09/Kurzfassung09.pdf.
[43] http://www.un.org/ageing/popageing.html.
[44] http://www.xsens.com/en/general/xbus-kit.
[45] http://www1.smart-senior.de/enEN/.
[46] http://www1.smart-senior.de/index.dhtml/304ced441a418651322t/-/enEN/-/CS/-/Konsortium/Partner.
[47] http://www1.smart-senior.de/index.dhtml/454c99d3196efe60778q/-/enEN/-/CS/-/.
[48] Inter alia, Web 2.0 und die Generation 50+ 2007; EIAA Mediascope Europe 2008, (N)ONLINER Atlas 2009.
[49] H. Klaus, Szenarien für innovative Sicherheitslösungen und Service-Portale, in: *Ambient Assisted Living 2010, 3. Deutscher Kongress mit Ausstellung, Assistenzsysteme im Dienste des Menschen – zuhause und unterwegs, 26–27 Januar 2010 in Berlin, Tagungsbeiträge*, VDE, Berlin, 2010.

[50] I. Korhonen, J. Parkka and M. Van Gils, Health monitoring in the home of the future, *IEEE EMB* **22** (2003), 66–73.
[51] L. Lee, A. Arthur and M. Avis, Using self-efficacy theory to develop interventions that help older people overcome psychological barriers to physical activity: A discussion paper, *Int. J. Nurs. Stud.* **45**(11) (2008), 1690–1699.
[52] S.F. Lerman, Z. Rudich and G. Shahar, Distinguishing affective and somatic dimensions of pain and depression: A confirmatory factor analytic study, *J. Clin. Psychol.* **66** (2010), 456–465.
[53] K.E. Lewis, J.A. Annandale, D.L. Warm, C. Hurlin, M.J. Lewis and L. Lewis, Home telemonitoring and quality of life in stable, optimised chronic obstructive pulmonary disease, *J. Telemed. Telecare* **16**(5) (2010), 253–259.
[54] B. Littig and E. Grießler, *Soziale Nachhaltigkeit*, Kammer für Arbeiter und Angestellte für Wien, Vienna, 2004.
[55] P. Lugert, *Weiblich, alt und chronisch krank? Die Inanspruchnahme medizinischer Leistungen von chronisch kranken Versicherten*, Statistisches Bundesamt, Wuppertal, 2009.
[56] J. Mao, M.S. Gold and M.M. Backonja, Combination drug therapy for chronic pain: A call for more clinical studies, *Eur. J. Pain.* **12**(2) (2010), 157–166.
[57] S. Meyer and E. Schulze, *Smart Home für ältere Menschen. Handbuch für die Praxis*, Fraunhofer IRB Verlag, Stuttgart, 2009.
[58] S. Meyer, E. Schulze, F. Helten and B. Fischer, *Vernetztes Wohnen. Die Informatisierung des Alltagslebens*, edition Sigma, Berlin, 2001.
[59] S. Meyer, E. Schulze and P. Müller, *Das intelligente Haus – Selbständige Lebensführung im Alter. Möglichkeiten und Grenzen vernetzter Technik im Haushalt alter Menschen*, in: *Reihe Stiftung Der Private Haushalt*, Vol. 30, Campus Verlag, Frankfurt/New York, 1998.
[60] M. Noble, J.R. Treadwell, S.J. Tregear, V.H. Coates, P.J. Wiffen, C. Akafomo and K.M. Schoelles, Long-term opioid management for chronic noncancer pain, *Cochrane Database Syst. Rev.* **20**(1) (2010), CD006605.
[61] M. Nöthen and K. Böhm, Krankheitskosten in Deutschland: Welchen Preis hat die Gesundheit im Alter?, in: *Beiträge zur Gesundheitsberichterstattung des Bundes, Gesundheit und Krankheit im Alter*, K. Böhm, Statistisches Bundesamt, C. Tesch-Römer, Deutsches Zentrum für Altersfragen and T. Ziese, Robert Koch-Institut, eds, Berlin, 2009, pp. 228–246.
[62] OECD, *Key Environmental indicators 2008*, 2008.
[63] OECD, *Towards Sustainable Development – Environmental Indicators*, Paris, 1998.
[64] Population Division, Department of Economic and Social Affairs, United Nations Secretariat, the Ageing of the World's Population, http://www.globalaging.org/waa2/documents/theagingoftheworld.htm.
[65] E. Rosqvist, E. Heikkinen, T. Lyyra, M. Hirvensalo, M. Kallinen, R. Leinonen, M. Rasinaho, I. Pakkala and T. Rantanen, Factors affecting the increased risk of physical inactivity among older people with depressive symptoms, *Scand. J. Med. Sci. Sports* **19**(3) (2009), 398–405.
[66] C. Scanaill, S. Carew, P. Barralon, N. Noury, D. Lyons and G. Lyons, A review of approaches to mobility telemonitoring of the elderly in their living environment, *Annals of Biomedical Engineering* **34**(4) (2006), 547–563.
[67] S. Schmidt, B. Beil, M. Patten and J. Stettin, Acceptance of telemonitoring to enhance medication compliance in patients with chronic heart failure, *Telemedicine and e-Health* **14**(5) (2008), 426–433.
[68] J.H. Spangenberg, A. Femia, F. Hinterberger and H. Schütz, *Material Flow-Based Indicators in Environmental Reporting*, European Environment Agency, Luxembourg, 1999.
[69] Statistisches Bundesamt, *Nachhaltige Entwicklung in Deutschland Indikatorenbericht 2008*, Wiesbaden, 2008.
[70] The Privacy Act of 1974, 5 U.S.C. §552a, http://www.justice.gov/opcl/privstat.htm.
[71] A. Tinker, Housing for elderly people, *Reviews in Clinical Gerontology* **7** (1997), 171–176.
[72] A. Traganitis, D. Trypakis, M. Spanakis, S. Condos, T. Stamkopoulos, M. Tsiknakis and S. Orphanoudakis, Home monitoring and personal health management servies in a regional health telematic network, in: *Engineering Medicine and Biology Society. Proceedings of the 23rd Annual International Conference of the IEEE*, Vol. 4, 2001, pp. 3575–3578 [online available on: http://www.dtic.mil/cgi-bin/GetTRDoc?AD=ADA411266&Location=U2&doc=GetTRDoc.pdf].
[73] T. Tsutsumi, B.M. Don, L.D. Zaichkowsky and L.L. Delizonna, Physical fitness and psychological benefits of strength training in community dwelling older adults, *Appl. Human Sci.* **16**(6) (1997), 257–266.
[74] UNECE, Measuring sustainable development, New York/Geneva, 2009.
[75] United Nations, *Indicators of Sustainable Development: Guidelines and Methodologies*, New York, 2007.
[76] United Nations, The millennium development goals report 2009, New York, 2009.
[77] US – European Union Safe Harbor, http://www.export.gov/safeharbor/eu/index.asp.

[78] R.A. Winett, D.M. Williams and B.M. Davy, Initiating and maintaining resistance training in older adults: A social cognitive theory-based approach, *Br. J. Sports Med.* **43**(2) (2009), 114–119.
[79] A.K. Woodend, M. Fraser, H. Sherrard and L. Stueve, Readmission and quality of life: The impact of telehomecare in heart failure, *J. Card. Fail.* **8** (2002), 98.
[80] C. Zugck, M. Nelles, L. Frankenstein, C. Schultz, T. Helms, H. Korb, H. Katus and A. Remppis, Telemedizinisches Monitoring bei herzinsuffizienten Patienten, *Herzschrittmachertherapie und Elektrophysiologie* **16**(3) (2005), 176–182.

Handbook of Ambient Assisted Living
J.C. Augusto et al. (Eds.)
IOS Press, 2012

doi:10.3233/978-1-60750-837-3-693

R&D Projects Related to AAL in TECNALIA's Health Technologies Unit

Michael OBACH[a,*], Pierre BARRALON[a], Enrique LEÓN[a], Leire MARTÍNEZ[a], Javier ARCAS[b], Igone IDÍGORAS[b], Alberto MARTÍNEZ[b], Arantxa RENTERÍA[b] and Carmen PASTOR[b]
[a] *TECNALIA Research & Innovation, Health Technologies Unit, Donostia – San Sebastián, Spain*
[b] *TECNALIA Research & Innovation, Health Technologies Unit, Zamudio, Spain*

Abstract. Ambient Assisted Living (AAL) is a key research topic in TECNALIA's Health Technologies Unit. The present chapter gives an overview over the ongoing research and development projects of the biggest private research alliance in Southern Europe in this field.

Keywords. Fall detection, fall prevention, service robotics, low cost devices, training and rehabilitation at home, ambient assisted emotional regulation, user centred design, emotion detection, affective wearables, assistive technology

Introduction

The present chapter gives an overview over the ongoing and recently closed research and development activities of the Health Technologies Unit in TECNALIA Research & Innovation – in the sequel short *TECNALIA* – that are related to Ambient Assisted Living (AAL). TECNALIA is the largest private Research, Development and Innovation (R+D+i) group in Spain and one of the leading ones in Europe after a merging process of eight technology centres located in the Basque Country (Spain). TECNALIA's mission is to offer value and wealth to society in general, and to the business community in particular, by means of Research and Innovation. The operation model of TECNALIA is based on five sector-based multidisciplinary business divisions, with a strong focus on the market: Health and Quality of Life, Sustainable Development, ICT, Industry and Transport, and Innovation and Society [14].

AAL is one of the most important research fields of the Health Technologies Unit, which includes research, development, prototyping and testing of solutions on Assisting Independence and Maintaining Well-being.

The overall aim of *Assisting Independence* is thus to investigate and develop assistive devices and systems that can be used by disabled and ageing people to enable them to safely attempt and successfully complete Activities of Daily Living (ADL), both Basic and Instrumental (BADL and IADL), including mobility activities in and around the home. The principle of support is that it should reduce the hazards and risks involved in engaging in the daily activity, but it should not remove the activity nor transform it into some other activity. The standard set of BADLs and IADLs requires a

[*]Corresponding Author: Michael Obach, TECNALIA Research & Innovation, Health Technologies Unit, Paseo Mikeletegi 7, E-20009 Donostia – San Sebastián, Spain. E-mail: Michael.obach@tecnalia.com.

range of actions, movements, and postures that can be difficult or impossible to produce or maintain safely as a result of a lack of strength, stability, reach, range of movement, and manipulation dexterity. The provision of safe and effective physical forces, torques, extensions and manipulations can restore a person's ability to safely attempt and successfully complete BADLs and IADLs.

The purpose of *Maintaining Well-being* is to develop mechanisms to assist formal and informal caregivers in supporting the physical and emotional well-being of the impaired and elderly at home thereby deferring nursing home admission and facilitating the conditions for "ageing in place". The principle of support consists in the identification and the implementation of simple, inexpensive data management solutions that are sufficiently sophisticated to support decision making of the caregivers. The approach adopted to design usable devices is given by an intensive stakeholder consultation to identify specific needs and niche markets, user centred design, innovation and low-cost and a progressive development building up from the monitoring and persuasive tools.

Existing research approaches aimed at measuring the various constituents of well-being rely heavily on the observation of user's activities. User monitoring provides the tools and mechanisms to acquire data from the environment and the user through an orchestrated, thoughtful utilization of sensors embedded in common objects or clothes, attached to the body, or located in places around the living space. Systems that detect affective states based on bodily measures offer the possibility of taking actions aimed at reducing the impact of negative emotions on the physical and psychological health of older persons. To this end, the operation of such systems is based on an amalgamation of design principles employed in affective and pervasive computing applying Affective wearables, pattern recognition in vital signs, Affect/ambient-aware feedback and biofeedback.

Interactive communication systems involve the use of techniques and instruments like Pervasive technologies and Ubiquitous computing to facilitate daily activities and allow self-awareness. Therefore, "just-in-time" context-aware information is provided as a strategy to motivate behaviour change with the aim of promoting a healthy ageing.

One main principle of TECNALIA's Health Technologies Unit is to involve potential final users and all major stakeholders in the different phases of each project. This means involving older people, people with cognitive or physical disabilities, their relatives and caregivers, clinical experts and medical professionals in the project development.

The following sections give a chronologically ordered overview over some outstanding projects of the research groups of the Business Unit in the field of AAL and related research domains. Table 1 shows which "key areas of needs of the AAL target group" (see [5]) these projects mainly address.

1. The VIDA Project

1.1. Overview

- Short name of project: VIDA;
- Full name of project: *Vivienda Domótica Accesible* (Accessible Home Control System);
- Author: Igone Idigoras;

Table 1. AAL-related projects of TECNALIA in chronological order of their start date, and addressed key areas of needs of the AAL target group

Short name	Start date	Mobility	Health/ Wellness	Hobbies	Social Interaction	Home Care	Safety, Secur., Privacy
VIDA	2006-01-01					X	X
SOPRANO	2007-01-01					X	X
AmIE	2007-05-01		X		X	X	X
ELISA	2007-07-01	X			X		
AUZOLAN	2008-01-01		X		X	X	X
CompanionAble	2008-01-01		X		X	X	X
ShowerRug	2008-01-01		X				X
HAPTIMAP	2008-09-01	X		X			
TeleREHA	2009-01-01					X	
BEDMOND	2009-06-01		X			X	X
HearMeFeelMe	2009-06-01		X			X	
SENTIENT	2009-06-01		X				
Florence	2010-02-01		X		X	X	X

- Call identifier: Spanish R&D project funded by the Spanish Government within the AVANZA Programme;
- Consortium member: TECNALIA Research & Innovation (formerly ROBOTIKER-Tecnalia);
- Start date: 1st January 2006;
- End date: 31st December 2008.

1.2. Summary

The VIDA system is an accessible home control solution developed by TECNALIA. It allows monitoring, control and supervision of all electronic and electrical equipment of the home. The system was developed focusing on different groups of people with disabilities and is fully accessible for everybody regardless of their physical or sensory impairments.

The VIDA project addressed the lack of autonomy in the home of people with disabilities. VIDA is a comprehensive solution that supported remote control of light switches in each room, opening and closing of blinds, door opening and closing image access, and entertainment equipment like TV sets, CD and DVD players, and the radio. Furthermore, it allowed detecting incidents like water spills, smoke, gas, intrusion alerts, and alarms and it had a panic button.

Based on commercially available and standardized domotic networks, VIDA used a Smart phone or a PDA as universal remote control and user interface. The system was composed of the following elements:

- communications platform (gateway): a specific gateway based on the integration of standard communication protocols: Wi-Fi, IRDA, modem, USB, X10, ENX (EIB-KONNEX);
- software for device management, i.e. a PDA/Smartphone interface and a monitoring application for the PC.

There are a large number of home automation and domotic solutions on the market. However, such solutions often are not designed to be used by people with disabilities.

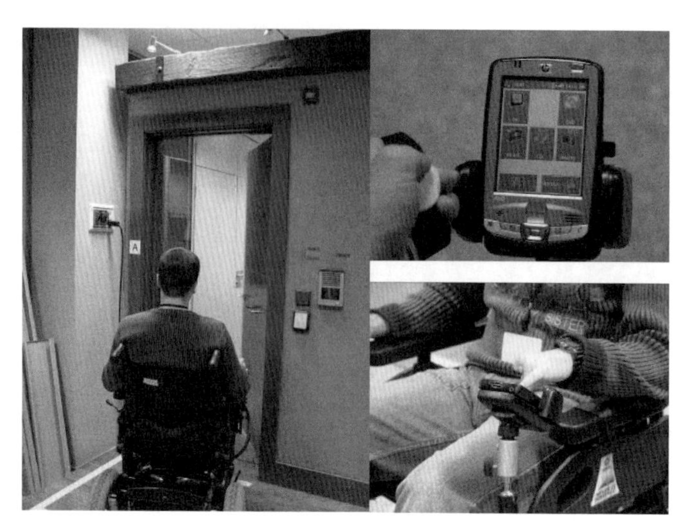

Figure 1. Some details of the VIDA system.

In Spain, for instance, small businesses sell some specially adapted solutions. There are an increasing number of controls and terminals in daily activities. Many of these devices however are a barrier for people with disabilities, because the devices are not adapted for special needs. Designers of many devices do not take into account the problems of mobility, dexterity, coordination and strength of people with physical disabilities, or problems with vision, hearing and language of people with sensory disabilities.

VIDA was designed starting from the real needs of different groups of people with disabilities, compiled from interviews at the first stages of the project. People with physical disabilities benefit from having a mobile device integrating those utilities of domotics that reduce or avoid displacements and facilitate the use of everyday elements, e.g. lighting, shutters, gate. People with mobility impairments receive a message through the PDA or Smartphone when the bell is ringing and without moving to the door the image of the person who rings the bell is shown on the display. Finally, the front door can be remotely opened, see Fig. 1.

Considering users with hearing impairments or visual impairments, multimodal event communication has been implemented in the VIDA system. Light, vibration, and text are used to inform hearing impaired people about any event detected at home, and text to speech features are included to inform about the detected events to visually impaired people. Events detected at home include technical alarms (smoke, water damages, gas), door bells, front door openings and phone calls. When any of those events are detected, the user is informed through different modalities: vibration, light, text and voice.

Text-to-speech and speech recognition features are also included in the solution oriented to help visually impaired people. All text and graphical options supported by the VIDA system can be accessed by visual impaired people using voice messages. Moreover, additional screen reading options have been implemented in the VIDA system to improve accessibility of blind people to the touch-screen-based graphical user interface.

2. The SOPRANO Project

2.1. Overview

- Short name of project: SOPRANO;
- Full name of project: Service-oriented Programmable Smart Environments for Older Europeans;
- Author: SOPRANO consortium (corresponding author: Igone Idigoras);
- Call identifier: Integrated Project, co-funded by the EC under FP6. Strategic Objective 6.2.2: Ambient Assisted Living for the Ageing Society;
- Consortium members (leader first): EXODUS S.A., Tunstall Telecom Ltd, SingularLogic Software Anonymos Etairia Michanografikon Efarmogon, CAS Software AG, empirica Gesellschaft für Kommunikations- und Technologieforschung mbH, PROSYST SOFTWARE GmbH, Dialoc ID Technology BV, Smart Homes – Dutch Expertise Centre for Smart Technology and Smart Living, TECNALIA Research & Innovation (formerly ROBOTIKER-Tecnalia), Institute of communication and computer systems, Netherlands organisation for applied scientific research TNO, Institute for Language and Speech Processing, Forschungszentrum Informatik an der Universität Karlsruhe, University Stuttgart, Institute for Human Factors and Technology Management, VICOMTech, Zentrum für Graphische Datenverarbeitung e.V., University of Ljubljana (Faculty of social sciences), INGEMA, University of Liverpool, Stichting Verzorging En Verpleging Eindhoven E.O. De Archipel, FASS – Andalusian Social Services Foundation, Work Research Centre Ltd., London Borough of Newham, West Lothian Council, Simon Fraser University;
- Start date: 1st January 2007;
- End date: 31st March 2011.

2.2. Summary

SOPRANO aims at designing a system that assists older people in coping with everyday life in greater comfort and safety, with integrated delivery of high quality support and care. The project also aims to help all Europeans to continue to live independently and play a full role in society. SOPRANO develops and adapts to normal home environments a sophisticated range of suitably unobtrusive components seamlessly linked to external service provision [22].

A major objective of SOPRANO is to take a leap forward in the way users can interact with and take charge of their living environment, as well as to develop the way professional care personnel can support the SOPRANO users when called on to do so. The SOPRANO system acts not as a traditional "smart home", passively receiving user commands, nor as pure "remote care", by alerting outside staff to act in case of an alarm. Instead, SOPRANO acts as an informed, friendly agent, taking orders, giving advice or reminders and ready to help, and get help when needed.

SOPRANO has been highly innovative both in terms of its approach to the research and development process and in terms of the social and technical work being carried out. An extensive program of research was carried out involving users at all stages of the R&D process.

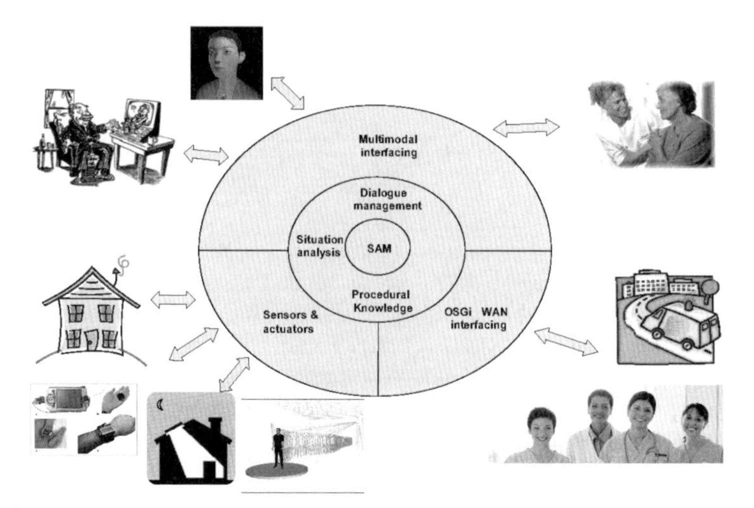

Figure 2. Use contexts in SOPRANO.

One of SOPRANO's main aims is to move away from technology-push and problem-focused development approaches towards more user-centred and user-driven design approaches. Such as system design is based upon well identified needs and requirements of older people. SOPRANO adopted the so-called Experience and Application Research (E&AR) design methodology which involves research, development and design by, with and for users. An extensive program of research was carried out involving users at all stages of the R&D process, which can be subdivided in several stages of user involvement. The aim of the first phase was to understand and to specify the context of use and to also specify user and organisational requirements. The gathered information was transformed into use cases. Then, three more cycles of user interaction have been realised following an iterative multilevel prototyping approach.

In the first cycle use cases were transformed into multimedia demonstrators and scenarios were presented to users by a theatre group. User feedback was reflected in the prototypes of the next cycle. The use cases selected and developed in the project are the following, see also Fig. 2:

- Medication 1: medication compliance support with nearby informal caregiver;
- Medication 2: medication compliance support with distant informal caregiver;
- Fall: adjusting care to increasing frailty;
- Safe: monitoring activity for signs of problems;
- Exercise: helping older people recover from hospital on their own;
- Activity: keeping healthy and active;
- Remembering: coping with cognitive ageing;
- Entertainment: countering boredom.

The second cycle aimed at testing real component prototypes of the SOPRANO system with end users for the very first time and to help technical designers to improve the prototype components and overall system.

In a third cycle the integrated SOPRANO system as a close-to-final prototype will be tested both in demonstration homes and in large scale field trials in order to evaluate the system's impact in real-life situations.

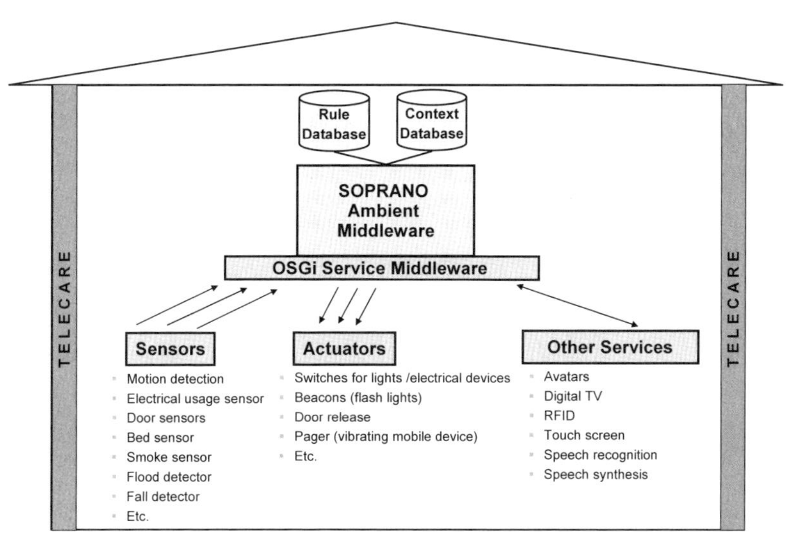

Figure 3. SOPRANO software components.

In every stage of the user involvement, the user feedback has been analysed and evaluated according to its value for SOPRANO (criteria are acceptability, perceived usefulness, usability, etc.), according to its cross-cultural validity and in stages of prototyping according to the feasibility of the idea.

The SOPRANO system comprises a central operating unit, peripheral devices, sensors and services for communication with external devices. A set of different services are supported by the system including:

- speech synthesis and speech recognition;
- touch screen for user graphical interface;
- digital TV service and graphical interaction with the user through the TV;
- RFID identification service;
- avatar service.

TECNALIA has participated in the graphical user interface design and development, both for TV and for touch screen interaction devices.

As shown in Fig. 3, all software components of SOPRANO are implemented or encapsulated as OSGi bundles and they operate in an OSGi application framework running in a Linux PC. The core, SAM Soprano Ambient Middleware, is a rule-based system working on an ontology model containing information about the assisted person and the environment. These research results have been used by FZI Research Centre for Information Technologies, CAS Software AG and Friedrich-Schiller-University of Jena in the openAAL joint open source initiative, which is available under the very flexible and industry-friendly LGPL-license [13].

Moreover, SOPRANO is one of the original projects integrating the universAAL initiative. The universAAL project (www.universaal.org) is an EU-FP7-funded project which aim is at consolidating different platforms in the field of AAL with the objective to provide a common Reference Architecture for AAL and also a Reference Open Source implementation that gets the better solutions from each source project. Other original projects were PERSONA, MPOWER, OASIS, GENESYS, AMIGO and

VAALID. Starting from the different semantic platform solutions in the field of AAL and semantic approaches obtained in those source projects, the current process in universAAL is consolidating the engineering decisions and concepts for a common reference solution. universAAL is also actively supporting the AAL Open Association (AALOA) activities using it as a tool for promotion and community creation around technical aspects of AAL systems [1].

3. The AmIE Project

3.1. Overview

- Short name of project: AmIE;
- Full name of project: Ambient Intelligence for the Elderly;
- Author: AmIE consortium (corresponding author: Alberto Martínez);
- Call identifier: ITEA 2 – 06002;
- Consortium members (leader first): Telefónica I+D, Alcatel Bells, Audio Riders, City of Oulu, Fagor Electrodomésticos, Ikerlan, Inabensa, Indra, INGEMA, In-Ham, Mawell, Mextal, Mobilera, Philips CE iLab, RBG Medical Devices, TECNALIA Research & Innovation (formerly ROBOTIKER-Tecnalia), Soneco, Technische Universiteit Eindhoven, Vrije Universiteit Brussel, VTT, Yrjö ja Hanna – Säätiö/Yrjö & Hanna, Zuidzorg, Incode;
- Start date: 1st May 2007;
- End date: 1st June 2010.

3.2. Summary

Europe is currently the continent with the highest proportion of elderly citizens, what also means people with impairments, disabilities or chronic diseases. As a result, European governments are facing challenges like providing assistance, medical support and a sustainable economy of the welfare state. The AmIE project responded to some of these challenges with a complete, intelligent, distributed system providing customized adaptive support to all people in need of assistance, according to their own specific situation, and in a non-intrusive and respectful way.

The AmIE project was a solution where the interaction with the user was not a standard or a roughly configured one, but adapted to each user and to each situation for an optimal acceptance and understanding, and where the design was based in the principle of non-intrusiveness so that the daily life of the user was not affected by the system elements. More specifically, the system was able to adapt to the user needs and character, helping them in getting through their daily routine in a way that was effective in providing support where needed without making them feel humiliated by excessive attention.

Individual users are the main focus of AmIE. They should perceive the intelligent ambience as a friendly, reliable and useful context in which to develop their daily activities, and neither as a handicap due to its difficulty of use nor as an intrusion.

AmIE was not just another tele-care system; it was designed to be a part of the users' way of life, offering a simple interactive interface in a nonintrusive way. The AmIE system enables the user to have a totally autonomous life style by providing cus-

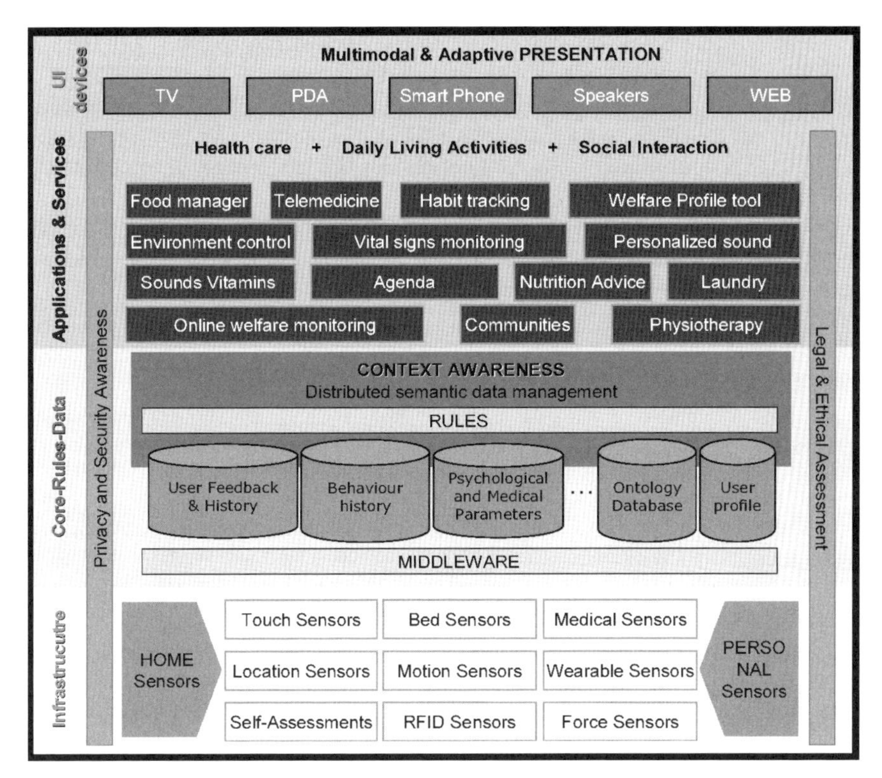

Figure 4. Architecture layers of the AmIE system.

tomised solutions for his/her particular needs and preferences, daily activities and close ambience, respecting his/her privacy and taking into account all legal constraints.

While primarily addressing older people, the results of the project can be extended to other target groups, such as: people with disabilities, patients waiting for transplants, patients with muscular dystrophy or sleep apnoea, pregnancy at risk, patients in prison facilities and people in drug rehabilitation programmes.

AmIE provides new approaches to and important tools for non-intrusive sensing and intelligent monitoring addressing context awareness, future ambient-intelligence solutions, integrating sensitive and cognitive capacities, intelligence and self-learning abilities, ontologies and actuation rules, design of self-configurable and user-adapted interfaces through user profiling tools, domotics, new user and context models, innovative security and privacy approaches, etc.

Figure 4 represents all the modules considered in the AmIE architecture to identify the different modules developed in the different scenarios considered in the project. The picture sums all the developments and functionalities implemented by all partners in the AmIE project. The different blocks are distributed in several layers according to the functionality implemented in each of them.

The lower layer represents the sensors and devices which generate information related to user context within the AmIE scenario.

In a first intermediate level, the information will be processed and used to adapt the system to user needs.

In a higher intermediate level, there are many services that interact with the user in many different ways according to the situation.

The Human Computer communication is managed with the HCI module which manages the devices in the presentation layer [15].

TECNALIA contributed to the project part of the design and development, from the definition of user requirements to the dissemination and exploitation activities, going technically through the selection of the smart home sensor network and the design and development of the algorithms to monitor the nightly activities of the elderly person to remotely inform the medical doctor.

4. The ELISA Project

4.1. Overview

- Short name of project: ELISA;
- Full name of project: Intelligent Localization Environment for Assisted Services;
- Author: ELISA consortium (corresponding author: Arantxa Rentería);
- Call identifier: *Proyecto Singular Estratégico* funded by Spanish Government and European FEDER Programme;
- Consortium members (leader first): CreativIT (formerly Apif Moviquity), TECNALIA Research & Innovation (formerly ROBOTIKER-Tecnalia), Universidad Politécnica de Madrid, EARCON, Intelligent Data, VICOMTech, Gowex, INGEMA, Edosoft Factory, MICROGÉNESIS;
- Start date: 1st July 2007;
- End date: 31st December 2009.

4.2. Summary

The ELISA project addressed the problem of personal localization and guidance in indoor and outdoor environments. The goal was to provide users with the most accurate and reliable technology depending on their profiles. The authors analyzed different technologies for these purposes. Relevant parameters which finally drove the overall system performance were highlighted. In particular, the indoor technologies studied were Bluetooth, Wi-Fi, RFID, UWB, and ultrasounds. With the aim to cover outdoor environments the project analyzed technologies such as WiMAX and GPS. Finally, the indoor location system was integrated with a GPS based outdoor localization system to provide global coverage.

When focussing on a collective of citizens with special needs, either sensorial, motor or cognitive (dependent, disabled and elderly people), location-based services can provide final users with a high level of autonomy and safety through the assistance these services can supply. Thus, they promote their social inclusion and the ability to avoid physical obstacles by appropriate guidance. Upon this motivation, the ELISA services were location based and personalized in function on the users' profiles.

The following *indoor services* were provided:

- Access control. This service prevents unauthorized personnel (patients) from entering restricted areas or leaving the place, e.g. a hospital or a nursing home.

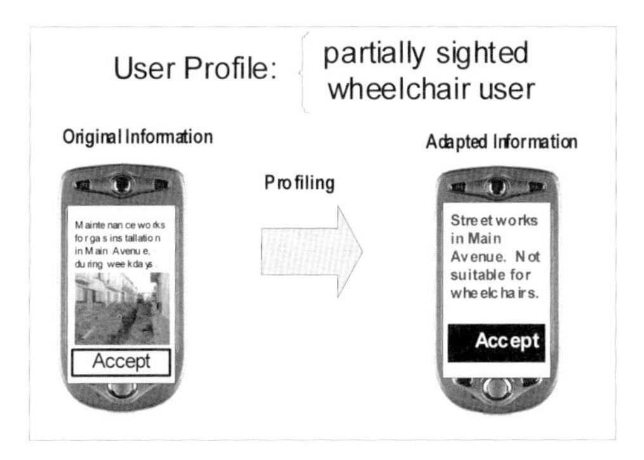

Figure 5. ELISA interface for localisation and guidance services [18].

When the patient enters a restricted area, the system activates the automatic protection for this area and the caregiver receives an advice on his or her PDA.

- Equipment location. This service allows the caregivers to locate free wheelchairs.
- People search and location. The main aim of this service is to provide a support tool to caregivers. Through this service caregivers are allowed to locate any patient within the centre.
- Guiding service. This service guides the users from their current position to the desired one. After the user has selected where to go, the service provides a map of the centre with the position and the destination and the route according to his or her profile.
- Alarm. Any patient having a PDA is able to inform the caregivers by an alarm in the caregiver's PDA that they need some help.

The *outdoor services* that were developed are listed below:

- Generate user content. Users are able to create their own content with their mobile devices, annotating, uploading and sharing it with the community.
- Alarm. This service is equivalent to the provided at indoor locations.
- Personalized routes. The objective of this service was to create a route allowing users to visit the destination points they want. The route takes into account possible disabilities users could have. Besides, routes use public transportation when it is adapted to user's special needs.
- Public transportation. This service focuses on helping users to move by means of public transportation.

The role of TECNALIA in this project was the data filtering and the user configuration facilities, in order to adapt the information provided to the user on the screen to his or her specific impairments or preferences, see Fig. 5.

Other, similar projects, e.g. ENABLED, MAPPED, ASK-IT, GiMoDig, dealt with similar objectives as ELISA, but did not cover indoor and outdoor applications at the same time.

5. The AUZOLAN Project

5.1. Overview

- Short name of project: AUZOLAN;
- Full name of project: Integrated care and support for elderly people living in remote rural areas;
- Author: Igone Idigoras;
- Call identifier: national R&D project founded by the Spanish Government under the AVANZA Programme;
- Consortium members (leader first): TECNALIA Research & Innovation (formerly ROBOTIKER-Tecnalia), Residence ORUE, IKUBO;
- Start date: 1st January 2008;
- End date: 31st December 2009.

5.2. Summary

The main objective of the AUZOLAN project was the provision of an integrated care and assistance service for elderly people living at home in rural areas. The developed solutions respond to this need by integrating several services into a common platform covering social care (tele-care) and health care (tele-health) domains.

The AUZOLAN system is the result of two Spanish projects carried out during 2008 and 2009 by ROBOTIKER-Tecnalia (now TECNALIA), the residence ORUE (company providing health and social care services located in a rural area) and the telecommunications engineering company IKUBO. The specific role of TECNALIA was the development of the services provided at home and at the care centre. The integration with the existing social alarm call centre was also led by TECNALIA.

Using the AUZOLAN system, the residence centre ORUE provided integrated care services to all elderly people living in the rural area nearby. The system offered:

- customized services adapted to local needs and conditions;
- preventive programmes in addition to alarm and care services;
- the support from an existing socio-medical care centre already equipped with suitable professional and technical resources;
- the attention from a care centre located very locally offering a closer attention and shorter reaction time in emergencies;
- a mixture of remote and face-to-face services.

Another innovative aspect of the project has been the application of user-driven open innovation methodologies in order to engage the users early into the human-centric and participatory design process. Living Lab methodology was applied to ensure the proactive and continuous involvement of the users during all stages of the project development.

The three main components of AUZOLAN consisted of a Care Centre, a Communication Network and the home of the elderly people. In particular, a 24/7 tele-care call centre was located at ORUE, where care assistants attending the call centre used multimedia equipment (webcam, microphone and speakers) to attend the user alarms and provide the remote care and health services of the AUZOLAN system.

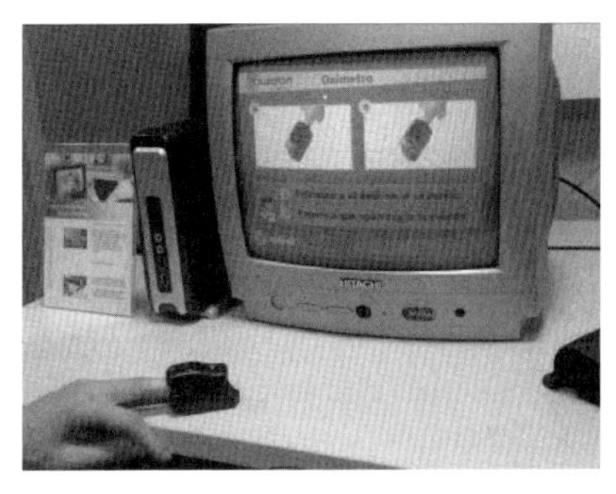
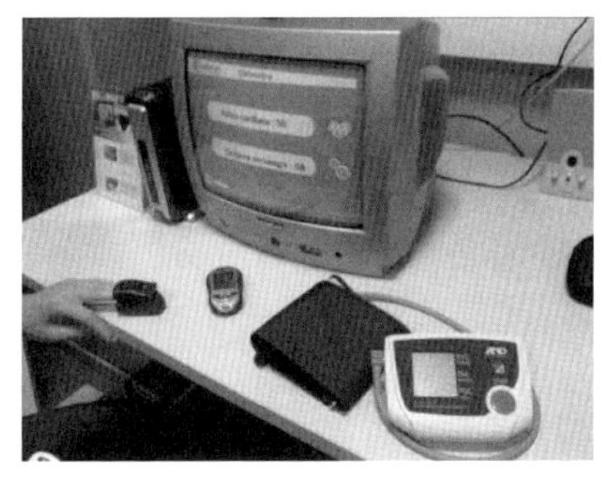

Figure 6. Health monitoring services of AUZOLAN.

The AUZOLAN project was focused in a rural area without any broadband communications infrastructure. So deployment of the communication infrastructure was necessary. A private broadband network was installed that combined WiMAX and Wi-Fi technologies.

Eight pilots were tested in the homes of elderly people living in the far-flung neighbourhood of ORUE. The equipment installed in the homes included social alarm and emergency sensors, a residential gateway as the central operating unit at home managing all the services offered to the end user through the TV including a webcam and microphone devices used for video and audio connection with the care centre and finally some health monitoring devices, i.e. portable wireless health monitoring devices were also provided to the end users to be used by elderly people in their own home to measure and monitor their health by themselves and also to transmit this information to the care centre. Devices to monitor blood pressure, blood glucose and weight were supported by the AUZOLAN platform.

The AUZOLAN system has been designed to be easy to use by elderly people at home. All services were provided through the TV set. End users could access AUZOLAN services using their own TV set and a very simple remote control as shown in Fig. 6. The services included personal and technical alarm detection, remote visits as daily or weekly audiovisual communication with staff from the health-social care centre by means of the domestic television set, rehabilitation exercises in the home through the TV, and vital data acquisition at home and transmission to the care centre.
The requirements which the project addressed included:

- Increase in security and attention in case of alarm or emergency. The users have a technical alarm management system (gas, smoke and inactivity detection) and a personal alarm to communicate directly with a nearby care centre;
- Many elderly people suffer from chronic illnesses (e.g. diabetes and hypertension) needing a regular follow-up and occasional transport to the health centre or chemist. The system offers supervision and measurement of vital signs in the home either carried out by the users themselves or supported by informal caregivers;
- Physical exercises, including keep-fit exercises, are beneficial for the elderly. The system offers customised videos for physical exercises that users can do at home. A physiotherapist evaluated the needs of each user and created a customised exercise plan;

- Another important problem of the elderly people living on their own in rural areas and suffering from mobility problems is the reduction of social interaction activities. The system provided different social interaction activities including daily or weekly face-to-face contact with the staff of the tele-care centre and video-conferencing contact both with the care centre and with other users in the neighbourhood.

After the eight pilot studies in real homes, which are running since October 2009, more end users have been incorporated during the first months of 2010. The AUZOLAN solution is currently being provided with new functionalities aiming at developing an integrated platform. To this end the number of pilot installations will increase up to 20 homes. The three most important new services developed are the home delivery of catering services, allowing the users to choose meals using the TV set, the home delivery of medication, and the services for the encouragement and promotion of social interaction of elderly and disabled people with mobility problems living on their own in urban city area.

6. The CompanionAble Project

6.1. Overview

- Short name of project: CompanionAble;
- Full name of project: Integrated Cognitive Assistive & Domotic Companion Robotic Systems for Ability & Security;
- Author: Companionable consortium (corresponding author: Arantxa Rentería);
- Call identifier: ICT-2007.7.1 ICT and Ageing;
- Consortium members (leader first): The University of Reading, Ilmenau University of Technology, Assistance Publique – Hôpitaux de Paris, Groupe des Écoles des Telecommunications, TECNALIA Research & Innovation (formerly ROBOTIKER-Tecnalia), Austrian Institute of Technology GmbH, Legrand France SA, AKG Acoustics GmbH, Chambre de commerce et d'industrie de Paris, AG ESIGETEL, Université d'Evry-Val d'Essonne, MetraLabs GmbH Neue Technologien und Systeme, Stichting Smart Homes, Center for Usability Research and Engineering, University of A Coruña, Innovation Centre in Housing for Adapted Movement, Verklizan, Ingema;
- Start date: 1st January 2008;
- End date: 31st December 2011.

6.2. Summary

There are widely acknowledged imperatives for helping the elderly living at home (semi)-independently for as long as possible. Without cognitive stimulation support the elderly dementia and depression sufferers can deteriorate rapidly and the caregivers will face a more demanding task. Both groups are increasingly at the risk of social exclusion.

CompanionAble is providing the synergy of Robotics and Ambient Intelligence technologies and their semantic integration to provide a care-giver's assistive environment. This will support the cognitive stimulation and therapy management of the care-

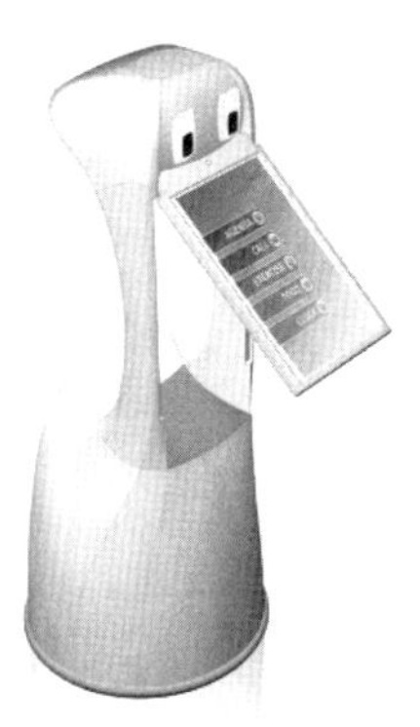

Figure 7. CompanionAble mobile robot [23].

recipient. This is mediated by a robotic companion (mobile facilitation), see Fig. 7, working collaboratively with a smart home environment (stationary facilitation).

The distinguishing advantages of the CompanionAble Framework Architecture arise from the objective of graceful, scalable and cost-effective integration. Thus, CompanionAble addresses the issues of social inclusion and homecare of people suffering from chronic cognitive disabilities prevalent among the increasing European older population. A participative and inclusive co-design and scenario validation approach will drive the RTD efforts in CompanionAble; involving care recipients and their close caregivers as well as the wider stakeholders. This is to ensure end-to-end systemic viability, flexibility, modularity and affordability as well as a focus on overall care support governance and integration with quality of experience issues such as dignity-privacy-security preserving responsibilities fully considered [17].

TECNALIA's role within the CompanionAble project is the design and implementation of the graphical user interface, to be mounted on a tactile display in the robot, and the development of a software module to monitor the night habits of an elderly person, in order to detect potential diseases. In addition, TECNALIA is the responsible partner for dissemination activities.

7. The ShowerRug Project

7.1. Overview

- Short name of project: ShowerRug;
- Full name of project: Fall detection in specific indoor environment;
- Author: Pierre Barralon;
- Internal project;
- Start date: 1st January 2008;
- End date: 31st December 2010.

7.2. Summary

Two important problems of ageing which relate to physical and cognitive disability are falls and dementia. Falls are a very common problem in the older population with 30%

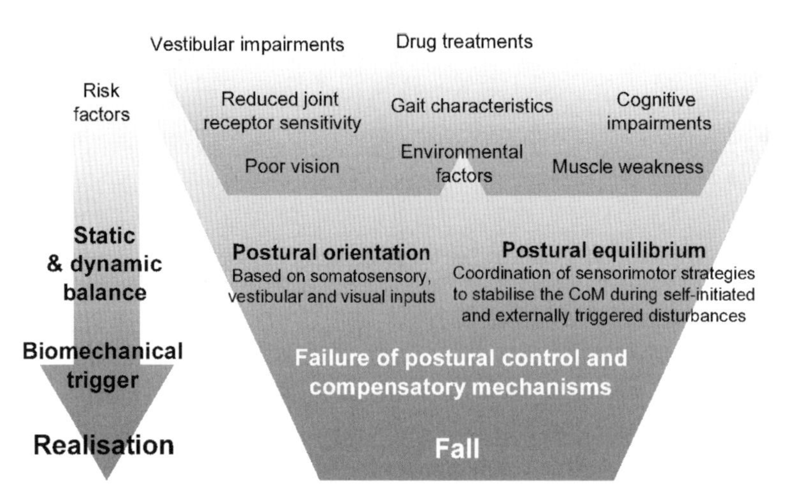

Figure 8. The chain of factors of the phenomenon of fall.

of community dwelling older people above 65 years of age falling each year and 12% of these falling at least twice [9]. Depending on the population studied, between 22%–60% of older people suffer injuries from falls, 10%–15% suffer serious injuries, 2%–6% suffer fractures and 0.2%–1.5% suffer hip fractures specifically incurring high costs in terms of quality of life as well as significant health and social care expenditure. Even non-injurious falls have significant negative consequences for the individual because of fear of falling, functional deterioration, anxiety, depression and loss of confidence and hence independence.

The Prevention of Falls Network Europe (ProFaNE) collaborators, in conjunction with international experts in the field and using consensus methodology define a fall as "an unexpected event in which the participant comes to rest on the ground, floor or lower level" [6]. Under the assumption that a fall can be described as a mechanical phenomenon, biomechanics is the science needed for addressing this problem. Additionally, in theory, a fall can be detected with 100% accuracy only after its end and any attempt to detect it before its completion will introduce a risk of being wrong. This is because the fall is the last element of a chain of conditions (Fig. 8).

In the EU-27 countries lived 495 million habitants in 2007 [3]. 16.7% of the population, i.e. 82.6 million people, were over 65 years old. Considering that 33% of them fall at least once a year [6], this corresponds to 27.3 millions people who experience a fall. Moreover, 6% of the falls happen in the shower or the bathtub [6,9,10]. This suggests that there may be as many as 1.6 million older people in Europe who fall each year in the shower or bathtub.

Fall detectors are mainly divided into two categories: wearable and external devices. Wearable fall detectors were suggested not to be well accepted by users when having shower [12]. The problem was, therefore, to detect falls in the context of the shower using a non-wearable solution.

TECNALIA's suggested solution to fall detection and fall prediction in the bathtub was a sensorised rug, see Fig. 9, which continuously monitored the plantar pressure distribution of the user. Figure 10 shows illustrations of the plantar pressure distribution measured together with the detection and orientation of the feet, Base of Support,

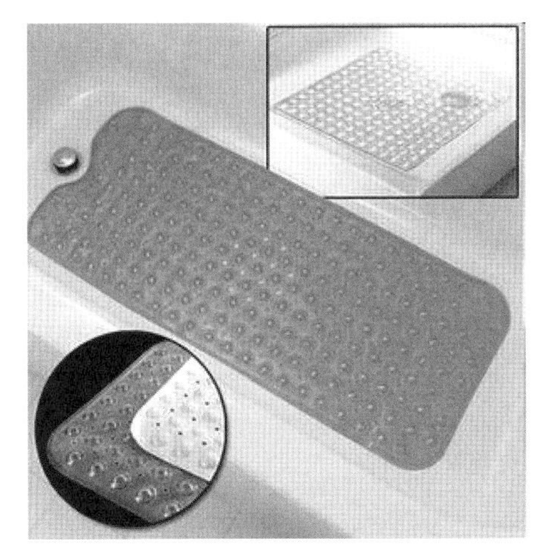

Figure 9. Illustrative solution of the ShowerRug.

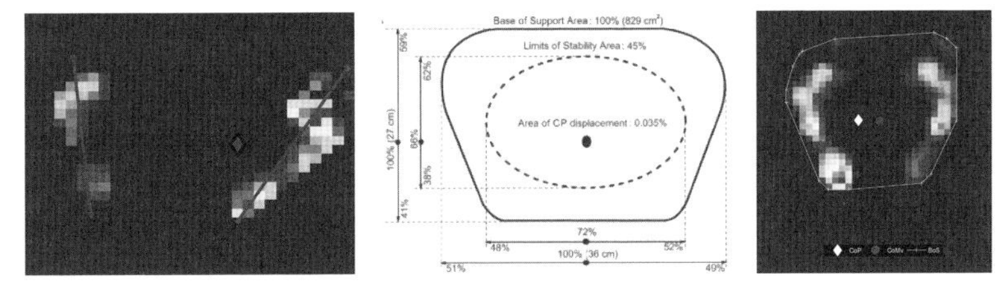

Figure 10. Plantar pressure distribution.

Centre of Pressure (CoP) and the vertical projection of the Centre of Mass (CoMv). Machine learning techniques were developed and implemented to extract and analyse postural stability features which are the required indicators.

Tests with 10 healthy subjects were performed who replicated shower activities and various types of falls. The algorithm used achieved detections with a sensitivity and specificity of 80%.

8. The HAPTIMAP Project

8.1. Overview

- Short name of project: HAPTIMAP;
- Full name of project: Haptic, Audio and Visual Interfaces for Maps and Location Based Services;
- Author: HAPTIMAP consortium (corresponding author: Arantxa Renteria);
- Call identifier: ICT-2007.7.2 target a): "ICT – Independent living and inclusion";
- Consortium members (leader first): Lund University, Navteq, Siemens, BMT Group, CEA, ONCE, Finnish Geodetic Institute, University of Glasgow, OFFIS, Queen's University, TECNALIA Research & Innovation (formerly ROBOTIKER-Tecnalia), Kreis Soest, Lunds Kommun;

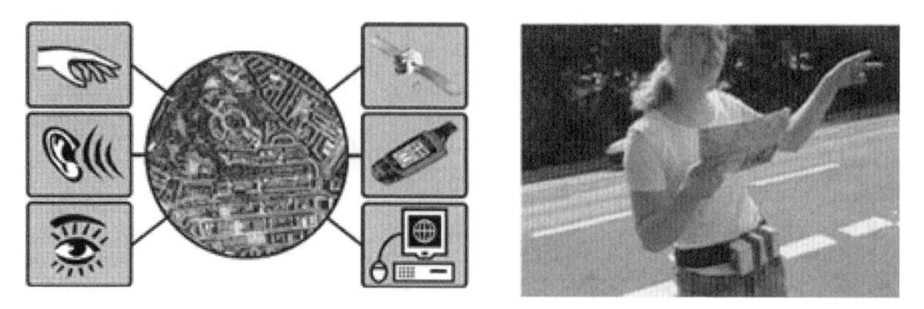

Figure 11. The HAPTIMAP concept.

- Start date: 1st September 2008;
- End date: 21st August 2012.

8.2. Summary

The HAPTIMAP project will enable digital maps and mobile location based services to be accessible to a wide range of disabled users [20]. The strategy is twofold, firstly to develop tools that make it easier for developers to add adaptable multimodal components (designed to improve accessibility) into their applications and, secondly, to raise the awareness of these issues via new guidelines and to suggest extensions to existing design practices so that accessibility issues are considered throughout the design process.

The HAPTIMAP project will make use of an Inclusive Design/Design for All approach where the goal is to increase the number of persons who are able to use mapping services by making these types of application easier to use by all people, including those with visual impairments. Thus the user groups contain both sighted persons and persons with visual impairments, including the elderly.

Multi-modality is a useful addition for navigation applications, allowing transfer of information from the relatively overloaded visual sense to hearing and touch. However, if not sufficiently well understood by designers, the use of touch and sound can be annoying. HAPTIMAP is analysing ways to effectively employ touch and hearing to make map and navigation applications more useful and engaging as well as more accessible to users with impairments, see Fig. 11.

With the Toolkit API, developers of mobile navigation programs wishing to endow their software with the capability of user-interaction through the senses of touch and sound, as well as visually, will be able to do this. The toolkit will be able to adapt to the capabilities of the device on which the program is working, and to the sensor information that the device can provide (such as location) to intelligently suggest what that user is doing, and in what context he or she is doing it.

The specific role of TECNALIA is the development and implementation of data filtering, route adaptation and user configuration facilities in order to adapt the information provided to the visually impaired users to their specific impairments and preferences. Main ways of interaction are through audio or vibrating modes.

Some other projects cover also mobile applications for navigation and mapping (Navteq, Google Maps), others use audio or haptic functionalities in order to improve accessibility to visually impaired users (IBM Websphere, MICOLE, Open Haptics, CHAI3d), even in mobile environments (Inmersion), but only HAPTIMAP deals in parallel with mapping, navigation, audio and haptic interfaces for mobile applications.

9. The TeleREHA Project

9.1. Overview

- Short name of project: TeleREHA;
- Full name of project: *Tele-rehabilitación efectiva en el hogar: investigación y desarrollo de sistemas, técnicas, métodos y mecanismos*;
- Author: Javier Arcas;
- Call identifier: Spanish Applied Research Subprogramme for Research Centres (MICINN – Ministry of Science and Innovation, Spain);
- Consortium members (leader first): TECNALIA Research & Innovation, IBV, CETEMMSA;
- Start date: 1st January 2009;
- End date: 31st December 2011.

9.2. Summary

The TeleREHA project is aimed at the research, development and evaluation of low-cost technologies focused on training and rehabilitation at home. Another objective is the remote supervision of people with motor or cognitive deficits. Rehabilitation is coordinated through a web platform where patients exercise their therapies using "serious" videogames, specifically designed to alleviate cognitive or motor diseases that are to be treated by means of low cost hardware devices adapted to those concrete treatments. Through the use of the platform, therapists are able to perform an integral management of the range of actions they have to undertake with their patients: monitoring, assessment, configuration of therapies etc.

The role of TECNALIA in this project embraces two different aspects. Firstly, the entire development of the web platform where the whole rehabilitation process takes place, intended to be used by patients (therapy sessions with games, rehabilitation calendar, consults about progress, communications...) and therapists (patients management, therapies configuration, therapy sessions assignment, session assessments, communications, monitoring…). Secondly, TECNALIA has designed a low cost hardware device for stroke rehabilitation that seamlessly integrates with rehabilitation games specifically created for the aforementioned web platform using the Bluetooth protocol.

Within the scope of AAL, the TeleREHA project involves some key factors:

- Increase in time spent by the patient at home: Frequent journeys to the hospital for the conduction of the therapy are now replaced by the rehabilitation exercises at home.
- A greater development of patient autonomy: The web platform has been designed having in mind the accessible and intuitive use of the interfaces, so no external help is needed for the navigation.
- Impact on the patient's health improvement: The main objective of the project is rehabilitation of motor and cognitive capabilities and promotion of recovery through individualized therapies and personalized monitoring.
- Emphasis on relatives' involvement: The multi-user option has been considered in the rehabilitation and training games, so that relatives are involved in the patient's therapy. This entails a beneficial increase in motivation and a better integration into the daily environment of the patient.

- Use of ICT: TeleREHA is a software platform on the Internet; communications between patient and therapists are made through videoconference; hardware devices are transparently connected via Bluetooth. Therapists can also tele-monitor patients' performance during rehabilitation sessions.
- Decrease of public expenses within the health infrastructure, and a better use of therapist's human capital, since their time is more valuably spent.

The TeleREHA videoconference system is always initiated by the therapist, after checking on the web platform that the patient is online. The videoconference can be started at any time, regardless of the activity the patient is carrying out. In order to preserve privacy, the patient is prompted with an on-screen alert, with the choice to accept or reject the call.

The TeleREHA platform provides two different ways to monitor patients' performance during a rehabilitation session:

- therapists can visualize the same 3D environment where patients are carrying out their rehabilitation sessions with the previously mentioned hardware devices;
- therapists can visualize through patients' webcam the movements they are doing with the affected limb.

Both cases are complemented with the posterior visualization on the web platform of the results from the therapy, e.g. trajectories, angles, and forces.

10. The BEDMOND Project

10.1. Overview

- Short name of project: BEDMOND;
- Full name of project: Behaviour pattern based assistant for early detection and management of neurodegenerative diseases;
- Author: BEDMOND consortium (corresponding author: Alberto Martínez);
- Call identifier: European R&D project, partly co-funded by the AAL JP Programme and the NFA from Austria, Portugal and Spain (AAL-2008-1-026);
- Consortium members (leader first): TECNALIA Research & Innovation (formerly ROBOTIKER-Tecnalia), Austrian Institute of Technology, Center for Usability Research and Engineering, IBERNEX, INGEMA and METICUBE;
- Start date: 1st June 2009;
- End date: 31st May 2012.

10.2. Summary

Healthcare professionals' research overwhelms with very convincing arguments that the detection of mild cognitive impairment (MCI) at an early stage supports a longer independent life at home for the patient because pharmacological treatment can be applied from the very beginning symptoms of such a critical disease. However, most relevant symptoms of MCI are related to behavioural changes while performing activities of daily living as a consequence of executive function deterioration (e.g. oversights and forgetfulness, disorientation, lack of abilities to manage with complexity). But physicians are in a need of on-time objective data about daily behaviour and activities of the person to infer robust conclusions about a possible cognitive decline related to neurodegenerative disease and not to the normal ageing process. The most valuable information about is subjective (face to face interview) and received normally late in the disease progression. This objective data can be provided by a non-intrusive sensor-based home and software for adaptive activity recognition and tracking, which later uses the health professional knowledge to interpret adequately that amount of information.

BEDMOND is an assistant for the health professional, a daily behaviour information provider to early diagnose MCI stages as a first step of neurodegenerative diseases, focused on elderly people while living at home. BEDMOND's system tools provide support in both stages: early diagnosis and disease tracking. For both stages, several tools are fitted for the specific needs of end users: health professionals, caregivers and the elder himself or herself.

During the early diagnosis, the following functions are relevant:

- The elder receives no support from the BEDMOND system in order not to disturb his or her daily life while still with no or only a few symptoms. A technical alarm system module can be installed at home as a non-MCI related support;
- The health professional receives, with the desired periodicity, a report which has processed intelligently the information gathered from sensors about the elderly person's activity and behaviour. He or she will obtain specific information about deviations on behaviours – strictly concerning the MCI appearance – biomedical parameters, daily routines and questionnaires fulfilment when requested. He or she can even check evolution and trends as relevant information;
- The caregivers are daily reported with the most important information about the activities of the previous day concerning meals, medications, and visits.

During the treatment process, these functionalities are relevant:

- The elder receives some support from the BEDMOND system prescribed by the health professional in order to facilitate daily life, now in a phase of cognitive decline: digital agenda to remind appointments and medication intakes, alarms not only technical but others related to the short-term memory loss (electrical appliances on, main door opened, etc.);
- The health professional receives a similar report to pre-diagnosis stage, with the desired periodicity, now normally shorter than in pre-diagnosis stage. This report is now focused on posterior steps of a global cognitive decline scale, just after MCI stage. At this stage, specific periodical questionnaires for cognitive decline progression screening are provided. New relevant information will be provided now to the doctor by the caregivers, thanks to the elder's behavioural diary tool. He or she will be able to not only monitor the treatment evolution but the decrease of the disease progression due to the early detection and subsequent early treatment;
- The caregivers are daily reported as usual, in addition to some disease concerned information. Besides the digital agenda as an aid for the elder, the caregiver will have now a tool for acquainting the doctor periodically with the elder's behavioural diary tool.

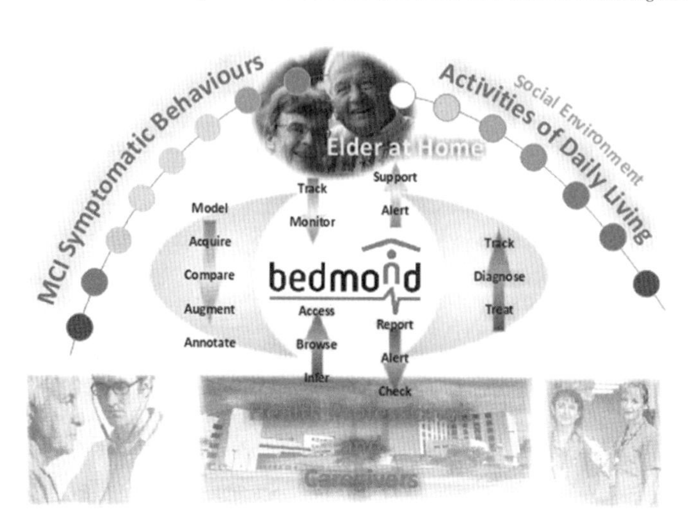

Figure 12. Overall concept of the BEDMOND project [16].

Hence, the system as shown in Fig. 12 consists of a support tool for medical experts addressed to the early diagnosis of neurodegenerative diseases in elderly people and posterior monitoring of user evolution after a treatment applied in such an early stage. The monitoring system should be used as a decision support system during the cognitive decline process by the medical experts, in order to make decisions about early treatments, which are mainly pharmacological, for the elders that could lead to a longer, independent stay at home on an e-Inclusion framework.

The smart home is equipped with integrated unobtrusive low-cost sensors. Data provided by the multimodal sensor network are then pre-processed to obtain comprehensible information about the daily routine of the person, which gathers a sequence of habitual activities of daily living and certain behaviours that might be related to the early appearance of MCI. The architecture follows a client-server (local-home and remote-centre) concept with a slim client side. To achieve a maximum of data security and a minimum amount of data transfer, the raw data is stored on the home side and only pre-processed data is transferred to the server. The server at the healthcare services centre has to handle a huge number of connected homes. The main gateway at the server side is a server interface. At home the architecture is based on Universal Control Hub technology (UCH) and an Apache Felix OSGi framework for Home Events Recognition (HOMER). HOMER integrates the local sensors (KNX and RF) and performs pre-processing for hardware independence and behaviour detection. UCH provides interoperability at the interaction layer, allowing the integration of devices and services using a unique communication protocol. Behaviour modelling and tracking is done by means of algorithms based on sensor data fusion techniques. International screening and scoring scales are used to interpret with professional criteria the deviations obtained when comparing the behaviour model and the daily performance. The access to information by caregivers and health professionals will be via browser-based interfaces [16].

The main role of TECNALIA in the BEDMOND project is the development of a behaviour model and a tracking system related to the daily activity of the user at home. At a higher level, TECNALIA processes intelligently the information acquired from the smart home multimodal sensor network to inform the neurologist and gerontologist for an early detection of a mild cognitive impairment. Finally, TECNALIA is deeply involved in the user interface development.

One similar North American project is *TigerPlace*, a project funded by the American NSF and carried out by the Sinclair School of Nursing (SON) and the Engineering Faculty, both at the Missouri University, in collaboration with the Americare Corporation of Sikeston [23].

11. The HearMeFeelMe Project

11.1. Overview

- Short name of project: HMFM;
- Full name of project: HearMeFeelMe – Compensating for eyesight with mobile technology;
- Author: HMFM consortium (corresponding author: Igone Idigoras);
- Call identifier: AAL-2008-1-041;
- Consortium members (leader first): VTT, ToP Tunniste, Caritas Foundation, FFVI and The 6. Joutsen apteekki, NCSR Demokritos, SSI and TECNALIA Research & Innovation;
- Start date: 1st June 2009;
- End date: 6th July 2011.

11.2. Summary

The HearMeFeelMe project (HMFM) aims at developing ICT-based systems that provide visually impaired elderly people with an easy, simple and intuitive way to access information and digital services in their home environment, allowing them to (1) have equal opportunities to participate in all aspects of the society, (2) maintain their independence, avoiding dependence on others when accessing information and services, and (3) improve the quality of life and individual wellbeing of the elderly [21].

HMFM deals with the chronic condition of vision impairment. Different degrees of vision impairments are inevitable results of growing old, as the physiology of our eyes changes with time when the eye tissues loose their flexibility and suffer from damages caused by everyday life and different health conditions (such as diabetes or high blood pressure). HMFM explores the possibilities for improving the quality of life by providing mobile service access for the visually impaired elderly using services related to medication, and health and medicine related information and services.

The technical solutions explored and used in HMFM are based on existing technological solutions available today, such as Near Field Communication technology (NFC). NFC provides an opportunity to build touch-based user interfaces especially suitable for elderly with decreased hand-eye coordination and vision.

The HMFM services constructed and piloted during the project allow the users to locate and identify medicine packaging, to obtain medication information and dosage instructions through audio, and receive instructions and reminders through an electronic medication plan. The services are piloted in Finland and Spain, whereas the localisation experiments are performed in Greece. Special emphasis is put on involving

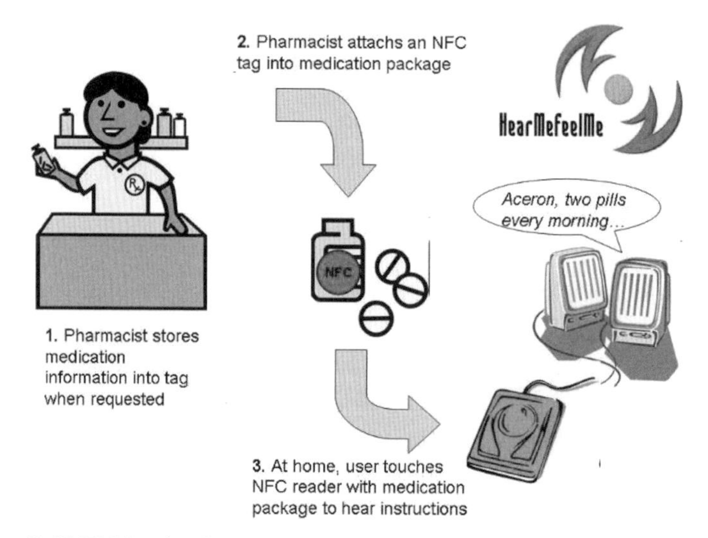

Figure 13. HMFM functionality used for identifying medication and related instructions [21].

the whole service chain, including pharmacy, home service providers, elderly users and their caretakers. Therefore, the focus is not only on technical constructions, but also on service design and planning of wide adoption in Europe.

The project partners include the small and medium enterprises (SMEs) ToP Tunniste and a pharmacy in Finland, the elderly care providers Caritas foundation in Finland and SSI (Servicios Sociales Integrados) in Spain, the end user organization Finnish Federation for Visually Impaired (FFVI), and the three research organizations VTT in Finland, TECNALIA in Spain and NCSR Demokritos in Greece. TECNALIA explores the NFC technology and related design issues, and has developed the prototypes and solutions used in some of the pilots. TECNALIA is also active in user involvement and field trials from research and methodological viewpoints, coordinating the field trials in Spain. During the iterative piloting phase, the service constructions are trials used through adoption involving all service chain partners in Finland and Spain.

The Finnish trial concentrates especially on the problem of identifying a medication package and reading the medication instructions. People with decreased vision may have difficulties in reading the textual information on medication packaging. Therefore, they might face problems in finding a correct medication package, and reading the related instructions related to dosage, recommended time for taking the medication, etc. In Finland, this information is already available in digital format, as pharmacies print it to a slip that is attached in the medication package. The service solution explored in HMFM stores this same data into an NFC tag that can then be read by any NFC enabled device, e.g. a computer attached with an external NFC reader, or an NFC enabled mobile phone. At the time of HMFM pilots, the availability of NFC enabled smart phones has been very limited, so the pilots have been implemented with a laptop computer with an external NFC reader. The concept of the service is illustrated in Fig. 13.

The experiences from pilots show that users have found the service easy and simple to use even for users with no or little prior experience with computers. The users found the service trustworthy and reliable, and most thought it increased their medical

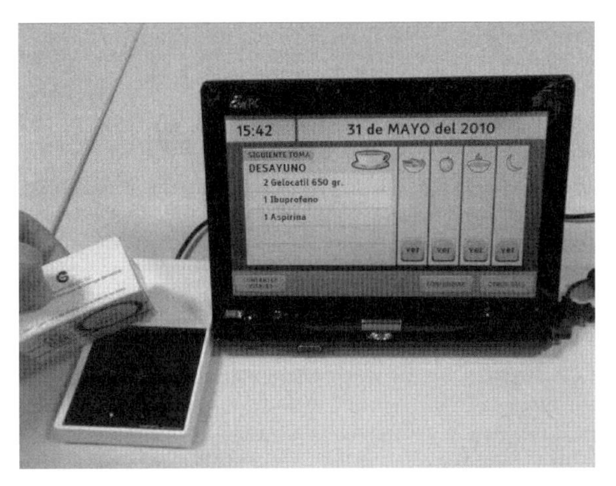

Figure 14. Spanish pilot setup: NFC reader and personal medication assistant.

safety and feeling of safety. However, many users had already established their own methods for medication management. For example, they relied on the help of their spouses, or organized the medication packages to help them in recognizing and scheduling medication taking. Many valued the independency and safety provided by the HMFM service, but they wished a more complete solution with additional features such as reminders. Solutions which serve as a reminder to take medication or about expiry dates were very highly rated by the user group involved in the user needs analysis. 96% of the 27 people interviewed in Spain considered useful any device providing medication reminders and medication plan information.

The Spanish trials have considered these results and the developed service solution provides not only medication identification options but also medication management, medication reminders and medication taking confirmation, see Fig. 14.

The system uses the same interfaces as the Finnish pilots allowing easy integration at the later phases of the project. The medication package is attached to a tag containing medication identification and prescription details.

Tags are read with an NFC reader, and the HMFM medication management service compiles a medication plan accordingly with the help of the user or caretaker. The small touch-screen computer can then remind the user about medication to be taken at the prescribed times. When receiving a reminder, the user will check the dosage instructions in audio format by bringing the package near the NFC reader. Simultaneously, the service can confirm that medication has been taken.

Tantamount to reading of information from a medication package is the ability to locate it first. The research performed by NCSR Demokritos aims at developing low cost RF methods for reading RFID tags from medication packages remotely and subsequently localising the package in indoor environments. In the later phases of the project, experiences from both countries will be used for building iterative integrated versions of HMFM service to be piloted. Furthermore, the work done at NCSR Demokritos in Greece on locating a medication package indoors will be evaluated through piloting [21].

12. The SENTIENT Project

12.1. Overview

- Short name of project: SENTIENT;
- Full name of project: Sensor Assisted Interface for Emotional Detection;
- Author: Enrique León;
- Internal project;
- Start date: 1st June 2009;
- End date: 1st March 2011.

12.2. Summary

There are numerous reasons why the identification of emotions has increasingly captured the attention of technology companies and research groups. Emotion recognition permits to establish relationships between the environment and the person's decisions, behaviour, and affects. This is particularly useful in areas related to human-computer interaction or tele-care. The SENTIENT project is an ongoing research endeavour which intends to detect negative emotional reactions using physiological signals, inform the user and/or the caregiver, and orchestrate a user-defined response from the environment to minimize the adverse consequences of said negative emotional states.

In its current version, SENTIENT comprises a commercial wearable sensor which sends the information onto a Smartphone, which in turn initiates an action based on the user's current emotional valence. Such action can take the form of light activation, music playing or phone calls and text messaging. The purpose of SENTIENT's approach is to enhance self-care and prevention while also enabling remote peer-support.

The algorithm is based on the combination of neural networks and statistical analysis while the design of the system is built on user consultation involving surveys and interviews with elderly groups and health care professionals, see [4,7,8,11].

There are a number of advantages of SENTIENT with respect to existing commercial and research approaches:

- SENTIENT can provide real-time indication of the polarity and intensity of the emotional valence;
- The system configuration is highly customizable to match the user's own coping strategy;
- The learning algorithm performs long-life learning and adaptation based on user feedback;
- The number of physiological signals can be adapted to include a number of Bluetooth commercial sensors;
- The system can operate in non-ambulatory conditions using heart rate monitoring only and still provide the same functionalities.

The ultimate goal of SENTIENT is to be able to offer a cross-platform portable system that can assist in providing care solutions that look after the person's emotional well-being.

13. The Florence Project

13.1. Overview

- Short name of project: Florence;
- Full name of project: Multi Purpose Mobile Robot for Ambient Assisted Living;
- Author: Florence consortium (corresponding author: Leire Martínez);
- Call identifier: FP7-ICT-2009-4;
- Consortium members (leader first): Philips Electronics B.V., NEC Europe LTD., OFFIS e.V., Stichting Novay, Telefónica Investigación y Desarrollo SA, TECNALIA Research & Innovation, Fundación Andaluza de Servicios Sociales, Wany SA;
- Start date: 1st February 2010;
- End date: 31st January 2013.

13.2. Summary

The background for the development of the Florence system is the slow but constant demographic change in many countries with an increasing part of elderly people while the number of younger people remains constant or even decreases. Due to the advances in health treatment, many previously fatal diseases have been turned into chronic conditions. This leads to an increasing demand for care, especially for the elderly. In addition to that, new family structures and more job-mobility make it more and more difficult to rely on volunteer care for elderly at home by family members. Hence, costs for both the society and the care provider are growing, which, at the end, may lead to potential undersupply of health care. Beyond the financial aspect, another problem is the increasing lack of social inclusion due to less stable social networks, which leads to increasing loneliness of the elderly with negative impact on their health and safety.

The aim of the Florence project is to improve the well-being of the elderly (and that of their beloved ones) as well as improve the efficiency in care through AAL services, supported by a general-purpose mobile robot platform. The Florence project is investigating the use of such robots in delivering new kinds of AAL services to elderly persons and their care providers. Florence will put the robot as the connecting element between several stand alone AAL services in a living environment as well as between the AAL services and the elderly person. Through these care, coaching and connectedness services, supported by Florence, the elderly will remain much longer independent.

A key aspect for Florence is user acceptance. Florence aims to improve the acceptance of AAL (robotic) services by providing both assistance and fun oriented lifestyle services via the same means. The ambition of Florence is that the elderly should be proud of having a Florence robot. Florence positions robots as autonomous lifestyle devices. By re-using the same interaction mechanisms of lifestyle services, Florence will make the adoption of AAL services by elderly easier. In addition, by positioning robots as a new kind of consumer products, i.e. as a new lifestyle product, Florence will attract the attention of services providers and consumer electronic vendors to the senior market. This increase of user-acceptance will greatly alleviate the need for personal care for elderly, and therefore provide for significant cost-savings [19].

As expected results the Florence system will support lifestyle and AAL services in the following categories (from [19]):

- Family involvement: Florence will provide a non-obtrusive, intuitive way of asynchronous communication with family members by sending pictures to the family members' mobile phones or emails or getting pictures from the family members to Florence robot's screen;
- Video telephone: Implementing a video communication possibility enables the elderly person to participate in the family life e.g. by seeing the grandchild or daughter;
- Home observation: The Florence robot can be sent to other rooms to take a picture to see what is going on. Open windows and cupboards could be detected and lost objects can be found;
- Emergency Intervention: In case of an emergency situation, e.g. a detected fall, a mobile robot has the advantage that it is able to move towards the person. The robot can talk to the person first, and than take a picture, send it to caregivers and initiate an alarm. Furthermore, the fallen person could call the robot for help. The robot is able to bring communication means directly to the user and initiate a call to family members or caregivers;
- Direct coaching: Florence will be able to monitor several sensor data items. One possible application for coaching is to give advices for wellness or activities;
- Remote coaching: Remote diagnosis is an example application of remote coaching. The collected data from the monitoring, together with answered questions on the phone and symptoms shown via a video conference system, will lead to a clearer diagnosis of a remote caregiver or doctor;
- Communication among caregivers: Florence will support a blog-like system that enables caregivers to maintain a diary about their activities. This is especially useful in cases of mild dementia, where communication with the elderly themselves is not always reliable.

TECNALIA's main relevant expertise for the Florence project includes Intelligent Robotics and Aged living needs and Quality of Life issues. TECNALIA's main interest in Florence is to design and develop different strategies for a more intuitive and natural interaction with the user. TECNALIA and Wany help the consortium define the robotic requirements and architecture. Within the robotics architecture, TECNALIA is responsible for designing, developing and implementing of so-called enablers that will help the user to have a more pleasant experience with the mobile robotic platform's navigation. Gesture interaction with machine vision techniques and image processing technology are also realized in order to support the multimodality for an enhanced user experience.

Moreover, TECNALIA has a leading role in the scenario and use case definition. Starting from the scientific literature and previous experience of the project partners, a set of initial scenarios is being developed, that is further analysed through focus groups and Wizard of Oz tests. The specified set of scenario and use cases is going through a feasibility check before a final set of scenarios is defined. These scenarios are developed into services, where TECNALIA is responsible of designing, developing and implementing services related to collaborative activities in a social context.

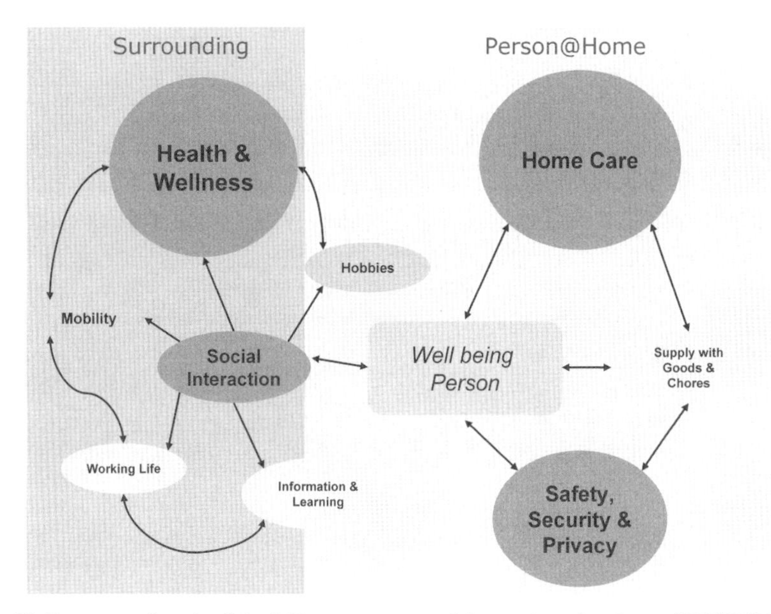

Figure 15. Key areas of needs of the AAL target group and the number of projects of TECNALIA that address each one of them; modified after [5].

14. Conclusions and Outlook

TECNALIA's Health Technologies Unit has been participating in at least 13 European, Spanish, regional and internal R&D projects related to AAL, which are summarized in the present chapter.

As shown in Table 2, these projects make use of many different enabling technologies. These are grouped following the classification published by van den Broek et al. [24].

TECNALIA has been working in several key areas of needs of the AAL target group as shown in Fig. 15 (compare [5]), where the font size and the size of ellipses are related to the number of projects that address each one of these areas, see Table 1. Most projects aimed at improving Home care, Health and Wellness, Safety, Security and Privacy, and Social Interaction, only a few Mobility and Hobbies. The areas Working Life, Information and Learning, and Supply with Goods and Chores will be addressed in future projects.

TECNALIA's projects in AAL cover a wide range of research lines, such as communication, rehabilitation, e-inclusion, cognitive decline and activities of daily living. All these efforts are improving the quality of life of the elderly, the dependent people, their families and their caregivers. Furthermore, they will lead to an enhancement of the functional independence and a reduction of the societal costs.

In addition to working in projects, TECNALIA is interested in contributing as an expert in technologies, business models and user needs to the definition of research, development and innovation in AAL and related areas in Europe in the future.

Table 2. Overview over a selection of enabling technologies used in TECNALIA's AAL-related projects

Short name	Sensing	Reasoning	Acting	Interacting	Communicating
AmIE	Technical alarms, ambient sensors in smart home; multi-param. physiolog. monitoring	Night Activity recogn. (modelling, tracking); deviation analysis	Information for health professional; domotic aids for laundry		KNX/EIB home network, IP connectivity
AUZOLAN	Tele-monitoring of weight, blood pressure, oximeter			Interactive TV based interface	WiMAX, Wi-Fi, Bluetooth, Ethernet
BED-MOND	Technical alarms and hazardous situations detectors, physiological activity detectors (sleep), others	Activity and behaviour recognition; deviation analysis	Risky situation mgmt. & reminders; behavioural deviation	UCH standard (Universal Control Hub for interaction)	KNX/EIB and RF home net, IP and telephone line conn.
Companion-Able	Sound identification, image analysis, bed and chair pressure detection, movement detection	Recognition of distress situations, emotions detection, habit tracking	Smart home and service (tele-)robotics	Multimodal: touch-screen, audio in/out; affective robot interface	ZigBee, RFID, KNX/EIB, Wi-Fi
ELISA	Location for outdoor & indoor navigation; sound; luminosity	User model and context model		Self-adaptive multi-modal (audio, graphical)	Wi-Fi, GSM, WiMAX
Florence	Infrared, compass, bumper, GPS, odometers, sound, motor encoders, laser range-finder; smoke; door/window; webcam; 3D-cam; indoor panic button; StarGazer; others	Context Management (CALA), data fusion Bayesian inference, image analysis/process; autonom. navig.; SLAM	Pekee II mobile robotic platform; window/door; remotely controlled: dimmable switches, power sockets, heater valve;	Multimodal: touchscreen, gestures, speech; Mobile phone interface	Wi-Fi, EIB, Miele@home, FS20, HomeMatic, GSM
HAPTI-MAP	Location technologies for outdoor, compass and gyroscope	User model and context model		Self-adapt. multimodal (audio, haptic, graph.)	Wi-Fi, GSM
HearMe-FeelMe	RFID for object location, NFC for object identification			Multimodal: audio, graphical, haptic, touch	
SENTIENT	Physiological data (heart rate)	Autoassoc. Neural Nets	Visual for self-regulation	Visual on Smartphone	Bluetooth
ShowerRug	Plantar pressure	Stability index; rule based on posture control	Sensory feedback	–	External alarm module
SOPRANO	Sensors for safety and security (smoke, door/window opening and closing), monitoring of heart rate and breathing rate in rest (radar sensor)	Ontologies; semantic service descript.; OSGi; context reasoning; rule based; semantic uplifting		Rich interaction, distrib. interfaces: touch-screen, TV set; voice synthesis, voice recogn., avatar, …	Home control: X-10, KNX, RF and Wi-Fi; SMS
TeleREHA			Home tele-rehab. hardware; comm. w. med. professionals	3D environments for rehab.; Internet platform	Bluetooth home network
VIDA	Safety and security: smoke, door/window; context sensing		Home automation: comfort, comm. and security domotic acting	Multimodal, accessible, mobile: audio, voice in/out, graphical, haptic	KNX/EIB, X10 home control nets, Wi-Fi, IR and RF

References

[1] AAL Open Association (AALOA), http://www.aaloa.org.
[2] AUZOLAN project, http://www.auzolan.org, last access: 2010-09-15.
[3] Eurostat, Europe in figures – Eurostat Yearbook 2008, http://epp.eurostat.ec.europa.eu/cache/ITY_OFFPUB/KS-CD-07-001/EN/KS-CD-07-001-EN.PDF, last access: 2010-12-02.
[4] A. Garzo, I. Montalban, E. León and S. Schlatter, Sentient: An approach to ambient assisted emotional regulation, in: *Proceedings of the International Symposium on Ambient Intelligence*, Guimarães, Portugal, June 2010 (Winner of Best Poster Award).
[5] M. Huch, Ambient Assisted Living Joint Programme, *mst/news*, 6/07, Dec. 2007, 7.
[6] S.E. Lamb, E.C. Jørstad-Stein, K. Hauer and C. Becker, Prevention of falls. Network Europe, and outcomes consensus group. Development of a common outcome data set for fall injury prevention trials: The prevention of falls network Europe consensus, *J. Am. Geriatr. Soc.* **53**(9) (2005), 1618–1622.
[7] E. León, G. Clarke, V. Callaghan and F. Sepulveda, A user-independent real-time emotion recognition system for software agents in domestic environments, *Engineering Applications of Artificial Intelligence, The International Journal of Intelligent Real-Time Automation* **20**(3) (2007), 337–345.
[8] E. León, I. Montalban, S. Schlatter and I. Dorronsoro, Computer-mediated emotional regulation: Detection of emotional changes using non-parametric cumulative sum, in: *Proceedings of the 32nd Annual Conference of the IEEE Engineering in Medicine and Biology Society*, Buenos Aires, Argentina, August 2010.
[9] S.R. Lord, *Falls in Older People: Risk Factors and Strategies for Prevention*, Cambridge University Press, Cambridge, 2007.
[10] S.R. Lord, J.A. Ward, P. Williams and K.J. Anstey, An epidemiological study of falls in older community-dwelling women: The randwick falls and fractures study, *Aust. J. Public Health* **17**(3) (1993), 240–245.
[11] I. Montalban, A. Garzo and E. Leon, Emotion-aware intelligent environments. A user perspective, in: *Proceedings of the 5th International Conference on Intelligent Environments*, Barcelona, July, 2009.
[12] N. Noury, A. Galay, J. Pasquier and M. Ballussaud, Preliminary investigation into the use of autonomous fall detectors, in: *Conf Proc IEEE Eng Med Biol Soc*, 2008, pp. 2828–2831.
[13] openAAL joint open source initiative, http://www.openaal.org, last access: 2010-10-15.
[14] TECNALIA's homepage, http://www.tecnalia.com, last access: 2011-02-15.
[15] The AmIE project consortium, AmIE project homepage, http://www.amieproject.com/, last access: 2010-08-24.
[16] The BEDMOND project consortium, BEDMOND project homepage, http://www.bedmond.eu/, last access: 2010-08-20.
[17] The CompanionAble project consortium, CompanionAble project homepage, http://www.companionable.net/, last access: 2010-08-06.
[18] The ELISA project consortium, ELISA project homepage, http://www.elisapse.es/, last access: 2010-08-06.
[19] The Florence project consortium, Florence project homepage, http://www.florence-project.eu/, last access: 2010-08-06.
[20] The HAPTIMAP project consortium, HAPTIMAP project homepage, http://www.haptimap.org/, last access: 2010-08-06.
[21] The HMFM project consortium, HMFM project homepage, http://ttuki.vtt.fi/hmfm/, last access: 2010-08-20.
[22] The SOPRANO project consortium, SOPRANO project homepage, http://www.soprano-ip.org/, last access: 2010-08-18.
[23] TigerPlace, http://www.tigerplace.net, last access: 2010-08-28.
[24] G. van den Broek, F. Cavallo and C. Wehrmann, *AALIANCE Ambient Assisted Living Roadmap*, IOS Press, Amsterdam, The Netherlands, 2010.

Novel Developments and Visions for the Area

Handbook of Ambient Assisted Living
J.C. Augusto et al. (Eds.)
IOS Press, 2012

doi:10.3233/978-1-60750-837-3-727

Introduction to Section on Future Developments and Visions for the AAL Area

Juan Carlos AUGUSTO [a,*] and Julie MAITLAND [b]
[a] *School of Computing and Mathematics, University of Ulster, UK*
[b] *National Research Council of Canada, Canada*

Abstract. The chapters in this last section of the handbook are gathered around two themes. The first four chapters consider the non-technical challenges that must be addressed if the field of Ambient Assisted Living is to realise its full potential. The last three chapters are similarly forward looking, providing alternative views on the possible future directions for the area. This introduction to the section includes a reflection from the section editors on the state of the art of the Ambient Assisted Living area as a whole as well as a brief description of the contributions included in this section.

Keywords. Ambient Assisted Living, user centered design, innovation

Introduction

This section of the Handbook offers a forward looking view on the area, its current capacity to deliver services and some of the main issues which need careful consideration to facilitate a successful immersion of AAL in our society. These chapters represent the opinion of experienced organizations and professionals who have developed and deployed AAL systems and explored their feasibility and their potential to match the expectations raised in previous years by academia, industry and governmental organizations.

Social Spaces for Reseach and Innovation (SSRI): Users leading Research and Innovation in Ambient Assisted Living by Ana Garcia Robles, Javier Garcia Guzman, Lorena Bourg, Jose Manuel Ojel and R. Ignacio Madrid, describes a new holistic approach to AAL deployment, which is growing out of pre-existing strategies like Open Innovation, User centred Innovation, Human Centred Design, and Living Labs models, and takes into consideration all of the different stakeholders.

New Ambient Assistive Technologies: The user' perspectives by Elisabeth Mestheneos, highlights the issues which need to be addressed to increase the chances to succeed in delivering benefits for our society.

Beyond System Integration: Who, What, How, and When by Lenka Lhotska, Jaromir Dolezal, Vaclav Chudacek, Michal Huptych and Miroslav Bursa, emphasizes the importance of making systems more flexible and adaptable to make the services delivered by the system more meaningful to individuals and their own circumstances.

*Corresponding Author: Juan Carlos Augusto. E-mail: jc.augusto@ulster.ac.uk.

Housing, gerontology and AAL: New services development by Javier Yanguas and Elena Urdaneta, examines different strategies to deploy AAL services which are effective and shaped by the user's needs.

Connecting Communities: The role of design ethnography in developing social care technologies for isolated older adults by David Prendergast, Claire Somerville and Joe Wherton, focuses on the importance to explore means by which technology can enhance social life for an important segment of our society. This chapter focuses on older adults but the potential scope of impact is much broader when you consider the potential benefit to people who experience barriers to social interaction through physiological conditions, cognitive conditions, and environmental factors.

Innovative rehabilitation technologies for home environments: An overview by Michael John, Beate Seewald and Stefan Klose, advocates for a more holistic integration of rehabilitation services which can connect isolated therapies amongst themselves and perhaps more importantly integrate them naturally with the daily life of those under rehabilitation, in their lives at home and their time at work.

Growing older together: When a robot becomes the best ally for ageing well by Francesca Irene Cavallaro, Arantxa Renteria, Anthony Remazeilles, Gabriel Gaminde, Ainara Garzo and Fabrice O. Morin, examines the prospects of robotics as personal assistants at home. The analysis is focused on social and ethical issues, rather than technical, which can guide the design and development of such applications.

Reflection

Work in the area has been mainly focused on older adults but much of this technology and solutions can be adapted to other segments of our society.

More integration between the health system and life at home and at work will benefit everybody as people will be able to enjoy a more holistic health system and a more fulfilling reintegration to normal life.

One area which is being increasingly considered in relation with home services and daily life is robotics. There are still significant technological challenges but it is also the right time to look carefully to the way such technology can be integrated to human's lives and the social and ethical implications of that development.

Our society is a complex mix of individuals; it represents a wide range of attitudes towards technology, level of knowledge and information, health, and cultural preferences. Developing technology which caters for such a broad range of individuals is a grand challenge that poses practical problems which so far have not been addressed, perhaps reflecting the fact that developments in the area are mostly a collection of isolated and unconnected efforts.

The development of spaces of innovation where users can lead research and innovation to contribute on making AAL technology meaningful to their context is a promising way ahead. End-User Led Innovation and Human Centered Design may hold the key for success in this area.

Work in this section, and in the rest of the Handbook, recognize there has been considerable advances but acknowledge some considerable hurdles that are yet to be overcome in the road to a succesful widespread insertion of AAL in our society. The content of this section put forward ideas and experiences which are exploring the frontiers of deployment of AAL services, and it indicates a promising and exiting future for the area.

Handbook of Ambient Assisted Living
J.C. Augusto et al. (Eds.)
IOS Press, 2012

doi:10.3233/978-1-60750-837-3-729

Social Spaces for Reseach and Innovation (SSRI): Users Leading Research and Innovation in Ambient Assisted Living

Ana GARCIA ROBLES[a,*], Javier GARCIA GUZMAN[b], Lorena BOURG[c], J. Manuel OJEL[a] and R. Ignacio MADRID[a]
[a] *Institute of Innovation for Human Wellbeing, Innovation Unit, Málaga, Spain*
[b] *Carlos III University, Computer Science Department, Getafe, Spain*
[c] *Ariadna Servicios Informáticos, R&D Department, Madrid, Spain*

Abstract. This paper introduces and describes with several examples a new research and innovation instrument and approach called Social Space for Research and Innovation (SSRI) that is generating good results in rural and urban communities working on ehealth and independent living. The SSRI is a multi-agent approach that places the beneficiary social communities at the forefront of the research and innovation process and where human, social, technological, economical, ethical and legal factors are considered all the way through said process. SSRI approach is growing rapidly at a national level in Spain and it is rapidly moving into the European and International scene.

Keywords. Social spaces for research and innovation, open innovation, people led innovation, social innovation, AAL, eHealth and independent living, living labs, user-centric innovation, human centred design

Introduction

In the European AAL program, AAL scope is defined as "cultivating the development of innovative ICT-based products, services and systems for the process of ageing well at home, in the community and at work, therefore improving the quality of life, autonomy, the participation in social life, skills and the employability of elderly people and reducing the costs of health and social care" [23].

There are many different stakeholders involved in the deployment of Ambient Assisted Living such as users and their caregivers, service providers, either public or private, technology and solution providers, and all the different stakeholders that define the legal, regulatory and economical context. The AAL Roadmap classifies these stakeholders in different groups: primary stakeholders or target group (users and their caregivers), secondary (service providers to the target group), tertiary (industries and companies that supply goods and services) and quaternary stakeholders (organizations and institutions that work in the economical and legal context) [23].

The direct involvement of users in the development of AAL products and services has been clearly identified as a key factor to reduce or even eliminate barriers for AAL deployment related to primary stakeholders. These barriers exist due to the lack of

---

*Corresponding Author: Ana Garcia Robles. E-mail: anagrobles@gmail.com.

effectiveness of the current AAL solutions as well as the reduced capacity of older people (and sometimes their caregivers) to use new technologies [23]. This difficulty regarding efficient access and use of technology is due to factors of several types, such as:

- Restrictions related to the usage of technology, physical conditions and social issues that prevent a quick and efficient adoption, specifically in difficult contexts such as rural environments or social communities of disabled people.
- Usability and human factors of several social groups (i.e. physical or intellectually disabled; or marginalised social groups) prevent the accessibility of technological solutions to these conditions that are very common in real life.

There is however many other technological, organizational, legal, ethical and economical challenges that affect all the different stakeholders and that, in general, are linked to a particular context; in many cases the context is a specific territory.

Furthermore, an important amount of ICT and e-learning research projects (for example, those supported by European Technology Platforms) have provided concrete, correct and very promising results for society. Nevertheless, once these results have been obtained there still remains a great amount of work in order to enable them to provide the excepted benefits to the societal communities [5,18]. Moreover, the results of ICT research projects are usually employed by enterprises in their commercial and industrial activities, but usually these results are not accessible to several societal communities [6].

This paper describes a new approach to potentially help reduce the various barriers that impede the AAL deployment: Social Space for Research and Innovation (SSRI). An improvement in the effectiveness of the AAL solutions as well as a friendly and personalized introduction of these technologies can be achieved through the use of Social Spaces for Research and Innovation. In these environments the daily context of the end user becomes the research, development and innovation scenario, and the user becomes the leader of the process. The use of this approach requires the development of specific methodologies, tools and evaluation procedures.

A description of the SSRI concept as well as its background is initially introduced followed by a description of its ongoing developed methodological framework. Furthermore, some examples of existing SSRI in the AAL field are presented. The paper ends introducing new developed AAL SSRI scenarios.

1. Social Spaces for Research and Innovation: Concept and Background

Social Spaces for Research and Innovation[1] (SSRI) are defined as organizational ecosystems in which the research and innovation activities are guided by the necessities and constraints of the social communities that benefit from the results, involving, in a balanced way, all the actors present in the research and innovation value chain such as social communities, technology and solution suppliers, service suppliers, funding organizations and members of the local, regional and national legal, economical and political scene.

[1] From the original name in Spanish: "Espacio Social de Innovación (ESdI)".

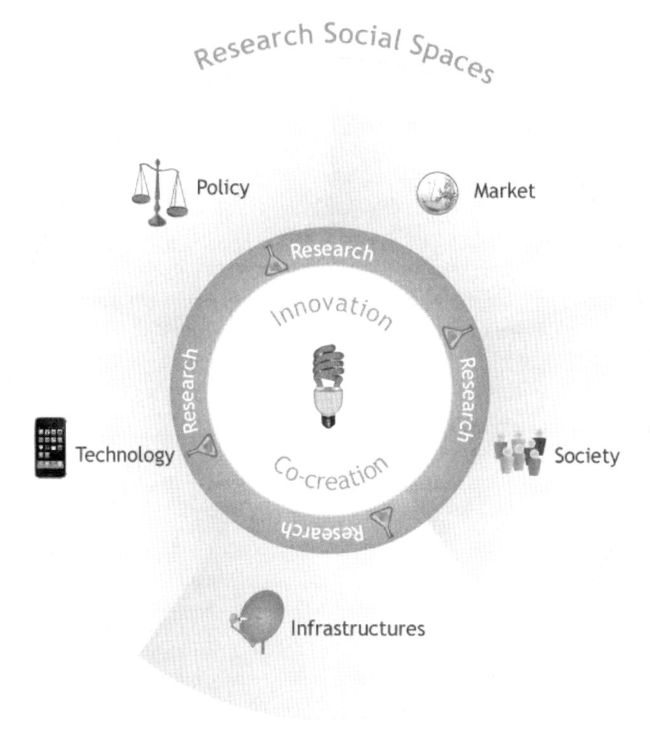

Figure 1. SSRI's main pillars.

SSRIs are linked to a specific context or territory whose main pillars or foundations are society, market, policy, technology and infrastructure (see Fig. 1).

SSRI is a very recently created concept and instrument but it has already achieved some success in the AAL field although it is in the area of Rural Development where the SSRI approach is really booming[2]. The first conference on Social Spaces for Research and Innovation held in Zaragoza (Spain) in 2008 was the scenario for the official national[3] launch of the Social Spaces of Research and Innovation community. During this conference a set of strategic objectives and a roadmap were defined. The main strategic objective was for SSRI to become an important instrument for the emancipation and independency of the society, promoting new models of governance and relationships between society, national institutions and companies and democratizing the process for innovation. The main steps to reach this objective at a national level included cooperation agreements, establishment of networks to share knowledge and good practices, constitution of the Spanish national network with an international perspective, official public calls for SSRI's and annual meetings[4].

The second annual conference on Social Spaces for Research and Innovation, that took place in Malaga in October 2009, meant an important step towards the consolida-

---

[2] 14 of the 19 officially recognized SSRIs in Spain are oriented to rural development and territorial cohesion (Oct 2010).

[3] Spanish launch.

[4] http://www.espaciossociales.es/index.php/en/objectives, Oct 17th 2010.

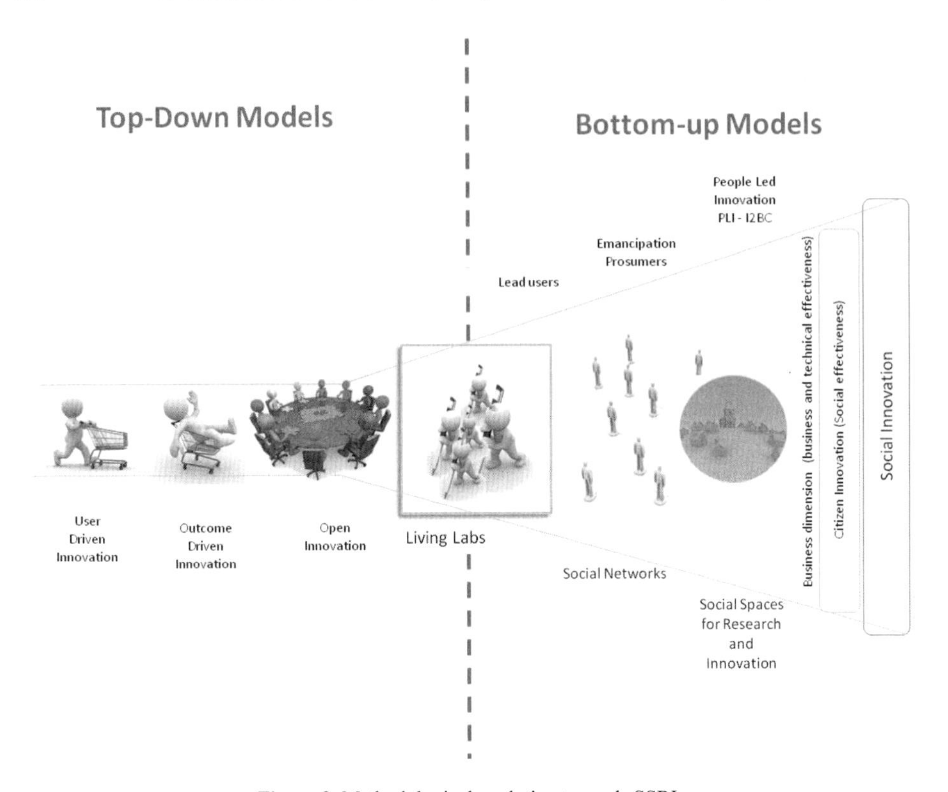

Figure 2. Methodological evolution towards SSRI.

tion of SSRIs. 19 SSRIs were officially recognized (3 of them in the domain of Health and Independent Living) and a first methodological framework was presented.

2010 has been a very active year in the consolidation of the national network, improvements of the methodological framework, success stories in existing SSRIs and active projects, and deployment of new SSRIs. At the end of 2010 the 3rd annual conference will take place with the recognition of new SSRIs and 2011 will be a decisive year in its internationalization, starting with the International Conference on SSRI to be held in Rome at the beginning of the year.

From a methodological perspective SSRI integrates well-known concepts such as Open Innovation promoted by Henry Chesbrough [2], Living Labs [19], user-driven innovation and Social Innovation [24] (see Fig. 2).

Open Innovation is defined as a paradigm where ideas, inventions and innovations are not internal to a single company anymore but there is a flow of knowledge and value in between a company and its environment [2].

User driven innovation refers to the definition of new products and services developed by consumers and end users, rather than manufacturers. Eric von Hippel of MIT [24] analyzed that most successful ICT products and services are actually designed by users, who then give ideas to manufacturers. This way the product is developed by the same people who are actually using it, resulting in a product much better suited to their needs.

User innovation principles are based on the idea that technology providers possess a deep knowledge of the technology's possibilities and solutions, while the users possess the knowledge about the needs and the restrictions of the operation environment [24].

Social Spaces for Research and Innovation (SSRI) is a specific and practical approach to implement open and user driven innovation [18].

Living Labs are "collaborations of public-private-civic partnerships in which stakeholders co-create new products, services, businesses and technologies in a real-life environment and virtual networks in multi-contextual spheres" [19]. There are many similarities between the Living Lab and SSRI approach[5] and although in some cases both methods are used in a complementary way there exist important differences from the conceptual point of view[6]: in the SSRI approach persons (citizens) lead the innovation process (they do not act only as participatory users), SSRI is a bottom-up approach and the governance model is implemented in such a way that all the research and innovation activities should be guided by the benefits and constraints of the social communities who can benefit from the results.

According to the dual view of a SSRI, both as a sustainable organization for networked ICT related innovation and as an organizer of innovation projects [18], the SSRI related challenges should be considered at two levels: strategic and operational.

At the strategic level, the analysis focuses on the effectiveness and performance of an SSRI as a strategic instrument to launch an independent and sustainable organization for open and user-driven innovation. The main challenges to consider in this category are:

1. Constitution of the SSRI community.
2. Implementation of a self-sustainability model.
3. Definition of the SSRI's innovation strategy.
4. Access to the required infrastructures for ICT related innovation.
5. Use of mechanisms to evaluate the performance of a SSRI as innovation ecosystem.
6. Implementation of mechanisms for enabling the learning process towards a mature SSRI.

At the operational level, the focus is on the activities required to properly manage each independent innovation project launched in the scope of a SSRI, and developed by a network of independent organizations. The main challenges to consider in this category are:

1. Active involvement of user communities in the innovation project from its inception.
2. Adaptation to the changing needs of the user communities.
3. Coordination of SSRIs members from different disciplines and academic background.
4. Correct application of techniques for developing and validating new ICT products and services.
5. Evaluation of technological effectiveness of products and services developed.

---

[5] Some of the existing SSRIs are also considered Living Labs and therefore are part of both the Spanish National Network of SSRI and the European Network of Living Labs (ENoLL).

[6] From a practical point of view, Living Lab is currently a wider used concept and some practical current implementations could be actually classified as SSRI.

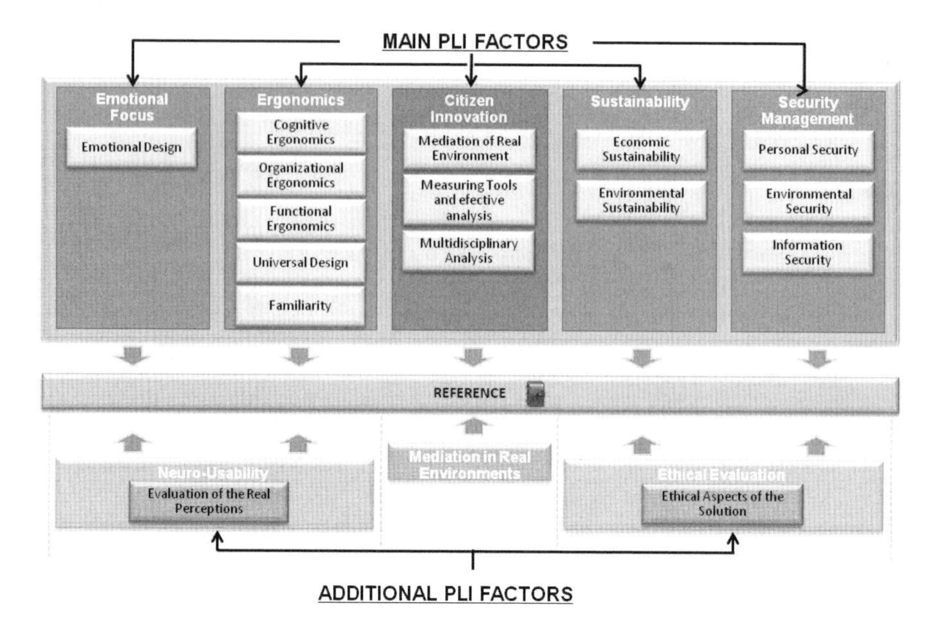

Figure 3. PLI factors.

2. Methodological Framework: PLI Approach for the Design and Validation of AAL Solutions

The SSRI methodological framework is being currently deployed by several Spanish organizations and research groups that foster the SSRI model[7]. The methodological framework intends to deliver methodologies to support and guide SSRIs along the eleven strategic and operational challenges described in Chapter 2. This chapter describes one of the already applied methodologies within this framework (PLI or People Led Innovation) that is demonstrating to be a practical tool to face some of the SSRI operational challenges [17].

PLI (People Led Innovation) is a conceptual model elaborated by I2BC by which the situating of people as leaders in the innovation process of any product or service that directly or indirectly influences their quality of life is promoted, integrating previous approaches such as "Customer Driven Innovation", "Outcome Driven Innovation", "Voice to Consumer", "Open Innovation" or the approximations related with the innovation based on social networks (prosumers) [9]. From the practical perspective, PLI is used as a Human Centred Design (HCD) approach [21] which combines Ergonomics and Emotional evaluation techniques (e.g. user experience testing) with participatory techniques (e.g. co-design sessions) in the context of the specific 'form of life' of potential users [17]. PLI is also used to evaluate the technical effectiveness of a solution, defining 'technical effectiveness' the ability of a solution to be effective, efficient and to solve the real problems of the target population within a real environment [9].

PLI is made up of seven different factors (see Fig. 3):

[7] This methodological framework is being developed under the umbrella of the CISVI project described in Chapter 3.

- Emotional focus.
- Ergonomics (including cognitive, functional and organizational ergonomics, universal design and familiarity).
- Citizen innovation.
- Sustainability (social, economical and environmental).
- Security management.
- Ethics.
- Neuro-usability (evaluation of real perceptions).

All these factors are considered (when appropriate) in the different innovation phases (from needs to market), especially in the design and evaluation part of the innovation cycle.

Detailed examples in the usage of the PLI methodology in the context of AAL SSRI and its results can be found in the referenced bibliography [17].

3. Some Living Examples of AAL SRRIs

3.1. CISVI Project

The CISVI project (Societal Communities for Research in eHealth and Independent Living)[8], a strategic project funded by the Ministry of Industry, Commerce and Tourism, has as main goal to validate the approach of SSRIs to create a new organizational model for innovation led by end-users and societal communities.

The project provides examples on lessons learnt and results of the application of the SSRI conceptual approach and methodologies to create sustainable organizations to enhance the collaboration of different organizations interested in the research and innovation on the eHealth and Independent Living areas. The examples are taken from the 4 SSRIs considered in the project.

3.1.1. Labour/Working Integration (Madrid)

The main purpose of this SSRI is to research on basic technologies that support young people with disabilities in performing their daily work. These technologies allow them to remember how to do any of the tasks that they have to carry out when they are confused, as well as to communicate audio visually with the labour mediator who monitors them (see Fig. 4) [12].

The main goal of this SSRI is to research and develop technologies that provide advanced support to:

- Previous training of the labour/working integration in a personalized and individual way, by means of the application of e-learning technologies, environmental intelligence technologies for tracking training activities and virtual systems for physical space representation, in an integrated and joint way.
- Training during the labour/working integration taking into account the special features of the job, enterprise and task.

[8] www.cisvi.es

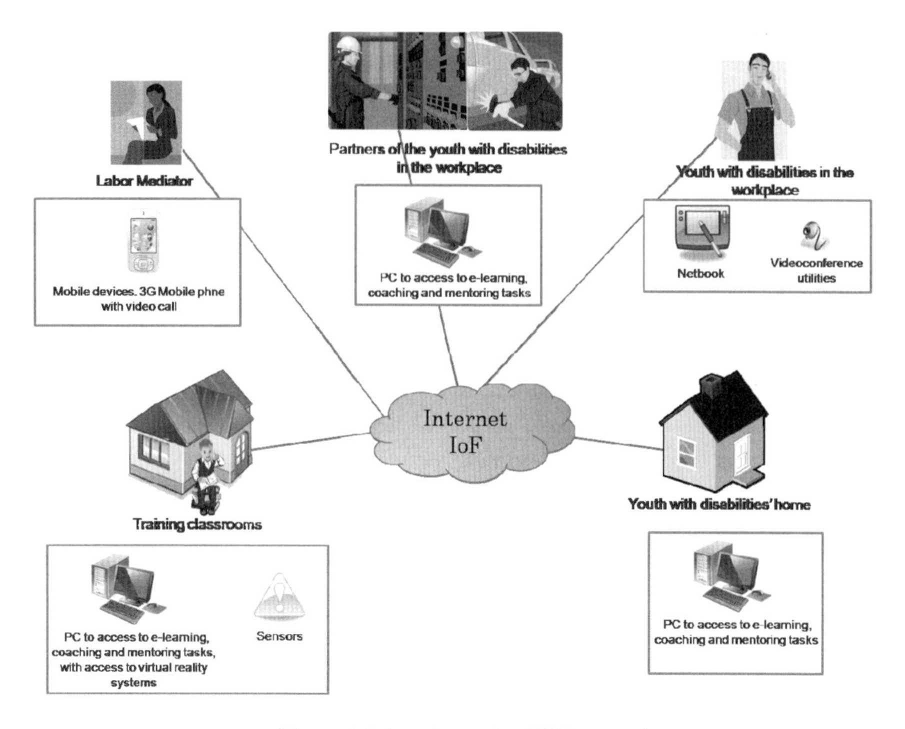

Figure 4. Labour integration SSRI's scenario.

- Conflict resolution that the young people with disabilities may have while performing their daily work.

3.1.2. Home Health Care for Older People (Madrid)

The main purpose of this SSRI is to research basic technologies that allow doctors to monitor elderly patients from their home, preventing that the elderly have to move to primary care centres or hospitals (Fig. 5).

The specific goals of this SRRI include:

- Make surgeries in the patient's home using high quality video-conference technologies due to the quality of the picture is a key success factor so that the doctor can diagnose to the patient from his home.
- Wireless sensor networks for continuous monitoring of patient.
- Technologies for learning and monitoring the healthy lifestyles recommended by the doctor to each patient in a personalized way.

3.1.3. Home Independent Life (Zaragoza)

The main purpose of this SSRI is to research and provide ICT solutions based on different technological areas of the so called "Internet of the Future", that would encourage an independent life at home (see Fig. 6).

The main objective of this SSRI is "to provide people with cognitive disabilities a higher level of autonomy enhanced security and improvement of their quality of life through the use of new technologies" [14].

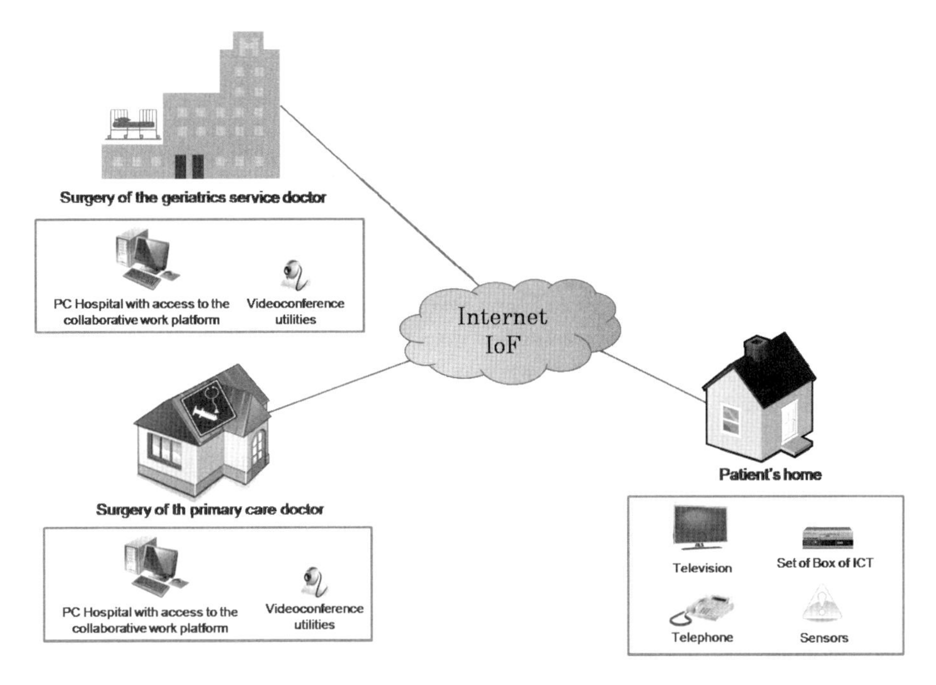

Figure 5. Home health care SSRI scenario.

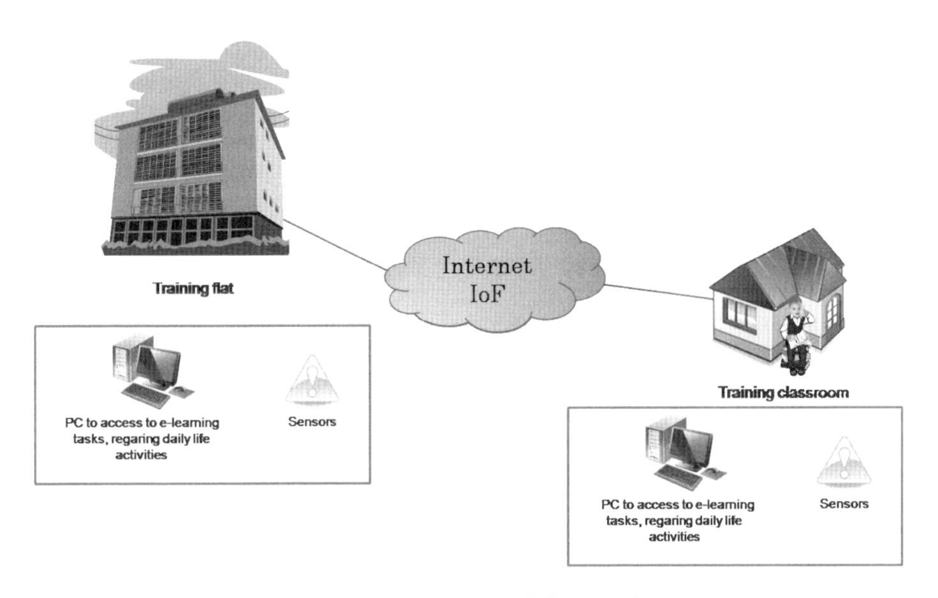

Figure 6. Home independent living scenario.

In order to achieve the general objective, the SSRI activities are focused on the following areas [12,14]:

- Support of daily activities (ADL) by means of context information and e-learning systems.

- Promotion of an open accessible community in which users (families, carers, educators, etc.) create and share educational content for learning activities of daily living.
- Support user cognitive training through entertainment activities such as memory and reasoning games.
- Enhance user safety by personal monitoring of unusual behaviours, lack of activity, etc. and by ambient monitoring such as fire warnings, "fridge door oversight" warnings, etc., fridge door oversight sound a bit weird.
- Easy communication through adapted teleconferences.

3.1.4. Development of Societal Communities in Rural Areas (Abla, Almería)

The main goal of this SSRI is to contribute and promote the social inclusion of older citizens in a rural area (ABLA municipality) through the application of open and user driven principles to research on adapted ICT solutions in the area of health (remote and monitoring control of people suffering COPD[9]), e-administration (use of e-ID) and independent living[10].

3.2. Fundacion PRODIS

Prodis Foundation is a non-profit Spanish organisation for the mental disabled people's welfare and leads Prodis' Social Space for Research and Innovation (SSRI), an important space for ICT innovation in the inclusion sector. Along with technological partner Ariadna Servicios Informáticos, this SSRI is working for the ICT application in areas such as education and work integration for people with intellectual disabilities. Prodis Foundation provides the end user with a vision of the inclusive scenarios where ICT can be used to substantially improve their quality of life.

3.2.1. General Description

Prodis Foundation implemented an educative program for the work integration of mentally disabled people called PROMENTOR. The PROMENTOR Program deals with several subjects and technical skills such as banking and accounting documentation, filing and organization, new technologies, and thinking strategies.

Prodis Foundation works to fulfil the social commitments of potential companies in which the students can be integrated. Once the new employee starts his tasks, Prodis' specialized personnel provide him with intensive coaching and mentoring to help adapt the acquired general skills to specialized and context dependent one. After the coaching stage, a labour mediator keeps in touch with the worker in case an intervention is in order to resolve any emotional or conflicts. Once a week, the workers attend follow-up meetings with Prodis' personnel and fellow students.

3.2.2. Prodis' Social Space for Research and Innovation

Prodis' SSRI aims to provide suitable technological solutions for work integration and education of people with intellectual disabilities.

---

[9] COPD Chronic obstructive pulmonary disease.

[10] More details about this SSRI can be found in Chapter 3.3.

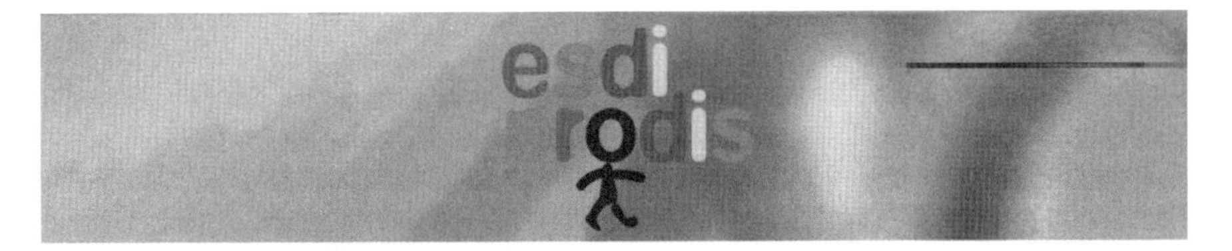

INNOVATION SCENARIOS

WORK INCLUSION	EDUCATION

INNOVATION ACTIVITIES

Mobile videoconference system for worker/labor mediator communication (CISVI) Digital didactic units' generation for knowledge reinforcement (CISVI) Tool for didactic units generation (CISVI) Indoor positioning system for internal mail delivery at the company (CISVI)	Didactic resources e-learning platform based (AMI4INCLUSION) RFID for ordering exercises' validation (AMI4INCLUSION) Accesible platform generation for mentally disabled people's education (eduWAI)

Figure 7. Prodis SSRI's innovation scenarios and activities.

At this moment, Prodis' SSRI is working in two innovation scenarios (Fig. 7), *work inclusion* and *education*, and they are considering the creation of one or two new transversal scenarios in the next few months. Under the scenarios already established, several innovation activities are being carried out, usually under the umbrella of international and national R&D projects. Prodis' SSRI structure is presented below detailing the innovation activities being carried out and the name of the projects that provide funding for these activities.

3.2.3. Success Cases

Up to now Prodis' SSRI has been working in several technological developments using short innovation cycles' implementing co-design sessions with users.

A few of the success stories of this methodology:

- The development of an RFID System for auto-evaluation of ordering exercises in order to improve the learning experience of students in filing and organizational tasks (needed for their work integration at the companies).
- A mobile video conference system aimed at providing the needed visual communication between specialized personnel and the employees to manage emotional conflicts usually arising at work.

Prodis' SSRI is also working, at this moment, in co-design sessions with users (teachers, labour mediators and intellectual disabled people) in order to successfully develop and validate the following products and services:

- A navigation system using augmented reality for internal and ubiquitous localization to help the worker in mail delivery tasks around the company's building
- Didactic units for helping mentally disabled people cope with the difficult aspects of their schedule and work tasks.
- An didactic system for teaching various methods of improving the emotional skills of people with intellectual disabilities.

3.3. Abla

3.3.1. General Description and Abla as Living Lab

Abla is a small village whose population is fewer than 1,500 inhabitants and is situated on the northern side of the Sierra Nevada range. Abla belongs to the Rio Nacimiento County. Abla is the heart of Rio Nacimiento Living Lab (RioNLL), a Rural Living Lab part of ENoLL since 2008 (3rd ENoLL wave). The Living Lab was set up oriented towards the creation, deployment and testing of Internet and ICT products and services, as a useful tool to improve the quality of life of their citizens, as well as to promote social innovation and a socio-economic development of the area. The main objectives of Rio Nacimiento Living Lab are:

- Acquire better knowledge and open people's minds to new experiences related to social and medical care for the rural population.
- Economical stimulation of new sectors related to ICT in the rural environment.
- Create new forms of citizen communication and participation.
- Promotion of Abla's culture and heritage as a way to boost Abla's tourism.
- Improvement of water and natural resources management (organic agriculture, renewable energies, natural areas, etc.).
- Improvement of educational resources in rural areas.

The main areas of interest to apply Future Internet technologies are related to the domains of Ambient Assisted Living (such as health and care of elderly people), education, and socio-economic development in a rural context, boosting tourism and the management of local natural resources.

RioNLL Future Internet current strengths relate to *Internet of the People and Internet of the Contents in Rural areas*, hosting events related to ICTs such as meeting of Rural Blogs, Annual Rural Party, Rural Innovation Fairs, workshops on Living Labs and the creation of a Social network for Abla citizens and more than 40 blogs. All public places such as restaurants, pubs, and the city council have free Wi-Fi Internet connection available. Available access technologies are DSL, 3G and radio satellite connection. The local health services are testing new formulas using the Internet technologies for patients' attention like *telemedicine*, home monitoring of patients with chronic diseases, and a social network to give support to professional and familiar care providers.

3.3.2. Abla SSRI

The initially adopted bottom-up approach (from the community to the technology and the projects), the strength of the social innovation movement in Abla and its initial focus on improving the quality of life of its citizens involving all the affected stakeholders (citizens, public institutions, research groups, SME's and others) are the main factors that helped in the promotion and recognition of Abla as a Social Space for Research and Innovation. Abla is one of the SSRIs of the CISVI project described in Chapter 4.1 of this paper. This chapter gets deeper into some of the details of the activities and results, emphasizing two aspects: the usage of the PLI methodology in the operational aspects of the SSRI and the lead of the social community in the definition and execution of the project.

The People Led Innovation (PLI) methodology is used in this SSRI combining participatory design of new products and services and evaluation of results to ensure that technological solutions fit user's needs. One of the objectives of the CISVI project in Abla SSRI was to identify older user's needs and barriers during the interaction with the existing electronic identity card system (eID). The national legal context encourages the implementation and use of eID forcing to adequate services in terms of usability and accessibility and prioritizing the digitalization of administration services. However the technological, infrastructure and societal contexts are not so favourable especially in rural areas (poor accessibility to certain infrastructure, low internet literacy in elderly populations, etc.) despite of the fact that it is in these rural remote areas where the eID could bring the most benefit (independent living). The usage of an iterative approach combining participatory design and evaluation with users are the key factors to detect user's barriers, produce and test new prototypes and to identify and correct mistakes as early as possible in the design and development cycle[11]. Citizen innovation and ergonomic and emotional factors are being used as part of the PLI methodology [17]. This SSRi also provides some examples in the redefinition of project objectives according to real community needs: The objective of the CISVI project in Abla SSRI was initially set (according to community needs) to social inclusion of elderly people in remote rural areas with special focus on e-Administration. The ongoing contact between research, social communities and other stakeholders (such as local health services) helped to identify new needs of the community (eHealth services for chronic disease monitoring and control) that were incorporated in the project objectives. The iterative, flexible and cooperative nature of SSRIs (and the projects executed in these contexts) allowed not only the incorporation of these new project objectives, but to reuse technological components already tested in other SSRI, accelerating the time-to-market and demonstrating that SSRI is an instrument to create real value in society with economies of scale.

4. Recently Deployed AAL SSRIs (New Scenarios)

The creation and consolidation of the SSRI Spanish National Network, the ongoing support of the Spanish Technological platform for Health, Wellbeing and Social Cohesion (eVIA) and some other organizations (e.g. i2BC), the success stories of SSRI in the AAL field and the ongoing searching of some social communities of formulas to improve their quality of life, are key factors that explain the increase of new SSRIs in the Spanish territory. This chapter describes three new SSRIs whose main objectives

[11] The 2nd participatory design and evaluation sessions that took place in June 2010 as part of the 2nd project iteration (not published yet) clearly showed that prototypes defined by the researchers based on 1st iteration results were wrongly designed and this allow a rapid re-definition of the solution. These findings are being considered great successes from the methodological point of view.

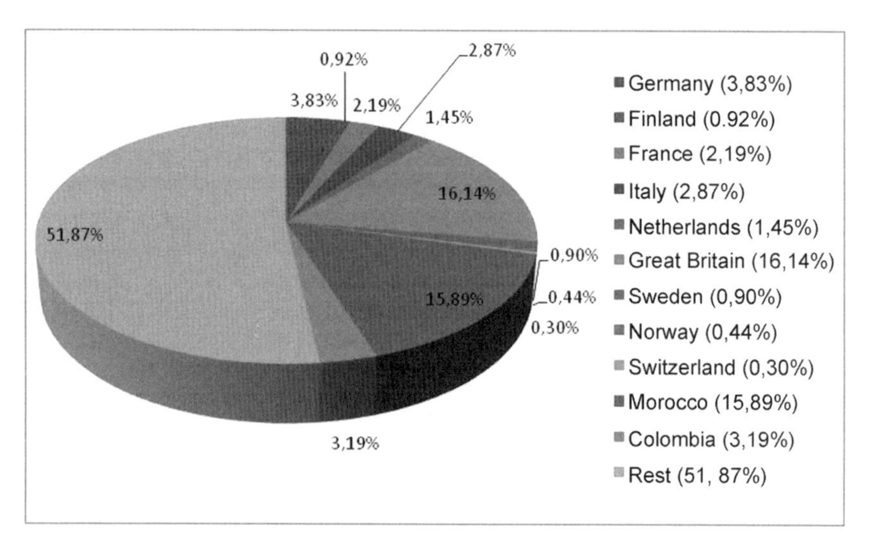

Figure 8. Percentage of foreigners by nationality.

are aligned with the AAL scope and definition [23]. The new AAL scenarios have been classified according to the areas defined in the AAL Roadmap [23]: AAL4persons (AAL@home and AALon_the_move), AAL@community and AAL@work.

4.1. AAL4persons in Costa del Sol SSRI (Málaga)

4.1.1. The Context: Costa del Sol as a International Retirement Migration (IRM) Scenario

The Costa del Sol (or "Coast of the Sun") stretches along 150 kilometres of Malaga province and it is one of Spain's most popular tourist destinations. The area's mild climate is the main attraction that makes it possible to enjoy the beaches and a wide variety of outdoor activities year round. Fuengirola is a large town and municipality on the Costa del Sol with 71,482 inhabitants (2009)[12] including 25,259 foreign residents (2009).

In Spain and several other Southern European countries such as Italy, Portugal and Greece, in recent decades have seen an increase in the number of foreign residents from northern Europe, especially the United Kingdom and Germany [1]. According to the 2010 Population Census[13], there were more than 308,745 foreigners aged 65 or living in Spain, and 78 per cent came from the European Union[14]. Some references estimated 240,794 aged at least 65 years, of whom 43,100 lived in the Costa del Sol area[14]. Other estimates indicate that there are more than 140,000 Britons aged over 60 years living in Spain[14].

According to the National Institute of Statistics (2010) Great Britain, Germany, Finland and Sweden make up the 21.79% of foreigners that live in the Costa del Sol (see Fig. 8). Costa del Sol is the area where the greatest number of Finns live abroad

---

[12] Multiterritorial information system of Andalusia (http://www.juntadeandalucia.es:9002/sima/htm/sm29054.htm) (2009).

[13] Instituto Nacional de Estadística, Censo Poblacional 2010, Madrid, 2010. Available at www.ine.es.

during the winter, around thirty thousand, of whom 10,000 thousand live all year long[14].

Increases in life expectancy in recent decades have come about through declines in later life mortality, so extending the length and health of retirement. Given that in recent years in developed countries, retired people have had increased purchasing power and rising housing assets, giving them a greater capacity for residential mobility and the choice to live in areas with good environmental conditions, one readily understands the growing importance of international retirement migration (IRM). This is one of the several residential strategies available to a household when its members leave the labour market or when individual, social or family circumstances change [16].

The climate of the receiving region has been considered in many studies to be the most important pull factor [10,11,16]. It is sometimes related to other environmental features [3,16], and sometimes to previous migratory experience or holidays in the destination area. The link between climate and health problems is also noteworthy. The other main set of reasons refers to the standard of living and economic features, including income levels and house ownership rates [10,16]. There are also frequent references to social factors, family relationships and distance [8,16].

A further aspect of this discourse is the evaluation of the migrant's influence on the destination region, which the retired person perceives and measures in several ways.

Apart from this, the migration of retired Europeans to Spain has shared characteristics with other large 'sunbelt' migrations. The specific configuration of Southern Spain's economic, social and environmental conditions, and its accessibility to the Northern European countries of origin, has made the region one of the most popular destinations for this type of migration. The image of the Costa del Sol has been based on three features of its pleasant climate: the high average winter temperature, the many hours of sunshine per year, and the number of rain-free days. Other factors (culture, folklore, resort facilities) are less important in popular perception of the region [16] although interest in these elements is increasing because of greater institutional support. The attractions of the Costa del Sol, as demonstrated by various tourist surveys, confirm the considerable importance attached to basic features such as the climate, the beach, and safety [16,22]. Also valued are the area's cleanliness, low prices, standard of living, and the beauty of the landscape. Commercial tourism increasingly stresses products that link the environment to 'quality of life' activities, the notable examples being golf courses and access to a romanticised, exotic landscape as with the *pueblos blancos* (white villages) of the interior of Andalusia. The Costa del Sol's successful combination of environmental attractions and a well-developed urban and tourist infrastructure attracts large numbers of retired Europeans alongside 'ordinary' tourists [4,13,16,20].

4.1.2. Drivers for the SSRI Deployment

Researches from I2BC and the Work Science Lab of the University of Oulu performed interviews with Finnish and Spanish associations of retired people during 2009 and 2010. During the same period I2BC's researchers also carried out a well-being and

---

[14] http://palaciocongresosdetorremolinos.wordpress.com/2010/12/07/la-comunidad-finlandesa-de-la-costa-del-sol-celebra-con-un-acto-en-torremolinos-el-93-aniversario-de-su-independiencia/ (2010).

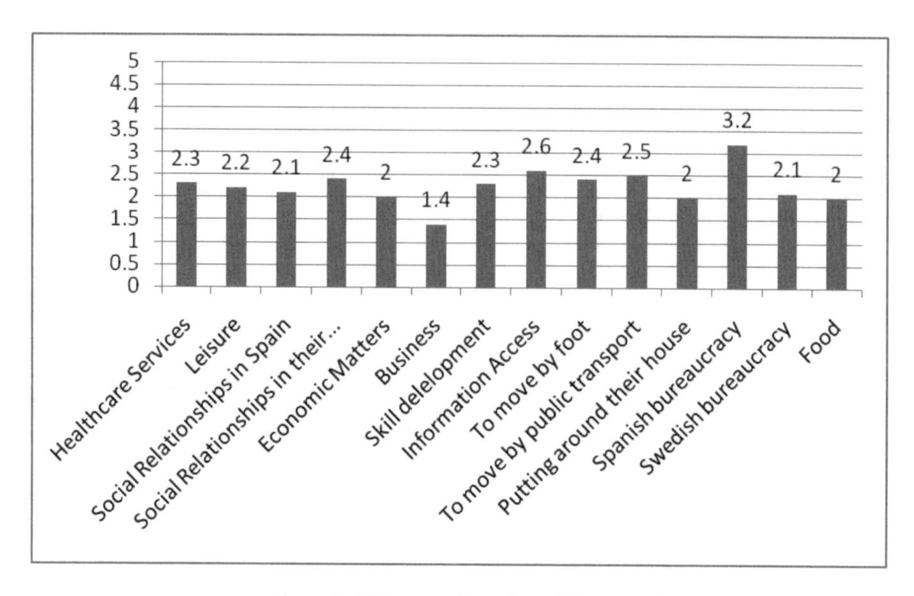

Figure 9. Main necessities of Swedish population.

needs analysis among the retired Swedish population in several communities along the Costa del Sol.

The main findings of the research conducted within the Finnish community were related to security problems, mobility problems (transportation and independent driving as they don't understand local signs), language issues, access to local finance services, and problems with Spanish bureaucracy. A lack of integration with local communities was also highlighted in the research[15].

Regarding the Swedish community, the research[16] performed in the area of wellbeing showed interesting results: the level of perceived wellbeing of this community is really high (7,8 over 10) and wellbeing was described as a combination of different factors such as health, leisure and culture, social relationships, economy, integration and participation, and, training and knowledge. The main necessities found among the Swedish Population in the Costa del Sol area relate to Spanish bureaucracy, information access and pedestrian mobility (see Fig. 9).

The result of these studies and further interviews and conversations with the Fuengirola City Council, local SMEs and entrepreneurship associations was the signing of a Memorandum of Understanding (MoU) for the establishment of an SSRI (initially located in Fuengirola but with the objective to geographically incorporate other villages and communities along the Costa del Sol). New participants such as several Spanish and Finnish universities, Finnish research and development centers, and local, national and international SME's and firms have recently joined the Costa del Sol SSRI during 2010.

The main objectives of Costa del Sol SSRI, agreed and defined by the MoU, are to establish a participatory model to improve the quality of life and wellbeing of citizens, promoting tourism potential of Costa del Sol, promoting cultural exchange, enhancing the knowledge of other European Union languages, promoting the incorporation of new

[15] Results not published yet.
[16] Results not published yet.

technologies to enhance citizen's lives (foreign and local), generating new employment opportunities within the Quality of life and Wellbeing sector.

4.1.3. Costa del Sol SSRI: Present and Future

Research and innovation AAL topics already identified in this SSRI are [23]:

- AAL for health, with especial focus on person-centred health management at home and away from home, tele-monitoring and self-management of chronic diseases and support for caregivers and care organizations;
- Personal and home safety and security (general requirements of feeling secure at home);
- Personal activity management;
- Bio-robotic systems;
- Person-centred services (shopping, feeding, personal care, social interaction and communication);
- Social inclusion;
- Entertainment and leisure; and
- Mobility (supporting individual physical monitoring, AA-driving and public transport).

This SSRI, still in its initial stages, is envisaged to grow in the coming months with the incorporation of new partners, the launching of projects in the AAL technological field, and the performing of several experimentation actions to promote social innovation and participation.

4.2. AAL@community in Lebrija (Seville)

One of the three areas in which the AAL approach is focused on is to promote the social participation of the elderly, allowing older people to be active members in their communities (not only as a passive subject or beneficiary, but also as a productive member). This section describes the Lebrija SSRI, which can be considered an attempt to explore opportunities and develop innovations in the area of AAL@community.

Lebrija is a city with 26,000 inhabitants, located between two highly populated cities in Andalusia: Sevilla and Jerez. Traditionally, main activities in Lebrija have been related with agriculture and construction (both are areas that will probably no longer be suitable to support Lebrija's economy). Additionally, Lebrija is facing the consequences of social and economic changes linked to the ageing of the population. In this context, the Lebrija SSRI has been initially promoted by UGT-Lebrija[17], the Lebrija city council and i2BC with the objective of promoting elderly people´s health and independent living in their own local context, focusing on areas such as the communication and participation of its inhabitants.

Lebrija SSRI is also a scenario in which AAL and other related projects can be piloted. An example of this is the WeCare 2.0 project[18], funded under the AAL-JP Call 2, which plans to set up technology pilots in four countries: Finland, The Netherlands, Ireland and Spain. WeCare 2.0 key goal is to prevent the elderly from feeling lonely through the provision of a support structure whereby they participate in social net-

[17] UGT is one of the main labour unions in Spain.

[18] WeCare 2.0 http://www.wecare-project.eu/.

works. The goal is to support and empower elderly people to participate in social networks as early as possible, before they start to suffer from ill health, isolation or loneliness. When or if people start to suffer from ill health, these social networks are already 'in place' and can function beneficially. The objective is to empower senior citizens to engage in active, two-way relationships of receiving help and offering help (interdependency), as much as possible and for as long as possible. Family, friends and neighbours (i.e. the community) create 'connected groups' of mutual care: receiving care and providing care to each other.

Planning and recruitment and user studies are the two main WeCare 2.0 tasks that have been performed in the Lebrija SSRI at this moment:

1. Planning and recruitment: During this phase, the Lebrija context was analyzed in order to plan user involvement and pilot activities. To do so we did not only adopt the traditional approach of bringing users to our labs and asking them what they needed, but moving ourselves (researchers and designers with different backgrounds and lifestyles) to their environment, the real context of old people in rural areas with their own lifestyles and needs. This SSRI approach intends to pay more attention to the analysis of daily living and its implication to the innovation process. In order to come together with the community, we organized a two-day event in Lebrija including general participatory talks in which citizens discussed about their status, daily life problems and (non-technological) needs in the education, health or well-being areas. There was also a leisure part of the event including coffee breaks, tapas tasting and a flamenco play. After this opening, we got introduced into the Lebrija community 'way of life', several associations and citizens were recruited to participate actively in the project and an atmosphere was created in which we were able to collaborate to reveal their technological problems and needs.
2. User studies: The needs and preferences of senior citizens in Lebrija have been investigated via interviews, focus groups, observation of participants' daily lives and desk research. Using the information collected, a set of user requirements for the WeCare 2.0 solution is been produced. These requirements include information about what kind of application they need and would like to use in order to promote their social lives by participating in community activities and fostering the exchange of cultural experiences and hobbies.

Next step for the Lebrija SSRI in this project is to involve users in the design process of the WeCare 2.0 solution, through co-design sessions in which they will be able to co-create together with researchers and developers the technology they need to improve their wellbeing in their community.

5. Conclusions

Social Space for Research and Innovation (SSRI) is a new approach and tool to accelerate AAL deployment taking into consideration all of the different aspects (personal, social, technical, ethical, economical and legal) and all the stakeholders that matter in the challenge of an ageing society in which Europe is presently facing. The positioning of users as leaders of the research and innovation activities, and the shift of such activities to their daily-life environments are some key characteristics of this approach.

SSRI concept and approach was born in Spain, and incorporates many aspects of the Open Innovation, User centred Innovation, Human Centred Design, and Living Labs models. Despite being a recently created and implemented approach (2008), Spain already boasts a national network of 19 recognized SSRIs, as well as a few more which will be incorporated at the end of 2010. There are also important national projects using SSRI as a research and innovation instrument in the AAL field (CISVI) and this trend is rapidly moving to the international sphere. There are already some success stories in the field of health and independent living and the number of newly developed AAL SSRIs and scenarios is increasing rapidly.

Some Spanish organizations are working in the development of the methodology framework, methodologies and tools that have already been put into practice with favourable results. However there is still work to be done and many improvements to be made, both in the methodology framework and sustainability aspects, improvements which will be incorporated in this model in the months to come. It is also foreseen that the upcoming rapid growth in the number of AAL projects that will use this approach in the next years which will help to evaluate and improve the model.

Acknowledgements

We'd like to thank the Spanish Ministry of Industry, Tourism and Commerce, the PNICDT 2008-2011 program and the European Fund for Regional Development (FEDER) for the grant TSI-020301-2008-21 that aids in co-funding the CISVI project.

We'd also like to thank Gemma Risquez at I2BC for her contribution in providing research material not published yet (results of questionnaires given to the Norwegian communities in Costa del Sol) and Mark L. Finlay for his help with the English version of this paper.

References

[1] M.A. Casado-Díaz, C. Kaiser and A.M. Warnerss, Norther European retired residents in nine southern European areas: Characteristics, motivations and adjustment, *Aging & Society* **24** (2004), 353–381.
[2] H.W. Chesbrough, *Open Innovation: The New Imperative for Creating and Profiting from Technology*, Harvard Business School Press, Boston, 2003.
[3] L. Cuba and C.F. Longino, Regional retirement migration: The case of Cape Cod, *Journal of Gerontology* **46** (1991), 533–542.
[4] R. Díaz, La inmigración de extranjeros en las Canarias Orientales. Una valoración global, in: *III Jornadas de la Población Española Editores*, Torremolinos AGE, 1991.
[5] European Commission, Living labs for user-driven open innovation, Directorate General for the Information Society and Media, Unit F4: New Infrastructure Paradigms and Experimental Facilities, 2008. Available at: http://ec.europa.eu/information_society/activities/livinglabs/docs/brochure201108.pdf.
[6] Evia Steering Committee, Strategic research roadmap for technologies to support accessibility and ambient assisted living, Spanish Technological Platform for ICT Support to Accessibility and Independent Life, 2009. Available at: http://www.evia.org.es/documentos.aspx [downloaded January, 2009].
[7] J.A. Fernández, D. López and C. Aparicio, *Extranjeros de Tercera Edad en España, Características Demográficas*, Instituto de Demografía, Madrid, 1993.
[8] R. Ford, The process of mobility decision-making in later old age: Early findings from an original survey of elderly people in South East England, *Espace, Populations, Sociétés* **3** (1993), 523–532.
[9] I2BC and SGS ICS, Reference of certification for solutions designed under the principles of technological effectiveness, I2BC Technical Report, 2008.
[10] J.E. Kallan, A multilevel analysis of elderly migration, *Social Science Quarterly* **74** (1993), 403–416.
[11] J.A. Krout, Seasonal migration of older people, *The Gerontologist* **23** (1993), 295–299.

[12] E. Mazzone, E. Gutiérrez, C. Barrera, C. Finat, O.C. Santos, J.G. Boticario, J. Moranchel, J.R. Roldán and R. Casas, Involving users in the design of ICT aimed to improve education, work and leisure for users with intellectual disabilities, in: *Proceedings of the 12th International Conference on Computers Helping People with Special Needs ICCHP'2010*, Lecture Notes in Computer Science, Vol. 6180/2010, Vienna, 2010, pp. 5–12.
[13] C. Montiel, Desarrollo turístico, promoción inmobiliaria y degradación medioambiental en el municipio de Benitachell (Comarca de la Marina), *Investigaciones Geográficas* **8** (1990), 113–129.
[14] J. Moranchel, R. Casas, J.R. Roldán, C. Barrera, J. García and J. Falcó, Social spaces for research and innovation for independent living, in: *The 25th Annual International Technology & Persons with Disabilities Conference*, 2010.
[15] A. Paniagua, Migración de no europeos retirados de España, *Geriatría y Gerontología* **26** (1991), 255–266.
[16] V. Rodriguez, G. Fernández Mayoralas and F. Rojo, European retirees on the Costa del Sol: A cross-national comparison, *International Journal of Population Geography* **4** (1998), 183–200.
[17] F. Sainz, R.I. Madrid and J. Madrid, Introducing co-design for digital technologies in rural areas, in: *Proceedings of the NORDICHI'2010 conference*, Reykjavik, Iceland, 18–20th October 2010.
[18] H. Schaffers, J. García Guzman, C. Merz and M. Navarro, eds, Living labs for rural development: Results from the C@R integrated project, TRAGSA and FAO, Madrid, 2009.
[19] J. Schumacher and V. Niitamo, *European Living Labs. A New Approach for Human Centric Regional Innovatio*n. Wissenschaftlicher Verlag Berlin, Berlin, 2008.
[20] J.M. Serrano, Residentes extranjeros en la región de Murcia: Aproximación inicial a su estudio, *Papeles de Geografía* **17** (1991), 227–253.
[21] M. Steen, *The Fragility of Human – Centered Design*, IOS Press, Amsterdam, The Netherlands, 2008.
[22] E. Torres and V. Granados, El sector turístico de la Costa del Sol, in: *Presente y Futuro de la Provincia de Málaga*, SODPE, 1996.
[23] G. van den Broek, F. Cavallo, L. Odetti and C. Wehrmann, eds, AALIANCE (2010) – Ambient Assisted Living Roadmap, Berlin, 2010. Available at: http://www.aaliance.eu/public/documents/aaliance-roadmap/aaliance-aal-roadmap.pdf.
[24] E. Von Hippel, *Democratizing Innovation*, The MIT Press. Cambridge, MA, 2005.

Handbook of Ambient Assisted Living
J.C. Augusto et al. (Eds.)
IOS Press, 2012

doi:10.3233/978-1-60750-837-3-749

New Ambient Assistive Technologies: The Users' Perspectives

Dr. Elizabeth MESTHENEOS*
President, AGE Platform Europe

Abstract. The effectiveness of new technologies from older people's perspectives depends on motivation, support, cost, safety, security and ethics. The human rights of older people inform approaches to the development and use of new AAL technologies.

Keywords. Overcoming older people's barriers in using Ambient Assistive Technologies, human rights, social inclusion

Introduction

Those of us old enough to remember the first PCs in the 1970s and early 1980s recollect that there was no compatibility between systems; that they were frequently difficult to set up and use unless you were really interested in the mechanics of the technology; they often assumed knowledge that was nowhere written down or else written in a way that was incomprehensible; they always needed advice and help from a few, more knowledgeable, friends to solve particular problems; they were expensive; they often did not coordinate with other appliances (e.g. printers); they needed good eyesight as they had black and white small screens; they required dexterity and nimble fingers (to screw in various components); and they assumed you could type. The Internet brought new problems of compatibility, bugs, systems that collapsed from overload, unreliability and unverifiable sources. Some of these problems for the users of the machines have been overcome, but they should still alert us to the kind of issues that new ICT (Information and Communication Technology) applications and their producers face and that all naïve, new and non-technical people using the ICT innovation confront. Assistive technologies for older people, currently under development, are designed both to aid them and the health and welfare systems in independent living; these can work well, effectively and profitably only if the needs of users are taken into consideration from the outset[1].

Digital illiteracy amongst older people, especially those who never had to learn it during their working lives, remains an issue throughout the European Union [10]. Familiarity with using digital technologies almost certainly aids in the acceptance of and skills in learning and adopting other similar or additional digital technologies. While some Member States have run awareness campaigns to try and raise digital literacy amongst all older people – backed by educational authorities, NGOs (Non

---

*Corresponding Author: Dr. Elizabeth Mestheneos. E-mail: alice.sinigaglia@age-platform.eu.
[1] This conclusion is the outcome of many European research projects such as FUTURAGE, ERA-AGE and FORTUNE-USEM.

Governmental Organizations) and self help learning groups – there remain large differences amongst Member States: the southern and eastern ones lag behind those in northern Europe, and rural areas lag behind urban ones, while differences in usage by age group reflect the same "digital divide". The recent report from the Commission [8] states that 43% of European households still do not have Internet access while the Expert Review [13] 2009 reported digital literacy as still a significant challenge, especially among those aged over 55. The 55 plus vary in their educational, economic and life experiences, more than any other age group. Their access to and level of digital competence also reflects their previous and current access to digital learning and the capacity to use ICT but also the actual availability and relative cost of broadband and the Internet. While this is a dynamic situation, there is no room for complacency as the European institutions, Member State governments, private services and producers shift to more of their services and functions being conducted through the use of ICT.

While these issues are well known, some other identifiable repercussions for and implications in using new digital assistive technologies in the homes of older people will impact on the development of AAL (Ambient Assisted Living). One should also note that the division between assistive technologies and "everyday/normal" technologies is sometimes quite difficult to pinpoint. It could well be argued that the more the assistive technologies resemble ones used more generally, the more acceptable they will be.

There is little original in discussing the problems, needs and reactions of older people as willing and unwilling users of new technologies. In 2008 the Australian government ordered a comprehensive scoping study on the use of assistive technologies by frail older people living in the community; they reviewed in full detail all the literature and research on the theme of this chapter, a majority of it originating in North America, the UK and Japan. It noted areas in which research evidence was unsatisfactory or lacking in demonstrating the effectiveness of assistive technologies [16]. However it also noted the positive research evidence for a wide range of issues: "improved safety and reduced falls; reduced hospitalisation; improved independence, mobility and physical function; improved well-being and quality of life, including an enhanced sense of safety and increased opportunities to continue living at home." The reader may access the detailed review of the literature on the evidence for the benefits of AAL as reviewed in 2008 which also mentions the lack of consultation with older people. Nearly three years later, further evidence of the effects of the use of AAL on the lives and well being of older people is slowly accumulating. However the point of this chapter is not to review all the literature – others have done this – but to present some of the obvious shortfalls in the approaches by AAL developers and industries as understood from older peoples' own perspectives[2] rather than that of the professionals.

Hence though placed amongst academic work on AAL, this chapter firmly takes the perspective of older people and, hopefully, this is its added value for the reader. The rapidity of change, the increasing use of the Internet for debates and references, means that readers can easily access the current state of debate and the findings of the many European funded programmes that support AAL.

What must be remembered when discussing "the perspective" of older people is that they are not in any sense homogenous; they have different capacities, biographies, and life experiences covering very different decades and politico-economic situations. This article introduces some of the main issues that confront older people including

[2] One must also include the family carer's perspective since many are themselves older people.

their motivation; costs in the use and take up of AAL technologies; accessibility to AAL technologies; support in using them and the ethical issues associated with older people using unfamiliar technologies, especially those who are frail or have serious problems related to dementia, depression and Alzheimer. It then continues by examining the appropriate areas in which ICT can help older people in the immediate and medium term.

1. Main Problems for Older People in the Use of ICT

1.1. Motivation

Those who have never used ICT technologies and the Internet remain unconvinced that it is essential to their lives; they have lived using other modes of communication successfully and can see little reason to change. The results from the recent 2010 European survey [14] (p. 72) shows that the first reason for not having a computer or the Internet is a lack of interest: this may confuse the different situations of having had no experience of them with having tried and genuinely not being interested, but the latter is likely to be less common. The difficulty here lies in the introduction of AAL at a time when it is judged that they are needed, into the homes of older people who have never learned any ICT skills. Receiving instructions over the internet, connecting with professionals for advice or ordering services into the home, may not be at all appealing to people – either because they have no experience of ICT or because often what they are seeking and need is personal contact. Loneliness in old age, especially amongst those most confined to their homes for reasons of health and frailty, remains a huge problem [4,19]. Another common problem relating to loneliness is the issue of depression, one of the most significant and under diagnosed and treated health problems that has a very large impact on the quality of life and well being of older people.

Motivation is a factor which plays an important role: the extent to which older people actively decide to purchase and use ICT equipment represents a very different set of attitudes from the common situation where others have forced or manipulated them into getting it. Attitudes to the adoption of innovations vary by people's character: some are innovators and like new gadgets and technologies, others are far more cautious. Innovation is something that we currently value, but older people have already experienced a large range of innovations: they may be tired of changing and learning new technologies again since they may have also to learn new skills – yet found the old solutions perfectly satisfactory.

Selling new technologies to people on the basis of fear is also a poor motivator. Variously policy makers and AAL developers mention older people being afraid of slipping and falling, of burglary and their safety in their homes, of being alone, of forgetting to switch off cookers, lights and appliances. Yet this approach or stressing the negative aspects associated with some ageing people, would appear to be a negative way of getting older people themselves interested and able to use new technologies. It is far better to motivate people positively and preferably before they need assistive technologies.

Indeed promoting AAL solutions as being purely useful cannot be a motive force for the uptake of new technologies by seniors; they need to be attractive and fun, too. Developing a phone with huge buttons in the user interface can give the impression of being user-friendly but may end up being rejected as older people find it adds little to their usual means of communication and may even find it stigmatizing. On the contrary offering amusing features, which are adapted for users of all ages is a strong stimulator. If older people are to genuinely embrace the developed technologies, the AAL/ICT developers have to pay attention to design and appeal to the basic need of everyone regardless of age to entertain themselves in everyday tasks. Can anyone think of today's smart phone users accepting in a later life a technology which is tiring and boring?

Again it needs to be noted that the motivations of older people for the take up of AAL/ICT are not necessarily those of carers or health and social service providers. How motivation can be generated for far more positive reasons is discussed below.

1.2. Costs

While the European Union is currently keen to underline the tremendous potential value that can come from developments of the knowledge society through new applications in the ICT industry (e.g. e-health, e-inclusion), the recent Commission research shows that the second most important reason for the non use of existing ICT remains its cost to the users both in terms of hardware and broadband access [9].

This flags a concern in the development of AAL: who will meet the costs of assistive technologies for older people in their homes? Some motivated older users with adequate incomes will pay; others will have to rely on their families who are concerned for them and are able to meet the costs. However, inadequate and underfunded health and welfare systems – common in many Member States – are going to face difficulties in meeting the capital and restructuring costs of new expensive technologies, even when they might save on staff and provide more support services in the long run. Private insurance policies will have to be radically altered if they are willing to cover some of the future risks and expenses for ageing customers who want to use AAL.

Another issue is that the costs of new assistive technology will not simply be those of the outlay on the original basic equipment but also those relating to its installation, maintenance, periodic upgrading and emergency support.

Though the assumption is that the use of assistive technologies will reduce the costs of care or make the existing available care personnel more able to service more people, there are severe limits on this projection.

Older people using new AAL technologies will need more training and support than younger users and one can predict that this will be strongly related to educational and income levels and mental health. Thus a fear is that de facto the cost of investing in and using AAL technologies will exclude some of the oldest, poorest, and most vulnerable throughout the European Union, typically those most in need of support for health and welfare services.

Efficiencies from the use of AAL technology in making the work of health care professionals more productive will still have to confront a reality that demand is likely to continue to rise as a result of increasing longevity[3]: this will be partly related to the success of new technologies in keeping people alive further, and hence contributing to an increase in demand and expectations.

[3] Increasing life expectancy is not necessarily accompanied by an increase in healthy life expectancy even though this is a current goal of European policies.

1.3. Accessibility

A lack of common standards in accessibility remains a critical problem in the development of AAL technologies. Though e- and web site guidelines exist under the W3c/Web-Accessibility Initiative/Web-Content Accessibility Guidelines (WAI/WCAG 2.0) that are commonly accepted as the reference point for web-accessibility, they are currently opaque and open to interpretation at local and national levels – leading to a fragmentation in implementation and in local legislation. Additionally, W3C web accessibility standards and guidelines do not address accessibility for older people particularly those, older and younger, with intellectual disabilities – something that should greatly concern designers of AAL systems, since these groups are supposed to be the prime beneficiaries of the AAL technologies.

If we are not to repeat the unsurprising variability of systems in the early years of computers, we need binding clear and consistent legislation and rules for AAL manufacturers and service providers. This would enable them to operate across national borders in Europe and encourage free competition between AAL–ICT producers and providers. The USA has already adopted section 508 in the Draft Accessibility legislation and demonstrated the business case for e- and web accessibility. The benefit for consumers of "designed for all" ICT products and services is that this enhances usability and creates a far wider market, reinforcing the competitiveness and Internal Market objectives of the European Union. Thus developing e- and web-accessibility is a win-win situation for all since they could support the social and economic inclusion of disadvantaged people.

Of course there need to be additional facilities and alternative content accessible to people with limited abilities to read and understand text. This is where the European Commission can help by encouraging the development of an evaluation and assessment methodology and conformity assessment methods, to complement the WAI guidelines, and to provide consumers with reliable information about the accessibility of websites they access. The use of automatic testing and human testing elements should also be systematically considered. When looking at external evaluations of websites, it must be made very clear that self-declaration of accessibility is not the best solution. The system put in place to judge compliance with accessibility standards should be made by a mixed group of experts, comprised of consumers, web designers and industry representatives. In this respect, phase 2 of the Standardisation Mandate 376 to CEN, CENELEC and ETSI in support of the European accessibility requirements for public procurement of products and services in the ICT domain, may deliver results but the process has not started yet.

1.4. Support

Whatever the forms of the AAL technology, there are issues for older people about the installation, maintenance and monitoring of the equipment. Who will look after it when it appears to have gone wrong? However good and reliable the equipment is, if it does not provide a quality service through professional support, it will be abandoned. Many older people do not have someone in their social network able to help them with the installation of new equipment, teach them the necessary skills and deal with problems. Interestingly most users of digital technology rely on informal hints, support and help from friends and peer users. One can argue that much knowledge about digital technologies is passed on by word of mouth, with people copying or demonstrating to each other appropriate actions for its full use. Many older people live on their own and cannot call on younger neighbours or their children to help them – in marked contrast to most young people who have access to such resources through their school or in their job. Additionally, if problems arise, then older people who look for assistance cannot easily discriminate between good, trustworthy technicians and bad yet expensive ones. Negative experiences – both personal and relayed – become a barrier to adoption of ICT.

As attitudes and experiences vary considerably amongst older people, so it becomes clear that some people will need more guidance than others. If the AAL technology is to work, training and support will be needed from the start of its introduction. Confidence enables the older person to approach new technologies without fear and thus to experience fewer problems. One major function of AAL will be to provide social and health support – yet ultimately it is the availability of the professional on the "other end" which will give the necessary reassurance and guidance and give value to the technology itself [4]. Especially at times when people feel physically, emotionally or mentally vulnerable, having to deal with unfamiliar technologies and new technologies can be frightening, and represent a new problem rather than a solution. There is some limited evidence that ensuring adequate training as well as providing personal support is valuable in ensuring that older people and their carers do not abandon the assistive technologies [6].

Older persons must know that they can contact directly a health care professional – preferably an organization or person they already know. In case they panic – e.g. when the equipment does not work, or when electronic contacts are not adequate – there must be personnel offering both technical and professional support. Older people should not feel neglected because of the use of technology, but should feel that it gives them additional possibilities. Technology can be helpful but it cannot replace direct contacts with health and social care workers or take over all their tasks.

Another aspect reflects the importance of taking into consideration the cognitive differences amongst older people e.g. variability in their attitudes, behavior, and subjective norms, and this may indicate why some become users and others abandon assistive devices [21].

The use of local technical assistants appears to be a good solution, judging from the experience of the recent European Dreaming project in the pilot site of Langeland in Denmark, where a technologically competent retired farmer helped older patients in the locality with the equipment [15]. They knew and trusted this person, he was competent and available, and his services were free during the lifetime of the project. Such support would need to be built into the design of new AAL applications.

1.5. Security and Ethics

Ethical issues are raised in the relationship of ICT to ageing reflecting the vulnerability of users, the changing characteristics of the user population, budget constraints and constant developments and innovations in science and technology. Ignoring or undervaluing ethical concerns can lead to the rejection of ICT by the older person and informal carers and this, in turn, creates a barrier to market uptake [7]. At the centre of ethical issues is the changing political and social situation of European citizens: human

---

[4] The ACTION European programme discussed the role of technical support in the adoption of ICT by older people and their families. http://www.ict-ageing.eu/?page_id=1632.

rights are not limited by age or other discriminating criteria. Each person, however frail or with whatever mental problems, cannot be deprived of these rights as well as their rights to human dignity e.g. they or their representative need to know the risks the technology generates, the choices they have [1,20]. Putting the older person at the centre of developments rather than treating them instrumentally as a means to the end of the developer, service provider or entrepreneur, represents an important shift in thinking about the nature of technology. It is important that it does not discriminate against any section of the community; generally, but particularly where public funding has been used in ICT development, there is also the issue of equity i.e. fair access for all the population to the benefits of technology.

An important issue that each AAL application may have to confront and consider is the degree to which it is secure for users. Research from the European Union suggests that in general the public are worried about data security. This also underlines the need for good training, awareness raising, and support activities, in line with the needs of older people and persons with disabilities, so they can not only use the system but can protect themselves. Training the trainers in informal, local, social and family networks, as well as local service providers, will be critical in supporting the introduction of AAL. Some good practice examples of ICT programmes exist already that take into consideration the ethical aspects of ICT usage with older people e.g. assessing risk, using ICT with people with dementia, informed consent [12]. Furthermore the standards of safety in and support for technical appliances is important, especially where systems fail. Who pays for failure or inadequacies in installation, system operations and maintenance? These issues are often not made clear to older persons relying on these technologies and indeed the legal implications, such as the liability of the manufacturer, is still not clear at the European level.

Specifically in AAL, privacy represents a quite different issue relating to security: for example, the idea that AAL can be used to constantly monitor people in their own home has some problems. Thus sensors to detect falls or a lack of movement may be more acceptable than more intrusive built in monitoring cameras. It requires the full consent of the persons concerned and certainly requires that when monitored persons want to have some privacy they are able to switch off the system. While this sounds easy, too often the mentally frail or forgetful may not be able to make sensible decisions about when to switch the technology on or off. This clearly indicates to the health care system that when people no longer have the capacity to wisely operate the electronic system, they should no longer rely on it, but employ other methods.

A further ethical issue that needs to be addressed and respected – whether at the research stage or in the use of AAL technologies – is that of informed consent. This is particularly tricky where the older person has mild dementia or is frightened of giving consent as they are unsure what this means.

AAL manufacturers and designers in isolation cannot overcome these main issues and known problems. Indeed, e-accessibility and the take up of the new AAL technologies will depend on their public acceptance amongst a non-technologically sophisticated set of users. This underlines the importance of ensuring the incorporation from the beginning of their inception and design of potential users and older people, something that will also help avoid costly future adaptations. One should also bear in mind that it is the right of all citizens to benefit from the new technologies, given that these initiatives are mostly financed from public funds.

2. Uses of ICT

The potentialities and already growing adoption of ICT are of huge potential benefit to all older people – in particular, the frail and more housebound. If we examine some of these, we can also learn how AAL technologies may need to integrate with these proven and valued existing technologies.

2.1. Access to and Use of Services

A wide gamma of private services e.g. banking, shopping, uses ICT. Additionally, many public services and increasingly voting systems are becoming geared to ICT users. The benefits for people living in remote areas or people with major mobility or health problems can be huge; but we can recognize that this trend creates considerable exclusion as systems are too rarely designed for all. Thus, solutions providing different options and choice and accessible to all users, should be encouraged and developed and mainstreamed – e.g. accessible cash machines, accessible ticket machines, accessible e-Banking systems, accessible voting systems.

2.2. Housing

ICT can help people to manage their energy usage, given that it is increasingly expensive and that global warming and energy resources have to be tackled. This is an issue for older people who tend to live in less modern houses and, especially amongst the frail, who have a need for more heating than the general population. In addition there are many ICT linked solutions that can make homes and the people in them safer – e.g. warning systems for cookers, automatic taps, or automatic lights. A major issue is how to make the current housing stock adapted to elderly needs in a useable, user-friendly and affordable manner.

2.3. Health

ICT Tools are well under development that can help avoid overmedication and can provide health professionals with immediate support in such fields as monitoring in the older person's home. They are already used in monitoring some diseases – e.g. cardio-vascular problems – and in improving record-keeping and feedback. This will provide a new and more expansive meaning to the term 'Outpatients and home care'.

ICT can help people suffering from Alzheimer's and other dementia diseases – one of the great scourges of our time and for the ageing population – bridging the gap between the home and care centres [2,5,18]. In this area, ICT provides good opportunities to relieve the heavy burden put on carers, giving them the possibility of communicating with the world outside the care setting. An important finding from the Eurofamcare research on family carers was the need they had for information, more effective ways of communicating with services, and finding social support [17]. The need for support related not only to their socio-demographic status (including age and gender) but also to their living arrangements, obligations and relationships in their families, and whether they were still in the labour market. Another phenomenon that impacts strongly on the use of ICT both for the older person and the family carer is proximity.

2.4. Social Inclusion

The alleviation of social isolation through ICT can be of real importance to the frail elderly. However in stressing this positive side and the role that it can play in boosting the capacity for independence, community living and self help, those providing ICT and AAL technologies should recognize that they are complementary and cannot replace human contact. Direct contact with a real person is essential otherwise the isolation of the elderly will increase and this has implications for the continuing need for a growing workforce in certain sectors like social and healthcare services.

Social network maintenance is an important potential tool for the frail and less mobile who through ICT can maintain the link between the generations, especially in our mobile societies. The constant growth in the numbers of older people living alone has a particular impact on the demand for new methods of social inclusion. One should also note that a disproportionate percentage of the older population are women, who tend to have had less education. Currently amongst those living alone in the European Union at aged 75+ more than 70% are women [11].

Another matter of considerable interest is the capacity that some ICT technologies have to allow some older people of working age to remain in the labour force. These can include telework facilities for themselves or health and social monitoring facilities for older dependents, better designed ICT tools that help compensate age related impairments, on-line help tailored to older workers, support to mobility, etc.

3. Ensuring Success for Users in AAL

The introduction of AAL technologies has begun with different degrees of success. Some of the guidelines that need to be taken into consideration have been indicated earlier in the chapter, but we can also postulate some of the other factors that can help make the technologies acceptable – some of these having been clearly set out by Age Platform Europe and the European Expert group[5].

3.1. Involve Users

Too often older people are designated as users of a technology or beneficiaries of a policy over which they have had no control nor has their opinion been solicited. It is clear that for AAL to be accepted users need to be involved in their design from the start. This sounds easy but there are specific difficulties. Firstly users are heterogeneous – and in the specific case of AAL they may well be people with special needs and difficulties whether these be frailty, a lack of mobility or mental problems such as dementia. In asking for opinions from users it is important that these more marginalized groups and, where appropriate their informal and formal carers be called on to discuss their needs and problems. Another problem lies in the variability of even frail and dependent users in terms of their ages (50–115 covers a lot of variability in life experiences and physical conditions) and educational levels, (from the almost illiterate and least educated, to the most educated and experienced) or even their

[5] See www.age-platform.eu; specifically joint responses by AGE-ANEC-EDF Answer to the Survey on E-inclusion Policy, April 2009, http://www.age-platform.eu/en/age-policy-work/accessibility/age-position-statements/540-age-joint-survey-on-european-e-inlcusion-policy.

previous experiences with ICT. Finally there is the issue of a more democratic approach to participation [3] since improving people's quality of life involves them making active, considered reflection on their current and future needs and experiences; their preferences need to be incorporated into current innovations and policy development and this in turn will change the social realities facing the different and coming generations of older people.

AAL is of interest to many disabled users and in this, as in other spheres, user needs are highly specific. The ageing of both the disabled population and later age onset of disabilities amongst the older population represent quite different user situations and this must be taken into consideration by AAL designers. The nature of the technology proposed will determine the type of user research and involvement that is needed and appropriate. It is also clear that one should try to ensure that user groups are in some way representative – though this depends on the objectives of the research and the nature of the proposed technology. This is not always easy e.g. recruitment; enabling people to use their own voice; engaging in a long-term creative dialogue with users and listening hard to what they are saying. From the perspective of AAL designers, genuine user involvement presupposes active participation at all research phases, from early on in the framing research questions, to disseminating results and being a part of a potential follow-up of the project. Of course there is no moral imperative to involve users, but it is highly likely that the technology will remain unused, fail or have a limited impact without such involvement, and this is bad for business[6]. Indeed it can be argued that under the right stimulus users can come up with new ideas and substantive involvement, but it does suppose that the professionals are truly interested and respectful of the user group. As yet one sees few signs of this e.g. in the funding institutions as well as the technical partners.

3.2. Motivate Potential Users

Fears – of failing, looking stupid, or "hurting" the equipment or technology – are common amongst older users. This lack of self-confidence in the ability to understand and handle the technology is addressed by many programmes designed for older users. It is important to note that it is preferable for older people to become confident in their use of ICT technologies, before they have to use assistive technologies. One of the hardest challenges is to convince people to try radical new technologies for the first time. Effective intermediaries seem to be people connected with the target community – for example, groups of older people being coached by retired ex-employees of technology. It is also effective to use existing networks attended or supported by older people e.g. older people's clubs and training or educational centres; more older people are enticed into learning and using ICT technologies by "word-of-mouth" through the club network. Motivation is more likely to come from contacts with extended families, with social groups and relevant health information. Family contacts (particularly children and grandchildren) have been found to be good intermediaries. One should also note that teaching older people is best done informally via both practical and personal face-to-face instruction i.e. learning by doing, though ensuring that where people are taught in groups they mix with those of similar skill or interest levels. Informal learning is also important for updating and upgrading skills. There is still a

[6] The inability of NGOs of older people or the disabled to participate in the AAL programmes because of the rules of funding and own contributions has not helped promote the issue of user involvement.

long way to go before the majority of older people are able to use the Internet and computers to the degree of comfort that will make them happy to use AAL.

Aspects rarely considered when designing technologies for users concern firstly their attractiveness: elderly ladies in the UK increasingly buy or decorate with flowers any walking stick that they need. This is an important – if traditional – type of assistive technology, but it took a long time until people realized that a lot of potential users were older people who liked to look smart. Alarm pendants and bracelets in dull grey colours are unlikely to be acceptable to many users and there is no reason why they cannot be made pretty and not just clinically functional. People do not change tastes just because they are more fragile. Additionally there is an emotional barrier for many older people – a pride, in not wanting to accept that they now need aids of any kind. Thus, disguising or mainstreaming them so they can be seen as normal or nice is an important way forward. A slightly different aspect is ensuring that design professionals and industry try as far as possible to use the principles of 'Design for all'.

Where alternative formats are needed for specific disablements then there is a strong case to be made for the European Union ensuring, through a copyright exception in the Single Market Directive, that the legal cross-border exchange of copyright-protected content is possible for non-profit purposes and at no extra cost.

Another aspect that does not motivate older people to use AAL technologies is that they may be too expensive or considered a 'luxury', something that no-one else can use after their death. Thus consideration of the varying use and the absolute costs of using the technologies have to be clear.

Ensuring that the AAL technology represents a genuine positive gain in their lives is essential for motivating the older person and their families to adopt it. Non-joined up technologies have the risk of easily being abandoned whereas an "add on" piece of technology – e.g. using existing technologies such as phones and TVs, and the Internet – has the capacity to enable the more frail and housebound to use the AAL for wider purposes than care. Thus they can order groceries, clothes etc., delivered to their homes – vital for people who are no longer able to do their own shopping. While independence may gradually decline, it is difficult for older people to acknowledge this: if they use the technology for pre-existing social reasons, then the additional recognition that it can serve care and support needs will make it more acceptable. Recognising that the technology may offer the least restrictive way of continuing an independent life may also be a factor in AAL's acceptance. If they have positively accepted a new device, they are likely to be more effective users.

Interoperability is critical, where applications are able to 'talk' to each other and that can operate when people travel, work, visit friends etc. in a seamless chain – i.e. without ruptures in service provision in case of failure of the system, or the internet not working, etc.

3.3. Ensure that Equipment Is Easy to Use

One of the major areas where AAL is seen as having a large potential value is in health applications. Where the health of an older person needs to be monitored by regular measurements (e.g. blood pressure, sugar level, cardio vascular functioning), electronic equipment that measures and sends the data to a medical office and allows videoconferencing with professionals about these outcomes and further treatment and care, there is a potential gain for all participants. However, this will necessarily require that the equipment is simple to use. Older people with chronic or acute health conditions may be stressed when they are alone and worried about their health; at such moments they may find it difficult to follow complex instructions or procedures.

Another simple innovation that may help AAL users will be the further development of voice activated solutions, since many older people have poor written word and typing skills. Other solutions such as Skype will be useful in that they allow people to see one another and talk more personally – something of particular interest to grandparents who like to see, as well as talk to, their grandchildren.

3.4. AAL Is Only Part of the Solution for the Frail

No AAL designer should imagine that any specific technology will solve the complex needs of older people. Independent living and social inclusion require not only keeping older people in good health and mobile but also reducing social isolation. Thus the risks arising from the physical environment of the house and local community have to be dealt with – frailty is all too often the result of falls in old age. Chronic illness or handicap cannot simply and exclusively be dealt with through new technologies nor can the common problem of dementia. All situations have to be analysed in terms of their risk and problems for the older frail person and how it can most effectively be prevented. ICT can play a role, but often there will be other and simpler solutions to be tried first. In other cases ICT alone will not suffice.

There are quite a few situations in which risks can be caused by more than one condition, indeed they probably are the majority of cases, and thus AAL has to be flexible enough to recognize these complexities. As already indicated, when people are frail or with chronic illnesses they also need personal contacts. Technology is supposed to help and assist patients and professionals but it can never replace family, friends, neighbours as well as health and social care workers who are all vital and central in the delivery of care and support.

4. Conclusions

Each year more people become more familiar with digital technologies and this will almost certainly help in the later acceptance of new high technology systems such as AAL. Each year the varied forms of assistive technologies become more diverse, easier to use and often more integrated with existing familiar technologies.[7] Yet there is a considerable danger, as outlined in this chapter, of many older people remaining excluded from the world of AAL and the potentialities it offers for a better quality of life in terms of social integration, participation, service access, health maintenance and well being.

The barriers to the use of these new technologies, discussed briefly, are not insurmountable. For them and for all with chronic conditions any ICT or AAL technology has to be made as easy as possible, fitting into their lives and homes. The only way in which this can be guaranteed is by ensuring that older people have a voice and choice in the development of these technologies. Despite mention or rather lip-service being made to the need for democratic participation and the human rights of

[7] The various new types of smart phones that incorporate many useful applications combined with high quality user interfaces can for instance provide solutions such as reminders and nutrition tips in a single mobile device.

older people, it is still common to find developers and policy makers keen on retaining their own perspectives. However the non adoption or abandonment of AAL technologies is an expensive and unhappy choice for all. There must be a reconciliation between the different interests and a recognition of the importance of including a growing section of the population who can benefit from these interesting innovations in technology that could aid their well being, their social inclusion, their care and comfort.

Particular attention needs to be given to those frail older people needing care and support from others who are socially and economically excluded; it is important that these needs and problems are not compounded by technological exclusion. There need to be general and targeted European efforts to overcome these e.g. European Year 2010 against poverty and social exclusion or EY 2012 on active ageing and intergenerational solidarity. Technologies represent an additional resource to meet the growing needs and demands for care and support for older people, especially the oldest and most frail, but they are and can only ever be a part of the solution.

Acknowledgements

Thanks to Nena Georgantzi and Ilenia Gheno, research project coordinators at AGE Platform Europe for their support, advice and encouragement: to Marja Pijl who inspired some of the approach taken in this article.

And to those friends who provide technical support for using a manuscript and an editing system that was not end user friendly. This leads to the important question as to whether the person paying the cost of the technology is the end user e.g. the publisher, or the real end user e.g. the writer, editor.

Reference

[1] AGE Platform Europe, Older People and Information and Communication Technologies: An Ethical Approach, http://www.age-platform.eu/images/stories/EN/pdf_AGE-ethic_A4-final.pdf.

[2] J.C. Augusto, S. Martin, M.D. Mulvenna, W. Carswell and H. Zheng, Holistic night-time care, in: *Proceedings of the 7th World Conference of the International Society for Gerontechnology, May 27–30, 2010, Vancouver, Canada.*

[3] P. Beresford, User involvement in research: Connecting lives, experience and theory, 2003, http://www.feantsa.org/files/Participation/Good%20Practice%20Compendium/User%20Involvement%20in%20Research.doc.

[4] A.P. Bowling, R.J. Edelmann, J. Leaver and T. Hoekel, Loneliness, mobility, well-being and social support in a sample of over 85 year olds, *Personality and Individual Differences* **10**(11) (1989), 1189–1192.

[5] W. Carswell, P.J. McCullagh, J.C. Augusto, S. Martin, M.D. Mulvenna, H. Zheng, H.Y. Wang, J.G. Wallace, K. McSorley, B. Taylor and W.P. Jeffers, A review of the role of assistive technology for people with dementia in the hours of darkness, *Technology and Health Care* **17**(4) (2009), 281–304. IOS Press.

[6] C.W.Y. Chiu and D.W.K. Man, The effect of training older adults with stroke to use home-based assistive devices, *OTJR, Occupation, Participation and Health* **24**(3) (2004), 113–120.

[7] Commission Staff Working document, accompanying document to the communication from the Commission to the European Parliament, the council, the European Economic and Social Committee and the Committee of the Regions, Ageing Well in the Information Society, SEC (2007) 811, Brussels, 14 June 2007.

[8] Digital Agenda for Europe, http://ec.europa.eu/europe2020/pdf/digital-agenda-communica-tion-en.pdf, May 2010.

[9] Eurobarometer, "E-Communications Household Survey", http://ec.europa.eu/information_society/policy/ecomm/doc/library/ext_studies/household_10/report_en.pdf.

[10] European Commission, Digital Literacy European Commission Working Paper and Recommendations from Digital Literacy High-Level Expert Group, 2008.
[11] http://ec.europa.eu/health/major_chronic_diseases/diseases/ageing_related_diseases/index_en.htm.
[12] http://ec.europa.eu/information_society/activities/einclusion/library/studies/docs/ageing_ict_good_1.pdf.
[13] http://ec.europa.eu/information_society/eeurope/i2010/docs/digital_literacy/digital_literacy_review.pdf.
[14] http://europa.eu/rapid/pressReleasesAction.do?reference=IP/10/1328&format=HTML&aged=0&language=EN&guiLanguage=en.
[15] http://www.dreaming-project.org/pilot_sites.html.
[16] http://www.health.gov.au/internet/main/publishing.nsf/Content/0D4884B9C73FBDD9CA25782B000030B7/$File/AssistiveTechnologyReport.pdf.
[17] G. Lamura, E. Mnich, M. Nolan, B. Wojszel, B. Krevers, L. Mestheneos and H. Döhner, Family carers' experiences using support services in Europe: Empirical evidence from the EUROFAMCARE study, *The Gerontologist* **48**(6) (2008), 752–771.
[18] P.J. McCullagh, W. Carswell, M.D. Mulvenna, J.C. Augusto, H. Zheng and W.P. Jeffers, Nocturnal sensing and intervention for assisted living of people with dementia, in: *Healthcare Sensor Networks – Challenges Towards Practical Application*, D. Lai, R. Begg and M. Palaniswami, eds, Taylor and Francis/CRC Press, 2010.
[19] L.C. Mullins and N. McNicholas, Loneliness among the elderly: Issues and considerations for professionals in aging, *Gerontology & Geriatrics 25 Education* 7(1) (1987), 55–66.
[20] A.-S. Parent and N. Georgantzi, Ensuring a fruitful future to innovation and research, 2010, http://www.age-platform.eu/images/stories/Paper_Confidence2010_AGE_FINAL.pdf.
[21] M. Roelands, P. Van Oost, A. Depoorter and A. Buysse, A social-cognitive model to predict the use of assistive technologies for mobility and self-care in elderly people, *The Gerontologist* **42**(1) (2002), 39–50.

Handbook of Ambient Assisted Living
J.C. Augusto et al. (Eds.)
IOS Press, 2012

doi:10.3233/978-1-60750-837-3-763

Beyond System Integration: Who, What, How, and When

Lenka LHOTSKÁ[a,*], Jaromír DOLEŽAL[a,b], Václav CHUDÁČEK[a], Michal HUPTYCH[a], Miroslav BURŠA[a] and Jan HAVLÍK[b]
[a] *Department of Cybernetics, Czech Technical University in Prague, Czech Republic*
[b] *Department of Circuit Theory, Czech Technical University in Prague, Czech Republic*

Abstract. The objective of AAL and home care is a better care for frail individuals (elderly chronic and disabled patients) in a home care setting. In principle it means to allow the citizens to stay at home as long as possible, delaying the institutionalization of people, possibly avoiding it for a high percentage of them. Recent development in ICT shows that it is almost impossible to design and implement an AAL system as fixed to certain hardware, operating system, and infrastructure. Thus it is necessary to develop such architectures that will be easily extensible and modifiable. We will discuss such approaches in the chapter. We will also analyze the social, legal and ethical issues connected with the technology issues.

Keywords. System integration, multi-agent system, user interface, usability laboratory, ethics, data privacy

Introduction

The objective of ambient assisted living (AAL) and home care is a better care for frail individuals (elderly chronic and disabled patients) in a home care setting. To improve this kind of care means to allow the citizens to stay at home as long as possible, delaying the institutionalization of people, possibly avoiding it for a high percentage of them. Institutionalized elderly citizens are at high risk of cognitive impairment, functional loss, social isolation, or death.

Integrating information deriving from different sources and implementing it with knowledge discovery techniques allows medical and social actions to be appropriately performed with reliable information, in order to improve quality of life of patients and care-givers. To stay at home means to keep independency, self-sufficiency, social network role.

Currently the mobile technologies, sensors and other devices enable collecting vast amount of data of individuals. This multi-parametric data may include physiological measurements, genetic data, medical images, laboratory examinations, and other measurements related to a person's activity, lifestyle and surrounding environment. There will be increased demand on processing and interpreting such data for accurate alerting and signalling of risks and for supporting healthcare professionals in their decision making, informing family members, and the person himself/herself.

---

[*]Corresponding Author: Lenka Lhotská, Department of Cybernetics, Faculty of Electrical Engineering, Czech Technical University in Prague, Technická 2, 166 27 Prague 6, Czech Republic. E-mail: lhotska@fel.cvut.cz.

Recent development in ICT shows that it is almost impossible to design and implement an AAL system as fixed to certain hardware, operating system, and infrastructure. Thus it is necessary to develop such architectures that will be easily extensible and modifiable. We will discuss such approaches in the chapter. They are mostly based on multi-agent architectures. Another important issue is data storage. The database system must be also designed in such a way that it allows storing new type of data when such need appears.

There are many questions linked with data collecting, storing, processing, access, and use. For example: Should all measured data be stored or only aggregated information? How long should the data be stored? Should the data be stored locally or in a central data storage? How long should be the data stored if no alarm or unusual situation occurs? Who has the right to access and use the data or part of it? We will try to answer these questions and also analyze the legal and ethical issues connected with them. The major ethical issues arise about the handling of sensitive data about health and data about everyday activity patterns.

1. Technology

1.1. Example of a Real-Life Scenario

Mike is a pensioner in his 80ies. He is living alone in his appartment. He suffers from a milder form of dementia, but he is able to care for himself to a certain degree. He has no serious motoric problems, he can go for shopping, cook, and perform other standard daily activities. However, he forgets from time to time to take his medicaments, to switch off the lights, to lock the door, close a window or turn off the water tap. Other family members do not share the appartment with him. They live not far from him.

In current circumstances he has reminders in form of post-fix sheets distributed in the rooms and at the appartment door. His children phone him regularly and check whether everything is going well.

Now let us transfer in (near) future. Mike is getting ready for his regular shopping. After having breakfast he is collecting the shopping bag, purse, shopping list, mobile phone and wants to leave. The PIR-based (Passive InfraRed) motion detectors placed in rooms and corridor identify his movement towards the appartment door. At the same time the sensors placed on the window in the bedroom signal that the window is open. His medicament box signals that the section for this morning is not empty. Nice voice from a small (almost invisible) loudspeaker reminds him gently to shut the window in the bedroom and to take his morning pill. He thanks and returns to do it. After shutting the window and taking the pill he goes for shopping. He shuts the door but he forgets to lock it. Before he moves towards the lift his mobile phone starts to beep. He takes it out of his pocket and reads the message: Please lock the door. After locking the door he finally goes for shopping.

This is not a science fiction story but an almost real scenario that can be realized even with current technology. The technology allows us to detect many situations and states especially in closed areas, such as houses, appartments, etc. where we can place fixed sensors and cameras. Another issue is how reliably we can evaluate the data collected from the sensors. The simplest situation is if there is only one person present. In case we have to distinguish two or more persons, their movements, other activities, we arrive at a more challenging task. Then we have to start detailed analysis of the data arriving from different types of sensors. Let us compare two types of sensors from the opposite ends of the scale: simple PIR-based motion detectors (PID) and cameras.

From PIDs we are able to detect motion, at best its direction. However it is difficult to distinguish if there is only one person moving or two very closely to each other. Moreover to distinguish two persons from the data sent from PIDs is almost impossible if their walking speed is similar.

Camera allows more detailed analysis of individuals. We can even use face recognition so that we are able to distinguish different persons in the room. There exist already software tools that can distinguish males and females with high success rate. Then many medical purposes can be found, for example detection of problems with walking, tendency to falls, behavioural patterns, temporal development (and comparison with previous states) leading to more precise evaluation of the health state (supported by measurement and evaluation of physiological values).

1.2. Existing Projects and Activities

With the development of technology in last two decades many projects have been developed in the area of assistive technologies, ambient assisted living, tele-care, and related fields. For example, in [17] there are listed more than 100 research and development projects or services relevant to these areas ongoing in the United Kingdom and Europe. They receive funding from different resources, as European Commission Framework Programmes 6 and 7, Ambient Assisted Living Joint Programme, companies, and national funding schemes.

Just for demonstration of growing number of publications on assistive technologies and ambient assisted living we did search in indexed databases using 360Search metasearch engine available at the Czech Technical University in Prague (http://knihovny.cvut.cz/information-resources/e-databases/). First using the keywords "assistive" and "technology" the engine returned 209 publications. Out of this number 157 were published in 2008 – February 2011. The oldest article was published in 1994. Using "ambient" and "assistive" and "living" we got 181 publications. Out of them 149 were published in 2009 – February 2011. The oldest paper was published in 2000. That shows immense growth of interest and applications in both areas.

During last five years many conferences and workshops focused on assistive technologies and ambient assisted living have been organized, e.g. AAL-Forum, ICOST (International Conference on Smart Homes and Health Telematics). In addition, other conferences ranging from information and communication technologies over sensor technology to biomedical engineering have had assistive technologies and ambient assisted living among the main topics and organized special sessions.

The variety of topics of the projects [17] and publications is quite large and covers many different problems of applications of assistive technologies for people with special needs. More and more they are focused on supporting elderly people afflicted by Alzheimer disease and related dementias. The reason is quite simple: people are living longer and therefore more people are experiencing cognitive problems, in particular dementia. The estimation is that approximately 28 million persons worldwide suffer from dementia and direct care costs are in order of hundreds of billions of dollars annually. The motivation of all these projects is very similar: to design and develop technologies that enable people with dementia to remain in their own home. There is also a certain shift from monitoring only daily activities to assistance over night [3,5,16]. There is also another shift in the projects observable – technology is used not only for monitoring but also as support of various therapies [4,5]. Therapies include the provision of mental tasks to stimulate the brain and maintain activity levels, the delivery of music and familiar pictures for memory training, and the use of light therapy to enhance wellbeing.

Recently there have been initiated projects in many EU countries that do not focus only on medical or health care aspects of AAL, but also on additional functions and services the systems may offer to their clients. Let us demonstrate the scope of possible functions on the HomeBrain – TV Computer project although the list of functions may not be completely exhaustive. HomeBrain – TV Computer is a new project initiated by a Czech company High Tech Park in cooperation with several other companies (http://www.htpark.eu/en/solutions/r1-project3b-homebrain/). The main idea is to integrate many different functions and unify the control interface. Actually the user inteface is the core of the project. A TV computer serves as the user interface and can be easily controlled in the same way as a standard TV set. It fulfils several main functions, namely gate to the internet, multimedia services, senior monitoring, health state monitoring, social networking of HomeBrain users, remote control of home devices, intelligent security system. Additionally, it can be connected to telebanking, e-services (including e-government), and other electronic services. HomeBrain is an example of an integration platform that provides the user with a relatively simple interface. It can be easily extended by newly developed modules. This feature also means that the configuration can be designed on demand based on the user requirements because not everybody wants to have complete set of all possible functions and installed devices.

The designers have defined several basic requirements on the HomeBrain. It must be small, having the size of a common TV set-top box and being easily controllable without any need to study a long and complex manual. The HomeBrain device installation is simple – it only needs to be connected to the TV set and internet. Microsoft environment is used for development of applications and interconnection with other technologies.

Let us focus now on the typical functionalities of the HomeBrain system. In addition to classic TV programs it is possible to watch programs on Internet TV. Search for selected music can be easier – no need to try to find a particular CD or DVD in boxes or stands. Music can be downloaded from the internet (using legal way), or from a storage on the hard disk and stored in the catalogue. Movies can be lend in a virtual rental store. Browsing digital photographs, creating albums and sharing them with friends is another pre-defined function.

If the user wants to control home appliances remotely on the TV, phone, or via internet the system is easily extensible. The only condition is that the home appliances have the option of remote control. Another possible function is intelligent security. The user interface is interconnected with the installed security system and allows intelligent evaluation.

Eshop is another option. It can be comfortable for elderly people, for people with motoric disabilities or even for ill people. There is a special service that uses bar code reader. Thus regularly bought food can be easily ordered again. The information is sent from the reader to the HomeBrain and then the list of required items is sent to the particular eshop. Of course, necessary condition is existence of such a shop in relatively close distance so that the delivery costs do not exceed certain reasonable level.

Health state monitoring is becoming more and more important area of AAL applications. Heart-attacks, diabetes, increased cholesterol are typical manifestations of unhealthy lifestyle at present time. Timely anticipation of such state can save lives.

Another group is represented by chronically ill persons who must be regularly checked (or even monitored over longer time span). There have been developed many different applications using various sensors and devices for measurement of physiological values. The HomeBrain has an interface for data transfer from such sensors or devices. The user can decide whether the health state information is only stored locally or also sent to his/her family doctor. The system also offers a similar function to Skype, namely remote contact with other family members or friends living in distant places. There are more functions ready, i.e. calendar, e-mail, video calls, sms messaging, telebanking, e-services (e.g. contact with local authorities), monitoring elderly family members remotely, internet browsing, games.

Functions that depend on external services can be active only if the services are available at the given location. This concerns, for example, delivery of food ordered in the eshop, electronic contact to local authorities. Introduction into routine operation is conditioned by satisfaction of several basic requirements, namely commitment by health and social care providers, concerted action between all stakeholders, and last but not least reasonable prices of paid services, including Internet connection.

1.3. Technological Trends

The technological development in recent decades has shown us that almost everything we considered some years ago as pure science fiction is possible.

In the AAL roadmap [1] there are the main technological trends listed and analyzed. Let us mention them briefly: availability of the Internet in devices (Internet of Things); RFID (Radio-Frequency Identification) capable devices; concepts of context awareness; integration of services; increasing networking capacity (enabling multimedia communication); broadband communication; robotics (especially autonomous mobile robots); advanced software systems (recognition of user states, ability to adapt to and learn from user behaviour and state); integration of entertainment devices; easy authentication systems; advanced security and privacy measures; communication capabilities in home artefacts; advanced sensor technology for as unobtrusive and non-invasive measurement of physiological parameters as possible.

We can see from this list that finding solutions in each separate area is probably an issue of near future. The key issue will be their integration in larger systems collecting and processing large volumes of data, evaluating more complex situations and scenarios, precise identification of potentially dangerous situations and finding solutions (e.g. alarms in case of health or life threatening events, access blocking in case of security attack).

Although many issues have been successfully solved and introduced either in applied research or in development of prototypes or final products there are still many problems on the waiting list.

Nowadays we can measure relatively unobtrusively many physiological parameters on a human body: electrocardiogram (ECG), heart rate, breathing rate, body temperature, blood pressure, energy output, etc. However not everything can be measured contactless. Still we need to fix electrodes on the skin or use at least sensors integrated in underware. However the task of data processing and especially evaluation and interpretation remains still challenging. We have to realize that the persons perform their daily activities in standard environment and not in a noise free laboratory. That means the data contain noise and artefacts, both from the body itself (movements, worse contact of sensors to body) and environment. Thus the task of noise and artefact removal is not yet fully solved and remains open for the future research and development.

Once we have clean signals and data the processing is rather straightforward. Naturally there must be clear specification of processing outputs. Based on our practical experience we can say that it is very important to develop this specification in close collaboration with medical doctors, psychologists, rehabilitation nurses, physiotherapeutists, etc. (all potential participants in health care, home care and well being activities). Only then we can design and develop useful and suitable applications with interpretable results. There have been developed many different methods in the area of biological signal processing, feature extraction and selection, data mining and knowledge discovery. But many times we came across the problem of not full understanding of input data by people who should perform the data processing. They only took the input data as large data sets without prior knowledge of their semantic content. We regard this as a serious fault. In addition to technological development it is necessary to keep this fact in mind all the time: We have to know what the meaning of input data is, what the meaning of extracted features is and finally what the meaning of the results is.

Concerning sensor technology (again in combination with data evaluation) there are other open issues. One such example is adequate nourishment and its control. Till now there is no simple way how to measure proper nourishment and hydration of people, especially in their home environment. If they share household with somebody who is aware of this problem the situation has a solution. But in case they live alone the problem may lead even to life threatening health state. There are no simple sensors that could measure the corresponding quantities. For medical use there are devices for analysis of body composition. They measure body impedance and based on that calculate content of body fat mass, fat free mass and also the amount of body water in intracellular and extracellular fluids in different body parts. But even in hospitals this device is not used for evaluation of hydration of elderly patients. The main use is in the treatment of obese patients or patients with metabolic disorders. Even more complex problem is proper composition of food and regular food intake. This problem becomes more serious for people with cognitive disorders who are not able to recognize vital consequences. These types of problems have also their social and ethical dimensions that will be discussed later in this chapter.

Using different combinations of sensors in the environment (e.g. cameras, PIR based motion detectors, detectors of open/closed windows and doors, sensors detecting switched on/off electric appliances) we can get rather detailed description of the environment. However, when we add persons to this environment the task becomes more complex. We have to find solution of the following items:

- Identification of individuals (possibly without any RFID or similar devices attached to each one) based on their behavioural patterns, faces, walking;
- Recognition of emotional states;
- Better identification and interpretation of health state (here additional data can be acquired from a body sensor network);
- Identification of a potential intruder (many elderly people are too gullible and let a stranger come in their homes).

Vitally important prerequisite for the deplyment of all these advanced technologies is broadband access and the ability of providers to enable full connectivity not only in cities, but also in rural or sparsely populated areas.

1.4. Software Solutions

The domain of AAL is inherently distributed both geographically and functionally. Thus in the software architecture design it can lead to application of multi-agent approach. The multi-agent technology has been recently considered to be much more suitable for creating open, flexible environment able to integrate software pieces of diverse nature written in different languages and running on different types of computers [15]. It enables to design, develop and implement a comparatively open multi-agent environment suitable for efficient creating of complex knowledge-based or decision support systems. Such an environment is able to integrate geographically distributed knowledge sources or problem solving units. The task under consideration is located just on the borderline between Software Engineering and Artificial Intelligence. The idea of software integration based on efficient communication among parallel computational processes as well as that of the open architecture (enabling to add new elements without any change in the others) has been provided by the Software Engineering area. On the other hand, the multi-agent approach stemming from the theory of agency, from behavioral models of agents and methods of agentification of stand-alone programs can be considered as a contribution of Artificial Intelligence. Multi-agent systems have useful properties, such as parallelism, robustness, and scalability. Therefore they are applicable in many domains which cannot be handled by centralized systems, in particular, they are well suited for domains which require, for example, resolution of interest and goal conflicts, integration of multiple knowledge sources and other resources, time-bounded processing of very large data sets, or on-line interpretation of data arising in different geographical locations. A multi-agent system is a collection of independent, autonomous agents that communicate, cooperate and coordinate their activities with the aim to reach solution of a complex task. Heterogeneity of individual agents and integration of legacy systems are further basic characteristics that are advantageous for many applications [9]. An agent is usually defined as an autonomous software entity that receives inputs and interacts with its environment (including other agents), performing tasks in the pursuit of a set of goals.

Healthcare and AAL applications have some characteristics that make multiagent systems a particularly appropriate model:

- Knowledge is distributed in different locations.
- The provision of services involves the coordination of the effort of different individuals with different skills and functions.
- Finding standard software engineering solutions for health care problems is not straightforward. Interaction of different software applications is sometimes required.
- In the recent years, there has been a shift towards health care promotion, shared patient-provider decision-making and managed care. Shared decisions and actions need to be coordinated to make sure that the care is efficient and effective.
- There is an increased demand for information and online systems providing access to the medical knowledge available on the Internet.

Multi-agent approach allows designing flexible hierarchical architectures that can offer answers to questions asked in the Introduction to this chapter, namely those on the data storage. For data storage there can be smaller local storages and a central data storage used for different types of data. Since there can be collected health state data and daily activities patterns the large volumes of data can be stored locally and based on the data analysis during system development the professionals (e.g. medical doctors) can define, which type of data should be sent to a central data storage maintaining electronic health care records [2]. In case of medical data storage legal regulations define the rules for handling the data (how long they have to be stored, who can access the data, etc.). Other types of data, as daily activities patterns, alarms are not so strictly regulated. However, similar rules as to medical data can and should be applied in order to reduce the possibility of misuse. That means that the client or his/her legal representative specifies who has the right to access the collected data and aggregated information. Similar document as informed consent should be developed. The data access rights must be structured. The issue of time period over which the daily activities or alarm data should be stored depends on the particular setting. That includes client physical and mental state and its evaluation by a professional. If there are no deviations in the data over months then assuming the system is adaptable the oldest raw data can be forgotten using exponential forgetting and only aggregated information is stored. In case of identified trends in the collected data it is preferable to keep the data stored over longer time period. Then it can be used for more detailed analysis since the analysis may reveal, for example, worsening cognitive abilities not observable in direct frequent contact with the client.

Definitely, user interfaces must remain in focus of attention. As the technology offers more and more possibilities of utilization the user interfaces must be designed with respect to large variety of users and especially with respect to their physical and mental abilities/disabilities. Control of individual devices or their complexes (e.g. smart home) must be user friendly, simple, allowing different modes of control (e.g. via PC and keyboard, TV set with remote control, voice control). The software should be adaptable to the user and to be able to learn from previous interactions with the user. That is closely linked with the requirements mentioned above, namely identification of behavioural patterns of individuals.

There remain other open issues in the technology part. The most important ones include requirements on standardization of data formats (i.e. the ECG, electroencephalography, and other medical devices measuring biological signals generate proprietary data formats which are usually not publicly known thus it is impossible to integrate such devices into larger systems because the signals can be processed only by software delivered by the device producer), data transfer protocols; security and data privacy. Recently there have been published many papers analyzing these problems, comparing existing standards and recommending future standardization activities [18]. There are defined standards for wired and wireless communication between electronic devices [10–12].

Most of the past and current projects have been focused on the technological issues. However, once we want to develop systems that will be surrounding us almost everywhere we have to discuss and try to solve psychological, social, ethical and legal issues emerging from the ubiquitous technology.

1.5. Standardization and Interoperability

If we want to develop flexible AAL systems we have to define standard interface that allows "plug-and-play" type of connection. AAL systems are composed of different hardware and software modules that must communicate. The basic condition is that the receiver understands correctly the content of the message. Thus it is not sufficient to be able to receive the message, i.e. to understand the syntax of the message, but it is necessary to understand the semantics. This requirement implies development of a data model that maps semantic content from the data received from the devices into an information system that is usually used for collecting and evaluating data from monitored persons. Current information systems in health care use mostly HL7 communication standard (http://www.hl7.org). It is based on several relatively simple principles: creation of formats and protocols for exchange of data records between health care information systems; format standardization and connected interface unification; improvement of communication efficiency; guide for dialogue between involved parties at interface specification; minimization of different interfaces; minimization of expenses for interface implementation. It is important that HL7 does not impose any limitation on the architecture of individual systems, operating systems, or programming languages for the implementation.

There exist examples of solutions where the models and modeling tools have been developed for exchange of data between devices and information systems. One of the examples is the iCARDEA project (http://www.srdc.com.tr/icardea/), in which the inteface Medical Device Modeling Tool has been designed and developed. It transforms measured data both from proprietary formats and from standard formats into IEEE 11073 format [13]. In the next step the data types from IEEE 11073 DIM (Domain Information Model) are mapped to HL7 v2.5 data types. Further there can be used mapping onto HL7 CDA (Clinical Document Architecture), HL7 PHMR (Personal Monitoring Report), HL7 v3 Observation message used in description of clinical processes, USAM (Unified Service Action Model) in GLIF (GuideLine Interchange Format) for clinical decision support, or any format of message/document based on HL7 RIM (Reference Information Model).

Another example is presented in [14] where the scheme for data exchange between HL7 and IEEE 1451 standards is proposed. The designed system monitors remotely the patient state and transmits measured ECG, temperature, glucose content and possibly other data. The sensors send data streams to a personal digital assistant (PDA) or smart phone. On the PDA there are implemented following functions: receiving commands from the server and responses to them, data collection from the sensors, and sending data to the server. Monitoring centre has the greatest number of functions in the proposed architecture. The basic functions are connected with data input and successive processing and control of subordinate units. The monitoring centre receives sampled data and responses to commands. The main commands serve for control of client devices. For each patient the XML data files are created. These files are defined according to HL7 v2.5 standard. Each patient has assigned one XML file. There are recorded personal information, symptoms, patient history, current illness and necessary sampled data.

From the above mentioned examples it is obvious that the greatest problems and at the same time the greatest space for future solutions are in the area of correct mapping of acquired data onto a data model that describes electronic patient record. Especially with respect to future development and possibility to sense and store far more larger volumes of heterogeneous physiological parameters the issue of interoperability becomes more and more important. Interoperability may significantly influence effectivity both at design and development of an integrated system and at its routine operation.

For the future it seems to be most advantageous to create an extension of basic standards and technologies that allow easier satisfaction of the requirement on interoperability than above described examples, in which it was necessary to define mapping of data types for used standards and implement corresponding interfaces.

2. Psychological Issues

Each of us is a personality with unique experience, background knowledge, emotional and psychological setup, acceptance and perception of other humans and also technology. Thus we will find high variation in attitude towards high tech installations, especially in our homes. Frankly speaking, how many of us would be happy to be monitored by cameras and other devices 24 hours a day without knowing who has access to this data? It recalls "big brother" from Orwell's 1984. However, the continuous monitoring is a standard at intensive care units in hospitals. Moreover, surveillance by cameras is nowadays used in many public places, e.g. airports, train stations, in some cities in public transport. Usually we are not aware of it or simply we do not care or sometimes we know that the technology is there for enhancing our safety. On the other hand being at work and having elderly grandparents or parents at their homes and knowing they have certain health problems it would be good to check from time to time what they are doing and whether there is no problem without instant phoning them (they might get the feeling they are permanently supervised). However, we have to explain them why the technology should be installed in their home.

As we are so different, it is difficult to design a general system that is easily acceptable for everybody. Therefore a lot of research must be done in interaction with as large set of potential users as possible. These users must be selected from a large variety of population, i.e. city/village, healthy / motoric disabilities / visual impairment / hearing impairment / cognitive disorders – all on different levels, male / female, different age, different experience with technology (none/weak/medium/intensive). Some studies have been already performed and provided interesting results, e.g. [19,21,22]. So they can serve as inspiration for the future ones. The key issue is also proper design of the experiments – real life scenarios. In this respect, popularization and introduction of these topics into public awareness and possibility of visiting such model homes are options that can make this technology more familiar to broader public.

Now we can only estimate what the results of new studies could be. But based on the recent studies it is obvious that the main and most important issue is human technology interface. It seems that it definitely must be adaptable to user needs, behaviour and abilities and it must be evolvable in time. That means when the user needs and abilities change (usually they worsen – deterioration of cognitive and/or motoric abilities) the system has to recognize it and adapt the interface and functions accordingly.

The designer must obtain a thorough understanding of the users, their disabilities, their environments, and their problems. The greatest challenge for the designer is not solving the problem but understanding the problem. User evaluation is an essential tool for obtaining proper understanding. Technology developed for use by lay users must have such control or user interface that is easily accessible, usable and useful for its intended users. Therefore the user-centered design process must be used.

In the development phase it is highly advisable to use a tool known as the Virtual Usability Laboratory for software development (http://openvulab.org). Such a tool is designed to unobtrusively monitor users of web-based applications remotely. At the same time the tool allows querying users after their interaction with the application. After experiments when a large number of users have tested the application the usability data is collected and analyzed. This data contains, for example, browsing patterns, system invocations, user interactions. Similar approach is used in standard Usability Laboratory (http://ulab.cz) where tangible devices and tools are tested from all aspects of their design, i.e. functions, ease of use, ergonomy, safety, demands on cognitive and motoric abilities.

3. Social Issues

Humans are social beings. Mostly they do not live as lonely survivors of a shipwreck on a waste island. However, many elderly people spend most of their time isolated in their homes, especially in winter when the weather conditions hinder them to go out. Great challenge is to offer them socializing virtually, in an unobtrusive way. There are, for example, projects using a TV set and a webcam for dialogue of a home care client and a nurse in a call centre. So why not using this idea for interconnecting people who know each other and want stay in contact? They could communicate among themselves remotely when their state does not allow them physical presence in one place. In this way they can organize a sort of a teleconference quite easily. The important feature is that they stay in contact with other people.

Technically capable people having Internet connection may use social networking on the Internet. However, it is necessary to stress that there might be a potential danger of misuse of information exchanged in the group. The elderly people are usually more gullible and in this respect fragile. Although there are quite regular warnings in TV and radio broadcastings there are new cases of wilful deception of elderly people. There should be a reliable person who will supervise such network and identify possible intruders. For the beginning, the simplest measure is that the participation is by invitation only, possibly confirmed by several trustful participants.

4. Ethical Issues

The major ethical issues arise about the handling of sensitive data about health and data about daily activities. Explicit informed consent must be asked to the participants in order to include their sensitive data in the EHR or local storage, and to their data being shared, transmitted and analyzed by authorized personnel within the designed system.

All the procedures must conform to relevant EU legislation (in EU countries) and to national legislations related to the principle of respecting confidentiality. Since a proportion of clients are presumably affected by some degree of cognitive impairment, special precautions must be taken as regards such patients. The restrictive rules applied in case of Clinical Trials must be used (Directive 2001/20/Ec of the European Parliament and of the Council of 4 April 2001): "In the case of other persons incapable of giving their consent, such as persons with dementia … omissis … the written consent of the patient's legal representative, given in cooperation with the treating doctor, is necessary before participation in any such clinical trial. The notion of legal representative refers back to existing national law and consequently may include natural or legal persons, an authority and/or a body provided for by national law".

The necessity of inclusion of such patients into AAL systems derives from: 1) the high prevalence of cognitive impairment among elderly patients (up to 50% in 85+); 2) the high correlation among cognitive impairment, chronic diseases, and functional disability; 3) the need of providing structured intervention plans for cognitively impaired patients.

When designing an AAL system all subjects must participate voluntarily after being informed of the objectives and methodologies of the project. Explicit informed written consent will be asked for. Since some difference in respecting privacy could arise between different subjects, two different forms for informed consent/authorization should be used: 1) subjects who will authorize treatment of personal data; 2) physicians who consent to use their information and knowledge about patients who already agreed to participate. To be enrolled, both consents are needed.

All the researchers involved who take part in the analysis of non-anonymous data must be asked for an explicit declaration of respecting confidentiality.

Personal data must not be used for commercial purposes.

In the management of sensitive data it is necessary to define some levels of security [9]: *confidentiality* (i.e. ensure that only those that are properly authorised may access the information), *integrity* (i.e. ensure that information cannot be altered by insertion, deletion or replacement), *authentication* (i.e. ensure that a correct identification of the user has been done), and *non-repudiation* (i.e. prevent some of the parts to negate a previous commitment or action). In most cases it is required to assure both secure transmissions and secure storing/management of data and knowledge. In the first case, there are approaches based on public key infrastructures (PKI) that allow different participants to exchange sensitive data covering all the security levels described in the above paragraphs. From a technical point of view, several solutions are available such as SSL (secure socket layer) and PGP (pretty good privacy) that relies over electronic certificates emitted by an authority certification. In the second case, the computer platform can establish different permission levels to access the data by authorised entities (policies of users) which will require secret identification by a password system.

5. Sustainability

The term sustainability is mostly referred to the environmental issues. In this case we speak about economic, health and social sustainability [8]. As many projects have already shown the design and development of assistive technologies or AAL systems have been performing well during the project duration but it has been difficult to continue further development or even maintenance of already developed applications without financial resources after project end. The most difficult task is to find stakeholders that will invest in such projects. It is necessary to present to health and social care providers, health and social insurance companies that such systems can reduce the costs of care because they can reduce or even avoid hospital stay of the aforementioned persons.

A solution might be a network (or consortium) of partners playing different roles in AAL, namely researchers (in technology, health care, social care), developers, industry, economy, caregivers, and users. There have been developed several projects [20], in which the technology has been installed in real appartments inhabited by senior persons. At the beginning the projects were financed through grants. After this financing finished, the technology has been used further and the project partners have tried to continue as volunteers. Obviously that is not a standard solution.

There might be developed different financial models depending on the offerred services, involved users, care and service providers. Taking into account the fact that the users are not only the senior persons, but also the care givers (medical, social), the community, the region, the social and health insurance companies. AAL systems can save expenses either through postponed or avoided hospital or senior home stay. Before introducing and installing such systems in people's homes following questions should be answered:

- Should the appartment / house owners be responsible for the infrastructure?
- Should the tenant pay (and how much)?
- Does the investment in AAL system pay off for large construction companies?
- Who pays for the additional services?
- Are health and social care givers involved?
- Are insurance companies participating in the activity?

Recent publication [7] presents interesting facts that confirm necessity of these questions. It has been already quantified that costs to provide nursing home care for an individual are $77,745 a year. A primary care service (regular visits by nurses and doctors at person's home) costs $13,121. And by contrast, telehealth service based on remotely performing as many of the tasks as possible costs $1,600. When we add more functions the difference might be even greater. For introduction to routine use there is remaining one important issue, namely approval by relevant authorities if the system has the health care related functions (monitoring, therapeutical support, etc.). In such cases the legal regulations of the relevant country must be followed.

The fact that the issues discussed in this and previous sections are important is also confirmed by many documents published by the European Commission and other authorities. Although the Communication [6] is mainly focused on telemedicine there are many statements that hold for the areas of AT and AAL as well. To summarize briefly, the document points out the strategic sets of actions that must be performed, namely building confidence in and acceptance of corresponding services, bringing legal clarity, and solving technical issues and facilitating market development.

Especially legal clarity is a key issue. Its lack, in particular with regard to licencing, accreditation and registration of telemedicine, AT and AAL services and professionals, liability, reimbursement, jurisdiction, is a major challenge. When we add cross border provision of services legal clarification concerning privacy is also required.

When checking the legal regulations in EU Member States we find out that only a few states have clear legal frameworks concerning telemedicine, but only it. There is no word about AT or AAL. Many states require physical presence of the patient and the health professional in the same place for a medical act to be legally recognized. Moreover, there are often limitations in legal regulations or administrative practice on reimbursement of telecare services (both medical and social). Again there is no notion about AT and AAL.

6. Conclusions

In this chapter, we have tried to address some of the technological, psychological, social and ethical issues that must be solved in the future. The technological development in recent years has brought many innovative sensor systems, devices and tools that can be utilized in the area of AAL. However, system integration is not fully solved yet. We propose using a multiagent system paradigm that facilitates the communication and coordination among the different users following some organizational rules, even if they are in different physical places. So, it is especially suitable for distributed systems, either at the level of users location or at the level of information location. The security and privacy preserving issues must be properly solved in the implementations in AAL since they are working with personal and medical data. Standardizing activities both on the hardware and software side must continue with the aim to reach better interoperability and integration.

One of the contributions of this work has been identification of non-technical problems linked with introduction of technology allowing continuous monitoring of persons' health state and activities in their homes. We have shown that before starting implementation of such systems it is necessary to perform detailed acceptance study with successive evaluation. The aim is that the lay users (mostly elderly people or people with different impairments) will be willing to use the technology, will accept it and it will not cause them any problems. The designers and developers have to have in mind that the design must be user centered.

Activities in medical area are well reflected in ethical and legal documents. Thus the part of AAL handling data about persons' health state can be approached in the same way. However, the daily activities monitoring and other activities must be described appropriately with respect to ethical and legal frameworks valid in correspondding countries.

As the areas of research and development of assistive technologies and ambient assisted living are growing, the need for interdisciplinary education supporting this development and practical application is continuously growing. Currently there is a lack of graduates having interdisciplinary theoretical education in the fields of electronics and information and communication technologies and simultaneously focusing on the whole complex of practical needs of applications related to assistive technologies (AT) and AAL. The same situation arises at producers of these technologies. There are very few graduates able to understand and realize complex applications as a whole. Most of the graduates are able to manage separate narrow applications without ability to interconnect them. Therefore the research activities must be followed by similar development in higher education and courses that will fill the gap in the education have to be prepared. The situation in the given field may be characterized in following way: there are no graduates specialized in AT and AAL; there is no complex educational program in AT or AAL; there exist a number of information barriers between disciplines that may be solved exclusively by consistent interdisciplinary integration; there exists social and objective demand for employees in AT and AAL; in most EU countries there are relatively numerous small and medium-sized enterprises and institutions focused on AT and AAL that need graduates and support for life long learning of current employees. The main aim is increase of competence and qualification for the interdisciplinary area of AT and AAL. An important feature is consistent interdisciplinary orientation with the aim of optimum balance between theoretical and application content. Very significant element is focus on system integration which is not contained in current educational programs though being very important.

Acknowledgements

This research has been financed by the research program MSM 6840770012 of the CTU in Prague, Czech Republic.

References

[1] Ambient Assisted Living Roadmap, VDI/VDE-IT AALIANCE Office, G. van den Broek, F. Cavallo, L. Odetti and C. Wehrmann, eds, 2010.
[2] P. Aubrecht, K. Matoušek and L. Lhotská, On designing an EHCR repository, in: *HEALTHINF 2008 – International Conference on Health Informatics*, IEEE, Piscataway, 2008, pp. 280–285.
[3] J.C. Augusto, S. Martin, M.D. Mulvenna, W. Carswell and H. Zheng, Holistic night-time care, in: *Proceedings of the 7th World Conference of the International Society for Gerontechnology*, Vancouver, Canada, 2010.
[4] A.J. Bharucha, V. Anand, J. Forlizzi, M.A. Dew, C.F. Reynolds 3rd, S. Stevens and H. Wactlar, Intelligent Assistive technology applications to dementia care: Current capabilities, limitations, and future challenges, *Am. J. Geriatr. Psychiatry* **17** (2009), 88–104.
[5] W. Carswell, P.J. McCullagh, J.C. Augusto, S. Martin, M.D. Mulvenna, H. Zheng, H.Y. Wang, J.G. Wallace, K. McSorley, B. Taylor and W.P. Jeffers, A review of the role of assistive technology for people with dementia in the hours of darkness, *Technology and Health Care* **17** (2009), 281–304.
[6] Communication from the Commission to the European Parliament, the Council, the European Economic and Social Committee and the Committee of the Regions on Telemedicine for the Benefit of Patients, Healthcare Systems and Society, COM (2008) 689 final, Brussels, 2008.
[7] P. Dempsey, Home diagnosis, *IET Engineering & Technology* **6** (2011), 83–85.
[8] S. Evans, S. Hills and L. Grimshaw, Sustainable systems of social care, SCIE Report 35, 2010.
[9] K. Gibert, A. Valls, L. Lhotská and P. Aubrecht, Privacy preserving and use of medical information in a multiagent system, in: *Advances in Artificial Intelligence for Privacy Protection and Security*, Intelligent Information Systems, Vol. 1, World Scientific, London, 2010, pp. 165–193.
[10] Institute of Electrical and Electronics Engineers, IEEE Std. 802.11-2007, Wireless LAN Medium Access Control (MAC) and Physical Layer (PHY) Specifications, 12 June 2007.
[11] Institute of Electrical and Electronics Engineers, IEEE Std. 802.15.1-2005, Wireless Medium Access Control (MAC) and Physical Layer (PHY) Specifications for Wireless Personal Area Networks (WPANs), 14 June 2005, URL http://standards.ieee.org/getieee802/download/802.15.1-2005.pdf.
[12] Institute of Electrical and Electronics Engineers, IEEE Std. 802.15.4-2006, Wireless Medium Access Control (MAC) and Physical Layer (PHY) Specifications for Low-Rate Wireless Personal Area Networks (WPANs), 8 September 2006, URL: http://standards.ieee.org/getieee802/download/802.15.4-2006.pdf.
[13] ISO/IEEE 11073-10201:2004(E) Health Informatics – Point-of-care medical device communication – Part 10201: Domain Information Model, ISO/IEEE Std.
[14] M. Lee and T.M. Gatton, Wireless health data exchange for home healthcare monitoring systems, *Sensors* **10** (2010), 3243–3260.
[15] L. Lhotská and O. Štěpánková, Agent architecture for smart adaptive systems, *Transactions of the Institute of Measurement and Control* **26** (2004), 245–260.
[16] P.J. McCullagh, W. Carswell, M.D. Mulvenna, J.C. Augusto, H. Zheng and W.P. Jeffers, Nocturnal sensing and intervention for assisted living of people with dementia, in: *Healthcare Sensor Networks – Challenges Towards Practical Application*, D. Lai, R. Begg and M. Palaniswami, eds, Taylor and Francis/CRC Press, 2010.
[17] Ofcom's Advisory Committee on Older and Disabled People: Next Generation Services for Older and Disabled People, ANNEX B: R&D Activities, 13th September 2010.
[18] Policy Paper on Standardisation Requirements for AAL, G. van den Broek, ed., AALIANCE, 2009.
[19] K. Renaud and J. van Biljon, Predicting technology acceptance and adoption by the elderly: A qualitative study, in: *Proceedings SAICSIT*, ACM, 2008, pp. 210–219.
[20] C. Saelzer, Besser wohnen mit Technik? (Better living with technology?), *Das AAL Magazin* **2** (2010), 12–16.
[21] A. Sixsmith, S. Meuller, F. Lull, M. Klein, I. Bierhoff, S. Delaney and R. Savage, SOPRANO – An ambient assisted living system for supporting older people at home, in: *ICOST 2009*, M. Mokhtari et al., eds, LNCS, Vol. 5597, pp. 233–236.
[22] L. Zaad and S.B. Allouch, The influence of control on the acceptance of ambient intelligence by elderly people: an explorative study, in: *AmI2008*, E. Aarts et al., eds, LNCS, Vol. 5355, pp. 58–74.

Handbook of Ambient Assisted Living
J.C. Augusto et al. (Eds.)
IOS Press, 2012

doi:10.3233/978-1-60750-837-3-778

Housing, Gerontology and AAL: New Services Development

Javier YANGUAS* and Elena URDANETA
Fundación INGEMA, San Sebastián, Spain

Abstract. The technological challenge to provide systems for senior citizens that could foster the different facets of life quality perception demand system architectures for applications and new services that overcome the isolated applications of the past. The new system would integrate customary sociosanitary care, with new devices to provide new services. Four categories of AAL Services are addressed: a) Social Integration; b) Daily Life Support; c) Feel safe and protected; and d) Mobility. The idea was to identify common functional components, and to offer new services integrated with new technologies to care older persons. The needs that the older person could satisfy with the Ambient Assisted Living System are four-fold. The users will determine who, when and for which purpose this information is shared with others. The knowledge about their functional status could be used by the elderly to increase or adapt the amount and type of care. This chapter has two aims: on one hand, the reflection about older person needs and requirements; on the other hand the reflection about new AAL Services on the top of a universal platform. Some platform components that manage basic information gathered from sensors and other information sources, such as clinical history and agenda of the user, and create a representation of the context of the person. Any software component in the platform can subscribe to context events in order to use this information to provide a better user experience and offer personalized services to the user in a proactive way. Finally, the open and distributed nature of the services should lead to more applied services that integrate all the care but also improved alternatives for different parts of the existing system, both at the level of application and the platform itself.

The AAL system could be a important part in the new design and offer of new services to care with and for older people and with high quality.

Keywords. New care services, older people, housing

Introduction

According to the European Union, the percentage of persons aged 60 years or more will be approximately 37% in Europe in 2050 [1].

In addition to larger numbers of older people, the population group known as the "Fourth Age" (The Oldest Old) will also grow significantly, ie the number of very elderly persons (80 years and over) will reach significant proportions from the current 3% to at least 10% of the population by 2050.

Care for elderly people is of increased importance nowadays, given the ageing population in Europe. An increased number of people spend a significant amount of their elderly life at home due to their frailty; separated from other family members or friends, they are deprived of the ever important feeling of comfort and security.

*Corresponding Author: Javier Yanguas. E-mail: Javier.yanguas@ingema.es.

In this respect, one of the strategies adopted by several International Agencies (World Health Organization, United Nations…), is the maintenance of older people for as long as possible in their own homes, mainly due to two main reasons: firstly, elderly people's reluctance to leave their homes and secondly, the unsustainable public cost of current nursing homes.

There is a growing interest in designing and developing human-computer interfaces that fit the needs of the aged users. The interfaces' specific characteristics have to conform to the performance of older users. Design considerations include variations of the visual, auditory, cognitive and motor functions associated with the process of aging, but other considerations such as emotional, health and social aspects have to be taken into account as well. It has been found that with aging, a decrease of human function takes place [18].

Indeed, several studies show how, when learning to use a computer, older adults take longer to master the system, make more errors, and require more help than younger people [15]. Since software applications tend to increase in complexity over time, they may overload the processing capacity of elderly people. However, according to some authors [16], technology has been identified as one tool that can be used to improve independent living, improve the safety and autonomy of people with dementia, and support their quality of life.

Pluggable user interfaces is a software concept that facilitates adaptation and substitution of user interfaces and their components due to separation of the user interface from backend devices and services [3].

Subjective evidence, based on our experience in the European i2home project, suggests that most of the claimed benefits of the pluggable user interface technology are evident [19].

Research challenges of the user requirements research was to find out the needs and requirements of older people as well as to collect the data that will help to optimize the technological specifications for detecting and collecting daily patterns [4].

Another European project is UniversAAL, which stands for UNIVERsal open platform and reference Specification for Ambient Assisted Living. It is an FP7 project aiming at creating an open platform and standards which will make it technically feasible and economically viable to develop Ambient Assisted Living (AAL) solutions.

The UniversAAL project aims to make it a lot easier to develop and successfully deploy AAL solutions, by providing a standardized "universal" approach to developing them. By simplifying the task of creating AAL solutions, the project will make it more commercially attractive to develop them, thereby reducing costs and increasing uptake [5].

In the United Kingdom there are several projects developed by the Housing Learning and Improvement Network, related to extra care housing [7]. The word 'home' no longer defines a building where older people go to end their days; it is now a place where older people go to make the most of the next phase of their lives. Older people want homes that give them independence, choice and the ability to maintain their friendships and family contacts. They do not see their homes simply as a place where they receive health or social care.

Also the program *Lifetime Homes, Lifetime Neighbourhoods* [13], which sets out plans for both shortand medium-term building of specialized housing for older people and for ensuring older people can move around and feel safe in their communities.

About the new services, there is a need of the Market analysis. In the European Project SOPRANO the market analysis carried out has revealed that there are four different markets or domains that – in one way or other – target older people and in which SOPRANO could be economically exploited [14]. The term "domain" was used rather than "market" since the areas in question are often quite different from classical markets (such as the market for consumer electronics) in terms of structure, players involved, ways of payment etc. and also because the areas are not recognised as "markets" by many people. These are:

- The *social care domain* with a focus on the non-medical aspects of care for older people.
- The *medical care domain* in so far as of relevance for SOPRANO, i.e. dealing with integrated social and medical care and systems like remote consultation, remote patient monitoring, rehabilitation and prevention.
- The *housing domain* encompassing both mainstream housing for older people (privately owned homes, rented homes) and specialist/supportive housing for older people.
- The *informal-care / family-care / self-care domain*, incl. both care schemes that are supported by – for instance – the state and the potential market for self-purchased solutions.

Social harmonizing for room at welfare centres: The County Council sets the conditions for provision of the service, sets the number of beds and room with public funding, sets a maximum annual applicable rate, and regulates the input of the user.

In Spain, and more in detail in the Basque Country, the situation could be described as follows:

Nowadays the institutionalized beds harmonized by the County Council represent 90% of the actual places for day care centres and the 85% of residential beds. In 2010 it is intended that the percentage of social harmony is reduced to get a more balanced model between public and private offer.

Home help service: Town Councils manage this service, so they establish the terms of the service. However, because of the actual low, the funding of the service for dependent people falls to the County Council. This situation requires a review of the legal framework, since the asymmetry between competence and management is a constant source of problems.

The user's contribution: The County Council's model is characterized by the following:

- It takes into account the individual applicant and her or his family unit, not the descendants. The family unit is composed of the individual user, the spouse or partner, children under age or disabled children. Whether the elderly person lives with other relatives is not taken into account.
- It takes into account personal assets, not just income, establishing a level of wealth above which the user has to pay the full cost of services. The main dwelling shall not be counted as scheme.
- Below that level of wealth, the individual user pays a percentage of his/her monthly income, which in residential services is 85% and in other services varies according to a graduated scale. When the patient lives in a family unit the income "*per capita*" is considered according to the number of people.
- It is established a self available amount equivalent to the Minimum Inter professional Wage (in services for people living at their own home), or to the

20% of the same reference (for residential services), which is free of charge in any case.

- The reduced number of beds in hospitals and in residence of short, medium and long stay, makes of this group an excellent field for development of applicable technology to help in basic and instrumental activities of daily living and reminders, either to take medication, or recipes for cooking or appointments are essential to enhance the quality of life.
- Implement technology with the elderly should take into account the broad level of ignorance and sometimes lack of interest that generate new technologies in older adults. We also find that we have a number of disabilities that interfere with technological applications, such as those oversights by dementia, mobility deficit for vascular sequels, gait disorder for osteoporosis, falls and fractures. They also present difficulty in gaining access to technology, often for lack of information and many other times by the high economic cost that they possess.
- In the Basque country the use of technology by persons with disabilities is higher than the average population, but in the elderly is very low. The 74% of older adults do not use technical services for remote, the 22.1% use in low grade and 3.9% in high grade.
- In this way Public Administrations are the most interested in promoting ICTs among the elderly people. For this purpose the Basque Country has designed a plan: Euskadi, Information Society 2010, also called Euskadi's Digital Agenda whose main goal is to bring the ICTs closer to those elderly who want to know, learn and enjoy the improvement in quality of life that their use and knowledge means.

The law on the Promotion of Personal Autonomy and Care for Dependent People (39/2006) established the cooperation between Spanish Government and Autonomous Communities, that led to the creation of the territorial council of the system for autonomy and care for the dependency. This law is the fourth pillar of the state of the welfare in our country, after de national system of health, the educative system and the system of pensions.

The care for the elderly dependents is the responsibility of the County Council, this has led to the end of 2005 to sign a bilateral agreement between the Basque Government and the Association of Basque Town Councils for the care of the elderly and the dependents.

The County council has jurisdiction on specialized services for the elderly dependents, those structures that require technical, physical and sufficient staff to provide a continuous attention to this group of patients and their families. This includes the residential places, day-care centres, and some models of cohabitation units with high levels of attention.

Local councils do not have the funding or the management for specialized services for older adults. The role of local councils is focused on basic social services (information, guidance and evaluation) and its programs are home help, programs for prevention and social integration and coexistence of alternatives in the community for the people.

The Basque Government is basically responsible for common legislation (enactment and vigilance for compliance) and the coordination of a harmonious development of social services in the 3 provinces of the Basque Country. Its role is basic to consolidate the assistential system.

The priority is the cooperation among administrators:

- With town councils: reaching consensus on a model of collaboration, mainly with regard to home help.
- With the Health Department of the Basque Government: the development of a socio-sanitary space is essential to give an integrated response to the needs of the dependent elderly.
- With the Housing and Social Affairs Department: promoting compliance with its legislative competences.

All the personal data is under the Spanish Organic Law 15/1999 of 13 December on the Protection of Personal Data (LOPD 15/1999) intends to guarantee and protect the public liberties and fundamental rights of natural persons, and in particular their personal and family privacy, with regard to the processing of personal data. This Organic Law shall apply to personal data recorded on a physical support which makes them capable of processing and to any type of subsequent use of such data by the public and private sectors.

Another important research projects related to AAL paradigm are:

CHRONIOUS primary goal is to define a framework for a generic health status monitoring platform schema addressing people with chronic health conditions by developing an intelligent, ubiquitous and adaptive chronic disease platform to be used by both patients and healthcare professionals [9]. Its solution will be applied to the chronic diseases of Chronic Obstructive Pulmonary Disease (COPD) and Chronic Kidney Disease (CKD) and Renal Insufficiency. The project will use wearable solution for monitoring not only vital parameter but also environmental parameters and social context parameters. CHRONIOUS will:

- empathise on designing customised and adaptive interfaces appropriate for each user category (patients, healthcare professionals etc.),
- create a repository (knowledge base) that will aid to derive the most accurate decision of learning process,
- exploit intelligent agent techniques coupled with intelligent indexing system, flexible search and retrieval of information,
- implement new algorithms and methods to perform perceptual and evaluation of the subject using information from multiple sensors. Research on multi-fusion algorithms that best integrate, analyze and combine data from the different sensors,
- interoperate with existing healthcare legacy systems based on standards such as HL7 etc.

HEARTCYCLE will provide a closed-loop disease management solution being able to serve both Heart Failure (HF) patients and Chronic Heart Disease (CHD) patients, including possible co-morbidities hypertension, diabetes and arrhythmias. This will be achieved by multi-parametric monitoring and analysis of vital signs and other measurements. The system will contain:

- A patient loop interacting directly with the patient to support the daily treatment. It will show the health development, including treatment adherence and

effectiveness. Being motivated, compliance will increase, and health will improve.
- A professional loop involving medical professionals, e.g. alerting to revisit the care plan. The patient loop is connected with hospital information systems, to ensure optimal and personalised care.

HEARTCYCLE project will design education and coaching services to promote self-behaviours in a closed loop monitoring system for patients with coronary heart diseases that suffered a myocardial infarction. The project will develop models for (i) predicting the short-term and long-term effects of lifestyle and medication and (ii) for obtaining an objective indicator of patient compliance.

HEARTCYCLE will develop a scalable open standard technological platform, i.e. the "e-ICCM" (Innovative Chronic Condition Management), which will enable the implementation and time to market deployment of remote management services, developing standard based interfaces with electronic medical records. The HEARTCYCLE system will be able to be integrated inside existing healthcare systems, by facilitating the tools for personalised management of chronic diseases and risk conditions. The system has identified the following modules:

- Medical Response Centre (MRC). This is the core of the continuous management process [6]. It performs: i) care plan assignment to every patient, ii) real-time continuous assessment of patient's health status, iii) short term decision support, iv) titration and decompensation management guideline, v) nurse and MRC manager intervention guideline, vi) referral to other care levels, and vii) patient-nurse communication. Self-Care Management Unit (SCMU). Located at the patient's home and enabling the connectivity of the monitoring devices. It performs: i) user interaction, ii) medication management, iii) vital signs monitoring and questionnaire management, iv) education and empowerment, v) social networking, and vi) communication with MRC.
- Education & Social connection. This is a web based each disease and risk condition, helping patients to live with chronic illness, ii) social network environment to enable experience sharing among patients, iii) diet programs, cooking guidelines and receipts, iv) physical activity guidelines and self-control measures.
- Logistic & Maintenance. This is a technical service that provides: i) SCMU configuration and assignment to patient, ii) SCMU installation, training and on-line support, and iii) maintenance.

HEARTCYCLE educational and coaching strategy comprises a set of tools that empower CHD patients during the rehabilitation process, giving them an active role in the management of their disease. The strategy has been implemented as part of a global system that covers the whole physical rehabilitation program, which comprises four phases, defined based on the standards followed in three countries: Germany, United Kingdom and Spain. Considered phases include assessment stage at the hospital, where the medical team evaluates the cardiac condition of patients and configures the exercise sessions accordingly, and three additional training stages in which the exercise sessions are increasing in difficulty (initial, improvement and maintenance stages). The proposed strategy depicts the specific education and coaching content and actions for each phase. More specifically, it includes tools like goals identification and setting, establishment of specific, measurable and time targeted objectives to reach a desired aim, and recording of accomplished targets using an electronic diary.

Category	ID	Function
Personal Health	PH.1	Account Holder Profile
	PH.2	Manage Historical Clinical Data And Current State Data
	PH.3	Wellness, Preventive Medicine, and Self Care
	PH.4	Manage Health Education
	PH.5	Account Holder Decision Support
	PH.6	Manage Encounters with Providers
Supportive	S.1	Provider Management
	S.2	Financial Management
	S.3	Administrative Management
	S.4	Other Resource Management
Information Infrastructure	IN.1	Health Record Information Management
	IN.2	Standards Based Interoperability
	IN.3	Security
	IN.4	Auditable Records

Figure 1.

Another important project, funded by the EPSRC and TSB under their Assisted Living Innovation Platform. NOCTURNAL (**N**ight **O**ptimised **C**are **T**echnology for **U**se**R**s **N**eeding **A**ssisted **L**ifestyles) project addresses the needs of people with the early stages of dementia at night, as well as those of their families and carers [12].

The project between Fold Housing Association and the University of Ulster is focusing on how the use of technology can enable discrete monitoring to detect risks at an early stage; encouraging and prompting the client to self manage within their own limitations. Whilst employing complex algorithms at the back end, it is evaluating therapeutic interventions such as the use of lighting guidance, simulated presence and verbal instruction, to assist those with dementia during the hours of darkness, enabling the client to remain in their own home safely [2].

With the last call of ICT Research Unit of the European Commission, launched in 2010, an important projects will be devoted to the use of Personal Health Record (PHR) is not a new concept. References to this extent can be even found from 1978. A PHR is defined as a health record initiated and updated by an individual. The "ideal" PHR will count with the updated and accurate information summarising the medical history and data of a person. The PHR belongs to the individual and is maintained by him/herself [8].

The representation of these PHRs throughout history has been done in different ways: paper, PC, Internet, Mobile Devices, etc. During the last decade the concept of PHR has been adopted by the software industries, something which has led to the creation of different PHR software application, currently available in the market. Standardisation is also an open issue in this kind of software. Since December 2008 it exists the so-called Personal Health Record System – Functional Model (PHR-S FM), released as Ballot Draft. The PHR-S FM Draft Standard for Trial Use (DSTU) is the industry's first draft of a technical standard to specify functionality for PHR systems. It defines the set of functions that may be present in PHR systems, and offers guidelines that facilitate health information among different PHR systems and between PHR and EHR systems. Above, in Fig. 1, it can be seen, the overview of the standard defined by a set of functions. These are categorised and listed hierarchically. (The highest level functions are shown.) Each function has an ID, Name, Statement, Description, Examples, and Conformance Criteria.

The PHR solutions in the market at the moment are:

Solution	Vendor	Description	Main gaps detected
HealthVault	Microsoft	Security-enhanced, flexible health solutions platform. Similar structure as DIABCONNECT but does not offer added value service or the use of modelling algorithms.	Closed to UK and US markets. Microsoft dependant software. Devices need to be certified by Microsoft to be considered compatible. Mobile devices containing non Microsoft OS cannot be integrated. Patient's data belonging to Microsoft web platform will involve severe privacy concerns.
Google Health	Google	Online PHR manager. Permits uploading information from scanned files or insert it manually. Free license of use and compatible with Google Accounts.	Connected only with a few related organisations in the USA. Not offering services. Very simple application.
Personal Health Solutions	Inter Component Ware – ICW Global	Global system including services, PHR management and using web interfaces or mobile devices for communication	Services do not offer the usage of predictive algorithms. Integration with external systems is not semantically applied but as a part of other ICW solution.

OMNIAHOMECARE was initially developed to provide remote assistance to elderly and to monitor their health status. The association "La casa dei sogni", which provides home assistance to elderly, was involved in the analysis and test from the first phases. OMNIAHOMECARE has been used in ADA Project, a national project dedicated to provide remote assistance to elderly, and in AID-Assistant project, dedicated to provide remote assistance to people with disabilities and chronic illnesses. In the latter case, the objective was to provide support for the assistants. It has been further enhanced with the results of LISCCO (Life Signs Continuous Control) project to provide continuous monitoring of health parameters in order to develop an Expert System capable of elaborating the information provided by the sensors and providing a reliable analysis of the health status of the elders.

The patient data can be remotely accessed by Tutors, which are the users designated to provide support and control of the patients' health status. Each tutor has access only to the data relative to the patient assigned to him/her in order to guarantee the respect of data privacy. Data contained in the PHR database are relative to the clinical history of the patient (blood group, trauma, disease, allergy, surgery, ongoing therapies, etc) and to the information collected by the sensors located at home or dressed by the patient. The PHR supports HL7 v3 standard to exchange medical information with other systems. Figure 2 represents a schema that shows the various OMNIAHOMECARE components.

The AAL terminology model captures the most important concepts used in the documentation of the AAL Reference Architecture. The AAL Layer model presents a generic pattern for organizing AAL software components.

Of key importance will be the ppromotion of the development of new technologies which improve people's accessibility, autonomy and opportunities during their ageing process, in conjunction always with the generation of innovative products and services.Currently, however, there is great confusion between WHAT and HOW to make things in the projects. Devices and technology has to help to develop new services.

Another important point to address is the confusion between the MEANS and the END. The User centered-design methodology, widely used in research and implemen-

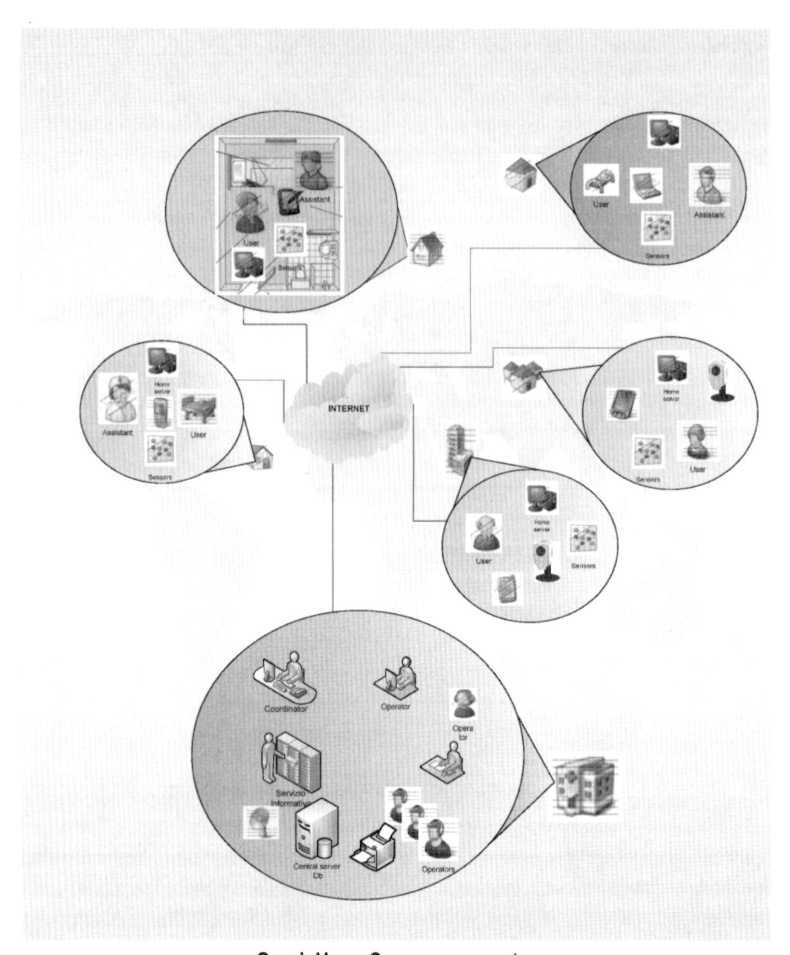

OmniaHomeCare components

Figure 2.

tation projects, is insufficient to develop a new gerontological service. Technological research has to be accompanied by the research of new services and care types. It is not enough to merely "technologize" our existing services the services that we have. Technology and gerontology has both to develop and to create new things together. Technology without GOALS (personal or therapeutic) or technology without SERVICE is putting the means before the END. The gerontology has demonstrated that general services are not optimal:

"*The change in the general care model for people suffering from dependency from "nursing home" to "living at home" is a good example*".

Furthermore, autonomy is an essential value. It is worthwhile to change the concept of the elderly as dependent to a new paradigm of autonomy. The assistive technology should emphasize this aspect.

Future

The person-centered point of view brings us closer to specificity. It offers us the possibility of working with the inter-individual variability and the intra-individual plasticity, that is, of working with the differences. Therefore, the person-centered approach in interventions and/or services based on technology should contain the capacity to adapt them to the specific person and to the specific context.

At the moment, we cannot make the mistake of confusing a part with the whole. Consider the analogy of a trip. The car, the colleagues, the landscape, the motorway, the engine are all elements that offer us the possibility of taking a trip but they are not the trip itself. A person is not only a brain or a mind or behavior or physiology. A person is not the car, is not the engine or the landscape. The person with its inherent complexity is the trip.

We believe that in the near future ageing will not only require, but also demand new strategies and approaches. A complete overhaul of the mainstay of attention and care is now necessary. The different ageing policies that have been implemented across the European Union in recent years, in general terms, have been unable to combine and coordinate accurately the wishes and the needs of the Elderly. This refers to the development of new types of services – both social and health services – and the necessary inclusion of the knowledge and developments that are emerging from R&D in various fields.

At this point in time, there are three questions to consider on the AAL paradigm:

a) The question of personalization. Understanding personalization as the possibility of incorporating the differences based on an individual's needs. Nowadays, most of the resources, services and products that have been planned and designed for older people and the disabled have not been widely embraced by these two groups. There is little variation in resources for people with a large number of differences. It is necessary to inspire the science of personalization, at least when we are talking about people, personalization that increases autonomy and independence (that gives to the elderly a voice).
b) Cognition, behavior and function are not enough. The inclusion of the subjective point of view (such as emotions or values or opinions) that can result in a complete turnaround is an unavoidable demand. If we would like to add life to the years and not only years to life, we cannot look the other way. While the empirical evidence underlines the relationships between the following: emotions and cognition; emotions and health; and cognition and health, the real gerontological world ignores this situation. It is not only one improvement; it is a request and a necessity.
c) The last question: the interdisciplinary. It is essential to open the doors between disciplines, exploring new paths and simultaneously incorporating new visions. The reality of ageing comes without an instruction manual but is, all the same, complex. A transverse point of view is essential, one that is based on a well built disciplinary development that can offer society new knowledge, based on a broader view of the process of ageing.

If people come first and taking apart from the whole is not the solution, the future must develop an "interdisciplinary" track and move forward to searching for the things that are interwoven. We are not speaking about abandoning the disciplinary development at all. We are talking about the need to open new doors between disciplines exploring new paths.

Finally, and in this respect, a new characterization of the new model of intervention with the elderly is essential. Concepts such as autonomy, participation, all-round point of view, individuality, social integration, independence, continuity of care and dignity should lead the future. The ageing social construction based on the idea of dependency is obsolete. Older people now and in the future require diverse new approaches based on a realistic, but at the same time, positive point of view.

Moreover, the current demographic transition will lead to increasing demands on health services. However, debate exists as to the role age plays relative to co-morbidity in terms of health services utilization. While age has been identified as a critical factor in health services utilization, health services utilization is not simply an outcome of ill health, nor is it an inevitable outcome of aging. Most data on health service utilization studies assess utilization at one point in time, and does not examine transitions in health service utilization. We sought to measure health services utilization and to investigate patterns in the transition of levels of utilization and outcomes associated with different levels of utilization [11].

Another challenge, the impact of scientific and technological development has to be considered. This is a cross-cutting factor which has special relevance in old age, because the opportunities and capacities to adopt, and to adapt to, new developments change considerably over the course of life with aging and depend on previous learning experiences. Moreover, it is more and more difficult to harmonise the increasing pace of innovations with the rhythms of life in old age producing "lost generations" and dependencies rather than independence in "ambient assistive living".

For older people that do suffer from a loss of function innovation, for example in the application of new technologies, it is possible to offset some of this loss and enable people to live fulfilled lives. What we do know from research already is that social engagement, with family and wider society, is vital for the quality of life of older people in all European countries. Therefore it is essential that research and innovation are focused on subjects that will lead to real quality of life gains for the ageing population [17].

Finally, regarding housing, there are some projects such as Service Flats, reviewing the modern technologies used in them to improve comfort, welfare, safety and energy efficiency. These service flats were built in Flanders (Belgium) by a company called Serviceflats Invest, a fixed capital investment company that was set up in 1995. This company has, to date, completed 46 projects comprising a total of 1,063 service flats specifically designed for the elderly. As a further indication of the demand levels, there are currently 4 projects under way with 99 flats under construction and 13 projects with 331 flats in the design stage.

Last year, the European Innovation Programme has launched several important initiatives.

The Assisted Living Innovation Platform is a £50m investment over five years by the Technology Strategy Board in the United Kingdom. More information about the innovation platform can also be found at http://www.innovateuk.org/ourstrategy/innovationplatforms/assistedliving.ashx. This Randomised Controlled Trial (RCT) has over 6,000 users.

Another interesting project is the CAPSIL Coordinating Support Action. It is a strategic international coalition of University and Industrial partners that already have extensive teams developing hardware/software/knowledge solutions to independent living based on user requirements. This support action is to launch initiatives, coordinated and disseminated by a series of workshops in the United States, European Union, and Japan, with three fundamental goals:

- To develop a detailed CAPSIL Roadmap for EU research to achieve effective and sustainable solutions to independent living based on an in-depth analysis of independent living requirements and the ICT scenarios developed or under development in the EU, as well as the US and Japan.
- To support aging research by proposing procedures to incorporate all of these diverse solutions. These CAPSILs will enable researchers and the information and Communication Technology industry to get the information they need to quickly and easily test solutions for prolonging independent living within the many and various heterogeneous communities. Only with this knowledge will the relevance and efficacy of technological solutions be maintained and be empowered with the capability to be adapted for various cultures.
- To use the CAPSIL Roadmap to help policy makers in the US and Japan coordinate research agendas and funding efforts across the three continents.

Finally, the open and distributed nature of the services should lead to more applied services that integrate not only all the care but also improved alternatives for different parts of the existing system, both at the level of application and the platform itself.

The AAL system has the potential of being an important part in the new design and offer of new services to care with and for older people and with high quality.

References

[1] A. Börsch-Supan, Longitudinal data collection in continental Europe: Experiences from the survey of health, ageing and retirement in Europe, in: *Survey Methods in Multinational, Multiregional and Multicultural Contexts*, J. Harkness et al., eds, John Wiley & Sons, Hoboken, NJ, 2009.

[2] W. Carswell, P.J. McCullagh, J.C. Augusto, S. Martin, M.D. Mulvenna, H. Zheng, H.Y. Wang, J.G. Wallace, K. McSorley, B. Taylor and W.P. Jeffers, A review of the role of assistive technology for people with dementia in the hours of darkness, *Technology and Health Care* **17** (2009), 281–304.

[3] Consortium URC, retrieved February 18, 2009, from http:// myurc.org/.

[4] C. Courage and K. Baxter, *Understanding your users. A practical guide to user requirements. Methods, Tools, and Techniques*, Morgan Kaufman Publishers, 2005.

[5] J. Goorman, UniversAAL project. Retrieved http://www.universaal.org/newsletter/newsletter_univers AAL_01d.pdf, 2010.

[6] S. Guillén, M.T. Meneu, R. Serafin, M.T. Arredondo, E. Castellano and B. Valdivieso, Disease management. A system for the management of the chronic conditions, in: *32nd Annual International Conference of the IEEE EMBS*, Buenos Aires, Argentina, August 31 – September 4, 2008, 20.

[7] Homes for our old age: Independent living by design, CABE, 2009.

[8] B.O. Hoppe, A.K. Harding, J. Staab and M. Counter, Private well testing in Oregon from real estate transactions: An innovative approach toward a state-based surveillance system, *Public Health Rep.* **126** (2011), 107–115.

[9] http://www.chronious.eu, Retrieved 30th January 2011.

[10] http://www.heartcycle.eu/, Retrieved 5th February 2011.

[11] R. Moineddin, J.X. Nie, L. Wang, C.S. Tracy and R.E. Upshur, Measuring change in health status of older adults at the population level: The transition probability model, *BMC Health Serv. Res.* **9** (2010), 306–312.

[12] M. Mulvenna, W. Carswell, P. McCullagh, J.C. Augusto, H. Zheng, P. Jeffers, H. Wang and S. Martin, Visualization of data for ambient assisted living services, *IEEE Communications Magazine feature topic on New Converged Telecommunications Applications for the End User, IEEE Communications Magazine* **49** (2011), 110–117.

[13] A. Shipley, Lifetime homes, lifetime neighbourhoods: A national strategy for housing in an ageing society, www.lifetimehomes.org.uk/pledge, Retrieved 2009.
[14] A. Sixsmith, S. Müller, F. Lull, M. Klein, I. Bierhoff, S. Delaney, P. Byrne, R. Savage and E. Avatangelou, A user-driven approach to developing AAL systems for older people: The SOPRANO project, In: *Intelligent Technologies for Bridging the Grey Digital Divide*, J. Soar, R. Swindell and P. Tsang, eds, 2010, pp. 30–45.
[15] K. Slegers, M.P. Van Boxtel and J. Jolles, The efficiency of using everyday technological devices by older adults: the role of cognitive functions, *Ageing & Society* **29** (2009), 309–325.
[16] P. Topo, Technology studies to meet the needs of people with dementia and their caregivers. A literature review, *Journal of Applied Gerontology* **28** (2009), 5–37.
[17] A. Walker, Why involving older people in research? *Age and Ageing* **36** (2007), 481–483.
[18] R. Witte, Shrinkage, neuron and synapse loss: Aging takes its toll on the brain, *Geriatrics & Aging* **1**(1998), 14–15.
[19] G. Zimmermann, J. Alexandersson, C. Buiza, E. Urdaneta, U. Díaz, E. Carrasco, M. Klima and A. Pfalzgraf, Meeting the needs of diverse user groups: Benefits and costs of pluggable user interfaces in designing for older people and people with cognitive impairments, in: *Intelligent Technologies for Bridging the Grey Digital Divide*, J. Soar, R. Swindell and P. Tsang, eds, New York, 2010.

Handbook of Ambient Assisted Living
J.C. Augusto et al. (Eds.)
IOS Press, 2012

doi:10.3233/978-1-60750-837-3-791

Connecting Communities: The Role of Design Ethnography in Developing Social Care Technologies for Isolated Older Adults

David PRENDERGAST[a,*], Claire SOMERVILLE[b] and Joe WHERTON[b]
[a] *Health Research and Innovation, Intel Labs, Leixlip, Ireland*
[b] *Technology Research for Independent Living (TRIL) centre, Ireland*

Abstract. Social isolation and loneliness in old age can be caused by a variety of factors, including decline in physical and mental health, as well as changes in social environment. The Building Bridges projects explored how communication technology could be developed to reduce risks of loneliness and isolation among older adults. This paper provides an overview of the TRIL Building bridges system and a description of the design ethnography process involved. This paper illustrates the need to include potential users at different stages of the design process. It also demonstrates the benefits of using different methods for eliciting participation in a created social network.

Keywords. Ethnography, design, ageing, independent living, social connection, technology

Introduction

This paper describes the ethnographic design approach involved in the development of a communication technology to reduce risks of loneliness and isolation among older adults. The Building Bridges system was developed to encourage and support social engagement with both strangers and friends. It consists of a touch screen interface with speakers and a phone handset. A core characteristic of the device in its current form is its broadcasts feature (e.g. news, documentaries, health information), followed by the ability to host a group chat. In addition, participants can initiate calls, send virtual postcard messages and join the tea room, an audio chat room that is always open and can hold up to twenty people at any one time. The concept and design were grounded in an understanding of users' needs and wishes achieved through home visit interviews, focus groups and design workshops involving potential users. This paper provides an overview of the technology developed and the qualitative research that guided design efforts.

[*] Corresponding Author: David Prendergast, Health Research and Innovation, Intel Labs, Collinstown Industrial Park, Leixlip, Ireland. Email: david.k.prendergast@intel.com.

1. Technological Solutions to Loneliness and Social Isolation

Loneliness and social isolation are closely associated with mental and physical health. Older adults may lose social connections due to retirement, relocation or widowhood. It may also be a consequence of illness, depression, and lack of mobility.

Modern technology and the internet offer new ways to help older adults remain connected with peers and family members in a flexible and inexpensive way. However, these are often inaccessible to them due to decline in cognitive, sensory and physical abilities. Furthermore, many older people are unfamiliar with computers and may be reluctant to adopt such technologies. Despite this, numerous studies have demonstrated the potential role of internet communication technology in reducing loneliness and improving quality of life among older adults. White et al. [11] explored the effect of internet use in a retirement community and demonstrated through assessments that reconnecting social ties decreased levels of loneliness. Similarly, Groves and Slack [5] investigated the impact of a computer-training program with 20 nursing home residents. Pre- and post- evaluations showed an increase in independence and engagement in social activities. Such studies illustrate the potential benefit of existing technologies. However, in many cases this requires time and motivation for older adults to learn and adopt new technology and interface conventions.

Previous research has been carried out to improve the usability of email systems for older adults. Czaja, Guerrier, Nair and Landauer [1] developed an electronic messaging system for older adults to perform routine communication tasks. The system included a text editor, basic electronic mail functions and access to information (news, weather and health information). The technology included a CRT, monitor, keyboard, printer, modem and controller. To operate the system, the users typed the name of another participant, and the system dialled automatically. The user then pressed a boldly labelled Return key. They could then write the message and press boldly labelled Send key when complete. It was found that the participants could use the system with a minimal amount of difficulty. More recently, Hawthorn [6] developed a new email system (SeniorMail) which was designed through a series of focus groups, interviews and usability tests with older adults. Design modifications focused on visual presentation (e.g. bigger buttons and larger font) and simplifying navigation. Similarly, Dickinson et al. [3] developed an email system for older adults. The initial design phase reviewed existing recommendations to established guidelines for the software before development. This focused on functionality (e.g. each screen has a clear primary function and only a few buttons are available), accessibility (e.g. large clickable targets and high contrast between text and background), user interface paradigms (e.g. no scroll bars), terminology, and personalisation (customizable to match sensory impairment). The interface requirements were then explored further through design workshops with potential users that highlighted further requirements such as the need to avoid formal language, and increasing the salience of icons and buttons. Tests using the final prototype demonstrated that people with no experience of the internet found it significantly easier to use than a commercially equivalent design. The positive experience of the system also led participants to feel more confident about computer use.

The research conducted to date highlights the potential for developing technology to reduce risks of loneliness and isolation among older adults and the need to include potential users throughout the design process to establish interface requirements. This paper highlights the importance of involving potential users at the earliest stages of the

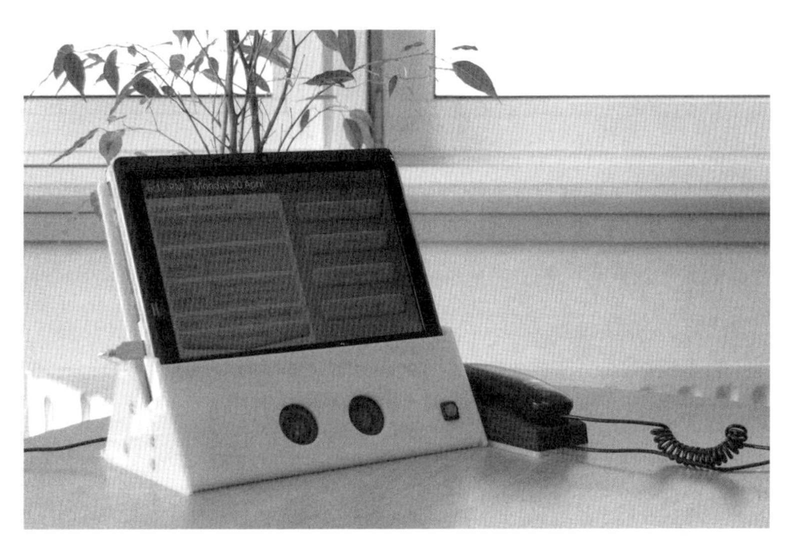

Figure 1. The Building Bridges device displaying the Main Menu screen.

design process to develop a concept that meets the needs and wishes of potential users, and suits real contexts.

2. System Overview

The aim of the Building Bridges project was to develop communication technology designed to encourage peer-to-peer social engagement among older adults and reduce risks of loneliness and social isolation. The project is part of the Technology Research for Independent Living (TRIL) Centre, which is a collaboration between the Intel Digital Health Group, Trinity College Dublin (TCD), University College Dublin (UCD), National University of Ireland Galway, and St. James Hospital, Dublin (www.trilcentre.org).

The device consists of a 12 inch touch screen computer in a custom made stand, a phone handset with functioning cradle, and speakers. The software uses Voice over IP (VoIP) protocol with a customised Flash based interface. The system features are briefly described below. See [12] for more details about the system features and interface design.

Broadcast and chat: Users can listen to regular broadcasts (e.g. news, documentaries, health lectures, stories and music). The broadcasts information (time, day and topic) is presented on the Main Menu screen. At the scheduled time, the user can choose to listen to the broadcast by pressing a button on the screen. During the broadcast, icons that represent other people (i.e. avatars) who are also listening are shown on the right of the screen. At the end of the broadcast the user can join a 'group chat' with the other listeners by lifting the phone handset on the device. During the group chat, visual cues are presented on the screen to support the conversation (e.g. who has entered/left the call, if someone wishes to interrupt the conversation and a counter representing how much time is left on the group chat). Figure 2 presents an example image of the 'group chat' display.

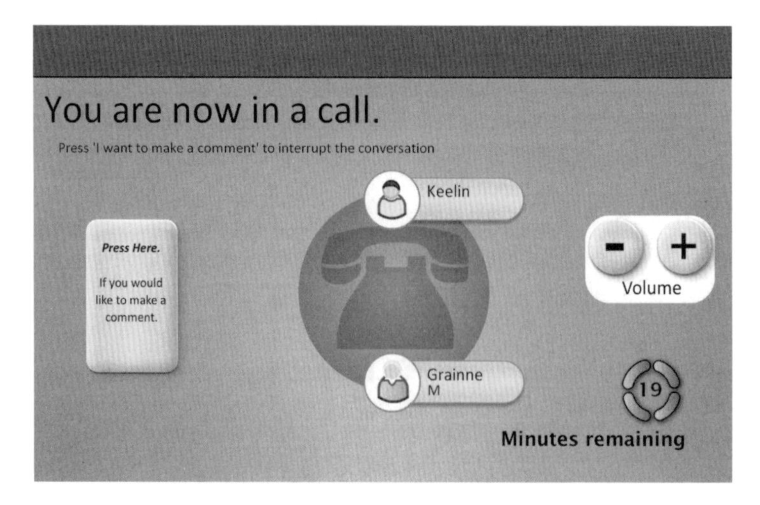

Figure 2. The screen display during a group chat.

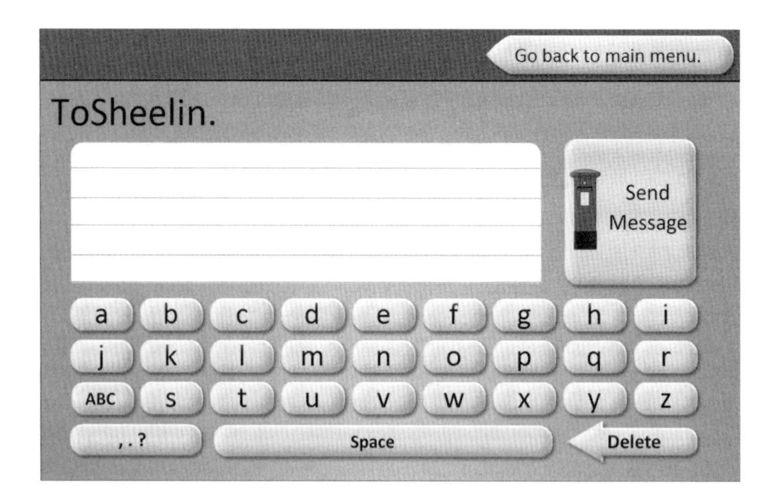

Figure 3. The touch screen keyboard.

Calls: Users can make one-to-one and group calls. The user simply presses the button labelled "Make a Call", which leads to another screen showing a list of the other people they can call. They then select the person(s) they wish to call and press the button labelled "Call". During the call the user is provided with the same display as the after-broadcast chat without the counter.

Messaging: To write a message the user first presses the button labelled "Write message" and selects the person(s) they wish to write. This leads to a screen presenting a simple touch screen keyboard (see Fig. 3).

Tea Room: The Tea Room is an audio chat room that users can access anytime day or night. The user enters this by pressing the button labelled "Visit Tea Room" on the main menu screen. If another person is in the tea room, their icon would show up on the screen. The user can then lift the handset to talk.

3. Design Process

The design process can be summarised under four main phases (see Fig. 4). Potential users were involved at each phase. The first phase of ethnographic fieldwork included in-depth interviews, a small-scale pilot trial accompanied by qualitative interviewing as well as focus groups and surveys with potential users. This research work provided an understanding of the problems being addressed. The second phase included a collaborative analysis of the ethnographic data by a multidisciplinary team (social scientists, designers, engineers and clinicians). This helped identify opportunities for technological support, which were discussed with potential users in order to refine ideas towards a unified concept. The third phase included an iterative process of establishing design requirements to ensure that the system suited the wishes of users. The final phase included home trials to refine the system features and interface design.

3.1. Phase One: Understanding the Problem Through Ethnography and Fieldwork

The first phase of the design process comprised of a broad multi-method ethnographic sweep of data collection that sought to identify the level of acceptability, technology competency and potential barriers to the introduction of a communication technology among older adults. The research design included the use of structured survey data from the TRIL Clinic Cohort of older adults; in-home qualitative interviews with older adults; focus groups; and a small pilot trial of an off-the-shelf communication technology. This multi-method approach of engaging potential users at the earliest point of the design process helped to build a holistic picture of the lives of older adults as well as clarify their needs and expectations of communication technologies.

Structured survey data from the TRIL Clinic quickly revealed the low levels of technology competency among the target population but also demonstrated that older adults were nevertheless enthusiastic about engaging with technologies and with the processes of designing a technology appropriate to their needs. Less than 10% of survey participants owned a computer and around one third had never used one at all. Nearly half did not own a mobile phone and of those that did only one third used the text messaging function. Despite these low levels of uptake, many of those interviewed spoke of a wish to be able to engage more fully with technologies. A 72 year old man said "*I'd love to be able to get on those sports websites – I think if they [computers] were easier looking I'd use them – they're a bit complicated looking.*"

Simplicity of use, look and design were clearly required if the technology was to meet with the needs of the target population.

The results of the data generated within the TRIL Clinic surveys were echoed during semi-structured interviews in their homes. For example, despite the presence of assisted-living technologies such as panic alarms and stair-lifts, few interviewees were able to navigate the contacts lists on their landline phones and frequently preferred to retain a written list of important telephone numbers close to their phones.

One of the benefits of undertaking interviews in the homes of participants was the opportunity to directly observe the spatial context of their living environment and explore potential locations of a new communication technology within their homes. The majority of older adults had lived in their homes for more than 30 years during which time the accumulation of photos, ornaments, furniture, books and the like often meant that open space for any new item might be problematic. Telephones were generally located in hallways with some people opting to have extensions located beside their beds or day chairs for easier access. The design of additional communication technologies in the home would need to take account of these restricted spaces as well as the hazards of trailing wires and power/broadband socket access if the device was to remain out of its box, plugged-in and activated to avoid the situation as described by one 76 year old female interviewee: "*I was given a DVD player but it's still in the box- and also an alarm but I can't remember the code.*"

These sources of data provided insights into the types of issues that might both discourage and stimulate technology uptake but further probing was necessary to delve into the *experience* of using a communication technology with more extensive functionality than most participants were familiar. At the time Skype had just launched a device that resembled a conventional corded landline telephone but operated VOIP and could facilitate a conference call with up to 5 users. Running a small scale trial using these devices with a group of older adults allowed three objectives to be explored. Firstly, concept testing: Would older adults be interested and willing to participate in a conference call with either friends or strangers? Secondly, technology testing: How stable was VOIP for these purposes and would 3G modems support such applications? Finally, how would communication emerge and what visual, acoustic or symbolic aids could be designed into the technology to help facilitate a flow of conversation?

Two groups of 4 participants were recruited to take part in the Skype trial. The devices were installed in their homes with technical problems resolved as they arose by visits from a technologist. The participants were not known to one another and had a range of technology competencies. Entry and exit interviews were conducted with each participant at their homes and conference calls were scheduled and facilitated by a researcher. A series of scheduled conference calls were achieved over the course of a few weeks lasting around 45 minutes each.

Five overriding themes emerged from this trial as well as a number of key design pointers related to the functioning of the technology.

i. Conversational Dynamics

It was apparent that there was a tendency for pairs of participants to dominate conversations blocking the engagement of others on the call. Without the visual cues of physical face-to-face interaction participants found it difficult to break into conversation or become aware that another person was trying to speak. The need for some level of graphical representation of non-verbal conversational cues would be necessary to facilitate flow and turn-taking.

ii. Scheduling and Timing

These calls were scheduled and it took some group negotiation to arrive at a convenient time that suited all participants. However, once this was agreed (6–7pm) participants felt they could accommodate the call as part of their routine and also commented that it was something to look forward to doing.

iii. Forming Relationships

Over time conversations over Skype began to flow better as participants became more familiar with one another. They expressed a desire to be able to see each other or at least put a face to a name and voice.

iv. Enjoyment

Views expressed at the exit interviews suggested that all of the older adults who took part enjoyed the experience. They all stayed on the call for the full duration of 45 minutes, even those who had previously indicated that they generally wouldn't spend more than 5 minutes on a telephone, and they expressed enjoyment with getting to know one another and finding common ground during their calls.

v. Understanding the Technology

Initially there were some difficulties in visualising what was happening and how the technology connected people. For example, it was confusing to figure out if someone, and who, had joined a conference call. They were not certain if others were together in the same room or if they were all sitting in their own homes. It took some time for participants to develop a mental model of how the technology was functioning. Beeps and flashing lights were interpreted as problems indicating something had gone wrong rather than positive feedback.

Results from these interviews, surveys and the Skype trial were fed back to interaction designers on the team who produced paper prototypes and initial storyboards of how a communication technology might look and what functions and visual representations might be appropriate in addressing the issues raised by the older adults. These were used to prompt discussions in further interviews and focus groups in phase two of the design process.

Conducting fieldwork with potential end users as the first step in the design process meant that the needs and requirements of older adults lay at the heart of the technology development. The use of multiple types and sources of data which were presented to the team meant that the designers and engineers were able to develop an ongoing dialogue with their users which in turn drove their decision-making. The enduring question that frequently propelled discussions in the later phases always centred upon: "How would an older adult respond to or feel about that?" The iterative nature of the design process, initiated in phase 1, facilitated those voices.

3.2. Phase Two: Developing the Concept: Workshops and Focus Groups

The second phase aimed to establish a concept based on the ethnographic data. This included 3 steps. Firstly, the ethnographic data was presented to the research team to identify opportunities for technology. Second, these opportunities were explored through focus groups with older adults. Third, feedback from focus groups were reviewed by the research team to establish a unified concept.

Step 1: Identifying opportunities for technology

The first step in this phase was to identify key themes within the ethnographic material that usefully summarised the problems to be addressed and opportunities for technological support. The methodological approaches taken here were designed to stimulate and support collaborative discussions about the ethnographic data across a multidisciplinary team. During presentation of field notes from Phase 1, other members of the research team wrote down key points that they felt were important. Each point was written on a single post-it note.

Once all the data had been presented, all the members of the team were required to stick all of the post-it notes onto large whiteboards. The researchers then collectively decided on post-it notes that were related. Those considered similar were placed next to each other on the board. This process continued until a number of clear categories emerged which were further discussed, grouped and re-grouped to form themes. The post-it notes and whiteboard allowed the notes to be arranged spatially to facilitate the group discussion. The various topics raised were summarised under six broad themes:

(i) *Learning curve* (e.g. training support, avoid dependency)
(ii) *Privacy and intrusion* (e.g. security, speaking with strangers)
(iii) *Joining conference calls* (e.g. timing/scheduling, reluctance to connect)
(iv) *Make it interesting* (e.g. gaming, competition, sharing)
(v) *Visualisation of others* (e.g. simulate physical presence, who is talking)
(vi) *Group generation* (e.g. common factor, snowballing contacts)

Step 2: Focus groups

The next step in this phase was to get input from older adults regarding the technological opportunities identified and the issues raised during the workshops. There were six focus groups in total. Four took place at Active Retirement Groups in Dublin (each including 10–20 participants). Two focus groups took place at St James's Hospital, Dublin (each including 5 participants), in which participants were recruited through the TRIL clinic.

The methodological approach at this stage was designed to stimulate and support discussions with older adults who may have little or no experience with computers and the internet. In order to achieve this, the various issues raised in the workshop were communicated through 'storyboards'. Each storyboard included 4 to 6 frames on a piece of board (42 × 32 cm) and was structured so that the first frame described the user and the last frame highlighted how the technology benefited the user whilst the middle frames described the concept. See below for an example storyboard representing a social isolation network.

The below scenario focused on connecting people with shared interests. Frame 1 introduces the character, who has an interest in canaries. In Frame 2 he registers his profile on system, including his personal interests. In Frame 3, he gets a response from someone in America who is also interested in canaries and would like to have a chat. Frame 4 describes them having a chat and sharing tips on looking after canaries.

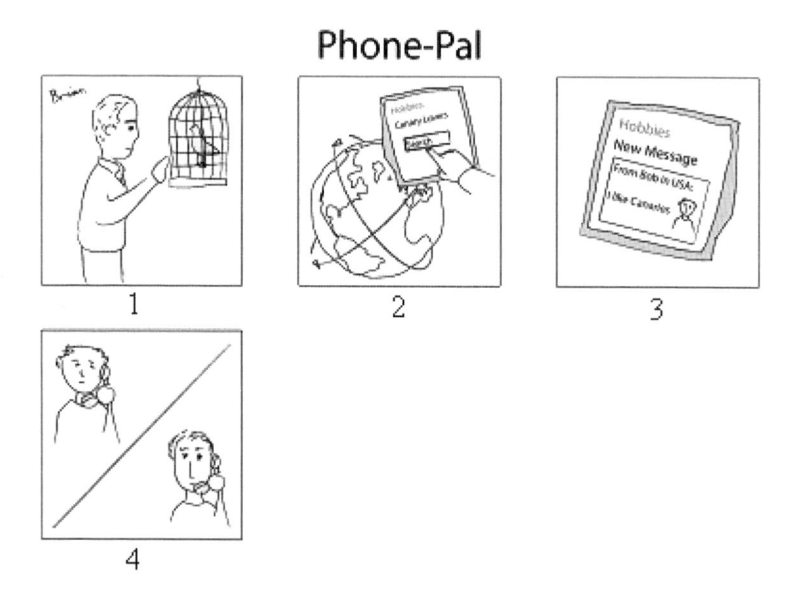

Figure 4. Example storyboard, 'Phone Pal'.

The key issues raised in the workshop were presented across 12 different storyboards. After each storyboard had been presented, the researcher asked what they thought about the scenario presented, what they liked or disliked and how it might be improved. The purpose of the storyboards was to stimulate discussion around various issues related to socialising through communication technology, as opposed to the technology involved. For this reason they were structured to be short, simple and ambiguous with regard to technology, in order to ensure that comments were not limited or biased by perceived knowledge or anxieties about computers. This allowed discussion to remain open-ended and reveal issues that were not already considered. For example, the main theme captured in the scenario presented in Fig. 4 includes the linking of strangers through shared interests. When discussing this scenario, participants commented that linking people in this way was limited, as they may not have interests to discuss with a stranger. However, the need for some common ground or shared experience was needed. It also cued discussion around being 'community contained', rather than global as there was the possibility of future face-to-face contact. This highlights how the storyboard reveals key issues that were not initially considered by the research team. Storyboards were broad and ranged from recreational interaction (e.g. games) to more instrumental interaction, such as peer-support (e.g. caregiver network) and formal health consultations (e.g. collaborative health check with consultants and family members).

Step 3: Establish a unified concept

In order to summarise focus-group discussions, positive and negative comments associated with each storyboard were reviewed. This helped direct decisions towards feature requirements to be included in the proposed concept. For example, particpants emphasized the need to have something to talk about. However, it was highlighted that shared hobbies or interests were too limited, instead they felt that most day-to-day conversations were based on shared experiences (e.g. visiting same places or memories) or some common ground (e.g. about people they know). Furthermore, concerns about being obliged to communicate with others were also expressed, and so the system should provide opportunities for meeting whilst avoiding the stress involved in feelings of social obligation or fear of intruding upon others.

Such issues were not initially considered by the research team, which highlights the value in openly discussing potential users' views about socialising through technology without focusing on the technical or usability issues. Drawing from their feedback it was evident that social encounters would need to be supported by a shared experience or common ground. It was also found that concepts that were educational were also popular as particpants could see an added benefit. Therefore, it was decided that a core feature in the design would be to provide 'broadcasts', which would be followed by a group chat. This would allow opportunistic social interaction as well as provide common ground through the broadcast topic.

3.3. Phase 3: Exploring Design Requirements Through Home Visit Interviews

After establishing the core features, the technical requirements for hardware and software were established in order to begin developing the prototype. It was decided that the main features (broadcasts, group calls and messaging) could be achieved through Skype which allows developers to create interfaces with an API (Application Programming Interface). It was also decided that a touch screen interface would be used as it avoided the need for a keyboard and mouse.

Existing design guidelines for accessible systems for the older adults were reviewed as a starting point [3,6–8]. Six of the participants who took part in the focus groups were visited in their own homes to discuss the concept and interface designs. Before visiting the participants, four of them took part in a short telephone conference call using standard telephones. The conference call started with a health broadcast (5 mins), followed a group chat. Unlike the previous telephone conference calls described in Section 2.1, the conversation was not facilitated by the researcher. This simulated the core feature in the technology concept in order to faciliate the interviews during the home visit, and provide the particpants with greater insight into how such technology should be developed.

During the home visit the researcher described the core feature of using a 'broadcast' followed by a group chat using the same storyboard format described in Section 3.2. The concept was then discussed to understand how the participants would use it and what difficulties or concerns they would have. For example, one of the participants who took part in the conference call stated that, "*I didn't know when it would be polite to interrupt. Usually with people I can look at you and interrupt in an appropriate way – I wasn't sure what I should do there...*" This highlights the need for additional features that compensate for the absence of physical cues. Another commented that, "*suppose you say you're listening into it and then something happens. Out of politeness, you should say if you're not attending*". Such concerns around commitment to join the 'broadcast' and 'group chat' highlight the need to include something flexible and that people did not feel committed, and could decide to listen as and when the broadcast commenced.

After discussing the concept, participants were shown different interface designs on a touchscreen. A 'think aloud' interview was conducted in which the participant was given a specific goals (e.g. send a message) without being given instructuctions on how to perform the task. When they appeared to struggle the researcher would ask them to describe what they were trying to do. This approach helped reveal aspects of the interface that are not intuitive and helped guide development of the interface structure. For example, when presented with a new interface, participants attended to all of the information on the screen, and so any information that did not support the interaction were removed. It also highlighted the importance of button affordances. It was necessary to give buttons a three-dimensional appearance and represent them consistently (shape, colour and sound). Boxed text should be avoided (e.g. screen titles) so that they do not resemble buttons.

Other interface issues were highlighted beyond usability. In the initial design users wrote messages directly onto the screen using a stylus. Although this was popular with many, some raised concerns about how their handwriting appeared to other people. After using the stylus, one particpant stated that "*my writing is a lot better than that on paper ... that looks like it's been written by a four-year old.*" Such factors would potentially hinder use of the system and so it was decided that a touch screen keyboard was more inclusive.

Involving older adults during this phase of the design was instrumental for guiding the prototype development so that it was easy to use and met the needs and wishes of potential users. However, it should be noted that conducting one-off interviews have limitations and are time/context-restricted. Therefore, a final phase was necessary in the design process, in which older adults used the system at home over a number of weeks. This allowed them to become familiar with the technology and identify more subtle design issues that would only emerge in real contexts amidst 'the messiness of everyday life'.

3.4. Phase 4: Iterative Development Through Home Trials

In the final phase the prototype devices were deployed in 35 homes in three separate home trials. The first home trial focused on usability. It included 5 healthy older participants and lasted 4 weeks. A 'think aloud' interview was conducted at the beginning and end of the trial. Additionally, a semi-structured interview was conducted at the end of the trial focusing on problems experienced and their perspective on how the device could be improved. The second home trial included two groups of 5 participants (Group 1 were 5 strangers and Groups 2 were 5 members of an Active Retirement Group). The home visit procedure was identical to that used in the first home trial however in this trial the semi-structured interview focused on usage of the system (e.g. reasons for calling other people and what they talked about), usage (e.g. when they use it), and how it fitted into daily routines (e.g. reasons for switching it off). Additionally, usage of the system features (time, frequency and duration) of each feature and screen presses were logged remotely on a server.

These initial two home pilot studies provided insight into subtle, but important, design issues that would only emerge after more lengthy use of the system in real contexts. Usability issues started to emerge as the participants started to use it more regularly. For example, the 'Go Back to Main Menu' button was located at the bottom of the screen, and so it would occasionally be hit inadvertently by the users knuckle or wrist when writing a message. To overcome this all navigation buttons were placed at the top of the screen so that they would not be pressed by mistake. It was also found that people started to use a chopstick or pencil as a stylus as this was found to be easier than using a figure: "*I use this chopstick to type messages, it makes it much easier. You can also see what letters are being pressed because your finger isn't covering the button.*"

The remote log data also helped understand how the system was incorporated into everyday routines. For example, it was noted from the remote data logs that just over a third (34%) of calls made were unanswered by the recipients. This issue was highlighted during exit interviews: "*When I did ring both of them, it seemed to ring out or I was wondering if they were out a lot and I sent them messages instead.*" It emerged that this occurred because people would leave the device on when they left the house. A related problem was that participants turned the device 'off' when they were in the house. For example, one female participant stated "*Everyone was [not available], so they were obviously off so I switched mine off too*." The need to guide users in turning the device on/off at appropriate times was evident. Subsequently, it was decided to locate the device in a prominent location in the house (e.g. in the lounge) and have it double up as a digital photo frame when not in use to encourage users to keep it switched on.

As participants became familiar with the system over time, they became more confident in suggesting how it should be improved to suit real situations. They requested a loud audio cue when a message was received, or when a broadcast was about to start, so that they could be alerted when away from the device.

Once the research and engineering team were confident in the stability and design of the prototype as a result of these initial iterative development cycles, it was decided

Table 1. Total Usage of the System and its Core Component Capabilities by primary group members

	Name	Loneliness (DeJong)	Initiate calls	Send messages	Tea Room	Broadcast attendance	Total
HIGH	Grace	Social	7.97%	3.66%	5.73%	0.64%	18.00%
	Joan	Social	3.50%	5.75%	3.58%	2.75%	15.58%
	Julia	Social/Emotional	5.78%	1.84%	3.96%	2.24%	13.82%
HIGH-MID	Alice	None	0.45%	1.89%	0.82%	2.82%	5.98%
	Louise	Social/Emotional	0.34%	1.68%	0.97%	2.75%	5.75%
	Karen	None	0.41%	1.99%	1.40%	1.66%	5.45%
	Grainne	Social/Emotional	1.53%	1.35%	1.31%	0.62%	4.82%
	Kevin	None	1.34%	0.31%	0.79%	2.35%	4.79%
	Emer	None	0.63%	1.83%	1.23%	0.97%	4.65%
LOW-MID	Theresa	Emotional	0.69%	1.21%	0.41%	2.17%	4.48%
	Sue	None	0.62%	0.69%	1.35%	1.35%	4.01%
	Martha	None	0.79%	0.74%	0.82%	1.23%	3.57%
	Sean	None	0.00%	0.75%	0.56%	1.99%	3.29%
LOW	Patrick	Social	0.19%	0.18%	0.53%	0.36%	1.25%
	Deidre	Emotional	0.34%	0.21%	0.37%	0.29%	1.21%
	Tim	None	0.38%	0.39%	0.29%	0.08%	1.14%
	Eamon	None	0.06%	0.25%	0.34%	0.36%	1.01%
	Liam	n/a	0.00%	0.28%	0.29%	0.22%	0.79%
	Bert	None	0.00%	0.00%	0.26%	0.14%	0.41%

to launch a third, more ambitious, home deployment involving 19 older households representing a range of social connection subtypes. These included people who felt socially isolated, others who were emotionally lonely due to lack or loss of attachment to a significant other, as well as participants who felt neither of these categories applied to them. A PC client version of the technology was also made available on disk for friends and family members nominated by those receiving the touch screen devices. The concept behind this pilot was to link each participant into two networks: a large circle of peers (primary group) that they had not met before and a small cluster of friends and family (secondary group). The aim of the study was to examine how individuals and groups utilised the four main features of the system over a time period of ten weeks in real world settings beyond the laboratory. Researchers conducted entry and exit interviews and made contact briefly once a week to give participants an opportunity to present problems, but the general approach of the project was to provide limited facilitation outside the provision of broadcasts.

The deJong-Gervield loneliness scale [2] was used get some indication of their degree of loneliness. This is a self report scale, which includes 6 items. Three items relate to social loneliness and three relate to emotional loneliness. The particpants were categorised as 'socially lonely' if they scored 2 or more on the social items, and 'emotionally lonely' if they scored 2 more on the emotional items. If they scored 2 or more for both, they were categorised as being both socially and emotioanlly lonely. Immediately most striking was the strong degree to which those classified as socially lonely made use of the Building Bridges technology. Only one individual in this category did not engage with the system, and his experience in the study was interrupted early by a prolonged and unexpected hospital stay. Overall, the socially lonely users became lead users and advocates of the platform, attempting to focus social interaction and encourage usage among other members. Those who felt emotionally isolated were generally more ambivalent about the system as were those who scored as not lonely. The majority of these participants reported that they had enjoyed the system because of the opportunity to meet new people, but several explained that they didn't yet have a need for it. This was frequently noted with the projection that they could perceive a use for it in the future, should they ever become housebound.

Usage was initially high for the first four weeks but waned as several of the more active participants went on holiday. Activity increased towards the end of the study, with a number of members deciding to go beyond the technology and meet in person for walks in the park. 'Perceived value' was another driver for activity. Whilst many participants were engaged in the study for altruistic reasons, periods of action were often initiated by provision of certain types of content. Analysis of usage data and logs suggest that health broadcasts were particularly popular, especially those the team created in the areas of falls prevention and memory training.

The exit interviews provided insight into issues to consider when developing communication technology for supporting social interaction among older adults. Firstly, problems arose due to *variability* of system use across participants. This led to the problem of frequent users becoming frustrated with the relative disengagement of others. For example, there were frustrations around getting no response, or delayed responses, to messages and missed calls: "*I make contact, send messages and people don't reply.*" Second, participants highlighted a need for greater *flexibility over privacy and personal identity*. During the design phase it emerged that some people had concerns around security, and so contacts were represented using a generic avatar and first names. However, as the trial progressed and users became familiar with each other, they requested some record of information about different people (e.g. interests, where they lived) as well as the ability to see each other via a webcam. More work is needed to see how information can be shared in a graduated way to maintain sense of privacy without hindering social relatedness as people get to know each other. Finally, it was repeatedly mentioned that the system would work best in conjunction with *meeting up face to face*. One participant said "*I think there comes a point where you do actually need to meet to become really friendly with somebody. It's a sight barrier, not being able to see their faces. I can't quite say why*" (Julia), while another suggested that for the trial to be more successful in engaging participants in socialising it "*would [have been] nice if we were met and went walking or to a pub*" (Louise). This leads us to believe that a technology of this kind would probably work better in conjunction with facilitating some personal, face-to-face interactions.

4. Conclusion

This paper illustrates the need to include potential users at different stages of the design process. It also demonstrates the benefits of using different methods for eliciting participation. A similar approach might be taken for developing ICT for other user groups at risk of loneliness and social isolation. Each phase of the development was necessary to ensure that the system matches what users need and want. The first phase helped understand the problems being addressed. The second phase involved the identification of technological opportunities based on the ethnographic data, which was analysed collectively by a multidisciplinary team. The storyboards used during the focus groups allowed these ideas to be communicated to seniors with different levels of experience with technology in order to establish the unified concept. The third phase involved home visits to identify design requirements. The 'think aloud' visit interviews guided the design towards an intuitive interface that could be easily used by older adults with little or no computer experience. The final phase allowed users to contribute to the design after using the device for a number of weeks. This was important for refining the prototype and revealing subtle but important design issues. The home trials also provide insight into how the technology should be implemented to improve its efficacy as part of a toolkit for supporting social connectedness.

Acknowledgements

This research was completed as part of a wider programme of research within the TRIL Centre, (Technology Research for Independent Living). The TRIL Centre is a multidisciplinary research centre, bringing together researchers from UCD, TCD, NUIG and Intel, funded by Intel, GE and IDA Ireland. http://www.trilcentre.org. The authors would also like to acknowledge the help and support of our colleagues, especially Brian Lawlor, Ben Arent, James Brennan, Vanessa Buckley, Julie Doyle, Ronan McDonnell, Blaithin O'Dea, Simon Roberts, Cormac Sheehan, David Singleton, Chiara Garattini, Zoran Skrba, Susan Squires, Maurice ten Koppel, Flip van den Berg and Ciaran Wynne.

References

[1] S.J. Czaja, J.H. Guerrier, S.N. Nair and T.K. Landauer, Computer communication as an aid to independence for older adults, *Behaviour and Information Technology* **12**(4) (1993), 197–207.
[2] J. de Jong Gierveld and T. Van Tilburg, A 6-item scale for overall, emotional and social loneliness, *Research on Aging* **28**(5) (2006), 582–598.
[3] A. Dickinson, A.F. Newell, M.J. Smith and R.L. Hill, Introducing the Internet to the over-60s: Developing an email system for older novice computer users, *Interacting with Computers* **17**(6) (2005), 621–642.
[4] J. Drennan, M. Treacy, M. Butler, A. Byrne, G. Fealy, K. Frazer and K. Irving, The experience of social and emotional loneliness among older people in Ireland, *Ageing and Society* **28**(8) (2008), 1113–1132.
[5] D.L. Groves and T. Slack, Computers and their application to senior citizens therapy within a nursing home, *Journal of Instructional Psychology* **21**(3) (1994), 221–227.
[6] D. Hawthorn, How universal is good design for older people?, in: *Proceedings of the ACM Conference on Universal Usability*, Vancouver, Canada, 2005, pp. 38–45.
[7] B.J. Holt and R.W. Morrell, Guidelines for web site design for older adults: The ultimate influence of cognitive factors, in: *Older Adults, Health Information and the World Wide Web*, R.W. Morrell, ed., Lawrence Erlbaum Associates, Mahwah, 2002, pp. 109–132.
[8] M. Inoue, A. Suyama, Y. Takeuchi and S. Meshitsuka, Application of a computer based education system for aged persons and issues arising during the field test, *Computer Methods and Progress in Biomedicine* **59**(1) (1999), 55–60.
[9] M.A.R. Tijhuis, J. de Jong-Gierveld, E.J.M. Feskens and D. Kromhout, Changes in and factors related to loneliness in older men: The Zutphen Elderly Study, *Age and Ageing* **28**(5) (1999), 491–495.
[10] S.J. Westerman, D.R. Davies, A.I. Glendon, R.B. Stammers and G. Matthews, Age and cognitive ability as predictors of computerised information retrieval, *Behaviour and Information Technology* **14**(5) (1995), 313–326.
[11] H. White, E. McConnell, E. Clipp, L. Bynum, C. Teage, L. Navas, S. Craven and H. Halbrecht, Surfing the net in later life: A review of the literature and pilot study of computer use and quality of life, *Journal of Applied Gerontology* **18**(3) (1999), 358–378.
[12] J.P. Wherton and D.K. Prendergast, Building Bridges: Involving older adults in the design of comunication technology to support peer-to-peer social engagement, in: *HCI and Usability for E-Inclusion*, A. Holzinger and K. Miesenberger, eds, Springer-Verlag, Berlin, 2009, pp. 111–134.

Handbook of Ambient Assisted Living
J.C. Augusto et al. (Eds.)
IOS Press, 2012

doi:10.3233/978-1-60750-837-3-805

Innovative Rehabilitation Technologies for Home Environments – An Overview

Dr. Michael JOHN[a,*], Stefan KLOSE[a] and Beate SEEWALD[b]
[a] *Fraunhofer Institute for Computer Architecture and Software Technology, Munich, Germany*
[b] *Rehabilitation Center Lübben, Fraunhofer Gesellschaft, Munich, Germany*

Abstract. A significant number of studies show the positive effects clinical rehabilitation programs have on improving patients' health. However, these studies also, often mention that these health benefits decrease if a post-therapeutic regimen is not integrated into a patients' daily routine. Existing barriers such as travel times to sports facilities, irregular working times, caring for family members or a simple lack of desire are reasons why good intentions quickly fade and the aftercare recommendations are not put into practice. The necessary changes in behaviour and in the mind set of a patient that are reached during the clinical rehabilitation process often disappear. The motivation to continue the rehabilitation program at home is low, even if further therapy is necessary for the stabilization of the patients' health. In this paper we describe the need for innovative rehabilitation technologies for home environments after a clinical rehabilitation phase. First we introduce the therapeutic applications like cardiovascular training, fall prevention and stroke rehabilitation as well as the corresponding options for interactive multimedia training devices. After that we describe the stakeholder and system requirements for new prevention and rehabilitation technologies. We give an overview over current projects and ambient technologies enabling health prevention and home rehabilitation. At the end of the paper we argue that these technologies should be integrated into the health systems.

Keywords. Interactive multimedia training devices and applications, assistive technologies for prevention and rehabilitation, telerehabilitation, exergames

Introduction – The Need for a Sustainable Rehabilitation in the Home Environment

The term Rehabilitation takes its origin from the Latin rehabilitatio = 'restoration', and can be translated as 'making fit again'. According to the WHO (World Health Organisation), rehabilitation of people with disabilities is a process aimed at enabling them to reach and maintain their optimal physical, sensory, intellectual, psychological and social functional levels. Rehabilitation provides disabled people with the tools they need to attain independence and self-determination [88].

The essence of medical rehabilitation is the restoration of performance after a serious illness or, in a situation of chronic illness, relearning and balancing skills that had been lost. In order to achieve this goal it is necessary to practice such skills as, for example, personal care, walking, driving a car, shopping, learning and many other activities in a rehabilitation environment. A summary of all rehabilitation activities can be found in the Classification List International Classification of Functioning, Disabilities

*Corresponding Author: Dr. Michael John. E-mail: michael.john@first.fraunhofer.de.

and Health (ICF) [89]. The financing of rehabilitation services is dependent upon national factors. Services related to rehabilitation are closely connected to developments in the labour market and employment policy. In accordance with each country's forms of financing its health system, generally speaking minimal tax resources and/or decreasing premium income are associated with restrictions with respect to rehabilitation services. In addition to acute care and nursing care, medical rehabilitation is part of the health care system that is influenced by the national capacities of each country in question. Numerous different systems of rehabilitative care exist in Europe. The differences according to per capita care between the individual member states are evident [29].

The demographic development in the EU will compel a paradigm shift. In wealthy industrial countries, average life expectancy is rising each century by one year. Increased life expectancy results in the necessity to adapt working lifetime periods. Currently, chronic diseases determine approximately three-fourths of all courses of disease in industrial nations. Within the EU-27, some 25% of employees complain of back pain and some 23% of muscular aches and pain. Musculoskeletal complaints are among the most frequently reported work-related health problems [22]. In view of their effects upon the health of individual employees, musculoskeletal diseases are a definite source of concern. Additionally, the economic effects for companies and the national insurance costs for the European countries are considerable. In the year 2006, altogether all responsible purchasers spent 7,411 billion euros for preventive and rehabilitation services in Germany [80].

Based on the current demographic developments, one can assume for the future that the need for preventive and rehabilitative services will increase significantly. In view of the paucity of available funds, the various states must of necessity make the preventive and rehabilitative services more flexible and reorganise them. It is to be expected that in the future more outpatient instead of inpatient services will be prescribed, and shorter treatment periods, higher personal shares in costs and obligatory private retirement plans for insured persons will commence. The way the current range of rehabilitative options will develop will depend upon the authorisation or responsibility for the provision of the necessary measures. If the employer is legally required to assume part of the risks, for example in case of industrially-related illnesses, this obligation will force preventively oriented industrial health management or the establishment of a system of Disability Managements [16]. The looming shortage of trained personnel is also forcing companies to keep their present employees fit. Where the responsibility for the provision of rehabilitation services lies with social insurance carriers or medical insurance companies, in financially challenged periods they must keep a close eye on budgets, flexibilisation of their range of products and collecting co-payments from the insured. The better the rehabilitation system is developed in a country, the greater will be the pressure in the years to come to make the system affordable. Then the objective will be to offer modularly constructed, cost-efficient therapeutic options over an extended period, including in the home environment, thus ensuring sustainable efficiency in times of stagnating or indeed decreasing financial resources.

Numerous studies have demonstrated that regular, moderate strength and endurance training represents an excellent chance to remain healthy while ageing. The positive effects on the physical and mental wellbeing that patients perceive through quality-secured, multimodal therapy to activate mobility has been demonstrated in studies [19]. The latest results were recently published in the 'Archives of Internal Medicine'. An analysis of the Nurses' Health Study with statistics concerning more than 13,500 women impressively shows that regular mobility training serves not only the individual but also society as a whole by obviating health-related expenses. In total only some 1450 women age healthily, that is to say just less than ten percent. In the group with the highest physical activity the score for healthy ageing was twice as high as in the group with the least activity. Or, in other words: a person that exercises a great deal in his middle years doubles his chances of remaining healthy into his old age. And in this case, a great deal of exercise means swimming or cycling for some five hours per week [81].

Therefore, an individual and personally responsible medical impetus to more exercise and regular monitoring of vital signs has the following positive effects:

Regular and Controlled Fitness and Strength Training Protects Against Cardiorespiratory Diseases

The less fit a person is and the more circulatory risks apply to him, the more he will benefit from a progressive regular programme of physical activity. Not only in terms of prevention but also of therapy, a customised programme of regular physical exercise yields excellent results in the treatment of coronary disease. Intensive physical training will already improve the capacity to repair diseased coronary vessels by improving the inner lining of the arteries after only four weeks.

By now, the effectiveness of physical activity with regard to chronic myocardial insufficiency has also been confirmed: in the ExTraMATCH study with a total of 801 patients, there was noted to be a significant decrease in the relative risk for total morbidity by 35 percent and in the frequency of hospitalization by 28 percent [23].

Special Training Measures Have a Positive Influence on Preventing Falls

That a great deal of exercise has by now been noted to keep people healthy to a even later age as well as possibly saving money, was demonstrated in a study by Dr. Wolfgang Kemmler at the University of Erlangen. In this study, women over 65 years of age were monitored during 18 months of continuous special training in terms of bone density, risk of fall and cardiovascular risk. Of these 246 women, one-half underwent aerobic and balance training (four times a week, a total of 160 minutes per week), the other half a wellness programme. After 18 months, the bone density in the training group was significantly higher (increase of just under two percent) than in the wellness group, and the number of falls was two-thirds fewer. On the cardiovascular risk level alone, determined with the Framingham score, the training had no significant effect [43]. These data are relevant insofar as they make it clear that women can avoid expensive and prognostically unfavourable hip fractures through physical activity.

Improvement of Cognitive Skills

An increasing number of studies is demonstrating that regular moderate endurance training and coordination training can further the brain function of older people. Analyses have shown that physical fitness can determine up to 20 percent of cognitive performance. The group of researchers with Arthur F. Kramer of the Beckman Institute of the University of Illinois used a procedure for measuring brain activity (magnetic resonance tomography) to study the effects of a six-month programme of endurance training (walking programme) on the brain. The results are impressive: the test persons in the endurance programme demonstrated better performance in carrying out the task of goal-directed steering of concentration than those that had only participated in the stretching programme [21].

Wildor Hollmann of the German Sports Academy in Cologne demonstrated that after endurance training, older persons demonstrated a brain activation pattern that was similar to that of younger persons. These results indicated that focused endurance training for older persons – even after a relatively short time – furthers the effective and flexible utilisation of cognitive resources.

A bit more activity can also improve their lives, was the conclusion of a French study at a nursing home with 160 patients that were still able to move and understand simple requests. They could either participate in special Tai Chi exercises, in communication training with balance exercises, or they received only the usual care. After six months, such everyday skills as washing, dressing or using the toilet were significantly better in the two intervention groups than in the control group, while the clearest improvement was observed in the Tai Chi group. This group also demonstrated the fewest behavioural disturbances [18].

Decreasing Depression

The effect that endurance sports have an antidepressive effect has been described for many years. In a project of the University Clinic of Tübingen, physicians were able to prove this fact: in recurrent depression, endurance training led to a release of nerve growth factors that had until then been decreased. For one study, older women with recurrent depression underwent 30 minutes of endurance training on a cycle ergometer. Before and after the stress, the concentration of the nerve growth factor BDNF (brain-derived neurotrophic factor) in the blood, which plays a central role in the development of depression, was measured. It was noted that the BDNF level, in comparison with that of non-depressive women, was decreased prior to the stress. However, the value stabilised in the depressive participants after the stress phase (The International Journal of Neuropsychopharmacology 2010, online). Thus it was first of all possible to show that endurance training normalises the concentration of the nerve growth factor. This could also be the reason why endurance sports have a stabilising and mood-lifting effect on people with depression. Further studies are planned with people with early memory disturbances in old age [50].

Effects on the Health Care Industry

These studies demonstrated impressively that the financeability of the European health care industry in times of a greying society will be considerably dependent upon the extent to which it will be possible to limit avoidable chronic diseases through suitable preventive measures. Ceasing or even simply changing lifelong behavioural patterns of health-threatening living habits is as difficult for the persons concerned as it is for their treating therapists. Setting a 'chronically' lazy society in motion demands, in today's world, an innovative, target group oriented system of incentive system. More personal responsibility must be demanded and supported with bonus systems. However, the most important thing appears to be to awaken the desire to take more exercise.

It could also be demonstrated that these measures have an effect upon such economic parameters as the duration of disablement or the need to use medical services [19]. Nonetheless, in terms of the sustainability of achieved rehabilitation success, the results still show considerable deficits. A regional survey of 1200 projects and scientifically monitored model plans carried out in Germany involving aftercare in rehab carriers and clinics of the national old-age pension fund demonstrated the need for systematically aftercare and the associated reinforcement and lengthening of the health-furthering effects of rehabilitation [46].

Numerous statistical figures show that the rehabilitation success achieved in most patients is used up in most of them by 12 months later at the latest. 48% of those interviewed state that they no longer felt any positive effects of the rehabilitation as early as after three months. The main reasons why the participants did not continue their good intentions such as, for example, more exercise or a healthier diet were explained as: 'No time', 'lacking ambition', 'cannot do it for myself' and 'it's too expensive' [26]. Infrastructural weakness in structurally weak areas or a shortage of persons in the area that support changed living habits can explain why offers were not utilised and many patients lacked sufficient perseverance. This is why, in this context, viable alternatives must be found that are suitable for overcoming such barriers. Sports activities can decrease the recurrence of back pain and pain in the neck-shoulder area. In order to be effective, activity should, however, comprise intensive exercises and be repeated at least three times a week.

As numerous studies have shown, willingness to pay for health services increases with rising income. The more a person earns, the more prepared he is to spend money on his health. Indeed, certain studies have concluded that willingness to pay rises disproportionately [17]. Subsequent to demographic developments, medical-technical progress and the increased awareness of health the demand for products and services in prevention, therapy and care are increasing rapidly (cf. Ill. 1 Development of Health Expenditures in Germany). Linked to this are tremendous innovative and value added potentials in the health care sector.

In Germany two examples of success have shown how people from all areas of the population can be encouraged to exercise more. 'Telegymnastics' in the West of Germany and 'Medicine by notes' in the East of Germany resulted in living rooms being converted to fitness rooms for the first time in the 1970s. Four decades later, hosts of (formerly) sluggish 'couch potatoes' have begun to rise from their sofas in order to outdo even themselves by way of such suitable physical exercise as slalom skiing. As of 31 December 2009, Nintendo announced that 9.6 Wii owners in Europe had purchased one of the two training programmes Wii Fit or Wii Fit Plus. Wii Fit Plus has been available in Europe since October 2009 and supplements Wii Fit by a few new exercises and features [59]. This type of exercise involves no financial contributions at all on the part of statutory health insurers and motivates the end user, as an extra benefit, to adopt behaviour more beneficial to health even without the usual exercises.

However, studies with the Wii have shown that this type of training support only motivates sufficiently at the beginning. Imprecise measurements, the lack of monitoring of movement, the fear of doing something wrong and exhausting commentary decrease the fun of the game or the exercise even after a relatively short time [40]. To reinforce sustainability, therefore, systems are called for that offer medically efficient exercise programmes, provide an optimised exercise analysis, therapeutic support and facilitate monitoring of the vital signs. Incorrectly carried out exercises can be more damaging, in the long run, than they are useful.

1. Areas of Application for Multimedia Rehabilitation and Prevention

Some of the most challenging focal topics and themes in Europe at the moment include healthy ageing, prevention research, nursing care research, research related to the care of the chronically ill and patient orientation, innovative assistance in rehabilitation and for the disabled, barrier-free living and the sustainable integration of disabled persons

[15]. Interactive, multimedia training applications are intrinsically suitable in the context of health care services. The opportunities lie in holistic solutions. This will ensure that interactive multimedia training applications can be utilised both in the clinical environment and the residential one, and guarantee seamless transition from inpatient to outpatient care in everyday life.

Table 1. Application areas for interactive multimedia training environments

Type of health service	Options for interactive multimedia training applications
Outpatient/inpatient rehabilitation In the context of outpatient or inpatient rehabilitation, the patient receives treatment tailored to his individual current needs including, in addition to physiotherapy and psychological monitoring, various types of training, advisory services for his relatives and the prescription of medications and other auxiliary medical supplies. Clients for these services can be old age pension schemes, national insurance companies, accident insurers or sole or joint liability companies. Treatment can be implemented in outpatient rehabilitation facilities closest to the patient's residence in special rehabilitation clinics, nursing homes or acute care hospitals. Depending on the indication and degree of severity of the case, treatment can last from 2 weeks to several months.	In this phase, interactive multimedia training equipment can be used for documentation, proof of training results and to offer additional training units (treatment location room). Patients are familiarised with the use of such equipment. During follow-up care in a home setting the patients can maintain contact to the physicians or other patients. There are options for application in • Physiotherapy • Sports therapy • Psychology • Occupational therapy • Health training
Geriatric rehabilitation Geriatric rehab facilities are particularly equipped for multimorbid patients. Geriatric rehabilitation is available both on an in- and outpatient basis. According to individual requirements, geriatric rehabilitation can comprise such measures as the following: continuous medical diagnostics, activating therapeutic care, physiotherapy, exercise and occupational therapy, speech therapy (neuro-)psychological and psychotherapeutic treatment and social counselling. In addition to preventing dependency on care, the goal of geriatric rehabilitation is to help older people achieve or maintain the greatest possible degree of independence despite their illnesses and limitations [6].	Interactive multimedia training support can be used in order to support frequently recurring treatment routines or medical assessments. The barrier-free operability of such devices is the first requirement. Increasing training motivation and the option of the documentation of training results are particularly important aspects in order to increase self-motivation. Useful training support is required for • Exercises on muscle build-up • Coordination exercises • Speech therapy • Mental fitness training
Mobile rehabilitation Mobile rehabilitation is a new, future-oriented concept in outpatient rehabilitation close to the patient's home. Outpatients receive rehabilitation services from an interdisciplinary team (physiotherapy, occupational therapy, speech therapy and social counselling) under medical supervision based on previously established rehabilitation planning, in their own home environment). In his own familiar surroundings, the patient no longer need face the difficult task of dealing with the familiarisation and transfer processes encountered upon their transition from inpatient rehab to home rehab. Based on its resource-oriented and socio-ecologic approach, home visit therapy reaches people requiring rehabilitation that had up to then not yet benefited from any rehab measures or that cannot receive optimal care by means of other forms of rehabilitation [38].	In terms of time, therapy with an existing actual therapist is clearly limited in terms of mobile rehabilitation. The time frame of one session to the next could be optimally used with independent training under controlled conditions. Interactive multimedia training support should be developed that support motion and strength training on an individual basis. The barrier-free operability of such devices is the first requirement. Increasing the training motivation and the option of documenting training results are particular important aspects. Useful training support is necessary for • Exercises to build up muscle • Exercises to improve fitness • Coordination exercises • Speech therapy • Health courses • Mental fitness training

Table 1. (Continued)

Type of health service	Options for interactive multimedia training applications
Mobile geriatric rehabilitation Mobile geriatric rehab is a special form of outpatient geriatric rehab. It is provided by an interdisciplinary team in the home environment. Mobile geriatric rehabilitation differentiates itself from other forms of rehabilitation by such facts as that it treats the older person in his familiar surroundings. The number of days of treatment is generally up to 20, and per treatment day in terms of all measures the patient receives an average of at least 2 therapy units [76].	In the context of mobile geriatrics, therapy with an actually present therapist is clearly limited in terms of time. The time frame from one session of therapy to the next could be optimally used with independent training under controlled conditions. Interactive, multimedia training support should be developed that can individually support movement and strength training. The barrier-free operability of such devices is the first requirement. Increasing training motivation and the option of documenting training results are particularly important aspects. Useful training support is required for • Exercises to build up muscle • Exercises to improve fitness • Coordination exercises • Speech therapy • Health courses • Mental fitness training
Rehab sports Rehabilitative sports is useful for disabled people or those at risk to become disabled in order to integrate them into society and the employment environment, if possible in the long term, in the context of the specific tasks of the current rehabilitation provider. Rehab sports comprise exercises provided in a group in the context of regularly held exercise events in suitably equipped facilities under the supervision of qualified therapists. Rehab sports help people help themselves and aims to motivate them with regard to long-term, independent exercise training under their own responsibility [67].	Participation in Rehab sports presupposes the mobility of participants. Often relatives requiring care have family obligations such as child care; they have no transportation options or professional obligations that stand in the way of regular participation in rehab sports. In these cases the use of interactive, multimedia training systems could at least facilitate remote participation in training.
Activating care Activating care means more than simply mobilising patients; another of its goals is to make them as independent of the therapist as possible. The resident of a nursing facility is to have the feeling that he is receiving guidance – not that he is dependent. To begin with this concerns advice, instruction and support. Activating care is understood to mean ordinary nursing care that furthers the autonomy and independence of the patient. It considers the capacities of the patient so that he can be active on his own while receiving supervision and motivation. The goal is to acquire or restore the independence of the person receiving care. The patient receives assistance in becoming able to carry out personal care activities or reactivate skills that have been lost.	Assistance systems that helps the person concerned remain independent for as long as possible, preferably to live in his own home environment are also useful in terms of activating care. In the context of activating care, the use of assistance systems could be facilitated and an introduction could follow. Passive support can offer • Strength improvement (stand-up aids, walkers etc.) • Feedback mechanisms (warning signal when devices are not switched off, open doors, reminders to take medicines etc.) • Speech recognition and analysis • Intensification of sensory perception (hearing aids, visual aids, optical warning of hot and cold, colour recognition; Activating support can offer • Interactive multimedia training equipment for muscle build-up, increasing physical condition, fitness Visual and auditory communication aids to participate in a social life

Table 1. (Continued)

Type of health service	Options for interactive multimedia training applications
Functional training Functional training is a choice for the disabled and those at risk of becoming disabled in order to integrate them into society and the employment environments bearing in mind the specific tasks of the current rehabilitation provider, if possible for a long-term perspective. Functional training may be indicated particularly in instances of illness or functional limitation of the organs of support and mobility. The effects of functional training, particularly using the resources of physiotherapy and/or occupational therapy, focus on the specific bodily structures (muscles, joints etc.). of a person that is disabled or at risk of becoming disabled. Functional training comprises exercises provided in a group in the context of regularly held exercise events in suitably equipped facilities under the supervision of qualified (physio-) therapists. Functional training also includes practice in joint protection measures and the use of technical aids and objects utilised in daily life. Functional training helps people help themselves and aims to motivate them with regard to long-term, independent exercise training under their own responsibility [67].	In the context of function training, the use of interactive, multimedia training applications is above all useful in the interest of continuing additional therapy units outside the personal therapeutic sessions independently in the home environment under supervision. In this type of setting the focus lies above all on the monitoring of movements, the documentation of training results and the support of training motivation.
Workplace health promotion Workplace Health Promotion (BGF) comprises all joint measures of employers, employees and society for the improvement of health and wellbeing at the workplace. This can be achieved by linking the following approaches: improving the organisation of work and working conditions, encouraging active employee participation, reinforcing personal competencies [51]. Numerous large companies and administrations have signed the Luxembourger Declaration in the last few years and committed themselves to active realisation of its contents [84]. In Germany protection against work-related threats to health is anchored in the SGB (German Social Security Code) VII as a task of national health insurers. The SGB V obliges medical insurance companies in § 20 to provide services on behalf of primary prevention. In Germany, industrial health care is also financially supported by the federal government. Certain services are tax-free up to the sum of € 500 per employee and calendar year.	This relatively new form of improving health offers numerous options for the application of interactive multimedia training devices. Prevention is the core concept. The main goal is the prevention of missed work due to illness. Therein lies the predominant interest of the company. Multimedia, interactive training applications can establish a link between training workplace and training location. Training facilities independent in terms of time and location facilitate access to fitness services.

These possible areas of application areas for interactive, multimedia training systems show the relevance and importance of new rehabilitation services for the ageing society. Nevertheless anyone seeking innovative ideas or already involved in the development of a prototype should free himself of the usual cliché of old or disabled persons in wheelchairs. Many conditions and handicaps not always visible to others at first glance are accompanied by pain that is similarly invisible to the outside world. Most of these conditions concern the motor system. As is the case with respiratory diseases, allergies and serious obesity, psychologically-oriented limitations are becoming increasingly prevalent. Causes of chronic conditions are frequently accidents, injuries at birth, congenital diseases, old age or acute illness. Usually these conditions arise at least during middle to late adulthood. Hereinafter we shall use some case studies to clarify the broad spectrum and the complexity of possible indications for rehabilitation services:

Case Study 1. Rehabilitation After Hip Surgery

After years of constant worsening of her health condition, with severe pain every day, a 70-year old female suffering from osteoarthritis of the hip joint underwent total hip arthroplasty. At the time of the operation she could neither walk, bathe, nor, at the very last, even shower on her own anymore. She had long been unable to tie her shoes. With only slippers on her feet, she no longer wished to leave her home. Additionally, taking pain medication affected her ability to drive. The car stayed in the garage. She visited her doctor by taxi, and occasional shopping for groceries was one of her only activities outside her home. She suffering increasingly from loneliness. Mrs K underwent surgery in October. The operation was without complications. The postoperative programme planned by the acute clinic in collaboration with the rehabilitation facility comprised a 3-week course of inpatient rehabilitation in a specialised orthopaedic clinic. The follow-up programme for her everyday life was to include physical exercises for at home that would enable her to function without restriction both inside and outside her home within the medium term. Back at home, despite her good intentions Mrs K found it difficult to carry out the recommended exercises. She had already forgotten many of them. She felt increasingly uncertain as to whether she was doing the exercises correctly. She missed the instructions, the encouraging words and also the strictly followed therapeutic plan that she had learned to appreciate more and more during her rehab admission. After only a few weeks she returned to her family practitioner who finally prescribed therapy for her and referred her to a physiotherapist. Despite an urgent desire to be once more capable of living independently in her own four walls, Mrs K found herself unable to continue her training programme without additional support. Her case called for a monitored, barrier-free interactive multimedia follow-up programme for every day was to help her sustainably improve the rehabilitation results that she had achieved. Using easy messaging tools could help to stay in contact with her physiotherapist.

Case Study 2. Rehabilitation After Leg Amputation Associated with Type II Diabetes Mellitus

Mr O, employee, 55 years old with Type II diabetes mellitus and a gangrenous foot had his leg amputated at the tibia. The treating physician explained to the changes the patient would experience postoperatively and, specifically, post-amputation. Dr G told him about the experience of other patients that had encountered postoperative problems with their equilibrium, dealing with their altered self-image and being confronted with sensory changes. She also explained the increased risk of possible wound healing problems due to the diabetes mellitus. She presented numerous possibilities for dealing with these matters and advised him at length to take the time for comprehensive rehabilitation. While still in the acute clinic, Mr O received physiotherapeutic therapy and prophylactic measures were taken against thrombosis and contractures. Bandages were used to help establish a functional amputation stump and to reduce any possible stump oedema. Mr O first attempted to walk postoperatively using a provisional prosthesis while still in the acute care clinic. During his inpatient rehabilitation period, his leg was measured with a view to a permanent prosthesis. The rehabilitation physician discussed various therapeutic measures with him (physiotherapy, occupational therapy, gait training, coordination exercises, dietary advice etc.) and consulted with him to formulate a therapeutic goal. Mr O's greatest wish was to be able to practice his profession again. With this in mind, in principle he was prepared to agree to a stringent exercise programme and change the unhealthy lifestyle he had led up to that time. Without assistance, he agreed, he would not achieve his therapeutic goal. In the context of his discharge examination following inpatient rehabilitation, he told the physician about his concern that he would lack the motivation when back at home alone to continue his exercises properly. Without therapeutic support, he felt he would probably not make it. What he would most appreciate would be sporadic continued follow-up by his treating therapists.

These examples demonstrate that the course of rehabilitation can be long and drawn out as well as intensive in terms of their effects upon the personality. In general, the more time and therapy units are at the disposal of a patient, the better rehabilitation results can be anticipated. Considerations of efficiency, in particular, are a clear argument in favour of using multimedia, interactive therapeutic intervention with the potential to achieve sustainable rehabilitation results. In the following chapter we discuss the user and system requirements for such therapeutic applications.

2. Stakeholder and System Requirements for New Prevention and Rehabilitation Technologies

The demands of individual user groups (stakeholders) derive from the realms of application of rehabilitation technologies. These demands can be classified and weighted in terms of individual end user groups (patients, therapists, physicians, relatives). In the context of a user-centred development process, technical system requirements can be derived from these in a second step.

Some studies show that interactive multimedia training environments for the motor and equilibrium training of patients with brain injuries and older people are equally effective and they help support the healing process. An American study by Maureen and Holder shows, for example, that virtual exercises are just as effective for the motor and equilibrium training of patients with brain injuries and older people, and that they support the healing process [34]. In a case study concerning virtual training of the upper extremities post-CVA it became clear that patients tolerate this type of training very well and, in addition, it leads to significant improvement in motor skills both in the virtual and the real world [83]. The Results also showed that patients tolerate this type of training very well and it leads to significant improvement in their motor skills in both the virtual and the real world

Studies have indeed demonstrated that energy and calorie consumption during active computer games, such as the Wii Fit, is significantly greater than during traditional game environments [11,28]. A study by Mellecker et al., that assessed calorie consumption by comparing traditional and activating games based on the system XaviX J-Mat, came to similar conclusions [54]. The American College of Sports Medicine (ACSM) and the American Heart Association (AHA) have stated that increasing units of balance exercises with the Wii Balance Board are suitable for training the perception of the body and thus decreasing the threat of falling in people over 60 years of age [30].

A study of persons using Wii Fit involved aspects of weight reduction and calorie consumption. Although indeed, on a worldwide level it is a fact that a high potential degree of willingness to participate in activating games (approximately 100 million game programmes sold) using the technical platforms of the game company, it must be said limitatively that thus far only a few significant studies have been carried out that would justify its use for medical purposes alone. A study in the British Medical Journals shows that, in any case, Wii-tennis does not represent a substitute for the actual game of tennis [14]. Scott Owens, Professor of Health and Exercise at the University of Mississippi, carried out a study with eight families to determine whether Nintendo' Wii Fit has a positive effect on fitness. The study lasted for 6 months and the families were monitored in a three-month cycle (each family used the device for three months). The study demonstrated that young people can profit most from the Wii Fit, since the greatest improvements in terms of overall fitness are demonstrated in them. In older and heavier family members the Nintendo Wii Fit leads to fewer changes or indeed no changes at all. It appeared that the families became bored with the games over the course of the study. In the first month and a half, family members spent an average of 22 minutes of game time with the Nintendo Wii Fit, whereas in the course of the study this time went down to a scant four minutes [72].

In order to determine which criteria and technical demands should be applied to game-based, interactive therapeutic support on behalf of the increased efficiency of rehabilitative measures, a study was carried out at the Rehab Centre Lübben, a specialised clinic for orthopaedics and oncology, involving a total of 60 patients over a period from 2007 through 2009 [40]. During their inpatient rehabilitation admissions, patients chosen during a random sampling underwent specific exercises to build up the muscles using a conventional footstepper or a balanceboard of Nintendo's Wii in their rooms twice a day, independently.

Based on empirical data, the question was explored of to what extent the technical and motivational functions of the Wii are sufficient to guarantee efficient and valid follow-up in terms of rehabilitation measures in the home environment. An analysis determined whether willingness to carry out muscle-strengthening exercises in the home environment using games with real-time visualisation of exercises could be increased, thus improving training results as a whole. To establish and evaluate the data, a combined quantitative/qualitative approach was chosen. In addition to measuring efficiency (improved muscular strength through biodex measurements) after an interview patients completed a quantitative and qualitative questionnaire.

The assumption that training results achieved with the Wii Fit differentiated positively in comparison with training results achieved by the footstepper group could not be confirmed based on examinations. Biodex measurements of improvement in muscular strength showed better results, on the whole, for participants in the stepper group. On closer perusal, however, it was noted that participants that said they exercised minimally or more actively using the Wii training device achieved results that were equal to, or better than, those of participants in the footstepper group. People that did not practice sports showed significantly better training results after muscle strength measurement having used the conventional footstepper, although those that exercised with the Wii generally demonstrated an average of 30% longer training time. This result demonstrates that while indeed motivation to exercise definitely increased for people using the Wii, the correct implementation of exercises is, nonetheless not optimally supported. People with a good sense of their bodies can apparently compensate for this deficiency. The 'anti-sports' group apparently require goal-oriented training support demanding precise exercise monitoring.

In summary, the abovementioned study results yield significant specifications for product design for multimedia, interactive training support systems suitable for rehabilitation and prevention.

2.1. Demands of Patients and Family Members

Being personally seen and able to perceive oneself as competent are significant building blocks of successful rehabilitation. These criteria should be applied in the establishment of a telemedical rehab application. Here it frequently applies that several target-group specific environments must be established for one and the same training programme. Even early consideration of such aspects as gender, age, social status or migration background contributes considerably to the rehabilitative success. Therefore, these interfaces must be adapted to age, degree of physical disablement and preferred design style of user groups. This should be borne in mind during the conception of training programmes, interfaces and the development of a multimedia environment and audio design.

From the point of view of the end user a predominant goal is to carry out rehabilitation exercises in the home environment to minimise the time necessary to visit a physician or therapist. Indeed, however, in this context contact should be maintained with the physio- or sports therapist. Similarly, study participants wanted their therapists to correct them in terms of the way they carried the exercises and assist them in establishing and adapting training units.

Because the use of computers and games is entirely new for most of the – above all older – study participants, the exercise device must be easy to operate and barrier-free, this is to say it must not have any cables, components over which one might trip, etc. Menus and text fields should be clearly organised and easily legible (in large print). Just as important is that the user not be cognitively overloaded by too many information and measurement devices or excessive demands placed on him through an overly complicated system of dealing with input devices.

Illustrating movements in a 'multimedia environment', for example with the aid of an avatar, should be feasible and realistic. The documentation of training units is helpful to the user in order for him to visualise success. The possibility of visualising one's results and one's own progress was important to everyone interviewed.

Every person brings along different requirements when it comes to training therapy. In this context therapy and training programmes must be adaptable to individual considerations. Individual therapeutic recommendations are based on a combination of therapeutic background knowledge and patient history. Generally applicable therapeutic recommendations, as one sees, for example, with the Wii Fit, represent more uncertainty than assistance. Beyond this, therapy in terms of stated medical criteria must be adapted to the individual performance capacity of the patient.

In the context of the interviews, the answers of everyone interviewed made it clear that they wished the game characters, combined with joint game and competitive situations, to be associated with unique and positive charm because, in the long run, these characters were actually the impetus for additional training units. The integration of patient training can also have a positive effect on motivation. Recognisable links between exercise, relaxation, nutrition, mental fitness and stress are a significant building block in the interest of a healthy lifestyle.

Most patients felt particularly positive regarding the transfer of exercise data to their treating facility, for example in order for the course of therapy to be professionally monitored. Some of them could imagine making these data available to medical insurance companies, for example in order to be allowed to participate in bonus programmes. Possible sanctions on behalf of the assessibility of individual training programmes such as, for example, no share in costs, were viewed by some as an explicit impetus for training.

2.2. Demands of Therapists and Physicians

In order to take the broadest possible view of the theme, interviews and questionnaires were implemented with therapists. The goal was to establish their view of the demands upon telemedical remote monitoring by way of a sensory-based multimedia training programme. An interview guideline comprising 21 open questions was developed for the interviews, which would serve for the ongoing establishment of demands upon a telemedical rehab programme. From the point of view of physicians and therapists, the following demands on the system have been established.

Treatment success realised on an inpatient basis is to be secured in a sustainable manner by continuing constructive therapy in the home environment. Therapy in the home environment can, nonetheless, only develop its full positive effect if a training device is recommended by a trusted therapist and its initial introduction effected by a therapist. In this way the patient is already familiar with the device when he begins using it at home. An introduction and initial exercises under supervision also help prevent beginners' errors.

It appears to be a prevailing wish of physiotherapists and sports therapists to maintain contact with their patients after inpatient therapy, insofar as they can indeed integrate such additional monitoring work into their shifts and working days. In order to optimally integrate patients into the treatment process, it is of great significance that they be given a feeling of security and therapeutical guidance. This requires clear specifications in the form of therapy goals that can ideally be agreed upon in advance in consultation with the patients and which are monitored by supervising therapists. To evaluate the correctness of exercises that have been carried, the steps of that exercise must be precisely illustrated and the therapist must be able to intervene to make corrections. Medical or therapeutic specialists must be able to prescribe the exercises. Documentation of training results must be available for the perusal of the user and the therapist.

For therapists, it is of utmost importance that they be able to establish such basic parameters of a course of training as the number of repetitions, the patient's recovery phases and the course of his heart rate. The user should also have the option of setting the recovery phases himself. Measuring such vital parameters as the pulse is important in order to determine how much stress is being placed upon the patient. Similarly useful for therapists are scales for self-assessment of the personal condition to help them evaluate how the patient feels during exercise at home. Based on their knowledge and experience, physiotherapists feel confident enough to assess a patient's condition by taking his pulse and making video recordings of the course of exercise. This means that values in terms of strength need not be measured immediately.

Stated to represent a sensory measure with a high degree of acceptance was the visual sensor, possibly even in combination with a pressure mat on which isometric measurements could be carried out. Therapists assess the degree of acceptance of a sensor near their body, such as for example a t-shirt or a training outfit, as relatively low on the part of patients, since this would involve a preparatory phase prior to every training unit. Additionally the advantage of additional sensors was not recognised, if one could already determine the correctness of exercise performed by means of visual information. Therapists did, however, consider it important that the visual sensor take measurements continually during training.

In response to the question of how frequent direct contact between therapist and patient should be after the latter's discharge from an inpatient rehabilitation facility in order to guarantee smooth continuation of his training in the home environment, physiotherapists agreed that to begin with there should be close control time intervals between 3 and 6 days. Later two- to four-week contact was considered to be sufficient. However, the patient must have the option of receiving immediate answers to any questions he might have, and solutions to any problems, from the treating physiotherapist. Email was listed as the preferred contact medium, which one could read in the course of a workday and then integrate into his workday for example by telephone during the course of the day. Physiotherapists considered communication by videoconferencing to be particularly effective. The advantage of this form of communication is that patients can be coached and supervised directly in front of a TV screen.

Training results can be documented both in the home environment and the clinic. For the presentation of data, therapists envisage a preliminary evaluation first, for example the deviation of actual values from normative values. It would, however, be a challenge to establish a dependable standard exercise sample, since individual exercise patterns differ considerably from one another.

Therapists considered a notification function a useful tool for them that could be activated at any time that an actual value of the patient dropped below the target value. Thus one could control remotely whether a patient is even doing the exercises at all and, in this case, if necessary take suitable measures to motivate him. In the home environment, the living area in front of the television is considered to be the best location for a training device.

Therapists stated that they were prepared to assume responsibility for telemedical monitoring if the system offered the specified control and intervention mechanisms. Additionally, they consider it a relevant condition that the patient use the device correctly and regularly and not carry out any exercises that the therapist cannot monitor. Therapists were interested in the possibility of also having contact with the treating physician using an electronic patient dossier, for example to use supplementary measurements to determine the vital capacity of the patient or initiate additional EKG or lactate measurements. Therapists found it equally interesting to receive information on medication values, for example when a treating orthopaedist administers pain medication, reflecting the condition of the patient.

2.3. Demands of Medical Insurance Companies and Insurers

Of supreme important to medical insurance companies and insurers is the increase in sustainability of rehabilitation results that have been achieved. In the context of rehabilitation, the purchaser has striven for the conceptual anchoring of the bio-psychosocial model of components of health in everyday clinical practice, whereby the social environment or the family members should be included in terms of their co-therapeutic function.

At the 4th National Congress for Rehabilitation and Participation of the BAR on 7 November 2007 in Nuremberg, Professor Schwartz of the Medical Academy in Hannover made the statement that 'in follow-up care, based on the limited rehabilitative competency of physicians there is a clear potential for improvement'. This statement indicates that in Germany, no comprehensive quality-assured rehab competency exists amongst physicians. This makes it all the more important that the therapeutic module for the home environment be organised such that quality assurance can be guaranteed through the treating rehabilitation facilities.

In comparison with such other follow-up care programmes as IRENA [39] or prevention programmes of medical insurance companies, the system must demonstrate a favourable price/performance ratio. Offers of services in the home environment must be oriented to prices that are paid for similar outpatient rehabilitation offers. The expenditures that, in total, are available for rehabilitation from old-age insurers have a ceiling. In terms of demographics it must be possible in the future to guarantee more services for more people at equal, possibly lower costs while maintaining the same high level of quality [10]. The quality of results and the sustainability of rehabilitation measures will be the predominant driving factors in this context.

Therapeutic modules must meet medical and therapeutic standards. For balancing with providers of services it must be possible to document therapy units that have been carried out. The measurement of results, registration and documentation of courses of exercise and practice must be guaranteed. Without this information, the correct implementation of therapeutical units in terms of the correctness of execution and regularity of training cannot be determined. Tele-Rehab would be, similarly to other follow-up care offers (IRENA, Reha-Sport etc.) a professional medical service according to SGB IX, for which quality assurance is urgently necessary. The documentation of services is a fixed component of quality assurance. To lower costs, therapeutic devices might possibly be conceived as lease models.

A few medical insurance companies have already set out on this route of new, innovative forms of medical care. For example, the company Barmer Ersatzkasse is currently offering a module on mobile fitness. For the chest belt required for this the insured person must pay 93 euros one time and pay an annual fee of 66 euros. A link to bonus programmes as per the specifications of the BEK might be possible [8].

2.4. Demands on the User Interface and the Technical System

According to information from Deutschen Rentenversicherung (German old-age pension) some 60 % of all therapeutic services fall in the category of exercise therapy. Recording movements is the key to the success of an interactive training programme. To record the correctness of movements, suitable sensors such as visual, pressure or motion sensors must be used. Such sensors must be as precise as possible to document the correctness of movement in an exercise. To increase the accurate perception of body movements a real-time correction is required to point out indications of erroneous movement. Only immediate feedback demonstrates strengths and weaknesses. In the interest of maintaining motivation, the illustrations should take place in a motivating environment that can be used both on a mobile and stationary basis.

A sensor close to the body, however, is only acceptable in the clinical realm and for focused training of relatively minimal courses of motion. In the home environment the placement of an additional sensory unit is difficult for most patients to handle. This also applies to the registration of vital signs, insofar as patients are not already using a body near sensor over the long term.

In the interest of the dependable registration of movement, in some instances a combination of several different types of sensors is required. It must be borne in mind that the sensors are to be used not in a laboratory environment but in a home environment by lay persons. Therefore, sensors must not be attuned to special environmental conditions that are not common to the home environment. A camera-based recording of the course of motions without contact with the body offers optimal conditions for training at home. Indeed supplementary sensory materials are likelier to be accepted if they are integrated into already familiar objects such as therapy and training devices. Additionally, they offer an excellent opportunity to make a programme of exercise varied.

Software must be capable of analysing data from various sensors in real time, if necessary merging them and interpreting them. For this, special algorithms adapted to the context of motion recognition must be developed. In order to be able to evaluate the correctness of movements during exercise, motion models must be available that permit normative-actual comparisons.

Both the exercises to be carried out and the actual movements of the person being rehabilitated must be visualised. This can be done with the aid of 3D avatars or videos of the physicians. There must be audiovisual information about deviations from the norm. The possibility of joint virtual group exercise is also conceivable in this aspect.

The user interface must be constructed simply and attractively and be intuitively useable. The manner in which patients experience the feedback mechanisms through sensory and multimedia presentation devices lays the cornerstones for long-term use of the system.

The use of the TV as a presentation device for reproduction proves advantageous because it involves a cost-effective device that is available in virtually all households and is also suitable for small residential units. It is easy to ensure that the system is convenient to handle in terms of its everyday use. It must be easy to handle the remote control for programme operation. Ideally, additional devices or sensors should have plug-and-play functions according to the motto 'plug in, switch on, take off'.

Training devices for the home environment will probably have to be financed by patients for the most part. For this reason, particular attention should be paid to the durability, appearance and handling of the hardware to be used, including in order to achieve the necessary user acceptance. Expenditures should not lie above the normal commercial prices that are paid for TV games such as the Wii Fit. Optionally the devices should also be usable on the basis of a lease model.

As is the case regarding the correction of movements, the visualisation of results of movement and the measurement of vital signs yield a learning effect in terms of body perception. They must be understandable to the physiotherapist and/or physician and, if indicated, comply with medical standards in terms of visualisation. Additionally, an instrument for achieving the goal, for example in the form of an intermediate result (training performance) would be a direct instrument of motivation for the continuation of training and therapy units.

Training measures must usually be implemented daily over an extended period. After a while exercises will become boring. This monotony can be broken by way of so-called 'serious games'. By integrating structured and target group oriented serious games into the application logic of a therapy module, frequently abstract, faraway therapeutic goals can be translated into entirely concrete goals achieved during a single therapeutic session.

An integrated notification system is important. For example, the option of image telephony can help maintain direct contact with a familiar therapist. For example, such an audiovisual communication option as telephony can serve to maintain contact with the monitoring therapist or former fellow patients. This ensures a comfortable atmosphere and the often necessary training pressure.

All medical and personal data set high demands in terms of data protection. In this context, tele-rehabilitation systems must meet stringent security requirements and protect against access by outsiders or the divulgence of training and therapy data.

3. Ambient Technologies Enabling Health Prevention and Home Rehabilitation

Recently, there has been increasing demand for telemedical applications for activity monitoring and rehabilitation with the aid of multimedia technologies. These innovative, multimedia, sensor-based forms of training and therapy have in principle brought about the option of transferring rehabilitation and prevention measures to the home environment. In rough terms, here one can differentiate sub-systems used on a mobile or stationary (or ambient) basis. For the activation of movement in daily life or in rehabilitation there are purely mechanical systems such as, for example, the home or cycle trainer, as well as an increasing number of telemedical applications for monitoring movement in daily life or, as a mobile accompaniment to physical training, using the mobile phone.

3.1. Conventional Training Devices

In clinical rehabilitation facilities and physiotherapeutic practices, various mechanical training devices are used that are suitable for supporting physio- and pain therapy. Topping this list might be that of Medical Training Therapy (MTT) [44]. Medical training therapy is a form of therapy that accompanies a patient from the beginning of his rehabilitation programme onward. It offers the option of activating motion patterns, initiating functional patterns, effecting mobilisation in the sense of auto-mobilisation, exercising patients to build muscular endurance and muscular strength and improving muscle function in the sense of coordination. The goal is clear improvement in muscular and physical capacity in the professional and sports areas.

The MTT provides particular motivation for many patients, because the increase in innate capacity can be impressively experienced and showcased not only in terms of an increase in strength and endurance but also, and above all, in terms of improvement in general coordinative skills on the exercise devices used. As a patient, one can always objectively evaluate his own level of performance and its development using the MTT. Such stress parameters as stimulation density, intensity and duration can be dosed precisely with the MTT according to the scientific criteria of training theory and adapted to the training goal of therapy. Herein lie the significant advantages in comparison with traditional methods of physiotherapy, such as for example strength exercises with manual counter-pressure.

These rehab training devices have nothing in common with the technically simplest strength machines, as these are generally used in fitness studios. It requires considerable know-how to work with these devices. Particularly complex and cost-intensive devices such as, for example, the Biodex [12] are able to visualise and document training results. As a rule, these devices are quite well accepted by patients. Their disadvantages lie particularly therein that their cost makes them unsuitable for home use, as does their considerable weight and space requirements and the complexity of their use.

On the health market, particularly in the area of wellness, one can find numerous aides with the objective to equip the fitness fan with modern, trendy technical tools. For building up muscles, vibration devices have been on the open market since 1996. A person using these can stand on a platform and undergo comprehensive training of both the extremities and the trunk musculature. The terms *Whole Body Vibration (WBV), Vibration Training, Acceleration Training* and *Stochastic Resonance Training* have been applied to training with this group of devices. There have been numerous studies concerning vibration training, usually involving quite small groups of subjects or patient groups. The vibration technology of Galileo [27] or PowerPlate [66] is hotly debated in professional circles. The absence of activating components is a weak point of this technology. Many of these fitness devices are left forgotten in a corner after a brief period of use. They frequently prove unsuitable for integrated use in various areas of life, such as for example at home, in rehabilitation facilities or during sports.

The reason for this is above all the fact that the existing systems are isolated solutions that exist without linkage to one another and encompass no motivating feedback properties. The devices prescribe the course of motion, and monitoring and remote management by therapists and physicians is not possible, nor do they possess options for a link to a community.

3.2. Mobile Systems

To evaluate daily and motion activities, a series of technologies exists that are already available on the market today. Some standard ones include the new pedometers and activity meters from such companies as Omron Medical Engineering or Aipermon. The module AiperMotion [2] from the German company Aipermon is used to assess daily motions. A small motion detector is attached to the belt. It contains a sensor that continuously measures acceleration in all three directions in space. These smallest movements allow the calculation of the nature and intensity of motion and compare this with stored motion samples. Additionally, the pedometer Walking Style Pro [62] calculates individual calorie and fat burning. With the Beurer AS50, the Beurer Company has placed a type of device on the market that brings together many functions in the form of a small wrist watch: pedometer, calorie consumption, fat burning, activity time, and distance and feedback mechanisms such as a smiley face that displays how the exercise has gone. For purposes of evaluation, data can be transmitted with the aid of software on the PC [78]. For persons involved in extreme sports such as, for example, triathletes, with such exercise scenarios as swimming, cycling and running, the Forerunner 310XT by Garmin provides a GPS-capable training tool that also records distance, step and heart rate, performance data during cycling and running sports, and then wirelessly transmits these data to a computer. If the Forerunner 310XT is coupled with an optional wireless heart frequency sensor, the device constantly records heartbeats per minute and uses the heart rate for a more detailed calculation of calorie consumption [24].

Outdoors, localisation via the GPS is now state-of-the-art, and it will be expanded in the future by Galileo localisation system. Indoors, the GPS signal is compromised to such an extent through ceilings and walls that it can no longer be utilized. For this reason, other localisation methods must be used (such as infrared, Bluetooth, RFID, WLAN). To detect motion, so-called acceleration sensors (accelerometer/gyroscope) are used. Suitable commercially available acceleration sensors include, for example, the Wii Remote [4], MicroStrains G-Link [57] and SparkFun WiTilt [77], which comprise a wireless interface that can be used for data utilization. A sensor that can be used in this environment is the motion sensor by the company Actigraph [1].

A few mobile systems can be found in the area of measurement systems for the manufacture of orthopaedic products or gait analysis. The company Xybermind GmbH has had a device called Achillex [90] that uses acceleration sensors and a gyroscope for the measurement of running style on the market for four years. The measurement range of the acceleration sensors (+/– 20 g) and the gyroscope (+/– 20 rad/s) is necessary for measuring sports motion. Electronic measurement components are integrated into fabrics. The company Novel has developed a broad palette of sensors for the measurement of pressure distribution in medical and technical/industrial areas. Emed pedography systems are used for the exact measurement and analysis of planar pressure distribution [60]. The pedar system is a pressure distribution measurement system for determining local forces generated between the foot sole and shoe. The company GeBiom sells systems for measuring pressure distribution in bicycle seats [25]. However, frequently such expensive CNC (computerized numerical control) solutions are only available to the health trade professions and associated sectors and not the end customer market.

Thus far, equipment for monitoring motion in the realm of prevention has been limited to the ICT-based recording of daily motion activities for overweight children and young people [74]. In Germany a series of tests and studies have been carried out that introduce motion-activating systems into the broader population. The InPriMo consortium (InPriMo: individualised prevention with mobile end devices) promoted by the National Ministry for Economics and Technology has since 2005 been developing new forms of individualised preventive health methods using mobile end devices that facilitate an impetus to resume participation in sports using instructions attuned to each individual person. These devices comprise a combination of sports and prevention programmes with mobile end devices that allow participants to monitor their own activities [37]. The first studies were carried out in young people with asthma [36].

Especially for the area of high performance sports, for example, a sensor bandage was developed at the Australian Institute of Sport. Integrated into the fabric are motion and stretch sensors including a small electronic unit that transmits measurement values wirelessly to a computer. The system converts bending and stretching of the hand and elbow joints into various drum sounds, ideally finally resulting in a driving rhythm. The resulting rhythm shows sports practitioners and trainers whether they have implemented a motion sequence cleanly and smoothly [73].

At the School of Electronics and Computer Science of the University of Southampton, an underarm crutch has been developed that can monitor, thanks to popular sensors, whether it is indeed being used correctly. In this way, researchers in the field of physiotherapy can take corrective measures for patients with leg injuries that are frequently unable to distribute stress correctly. The intelligent crutch uses three acceleration samples to monitor motion. A pressure sensor measures how strongly the crutch, and thus the leg of the patient, is being placed under stress. Additional sensors determine whether the user is holding the grip correctly. These data is transmitted wirelessly to a PC. If the crutch is used incorrectly, an optical warning is displayed on the crutch. The translation of the underlying concept is thus relatively favourable, since it is based on standard commercial technology and sensory features – similarly to that which is used in Nintendo's Wii [42].

The mobile devices for motion and vital data measurement currently on the market, however, appeal to above all high performance sportspersons, aficionados of technological affine sports, and highly-paid risk patients. People for whom sports is part of their life prefer devices, above all, that support them in measuring and comparing their performance. Higher, faster, further are their criteria. The abovementioned devices by Polar and Garmin are attuned precisely to this objective. Notwithstanding this, for a target group that is less than mobile that is forced, for health reasons, to integrate more activity into their everyday life, these devices do not provide suitable support. With regard to many of these patients, the baseline is a lacking sense of their bodies along with motor weakness. Incorrect motion sequences leading to pain after exercise are often why people stop exercising. In this context, beyond simply recording physical activity and calorie consumption, suitable mobile analysis components for motion correction as well as relevant feedback forms still need to be developed, so that these systems can be used in the context of medically recognised therapy.

3.3. Motion Tracking Technologies in Home Environments

Uses in the home environment have thus far been limited to initial attempts to delineate and visualise daily activities. However, these uses are based on the assumption that a home is equipped with a sensory system [32]. Sensors to detect motion, however, can also be installed in a stationary manner in an environment (e.g. cameras, sensory mats). Stationary sensor systems frequently require that the subject wears additional sensory components close to his body (e.g. reflectors or tags) in order to yield greater precision. A disadvantage is that these components require additional electronic features, batteries etc. in order to transmit data obtained wirelessly. Permanent cable connections obstruct the motion sequence, create acceptance problems and increase the system's sensitivity to disturbances. In the sense of usability and acceptance in the target group, stationary sensors with or without lightweight components near the body are preferable.

In the realm of medical and rehabilitative technology, sensors have been developed that measure various sensory principles (resistive, capacitive, inductive) of the mechanical pressure divided between the body of the patient and the floor at high resolution (with up to approximately 1 sensory element per cm^2). A pressure measurement plate by the company Medilogic represents a quadratic measurement field with 4,096 pressure sensors (external diameter 530 × 540 mm). The data is transferred wirelessly from this measurement field via a data transmission modem to the computer [52]. Additionally, the flexible variant of the Medilogic pressure measurement mat facilitates the determination of pressure distribution during sitting, for example on seat cushions or seat frames. According to varying dimensions (305 × 200 mm to 758 × 808 mm with 240 to 480 sensors) of the flexible measurement mat, a broad spectrum of applications is opened [53]. These sensors in principle offer sufficient precision and sampling rate for motion analysis, though they are indeed – particularly for their application in the home setting – much too expensive. An interesting newer development line is currently that of 'intelligent textiles' developed for technical safety applications, for example carpets (SensFloor by Future-Shape GmbH, 'sensor sheets' by Elsi Technologies), which electromagnetically or electrostatically record, with high spatial resolution and with high precision, the effect of parts of the human body on sensory elements.

In order to correctly observe human motion sequences, a model of the human body that sufficiently reflects the principal anatomy and physiology at any given time must be established digitally and continued to be written with a sufficient update rate in real

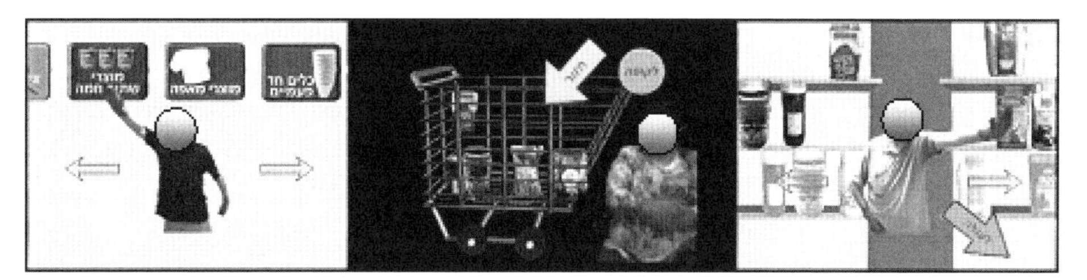

Figure 1. Screen shots of the application Vmall that show how a patient that has suffered a stroke practices shopping in a supermarket [87].

time. The sensors used for this can be placed near the body (that is to say, on body parts or on clothing) (such as strain gauges, in order to determine angle parameters of the limbs). To detect position and motion, one can also use Motion Capturing or Tracking Methods. Motion Capturing Methods, which have been in use since the 1970s, are used extensively in the film and computer game industries. However, they are also utilised for motion analysis in the field of Life Sciences [85]. During (optic) Motion Capturing, mostly retroreflective markers that are attached to clothing are detected with the aid of several cameras (mostly HighSpeed cameras). With the aid of these images, one can determine the positions of markers in three-dimensional space and with respect to one another. Other Motion Capturing or Tracking Systems are based on magnetic, mechanical or acoustic methods. The use of AR [5] methods (such as the ARToolkit) for monitoring motion is also conceivable. Disruptive, however, with regard to this method are the markers (size, cost of establishment) or the occasionally used 'exoskeletons' [55]. A new approach to the detection of motion is optic markerless tracking. Markerless systems have been developed by MIT Stanford [79] and the Max Planck Institute in Saarbrücken [82]. A commercial system is available from Organic Motion [63]. Another commercial system will be available from Microsoft commencing in November 2010 [56]. To what extent these technologies can be used for precise motion detection in a context of home rehabilitation must still be evaluated.

3.4. Current Multimedia Rehabilitation Applications

For rehabilitative purposes, some of the applications being developed include ones that exercise the upper or lower extremities [48]. NeuroVR is an example of a freely accessible Virtual Reality Platform designed for users without specific computer knowledge in order to adapt the virtual environment to the training situation of the patient. The platform is delineated by the fact that it is economical and easily accessible. Thus far input has still been effected by mouse and joypad. Currently, however, responding to the requirements of people with compromised mobility, work is being done on gesture steering with webcams [3].

In newer approaches, motion games for therapeutic purposes with regard to heart diseases [49] or mobility limitations, for example after a stroke, are being tested [20]. Thanks to the options of immersive media environments, it is possible to stimulate dysfunctional parties via multimodal sensory channels (surface feel, hearing, vision) [33]. To restore coordination skills after a stroke, recent concepts from the realm of neuropsychology use virtual environments for the cognitive training of functionally compromised body parts. A person's motion can be projected into a game-like virtual reality environment in which he can carry out such everyday activities as shopping or play-

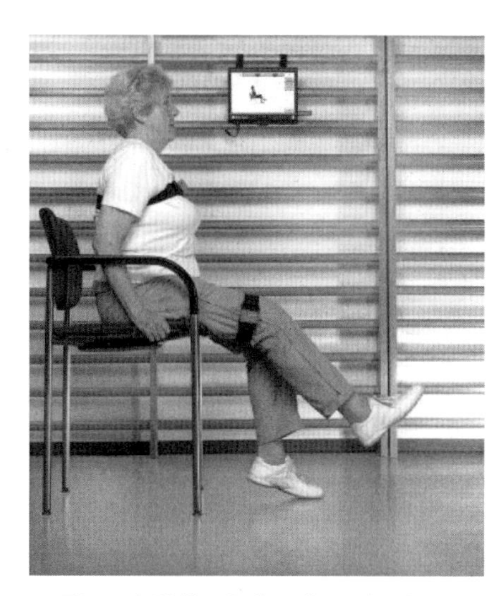

Figure 2. Philips Orthopedic Trainer [13].

ing football, whereby functionally compromised body parts receive cognitive stimulation.

The project Gaming Rehabilitation System uses a marker-based approach in which the patient puts on a glove that the camera can follow more easily [68]. The arms that the patient must use to catch a ball are projected into a virtual reality environment. The Philips Company has an orthopaedic trainer on the market that consists of a central unit with a touchscreen, two wireless motion sensors and wireless headphones [65]. It supports the patient's self-training by way of video instructions and audio-feedback. This allows the therapist to compose individual training programmes for his patients and adjust these to his requirements. While the patient carries out the exercises under the direction of videos, the sensors measure his motions on his thighs and upper body Sensors similar to those of the orthopaedic trainer are also used in stroke rehabilitation.

Applications of telerehabilitation are based on the infrastructure of telemedicine. On the one hand, they record a patient's state of health in a divided environment in which the physician uses a video conference system to communicate with patients or in which vital signs are automatically recorded using embedded medical end devices. Through the available communication medium of a video conference system, physicians and caregivers can also give patients instructions.

In the project Teletherapy – Subsystems Neurolinguistic Module [9] an expandable computer-driven speech training programme for neurological patients with speech disturbances was developed and tested in the telemedical area. In this project, concluded in 2004, aphasia (speech disturbances) patients at the Specialised Clinic Herzogenaurach learned to work with the speech programme on a PC, so that they could carry out exercises independently on a PC and continue practicing them at home. Via the server and using integrated system software, a therapist could automatically call up data on exercise times, exercise duration and exercise results and steer the patient's training process as well as adapting his exercises individually in accordance with speech progress. In the Evocare project, participating stroke patients with aphasia have the possibility of using neurolinguistic therapy software in their own homes and transmitting the data to their treating physician. The physician can use this information to steer the con-

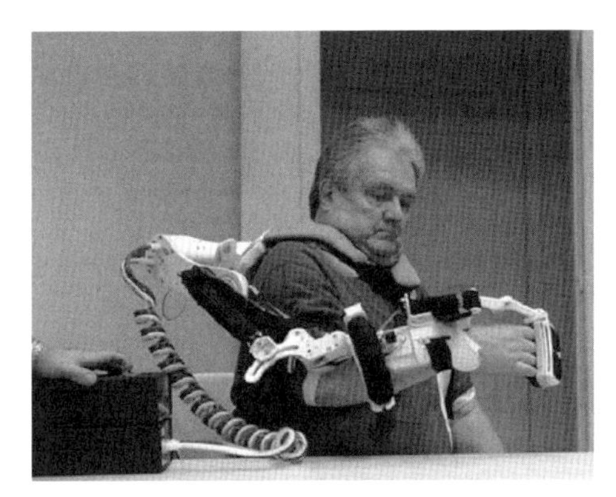
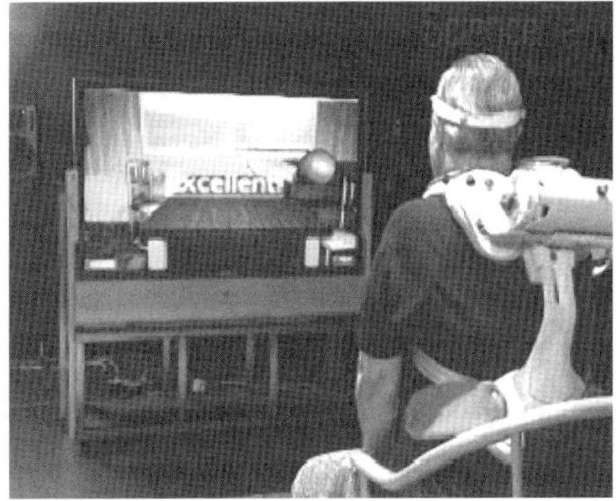

Figure 3. RUPERT system in use [71].

tinued course of therapy better, without the patient being burdened with additional surgery visits [91].

For acute or early rehab, for example after a stroke, exoskeletons are currently being used in clinics. The company Hocoma is producing an exoskeleton-like motion system that, via sensory stimulation, enables a patient to relearn his functional motions. A comparable system for neurological gait rehabilitation is the haptic walker [70]. Presently a home trainer for the therapy of the lower extremities is being developed at the Orthopaedic Clinic of the University of Heidelberg. A hollow tube that is filled with air by an electric motor moves the knee and ankle joints. The patient sits or lies in the trainer, because a weight relief system such as in the Lokomat for walking upright would be too expensive for home use [45].

Robot-assisted therapy approaches, such as for example combining the MIT-Manus system, combine multimodal learning environments with physical interactions that are supported by a robot [47]. The coordinative skills are trained through the combination of haptic and visual stimuli. With the portable RUPERT system developed at the University of Arizona, the motions of the upper extremities can be trained after a stroke [31]. With a combination of a virtual reality environment and a robot arm, actual motions are imitated, visualised on a screen and evaluated in terms of their implementation. The patient uses the visual feedback to relearn the various types of motion.

In recent times, as an option of the recreational transmission of motions, sensor-based game environments have gained ground in terms of consumer application [64].

So-called Exergames (from the English *exercising*) allow patients on their own to use a multimedia training programme and a personal adviser to complete physical training programmes, which can also be done by several participants that come together in a virtual community and exercise or compete with one another. Some of these include virtual bicycle and rowing trainers, Pilates, yoga or cardio-fitness courses. Frequently in such multimedia fitness and training programmes a conventional training device (such as a bicycle) is connected to a multimedia training environment [86]. Also very popular are dance and motion games for platforms from such well-known game manufacturers as Sony, Nintendo and Microsoft.

With these innovative, multimedia, sensor-based forms of training, such as for example the Wii by the game manufacturer Nintendo, Move by Sony or Kinect by Microsoft, it appears that the option is arising of relocating rehabilitation and prevention measures under controlled conditions to the home environment. Indeed, initial studies have already shown that commercially utilised sensory features do not meet medical requirements in terms of precision of motion monitoring and those concerning the individual adaptability of therapy concepts for the patient. After a time, the initial enthusiasm has begun to wear off, so that the training effect does not meet expectations in the long run. What are lacking are sustainably effective motivation strategies and improved feedback mechanisms.

In summary, it can be stated that it is true that a few solutions have been developed in individual sub-areas. However, a total system that supports individual and barrier-free rehabilitation activities based on medical sensory features and continues inpatient rehabilitation processes with the aid of a motivating multimedia environment does not yet exist. Indeed, several projects have currently assumed this task and are developing home applications for orthopaedic prevention and rehabilitation. For example, currently, in the project SmartSenior, in the area of multimedia and interactively intertwined therapy, individual approaches to stroke rehabilitation and fall prevention are being developed that are to make it possible to shift rehabilitation to the home environment [75]. The Fraunhofer FIRST is presently developing, in the project 'MyRehab' jointly with the Rehab centre Lübben, a telemedical assistance system for the continuation of rehabilitation in the home environment [41].

4. Summary and Forecast

As time goes on, demographic developments in the EU and the increase in chronic diseases will force a paradigm shift. After all, those diseases are incurable and require permanent medical monitoring that should optimally be supplemented by preventive measures. The prevalence of chronic diseases and multimorbidity increases with age [7]. It must also be remembered that chronic diseases and multimorbidity increase significantly at decreasing socio-economic levels [58]. Chronic and degenerative diseases represent 80% of all costs of disease and are spent for 20% of those insured by GKV [61]. These points clearly demonstrate the economic brisance and the substantiation for an expansion of preventive measures.

Nearly all EU member states are reforming their social security systems in the context of a longer working life. And they all view an increase in the actual retirement age as a major tool for the adjustment of the old age pension system to the ageing population. These facts represent significant perspectives for the establishment of innovative preventive measures that make sense in any stage of life. Focal points for action, therefore, lie in improving the health of children and young people, in older people and employees or their companies.

Based on this demographic development, the costs of medical care and rehabilitation will continue to rise, and politicians and purchasers will force the providers of services in the realm of medical care to decrease their expenditures and to demonstrate that they are providing efficient care. In addition to the necessary rehabilitative measures, preventive health measures and preventive medicine will acquire greater relative importance in the future.

The interlocking of preventive and rehabilitative measures with the aid of information and communication technology is one of the most significant and promising areas of research. In this context, it is the task of IKT to facilitate the trans-sectoral provision of services and optimal communication on the part of providers and purchasers. The transmission possibility of vital signs has thus far met with interest in only heart specialists, high-risk patients and persons practicing extreme sports. In combination with further measurement data such as, for example, daily activities or individual movement behaviour that represents directly recognisable value for the user, this technology could bring about a thus far unprecedented degree of acceptance.

Capacities in the areas of sensor technology already exist; processing computer units such as, for example, PCs continue to become smaller, less expensive and more efficient. Frequently households already contain a computer or comparable hardware platform. Add to this the increasingly optimal spread even throughout the more rural regions of Europe of high-performance, broadband internet connections. Similarly, at least in the area of medicine the standardisation plans of the Continua Health Alliance and HL7 are displaying growing interoperability of medical data and documentation systems.

The possibility of transferring rehabilitative and preventive measures, under controlled conditions, to the home environment by means of virtual applications can signify a low-threshold initiation of exercise and sports even outside the home environment. Nonetheless this presupposes that suitable quality exists not only in technical areas but, in particular, that of communication. Only with suitably qualified introduction and communication of technical systems can the goal of the preparation of exercise activation under individual responsibility be realised individually or in groups. Lacking in currently available systems are sustainably effective motivation strategies and improved feedback mechanisms that are specifically attuned to the needs of the target group of users.

In the area of mobile rehabilitation, such products as pedometers, heart rate monitors and sphygmomanometers have already made their way to the general public. Options for their use, however, thus far remain limited, because they do not possess open interfaces with existing diagnostic, therapeutic and clearing systems. Efficient therapy and training support that can be measured via personal therapeutic monitoring requires additional technologies that permit support of the course of therapy and exercise in a corrective, motivating manner that takes heed of high-risk cases. In practice there are already numerous types of sports, as well as therapeutic and training methods that demonstrably help prevent chronic diseases.

If we can succeed in integrating these modularly composed exercise procedures in a mobile, multimedia and medically valid therapeutic and training environment, it may be possible to reactivate many people. Through the option of movement assistance and medical vital signs diagnosis, multimodal therapeutic and training programmes are in principle suited for use in the context of rehabilitative aftercare in the home environment. The health economic use of such sensor-assisted condition, coordination and strength training in the various living areas in the home, the clinic or the workplace lies in its motivational orientation. Similarly to the current IRENA aftercare programme [35] of old-age pension insurers, through this type of multimedia therapeutic support the sustainability of achieved prevention and rehabilitation results could be improved. Further areas of use for such programmes can be identified in that of rehab sports co-financed by health insurers [69] and the original bonus programmes in the context of prevention.

The goal of future developments must be to establish, and adjust, all such systems individually according to the capacity of patients. In this context physiotherapists and treating physicians will prepare precisely tailored therapeutic and training plans that the person exercising can continue and modify under his own responsibility. During independent training the patient must receive feedback if he implements movements incorrectly, regarding his vital signs and his training results. The therapist need only contact the patient in case of major deviations from the training plan. The patient will acquire the competence to develop his own motivation strategies to realise more movement in his daily life.

A positive remark that one can make is that the already quite advanced developments in technology possess fundamental potential for use, for example, for people with disabilities to motivate them to exercise or in the field of sports for the disabled. Nonetheless this presupposes that suitable modules, both in technical terms and in terms of content, are adapted to the individual conditions of certain types of disablement.

Essential to the use of these technologies in an integrated prevention and rehabilitation programme is, after all, the demonstration of efficiency in terms of the authorisation of preventive and rehabilitative technologies and multimedia forms of therapy in accordance with the latest legislation on medical products. Although, indeed, with the technical platforms of game manufacturers a great potential degree of distribution of activating games and mobility options already exists worldwide, thus far meaningful studies that would secure and justify the use of these devices for medical purposes are lacking. For innovative products in the area of motivating movement and multimedia rehabilitation, therefore, further studies to gather evidence of the efficiency of mobile and multimedia training support are necessary that must be carried out jointly with health insurers and old-age pension carriers.

References

[1] ActiGraph Activity Monitor Devices, http://www.theactigraph.com/ (last visited: 02/24/2011).

[2] Aipermon, A world's first. Activity motivation and conscious nutrition in one device, http://www.aipermon.com/eng/produkte-aim-start.htm (last visited: 02/24/2011).

[3] D. Algeri et al., *A free tool for motor rehabilitation: NeuroVR 1.5 with CamSpace*, Istituto Auxologico Italiano, Applied Technology for Neuro-Psychology-ATNP Lab, Milan, Italy. Universita' Cattolica del Sacro Cuore, Department of Psychology, Milan, Italy.

[4] Amazon.de, Nintendo Wii-Remote, http://www.amazon.de/Nintendo-Wii-Remote/dp/B000IMWK2G (last visited: 02/24/2011).

[5] AR: Augmented Reality.

[6] Arbeitshilfe zur geriatrischen Rehabilitation, Schriftenreihe der Bundesarbeitsgemeinschaft für Rehabilitation Heft 6, www.bar-frankfurt.de/upload/Arbeitshilfe_Geriatrie_166.pdf (last visited: 02/24/2011).

[7] M. Arnold, M. Litsch and F.W. Schwartz (Hg.), Krankenhaus-Report 1999, Schwerpunkt: Versorgung chronisch Kranker. Verlag Schattenauer, Stuttgart, 1999.

[8] Barmer GEK Bonusprogramm, http://www.barmer-gek.de/barmer/web/Portale/Versicherte/Leistungen-Services/Leistungen-Beitraege/Bonusprogramm/Bonusprogramm.html (last visited: 02/24/2011).

[9] Bayerisches Staatsminesterium für Umwelt und Gesundheit, Telemedizin, http://www.stmug.bayern.de/krankenhaus/telemedizin/projekte_detail.htm?ID=AAEYIEwkrRir%2BXT9PY%2FmuA%3D%3D (last visited: 02/24/2011).

[10] B. Beyrle, Rehabilitations-Versorgungskonzepte in der GKV, 1. Fachtag der katholischen Rehabilitations-Einrichtungen, Frankfurt, http://www.kkvd.de/aspe_shared/form/download.asp?nr=232728&form_typ=115&acid=63F3B0F531B141B2AC4BD5848C3AE331FF4&ag_id=5308, 19.2.2009 (last visited: 02/24/2011).

[11] E. Biddiss and J. Irwin, Active video games to promote physical activity in children and youth. A systematic review, *Archives of Pediatrics & Adolescent Medicine* **164(**7) (July 2010), http://www.aahf.info/pdf/youth_articles/exergamesjournalarticlepdf.pdf (last visited: 02/24/2011).

[12] Biodex Medical Systems, http://www.biodex.com/ (last visited: 02/24/2011).

[13] Charité, Forschungsgruppe Geriatrie, Durchführung eines sensorbasierten häuslichen Schlaganfall-Rehabilitationssystems für die Arme, http://geriatrie.charite.de/forschung/ausgewaehlte_abgeschlossene_projekte/sensorbasierte_schlaganfallrehabilitation/ (last visited: 02/24/2011).

[14] R.A. Clark, A.L. Bryant, Y. Pua, P. McCrory, K. Bennell and M. Hunt, Validity and reliability of the Nintendo Wii Balance Board for assessment of standing balance, *Gait & Posture* **31**(3) (March 2010), 307–310.
[15] Council of Europe Disability Action Plan 2006–2015, http://www.coe.int/t/e/social_cohesion/soc-sp/integration/02_Council_of_Europe_Disability_Action_Plan/ (last visited: 02/24/2011).
[16] Countries in which Disability Management is significant include Australia, New Zealand, Canada, Hong Kong, Germany, Switzerland, the Netherlands, Great Britain, Scandinavia and Finland, Ireland.
[17] L.J. Damschroder, P.A. Ubel, J. Riis and D.M. Smith, An alternative approach for eliciting willingness-to-pay: A randomized Internet trial, *Judgment and Decision Making* **2**(2) (April 2007), pp. 96–106.
[18] A. Dechamps, P. Diolez, E. Thiaudière, A Tulon, C. Onifade, T. Vuong, C. Helmer and I. Bourdel-Marchasson, Effects of exercise programs to prevent decline in health-related quality of life in highly deconditioned institutionalized elderly persons, *Archives of Internal Medicine* **170**(2) (2010), 162–169.
[19] S. Dibbelt et al., Das Integrierte orthopädische-psychosomatische Behandlungskonzept – IopJo, Studie, Die Rehabilitation 845. Jahrgang, Heft 6, Stuttgart, Thieme Verlag, Dezember 2006.
[20] Entertainment Robotics, Modular interactive tiles, http://www.e-robot.dk/therapy.html (last visited: 02/24/2011).
[21] K.I. Erickson and A.F. Kramer, Aerobic exercise effects on cognitive and neural plasticity in older adults, *British Journal of Sports Medicine* **43**(1) (2009), 22–24.
[22] European Agency for Safety and Health at Work, Arbeitsbedingte Musculoskeletal Krankheiten: Präventionsbericht, Fachtsheets (Ausgabe 78, Februar 2008), Bilbao, Eigenverlag, 2008.
[23] Exercise training meta-analysis of trials in patients with chronic heart failure (ExTraMATCH), *BMJ* **328** (2004), 189, EE originally published online 16 Jan 2004, http://bmj.com/cgi/content/full/328/7433/189 (last visited: 02/24/2011).
[24] Garmin, Forerunner® 310XT, https://buy.garmin.com/shop/shop.do?cID=142&pID=27335 (last visited: 02/24/2011).
[25] gebioMized – Die Sportmarke der GeBioM, www.gebiomized.de (last visited: 02/24/2011).
[26] N. Gerdes, B. Bührlen, S. Lichtenberg and W.H. Jäckel, Rehabilitationsnachsorge – Analyse der Nachsorgeempfehlungen und ihrer Umsetzung. Rehabilitationswissenschaften, Rehabilitationspsychologie, Rehabilitationsmedizin, Bd. 10. Regensburg: S. Roderer, 2005.
[27] Gesundheit, Fitness & Prävention – formed – Galileo-Vibrationstraing – Bodyanalyzer, http://www.galileo4you.de/ (last visited: 02/24/2011).
[28] L. Graves, G. Stratton, N.D. Ridgers and N.T. Cable, Comparison of energy expenditure in adolescents when playing new generation and sedentary computer games: Cross sectional study, *BMJ* **335** (2007), 1282–1284.
[29] C. Gutenbrunner, *Weißbuch Physikalische und Rehabilitative Medizin in Europa*, Thieme Verlag, Stuttgart, New York 2006.
[30] W.L. Haskell, I.M. Lee, R.R. Pate, K.E. Powell, S.N. Blair, B.A. Franklin, C.A. Macera, G.W. Heath, P.D. Thompson and A. Bauman, Physical activity and public health: Updated recommendation for adults from the American College of Sports Medicine and the American Heart Association, *Med. Sci. Sports Exerc.* **39**(8) (2007), 1423–1434.
[31] J. He et al., RUPERT: A device for robotic upper extremity repetitive therapy, in: *Proc. IEEE Eng. Medicine Biol.* Shanghai, China, Sept. 2005, pp. 2384–2387.
[32] A. Hein and T. Kirste, *Activity Recognition for Ambient Assisted Living: Potential and Challenges*, AAL Congress, 2008.
[33] M.K. Holden, Virtual environments for motor rehabilitation: Review, *CyberPsychology & Behaviour* **8**(3) (2005), 187–211.
[34] M.K. Holder, Functional balance and dual task reaction times in older adults are improved by virtual reality and biofeedback training, *CyperPsychology & Behaviour, M. Bebr.* (2007), 15–23.
[35] http://www.deutsche-rentenversicherung-bund.de/DRVB/de/Inhalt/Zielgruppen/Infos_fuer_Rehaeinrichtungen/nachsorgeprogramm/nachsorge_irena_karena.html?nn=37110 (last visited: 02/24/2011).
[36] http://www.nextgenerationmedia.de/documents/Inprimo_Asthma.pdf (last visited: 02/24/2011).
[37] http://www.nextgenerationmedia.de/documents/Inprimo_Profil.pdf (last visited: 02/24/2011).
[38] In Germany, mobile rehabilitation is part of medical rehabilitation as delineated in the Social Security Code V (compulsory health insurance). It is administrated and reimbursed according to § 40 Par. 1 SGB V concerning compulsory health insurance. This makes it a regulatory service that has, as is the case with other forms of outpatient rehabilitation, precedence of statutes over inpatient care.
[39] Intensivierte REhabilitationsNAchsorge der Deutsche[n] Rentenversicherung Bund.
[40] John et al., Rehabilitation im häuslichen Umfeld mit der Wii Fit – Eine empirische Studie, in: *Tagungsband 2. German Ambient Assisted Living Congress*, 27–28 January 2009, Berlin, pp. 238–245.

[41] M. John, T. Ernst, S. Klose, B. Häusler, M. Frenzel and T. Michaelis, Reha@home – Technisches Konzept und Prototyp für ein telemedizinisches Übungsprogramm im häuslichen Umfeld, in: *Tagungsband 3. Deutscher Ambient Assisted Living Kongress*, 26–27 January 2010, Berlin, p. 6.

[42] journalMED, "Intelligente" Krücke überwacht über Beschleunigungsmesser und Drucksensoren die richtige Verwendung, http://www.journalmed.de/newsview.php?id=26705, 26.08.2009 (last visited: 02/24/2011).

[43] W. Kemmler, S. von Stengel, K. Engelke, L. Häberle and W.A. Kalender, Exercise effects on bone mineral density, falls, coronary risk factors, and health care costs in older women. The randomized controlled senior fitness and prevention (SEFIP) study, *Archives of Internal Medicine* **170**(2) (2010), 179–185.

[44] O. Kieffer, Optimierung qualitätssichernder Prozesse am Beispiel der trainingstherapeutischen Behandlung von Rückenschmerzen, Dissertation, Deutsche Sporthochschule Köln, http://zb-sport.dshs-koeln.de/Hochschulschriften/Dissertationen-Internet/2007/Oliver_Kieffer/Dissertation-Oliver-Kieffer.pdf, 2007 (last visited: 02/24/2011).

[45] KNESTEL Firmengruppe – Ihr Dienstleister für intelligente Sonderlösungen, http://www.moregait.de/geraet.html (last visited: 02/24/2011).

[46] K.-H. Köpke, Wirksame Rehabilitation durch systematische Nachsorge, Soziale Sicherheit (Heft 7, 2004), Frankfurt am Main: AiB 2004.

[47] Krebs et al., Rehabilitation robotics: Pilot trial of a spatial extension for MIT-manus, *Journal of NeuroEngineering and Rehabilitation* **1** (2004), 5.

[48] H.E. Krüger-Brand, Telerehabilitation: Sensoren helfen beim Training, *Deutsches Ärzteblatt* **105**(18) (2008), http://www.aerzteblatt.de/v4/archiv/artikel.asp?id=59950, 2008 (last visited: 02/24/2011).

[49] S. Lakshmi, Robotic therapy tiles: Playing your way to health, http://www.wired.com/medtech/health/news/2007/10/therapy_tiles, 10.02.2007 (last visited: 02/24/2011).

[50] C. Laske, S. Banschbach, E. Stransky, S. Bosch, G. Straten, J. Machann, A. Fritsche, A. Hipp, A. Niess and G.W. Eschweiler, Exercise-induced normalization of decreased BDNF serum concentration in elderly women with remitted major depression, *The International Journal of Neuropsychopharmacology* **13** (2010), 595–602, http://journals.cambridge.org/action/displayAbstract?fromPage=online&aid=7748372 (last visited: 02/24/2011).

[51] Luxembourger Deklaration zur Betrieblichen Gesundheitsförderung des Europäischen Netzwerkes für BGF (ENWHP) von 1997.

[52] medilogic, DruckMessPlatte (drahtlos): http://www.medilogic.com/index.php?id=52&L=0 (last visited: 02/24/2011).

[53] medilogic, Sitzdruckmessung Dynamische Druckmessung beim Sitzen, http://www.medilogic.com/index.php?id=56 (last visited: 02/24/2011).

[54] R.R. Mellecker and A.M. McManus, Energy expenditure and cardiovascular responses to seated and active gaming in children. *Arch Pediatr Adolesc Med.* **162**(9) (2008), 886–891.

[55] MetaMotion, Gypsy 7™ Motion Capture Systems, http://www.metamotion.com/gypsy/gypsy-motion-capture-system.htm (last visited: 02/24/2011).

[56] Microsoft, Kinect für Xbox 360, http://www.xbox.com/de-de/kinect (last visited: 02/24/2011).

[57] MicroStrain, G-Link® -mXRS™ Wireless Accelerometer Node, http://www.microstrain.com/g-link.aspx (last visited: 02/24/2011).

[58] A. Mielk, Soziale Ungleichgewicht und Gesundheit. Einführung in die aktuelle Diskussion. Berlin: Hans Huber, 2005.

[59] Nintendo mit guten Verkaufszahlen in Europa, http://www.big-screen.de/deutsch/pages/news/allgemeine-news/2010_01_06_3270_nintendo-mit-guten-verkaufszahlen-in-europa.php, 06 Januar 2010 (last visited: 02/24/2011).

[60] Novel – Produkte – Sensoren, http://www.novel.de/ger/productinfo/sensors.htm (last visited: 02/24/2011).

[61] W. Olaf, U. Miegel and K. Thormeier, Die personell Verteilung von Leistungsausgaben in der gesetzlichen Krankenversicherung 1998 und 1999. Konsequenzen für die Weiterentwicklung des deutschen Gesundheitssystems, *Sozialer Fortschritt* **51**(3) (2002), 58–61.

[62] Omron Medizintechnik, Thema Bewegung, http://www.omron-medizintechnik.de/gesundheitsthemen/thema-bewegung.html (last visited: 02/24/2011).

[63] Organic Motion, Markerless Motion Capture, http://www.organicmotion.com (last visited: 02/24/2011).

[64] M. Pasch, N. Bianchi-Berthouze, B. van Dijk and A. Nijholt, Movement-based sports video games: Investigating motivation and gaming experience, *Entertainment Computing* **1** (2009), 49–61.

[65] Philips, Philips Orthopädie-Trainer, http://stream.hightechcampus.nl/orthopedictrainer/200904-orthopedictrainer.wmv (last visited: 02/24/2011).

[66] Power Plate Schweiz, http://www.powerplate.ch/ (last visited: 02/24/2011).

[67] Rahmenvereinbarung über den Rehabilitationssport und das Funktionstraining vom 01. Oktober 2003, www.bar-frankfurt.de/upload/Rehabilitationssport_314.pdf, Januar 2007 (last visited: 02/24/2011).

[68] Rehabilitation Gaming Systems, http://specs.upf.edu/rgs/ (last visited: 02/24/2011).

[69] RehaSport Deutschland e.V., Rehabilitationssport, http://www.rehasport-deutschland.de/rehasport.html (last visited: 02/24/2011).

[70] H. Schmidt, C. Werner, R. Bernhardt, S. Hesse and J. Krüger, Gait rehabilitation machines based on programmable footplates, *Journal of NeuroEngineering and Rehabilitation* **4** (9 February 2007), 2.

[71] ScienceDaily, Robotic Arm for Stroke Victims, Doctors and Engineers Develop Virtual-Reality Recovery for Stroke Victims, http://www.sciencedaily.com/videos/2005/0607-robotic_arm_for_stroke_victims.htm, June 1, 2005 (last visited: 02/24/2011).

[72] Science Daily, Wii Fit May Not Help Families Get Fit, http://www.sciencedaily.com/releases/2009/12/091218125110.htm, Dec. 25, 2009 (last visited: 02/24/2011).

[73] Scienceticker, Sensor-Bandage stimmt Sportler ein, http://www.scienceticker.info/2008/04/04/sensor-bandage-stimmt-sportler-ein/, 4 April 2008 (last visited: 02/24/2011).

[74] Selecting an appropriate motion sensor in children and adolescents, S. de Vries, I. Bakker, M. Kopman-Rock, R.A. Hirasing and W. van Mechelen, Selecting an appropriate motion sensor in children and adolescents, TNO Knowledge for business, http://www.ipenproject.org/pdf_file/hand-out%20poster%20beweegmeters%20satellite%20ICDAM%2006.pdf (last visited: 02/24/2011).

[75] SmartSenior, Selbstständig, sicher, gesund und mobil im Alter, www.smart-senior.de (last visited: 02/24/2011).

[76] Sozialverband VdK Rheinland-Pfalz e.V., Thema des Monats Dezember 2009/Januar 2010, Geriatrische Rehabilitation, www.vdk.de/cms/mime/2460D1259231727.pdf, November 2009 (last visited: 02/24/2011).

[77] Sparkfun Electronics, WiTilt v3.0, http://www.sparkfun.com/commerce/product_info.php?products_id=8563 (last visited: 02/24/2011).

[78] Sports Insider, Beurer AS50 – Tägliche Bewegung kontrollieren und protokollieren, http://www.sports-insider.de/1161/beurer-as50-tagliche-bewegung-kontrollieren-und-protokollieren/ (last visited: 02/24/2011).

[79] Stanford Markerless Motion Capture Project, https://ccrma.stanford.edu/~stefanoc/Markerless/Markerless.html (last visited: 02/24/2011).

[80] Statistisches Bundesamt, Gesundheitsausgabenrechnung für 2007, Vorsorge-/Rehabilitationseinrichtungen, Ausgabenträger insgesamt, Dokumentationsstand 28.04.2009.

[81] Q. Sun, M.K. Townsend, O.I. Okereke, O.H. Franco, F.B. Hu and F. Grodstein, Physical activity at midlife in relation to successful survival in women at age 70 years or older, *Archives of Internal Medicine* **170**(2) (2010), 194–201.

[82] The Marker-less MoCap Research group, http://www.mpi-inf.mpg.de/~rosenhahn/PostDocMPI.html (last visited: 02/24/2011).

[83] C. Trotti et al., Virtual reality for the upper limb motor training in stroke: A case report, *Cyberpsychology & Behavior* **12**(5), 2009. Department of Neurology and Neurorehabilitation, IRCCS Istituto Auxologico Italiano Verbania, Italy. Bioengineering Department, Politecnico di Milano, Milan, Italy. Department of Neurosciences, Universita' di Torino, Turin, Italy.

[84] Unternehmensnetzwerk zur betrieblichen Gesundheitsförderung in der Europäischen Union e.V., www.enwhp.de, www.netzwerk-unternehmen-fuer-gesundheit.de (last visited: 02/24/2011).

[85] Vicon, Motion Capture Systems from Vicon, http://www.vicon.com/ (last visited: 02/24/2011).

[86] Virtual Interactive Fitness and Web Racing, http://www.fitcentric.com/ (last visited: 02/24/2011).

[87] Weiss et al., Video capture virtual reality as a flexible and effective rehabilitation tool, *Journal of NeuroEngineering and Rehabilitation* **1** (2004), 12.

[88] WHO, Health Topics Rehabilitation, http://www.who.int/topics/rehabilitation/en/ (last visited: 02/24/2011).

[89] WHO, International Classification of Functioning, Disability and Health (ICF), http://www.who.int/classifications/icf/en/ (last visited: 02/24/2011).

[90] Xybermind, Das System Achillex, http://www.xybermind.net/products/main.htm (last visited: 02/24/2011).

[91] Zentrum für Telematik im Gesundheitswesen GmbH, ZTG-Newsletter Nr. 56, http://www.ztg-nrw.de/ZTG/content/e129/e1689/e6506/object7368/ZTG_NewsletterAusgabe56Juni2008_web_ger.pdf, Juni 2008 (last visited: 02/24/2011).

Handbook of Ambient Assisted Living
J.C. Augusto et al. (Eds.)
IOS Press, 2012

doi:10.3233/978-1-60750-837-3-834

Growing Older Together: When a Robot Becomes the Best Ally for Ageing Well

Francesca Irene CAVALLARO[a,*], Fabrice O. MORIN[a], Ainara GARZO[a], Anthony REMAZEILLES[a], Arantxa RENTERÍA[b] and Gabriel GAMINDE[b]
[a] *Tecnalia, Health Technologies Unit, Paseo Mikeletegi 7, E-20009 Donostia, San Sebastián, Spain*
[b] *Tecnalia, Health Technologies Unit, Parque Tecnológico 202, E-48170 Zamudio, Spain*

Abstract. While recent technological developments increasingly bring robots into people's life, improving individuals' productivity at work or easing their life at home, many elderly adults have not benefited of that societal change yet, therefore remaining excluded from the information society. Against this phenomenon, several innovative products have been recently proposed in assistive technology: among them, multipurpose robotic systems certainly represent the most appealing solution designed to improve elderly people quality of life. However, for robots to truly become part of the life of elderly people, essential usability, acceptance and ethical issues need to be addressed and solved by robotics researchers.

Keywords. Assistive Robotics, usability, acceptance of technology, ethics

Introduction

In his provocative book *Natural-Born Cyborgs* [13], Andy Clark claims that human beings are already cyborgs "in the more profound sense of being human-technology symbionts". In the present world, the author says, the power of our mind is no more confined to its "biological skin bag": we are "wired" and "merged" to external and non-biological tools enabling our brain to experience the life through augmented capabilities. But in this amazing world that according to Clark we live in, a world made of beings moving freely in intelligent environments, searching for sensory augmentation or taking advantage of futuristic thought-controlled prosthetics, there are some so unlucky to be still "unplugged": elderly individuals that, because of the digital divide, do not belong yet to the ICT society.

Nowadays, the relationship of older adults with technology cannot be compared with the relationship that younger adults experience: they don't share the same technological education and culture as younger users and, furthermore, the majority of ICT products have not been designed to suit them. For a large part of the old population, technology is unfamiliar, difficult to access and thus cannot be used. Indeed, most elderly users do not buy new products or even consider the adoption of new technologies potentially beneficial, because the learning process involved in using a new artifact can be too costly for them.

[*] Corresponding Author: Francesca Irene Cavallaro. E-mail: francesca.cavallaro@tecnalia.com.

However, despite this problematic relationship between elderly and technology, the critical demographic change forecasted, according to which twenty eight per cent of the European population will be over 65 by the year 2050 [35], makes improvement in assistive technology urgent and necessary.

The aging process often results in the need of physical and cognitive assistance: individuals become less physically fit and frailer, sometimes experiencing annoying memory problems. The greatest need for assistance comes when those elders wish to live independently in their home as long as they can. Providing all the care required at this stage as an informal caregiver, often a family member with a professional activity and personal family life, is not tenable. According to the American National Institute on Aging (NIA), having a full time job is nowadays incompatible with caring for an elder person who is not physically independent. Family life, health and professional career are at high risk when deciding to take care of elder parents.

If being an informal caregiver for a loved one is a feasible solution only at the price of devoting one's entire life to the caring task, nursing and care homes are not viable solutions to face the increase of assistance needs either. The corresponding financial cost, the significant space and staff shortages are already a critical issue that our society will not be able to overcome if strong changes are not realized. Technological advances should be directed to assist the senior population and those who provide care. This is a usual starting point for justifying the development of new robotic solutions. The recent advances in several scientific areas (such as computer science, automation, sensors and actuators design) have enabled to start moving the robots out of the industrial buildings, towards people's home, employing their skills to provide assistance to the individuals (Fig. 1 shows the statistic data for personal/domestic use of service robots). Nowadays there are several projects and expositions showing robotic systems able to act autonomously in home-like environments, verbally and physically interacting with end-users. These robots are designed as means to provide support for basic activities, like eating, bathing, dressing, and toileting, to assist in mobility and ambulation or rehabilitation activities, or simply to offer some companionship [50].

Nevertheless, even if the scientific technology seems to be ready to answer the specific user needs, very few robotic systems have been really accepted by the population and can be considered as commercial successes [34]. This aspect cannot be only justified by the price issue (any robotic system addressing a consequent market could indeed benefit from mass production) and it demonstrates that providing technical solutions is not enough to get robotic systems accepted by non-specialist users.

Socially Assistive Robotic (SAR) is the current and promising answer to this problem. SAR, indeed, is grounded on a user-centered point of view, in which aspects of usability and acceptance become predominant. The elderly person is not only considered as an end-user, but also as a key partner along the design process and the development of the robotic system.

This chapter is an overview of two non-technological factors in Human Robot Interaction, usability and acceptance, which are essential for the development of successful social assistive robots. Ethical concerns, inherent to the cohabitation of socially interacting robots and humans, will be also addressed at the end of the chapter, also pointing at key projects focusing on the creation of a new ethical framework for technology developers and users.

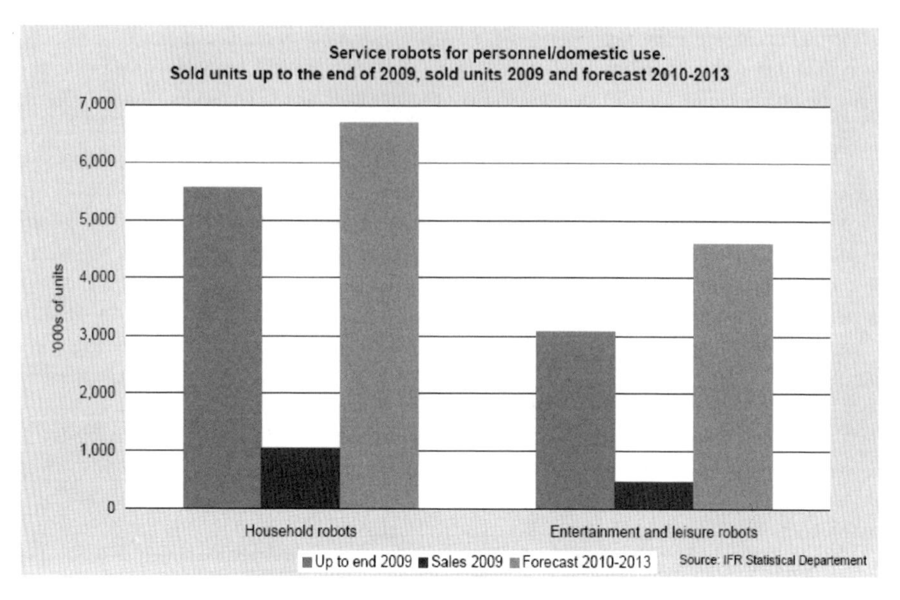

Figure 1. Statistics for service robots for personal/domestic use.

1. A Brief Overview of Social Assistive Robots

The proportion of elderly people living with limitations in mobility, dexterity and mental capacity, is expected to increase. In spite of their needs, it was reported that this population segment would hesitate to use technology owing to limitations in dexterity and/or sensory acuity [4]. However, through technological improvements of the past years, Assistive Technology is now able to support people. Robots, especially, can provide not only assistance in daily activities but also safety monitoring, thus improving their independent living. Nonetheless, many of these products have been so far designed with little consideration of the social, aesthetic, and emotional relations that elders will form with them. For a full social interaction with users, robots' features should take in consideration embodiment, emotion, dialog, personality, human-oriented perception, user modeling, socially situated learning and intentionality [31].

As the general population grows older, the need for long-term care increases, and the pool of potential caregivers declines, assistive robots acquire a further role in the provision of healthcare, supplementing the functions of caregivers. Socially interacting robots, thus, are becoming a reality and they can perform tasks related to tutoring, education, physical therapy, daily life assistance, emotional expression, entertainment, and many others (Fig. 2 shows some examples of social robots).

It has to be said that the term of "Social Assistive Robotics" is not yet referenced by international reports mainly focusing on the robotics systems already economically established. Social Assistive Robotics can be included within the Healthcare Robotics as defined in the US Robotic Roadmap [12] and within the report "Robotics for Healthcare" commissioned by the European Commission [7], but it is more precisely related to the Assistive Robotics group as defined by the International Federation of Robotics [39]. "Assistive Robotics" is a term that has been broadly used to designate all systems providing assistance to the person, in order to compensate disabilities due

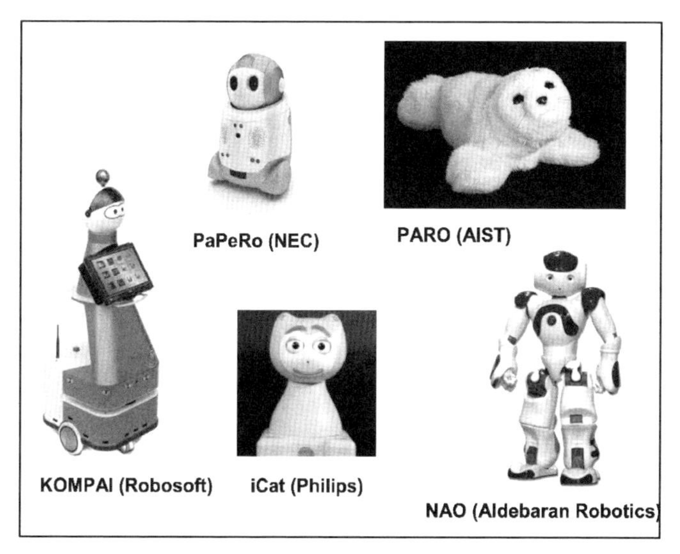

Figure 2. Examples of social robots.

to aging, acquired brain injury, stroke or neurodegenerative diseases. Initially, this term thus mainly designated systems dealing with physical assistance, such as rehabilitation robots, wheelchair robots, manipulator arms or robotic platform for physical rehabilitation training.

Within the Assistive Robotics group and at variance with the standard physical robot assistants previously mentioned, SARs adopt a contact-free assistance [72] and embed social features to improve the human-robot interaction [29]. The social emphasis of SAR also demonstrates its close relationship with Socially Interactive Robots (SIR), for which the robot is embodied within its societal environment, being able to recognize agents, understand its surrounding world, and engage in social interaction [31]. SAR can be considered as the projection of the generic SIR domains onto the Healthcare area: SAR aims at providing assistance trough social interaction.

The systems labeled as SAR robots are various, however, considering their main characteristics Broekens et al. [6] have divided them into two main groups of SAR: *service robots* and *companion robots*.

Service robots provide the user with a functional assistance that is strongly related to the good accomplishment of Basic or Instrumental Activities of the Daily Living [40], such as feeding, dressing, ambulating, meals preparation, taking medicines and so on. As an illustration, the Pearl robot from the Carnegie Mellon University [53] provides routine activities reminder (eating, drinking, taking medicine) as well as some walking guidance. The interaction is realized through speech synthesis, visual display onto a touch screen, and motions of an actuated head unit. Other relevant systems are the Care-o-Bot from Fraunhofer [37], the Cero robot from the IPLab of Stockholm [61], or the ROBOCARE robot [9].

Companion or pet-like robots rely on the assumption that the companionship can influence the psychological, physiological and even social health of the person [45]. Most of these systems are designed to be very similar to pets, in order to reproduce the same relationship the elderly could have with such animal. The seal Paro from the National Institute of Advanced Industrial Science and Technology (Japan) is one of the most famous companions developed. The interaction with the person relies on the use of light sensors, speech recognition systems, balance and tactile sensors. Actuators in the body enable to reproduce some light movements, and the eyelids permit to create face expressions. This system has been extensively tested, with people suffering from dementia [82], or with persons living in care centers, and these studies demonstrated positive influence on the patient social interaction with relatives, while reducing the presence of stress [84]. Another similar robotic system that could be also mentioned is the Huggable robot from the MIT Media Lab [69]. Using similar assumptions, several toys-like systems have been also tested as assistive devices for the elderly. The interested reader can refer to robots like the AIBO from Sony [71], the electronic device Nabaztag [41], the iCat from Philips Electronics [83] or the Pleo dinosaur [20].

The added value of the social component in assistive robots has also been investigated in rehabilitation, which is a field usually addressed by assistive robots. It was demonstrated, indeed, that the use of a robot with a sort of personality (like an avatar on a screen, or some physical limbs) that provides feedbacks to the user improves the involvement of the person within her rehabilitation activity [46].

Finally, other elements that have been proposed to define social assistive robots are: the user population addressed, the description of the task to realize, the type of the interaction and the role of robot [31].

Beyond the definition of all these key aspects, anyway, there are two transversal themes that should guide researchers' and designers' choices in developing a social assistive robot within a user-centered framework, and these are also the themes on which this chapter evolves: the usability and the acceptance of this kind of technology by elderly individuals.

2. Improving Usability for the Elderly

Designing technologies for older adults means, among other things, carefully taking into consideration all the changes in perceptual, motor and cognitive capabilities. Indeed, usability problems often lead older people to experience dissatisfaction when operating with technologies, with the eventual consequence of technology abandonment.

2.1. Definition and State of the Art

Assistive technology often fails to be adopted because of inadequate training on how to use it. The potential benefits to people's independence are not understood or the design of the device appears cumbersome and is unfamiliar. Robots cannot only be simply considered as assistive devices; they are also perceived by the user as entities to interact with.

The term *usability* describes the ease of using an object. The ISO 924111:1998 defines usability as "the extent to which a product can be used by specified users to achieve specified goals with effectiveness, efficiency and satisfaction in a specified context of use". The term *effectiveness* describes the accuracy and completeness with which users achieve specific tasks, while the term *efficiency* characterizes the resources expended in relation to the accuracy and completeness with which the users achieve goals.

When considering assistive robots, additional factors need to be taken into account to describe usability [86]:

- *Learnability*: how easy a system can be learned by novice users. In the case of assistive robots, people have not previous experience with them, so this is a key indicator. It includes issues like familiarity, consistency, generalizability, consistency and simplicity.
- *Flexibility*: it describes the number of possible communication flows in between the user and the system.
- *Robustness*: an efficient human-robot interaction should allow the user to correct its faults, and the system should be stable and able to prevent user errors.
- *Utility*: it refers to how an interface can be used to reach a certain goal or to perform a certain task.
- *Consistency*: is related to the cues provided to the users in order to help them predicting the system's way or working.

2.2. Main Results Up to Date

The experience gained with the design of industrial robots cannot be transferred to the assistive field. Industrial systems concentrate on precision, accuracy and repetition. However, domestic environments are unstructured and variable, and they require a high level of adaptability. The needs of assistive users are often much more complex than those for industrial tasks, but this fact is not always recognized by root designers, who concentrate on product design but tend to ignore social and human aspects. Another problem is that the aim of an assistive robot is not to replace an existing human, but rather to support and enhance the user's abilities, therefore a careful balance must be set between users and robot.

A model for human-robot interaction usually employed in elder care institutions is based on the model named UTAUT (Unified Theory of Acceptance and Use of Technology) [77]. The UTAUT is a model that consider influences on acceptance of technology mainly for the workplace, that take into account factors like performance expectancy, effort expectancy, attitude towards using technology, self-efficacy, anxiety, enjoyment, social presence and social abilities. According to this model, design for system usability should be rest on users preferences and understanding of their needs, furthermore, it should be customizable to accommodate with different levels of user abilities. Any complexity should be hidden and the system must have operational modes. The user interfaces must be intuitive and responsive, and user communications for control or training must be simple and direct.

The type of interaction will also be influenced also by how many different kinds of robots we expect people will interact with.

In the 6th and 7th Framework Programmes, the European Commission has provided funding for various projects dealing with ICT for senior citizens. All of them consider the concept of usability while designing robotic systems:

- HERMES [38] aims to develop assistive technology for older people to reduce age-related decline of cognitive capabilities. Based on an intelligent audio and visual processing and reasoning, the project results in a combination of a home-based and mobile devices to support the user's cognitive state and prevent cognitive decline, increasing her ability to cope with everyday life and to live independently.

- COMPANIONABLE [42] addresses the issues of social inclusion and homecare of persons suffering from chronic cognitive disabilities prevalent among the elderly population. The project focuses on combining the strengths of a mobile robotic companion with the advantages of a stationary smart home. Assistive effects of both individual solutions shall be combined to demonstrate how the resulting synergies can make the care and the cared person's interaction with her assistive system significantly better.
- Robot@CWE [55] demonstrates integrative concepts of advance robotic systems, to be seen as collaborative agents, in various environments and working together with humans. They propose evolution strategies toward "collaborative-working-centered" design of robotic systems and "IST robotics" concepts on the basis of sound collaborative practices and new technologies such as virtualized mixed environments, multimedia communication, ubiquitous environments, teleworking schemes, etc.

2.3. Identified Needs for Future Developments

While modern robotics has come a long way, there is still a considerable work to be done in various fields. New developments in other technologies such as Automatic Speech Recognition (ASR), Text to Speech (TTS), advanced non intrusive sensors, wireless communications and computer vision can be adapted and integrated in the design of state of the art robotic systems. Current trends and future research areas are:

Telerehabilitation robotics: Robotic-assisted telerehabilitation offers innovative, interactive, and precisely reproducible therapies that can be performed for an extended duration and be consistently implemented from site to site [8]. Robot-assisted therapy emphasizes the central role of the patient during the motor exercise. This poses major technical challenges for the design of safe and effective robotic platforms. The therapist has the ability to track their patient progresses remotely, as well as to change some settings remotely, based on their performance. Haptic devices, which takes advantage of a user's sense of touch by applying forces, vibrations and/or motions onto the user, could also be used in physical rehabilitation. Users can be challenged according to their specific abilities and be rewarded with graphics and sound, making that way the exercises more fun and rewarding.

Intelligent and natural interfaces: We cannot consider the elderly population as a homogeneous group in which all present the same health problems and needs. We must create systems capable to interact with each user adapting to the specific profile each user will have. Besides these individual user characteristics, cognitive as well as motor skills of older users do not remain constant, which requires an additional adaptation over time [57].

Game-based technologies: Several recent studies have examined video games as a new way to challenge the brain, keep it young, and promote healthy aging. According to [11], playing games could efficiently enhance seniors' health both physically and mentally [11]. Many skills can be enhanced through video games and can help the older people in their daily activities, for example by improving their attention span, training them to manage several tasks simultaneously, sharpening their reflexes and retaining memory. With the use of recent game control devices such as Nintendo Wii's innovative remote control and balance board or XBOX Kinect, the user could also perform physical exercises from their own homes [73].

Natural dialogue capabilities: Social Assistive Robots must provide dialogue capabilities based on the user's profile. As each user will have different characteristics, the dialogue needs to be based on a multimodal approach, using sound (text to speech), vision and touch interfaces. Spoken Dialogue Systems (SDS) allows users to interact with machines by means of spoken dialogues in natural language. These systems would be particularly suitable because older people usually have little or no computing experience [68].

Implicit communication (person's affective state): A standard communication is one in which the message to transmit is expressed explicitly, through speech or writing. The latest scientific findings indicate that emotions play an essential role in rational decision-making, perception, learning, and various cognitive tasks. Therefore, endowing machines with a degree of emotional intelligence should permit more meaningful and natural human-machine interaction [54]. Emotions can be detected using peripheral physiological signals obtained from sensors: monitoring activity, temperature sensors and cameras, using gesture recognition techniques, possibly giving an insight of the feelings a user has at a certain moment.

Behavioral anticipation: The detection and understanding of the behavior of external agents is mandatory to perform fluid interaction. Through learning a robot could reuse this knowledge in future tasks. This prediction can also be used to adapt its movements and actions. Robots should predict the actions of the user based on the monitoring of user's daily habits. They should also anticipate their needs studying their behavior [68].

Challenges related to regulations, laws, responsibility and insurance: Social assistive robots are to perform their activities with a certain autonomy, which naturally raises some evident security matters that need to be addressed. In [93] the authors propose a framework for a legal system for the so-called Next Generation Robot. Their goal is to ensure safer robot design through "safety intelligence" and provide a method for dealing with accidents when they do occur. One guiding principle of the proposed framework relies on the categorization of robots as "third existence" entities, since Next Generation Robots are considered to be neither living/biological (first existence) nor non-living/non-biological (second existence). The proposed third existence entity resembles living things in appearance and behavior that are not self-aware. While robots are currently legally classified as second existence (human property), the authors believe that a third existence classification would simplify the management of accidents in terms of responsibility distribution [53].

Component standardization (software and hardware): Currently, robots are built with proprietary technologies which tend to amplify the number of solutions without ensuring a general compatibility. This can be considered as counterproductive for the scientific progress as well as for the development of new robotic products. The standardization of robotic architectures and middleware has become a prime topic in order to obtain the expected performances. The emergence of a robotic supply industry is seen as a critical factor for reducing high development costs.

This requires interoperability of hardware and software components, which cannot be obtained without the standardization of robot architectures and middleware. Following the first standard for robotic components defined in 2008 [50], the world's first standard aimed specifically for service robots has just been published in February 2010 [51]. This specification document defines a Robot Localization (RoLo) service that can handle data and usages specific to use in robotics. It includes a platform independent model (PIM) as well as a mapping of this PIM to platform specific model (PSM) defined within the C++ programming language.

3. Elderly People Acceptance of Robots

3.1. Definition of Technology Acceptance

According to one of the most quoted definition of acceptance stated by [19], user acceptance of technology can be defined as "the demonstrable willingness within a user group to employ information technology for the tasks it is designed to support".

The increasing need of older people for physical and cognitive assistance is one of the leading drives for the development of novel and versatile robotic systems that support and promote aging in place. Several robotic systems have been developed with the aim of supporting frail elderly in their homes and reducing their dependence for routine tasks and activities. The solutions offered range from enhancing mobility and improving communication capabilities to supporting the continuity of care and sharing routine repetitive tasks with caregivers. However, no matter how sophisticated the system proposed could be, the lack of positive user acceptance can lead to assured abandonment of the system itself. Indeed, not even making a product highly usable guarantees that it will be accepted by its intended users [65], since even if usability and ease of use are essential conditions, and are often considered as prerequisites to end-user acceptance of technology, they don't entirely fulfill the definition of user's acceptance.

3.2. Models of Technology Acceptance

Acceptance is a core topic in human factors research, and one of the issues belonging to the research in Human-Robot Interaction. Due to the complexity of the concept, literature on acceptance provides some understanding of what makes users accept or reject a system but cannot identify a single-variable explanation of the level of acceptance any information technology will receive among its intended users [19].

One of the models trying to explain and assess acceptance of technology that has received considerable attention from researchers in the information systems field is the Technology Acceptance Model (TAM) proposed by Davis [17]. TAM models actual individual's behaviors or behavioral intentions, based upon the user's perception of the usefulness and ease of use of a particular technology since both (user's perception and ease of use) drastically influence the individual's attitude towards the technology, their intentions to use it, and their actual use. Many subsequent studies have extended the original version of TAM to incorporate additional variables within specific contexts [62]. Alavi and Joachimsthaler [1] propose, for example, that the most relevant user factors determining technology acceptance are *cognitive style*, *personality*, *demographics* and *user-situational variables*. Recently, despite a certain agreement on the individual and situational factors influencing the acceptance of new technologies, evidence has been collected that suggests that context of use might be more important than personality or individual psychological factors alone [19].

With the aim to propose a model that incorporates the most widely used models on acceptance of technology, Venkatesh et al. [77] integrated the theoretical models that employ intention and/or usage as the key dependent variable. The result of this process is the UTAUT model which has also been used in several studies on acceptance of robots. The key factors for acceptance of technology according to the UTAUT model are the following constructs: *performance expectancy*, *effort expectancy*, *attitude toward using technology*, *self-efficacy*, *anxiety* and *behavioral intention to use*.

3.3. Acceptance of Robots

Even if the research on user acceptance of technology has produced numerous studies and models, robots represent a very special kind of technology implying a new form of interaction not fully and perhaps not adequately addressed by previous acceptance models. The UTAUT model and the way it is used could be subject to discussion in the case of acceptance of robots, since it is neither developed for elders nor for a technology that performs as a conversational partner, like a robot is envisioned to do. Furthermore, acceptance of robots that would carry out daily tasks is largely dependent upon user's subjective perceptions of what robots are, how they work and what exactly they are and are not capable of doing in a domestic environment. Besides, researchers cannot expect that people will respond to the introduction of robots in their life in the same way they do for other technologies.

Robots can be complex and autonomous systems with endowed cognitive capabilities, and the interaction with them will change according to the physical nature of the robot, the number of systems a user may be called to interact with simultaneously, and the environment in which the interactions occur. Assistive robots, especially, are meant to actively and physically share spaces with people and display a level of autonomy and intelligence. Unlike the PC, which stays where it is placed and must be actively engaged and enabled, a robot will physically interact with and alter its surroundings and may not remain in a specific and single allocated space. The robot may move unexpectedly, users must follow its motion cues and physical state, and may not have direct access to orthodox interfaces such as a keyboard or display panel. Finally, depending on the role the robot is supposed to assume, the system could be an operator, a peer or a supervisor [58]. Consequently, a user could accept the robot as a conversational partner, find the robot's social skills credible, see the robot as an autonomous social being and therefore would be more likely exhibiting natural verbal and nonverbal conversational behavior as well as feeling comfortable in interacting with the robot. A user could also demonstrate more conversational engagement by being more expressive and thus behavioral clues can be used as an indication of conversational acceptance. Therefore, when dealing with acceptance of robots, it is advisable to not only address acceptance in terms of the usefulness and ease of use of a system, but to consider also relational or social acceptance issues.

In their review of Healthcare robot, Broadbent et al. [5] further develop Dillon's definition of acceptance stating that for acceptance of robots to occur, there are three basic requirements to be satisfied: a motivation for using the robot, sufficient ease of use, and comfort with the robot physically, cognitively and emotionally. According to the authors the relevant factors influencing user acceptance of robots can be grouped in

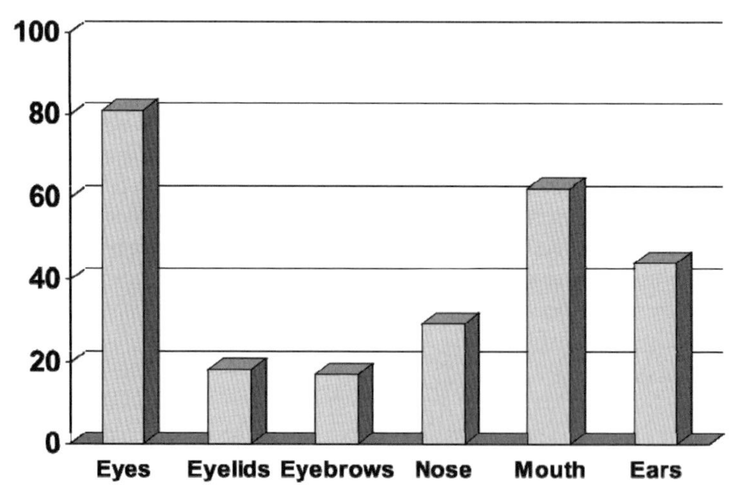

Figure 3. Features of robot's face contributing to its humanness [21].

two different clusters: *end-user factors* and *robot factors*. End-user factors are user's age and gender, user's needs, user's experience with technology or robots, user's cognitive ability and education, user's cultural background, user's role respect to the robot personality, user's anxiety and at last attitude toward robots. Factors that are strictly related to the robot are, instead: appearance, humanness, size, gender, facial dimensions and expressions, personality and adaptability.

Further on, research has shown that people respond to robots in unique ways, and often in ways similar to how they respond to living entities [80]. Appearance of robot, in this sense, has been always considered as a highly relevant factor, since the formulation of the *Uncanny Valley* hypothesis [48]. Recently this hypothesis has been developed and tested in studies intended to demonstrate that users prefer a more human-like appearance for the robot to perform jobs that are more, rather than less, social in nature [36]. Besides, there have been attempts [21] to identify which are the features and dimensions of a robot´s face that mainly contribute to people's perception of its humanness (see Fig. 3).

According to another way of classifying results from research on robot and agent acceptance, two are the meaning of acceptance that can be identified: acceptance of the robot in terms of usefulness and ease of use (*functional acceptance*) and acceptance of the robot as a conversational partner with which a human or pet-like relationship is possible (*social acceptance*). Ezer and colleagues [28] used a questionnaire to compare the results from elderly users and younger users about the types and characteristics of tasks that two types of population would be willing to let a robot perform. According to their results, respondents of both groups were more willing to have robots performing infrequent, albeit important, tasks that required little interaction with the human compared to service-type tasks with more required interaction. Respondents were less willing to have a robot performing non-critical tasks requiring extensive interaction between robot and human. Older adults reported more willingness than younger adults in having a robot performing critical tasks in their home. The results suggest that both younger and older individuals are more interested in the benefits that a robot can provide than in their interactive abilities.

So far, no unique and standard tool to assess elderly user's acceptance of robots seems to have been used. Besides, the existence of differing types of robots, with different shapes, design and various forms of interaction and feedback, represents one of the main methodological difficulties in the evaluation of social acceptance of robots [85]. Some of the available means the HRI researchers adopt to assess end-user acceptance of technology are ethnographic observation, system response-time analysis, common ground analysis, embodiment measurement, perceived enjoyment analysis, comfort level analysis, interaction profile analysis, and others. Recently, Riek and Robinson [56] proposed a new toolset named "Classification Ease", in which the assessment is made through a preliminary classification of the robot type, role and behavioral function. Finally, having found that Venkatesh UTAUT model has a low explanatory power and that it is not sufficiently addressing the social aspects of the interaction, Heerink and colleagues [39] have also proposed a toolkit to assess elderly users acceptance of social assistive robots that they consider suitable for repetitive testing and adequate to assess factors like attitude and trust.

4. Ethical Issues in Social Assistive Robotics

4.1. General Considerations

Employing robot-based AT solutions represents a potential option to improve elderly people life at home and to enhance eldercare in general, but, as for any ICT, several ethical implications must be taken into account before designing and adoption of new solutions. Although, as Tiwari et al. remark [80], a much-needed ethical framework for AT is virtually non-existent, especially for vulnerable and dependent people like elderly individuals, the research community is becoming more and more aware that the introduction of new technology in elderly users' life shall respect and, if possible, improve their autonomy, be beneficent under all possible conditions of use, and not infringe on their privacy [49]. These considerations generate a set of constraints with respect to the design and conditions of adoption of a robotic system collected and presented by the authors of the European project *Senior* [66] and that we can summarize as the following:

Adoption of the system must respect the user's freedom of choice: it must not be imposed, but proposed. It should be presented as an alternative to or an improvement over the existing service provided to the user, and if the system provides a novel service, care must be taken not to present such service as an obligation, but as a chance.

The system must reinforce personal autonomy: functional performance of a robotic system must not become an incentive for the user to become dependent upon the system. This may indeed precipitate the decline of the precious innate abilities of the user, or lead to dire consequences in case of system failure, for example. Designers are thus faced with an interesting dilemma insofar as there may be instances where optimal performance of a system with respect to a given task is not desirable.

The system must respect and guarantee privacy: it is easy to imagine scenarios, especially with systems that deal with medical data, where access to user data by malicious agents may lead to its inappropriate use and thus have very negative consequences for the user of the system. In particular, the use of wireless connectivity for semi-autonomous mobile agents opens many attractive possibilities in terms of assistive applications, but it requires appropriate communication protocols to ensure that personal data can only be accessed by those authorised to do so, similarly to any other electronic health data exchange and communication platforms.

The system must safeguard dignity and self-esteem: functional performance of a system should not come at the expense of the user's sense of self-worth and dignity. Besides the increased likelihood of abandonment this would generate, the psychological repercussions of any perceived loss of dignity should be considered as a threat to the general health of the user.

The system must emphasise user safety: while a priori obvious, this consideration touches an interesting ethical question insofar as it may require the designers of a given system to voluntarily limit the control given to the user over that system. The line separating a valid security measure to an ethically reprehensible hindrance to user freedom may thus become difficult to identify in some cases.

4.2. Summary of EU Efforts so Far

Perfectly aware of the possible ethical issues in AT, the European Commission has published some ethical recommendations for the researchers that work in the projects included in FP7 [57]. The ethical issues included in this document are evaluated in every projects presented to this program. The EU has also directly funded a few projects – in FP6, 7, CIP and AAL – focussing on ethical, social, legal and human right implications of ICT for ageing. We will list some of them below.

Under the 6th Framework Programme, the ETHICBOTS [24] project has been funded to promote and coordinate a multidisciplinary group of researchers in artificial intelligence, robotics, anthropology, moral philosophy, philosophy of science, psychology, and cognitive science, with the common purpose of defining a methodology for the identification and analysis of ethical issues related to human interaction with robotic, bionic, and AI systems for communication [23]. One of the main objectives of this project was to generate inputs to EU for techno-ethical monitoring, warning, and opinion generation. Another project explicitly devoted to social and ethical issues is SENIOR [66] closed in 2009, which was a support action that has provided a systematic assessment of the social, ethical, and privacy issues involved in ICT and Ageing.

Funded under the 7th Framework Programme, the ETICA project [22] and the Value Ageing IAPP [82] action have just started. ETICA aims at the identification and evaluation of emerging ICTs and their related potential ethical issues. This will lead to policy advices on appropriate governance structures and/or processes of ethics of future technologies that ETICA will recommend for consideration to the European Commission. Value Ageing, instead, is a joint research project about the incorporation of fundamental values of the EU in ICT for ageing. Among the actions foreseen in this project, a specific research effort will be devoted to identify social, psychological and ethical issues of assistive robotics for elderly.

With the first International Symposium on Roboethics (2004), the word "roboethics" has been coined to define principles and general ethical issues of ethics applied to robotics. Afterward the EURON network, European Robotics Research Network, has been created with the aim of drawing the first roboethics roadmap [85].

EU presented in 1995 the directive on personal data protection [27] which should be adopted by all the countries in the EU and which should ensure the quality of the data and their appropriate use. Also we can find some recommendations, given by Council of Europe [14], about the medical data acquired to assistive robotics in healthcare. Recommendations about personal data protection should be converted in mandatory actions [16,52] to assure the respect of privacy.

Recognized as "one of the most important human rights of the modern age" [35], privacy might be at risk due to the impact that new technologies have in our daily life. As a matter of fact, the ability to transmit, process and store personal information proper to new monitoring, location, and eHealth technologies potentially exposes the user to the risk of accidental or intentional disclosure of private information to a third party [40,58]. Personal robots can indeed become privacy intruders, mainly because of the vulnerability of their security system [18], which may lead to accidental or intentional disclosure of private information [76].

Finally, another ethical concern that has to be mentioned, considering the psychological and social aspects of care of aging people, is the perceived threat from technology by the existing care giving workforce. Technology is perceived as a threat that will take away their jobs while not to being able to meet the social and emotional needs of older persons in the way that human caregivers do [73]. Some researchers are actually warning against the risk of leaving elderly in the exclusive care of a machine [69].

5. Conclusions

Advances in medicine research are postponing the term of our life-end, but they are not sufficient to prevent physical and cognitive decline to appear, sooner or later. Emergent assistive technology can be the way to ageing well, with dignity, and helping elderly individuals to remain autonomous, experience personal growth in the later part of their life, maintain social ties, and enjoy the pleasures that life may offer. However, the positive contribution of the assistive technology can only be obtained if elderly users are willing to use it, which in turn depends on several complex factors: the needs that people perceive, the safety of the interaction, the perceived usefulness of the technology, and whether the individual feels that use of the device either supports or undermines their sense of personal identity. It has been shown that acceptance of home care technology by older people has not been a serious problem after proper introduction and training. However, important practical issues related to usability, acceptability as well as to specific ethical issues like privacy, autonomy and responsibility are still open challenges for technology developers.

In this chapter we have introduced one of the promising products of robotics for eldercare enhancement, Assistive Social Robotics, and we have discussed some of the main non technological issues proper to human-robot interaction because for a new attitude toward robotics to take place and for robots to finally become part of our life, researchers shall take into account usability, acceptability and ethical issues at the very first stage of the design of a new robotic assistant.

References

[1] M. Alavi and E.A. Joachimsthaler, Revisiting DSS implementation research: A meta analysis of the literature and suggestions for researchers, *MIS Quarterly* **16**(1) (1992), 95–116.

[2] P.M. Asaro, What should we want from a robot ethic?, *International Review of Information Ethics* **6** (2006), 9–16.

[3] S. Blackburn, *Oxford Dictionary of Philosophy*, Oxford University Press, 1996.
[4] K.H. Bowles and A.C. Baugh, Applying research evidence to optimize telehomecare, *Journal of Cardiovascular Nursing* **22** (2010), 5–15.
[5] E. Broadbent, R. Stafford and B. MacDonald, Acceptance of healthcare robots for the older population: Review and future directions, *International Journal of Social Robotics* **1** (2009), 319–33.
[6] J. Broekens, M. Heerink and H. Rosendal, Assistive social robots in elderly care: A review, *Gerontechnology* **8** (2009), 94–103.
[7] M. Butter, A. Rensma, J. van Boxsel, S. Kalisingh, S. Schoone, M. Leis, G. Gelderblom, G. Cremers, M. de Wilt, W. Koertkaas, A. Thielmann, K. Cuhls, A. Sashinopoulou and I. Korhonen, Robotics for healthcare, Final report, European Commission, DG Information Society, 2008.
[8] C. Carignan and H. Krebs, Telerehabilitation robotics: Bright lights, big future?, *Journal of Rehabilitation Research & Development* **43**(2006), 695–710.
[9] A. Cesta, G. Cortellessa, M.V. Giuliani, F. Pecora, M. Scopelliti and L. Tiberio, Psychological implications of domestic assistive technology for the elderly, *Psychology Journal* **5** (2007), 229–252.
[10] Charter of fundamental rights of the European Union (200/C 264/01), 2000.
[11] A. Cheok, S. Lee, S. Kodagoda, K. Tat and L. Thang, A social and physical inter-generational computer game for the elderly and children: Age invaders, in: *Wearable Computer*, 2005, pp. 202–203.
[12] H. Christensen, ed., A roadmap for US robotics: From internet to robotics, 2009.
[13] A. Clark, *Natural-Born Cyborgs: Minds, Technologies, and the Future of Human Intelligence*, Oxford University Press, 2003.
[14] Council of Europe, Committee of Ministers, Recommendation No. R (97) 5 on the Protection of Medical Data (1997).
[15] A. Damasio, *Descartes' Error: Emotion, Reason, and the Human Brain*, Avon Books, 1994.
[16] Data Protection Working Party. The Future of Privacy. Joint contribution to the Consulation of the European Commission on the legal framework for the fundamental right to protection of personal data, Article 29. Adopted on 01 December 2009, 02356/09/EN, WP 168, paragraph 46.
[17] F.D. Davis, Perceived usefulness, perceived ease of use, and user acceptance of information technology, *MIS Quarterly* **13** (1989), 319–340.
[18] T. Denning, C. Matuszek, K. Koscher, J.R. Smith and K.A. Tadayoshi, Spotlight on security and privacy risks with future household robots: Attacks and lessons, in: *International Conference of Ubiquitous Computing*, 2009, pp. 105–114.
[19] A. Dillon, User acceptance of information technology, in: *Encyclopaedia of human factors and ergonomics*, W. Karwowski, ed., Taylor and Francis, 2001.
[20] J. Dimas, I. Leite, A. Pereira, P. Cuba, R. Prada and A. Paiva, Pervasive pleo: Long-term attachment with artificial pets, in: *Workshop on Playful Experiences in Mobile HCI*, Lisbon, Portugal, 2010.
[21] C. DiSalvo, F. Gemperle, J. Forlizzi and S. Kiesler, All robots are not created equal: The design and perception of humanoid robot heads, in: *Designing Interactive Systems 2002 Conference Proceedings*, London, England, June 2002, pp. 321–326.
[22] Ethical Issues of Emerging ICT Application, ETICA, http://www.etica-project.eu/.
[23] ETHICBOTS: Emerging Technoethics of Human Interaction with Communication, Bionic and Robotic Systems, Project Deliverable 2, 2006.
[24] ETHICBOTS project, http://ethicbots.na.infn.it/.
[25] EUROP, Strategic Research Agenda, 2008.
[26] European Group on Ethics in Science and Technologies, http://ec.europa.eu/european_group_ethics/.
[27] European Parliament Council, Directive 95/46/EC on the protection of individuals with regard to the processing of personal data and on the free movement of such data, 1995.
[28] European Union, Charter of fundamental rights of the European Union, *Official Journal of the European Communities* **364** (2000), 1–22.
[29] N. Ezer, A. Fisk and W. Rogers, More than a servant: Self-reported willingness of younger and older adults to having a robot perform interactive and critical tasks in the home, *Human Factors and Ergonomic Society Annual Meeting Proceeding* **53**(2) (2009), 136–140.
[30] D. Feil-Seifer and M.J. Mataric, Defining socially assistive robotics, in: *IEEE International Conference on Rehabilitation Robotics*, Chicago, USA, 2005, pp. 465–468.
[31] D. Fiel-Seifer and M.J. Matarić, Human-Robot Interaction, *Encyclopedia of Complexity and Systems Science*, R.A. Meyers, ed., Springer Reference, 2009.
[32] T. Fong, O. Nourbakhsh and K. Dautenhahn, A survey of socially interactive robots, *Robotics and Autonomous Systems* **42**(3–4) (2003), 143–166.
[33] J. Forlizzi and C. DiSalvo, Service robots in the domestic environment: A study of the roomba vacuum in the home, in: *ACM SIGCHI/SIGART Conference on Human-Robot Interaction*, 2006.

[34] J. Forlizzi, C. DiSalvo and F. Gemperle, Assistive robotics and a ecology of elders living independently in their homes, Human-Computer Interaction Institute, 2004.
[35] M. Friedewald, A new concept for privacy in the light of emerging sciences and technologies, *Technikfolgenabschätzung – Theorie un Praxis* **19**(1) (2010), 71–74.
[36] K. Giannakouris, Ageing characterises the demographic perspectives of the European societies, *EUROSTAT Statistics in Focus* **78** (2008).
[37] J. Goetz, S. Kiesler and A. Powers, Matching robot appearance and behavior to tasks to improve human-robot cooperation, in: *IEEE International Workshop on Robot and Human Interactive Communication*, Millbrae, CA, 2003.
[38] B. Graf, U. Reiser, M. Hägele, K. Mauz and P. Klein, Robotic home assistant Care-O-bot® 3 – Product vision and innovation platform, in: *IEEE Workshop on Advanced Robotics and its Social Impacts*, Tokyo, Japan, 2009.
[39] M. Heerink, B.J.A. Kröse, B.J. Wielinga and V. Evers, Measuring acceptance of an assistive social robot: A suggested toolkit, in: *Proc. of the Third ACM/IEEE International Conference on Proceedings of Ro-man,* Toyama, 2009, p. 528.
[40] O.A.B. Henkemans, K.E. Caine and W.A. Rogers, Medical monitoring for independent living: User-centered design of smart home technologies for older adults, in: *Proc. of the Med-e-Tel Conference for eHealth, Telemedicine and Health Information and Communication Technologies*, 2007.
[41] HERMES project, http://www.fp7-hermes.eu/.
[42] http://www.companionable.net/.
[43] IFR world robotics – Service robots, statistics, market analysis, forecasts and case studies, IFR Statistical Department, 2009, http://www.worldrobotics.org/index.php
[44] S. Katz, T. Downs, H. Cash and R. Grotz, Progress in development of the index of ADL, *The Gerontologist* **10** (1970), 20–30.
[45] T. Klamer and S.B. Allouch, Acceptance and use of a social robot by elderly users in a domestic environment, in: *Pervasive Health*, Munchen, Germany, 2010.
[46] E.G. Krug, L.L. Dahlberg, J.A. Mercy, A.B. Zwi and R. Lozano, World Health Organization, Chapter 5 – Abuse of the elderly, in: *World report on violence and health*, 2006.
[47] S. Kulviwat, G.C. Bruner, A. Kumar, S.A. Nasco and T. Clark, Toward a unified theory of consumer acceptance technology, *Psychol. Market* **24** (2007), 1059–1084.
[48] E. Libin and A. Libin, Robotherapy: Definition, assessment and case study, in: *International Conference on Virtual Systems and Multimedia*, Seoul, South Korea, 2002, pp. 906–915.
[49] L. Magnusson and E.J. Hanson, Ethical issues arising from a research, technology and development project to support frail older and their family carers, *Health and Social Care in the Community* **11**(5) (2003), 431–439.
[50] M. Mahani and K. Severinson-Eklundh, A survey on the relation of the task assistance of a robot to its social role, Technical report NADA, April 2009 (Note: Presented at the 24th Annual Technology & Persons with Disabilities Conference, 2009).
[51] M. Matarić, J. Eriksson, D. Feil-Seifer and C. Winstein, Socially assistive robotics for post-stroke rehabilitation, *Journal of NeuroEngineering and Rehabilitation* **4**(5) (2007).
[52] E. Mordini and P. de Hert, *Ageing and Invisibility*, Vol. 7, IOS Press, 2010, pp. 195–218.
[53] M. Mori, Bukimi no tani "The uncanny valley" (K.F. MacDorman and T. Minato, Trans.), *Energy* **7**(4) (1970), 33–35.
[54] P. Newall, Ethics, The Galilean library, http://www.galilean-library.org/int11.html (2005)
[55] Object Management Group, Robotic Localization Service (RLS), Version 1.0 (2010).
[56] Object Management Group, Robotic Technology Component Specifiction (RTC), Version 1.0 (2008).
[57] E. Pauwels, Ethics for Researchers – Facilitating Research Excellence in FP7, European Commission, 2007.
[58] J. Pedersen, Privacy and location technologies, in: *Workshop Paper at the Workshop 'Location System Privacy and Control' at Mobile HCI 2004*, Glasgow, UK, September 2004.
[59] M.E. Pollack, S. Engberg, J.T. Matthews, S. Thrun, L. Brown, D. Colbry, C. Orosz, B. Peintner, S. Ramakrishnan and J. Dunbar-Jacob, Pearl: A mobile robotic assistant for the elderly, in: *AAAI Workshop on Automation as Eldercare*, 2002.
[60] P. Rani, N. Sarkar, C. Smith and J. Adams, Affective communication for implicit human-machine interaction, in: *IEEE International Conference on Systems, Man and Cybernetics*, Washington, DC, 2003.
[61] L. Riek and P. Robinson, Robot, rabbit, or red herring? Societal acceptance as a function of classification ease, in: *IEEE RO-MAN*, Munich, Germany, 2008.
[62] Robot@Cwe project, http://www.robot-at-cwe.eu/.
[63] C. Röcker, W. Wilkowska, M. Ziefle, K. Kasugai, L. Klack, C. Möllering and S. Beul, Towards adaptive interfaces for supporting elderly users in technology-enhanced home environments, in: *Conference*

of the International Communications Society: Culture, Communication and the Cutting Edge of Technology, Tokyo, Japan, 2010.
[64] J. Scholtz, Theory and evaluation of human robot interactions, in: *International Conference on System Sciences*, 2003.
[65] M. Scopelliti, M.A. Giuliani and F. Fornara, Robots in a domestic setting: A psychological approach, *Univ. Access Inf. Soc.* **4** (2005), 145–155.
[66] SENIOR project, http://www.seniorproject.eu/.
[67] K. Severinson-Eklund, A. Green and H. Hüttenrauch, Social and collaborative aspects of interaction with a service robot, *Robotics and Autonomous Systems* **42** (2003), 223–234.
[68] B. Shackel, Usability-context, framework, design, and evaluation, *Human Factors for Informatics Usability*, 1991.
[69] N. Sharky, The ethical frontiers of robotics, *Science* **322**(5909) (2008), 1800–1801.
[70] B. Siciliano and O. Khatib, *Handbook of Robotics*, Vol. 64, Springer, 2008, pp. 1499–1524.
[71] P. Slavini, C. Laschi and P. Dario, Design for acceptability: Improving robots' coexistence in human society, *International Journal on Social Robot* **2** (2010), 451–460.
[72] A. Sloman, Requirements for artificial companions, *Close Engagements with Artificial Companions: Key Social, Psychological, Ethical And Design Issues*, Y. Wilks, ed., John Benjamin Publishing Company, 2010.
[73] R. Sparrow and L. Sparrow, In the hands of machines?, The future of aged care, *Mind Mach.* **16**(2) (2006), 141–161.
[74] D. Spiliotopoulos, I. Androutsopoulos and C. Spyropoulos, Human-robot interaction based on spoken natural language dialogue, in: *European Workshop on Service and Humanoid Robots*, Santonini, Greece, 2001.
[75] W.D. Stiehl, J. Lieberman, C. Breazeal, L. Basel, R. Cooper, H. Knight, L. Lalla, A. Maymin and S. Purchase, The huggable: A therapeutic robotic companion for relational, affective touch, in: *IEEE Consumer Communications and Networking Conference*, 2006, pp. 1290–1291.
[76] D.S. Syrdal, M.L. Walters, N. Otero, K.L. Koay and K. Dautenhahn, He knows when you are sleeping. Privacy and the personal robot companion, in: *AAAI Workshop on Human Implications of Human-Robot Interaction*, Vancouver, Canada, 2007, pp. 28–33.
[77] T. Tamura, S. Yonemitsu, A. Itoh, D. Oikawa, A. Kawakami, Y. Higashi, T. Fujimooto and K. Nakajima, Is an entertainment robot useful in the care of elderly people with severe dementia?, *Journal of Gerontology: Medical Sciences* **59**(1) (2004), 83–85.
[78] A. Tapus and M.J. Matarić, Towards socially assistive robotics, *International Journal of the Robotic Society of Japan* **24**(5) (2006).
[79] Y.L. Theng, A.B. Dahlan, M.L. Akmal and T.Z. Myint, An exploratory study on senior citizens' perceptions of the Nintendo Wii: The case of Singapore, in: *International Convention on Rehabilitation Engineering & Assistive Technology*, 2009.
[80] P. Tiwari, J. Warren, K. Day and B. McDonald, Some non-technology implications for wider application of robots assisting older people, *Health Care and Informatics Review Online* **14**(1) (2010), 2–11.
[81] UNESCO, Universal declaration on bioethics and human rights, 2005.
[82] Value Ageing project, http://www.valueageing.eu/.
[83] A. van Breemen, X. Yan and B. Meerbeek, iCat: An animated user-interface robot with personality, in: *International Joint Conference on Autonomous Agents and Multiagent Systems*, 2005, pp. 143–144.
[84] V. Venkatesh, M.G. Morris, G.B. Davis and F.D. Davis, User acceptance of information technology: Towards a unified view, *MIS Quarterly* **27**(3) (2003), 425–478.
[85] G. Veruggio, The EURON roboethics roadmap, in: *Humanoids*, Genoa, Italy, 2006.
[86] G. Veruggio and F. Operto, Roboethics: A bottom-up interdisciplinary discourse in the field of applied ethics in robotics, *International Review of Information Ethics* **6** (2006), 2–8.
[87] K. Wada and T. Shibata, Living with seal robots – Its sociopsychological and physiological influences on the elderly at a care house, *IEEE Transactions on Robotics* **23**(5) (2007), 972–980.
[88] K. Wada, T. Shibata, T. Musha and S. Kimura, Evaluation of neuropsychological effects of interaction with seal robots on demented patients, in: *EuroHaptics*, 2006.
[89] K. Wada, T. Shibata, T. Saito and K. Tanie, Effects of robot assisted activity to elderly people who stay at a health service facility for the aged, in: *IEEE/RSJ International Conference on Intelligent Robots and Systems*, 2003, pp. 2847–2852.
[90] A. Weiss, R. Bernhaupt, M. Lankes and M. Tscheligi, The USUS evaluation framework for human-robot interaction, in: *AISB Symposium on New Frontiers in Human-Robot Interaction*, 2009.
[91] A. Weiss, R. Bernhaupt, M. Tscheligi, D. Wollherr, K. Kuhnlenz and M. Buss, A methodological variation for acceptance evaluation of human-robot interaction in public places, in: *IEEE International Symposium on Robot and Human Interactive Communication*, Munich, Germany, 2008.

[92] Y.H. Weng, C.H. Chen and C.T. Sun, Toward the human-robot co-existence society: On safety intelligence for next generation robots, *International Journal of Social Robotics* (2009).
[93] J.E. Young, R. Hawkins, E. Sharlin and T. Igarashi, Acceptable domestic robots: Applying insights from social psychology, *International Journal of Social Robotics* **1**(1) (2009), 95–108.
[94] L. Zyga, Living safely with robots, beyond Asimov's laws, *PhysOrg.com*, 2009, http://www.physorg.com/news164887377.html.

Indexes

Subject Index

Handbook of Ambient Assisted Living
J.C. Augusto et al. (Eds.)
IOS Press, 2012

Contributing Authors and Affiliations

A. Aftab 9
St. Luke's General Hospital
Kilkenny, Ireland

Foteini Agrafioti 178
University of Toronto
Toronto, ON, Canada

Javier Arcas 693
TECNALIA Research & Innovation
Zamudio, Spain

Juan Carlos Augusto 387, 727
University of Ulster
UK

Michael C. Balasch 652
Deutsche Telekom AG
Berlin, Germany

Pierre Barralon 693
TECNALIA Research & Innovation
Donostia – San Sebastián, Spain

Amritpal S. Bhachu 283
University of Dundee
UK

Jennifer Boger 304
University of Toronto
Toronto Rehabilitation Institute
Canada

Uta Böhm 652
SIBIS Institut für Sozialforschung
Berlin, Germany

Linda Boise 94
Oregon Health and Science University
OR, USA

Stephan Bosch 626
University of Twente
The Netherlands

Lorena Bourg 729
Ariadna Servicios Informáticos
Madrid, Spain

Francis M. Bui 178
University of Toronto
Toronto, ON, Canada

Miroslav Burša 763
Czech Technical University in Prague
Czech Republic

Clemens Busch 512
Schüchtermann-Schiller'sche Kliniken
Bad Rothenfelde, Germany

Irina Busch 652
Charité Universitätsmedizin
Berlin, Germany

Jens-Uwe Busser 652
Siemens AG
Munich, Germany

Vic Callaghan 408
University of Essex
UK

Christine Carius-Duessel 652
Charité Universitätsmedizin
Berlin, Germany

Aveline Casey 9
St. Luke's General Hospital
Kilkenny, Ireland

Francesca Irene Cavallaro 834
Tecnalia
Donostia, San Sebastián, Spain

Authors Index